Essentials of Strength Training and Conditioning

FOURTH EDITION

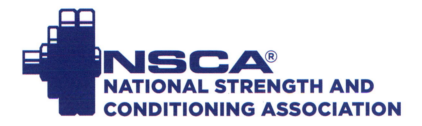

NSCA®
NATIONAL STRENGTH AND
CONDITIONING ASSOCIATION

G. Gregory Haff, PhD, CSCS,*D, FNSCA
Edith Cowan University, Western Australia

N. Travis Triplett, PhD, CSCS,*D, FNSCA
Appalachian State University, Boone, NC

EDITORS

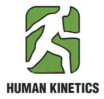

HUMAN KINETICS

Library of Congress Cataloging-in-Publication Data

Essentials of strength training and conditioning / National Strength and Conditioning Association ; G. Gregory Haff, N. Travis Triplett, editors. -- Fourth edition.

    p. ; cm.

    Includes bibliographical references and index.

    I. Haff, Greg, editor. II. Triplett, N. Travis, 1964- , editor. III. National Strength & Conditioning Association (U.S.), issuing body.

    [DNLM: 1. Physical Education and Training--methods. 2. Athletic Performance--physiology. 3. Physical Conditioning, Human--physiology. 4. Physical Fitness--physiology. 5. Resistance Training--methods. QT 255]

    GV711.5

    613.7'1--dc23

                     2014047045

ISBN: 978-1-7182-1086-8

Acquisitions Editor: Roger W. Earle; **Developmental Editor:** Christine M. Drews; **Managing Editor:** Karla Walsh; **Copyeditor:** Joyce Sexton; **Indexer:** Susan Danzi Hernandez; **Permissions Manager:** Dalene Reeder; **Graphic Designer:** Nancy Rasmus; **Cover Designer:** Keith Blomberg; **Photographer:** Neil Bernstein, unless otherwise noted; all photos © Human Kinetics, unless otherwise noted; Photo Asset Manager: Laura Fitch; **Visual Production Assistant:** Joyce Brumfield; **Photo Production Manager:** Jason Allen; **Art Manager:** Kelly Hendren; **Associate Art Manager:** Alan L. Wilborn; **Art Style Development:** Joanne Brummett; **Illustrations:** © Human Kinetics, unless otherwise noted; **Printer:** Walsworth

We thank The Fitness Center in Champaign, Illinois, and the National Strength and Conditioning Association in Colorado Springs, Colorado, for assistance in providing the locations for the photo shoot for this book.

Printed in the United States of America   10 9 8 7 6 5 4 3 2 1

The paper in this book was manufactured using responsible forestry methods.

Human Kinetics
1607 N. Market Street
Champaign, IL 61820
USA

United States and International
Website: **US.HumanKinetics.com**
Email: info@hkusa.com
Phone: 1-800-747-4457

Canada
Website: **Canada.HumanKinetics.com**
Email: info@hkcanada.com

E8489

Tell us what you think!
Human Kinetics would love to hear what we can do to improve the customer experience.
Use this QR code to take our brief survey.

CONTENTS

PREFACE

In 1994, the first edition of *Essentials of Strength Training and Conditioning* was published. After a second edition (in 2000) and sales of over 100,000 books, an expanded and updated third edition was published in 2008. This newest edition continues the tradition as the most comprehensive reference available for strength and conditioning professionals. In this text, 30 expert contributors further explore the scientific principles, concepts, and theories of strength training and conditioning and their applications to athletic performance.

The first edition grew out of an awareness that there was not a book about strength training and conditioning that captured the views of leading professionals in anatomy, biochemistry, biomechanics, endocrinology, nutrition, exercise physiology, psychology, and the other sciences and that related the principles from these disciplines to the design of safe and effective training programs. Also, the lack of relevant and well-conducted research studies had hindered earlier efforts to create an all-inclusive resource. Once it was finally developed, *Essentials of Strength Training and Conditioning* quickly became the definitive textbook on the subject.

The second edition, released six years later, was more than a simple freshening of the content; it was an overhaul of the scope and application of the first edition. Throughout the text and in the additional 100-plus pages, the chapter contributors used updated, relevant, and conclusive research and concepts to turn scientific information into information on performance. Many learning tools were added, such as chapter objectives, key points, application boxes, and sample resistance training programs for three different sports. These enhancements, plus the addition of a full-color interior and hundreds of color photographs, made the second edition truly exceptional.

The third edition, released eight years after the second edition, offered restructured chapters and expansions of other chapters complete with new photographs and updated terminology. In addition, the artwork was modernized and instructor and student resources were created to help keep this text the primary resource for the study and instruction of strength and conditioning.

Updates to the Fourth Edition

This fourth edition expands on the earlier editions and applies the most current research and information in a logical format that reaffirms *Essentials of Strength Training and Conditioning* as the most prominent resource for students preparing for careers in strength and conditioning and for sport science professionals involved in training athletes. The primary enhancements are as follows:

- Online videos featuring 21 resistance training exercises demonstrate proper exercise form for classroom and practical use.

- Updated research—specifically in the areas of high-intensity interval training, overtraining, agility and change of direction, nutrition for health and performance, and periodization—helps readers better understand these popular trends in the industry.

- A new chapter with instructions and photos presents techniques for exercises using alternative modes and nontraditional implements.

- Ten additional tests, including tests for maximum strength, power, and aerobic capacity, along with new flexibility exercises, resistance training exercises, plyometric exercises, and speed and agility drills, help professionals design programs that reflect current guidelines.

These enhancements, plus an expanded ancillary package for instructors including a new, robust collection of more than 60 instructor videos demonstrating resistance training, plyometric exercises, and alternative mode exercises, brings practical content to the classroom. Working along with the instructor guide and presentation package, a test package has been added to assist instructors in evaluating students' understanding of key concepts.

Each chapter begins with objectives and includes key points to guide the reader along the way. Key terms are boldfaced and listed at the end of the chapter. Chapters include sidebars that apply the content, and later chapters include sample resistance training programs for three different sports. Detailed instructions and photos are provided for testing, stretching, resistance training, alternative modes, plyometrics, agility training, and aerobic endurance exercise. Finally, chapters end with multiple-choice study questions, with an answer key at the end of the book.

Instructor Resources

In addition to the updated content, this edition includes newly created instructor resources:

- *Instructor Video.* The instructor video includes video of correct technique for 61 resistance training, alternative, and plyometric exercises. These can be used for demonstration, lecture, and discussion.

- *Instructor Guide.* The instructor guide contains a course description, a sample semester schedule, chapter objectives, chapter outlines, key terms with definitions, and application questions with answers.

- *Presentation Package and Image Bank.* This comprehensive resource, delivered in Microsoft PowerPoint, offers instructors a presentation package containing over 1,300 slides to help aug-

ment lectures and class discussions. In addition to outlines and key points, the resource contains more than 600 figures, tables, and photos from the textbook, which can be used as an image bank by instructors who need to customize their presentations. Easy-to-follow instructions help guide instructors on how to reuse the images within their own PowerPoint templates.

- *Test Package.* The test package includes a bank of 240 multiple-choice questions. The test package is available in multiple formats: HK*Propel* provides options for downloading the test files for integration with a learning management system or printing them as traditional paper-based tests. Instructors can also create their own assessments using the question bank within HK*Propel* and assign those assessments to students.

Instructor ancillaries, including an ebook version of the text that allows instructors to add highlights, annotations, and bookmarks, are free to adopting instructors. Please contact your Sales Manager for details about how to access instructor resources in HK*Propel*.

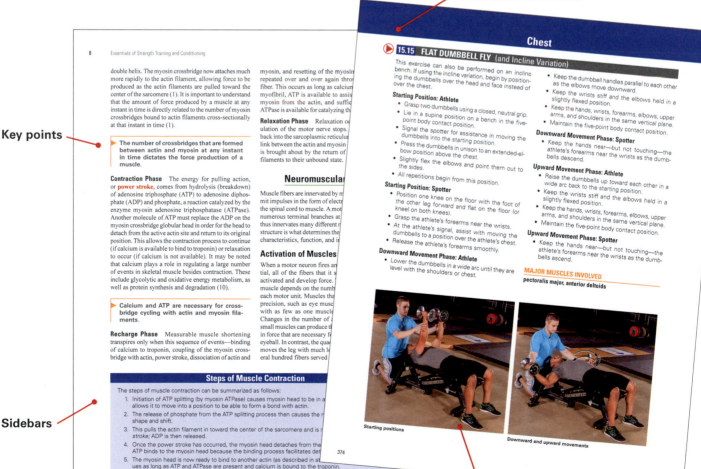

Video available online

Key points

Sidebars

Exercise photos

Student and Professional Resources

The learning content in HK*Propel* includes video of 21 resistance training exercises for use in understanding and performing correct exercise technique. Lab activities are provided to give students hands-on practice with testing and evaluation. The fillable forms make completing and submitting lab assignments easy. Your instructor may also assign you short quizzes to complete within HK*Propel* to demonstrate your mastery of each chapter's content.

See the card at the front of this book for your unique access code for HK*Propel*. For ebook users, reference the HK*Propel* access code instructions on the page immediately following the book cover.

Certification Exams

Essentials of Strength Training and Conditioning is the primary resource for individuals preparing for the National Strength and Conditioning Association's Certified Strength and Conditioning Specialist (CSCS) certification exam.

As a worldwide authority on strength and conditioning, the National Strength and Conditioning Association (NSCA) supports and disseminates research-based knowledge and its practical application to improve athletic performance and fitness. With over 30,000 members in more than 50 countries, the NSCA has established itself as an international clearinghouse for strength and conditioning research, theories, and practices.

The CSCS and NSCA-CPT were the first certifications of their kind to be nationally accredited by the National Commission for Certifying Agencies, a nongovernmental, nonprofit agency in Washington, DC, that sets national standards for certifying agencies. To date, more than 40,000 professionals residing in 75 countries hold one or more NSCA certifications.

Whether used for learning the essentials of strength training and conditioning, for preparing for a certification exam, or as a reference by professionals, *Essentials of Strength Training and Conditioning, Fourth Edition,* will help practitioners and the scientific community better understand how to develop and administer safe and effective strength training and conditioning programs.

Key terms

Study questions

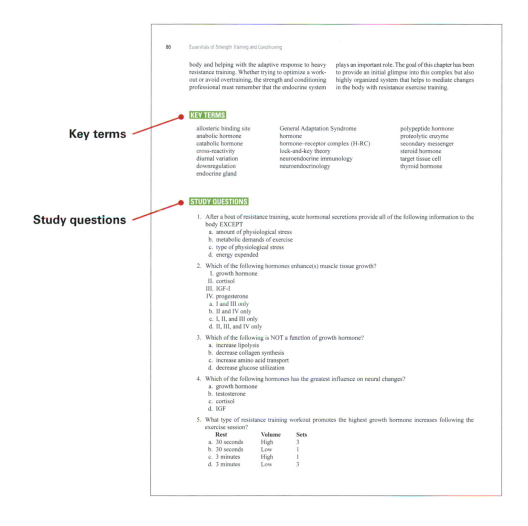

ACCESSING THE LAB ACTIVITIES

The lab activities are accessed through the HK*Propel*.

See the card at the front of this book for your unique access code for HK*Propel*. For ebook users, reference the HK*Propel* access code instructions on the page immediately following the book cover. Following is a list of the lab activities.

Lab 1: Anaerobic Capacity Testing

300-Yard (274 m) Shuttle Run

Lab 2: Aerobic Capacity Testing

1.5-Mile (2.4 km) Run

12-Minute Run

Lab 3: Anthropometry and Body Composition

Skinfold Measurements

Lab 4: Exercise Testing for Athletes

Test Selection and Order

Lab 5: Techniques of Exercise

Flexibility Exercise Techniques

Lab 6: Techniques of Exercise

Resistance Exercise and Spotting Guidelines

Lab 7: Muscular Strength and Power Testing

Vertical Jump Test

Standing Long Jump Test

1RM Bench Press

1RM Back Squat

Lab 8: Techniques of Exercise

Plyometric Exercise Techniques

Lab 9: Speed and Agility Technique and Testing

T-Test

Hexagon Test

Pro Agility Test

40-Yard (37 m) Sprint

Lab 10: Muscular Endurance Testing

Push-Up Test

YMCA Bench Press Test

Partial Curl-Up Test

Lab 11: Facility Layout Design

Facility Floor Plan

ACKNOWLEDGMENTS

The development of the fourth edition of the NSCA's *Essentials of Strength Training and Conditioning* was a massive undertaking that would not have been possible without the contributions of a vast number of people. The historic development of this iconic text has served as our guiding principle, and the hard work of the numerous authors who contributed to the three previous editions has established a strong foundation for this text. Therefore, we thank the previous editors, Thomas Baechle and Roger Earle, for their foresight over twenty years ago that has led us to where we are today and for their passionate work on all of the previous editions. This edition would not have been possible without the continued contribution of Roger Earle, who has gone beyond his role as a Human Kinetics representative. He is a true friend who has helped with many aspects of this book and our writing careers.

We would also like to thank Keith Cinea and Carwyn Sharp for their help throughout the process. These individuals have represented the NSCA well and positioned the science that underpins our profession as the standard that determines the content of this text. Because it is a key resource for current and future strength and conditioning professionals, it was essential for us to ensure that this text holds true to the NSCA mission of translating science into practice, and both Keith and Carwyn are ambassadors of this philosophy. Thanks also to the multitude of individuals at Human Kinetics who were essential to completing every phase of the publication of this book, from copyediting to graphic design. Probably the most important note of thanks goes to Chris Drews and Karla Walsh, our developmental editor and managing editor, who helped two novice book editors in countless ways. Without Chris and Karla, we would have probably been lost in the process.

G. Gregory Haff, PhD, CSCS,*D, FNSCA

To my coeditor and long-time friend, Travis Triplett: I could think of no one else I would want to edit a book of this magnitude with. Your kind heart and easygoing style is a perfect complement to my "bull in a china shop" methodology for processes like this. Thanks for always being one of my very best friends!

I have to thank my family. My wife Erin has sacrificed everything to allow me the ability to chase my dreams and undertake projects like this. Without her support I would merely be stuck under the heavy lifting bar of life. It is a blessing to have someone strong enough to spot you when times are tough, and for that I love you more than you know. For my father, Guy Haff—I doubt you ever thought that lifting weights would become my whole life's work when you took me to the West Morris YMCA at 11 years of age to teach me to lift. Without that I cannot imagine who I would be at this moment. Finally, I must dedicate my efforts to my mother, Sandra Haff. No matter where you are now, I hope you are still proud of the man I am and the man I strive to be each and every day. I miss you much, Mom, and I wish you were here to see all the great things that have happened.

N. Travis Triplett, PhD, CSCS,*D, FNSCA

I never dreamed that taking my first weight training class while at the university would have culminated in such a rewarding career in the field of strength and conditioning. It is difficult to thank every person who had a role in getting me to this point in my life and my career, which enabled me to enthusiastically embark on this project. I was fortunate to receive a strong foundation from my parents—I wish you could both be here to see that the example you set was followed. I also want to thank my brother and my circle of friends, who have always been supportive and have been there to brighten my day. Professionally, my two greatest influences have been Mike Stone and Bill Kraemer. I value your mentorship and friendship greatly. Numerous colleagues and former students around the world have contributed to my knowledge and success along the way, and I appreciate each and every one of you even if we don't see each other very often.

Finally, to my co-editor and good friend, Greg Haff: Who would have thought that sitting around at the lunch buffet as graduate students talking strength and conditioning would have led to this? I look forward to many more years of friendship and collaboration.

ACKNOWLEDGMENTS

CREDITS

Figure 2.5 Reprinted, by permission, from B.A. Gowitzke and M. Milner, 1988. *Scientific bases of human movement,* 3rd ed. (Baltimore, MD: Lippincott, Williams & Wilkins), 184-185.

Figure 2.10 Reprinted, by permission, from E.A. Harman, M. Johnson, and P.N. Frykman, 1992, "A movement-oriented approach to exercise prescription," *NSCA Journal* 14 (1): 47-54.

Figure 2.13 Reprinted from K. Jorgensen, 1976, "Force-velocity relationship in human elbow flexors and extensors." In *Biomechanics A-V,* edited by P.V. Komi (Baltimore, MD: University Park Press), 147. By permission of P.V. Komi.

Figure 4.5 Reprinted from *Steroids,* Vol. 74(13-14), J.L. Vingren, W.J. Kraemer, et al., "Effect of resistance exercise on muscle steroid receptor protein content in strength trained men and women," pgs. 1033-1039, copyright 2009, with permission from Elsevier.

Figure 4.7 Adapted from W.J. Kraemer et al., 1998, "Hormonal responses to consecutive days of heavy-resistance exercise with or without nutritional supplementation," *Journal of Applied Physiology* 85 (4): 1544-1555. Used with permission.

Table 5.3 Reprinted, by permission, from A. Fry, 1993, "Physiological responses to short-term high intensity resistance exercise overtraining," Ph.D. Diss., The Pennsylvania State University; Meeusen R, Duclos M, Foster C, Fry A, Gleeson et al., 2013, "Prevention, diagnosis, and treatment of the over training syndrome: joint consensus statement of the European College of Sports Science and the American College of Sports Medicine," *Medicine and Science in Sport and Exercise* 45: 186-205.

Figure 7.2 Reprinted, by permission, from A.D. Faigenbaum et al., 2013, "Youth resistance training: past practices, new perspectives and future directions," *Pediatric Exercise Science* 25: 591-604.

Figure 7.3a © Hossler, PhD/Science Source.

Figure 7.3b © SPL/Science Photo Library.

Figure 8.1 Reprinted, by permission, from R.S. Weinberg and D. Gould, 2015, *Foundations of sport and exercise psychology,* 6th ed. (Champaign, IL: Human Kinetics), 79.

Figure 8.2 Reprinted, by permission, from B.D. Hatfield and G.A. Walford, 1987, "Understanding anxiety: Implications for sport performance," *NSCA Journal* 9(2): 60-61.

Table 9.6 Adapted, by permission, from K. Foster-Powell, S. Holt, and J.C. Brand-Miller, 2002, "International table of glycemic index and glycemic load values," *American Journal of Clinical Nutrition* 76: 5-56. © American Society for Nutrition.

Table 9.10 Reprinted, by permission, from M.N. Sawka et al., 2007, "American College of Sports Medicine position stand. Exercise and fluid replacement," *Medicine and Science of Sport and Exercise* 39: 377-390, 2007.

Table 10.5 Reprinted, by permission, from National Heart, Lung, and Blood Institute, 1998, "Clinical guidelines on the identification, evaluation, and treatment of overweight and obesity in adults: The evidence report," *Obesity Research* 6: 464.

Table 10.6 Reprinted, by permission, from National Heart, Lung, and Blood Institute, 1998, "Clinical guidelines on the identification, evaluation, and treatment of overweight and obesity in adults: The evidence report," *Obesity Research* 6: 464.

Figure 13.6 Adapted, by permission, from G.M. Gilliam, 1983, "300 yard shuttle run," *NSCA Journal* 5 (5): 46.

Figure 13.11 Adapted, by permission, from D. Semenick, 1990, "Tests and measurements: The T-test," *NSCA Journal* 12(1): 36-37.

Figure 13.12 Adapted, by permission, from K. Pauole et al., 2000, "Reliability and validity of the T-test as a measure of agility, leg power, and leg speed in college age males and females," *Journal of Strength and Conditioning Research* 14: 443-450.

Figure 13.16 Reprinted, by permission, from M.P. Reiman, 2009, *Functional testing in performance* (Champaign, IL: Human Kinetics), 109.

Table 13.1 Adapted, by permission, from J. Hoffman, 2006, *Norms for fitness, performance, and health* (Champaign, IL: Human Kinetics), 36-37.

Table 13.2 Reprinted, by permission, from J. Hoffman, 2006, *Norms for fitness, performance, and health* (Champaign, IL: Human Kinetics), 36-37.

Table 13.3 Reprinted, by permission, from J. Hoffman, 2006, *Norms for fitness, performance, and health* (Champaign, IL: Human Kinetics), 38.

Table 13.5 Reprinted, by permission, from J. Hoffman, 2006, *Norms for fitness, performance, and health* (Champaign, IL: Human Kinetics), 58. Adapted from D.A. Chu, 1996, *Explosive power and strength* (Champaign, IL: Human Kinetics).

Table 13.6 Reprinted, by permission, from J. Hoffman, 2006, *Norms for fitness, performance, and health* (Champaign, IL: Human Kinetics), 58; adapted from D.A. Chu, 1996, *Explosive power and strength* (Champaign, IL: Human Kinetics).

Table 13.10 Reprinted, by permission, from American College of Sports Medicine, 2014, *ACSM's guidelines for exercise testing and prescription,* 9th ed. (Baltimore, MD: Lippincott, Williams, and Wilkins), 101.

Table 13.11   Source: Canadian Physical Activity, *Fitness & Lifestyle Approach: CSEP-Health & Fitness Program's Appraisal & Counselling Strategy*, Third Edition, © 2003. Reprinted with permission from the Canadian Society for Exercise Physiology.

Table 13.19   Adapted, by permission, from ACSM, 2014, *ACSM's guidelines for exercise testing and prescription*, 9th ed. (Philadelphia: Wolters Kluwer Health/Lippincott Williams & Wilkins), 88.

Table 13.22   Reprinted, by permission, from J. Hoffman, 2006, *Norms for fitness, performance, and health* (Champaign, IL: Human Kinetics), 113.

Table 13.25   Adapted, by permission, from V. H. Heyward, 1998, *Advanced fitness assessment and exercise prescription*, 3rd ed. (Champaign, IL: Human Kinetics), 155.

Table 13.26   Adapted, by permission, from V. H. Heyward, 1998, *Advanced fitness assessment and exercise prescription*, 3rd ed. (Champaign, IL: Human Kinetics), 12.

Table 16.1   Adapted, by permission, from D.T. McMaster, J. Cronin, and M. McGuigan, 2009, "Forms of variable resistance training," *Strength & Conditioning Journal* 31: 50-64.

Table 16.2   Adapted, by permission, from D.T. McMaster, J. Cronin, and M. McGuigan, 2010, "Quantification of rubber and chain-based resistance modes," *Journal of Strength and Conditioning Research* 24: 2056-2064.

Figure 17.1   Reprinted, by permission, from R.W. Earle, 2006, Weight training exercise prescription. In: *Essentials of personal training symposium workbook* (Lincoln, NE: NSCA Certification Commission), 2006

Figure 17.2   Reprinted, by permission, from R.W. Earle, 2006, Weight training exercise prescription. In: *Essentials of personal training symposium workbook* (Lincoln, NE: NSCA Certification Commission).

Figure 19.1   Reprinted, by permission, from K. Häkkinen, K. and P.V. Komi, 1985, "The effect of explosive type strength training on electromyographic and force production characteristic of leg extensor muscles during concentric and various stretch-shortening cycle exercises," *Scandinavian Journal of Sports Sciences* 7(2): 65-76. Copyright 1985 Munksgaard International Publishers, Ltd. Copenhagen, Denmark.

Figure 19.3   Reprinted, by permission, from K.P. Clark and P.G. Weyand, 2014, "Are running speeds maximized with simple-spring stance mechanics?" *Journal of Applied Physiology* 117(6): 604-615

Figure 19.11   Reprinted, by permission, from S.S. Plisk and V. Gambetta, 1997, "Tactical metabolic training," *Strength & Conditioning* 19(2): 44-53.

Table 19.4   Adapted, by permission, from S. Nimphius, 2014, Increasing agility. In *High-performance training for sports*, edited by D. Joyce and D. Lewindon (Champaign, IL: Human Kinetics), 194.

Table 19.5   Adapted, by permission, from S. Nimphius, 2014, Increasing agility. In *High-performance training for sports*, edited by D. Joyce and D. Lewindon (Champaign, IL: Human Kinetics), 185-198.

Table 20.2   Reprinted, by permission, from NSCA, 2012, Aerobic endurance training program design, by P. Hagerman. In *NSCA's essentials of personal training*, 2nd ed., edited by J.W. Coburn and M.H. Malek (Champaign, IL: Human Kinetics), 395.

Figure 21.1   Adapted, by permission, from G.G. Haff and E.E. Haff, 2012, Training integration and periodization. In *NSCA's guide to program design*, edited by J. Hoffman (Champaign, IL: Human Kinetics), 215.

Figure 21.2   Adapted, by permission, from G.G. Haff and E.E. Haff, 2012, Training integration and periodization. In *NSCA's guide to program design*, edited by J. Hoffman (Champaign, IL: Human Kinetics), 216.

Figure 21.3   Adapted, by permission, from G.G. Haff and E.E. Haff, 2012, Training integration and periodization. In *NSCA's guide to program design*, edited by J. Hoffman (Champaign, IL: Human Kinetics), 219.

Table 21.1   Adapted from G.G. Haff and E.E. Haff, 2012, Training integration and periodization. In *NSCA's guide to program design*, edited by J. Hoffman (Champaign, IL: Human Kinetics), 220.

Figure 21.4   Reprinted, by permission, from G.G. Haff and E.E. Haff, 2012, Training integration and periodization. In *NSCA's guide to program design*, edited by J. Hoffman (Champaign, IL: Human Kinetics), 223; adapted from figure 11.7, p. 2239. Reprinted from *Weight Training: A Scientific Approach*, 2nd edition, by Michael H. Stone and Harold St. O'Bryant, copyright © 1987 by Burgess.

Table 23.1   Adapted, by permission, from W. Kroll, 1991, "Structural and functional considerations in designing the facility, part I," *NSCA Journal* 13(1): 51-58, 1991

Figure 23.6   Adapted, by permission, from National Strength and Conditioning Association, 2004, *NSCA's essentials of personal training*, edited by R.W. Earle and T.R. Baechle (Champaign, IL: Human Kinetics), 604-606.

Table 24.1   Adapted, by permission, from NSCA, 2009, *Strength & conditioning professional standards and guidelines* (Colorado Springs, CO: NSCA), 17.

Figure 24.3   Reprinted, by permission, from R.W. Earle, 1993, *Staff and facility policies and procedures manual* (Omaha, NE: Creighton University).

Table 24.2   Adapted, by permission, from NSCA, 2011, *Performance training center emergency policies and procedures manual* (Colorado Springs, CO: NSCA), 3.

Structure and Function of Body Systems

N. Travis Triplett, PhD

After completing this chapter, you will be able to

- describe both the macrostructure and microstructure of muscle and bone,
- describe the sliding-filament theory of muscular contraction,
- describe the specific morphological and physiological characteristics of different muscle fiber types and predict their relative involvement in different sport events, and
- describe the anatomical and physiological characteristics of the cardiovascular and respiratory systems.

The author would like to acknowledge the significant contributions of Robert T. Harris and Gary R. Hunter to this chapter.

Physical exercise and sport performance involve effective, purposeful movements of the body. These movements result from the forces developed in muscles, which move the various body parts by acting through lever systems of the skeleton. These skeletal muscles are under the control of the cerebral cortex, which activates the skeletal muscle cells or fibers through the motor neurons of the peripheral nervous system. Support for this neuromuscular activity involves continuous delivery of oxygen and nutrients to working tissues and removal of carbon dioxide and metabolic waste by-products from working tissues through activities of the cardiovascular and respiratory systems.

In order to best apply the available scientific knowledge to the training of athletes and the development of effective training programs, strength and conditioning professionals must have a basic understanding of not only musculoskeletal function but also those systems of the body that directly support the work of exercising muscle. Accordingly, this chapter summarizes those aspects of the anatomy and function of the musculoskeletal, neuromuscular, cardiovascular, and respiratory systems that are essential for developing and maintaining muscular force and power.

Musculoskeletal System

The musculoskeletal system of the human body consists of bones, joints, muscles, and tendons configured to allow the great variety of movements characteristic of human activity. This section describes the various components of the musculoskeletal system, both individually and in the context of how they function together.

Skeleton

The muscles of the body do not act directly to exert force on the ground or other objects. Instead, they function by pulling against bones that rotate about joints and transmit force to the environment. Muscles can only pull, not push; but through the system of bony levers, muscle pulling forces can be manifested as either pulling or pushing forces against external objects.

There are approximately 206 bones in the body, though the number can vary. This relatively light, strong structure provides leverage, support, and protection (figure 1.1). The **axial skeleton** consists of the skull (cranium), vertebral column (vertebra C1 through the coccyx), ribs, and sternum. The **appendicular skeleton** includes the shoulder (or pectoral) girdle (left and right scapula and clavicle); bones of the arms, wrists, and hands (left and right humerus, radius, ulna, carpals, metacarpals, and phalanges); the pelvic girdle (left and right coxal or innominate bones); and the bones of the legs, ankles, and feet (left and right femur, patella, tibia, fibula, tarsals, metatarsals, and phalanges).

Junctions of bones are called joints. **Fibrous joints** (e.g., sutures of the skull) allow virtually no movement; **cartilaginous joints** (e.g., intervertebral disks) allow limited movement; and **synovial joints** (e.g., elbow and knee) allow considerable movement. Sport and exercise movements occur mainly about the synovial joints, whose most important features are low friction and large range of motion. Articulating bone ends are covered with smooth **hyaline cartilage**, and the entire joint is enclosed in a capsule filled with **synovial fluid**. There are usually additional supporting structures of ligament and cartilage (13).

Virtually all joint movement consists of rotation about points or axes. Joints can be categorized by the number of directions about which rotation can occur. **Uniaxial joints**, such as the elbow, operate as hinges, essentially rotating about only one axis. The knee is often referred to as a hinge joint, but its axis of rotation actually changes throughout the joint range of motion. **Biaxial joints**, such as the ankle and wrist, allow movement about two perpendicular axes. **Multiaxial joints**, including the shoulder and hip ball-and-socket joints, allow movement about all three perpendicular axes that define space.

The **vertebral column** is made up of vertebral bones separated by flexible disks that allow movement to occur. The vertebrae are grouped into 7 cervical vertebrae in the neck region; 12 thoracic vertebrae in the middle to upper back; 5 lumbar vertebrae, which make up the lower back; 5 sacral vertebrae, which are fused together and

What Factors Affect Skeletal Growth in an Adult?

There are several things that can positively affect the adult skeleton, and most are a result of muscle use. When the body is subjected to heavy loads (job tasks or resistance training), the bone will increase in density and bone mineral content. If the body performs more explosive movements with impact, similar changes can occur. Some of the higher bone densities have been seen in people who engage in gymnastics or other activities that involve high-strength and high-power movements, some with hard landings (11). Other factors that influence bone adaptations are whether the axial skeleton is loaded and how often this loading occurs (frequency). Since the adaptation period of bone is longer than that of skeletal muscle, it is important to vary the stimulus in terms of frequency, intensity, and type.

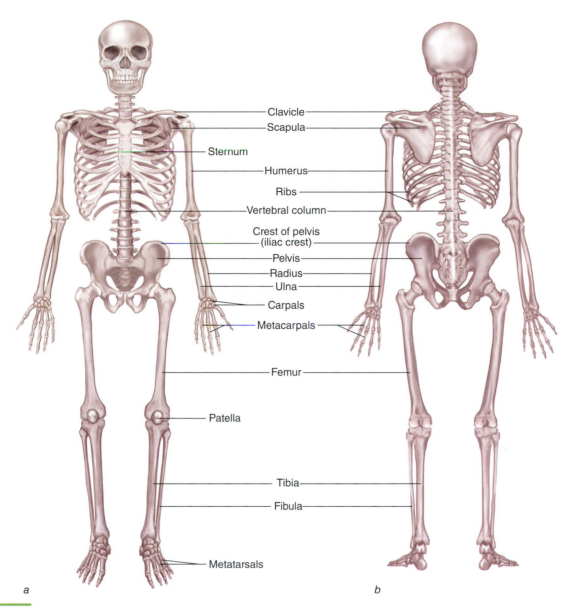

FIGURE 1.1 *(a)* Front view and *(b)* rear view of an adult male human skeleton.

make up the rear part of the pelvis; and 3 to 5 coccygeal vertebrae, which form a kind of vestigial internal tail extending downward from the pelvis.

Skeletal Musculature

The system of muscles that enables the skeleton to move is depicted in figure 1.2. The connection point between bones is the joint, and skeletal muscles are attached to bones at each of their ends. Without this arrangement, movement could not occur.

Musculoskeletal Macrostructure and Microstructure

Each skeletal muscle is an organ that contains muscle tissue, connective tissue, nerves, and blood vessels.

Fibrous connective tissue, or **epimysium**, covers the body's more than 430 skeletal muscles. The epimysium is contiguous with the tendons at the ends of the muscle (figure 1.3). The **tendon** is attached to **bone periosteum**, a specialized connective tissue covering all bones; any contraction of the muscle pulls on the tendon and, in turn, the bone. Limb muscles have two attachments to bone: **proximal** (closer to the trunk) and **distal** (farther from the trunk). The two attachments of trunk muscles are termed **superior** (closer to the head) and **inferior** (closer to the feet).

Muscle cells, often called **muscle fibers**, are long (sometimes running the entire length of a muscle), cylindrical cells 50 to 100 μm in diameter (about the diameter of a human hair). These fibers have many nuclei situated on the periphery of the cell and have a striated appearance

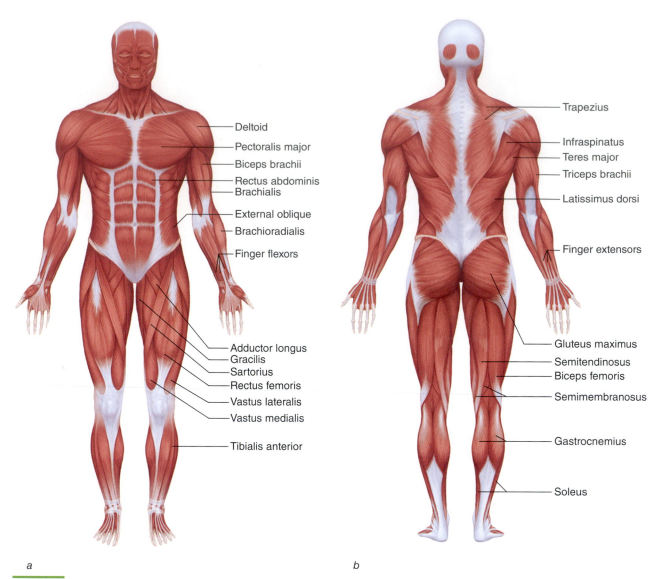

a

b

FIGURE 1.2 *(a)* Front view and *(b)* rear view of adult male human skeletal musculature.

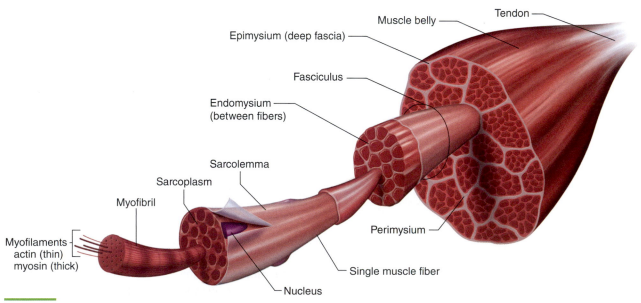

FIGURE 1.3 Schematic drawing of a muscle illustrating three types of connective tissue: epimysium (the outer layer), perimysium (surrounding each fasciculus, or group of fibers), and endomysium (surrounding individual fibers).

under low magnification. Under the epimysium the muscle fibers are grouped in bundles (**fasciculi**) that may consist of up to 150 fibers, with the bundles surrounded by connective tissue called **perimysium**. Each muscle fiber is surrounded by connective tissue called **endomysium**, which is encircled by and is contiguous with the fiber's membrane, or **sarcolemma** (13). All the connective tissue—epimysium, perimysium, and endomysium—is contiguous with the tendon, so tension developed in a muscle cell is transmitted to the tendon and the bone to which it is attached (see figure 1.3).

The junction between a **motor neuron** (nerve cell) and the muscle fibers it innervates is called the motor end plate, or, more often, the **neuromuscular junction** (figure 1.4). Each muscle cell has only one neuromuscular junction, although a single motor neuron innervates many muscle fibers, sometimes hundreds or even thousands. A motor neuron and the muscle fibers it innervates are called a **motor unit**. All the muscle fibers of a motor unit contract together when they are stimulated by the motor neuron.

The interior structure of a muscle fiber is depicted in figure 1.5. The **sarcoplasm,** which is the cytoplasm of a muscle fiber, contains contractile components consisting

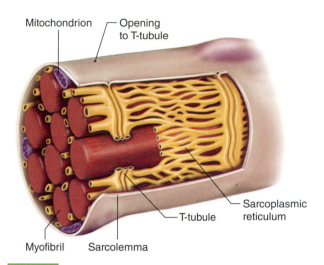

FIGURE 1.5 Sectional view of a muscle fiber.

of protein filaments, other proteins, stored glycogen and fat particles, enzymes, and specialized organelles such as mitochondria and the sarcoplasmic reticulum.

Hundreds of **myofibrils** (each about 1 μm in diameter, 1/100 the diameter of a hair) dominate the sarcoplasm. Myofibrils contain the apparatus that contracts the muscle cell, which consists primarily of two types of **myofilament**: **myosin** and **actin**. The myosin filaments (thick filaments about 16 nm in diameter, about 1/10,000 the diameter of a hair) contain up to 200 myosin molecules. The myosin filament consists of a globular head, a hinge point, and a fibrous tail. The globular heads protrude away from the myosin filament at regular intervals, and a pair of myosin filaments forms a **cross-bridge**, which interacts with actin. The actin filaments (thin filaments about 6 nm in diameter) consist of two strands arranged in a double helix. Myosin and actin filaments are organized longitudinally in the smallest contractile unit of skeletal muscle, the **sarcomere**. Sarcomeres average about 2.5 μm in length in a relaxed fiber (approximately 4,500 per centimeter of muscle length) and are repeated the entire length of the muscle fiber (1).

Figure 1.6 shows the structure and orientation of the myosin and actin in the sarcomere. Adjacent myosin filaments anchor to each other at the M-bridge in the center of the sarcomere (the center of the H-zone). Actin filaments are aligned at both ends of the sarcomere and are anchored at the Z-line. Z-lines are repeated through the entire myofibril. Six actin filaments surround each myosin filament, and each actin filament is surrounded by three myosin filaments.

It is the arrangement of the myosin and actin filaments and the Z-lines of the sarcomeres that gives skeletal muscle its alternating dark and light pattern, which appears as striated under magnification. The dark **A-band** corresponds with the alignment of the myosin

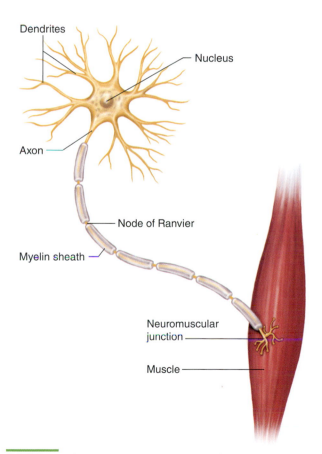

FIGURE 1.4 A motor unit, consisting of a motor neuron and the muscle fibers it innervates. There are typically several hundred muscle fibers in a single motor unit.

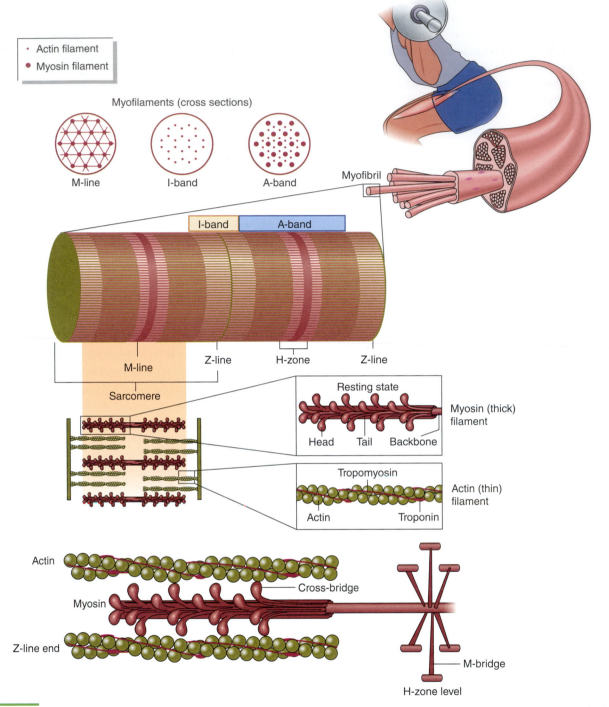

FIGURE 1.6   Detailed view of the myosin and actin protein filaments in muscle. The arrangement of myosin (thick) and actin (thin) filaments gives skeletal muscle its striated appearance.

filaments, whereas the light **I-band** corresponds with the areas in two adjacent sarcomeres that contain only actin filaments (13). The **Z-line** is in the middle of the I-band and appears as a thin, dark line running longitudinally through the I-band. The **H-zone** is the area in the center of the sarcomere where only myosin filaments are present. During muscle contraction, the H-zone decreases as the actin slides over the myosin toward the center of the

sarcomere. The I-band also decreases as the Z-lines are pulled toward the center of the sarcomere.

Parallel to and surrounding each myofibril is an intricate system of tubules, called the **sarcoplasmic reticulum** (see figure 1.5), which terminates as vesicles in the vicinity of the Z-lines. Calcium ions are stored in the vesicles. The regulation of calcium controls muscular contraction. **T-tubules**, or transverse tubules, run perpendicular to the sarcoplasmic reticulum and terminate in the vicinity of the Z-line between two vesicles. Because the T-tubules run between outlying myofibrils and are contiguous with the sarcolemma at the surface of the cell, discharge of an **action potential** (an electrical nerve impulse) arrives nearly simultaneously from the surface to all depths of the muscle fiber. Calcium is thus released throughout the muscle, producing a coordinated contraction.

> ▶ **The discharge of an action potential from a motor nerve signals the release of calcium from the sarcoplasmic reticulum into the myofibril, causing tension development in muscle.**

Sliding-Filament Theory of Muscular Contraction

In its simplest form, the **sliding-filament theory** states that the actin filaments at each end of the sarcomere slide inward on myosin filaments, pulling the Z-lines toward the center of the sarcomere and thus shortening the muscle fiber (figure 1.7). As actin filaments slide over myosin filaments, both the H-zone and I-band shrink.

The action of myosin crossbridges pulling on the actin filaments is responsible for the movement of the actin filament. Because only a very small displacement of the actin filament occurs with each flexion of the myosin crossbridge, very rapid, repeated flexions must occur in many crossbridges throughout the entire muscle for measurable movement to occur (13).

Resting Phase   Under normal resting conditions, little calcium is present in the myofibril (most of it is stored in the sarcoplasmic reticulum), so very few of the myosin crossbridges are bound to actin. Even with the actin binding site covered, myosin and actin still interact in a weak bond, which becomes strong (and muscle tension is produced) when the actin binding site is exposed after release of the stored calcium.

Excitation–Contraction Coupling Phase   Before myosin crossbridges can flex, they must first attach to the actin filament. When the sarcoplasmic reticulum is stimulated to release calcium ions, the calcium binds with **troponin**, a protein that is situated at regular intervals along the actin filament (see figure 1.6) and has a high affinity for calcium ions. This causes a shift to occur in another protein molecule, **tropomyosin**, which runs along the length of the actin filament in the groove of the

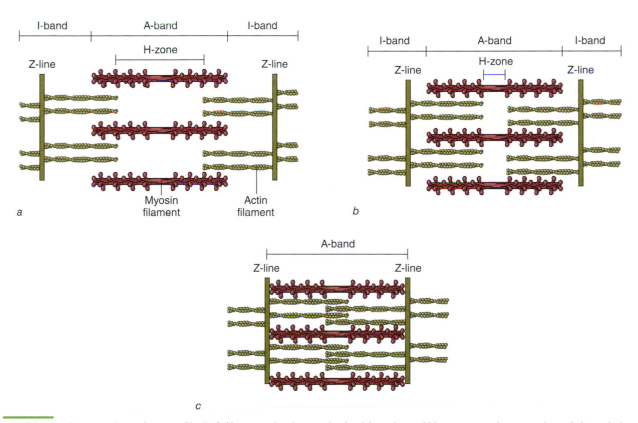

FIGURE 1.7   Contraction of a myofibril. *(a)* In stretched muscle the I-bands and H-zone are elongated, and there is low force potential due to reduced crossbridge–actin alignment. *(b)* When muscle contracts (here partially), the I-bands and H-zone are shortened. Force potential is high due to optimal crossbridge–actin alignment. *(c)* With contracted muscle, force potential is low because the overlap of actin reduces the potential for crossbridge–actin alignment.

double helix. The myosin crossbridge now attaches much more rapidly to the actin filament, allowing force to be produced as the actin filaments are pulled toward the center of the sarcomere (1). It is important to understand that the amount of force produced by a muscle at any instant in time is directly related to the number of myosin crossbridges bound to actin filaments cross-sectionally at that instant in time (1).

> **The number of crossbridges that are formed between actin and myosin at any instant in time dictates the force production of a muscle.**

Contraction Phase   The energy for pulling action, or **power stroke**, comes from hydrolysis (breakdown) of adenosine triphosphate (ATP) to adenosine diphosphate (ADP) and phosphate, a reaction catalyzed by the enzyme myosin adenosine triphosphatase (ATPase). Another molecule of ATP must replace the ADP on the myosin crossbridge globular head in order for the head to detach from the active actin site and return to its original position. This allows the contraction process to continue (if calcium is available to bind to troponin) or relaxation to occur (if calcium is not available). It may be noted that calcium plays a role in regulating a large number of events in skeletal muscle besides contraction. These include glycolytic and oxidative energy metabolism, as well as protein synthesis and degradation (10).

> **Calcium and ATP are necessary for crossbridge cycling with actin and myosin filaments.**

Recharge Phase   Measurable muscle shortening transpires only when this sequence of events—binding of calcium to troponin, coupling of the myosin crossbridge with actin, power stroke, dissociation of actin and myosin, and resetting of the myosin head position—is repeated over and over again throughout the muscle fiber. This occurs as long as calcium is available in the myofibril, ATP is available to assist in uncoupling the myosin from the actin, and sufficient active myosin ATPase is available for catalyzing the breakdown of ATP.

Relaxation Phase   Relaxation occurs when the stimulation of the motor nerve stops. Calcium is pumped back into the sarcoplasmic reticulum, which prevents the link between the actin and myosin filaments. Relaxation is brought about by the return of the actin and myosin filaments to their unbound state.

Neuromuscular System

Muscle fibers are innervated by motor neurons that transmit impulses in the form of electrochemical signals from the spinal cord to muscle. A motor neuron generally has numerous terminal branches at the end of its axon and thus innervates many different muscle fibers. The whole structure is what determines the muscle fiber type and its characteristics, function, and involvement in exercise.

Activation of Muscles

When a motor neuron fires an impulse or action potential, all of the fibers that it serves are simultaneously activated and develop force. The extent of control of a muscle depends on the number of muscle fibers within each motor unit. Muscles that must function with great precision, such as eye muscles, may have motor units with as few as one muscle fiber per motor neuron. Changes in the number of active motor units in these small muscles can produce the extremely fine gradations in force that are necessary for precise movements of the eyeball. In contrast, the quadriceps muscle group, which moves the leg with much less precision, may have several hundred fibers served by one motor neuron.

Steps of Muscle Contraction

The steps of muscle contraction can be summarized as follows:

1. Initiation of ATP splitting (by myosin ATPase) causes myosin head to be in an "energized" state that allows it to move into a position to be able to form a bond with actin.

2. The release of phosphate from the ATP splitting process then causes the myosin head to change shape and shift.

3. This pulls the actin filament in toward the center of the sarcomere and is referred to as the *power stroke;* ADP is then released.

4. Once the power stroke has occurred, the myosin head detaches from the actin but only after another ATP binds to the myosin head because the binding process facilitates detachment.

5. The myosin head is now ready to bind to another actin (as described in step 1), and the cycle continues as long as ATP and ATPase are present and calcium is bound to the troponin.

The action potential (electric current) that flows along a motor neuron is not capable of directly exciting muscle fibers. Instead, the motor neuron excites the muscle fiber(s) that it innervates by chemical transmission. Arrival of the action potential at the nerve terminal causes release of a neurotransmitter, **acetylcholine**, which diffuses across the neuromuscular junction, causing excitation of the sarcolemma. Once a sufficient amount of acetylcholine is released, an action potential is generated along the sarcolemma, and the fiber contracts. All of the muscle fibers in the motor unit contract and develop force at the same time. There is no evidence that a motor neuron stimulus causes only some of the fibers to contract. Similarly, a stronger action potential cannot produce a stronger contraction. This phenomenon is known as the **all-or-none principle** of muscle.

Each action potential traveling down a motor neuron results in a short period of activation of the muscle fibers within the motor unit. The brief contraction that results is referred to as a **twitch**. Activation of the sarcolemma results in the release of calcium within the fiber, and contraction proceeds as previously described. Force develops if there is resistance to the pulling interaction of actin and myosin filaments. Although calcium release during a twitch is sufficient to allow optimal activation of actin and myosin, and thereby maximal force of the fibers, calcium is removed before force reaches its maximum, and the muscle relaxes (figure 1.8*a*). If a second twitch is elicited from the motor nerve before the fibers completely relax, force from the two twitches summates, and the resulting force is greater than that produced by a single twitch (figure 1.8*b*). Decreasing the time interval between the twitches results in greater summation of crossbridge binding and force. The stimuli may be delivered at so high a frequency that the twitches begin

to merge and eventually completely fuse, a condition called **tetanus** (figure 1.8, *c* and *d*). This is the maximal amount of force the motor unit can develop.

Muscle Fiber Types

Skeletal muscles are composed of fibers that have markedly different morphological and physiological characteristics. These differences have led to several different systems of classification, based on a variety of criteria. The most familiar approach is to classify fibers according to twitch time, employing the terms **slow-twitch** and **fast-twitch fiber**. Because a motor unit is composed of muscle fibers that are all of the same type, it also can be designated using this classification system. A fast-twitch motor unit is one that develops force and also relaxes rapidly and thus has a short twitch time. Slow-twitch motor units, in contrast, develop force and relax slowly and have a long twitch time.

Histochemical staining for myosin ATPase content is often used to classify fibers as slow-twitch or fast-twitch. Although the techniques can stain for multiple fiber types, the commonly identified fibers are **Type I** (slow-twitch), **Type IIa** (fast-twitch), and **Type IIx** (fast-twitch). Another more specific method is to quantify the amount of myosin heavy chain (MHC) protein; the nomenclature for this is similar to that with the myosin ATPase methodology.

The contrast in mechanical characteristics of Type I and Type II fibers is accompanied by a distinct difference in the ability of the fibers to demand and supply energy for contraction and thus to withstand fatigue. Type I fibers are generally efficient and fatigue resistant and have a high capacity for aerobic energy supply, but they have limited potential for rapid force development, as characterized by low myosin ATPase activity and low anaerobic power (2, 8).

Type II motor units are essentially the opposite, characterized as inefficient and fatigable and as having low aerobic power, rapid force development, high myosin ATPase activity, and high anaerobic power (2, 8). Type IIa and Type IIx fibers differ mainly in their capacity for aerobic–oxidative energy supply. Type IIa fibers, for example, have greater capacity for aerobic metabolism and more capillaries surrounding them than Type IIx and therefore show greater resistance to fatigue (3, 7, 9, 12). Based on these differences, it is not surprising that postural muscles, such as the soleus, have a high composition of Type I fibers, whereas large, so-called locomotor muscles, such as the quadriceps group, have a mixture of both Type I and Type II fibers to enable both low and high power output activities (such as jogging and sprinting, respectively). Refer to table 1.1 for a summary of the primary characteristics of fiber types.

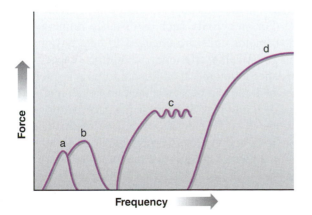

FIGURE 1.8   Twitch, twitch summation, and tetanus of a motor unit: a = single twitch; b = force resulting from summation of two twitches; c = unfused tetanus; d = fused tetanus.

TABLE 1.1 Major Characteristics of Muscle Fiber Types

Characteristic	Type I	Type IIa	Type IIx
Motor neuron size	Small	Large	Large
Recruitment threshold	Low	Intermediate/High	High
Nerve conduction velocity	Slow	Fast	Fast
Contraction speed	Slow	Fast	Fast
Relaxation speed	Slow	Fast	Fast
Fatigue resistance	High	Intermediate/Low	Low
Endurance	High	Intermediate/Low	Low
Force production	Low	Intermediate	High
Power output	Low	Intermediate/High	High
Aerobic enzyme content	High	Intermediate/Low	Low
Anaerobic enzyme content	Low	High	High
Sarcoplasmic reticulum complexity	Low	Intermediate/High	High
Capillary density	High	Intermediate	Low
Myoglobin content	High	Low	Low
Mitochondrial size, density	High	Intermediate	Low
Fiber diameter	Small	Intermediate	Large
Color	Red	White/Red	White

> **Motor units are composed of muscle fibers with specific morphological and physiological characteristics that determine their functional capacity.**

Motor Unit Recruitment Patterns

Through everyday experiences, we are quite aware that a given muscle can vary its level of force output according to the level required by a particular task. This ability to vary or gradate force is essential for performance of smooth, coordinated patterns of movement. Muscular force can be graded in two ways. One is through variation in the frequency at which motor units are activated. If a motor unit is activated once, the twitch that arises does not produce a great deal of force. However, if the frequency of activation is increased so that the forces of the twitches begin to overlap or summate, the resulting force developed by the motor unit is much greater. This method of varying force output is especially important in small muscles, such as those of the hand. Even at low forces, most of the motor units in these muscles are activated, albeit at a low frequency. Force output of the whole muscle is intensified through increase in the frequency of firing of the individual motor units. The

other means of varying skeletal muscle force involves an increase in force through varying the number of motor units activated, a process known as recruitment. In large muscles, such as those in the thigh, motor units are activated at near-tetanic frequency when called on. Increases in force output are achieved through recruitment of additional motor units.

The type of motor unit recruited for a given activity is determined by its physiological characteristics (table 1.2). For an activity such as distance running, slow-twitch motor units are engaged to take advantage of their remarkable efficiency, endurance capacity, and resistance to fatigue. If additional force is needed, as in a sprint at the end of a race, the fast-twitch motor units are called into play to increase the pace; unfortunately, exercise at such intensity cannot be maintained very long. If the activity requires near-maximal performance, as in a power clean, most of the motor units are called into play, with fast-twitch units making the more significant contribution to the effort. Complete activation of the available motor neuron pool is probably not possible in untrained people (4, 5, 6). Although the large fast-twitch units may be recruited if the effort is substantial, under most circumstances it is probably not possible to activate them at a high enough frequency for maximal force to be realized.

TABLE 1.2 Relative Involvement of Muscle Fiber Types in Sport Events

Event	Type I	Type II
100 m sprint	Low	High
800 m run	High	High
Marathon	High	Low
Olympic weightlifting	Low	High
Soccer, lacrosse, hockey	High	High
American football wide receiver	Low	High
American football lineman	Low	High
Basketball, team handball	Low	High
Volleyball	Low	High
Baseball or softball pitcher	Low	High
Boxing	High	High
Wrestling	High	High
50 m swim	Low	High
Field events	Low	High
Cross-country skiing, biathlon	High	Low
Tennis	High	High
Downhill or slalom skiing	High	High
Speed skating	High	High
Track cycling	Low	High
Distance cycling	High	Low
Rowing	High	High

▶ **The force output of a muscle can be varied through change in the frequency of activation of individual motor units or change in the number of activated motor units.**

Proprioception

Proprioceptors are specialized sensory receptors located within joints, muscles, and tendons. Because these receptors are sensitive to pressure and tension, they relay information concerning muscle dynamics to the conscious and subconscious parts of the central nervous system. The brain is thus provided with information concerning kinesthetic sense, or conscious appreciation of the position of body parts with respect to gravity. Most of this proprioceptive information, however, is processed at subconscious levels so we do not have to dedicate conscious activity toward tasks such as maintaining posture or position of body parts.

▶ **Proprioceptors are specialized sensory receptors that provide the central nervous system with information needed to maintain muscle tone and perform complex coordinated movements.**

Muscle Spindles

Muscle spindles are proprioceptors that consist of several modified muscle fibers enclosed in a sheath of connective tissue (figure 1.9). These modified fibers, called **intrafusal fibers**, run parallel to the normal, or **extrafusal**, fibers. Muscle spindles provide information concerning muscle length and the rate of change in length. When the muscle lengthens, spindles are stretched. This deformation activates the sensory neuron of the spindle, which sends an impulse to the spinal cord, where it synapses (connects) with motor neurons. This results in the activation of motor neurons that innervate the same muscle. Spindles thus indicate the degree to which the muscle must be activated in order to overcome a given resistance. As a load increases, the muscle is stretched to a greater extent, and engagement of muscle spindles results in greater activation of the muscle. Muscles that perform precise movements have many spindles per unit of mass to help ensure exact control of their contractile activity. A simple example of muscle spindle activity is the knee jerk reflex. Tapping on the tendon of the knee extensor muscle group below the patella stretches the muscle spindle fibers. This causes activation of extrafusal muscle fibers in the same muscle.

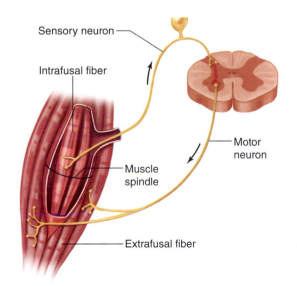

Sensory neuron

Intrafusal fiber

Motor neuron

Muscle spindle

Extrafusal fiber

FIGURE 1.9 Muscle spindle. When a muscle is stretched, deformation of the muscle spindle activates the sensory neuron, which sends an impulse to the spinal cord, where it synapses with a motor neuron, causing the muscle to contract.

How Can Athletes Improve Force Production?

- Incorporate phases of training that use heavier loads in order to optimize neural recruitment.
- Increase the cross-sectional area of muscles involved in the desired activity.
- Perform multimuscle, multijoint exercises that can be done with more explosive actions to optimize fast-twitch muscle recruitment.

A knee jerk occurs as these fibers actively shorten. This, in turn, shortens the intrafusal fibers and causes their discharge to cease.

Golgi Tendon Organs

Golgi tendon organs (GTOs) are proprioceptors located in tendons near the myotendinous junction and are in series, that is, attached end to end, with extrafusal muscle fibers (figure 1.10). Golgi tendon organs are activated when the tendon attached to an active muscle is stretched. As tension in the muscle increases, discharge of the GTOs increases. The sensory neuron of the GTO synapses with an inhibitory interneuron in the spinal cord, which in turn synapses with and inhibits a motor neuron that serves the same muscle. The result is a reduction in tension within the muscle and tendon. Thus, whereas spindles facilitate activation of the muscle, neural input from GTOs inhibits muscle activation.

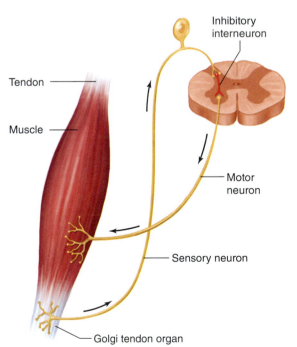

FIGURE 1.10 Golgi tendon organ (GTO). When an extremely heavy load is placed on the muscle, discharge of the GTO occurs. The sensory neuron of the GTO activates an inhibitory interneuron in the spinal cord, which in turn synapses with and inhibits a motor neuron serving the same muscle.

The GTOs' inhibitory process is thought to provide a mechanism that protects against the development of excessive tension. The effect of GTOs is therefore minimal at low forces; but when an extremely heavy load is placed on the muscle, reflexive inhibition mediated by the GTOs causes the muscle to relax. The ability of the motor cortex to override this inhibition may be one of the fundamental adaptations to heavy resistance training.

Cardiovascular System

The primary roles of the cardiovascular system are to transport nutrients and remove waste and by-products while assisting with maintaining the environment for all the body's functions. The cardiovascular system plays key roles in the regulation of the body's acid–base system, fluids, and temperature, as well as a variety of other physiological functions. This section describes the anatomy and physiology of the heart and the blood vessels.

Heart

The heart is a muscular organ composed of two interconnected but separate pumps; the right side of the heart pumps blood through the lungs, and the left side pumps blood through the rest of the body. Each pump has two chambers: an **atrium** and a **ventricle** (figure 1.11). The right and left atria deliver blood into the right and left ventricles. The right and left ventricles supply the main force for moving blood through the pulmonary and peripheral circulations, respectively (13).

Valves

The **tricuspid valve** and **mitral valve** (bicuspid valve) (collectively called **atrioventricular [AV] valves**) prevent the flow of blood from the ventricles back into the atria during ventricular contraction (**systole**). The **aortic valve** and **pulmonary valve** (collectively, the **semilunar valves**) prevent backflow from the aorta and pulmonary arteries into the ventricles during ventricular relaxation (**diastole**). Each valve opens and closes passively; that is, each closes when a backward pressure gradient pushes blood back against it, opening when a forward pressure gradient forces blood in the forward direction (13).

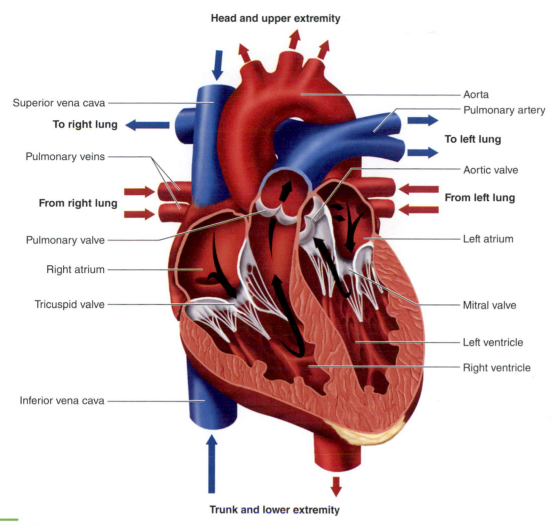

Head and upper extremity

Superior vena cava

To right lung

Pulmonary veins

From right lung

Pulmonary valve

Right atrium

Tricuspid valve

Inferior vena cava

Aorta

Pulmonary artery

To left lung

Aortic valve

From left lung

Left atrium

Mitral valve

Left ventricle

Right ventricle

Trunk and lower extremity

FIGURE 1.11   Structure of the human heart and the course of blood flow through its chambers.

Conduction System

A specialized electrical conduction system (figure 1.12) controls the mechanical contraction of the heart. The conduction system is composed of

- the **sinoatrial (SA) node**—the intrinsic pacemaker—where rhythmic electrical impulses are normally initiated;
- the internodal pathways that conduct the impulse from the SA node to the atrioventricular node;
- the **atrioventricular (AV) node**, where the impulse is delayed slightly before passing into the ventricles;
- the **atrioventricular (AV) bundle**, which conducts the impulse to the ventricles; and
- the **left bundle branch** and **right bundle branch**, which further divide into the **Purkinje fibers** and conduct impulses to all parts of the ventricles.

The SA node is a small area of specialized muscle tissue located in the upper lateral wall of the right atrium.

The fibers of the node are contiguous with the muscle fibers of the atrium, with the result that each electrical impulse that begins in the SA node normally spreads immediately into the atria. The conductive system is organized so that the impulse does not travel into the ventricles too rapidly, allowing time for the atria to contract and empty blood into the ventricles before ventricular contraction begins. It is primarily the AV node and its associated conductive fibers that delay each impulse entering into the ventricles. The AV node is located in the posterior septal wall of the right atrium (13).

The left and right bundle branches lead from the AV bundle into the ventricles. Except for their initial portion, where they penetrate the AV barrier, these conduction fibers have functional characteristics quite opposite those of the AV nodal fibers. They are large and transmit impulses at a much higher velocity than the AV nodal fibers. Because these fibers give way to the Purkinje fibers, which more completely penetrate the ventricles, the impulse travels quickly throughout the entire ventricular system and causes both ventricles to contract at approximately the same time (13).

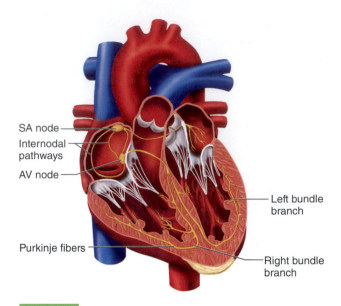

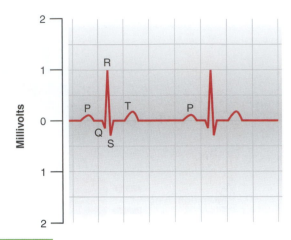

FIGURE 1.13   Normal electrocardiogram.

FIGURE 1.12   The electrical conduction system of the heart.

The SA node normally controls heart rhythmicity because its discharge rate is considerably greater (60-80 times per minute) than that of either the AV node (40-60 times per minute) or the ventricular fibers (15-40 times per minute). Each time the SA node discharges, its impulse is conducted into the AV node and the ventricular fibers, discharging their excitable membranes. Thus, these potentially self-excitatory tissues are discharged before self-excitation can actually occur.

The inherent rhythmicity and conduction properties of the **myocardium** (heart muscle) are influenced by the cardiovascular center of the medulla, which transmits signals to the heart through the **sympathetic** and **parasympathetic nervous systems**, both of which are components of the autonomic nervous system. The atria are supplied with a large number of both sympathetic and parasympathetic neurons, whereas the ventricles receive sympathetic fibers almost exclusively. Stimulation of the sympathetic nerves accelerates depolarization of the SA node (the chronotropic effect), which causes the heart to beat faster. Stimulation of the parasympathetic nervous system slows the rate of SA node discharge, which slows the heart rate. The resting heart rate normally ranges from 60 to 100 beats/min; fewer than 60 beats/min is called **bradycardia**, and more than 100 beats/min is called **tachycardia**.

Electrocardiogram

The electrical activity of the heart can be recorded at the surface of the body; a graphic representation of this activity is called an **electrocardiogram (ECG)**. A normal ECG, seen in figure 1.13, is composed of a **P-wave**, a **QRS complex** (the QRS complex is often three separate waves: a Q-wave, an R-wave, and an

S-wave), and a **T-wave**. The P-wave and the QRS complex are recordings of electrical depolarization, that is, the electrical stimulus that leads to mechanical contraction. **Depolarization** is the reversal of the membrane electrical potential, whereby the normally negative potential inside the membrane becomes slightly positive and the outside becomes slightly negative. The P-wave is generated by the changes in the electrical potential of cardiac muscle cells that depolarize the atria and result in atrial contraction. The QRS complex is generated by the electrical potential that depolarizes the ventricles and results in ventricular contraction. In contrast, the T-wave is caused by the electrical potential generated as the ventricles recover from the state of depolarization; this process, called **repolarization**, occurs in ventricular muscle shortly after depolarization. Although atrial repolarization occurs as well, its wave formation usually occurs during the time of ventricular depolarization and is thus masked by the QRS complex (13).

Blood Vessels

The central and peripheral circulation form a single closed-circuit system with two components: an **arterial system**, which carries blood away from the heart, and a **venous system**, which returns blood toward the heart (figure 1.14). The blood vessels of each system are identified here.

Arteries

The function of **arteries** is to rapidly transport blood pumped from the heart. Because blood pumped from the heart is under relatively high pressure, arteries have strong, muscular walls. Small branches of arteries called **arterioles** act as control vessels through which blood enters the capillaries. Arterioles play a major role in the regulation of blood flow to the capillaries. Arterioles have strong, muscular walls that are capable of closing

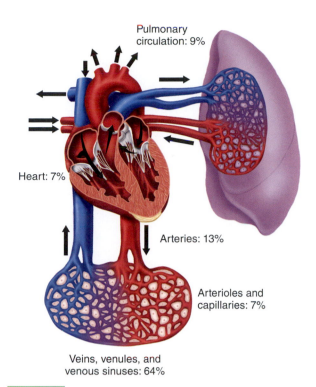

Pulmonary circulation: 9%

Heart: 7%

Arteries: 13%

Arterioles and capillaries: 7%

Veins, venules, and venous sinuses: 64%

FIGURE 1.14   The arterial (right) and venous (left) components of the circulatory system. The percent values indicate the distribution of blood volume throughout the circulatory system at rest.

the arteriole completely or allowing it to be dilated many times their size, thus vastly altering blood flow to the capillaries in response to the needs of the tissues (13).

Capillaries

The function of **capillaries** is to facilitate exchange of oxygen, fluid, nutrients, electrolytes, hormones, and other substances between the blood and the interstitial fluid in the various tissues of the body. The capillary walls are very thin and are permeable to these, but not all, substances (13).

Veins

Venules collect blood from the capillaries and gradually converge into the progressively larger **veins**, which transport blood back to the heart. Because the pressure in the venous system is very low, venous walls are thin, although muscular. This allows them to constrict or dilate

to a great degree and thereby act as a reservoir for blood, either in small or in large amounts (13). In addition, some veins, such as those in the legs, contain one-way valves that help maintain venous return by preventing retrograde blood flow.

> The cardiovascular system transports nutrients and removes waste products while helping to maintain the environment for all the body's functions. The blood transports oxygen from the lungs to the tissues for use in cellular metabolism; and it transports carbon dioxide, the most abundant by-product of metabolism, from the tissues to the lungs, where it is removed from the body.

Blood

Two paramount functions of blood are the transport of oxygen from the lungs to the tissues for use in cellular metabolism and the removal of carbon dioxide, the most abundant by-product of metabolism, from the tissues to the lungs. The transport of oxygen is accomplished by **hemoglobin**, the iron–protein molecule carried by the red blood cells. Hemoglobin also has an additional important role as an acid–base buffer, a regulator of hydrogen ion concentration, which is crucial to the rates of chemical reactions in cells. **Red blood cells**, the major component of blood, have other functions as well. For instance, they contain a large quantity of carbonic anhydrase, which catalyzes the reaction between carbon dioxide and water to facilitate carbon dioxide removal.

Respiratory System

The primary function of the respiratory system is the basic exchange of oxygen and carbon dioxide. The anatomy of the human respiratory system is shown in figure 1.15. As air passes through the nose, the nasal cavities perform three distinct functions: warming, humidifying, and purifying the air (13). Air is distributed to the lungs by way of the trachea, bronchi, and bronchioles. The **trachea** is called the first-generation respiratory passage, and the right and left main **bronchi** are the second-generation passages; each division thereafter is an additional generation (**bronchioles**). There are approximately 23

What Is the Skeletal Muscle Pump?

The skeletal muscle pump is the assistance that contracting muscles provide to the circulatory system. The muscle pump works with the venous system, which contains the one-way valves for blood return to the heart. The contracting muscle compresses the veins, but since the blood can flow only in the direction of the valves, it is returned to the heart. This mechanism is one of the reasons that individuals are told to keep moving around after exercise to avoid blood pooling in the lower extremities. On the flip side, it is important to periodically squeeze muscles during prolonged sitting to facilitate blood return to the heart.

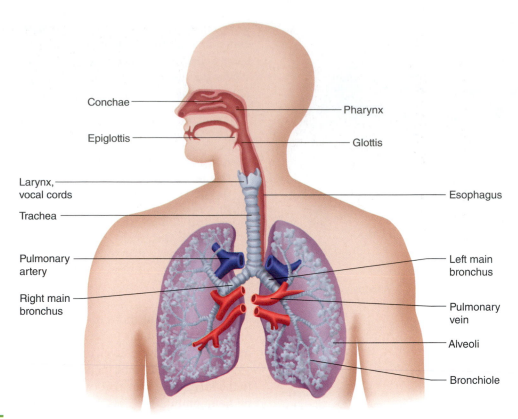

Conchae

Pharynx

Epiglottis

Glottis

Larynx, vocal cords

Esophagus

Trachea

Pulmonary artery

Left main bronchus

Right main bronchus

Pulmonary vein

Alveoli

Bronchiole

FIGURE 1.15   Gross anatomy of the human respiratory system.

generations before the air finally reaches the **alveoli**, where gases are exchanged in respiration (13).

> The primary function of the respiratory system is the basic exchange of oxygen and carbon dioxide.

Exchange of Air

The amount and movement of air and expired gases in and out of the lungs are controlled by expansion and recoil of the lungs. The lungs do not actively expand and recoil themselves but rather are acted upon to do so in two ways: by downward and upward movement of the diaphragm to lengthen and shorten the chest cavity and by elevation and depression of the ribs to increase and decrease the back-to-front diameter of the chest cavity (13). Normal, quiet breathing is accomplished almost entirely by movement of the diaphragm. During inspiration, contraction of the diaphragm creates a negative pressure (vacuum) in the chest cavity, and air is drawn into the lungs. During expiration, the diaphragm simply relaxes; the elastic recoil of the lungs, chest wall, and abdominal structures compresses the lungs, and air is expelled. During heavy breathing, the elastic forces alone are not powerful enough to provide the necessary respiratory response. The extra required force is achieved mainly by contraction of the abdominal muscles, which

push the abdomen upward against the bottom of the diaphragm (13).

The second method for expanding the lungs is to raise the rib cage. Because the chest cavity is small and the ribs are slanted downward while in the resting position, elevating the rib cage allows the ribs to project almost directly forward so that the sternum can move forward and away from the spine. The muscles that elevate the rib cage are called muscles of inspiration and include the external intercostals, the sternocleidomastoids, the anterior serrati, and the scaleni. The muscles that depress the chest are muscles of expiration and include the abdominal muscles (rectus abdominis, external and internal obliques, and transversus abdominis) and the internal intercostals (13).

Pleural pressure is the pressure in the narrow space between the lung pleura and the chest wall **pleura** (membranes enveloping the lungs and lining the chest walls). This pressure is normally slightly negative. Because the lung is an elastic structure, during normal inspiration the expansion of the chest cage is able to pull on the surface of the lungs and creates a more negative pressure, thus enhancing inspiration. During expiration, the events are essentially reversed (13).

Alveolar pressure is the pressure inside the alveoli when the glottis is open and no air is flowing into or out of the lungs. In fact, in this instance the pressure in all parts of the respiratory tree is the same all the way to the

How Important Is It to Train the Muscles of Respiration?

Regular exercise in general is beneficial for maintaining respiratory muscle function. Both endurance exercise, which involves repetitive contraction of breathing muscles, and resistance exercise, which taxes the diaphragm and abdominal muscles especially because of their use for stabilization and for increasing intra-abdominal pressure (Valsalva maneuver) during exertion, can result in some muscle training adaptations. This can help to preserve some of the pulmonary function with aging. However, it is generally not necessary to specifically train the muscles of respiration except following surgery or during prolonged bed rest when the normal breathing patterns are compromised.

alveoli and is equal to the atmospheric pressure. To cause inward flow of air during inspiration, the pressure in the alveoli must fall to a value slightly below atmospheric pressure. During expiration, alveolar pressure must rise above atmospheric pressure (13).

During normal respiration at rest, only 3% to 5% of the total energy expended by the body is required for pulmonary ventilation. During very heavy exercise, however, the amount of energy required can increase to as much as 8% to 15% of total body energy expenditure, especially if the person has any degree of increased airway resistance, as occurs with exercise-induced asthma. Precautions, including physician evaluation of the athlete, are often recommended, depending on the potential level of impairment.

Exchange of Respiratory Gases

With ventilation, oxygen diffuses from the alveoli into the pulmonary blood, and carbon dioxide diffuses from the blood into the alveoli. The process of **diffusion** is a simple random motion of molecules moving in opposite directions through the alveolar capillary membrane. The energy for diffusion is provided by the kinetic motion of the molecules themselves. Net diffusion of the gas occurs from the region of high concentration to the region of low concentration. The rates of diffusion of the two gases depend on their concentrations in the capillaries and alveoli and the partial pressure of each gas (13).

At rest, the partial pressure of oxygen in the alveoli is about 60 mmHg greater than that in the pulmonary capillaries. Thus, oxygen diffuses into the pulmonary capillary blood. Similarly, carbon dioxide diffuses in the opposite direction. This process of gas exchange is so rapid as to be thought of as instantaneous (13).

Conclusion

Knowledge of musculoskeletal, neuromuscular, cardiovascular, and respiratory anatomy and physiology is important for the strength and conditioning professional to have in order to understand the scientific basis for conditioning. This includes knowledge of the function of the macrostructure and microstructure of the skeleton and muscle fibers, muscle fiber types, and interactions between tendon and muscle and between the motor unit and its activation, as well as the interactions of the heart, vascular system, lungs, and respiratory system. This information is necessary for developing training strategies that will meet the specific needs of the athlete.

KEY TERMS

A-band	atrium	endomysium
acetylcholine	axial skeleton	epimysium
actin	biaxial joints	extrafusal fibers
action potential	bone periosteum	fasciculi
all-or-none principle	bradycardia	fast-twitch fiber
alveolar pressure	bronchi	fibrous joints
alveoli	bronchiole	Golgi tendon organ (GTO)
aortic valve	capillary	hemoglobin
appendicular skeleton	cartilaginous joints	hyaline cartilage
arterial system	crossbridge	H-zone
arteriole	depolarization	I-band
artery	diastole	inferior
atrioventricular (AV) bundle	diffusion	intrafusal fibers
atrioventricular (AV) node	distal	left bundle branch
atrioventricular (AV) valves	electrocardiogram (ECG)	mitral valve

motor neuron
motor unit
multiaxial joints
muscle fiber
muscle spindle
myocardium
myofibril
myofilament
myosin
neuromuscular junction
parasympathetic nervous system
perimysium
pleura
pleural pressure
power stroke
proprioceptor
proximal
pulmonary valve
Purkinje fibers

P-wave
QRS complex
red blood cell
repolarization
right bundle branch
sarcolemma
sarcomere
sarcoplasm
sarcoplasmic reticulum
semilunar valves
sinoatrial (SA) node
sliding-filament theory
slow-twitch fiber
superior
sympathetic nervous system
synovial fluid
synovial joints
systole
tachycardia

tendon
tetanus
trachea
tricuspid valve
tropomyosin
troponin
T-tubule
T-wave
twitch
Type I fiber
Type IIa fiber
Type IIx fiber
uniaxial joints
vein
venous system
ventricle
venule
vertebral column
Z-line

STUDY QUESTIONS

1. Which of the following substances regulates muscle actions?
   a. potassium
   b. calcium
   c. troponin
   d. tropomyosin

2. Which of the following substances acts at the neuromuscular junction to excite the muscle fibers of a motor unit?
   a. acetylcholine
   b. ATP
   c. creatine phosphate
   d. serotonin

3. When throwing a baseball, an athlete's arm is rapidly stretched just before throwing the ball. Which of the following structures detects and responds to that stretch by reflexively increasing muscle activity?
   a. Golgi tendon organ
   b. muscle spindle
   c. extrafusal muscle
   d. Pacinian corpuscle

4. From which of the following is the heart's electrical impulse normally initiated?
   a. AV node
   b. SA node
   c. the brain
   d. the sympathetic nervous system

5. Which of the following occurs during the QRS complex of a typical ECG?
   I. depolarization of the atrium
   II. repolarization of the atrium
   III. repolarization of the ventricle
   IV. depolarization of the ventricle
   a. I and III only
   b. II and IV only
   c. I, II, and III only
   d. II, III, and IV only

CHAPTER 2

Biomechanics of Resistance Exercise

Jeffrey M. McBride, PhD

▶ **After completing this chapter, you will be able to**

- identify the major components of skeletal musculature,
- differentiate the various types of levers of the musculoskeletal system,
- identify primary anatomical movements during sport activities and exercises,
- calculate linear and rotational work and power,
- describe the factors contributing to human strength and power,
- evaluate resistive force and power patterns of exercise devices, and
- identify factors of importance for joint biomechanics with exercise.

The author would like to acknowledge the significant contribution of Everett Harman to this chapter.

Knowledge of biomechanics is important for understanding human movements, including those involved in sport and exercise. **Biomechanics** focuses on the mechanisms through which the musculoskeletal components interact to create movement. Having insight into how body movements are carried out and the stresses that the movements place on the musculoskeletal system facilitates the design of safe and effective resistance training programs.

This chapter begins with an overview of skeletal musculature, body mechanics, and the primary movement patterns during sport activities and exercise, followed by biomechanical principles related to the manifestation of human strength and power. Next, the primary sources of resistance to muscle contraction used in exercise devices—including gravity, inertia, friction, fluid resistance, and elasticity—are discussed. Then we turn to concerns with resistance training that relate to joint biomechanics (with special emphasis on the shoulders, back, and knees).

Skeletal Musculature

To cause movement or to generate force against external objects, both ends of each skeletal muscle must be attached to bone by connective tissue. Traditionally, anatomists define the muscle's **origin** as its **proximal** (toward the center of the body) attachment, and its **insertion** as its **distal** (away from the center of the body) attachment. Sometimes the origin is defined as the more stationary structure to which the muscle is attached and the insertion as the more mobile structure. This definition can lead to a confusing reversal of the origin and insertion. For example, during a straight-leg sit-up, the origin of the iliacus muscle is the femur, because of its relative immobility. The pelvis, being more mobile, is the insertion. However, during the leg raise exercise, the pelvis is relatively immobile and would therefore become the origin, while the more mobile femur would become the insertion. The traditional definition therefore provides the most consistency.

Muscles are attached to bone in various ways. In **fleshy attachments**, which are most often found at the proximal end of a muscle, muscle fibers are directly affixed to the bone, usually over a wide area so that force is distributed rather than localized. **Fibrous attachments**, such as **tendons**, blend into and are continuous with both the muscle sheaths and the connective tissue surrounding the bone. They have additional fibers that extend into the bone itself, making for a very strong union.

Virtually all body movements involve the action of more than one muscle. The muscle most directly involved in bringing about a movement is called the prime mover, or **agonist**. A muscle that can slow down or stop the movement is called the **antagonist**. The antagonist assists in joint stabilization and in braking the limb toward the end of a fast movement, thereby protecting ligamentous and **cartilaginous joint** structures from potentially destructive forces. During throwing, for example, the triceps acts as an agonist, extending the elbow to accelerate the ball. As the elbow approaches full extension, the biceps acts as an antagonist to slow down elbow extension and bring it to a stop, thereby protecting elbow structures from internal impact.

A muscle is called a **synergist** when it assists indirectly in a movement. For example, the muscles that stabilize the scapula act as synergists during upper arm movement. Without these synergists, the muscles that move the upper arm (many of which originate on the scapula) would not be effective in bringing about this movement. Synergists are also required to control body motion when the agonist is a muscle that crosses two joints. For example, the rectus femoris muscle crosses the hip and knee, acting to flex the hip and extend the knee when contracting. Rising from a low squat involves both hip and knee extension. If the rectus femoris is to act to extend the knee as a person rises without inclining the trunk forward, then hip extensor muscles such as the gluteus maximus must act synergistically to counteract the hip flexion that would otherwise result from tension in the rectus femoris.

Levers of the Musculoskeletal System

Although there are many muscles in the body that do not act through levers, such as muscles of the face, tongue, heart, arteries, and sphincters, body movements directly involved in sport and exercise primarily act through the bony levers of the skeleton. In order to understand how the body effects such movements, a basic knowledge of levers is required. Several basic definitions follow.

first-class lever—A lever for which the muscle force and resistive force act on opposite sides of the fulcrum (see figure 2.2).

fulcrum—The pivot point of a lever.

lever—A rigid or semirigid body that, when subjected to a force whose line of action does not pass through its pivot point, exerts force on any object impeding its tendency to rotate (figure 2.1).

mechanical advantage—The ratio of the moment arm through which an applied force acts to that through which a resistive force acts (figure 2.1). For there to be a state of equilibrium between the applied and resistive torques, the product of the muscle force and the moment arm through which it acts must equal the product of the resistive force and the moment arm through which it acts. Therefore, a mechanical

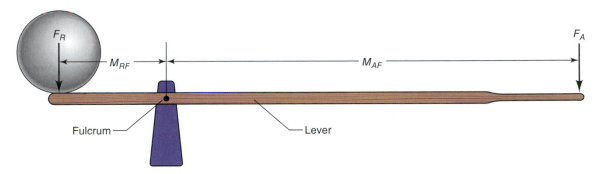

FIGURE 2.1   A lever. The lever can transmit force tangential to the arc of rotation from one contact point along the object's length to another. F_A = force applied to the lever; M_{AF} = moment arm of the applied force; F_R = force resisting the lever's rotation; M_{RF} = moment arm of the resistive force. The lever applies a force on the object equal in magnitude to but opposite in direction from F_R.

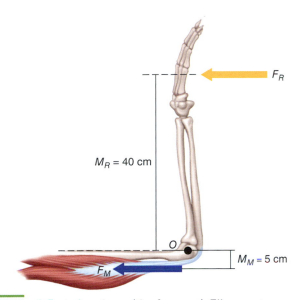

FIGURE 2.2   A first-class lever (the forearm). Elbow extension against resistance (e.g., a triceps extension exercise). O = fulcrum; F_M = muscle force; F_R = resistive force; M_M = moment arm of the muscle force; M_R = moment arm of the resistive force. Mechanical advantage = M_M/M_R = 5 cm/40 cm = 0.125, which, being less than 1.0, is a disadvantage in the common sense.

advantage, represented as a ratio greater than 1.0, allows the applied (muscle) force to be less than the resistive force to produce an equal amount of torque. Conversely, a calculated mechanical advantage of a ratio less than 1.0 indicates that one must apply greater (muscle) force than the amount of resistive force present, creating an obvious disadvantage for the muscle.

moment arm (also called force arm, lever arm, or torque arm)—The perpendicular distance from the line of action of the force to the fulcrum. The line of action of a force is an infinitely long line passing through the point of application of the force, oriented in the direction in which the force is exerted.

muscle force—Force generated by biochemical activity, or the stretching of noncontractile tissue, that tends to draw the opposite ends of a muscle toward each other.

resistive force—Force generated by a source external to the body (e.g., gravity, inertia, friction) that acts contrary to muscle force.

second-class lever—A lever for which the muscle force and resistive force act on the same side of the fulcrum, with the muscle force acting through a moment arm longer than that through which the resistive force acts, as when the calf muscles work to raise the body onto the balls of the feet (figure 2.3). Due to its mechanical advantage (i.e., relatively long moment arm), the required muscle force is smaller than the resistive force (body weight).

third-class lever—A lever for which the muscle force and resistive force act on the same side of the fulcrum, with the muscle force acting through a moment arm shorter than that through which the resistive force acts (figure 2.4). The mechanical advantage is thus less than 1.0, so the muscle force has to be greater than the resistive force to produce torque equal to that produced by the resistive force.

torque (also called moment)—The degree to which a force tends to rotate an object about a specified fulcrum. It is defined quantitatively as the magnitude of a force times the length of its moment arm.

Figure 2.2 shows a first-class lever, because muscle force and resistive force act on opposite sides of the fulcrum. During isometric exertion or constant-speed joint rotation, $F_M \cdot M_M = F_R \cdot M_R$. Because M_M is much smaller than M_R, F_M must be much greater than F_R; this illustrates the disadvantageous nature of this arrangement (i.e., a large muscle force is required to push against a relatively small external resistance).

Most human muscles that rotate the limbs about body joints operate at a mechanical advantage of less than 1.0 (that is, at a mechanical *dis*advantage). This is why internal muscle forces are much greater than the forces exerted by the body on external objects. For example, in figure 2.2, because the resistance moment arm is eight times longer than the muscle moment arm, muscle force must be eight times the resistive force. The extremely high internal forces experienced by muscles and tendons account in large part for injury to these tissues. During actual movement, the categorization of a lever as first, second, or third class often depends on the somewhat arbitrary decision of where the fulcrum lies. Therefore, understanding the principle of mechanical advantage is of much greater importance than being able to classify levers.

Mechanical advantage often changes continuously during real-world activities. The following are examples of this.

- For movements such as knee extension and flexion, where the joint is not a true hinge, the location of the axis of rotation changes continuously throughout the range of motion, affecting the length of the moment arm through which the quadriceps and hamstrings act. For knee extension, the patella, or kneecap, helps to prevent large changes in the mechanical advantage of the quadriceps muscle by keeping the quadriceps tendon from falling in close to the axis of rotation (figure 2.5).

- For movements such as elbow extension and flexion, there is no structure such as the patella to keep the perpendicular distance from the joint axis of rotation to the tendon's line of action relatively constant (figure 2.6).

- During resistance training with free weights, the moment arm through which the weight acts equals the horizontal distance from a line through the center of mass of the barbell or dumbbell to the body joint about which rotation of the limb occurs; the resistive moment arm thus varies throughout the movement (figure 2.7).

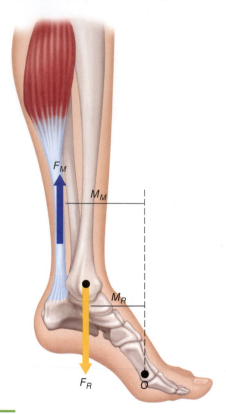

FIGURE 2.3   A second-class lever (the foot). Plantar flexion against resistance (e.g., a standing heel raise exercise). F_M = muscle force; F_R = resistive force; M_M = moment arm of the muscle force; M_R = moment arm of the resistive force. When the body is raised, the ball of the foot, being the point about which the foot rotates, is the fulcrum (O). Because M_M is greater than M_R, F_M is less than F_R.

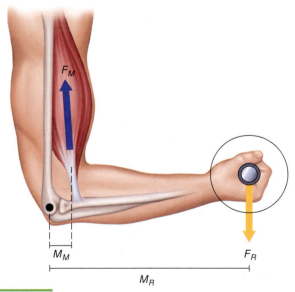

FIGURE 2.4   A third-class lever (the forearm). Elbow flexion against resistance (e.g., a biceps curl exercise). F_M = muscle force; F_R = resistive force; M_M = moment arm of the muscle force; M_R = moment arm of the resistive force. Because M_M is much smaller than M_R, F_M must be much greater than F_R.

> ▶ **Most of the skeletal muscles operate at a considerable mechanical disadvantage due to the lever arrangement within the body and relative to the external forces the body resists. Thus, during sport and other physical activities, forces in the muscles and tendons are much higher than those exerted by hands or feet on external objects or the ground.**

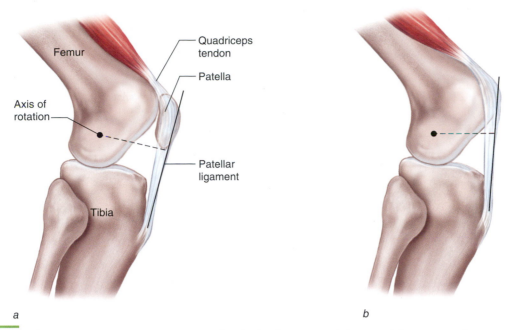

FIGURE 2.5 *(a)* The patella increases the mechanical advantage of the quadriceps muscle group by maintaining the quadriceps tendon's distance from the knee's axis of rotation. *(b)* Absence of the patella allows the tendon to fall closer to the knee's center of rotation, shortening the moment arm through which the muscle force acts and thereby reducing the muscle's mechanical advantage.

Reprinted, by permission, from Gowitzke and Milner, 1988 (12).

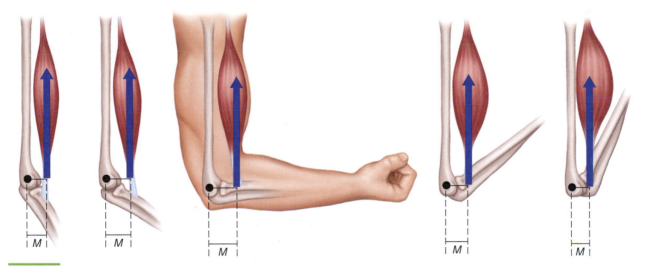

FIGURE 2.6 During elbow flexion with the biceps muscle, the perpendicular distance from the joint axis of rotation to the tendon's line of action varies throughout the range of joint motion. When the moment arm *(M)* is shorter, there is less mechanical advantage.

Variations in Tendon Insertion

Considerable variation in human anatomical structure exists, including the points at which tendons are attached to bone. A person whose tendons are inserted on the bone farther from the joint center should be able to lift heavier weights because muscle force acts through a longer moment arm and thus can produce greater torque around the joint. (In figure 2.6, for example, consider how the moment arm *[M]* would change if the tendon insertion

were farther to the right.) It is important, however, to recognize the trade-off involved in tendon insertion. The mechanical advantage gained by having tendons insert farther from the joint center is accompanied by a loss of maximum speed because, with the tendon inserted farther from the joint center, the muscle has to contract more to make the joint move through a given range of motion. In other words, a given amount of muscle shortening results in less rotation of body segments about a joint, which translates into a loss in movement speed.

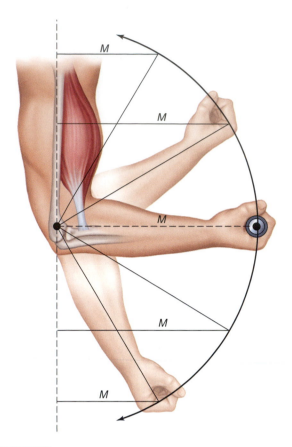

FIGURE 2.7 As a weight is lifted, the moment arm *(M)* through which the weight acts, and thus the resistive torque, changes with the horizontal distance from the weight to the elbow.

Figure 2.8*a* shows that, starting with the joint extended, when a hypothetical muscle shortens by a given amount, the joint rotates by 37°. However, if the muscle were inserted farther from the joint center, as in figure 2.8*b*, the same amount of muscle shortening would bring about only 34° of joint rotation because of the geometry of the dynamic triangle whose vertices are the muscle insertion and origin and the joint center of rotation.

To produce a given joint rotational velocity, a muscle inserted farther from the joint center must contract at a higher speed, at which it can generate less force due to the inverse force–velocity relationship of muscle (34) described later in this chapter. Therefore, such a tendon arrangement reduces the muscle's force capability during faster movements.

One can see how relatively subtle individual differences in structure can result in various advantages and disadvantages. Although these skeletal arrangements are nonmodifiable, it is important to understand that for slower movements, as in powerlifting, tendon insertion farther from the joint than normal can be advantageous, while for athletic activities occurring at high speeds,

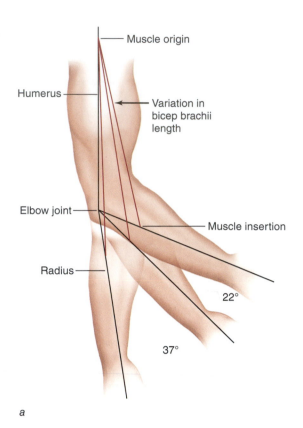

a

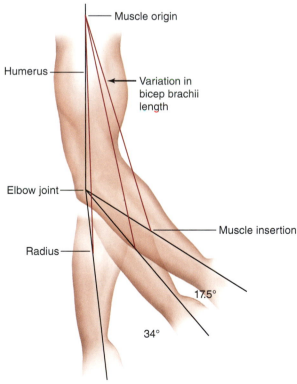

b

FIGURE 2.8 Changes in joint angle with equal increments of muscle shortening when the tendon is inserted *(a)* closer to and *(b)* farther from the joint center. Configuration *b* has a larger moment arm and thus greater torque for a given muscle force, but less rotation per unit of muscle contraction and thus slower movement speed.

such as hitting a tennis ball, such an arrangement can be disadvantageous.

Anatomical Planes and Major Body Movements

Figure 2.9 depicts a person standing in the standard **anatomical position**. The body is erect, the arms are down at the sides, and the palms face forward. Anatomical views of the body, as in magnetic resonance imaging, are generally shown in the **sagittal**, **frontal**, and **transverse planes**, which slice the body into left–right, front–back, and upper–lower sections, respectively, not necessarily at the midpoint. The anatomical planes are also useful for describing the major body movements. Examples of exercise movements that take place in these planes include standing barbell curl (sagittal plane), standing lateral dumbbell raise (frontal plane), and dumbbell fly (transverse plane).

Biomechanical analysis of human movement can be used to quantitatively analyze the target activity. In the absence of the requisite equipment and expertise, however, simple visual observation is adequate for identifying the basic features of a sport movement. Exercises can then be selected that involve similar movement around the same joints, thereby incorporating specificity of training. Slow-motion videotape can facilitate the observation. Also, commercially available software enables more detailed analysis of sport movements captured in digital video.

Figure 2.10 presents a simple list of possible body movements that provides a manageable framework for movement-oriented exercise prescription. Only movements in the frontal, sagittal, and transverse planes are considered because, although few body movements occur only in these three major planes, there is enough overlap of training effects that exercising muscles within the planes also strengthens them for movements between the planes.

Although a program providing resistance exercise for all the movements in figure 2.10 would be both comprehensive and balanced, some of the movements are commonly omitted from standard exercise programs whereas others receive particular emphasis. Important sport movements not usually incorporated into standard resistance training programs include shoulder internal and external rotation (throwing, tennis), knee flexion (sprinting), hip flexion (kicking, sprinting), ankle dorsiflexion (running), hip internal and external rotation (pivoting), hip adduction and abduction (lateral cutting), torso rotation (throwing, batting), and the various neck movements (boxing, wrestling).

Human Strength and Power

The terms *strength* and *power* are widely used to describe some important abilities that contribute to maximal human efforts in sport and other physical activities. Unfortunately, there is often little consistency in the way the terms are used. This section provides a scientific basis for understanding human strength and power and shows how various factors contribute to their manifestation.

Basic Definitions

Though it is widely accepted that **strength** is the ability to exert force, there is considerable disagreement as to how strength should be measured. The weight that a person can lift is probably the oldest quantitative measure of strength. Technological developments have popularized the use of isometric strength testing and also isokinetic strength testing. All sports involve **acceleration** (change in velocity per unit time) of the body and, for some sports, of an implement as well (e.g., baseball bat, javelin, tennis racket). Acceleration is associated with resistive force according to Isaac Newton's second law:

$$\text{Force} = \text{Mass} \cdot \text{Acceleration} \qquad (2.1)$$

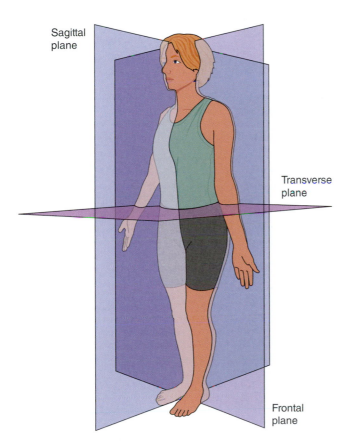

Sagittal plane

Transverse plane

Frontal plane

FIGURE 2.9   The three planes of the human body in the anatomical position.

Wrist—sagittal
Flexion
Exercise: wrist curl
Sport: basketball free throw

Extension
Exercise: wrist extension
Sport: racquetball backhand

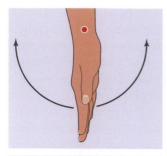

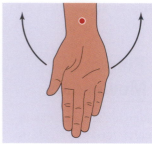

Wrist—frontal
Ulnar deviation
Exercise: specific wrist curl
Sport: baseball bat swing

Radial deviation
Exercise: specific wrist curl
Sport: golf backswing

Elbow—sagittal
Flexion
Exercise: biceps curl
Sport: bowling

Extension
Exercise: triceps pushdown
Sport: shot put

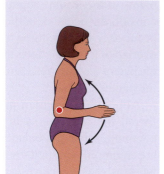

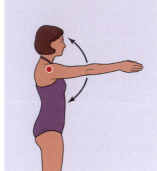

Shoulder—sagittal
Flexion
Exercise: front shoulder raise
Sport: boxing uppercut punch

Extension
Exercise: neutral-grip seated row
Sport: freestyle swimming stroke

Shoulder—frontal
Adduction
Exercise: wide-grip lat pulldown
Sport: swimming breast stroke

Abduction
Exercise: wide-grip shoulder press
Sport: springboard diving

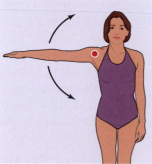

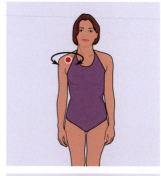

Shoulder—transverse
Internal rotation
Exercise: arm wrestle movement (with dumbbell or cable)
Sport: baseball pitch

External rotation
Exercise: reverse arm wrestle movement
Sport: karate block

Shoulder—transverse
(upper arm to 90° to trunk)
Adduction
Exercise: dumbbell chest fly
Sport: tennis forehand

Abduction
Exercise: bent-over lateral raise
Sport: tennis backhand

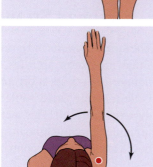

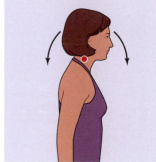

Neck—sagittal
Flexion
Exercise: neck machine
Sport: somersault

Extension
Exercise: dynamic back bridge
Sport: back flip

Neck—transverse
Left rotation
Exercise: manual resistance
Sport: wrestling movement

Right rotation
Exercise: manual resistance
Sport: wrestling movement

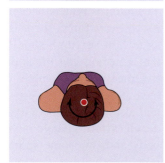

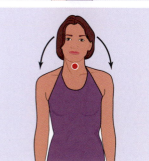

Neck—frontal
Left tilt
Exercise: neck machine
Sport: slalom skiing

Right tilt
Exercise: neck machine
Sport: slalom skiing

FIGURE 2.10 Major body movements. Planes of movement are relative to the body in the anatomical position unless otherwise stated. Common exercises that provide resistance to the movements and related sport activities are listed.

Reprinted, by permission, from Harman, Johnson, and Frykman, 1992 (16).

Lower back—sagittal
Flexion
Exercise: sit-up
Sport: javelin throw
follow-through

Extension
Exercise: stiff-leg deadlift
Sport: back flip

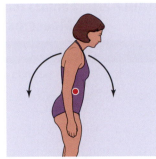

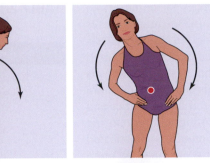

Lower back—frontal
Left tilt
Exercise: medicine ball
overhead hook throw
Sport: gymnastics side aerial

Right tilt
Exercise: side bend
Sport: basketball hook shot

Lower back—transverse
Left rotation
Exercise: medicine ball side
toss
Sport: baseball batting

Right rotation
Exercise: torso machine
Sport: golf swing

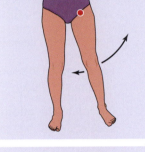

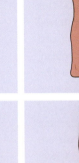

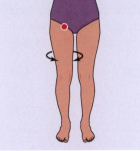

Hip—sagittal
Flexion
Exercise: leg raise
Sport: American football punt

Extension
Exercise: back squat
Sport: long jump take-off

Hip—frontal
Adduction
Exercise: standing
adduction machine
Sport: soccer side step

Abduction
Exercise: standing
abduction machine
Sport: rollerblading

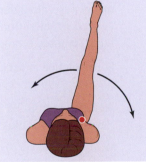

Hip—transverse
Internal rotation
Exercise: resisted internal rotation
Sport: basketball pivot movement

External rotation
Exercise: resisted external rotation
Sport: figure skating turn

Hip—transverse
(upper leg to 90° to trunk)
Adduction
Exercise: adduction machine
Sport: karate in-sweep

Abduction
Exercise: seated abduction
machine
Sport: wrestling escape

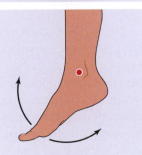

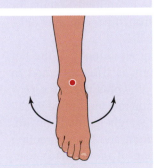

Knee—sagittal
Flexion
Exercise: leg (knee) curl
Sport: diving tuck

Extension
Exercise: leg (knee) extension
Sport: volleyball block

Ankle—sagittal
Dorsiflexion
Exercise: toe raise
Sport: running

Plantar flexion
Exercise: calf (heel) raise
Sport: high jump

Ankle—frontal
Inversion
Exercise: resisted inversion
Sport: soccer dribbling

Eversion
Exercise: resisted eversion
Sport: speed skating

Because of individual differences in the ability to exert force at different velocities (43), strength scores obtained from isometric and low-speed resistance tests may vary in predictive ability when the force is required with concomitant high velocity. Thus, testing an athlete's force capabilities at various loads may provide more insight into the person's sport-specific capabilities and weaknesses (6). Although controlling and monitoring velocity during strength testing require sophisticated equipment, the resulting strength scores may be more meaningfully related to sport ability than are static strength measures or maximum loads lifted.

Positive Work and Power

The curiosity about force capacity at particular velocities of movement or at high velocity has led to heightened interest in power as a measurement of the ability to exert force at higher speeds. Outside of the scientific realm, power is loosely defined as "explosive strength" (42). However, in physics, **power** is precisely defined as the *time rate of doing work,* where **work** is the product of the force exerted on an object and the distance the object moves in the direction in which the force is exerted. Quantitatively, work and power are defined as follows:

$$\text{Work} = \text{Force} \cdot \text{Displacement} \qquad (2.2)$$

and

$$\text{Power} = \text{Work} / \text{Time} \qquad (2.3)$$

Power can also be calculated as the product of force on an object and the object's velocity in the direction in which the force is exerted, or the product of the object's velocity and the force on the object in the direction in which the object is traveling.

For all the equations in this chapter to work out correctly, consistent units must be used. In the International System of Units (SI, abbreviated from the French), the worldwide standard, force is measured in newtons (N), distance in meters (m), work in joules (J, i.e., newton-meters, or N·m), time in seconds (s), and power in watts (W, i.e., J/s). The appropriate SI units for the equations can be obtained from other common units using the factors listed in table 2.1.

As an example of applying equation 2.2, the net work performed when a weight is lifted is equal to the magnitude of the weight (F_1) plus the force (F_2) required for a desired acceleration rate multiplied by the displacement (D) in which the weight is lifted upward. It should be noted that the weight and force direction must coincide with the direction of the displacement. The determination of this relationship is defined by the angle between the force vector and displacement vector (theta, θ). For example, the work involved in lifting a 100 kg (220-pound) barbell 2 m (6.6 feet) per repetition for 10 repetitions is calculated as follows:

TABLE 2.1   Factors for Conversion of Common Measures to SI Units

To get	Multiply	By
newtons (N)	pounds (lb)	4.448
newtons (N)	kilograms mass (kg)	local acceleration of gravity
newtons (N)	kilograms force (kg)	9.807
meters (m)	feet (ft)	0.3048
meters (m)	inches (in.)	0.02540
radians (rad)	degrees (°)	0.01745

1. Determine the **weight** (F_1) of the bar in SI units (newtons) by multiplying the mass of the bar in kilograms by the local acceleration due to gravity in meters per second squared. If the local acceleration due to gravity is not available, 9.8 m/s² is a good approximation. As stated earlier, theta (θ) is the angle between the force and displacement vector, which in this case is zero:

$$F_1^\uparrow F_2^\uparrow D^\uparrow \ \theta = 0 \text{ degrees}$$

Force applied to counter the weight of the bar (F_1) = 9.8 m/s² · 100 kg · cos 0° = 980 N

2. Calculate the additional force (F_2) required to accelerate the bar mass upward at a given rate. (Force required to lower the bar in a controlled manner is calculated later.) For example, if the desired acceleration rate upward is 2 m/s², the force required would be

Force applied to accelerate the bar upward (F_2) = 2 m/s² · 100 kg · cos 0° = 200 N

3. Apply equation 2.2 to calculate the work for 10 repetitions in Joules:

Work (positive) = (980 N + 200 N) · 2 m · 10 Reps = 23,600 J

This method of calculating work can be very useful for quantifying the volume of a workout. The work for each set is calculated as shown, and the total work for the whole workout is determined by addition. For free weight exercises, the vertical travel of the bar for one repetition of each exercise is measured for each individual by subtracting the height of the bar relative to the floor at its low position from the height of the bar at its high position. For weight-stack exercises, the vertical travel of the stack is measured. These measurements can be made with an empty bar or the lowest-weight plate on the stack, because the vertical distance traveled by the weight during a given exercise for an individual should be about the same regardless of the weight used. In the previous example, in which work was determined, if it takes 40 seconds to perform the 10 repetitions, the average power output in watts for the set is calculated using equation 2.3:

Power (positive) = 23,600 J / 40 seconds = 590 W

Negative Work and Power

Because power equals the product of force and velocity, when force is exerted on a weight in the direction opposite to the one in which the weight is moving (as when a weight is lowered in a controlled manner), calculated power has a negative sign, as does calculated work. All such "negative" power and work occur during eccentric muscle actions, such as lowering a weight or decelerating at the end of a rapid movement. Strictly speaking, there is no such thing as negative work or power. The term *negative work* really refers to work performed on, rather than by, a muscle. When a weight is lifted, muscles perform work on the weight, increasing the weight's potential energy. When the weight is lowered, its potential energy is used to perform an equal amount of work on the athlete. Thus, while repetitions are performed, the athlete and weight alternately perform work on each other, rather than the athlete's alternately performing positive and negative work. The rate at which the repetitions are performed determines the power output. The rate at which the bar would accelerate downward in free fall is 9.8 m/s². If the net force applied was 980 N (F_1), the acceleration rate would be 0 m/s². If we remove 200 N of force (200 N divided by the bar mass of 100 kg, $a = F/m$) the acceleration rate of the bar would be 2 m/s² downward (in other words, controlling the bar's rate of acceleration by decreasing the force applied).

1. Calculate the force (F_3) that must be removed to allow the bar mass to accelerate downward at a given rate. For example, if the desired acceleration rate downward is 2 m/s², the force required would be

   $F_1^\uparrow F_3^\downarrow D^\downarrow$ $\theta = 0$ degrees

   Force removed to accelerate the bar downward $(F_3) = 2$ m/s² · 100 kg · cos 0° = 200 N

2. Apply equation 2.2 to calculate the work for 10 repetitions in Joules:

   Work (negative) = (980 N + −200 N) · (−2 m) · 10 Reps = −15,600 J

3. Apply equation 2.3 to calculate the average power output for 10 repetitions in watts:

   Power (negative) = −15,600 J / 40 seconds = −390 W

Angular Work and Power

The work and power equations just presented apply to an object moving from one location to another in a straight line. Work and power are also required to start an object rotating about an axis or to change the velocity at which it rotates, even if the object as a whole does not move through space at all. The angle through which an object rotates is called its **angular displacement**, the SI unit for which is the radian (rad); 1 rad = 180° ÷ π = 57.3°, where π = 3.14. **Angular velocity** is the object's rotational speed, measured in radians per second (rad/s). Torque is expressed in newton-meters (N·m), but should not be confused with work, which is also expressed in newton-meters. The difference is that the distance component of the torque unit refers to the length of the moment arm (which is *perpendicular to* the line of action of the force), while the distance component of the work unit refers to the distance moved *along* the line of action of the force. Just as for movement through space, the work done in rotating an object is measured in joules (J), and power in watts (W).

This equation is used to calculate **rotational work**:

$$\text{Work} = \text{Torque} \cdot \text{Angular displacement} \qquad (2.4)$$

Equation 2.3 is used to calculate **rotational power**, just as it was used to calculate linear power.

> Although the word *strength* is often associated with slow speeds and the word *power* with high velocities of movement, both variables reflect the ability to exert force at a given velocity. Power is a direct mathematical function of force and velocity.

Strength Versus Power

The discrepancy between the common and scientific definitions of power has led to misunderstandings. For example, in the sport of powerlifting, which involves high forces but relatively low movement speeds, less mechanical power is produced than in several other sports, including Olympic lifting (6). Despite the discrepancy, the sport of powerlifting is unlikely to be renamed. In all other contexts, the strength and conditioning professional should use the word *power* only in its scientific sense to avoid ambiguity. Furthermore, although the word *strength* is often associated with slow velocities and the word *power* with high velocities of movement, both variables reflect the ability to exert force at a given velocity. Power is a direct mathematical function of force and velocity. Therefore, if at any instant, any two of the variables force, velocity, and power are known, the third can be calculated. If an individual can generate high force or high power at a particular velocity of movement, precisely the same ability is being described—that is, the ability to accelerate a mass at that particular velocity. Therefore, it is not correct to associate strength with low speed and power with high speed. Strength is the capacity to exert force at any given velocity, and power is the mathematical product of force and velocity at whatever speed. What is critical is the ability to exert force at velocities characteristic of a given sport to overcome gravity and accelerate the body or an implement. For a sport movement made relatively slow by high resistance, low-velocity strength is critical, whereas for a movement that is very fast due to low resistance, high-velocity strength is important. For example, when offensive and defensive American football linemen push against each other, their velocity of movement is slowed by the muscular force exerted by the opposing player as well as the inertia of the opposing player's body mass. Because the muscles are prevented from contracting at high velocity, the ability to exert force and power at low velocity is an important component of performance. In contrast, a badminton player's muscles quickly reach high velocity as a result of the minimal inertial resistance of the lightweight racket and the player's arm. Therefore, the ability to exert force and power at high velocity is critical to making rapid adjustments in a stroke.

> ▶ **The sport of weightlifting (Olympic lifting) has a much higher power component than the sport of powerlifting, due to the higher movement velocities with heavy weights of the weightlifting movements.**

Biomechanical Factors in Human Strength

Several biomechanical factors are involved in the manifestation of human strength, including neural control, muscle cross-sectional area, muscle fiber arrangement, muscle length, joint angle, muscle contraction velocity, joint angular velocity, and body size. These factors are discussed next, as are the three-dimensional strength relationship and the strength-to-mass ratio.

Neural Control

Neural control affects the maximal force output of a muscle by determining which and how many motor units are involved in a muscle contraction (**recruitment**) and the rate at which the motor units are fired (**rate coding**) (4). Generally, muscle force is greater when (a) more motor units are involved in a contraction, (b) the motor units are greater in size, or (c) the rate of firing is faster. Much of the improvement in strength evidenced in the first few weeks of resistance training is attributable to

neural adaptations as the brain learns how to generate more force from a given amount of contractile tissue (33). It is not unusual for novice resistance trainees to become discouraged when they cannot maintain the rate of increase of the first few training weeks. It is important for them to realize that continued improvement will result if they adhere to the training regimen, although via slower mechanisms such as muscle hypertrophy.

Muscle Cross-Sectional Area

All else being equal, the force a muscle can exert is related to its cross-sectional area rather than to its volume (11, 31). For example, if two athletes of similar percent body fat but different height have the same biceps circumference, their upper arm muscle cross-sectional areas are about the same. Although the taller (and therefore heavier) athlete's longer muscle makes for greater muscle volume, the strength of the two athletes' biceps should be about the same. With the same strength but greater body weight, the taller athlete has less ability to lift and accelerate his or her own body—for example, when performing calisthenics or gymnastics. This is why most elite gymnasts are not very tall. As described in chapter 1, resistance training increases both the strength and cross-sectional area of muscle.

Arrangement of Muscle Fibers

Maximally contracting muscles have been found capable of generating forces of 23 to 145 psi (16-100 N/cm²) of muscle cross-sectional area (21). This wide range can be partially accounted for by the variation in the arrangement and alignment of sarcomeres in relation to the long axis of the muscle (figure 2.11) (21). A **pennate muscle** has fibers that align obliquely with the tendon, creating a featherlike arrangement. The **angle of pennation** is defined as the angle between the muscle fibers and an imaginary line between the muscle's origin and insertion; 0° corresponds to no pennation.

Many human muscles are pennated (20, 39), but few have angles of pennation in excess of 15°. Actually, the angle of pennation does not remain constant for a given muscle, but increases as the muscle shortens. Any factor that affects angle of pennation would thus affect strength and velocity of shortening as long as the cross-sectional area remains the same. Muscles with greater pennation have more sarcomeres in parallel and fewer sarcomeres in series; they are therefore better able to generate force but have a lower maximal shortening velocity than nonpennate muscles. In comparison, lesser amounts of pennation can be advantageous for producing high velocities due to the greater number of sarcomeres in a row, at the expense of number of sarcomeres in parallel. The amount of pennation, however, has an effect on the muscles' ability to generate eccentric, isometric, or low-

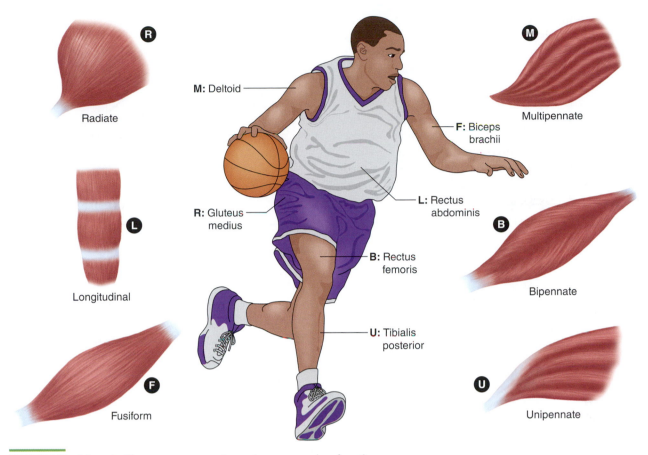

FIGURE 2.11   Muscle fiber arrangements and an example of each.

speed concentric force (40). Most importantly, although angle of pennation may vary depending on hereditary factors, it is modifiable through training, which could help account for some of the differences in strength and speed seen in individuals who seem to have muscles of the same size.

Muscle Length

When a muscle is at its resting length, the actin and myosin filaments lie next to each other, so that a maximal number of potential crossbridge sites are available (figure 2.12). Thus, the muscle can generate the greatest force at its resting length. When the muscle is stretched much beyond its resting length, a smaller proportion of the actin and myosin filaments lie next to each other. Because there are fewer potential crossbridge sites, the muscle cannot generate as much force as it can at its resting length. When the muscle contracts too much below its resting length, the actin filaments overlap and the number of crossbridge sites is reduced as well, thereby decreasing force generation capability.

Joint Angle

Because all body movements, even those occurring in a straight line, take place by means of rotation about a

joint or joints, the forces that muscles produce must be manifested as torques (recall that a higher torque value indicates a greater tendency for the applied force to rotate the limb or body part about a joint); consequently, we speak of torque versus joint angle rather than force versus joint angle. The amount of torque that can be exerted about a given body joint varies throughout the joint's range of motion, largely because of the relationship of force versus muscle length, as well as the ever-changing leverage brought about by the dynamic geometry of the muscles, tendons, and internal joint structures. This is shown in figures 2.2, 2.3, and 2.4. Additional factors include the type of exercise (isotonic, isometric, and so on), the body joint in question, the muscles used at that joint, and the speed of contraction (10).

Muscle Contraction Velocity

Classic experiments by A.V. Hill (19) on isolated animal muscle showed that the force capability of muscle declines as the velocity of contraction increases. The relationship is not linear; the decline in force capability is steepest over the lower range of movement speeds (see figure 2.13). Human movement technique can make the best of this relationship. For example, as a vertical jump begins, the arms swing upward, thereby exerting

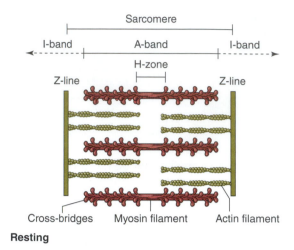

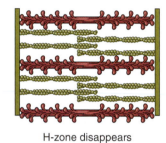

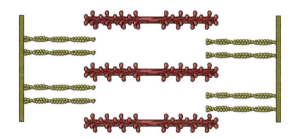

FIGURE 2.12 A schematic of the interaction between actin and myosin filaments when the muscle is at its resting length and when it is contracted or stretched. Muscle force capability is greatest when the muscle is at its resting length because of increased opportunity for actin–myosin crossbridges.

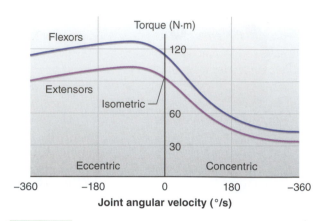

FIGURE 2.13 Force–velocity curve for eccentric and concentric actions.

Reprinted, by permission, from Jorgensen, 1976 (23).

downward force on the body at the shoulders, slowing the upward movement of the body, and forcing the hip and knee extensor muscles to contract more slowly than they otherwise would, enabling them to generate higher forces for longer times.

Joint Angular Velocity

There are three basic types of muscle action, during which forces are generated within the muscle that pull the muscle's ends toward each other if not prevented from doing so by external forces. The term *muscle action* is preferable to *contraction*, because the latter means "shortening," which does not accurately describe two of the three muscle actions.

- In **concentric muscle action**, the muscle shortens because the contractile force is greater than the resistive force. The forces generated within the muscle and acting to shorten it are greater than the external forces acting at its tendons to stretch it. Swimming and cycling involve concentric muscle action almost exclusively.

- In **eccentric muscle action**, the muscle lengthens because the contractile force is less than the resistive force. The forces generated within the muscle and acting to shorten it are less than the external forces acting at its tendons to stretch it (which increases the risk of soreness and injury). This occurs during the lowering phase of any resistance exercise. During standard resistance training, the eccentric force exerted by the muscle keeps the weight from being accelerated downward by gravitational force. Thus, the weight moves steadily downward rather than picking up speed and contacting the floor or the athlete's body.

- In **isometric muscle action**, the muscle length does not change, because the contractile force is equal to the resistive force. The forces generated within the muscle and acting to shorten it are equal to the external forces acting at its tendons to stretch it. During a sit-up with the trunk held straight, the abdominal muscles act isometrically to maintain the rigidity of the trunk, while the hip flexors carry out the sit-up movement. In contrast, the abdominal muscles act concentrically and eccentrically during the raising and lowering phases of the curl-up exercise, respectively.

Muscle torque varies with joint angular velocity according to the type of muscular action (figure 2.13). Tests have shown that during isokinetic (constant-speed) concentric exercise by human subjects, torque capability declines as angular velocity increases. In contrast, during eccentric exercise, as joint angular velocity increases, maximal torque capability increases until about 90°/s (1.57 rad/s), after which it declines gradually (4). That means that the greatest muscle force can be obtained during eccentric muscle action. This is exemplified by athletes who employ "cheating" movements when a weight cannot be lifted using strict form. For example, an individual who reaches a "sticking point" in the biceps curl exercise due to the limit of concentric elbow flexor strength usually leans the torso back, allowing the elbow flexors to exert increased force by operating isometrically or eccentrically and thereby enabling continued movement of the bar.

Strength-to-Mass Ratio

In sport activities such as sprinting and jumping, the ratio of the strength of the muscles involved in the movement to the mass of the body parts being accelerated is critical. Thus, the strength-to-mass ratio directly reflects an athlete's ability to accelerate his or her body. If, after training, an athlete increases body mass by 15% but increases force capability by only 10%, the strength-to-mass ratio, and thus the athlete's ability to accelerate, is reduced. A sprinter or jumper may benefit by experimenting with muscle mass to determine the highest strength-to-mass ratio, which would result in the best possible performance.

In sports involving weight classification, the strength-to-mass ratio is extremely important. If all competitors have close to the same body mass, the strongest one has a decided advantage. It is normal for the strength-to-mass ratio of larger athletes to be lower than that of smaller athletes because when body size increases, muscle volume (and concomitantly body weight) increases proportionately more than does muscle cross-sectional area (and concomitantly strength) (9). Trial and error can help athletes determine the weight category in which their strength is highest relative to that of other athletes in the weight class. Once an athlete finds his or her most competitive weight class, the object is to become as strong as possible without exceeding the class weight limit.

Body Size

It has long been observed that, all else being equal, smaller athletes are stronger pound for pound than larger athletes (9). The reason is that a muscle's maximal contractile force is fairly proportional to its cross-sectional area, which is related to the square (second power) of linear body dimensions, whereas a muscle's mass is proportional to its volume, which is related to the cube (third power) of linear body dimensions. Therefore, as body size increases, body mass increases more rapidly than does muscle strength. Given constant body proportions, the smaller athlete has a higher strength-to-mass ratio than does the larger athlete (9).

There has always been interest in comparing the performances of athletes in different weight categories. The most obvious method for doing so is to divide the weight lifted by the athlete's body weight. However, such an adjustment is biased against larger athletes because it does not take into account the expected drop in the strength-to-mass ratio with increasing body size. Various formulas have been derived to more equitably compare loads lifted. In the **classic formula**, the load lifted is divided by body weight to the two-thirds power, thus accounting for the relationship of cross-sectional area versus volume. Other formulas have since been developed because the classic formula seemed to favor athletes of middle body weight over lighter and heavier athletes (5). However, the determination by the classic formula that the performances of medium-weight athletes are usually the best may indeed be unbiased. Because of the bell-shaped curve describing the normal distribution of anthropometric characteristics among the population, the body weights of a majority of people are clustered close to the mean.

> In sport activities such as **sprinting and jumping**, the ratio of the strength of the muscles involved in the movement to the mass of the body parts being accelerated is critical. Thus, the strength-to-mass ratio directly reflects an athlete's ability to accelerate his or her body.

Sources of Resistance to Muscle Contraction

The most common sources of resistance for strength training exercises are gravity, inertia, friction, fluid resistance, and elasticity. This section provides information on the force and power required to overcome these forms of resistance. An understanding of the principles behind exercise devices using the various forms of resistance can provide insight into their effectiveness and applicability.

Gravity

The downward force on an object from the pull of gravity, otherwise called the object's weight, is equal to the object's mass times the local acceleration due to gravity:

$$F_g = m \cdot a_g \qquad\qquad (2.5)$$

where F_g is the force due to gravity (same as the object's weight), m is the object's mass, and a_g is the local acceleration due to gravity. The acceleration due to gravity can vary by geographic location. Weighing a barbell on a calibrated spring or electronic scale shows its actual weight. A balance scale determines only the object's mass, so its weight (F_g) must be calculated using equation 2.5 if a spring or electronic scale is not available.

Popular terminology for weight and mass is often incorrect. For example, some barbell and stack-machine plates are labeled in pounds. The pound is a unit of force, not mass. In actuality, only the mass of a barbell plate stays constant, while its weight varies according to the local acceleration due to gravity. The kilogram designation on a weight plate refers to its mass. It is not correct to say that an object weighs a certain number of kilograms, since weight refers to force, not mass. Instead, one should say "The mass of the barbell is 85 kg." The amount of mass an individual can lift will be slightly affected by terrestrial location because of variations in the acceleration due to gravity around the globe (see table 2.1). That same 85 kg barbell would feel like approximately 14 kg if it were on the moon, even though it did not physically change.

Applications to Resistance Training

The gravitational force on an object always acts downward. Since, by definition, the moment arm by which a force produces torque is perpendicular to the line of action of the force, the moment arm of a weight is always horizontal. Thus, torque due to an object's weight is the product of the weight and the horizontal distance from the weight to the pivot point (joint). During an exercise, although the weight does not change, its horizontal distance from a given joint axis changes constantly. When the weight is horizontally closer to the joint, it exerts less resistive torque; when it is horizontally farther from a joint, it exerts more resistive torque. For example, in an arm curl, the horizontal distance from the elbow to the barbell is greatest when the forearm is horizontal. Thus, in that position the athlete must exert the greatest muscle torque to support the weight. The moment arm decreases as the forearm rotates either upward or downward away from the horizontal, decreasing the resistive torque arising from the weight (see figure 2.7). When the weight is directly above or below the elbow pivot point, there is no resistive torque from the weight.

Exercise technique can affect the resistive torque pattern during an exercise and can shift stress among muscle groups. In the back squat, for example, a more forward inclination of the trunk brings the weight horizontally closer to the knees, thus reducing the resistive torque about the knees that the quadriceps must counteract. At the same time, the weight is horizontally farther from the hip, increasing the resistive torque about the hip that the gluteus and hamstring muscles must counteract. This resistive torque pattern is most often present when the barbell is positioned as low as possible on the upper back (often termed a low bar squat); the athlete must incline the trunk relatively far forward to keep the center of mass of body plus bar over the feet, thereby avoiding a fall. Because the bar is then horizontally far from the hip and close to the knee, stress is focused on the hip extensors and to a lesser extent on the knee extensors. The opposite of this resistive torque pattern would occur in a high bar squat, in which the bar is placed higher up on the back closer to the neck. As a result of this bar positioning, the torque distribution increases the resistive torque about the knees and concomitantly reduces the resistive torque about the hip (in contrast to what occurs with the low bar squat).

> **Exercise technique can affect the resistive torque pattern during an exercise and can shift stress among muscle groups.**

Weight-Stack Machines

As with free weights, gravity is the source of resistance for weight-stack machines. However, by means of pulleys, cams, cables, and gears, these machines provide increased control over the direction and pattern of resistance. Both free weights and stack machines have advantages and disadvantages. The following are some of the advantages of the stack machine:

- *Safety.* The likelihood of injury as a result of being hit by, tripping over, or being trapped under a weight is reduced. Less skill is required to maintain control of a weight stack than a free weight.
- *Design flexibility.* Machines can be designed to provide resistance to body movements that are difficult to resist with free weights (e.g., lat pulldown, hip adduction and abduction, leg curl). To some extent, the pattern of resistance can be engineered into a machine.
- *Ease of use.* Many people who fear that they lack the coordination or technique to safely lift free weights feel confident when using machines. Also, it is quicker and easier to select a weight by inserting a pin in a stack than by mounting plates on a bar.

Advantages of free weights include the following:

- *Whole-body training.* Free weight exercises are often performed in the standing position with the weight supported by the entire body, taxing a larger portion of the body's musculature and skeleton than a weight-stack machine would. Such weight-bearing exercise promotes greater bone mineralization, helping to prevent osteoporosis in later life (13). Moreover, the movement of a free weight is constrained by the athlete rather than by a machine, requiring muscles to work in stabilization as well as support. "Structural" exercises, such as the power clean and the snatch, are particularly useful in providing training stimulus for a major portion of the body's musculature.

- *Simulation of real-life activities.* The lifting and acceleration of objects represent a major part of sport and other physically demanding activities. Machines tend to isolate single muscle groups; the lifting of free weights involves the more "natural" coordination of several muscle groups.

Nautilus Sports/Medical Industries popularized the concept of tailoring resistive torque through the range of joint motion by creating an exercise machine that uses a cam of variable radius; this changes the length of the moment arm through which the weight stack acts (figure 2.14). The rationale was to provide more resistance at points in the range of motion where the muscles could exert greater torque, and less resistance where the muscles could apply less torque. For the system to work as planned, however, the athlete has to move at a constant, slow angular velocity, which is difficult to do consistently. Also, cam-based machines frequently fail to match normal human torque capability patterns (9).

Inertia

In addition to gravitational force, a barbell or weight stack, when accelerated, exerts **inertial force** on the athlete. Though the force of gravity acts only downward, inertial force can act in any direction. The upward force an athlete exerts equals the weight lifted plus any inertial force, which is the mass times the upward acceleration of the bar. Horizontal bar acceleration occurs if the athlete exerts net force on the bar directed to the front, back, left, or right. All exercises involve some acceleration at the beginning to bring the bar from a zero to an upward velocity, as well as some deceleration near the top of the exercise to bring the bar's velocity back to zero so that it does not continue its trajectory and fly out of the lifter's hands. With this acceleration pattern, the agonist muscles receive resistance in excess of bar weight early in the range of motion, but resistance less than bar weight toward the end of the range of motion (27). The athlete decelerates the bar by either (a) reducing upward force on the bar to less than bar weight to let some or all of the bar's weight decelerate it or (b) pushing down against

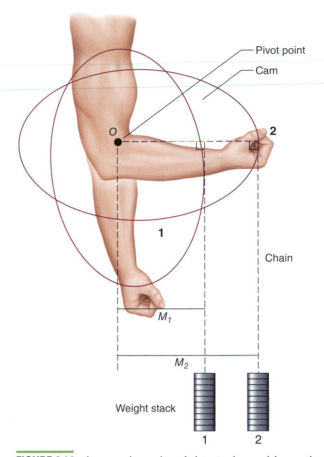

FIGURE 2.14   In cam-based weight-stack machines, the moment arm *(M)* of the weight stack (horizontal distance from the chain to the cam pivot point) varies during the exercise movement. When the cam is rotated in the direction shown from position 1 to position 2, the moment arm of the weights, and thus the resistive torque, increases.

the bar using the antagonist muscles. In either case, the deceleration has the effect of providing less resistance to the agonist muscles late in the range of motion.

Compared to a slow exercise with minimal acceleration of a given weight, an exercise involving higher acceleration (an "explosive" exercise) provides greater resistance to the muscles involved early in the range of motion and less resistance to the muscles involved toward the end of the range of motion. However, because of the addition of inertia, heavier weights can be handled in accelerative exercises than in slow exercises, allowing near-maximal resistance to be attained for all muscles involved in the exercise. During a power clean of a heavy weight, for example, the strong leg, hip, and back muscles accelerate the bar vertically to a high enough velocity that, even though the weaker upper body muscles cannot exert vertical force equal to the bar's weight, the bar continues to travel upward until the force of gravity decelerates it to zero velocity at the highest bar position.

Although acceleration changes the nature of an exercise and makes resistance patterns less predictable, acceleration in resistance training is not necessarily undesirable. Because acceleration is characteristic of natural movements in sport and daily life, resistance training exercises involving acceleration probably produce desirable neuromuscular training effects. Olympic lifting exercises such as the snatch and the clean and jerk are effective for improving the ability to produce high accelerations against heavy resistance (25).

Acceleration and deceleration are characteristic of virtually all natural movements. For example, sprinting requires the athlete's arms and legs to go through repeated cycles of acceleration and deceleration. Throwing a baseball, discus, shot, or javelin all involve sequences of body movements that accelerate the objects to high release speeds. Because acceleration is a particular kind of movement pattern, training with accelerative movements can provide specificity of training. That is why explosive exercises, such as the power clean and high pull, are used in training for many different sports in which the leg and hip muscles provide force for accelerating the body. The **bracketing technique**, in which the athlete performs the sport movement with less than normal and greater than normal resistance, is another form of acceleration training. According to the force–velocity relationship of muscle, a shot-putter who trains with an extra-heavy shot develops greater forces during the accelerative movement than when using the normal shot because the inertia of the heavier implement forces the muscle to contract at relatively low speed. When a relatively light shot is used, the lower inertia of the shot enables the putter to accelerate the shot more rapidly and to reach a higher speed of release, thereby training the neuromuscular system to operate within desired acceleration and speed ranges. Although the principle of increasing or decreasing the load during a movement as described has the theoretical basis for increasing acceleration capacity through the aforementioned methods, one should also consider the influence that such changes in loading have during highly specific or technique-oriented activities such as throwing or sprinting. For example, changing implement loading could have some negative consequences on technique since the body needs time to adjust the motor pattern for that particular movement with the new load.

Friction

Friction is the resistive force encountered when one attempts to move an object while it is pressed against another object. Exercise devices that use friction as the main source of resistance include belt- or brake pad–resisted cycle ergometers and wrist curl devices. For such devices,

$$F_R = k \cdot F_N \tag{2.6}$$

where F_R is the resistive force; k is the coefficient of friction for the two particular substances in contact; and F_N is the normal force, which presses the objects against each other.

The coefficients of friction for initiating and for maintaining movement are different. All else being equal, it takes more force to initiate movement between two surfaces in contact than to maintain previously initiated movement. Thus, a friction-resisted exercise device requires a relatively high force to initiate movement and a relatively constant force after movement has begun, no matter what the movement speed. Resistance provided by such devices is sometimes adjusted through a mechanism that alters the normal force that keeps the friction surfaces in contact with each other.

A weighted sled used in training for football or track is an example of a device that is resisted by both friction and inertia. The resistance due to the sled's inertia is directly proportional to both the sled's mass and its acceleration. The resistance due to the friction between the sled's runners and the ground is proportional to both the friction coefficient between surfaces in contact and the net force pressing the sled against the ground, which equals the gravitational force minus any upward force exerted by the individual pushing the sled. Mass can be added to the sled to increase the gravitational force. The friction coefficient varies with the surface on which the sled rests (e.g., sand, bare soil, dry grass, wet grass). Thus, for outdoor training, such devices do not provide consistently repeatable resistance. They are nevertheless useful in providing horizontal resistance, which cannot be directly provided by weights. It takes more force to get the sled moving than to keep it moving, because the coefficient of static friction is always greater than the coefficient of sliding friction. Once the sled is moving, the coefficient of sliding friction stays relatively constant. Therefore one should understand that friction resistance does not change as speed increases. However, in keeping with equation 2.3, power output increases with speed. Also, as expressed by equation 2.1, during the transition from a lower to a higher speed there is added resistance due to acceleration.

Fluid Resistance

The resistive force encountered by an object moving through a fluid (liquid or gas), or by a fluid moving past or around an object or through an opening, is called **fluid resistance**. Fluid resistance is a significant factor in such sport activities as swimming, rowing, golf, sprinting, discus throwing, and baseball pitching. (Except for swimming and rowing, in which the fluid is water, all these involve air resistance.) The phenomenon has become important in resistance training with the advent of hydraulic (liquid) and pneumatic (gas) exercise machines and with the increasing popularity of swimming pool exercise routines, particularly among older people and pregnant women. The two sources of fluid resistance are **surface drag**, which results from the friction of a fluid passing along the surface of an object, and **form drag**, which results from the way in which a fluid presses against the front or rear of an object passing through it. Cross-sectional (frontal) area has a major effect on form drag.

Fluid-resisted exercise machines most often use cylinders in which a piston forces fluid through an opening as the exercise movement is performed. The resistive force is greater when the piston is pushed faster, when the opening is smaller, or when the fluid is more viscous. All else being equal, resistance is roughly proportional to the velocity of piston movement:

$$F_R = k \cdot v \tag{2.7}$$

where F_R is the resistive force; k is a constant that reflects the physical characteristics of the cylinder and piston, the viscosity of the fluid, and the number, size, and shape of the openings; and v is piston velocity relative to the cylinder.

Because fluid cylinders provide resistance that increases with speed, they allow rapid acceleration early in the exercise movement and little acceleration after higher speeds are reached. Movement speed is thus kept within an intermediate range. Although such machines limit changes in velocity to a certain extent, they are not isokinetic (constant speed) as is sometimes claimed. Some machines have adjustment knobs that allow the opening size to be changed. A larger opening allows the user to reach a higher movement speed before the fluid resistive force curtails the ability to accelerate.

Fluid-resisted machines do not generally provide an eccentric exercise phase, but they may if they incorporate an internal pump. With a free weight, a muscle group acts concentrically while raising the weight and eccentrically while lowering it. With fluid-resisted machines without eccentric resistance, a muscle group acts concentrically during performance of the primary exercise movement, and the antagonist muscle group acts concentrically during the return to the starting position. In other words, whereas free weights or weight machines involve alternate concentric and eccentric actions of the same muscle with little or no rest in between, fluid-resisted machines generally involve alternate concentric actions of antagonistic muscle groups; each muscle group rests while its antagonist works. The lack of eccentric muscle action with fluid-resisted machines means that such exercise probably does not provide optimal specificity of training for the many sport movements that involve

eccentric muscle actions (e.g., running, jumping, and throwing).

Elasticity

A number of exercise devices, particularly those designed for home use, have elastic components such as springs, bands, bows, or rods as their source of resistance. The resistance provided by a standard elastic component is proportional to the distance it is stretched:

$$F_R = k \cdot x \tag{2.8}$$

where F_R is the resistive force, k is a constant that reflects the physical characteristics of the elastic component, and x is the distance that the elastic component is stretched beyond its resting length.

The most obvious characteristic of elastic resistance is that the more the elastic component is stretched, the greater the resistance. The problem with devices using elastic resistance is that every exercise movement begins with low resistance and ends with high resistance. This is contrary to the force capability patterns of virtually all human muscle groups, which show a substantial drop-off in force capability toward the end of the range of motion. Another problem with elasticity-resisted machines is that the adjustability of resistance is usually limited by the number of elastic components available to provide resistance to a movement. An effective resistance exercise device should incorporate enough variation in resistive force that the number of repetitions the trainee can perform is kept within a desirable range.

There are products that provide resistance to vertical jumping with elastic bands as a means of developing jumping power. However, the elastic bands provide little resistance early in the jump when the large gluteus and quadriceps muscles are capable of exerting great force. The bands provide the greatest resistance while the jumper is in the air—serving mainly to pull the jumper back to the ground, rather than resist the muscles, and to increase the speed at which the jumper hits the ground on landing, which may increase injury risk.

Joint Biomechanics: Concerns in Resistance Training

As with any physical activity, there is a degree of risk with resistance training. However, the risks involved are generally lower than for many other sport and physical conditioning activities (36, 37). Rates of injury are the highest for team sports; intermediate for running and aerobics; and lowest for cycling, walking, and resistance training, the latter of which has about 4 injuries per 1,000 hours of participation. A study of collegiate American football players showed only 0.35 resistance training–related injuries per 100 players per season. Injuries due to resistance training accounted for only 0.74% of the in-season injury-related time loss of the players (44). Despite the relatively low risk of resistance training, it is desirable to minimize the likelihood of injury through prudent risk management. The following are several factors to consider in avoiding resistance training injuries, with particular attention given to the back, shoulders, and knees.

> ▶ **The risk of injury from resistance training is low compared to that of other sport and physical conditioning activities.**

Back

In contrast to quadrupeds, whose vertebral columns hang like the cables on a suspension bridge, humans normally stand upright, with the vertebral bones stacked one on top of another, separated by rubbery disks. The advantage we gain from our upright posture and free use of the arms and hands is accompanied by the disadvantage of having our intervertebral disks under compressive force even when we are merely standing, sitting, walking, or running—and under even more compressive force when we are lifting and carrying (14). When we are in a standing position, any force we exert with the upper body must be transmitted through the back to the legs and ground. In addition, the back muscles act at a great mechanical disadvantage and must generate forces much greater than the weight of an object lifted. It is for these reasons that the back is particularly vulnerable to injury. It should be noted, however, that spinal internal loads are quite variable with varying postures during the lift (24) and that deep squatting positions with load are not necessarily associated with back injury (18).

Back Injury

Back injury can be extremely debilitating, persistent, and difficult to remedy. Thus, every effort should be made to avoid back injury during resistance training. The lower back is particularly vulnerable. It has been observed that 85% to 90% of all intervertebral disk herniations occur at the disk between the lowest two lumbar vertebrae (L4 and L5) or between the lowest lumbar and the top sacral vertebra (L5 and S1) (1, 3). This is not surprising, given the extremely high compressive forces on the disks during lifting. When a weight is supported in the hands or on the shoulders and the trunk is inclined forward, there is great torque about the lower intervertebral disks due to the large horizontal distance between the lower back and the weight. The back muscles operate at an extremely low mechanical advantage because the perpendicular distance from the line of action of the spinal erector

muscles to the intervertebral disks is much shorter (about 2 inches, or 5 cm) than the horizontal distance from the weight to the disks. As a result, the muscles must exert forces that frequently exceed 10 times the weight lifted (3). These forces act to squeeze the intervertebral disks between the adjacent vertebral bodies and can lead to injury.

The neutral back lifting posture has been found to be better overall than a rounded (opposite of arched) back in minimizing L5/S1 compressive forces and ligament strain (2). Therefore, a normal **lordotic** lumbar spine position is superior to a rounded back for avoiding injury to vertebrae, disks, facet joints, ligaments, and muscles of the back. In addition, the low back muscles are capable of exerting considerably higher forces when the back is arched rather than rounded (7).

The **vertebral column** is naturally S-shaped, being slightly rounded (**kyphotic**) in the thoracic spine and lordotic in the lumbar spine. The wedged shape of the vertebrae gives the spine its natural curve. However, the intervertebral disks are flat when the back is in its S shape. When the lower back is rounded, the **ventral** (toward the anterior) edges of the vertebral bodies squeeze the front portions of the intervertebral disks. In contrast, extreme arching of the back results in squeezing the **dorsal** (toward the posterior) portions of the disks. Such uneven squeezing of the intervertebral disks likely increases the risk of disk rupture (3). Thus, resistance training exercises should generally be performed with the lower back in a moderately arched position to reduce risk of damage to the disks.

Intra-Abdominal Pressure and Lifting Belts

When the diaphragm and the deep muscles of the torso contract, pressure is generated within the abdominal cavity. Because the abdomen is composed mainly of fluid and normally contains very little gas, it is virtually incompressible (3). The abdominal fluids and tissue kept under pressure by tensing surrounding muscle (deep abdominal muscles and diaphragm) have been described as a "fluid ball" (figure 2.15) that aids in supporting the vertebral column during resistance training (3). Such support may significantly reduce both the forces required by the erector spinae muscles to perform an exercise and the associated compressive forces on the disks (3, 30).

It is important to note that the Valsalva maneuver is not necessary for generation of intra-abdominal pressure. In the **Valsalva maneuver**, the glottis is closed, thus keeping air from escaping the lungs, and the muscles of the abdomen and rib cage contract, creating rigid compartments of liquid in the lower torso and air in the upper torso. An advantage of the Valsalva maneuver is that it increases the rigidity of the entire torso, making it easier to support heavy loads (15). For example, when lifting heavy loads in the back squat exercise, many athletes use the Valsalva maneuver, particularly when the trunk is most inclined forward, near the transition from the eccentric movement phase to the concentric movement phase. However, pressure in the chest associated with the Valsalva maneuver can have the undesirable side effect of exerting compressive force on the heart, making it more difficult for blood to return to the heart. Also, the Valsalva maneuver can transiently raise blood pressure to slightly elevated levels (15). The diaphragm and the abdominal muscles can contract *without* the glottis being closed, however, creating the fluid ball in the abdomen without pressurizing the chest compartment. This must be regarded as the safer way, of the two options, to add support to the lower spine without building up pressure in the chest, and is the technique that should be used for most resistance training. One can build up intra-abdominal pressure without building up chest pressure by consciously keeping the airway open. During a strenuous repetition, the abdominal muscles and diaphragm contract reflexively, even with the airway open. Athletes, particularly those who compete in Olympic lifting or powerlifting, may choose to use the Valsalva maneuver if they recognize and accept the risks involved and have the experience to avoid increasing pressure to the point of blackout.

Weightlifting belts have been shown to increase intra-abdominal pressure during resistance training and are therefore probably effective in improving safety when used correctly (17, 28). It has been cautioned, however, that if an athlete performs all of the exercises with a belt, the abdominal muscles that produce intra-abdominal pressure might not get enough training stimulus to develop optimally (17). It is particularly risky for an individual who has become accustomed to wearing a belt to suddenly perform an exercise without one, because the abdominal musculature might not be capable of generating enough intra-abdominal pressure to significantly reduce erector spinae muscle forces. The resulting excessive compressive forces on the disks could increase the chance of back injury. Conservative recommendations are as follows:

- A weight belt is not needed for exercises that do not directly affect the lower back.
- For exercises directly stressing the back, an individual should refrain from wearing a belt during lighter sets but may wear one for near-maximal and maximal sets. The beltless sets allow the deep abdominal muscles, which generate intra-abdominal pressure, to receive a training stimulus without placing excessive compressive forces on the intervertebral disks.
- Individuals may reasonably choose never to wear lifting belts if they build up the strength of their back muscles and the muscles that generate intra-abdominal pressure in a gradual and systematic manner and if they practice safe resistance training exercise techniques. Many world-class Olympic-style weightlifters never wear belts.

Shoulders

The shoulder is particularly prone to injury during resistance training, due to both its structure and the forces to which it is subjected during a training session. Like the hip, the shoulder is capable of rotating in any direction. The hip is a stable ball-and-socket joint, but the glenoid cavity of the shoulder, which holds the head of the humerus, is not a true socket and is significantly less stable. The shoulder joint has the greatest range of motion of all the joints in the human body; but the joint's excessive mobility contributes to its vulnerability, as does the proximity of the bones, muscles, tendons, ligaments, and bursae in the shoulder.

The stability of the shoulder largely depends on the glenoid labrum, the joint synovium, and capsules, ligaments, muscles, tendons, and bursae. The rotator cuff muscles (supraspinatus, infraspinatus, subscapularis, and teres minor) and the pectorals are particularly instrumental in keeping the ball of the humerus in place. With the shoulder's great range of motion, its various structures can easily impinge on one another, causing tendinitis as well as inflammation and degeneration of contiguous

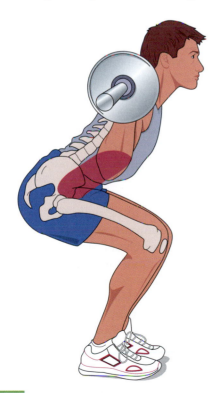

FIGURE 2.15   The "fluid ball" resulting from contraction of the deep abdominal muscles and the diaphragm.

tissue. High forces generated during resistance training can result in tearing of ligaments, muscles, and tendons. Athletes must take particular care when performing the various forms of the bench and shoulder press exercises because of the great stresses placed on the shoulder. For these exercises, it is particularly important to warm up with relatively light weights and to follow a program that exercises the shoulder in a balanced way, using all of its major movements.

Knees

The knee is prone to injury because of its location between two long levers (the upper and lower leg). Flexion and extension about the knee occur almost exclusively in the sagittal plane. Rotation in the frontal plane and transverse plane is prevented mainly by ligamentous and cartilaginous stabilizing structures. Frontal plane torque on the knee occurs, for example, when a football player is hit at midleg from the side while the foot is planted firmly on the ground. Fortunately, in training, resistive torques occur almost exclusively within the knee's normal plane of rotation.

Of the various components of the knee, the patella and surrounding tissue are most susceptible to the kinds of forces encountered in resistance training. The patella's main function is to hold the quadriceps tendon away from the knee axis of rotation, thereby increasing the moment arm of the quadriceps group and its mechanical advantage (see figure 2.5). If inappropriate load, volume, or recovery is introduced, repetitive high forces encountered by the patellar tendon during resistance training (as with any high-force activity such as running) can lead to tendinitis, which is characterized by tenderness and swelling. There is no inherent risk of tendinitis with performing these exercises; rather, tendinitis is simply a function of too much volume and intensity without appropriate progression.

It is not unusual for individuals to use knee wraps during training or competition in order to assist with maximizing performance or preventing injury. Wraps vary from the thin, elastic, pull-on variety that can be purchased in drug stores to the heavy, specialized wraps sold only through weightlifting supply houses. The use of knee wraps, particularly the heavy ones, is most prevalent among powerlifters. Very little research has been done on the efficacy of knee wraps. Detrimental side effects have been reported, however, including skin damage and chondromalacia patellae, the wearing down and roughening of the posterior surface of the patella (26). Through a spring effect alone, heavy wraps

around the knees added an average of 25 pounds (110 N) to squat lifting force. The notion that wraps work only by stabilizing the knee, lessening the athlete's fear of injury, or providing a kinesthetic cue is incorrect (26). The wraps actually provide direct help in extending the knee. On the basis of the lack of evidence that knee wraps prevent injury, athletes should minimize their use. If used at all, knee wraps should be limited to the sets with the heaviest loads.

Elbows and Wrists

The primary concerns with elbow and wrist injury involve overhead lifts (8). However, the risk with overhead lifting is quite small in comparison to the common source of injury of these joints, which includes participation in overhead sports such as throwing events or the tennis serve (8). Other examples of possible injury are elbow dislocation, sometimes observed in gymnastics (29), and overuse-related injuries such as traction apophysitis, sometimes observed in diving, wrestling, and hockey (29). One of the primary concerns is epiphyseal growth plate damage or overuse either in the posterior aspect of the elbow or in the distal radius in young athletes (29). The prevalence of elbow or wrist injury with weightlifting is very sporadic and often referred to in the literature only through case studies. One study indicated a tricep tendon tear in a middle-aged competitive weightlifter (35) and another a bilateral distal bicep tendon rupture in a recreational weight trainer (38). A study examining 245 competitive powerlifters found an extremely low incidence of elbow and wrist injury (41). Only very limited data have been presented to suggest possible distal radial epiphysis fracture in adolescent weightlifters (22). According to a recent study, which surveyed 500 experts in the field of sports medicine, most respondents indicated that avoiding resistance training before physeal closure was not necessary (32).

Conclusion

It is hoped that readers will apply the biomechanical principles discussed in this chapter to the selection of resistance exercise equipment and the design of exercise programs. Knowledge of how different types of exercise provide specific patterns of resistance to the body can aid in developing safe and effective programs to suit the specific needs of both athletes engaged in various sports and others who engage in resistance training for enhancement of physical performance, health, sense of well-being, and self-confidence.

acceleration
agonist
anatomical position
angle of pennation
angular displacement
angular velocity
antagonist
biomechanics
bracketing technique
cartilaginous joint
classic formula
concentric muscle action
distal
dorsal
eccentric muscle action
fibrous attachments
first-class lever
fleshy attachments
fluid resistance

form drag
friction
frontal plane
fulcrum
inertial force
insertion
isometric muscle action
kyphotic
lever
lordotic
mechanical advantage
moment arm
muscle force
origin
pennate muscle
power
proximal
rate coding

recruitment
resistive force
rotational power
rotational work
sagittal plane
second-class lever
strength
surface drag
synergist
tendons
third-class lever
torque
transverse plane
Valsalva maneuver
ventral
vertebral column
weight
work

STUDY QUESTIONS

1. Which of the following is the definition of power?
   a. (mass) · (acceleration)
   b. (force) · (distance)
   c. (force) · (velocity)
   d. (torque) · (time)

2. To compare performances of Olympic weightlifters of different body weights, the classic formula divides the load lifted by the athlete's
   a. body weight
   b. body weight squared
   c. lean body weight
   d. body weight to the two-thirds power

3. During a free weight exercise, muscle force varies with which of the following?
   I. perpendicular distance from the weight to the body joint
   II. joint angle
   III. movement acceleration
   IV. movement velocity squared
   a. I and II only
   b. I and IV only
   c. I, II, and III only
   d. II, III, and IV only

4. A vertical jump involves knee, hip, and shoulder movement primarily in which of the following anatomical planes?
   a. sagittal
   b. perpendicular
   c. frontal
   d. transverse

5. An athlete is performing a concentric isokinetic elbow flexion and extension exercise. Which of the following type(s) of levers occur(s) at the elbow during this exercise?
    I. first class
    II. second class
    III. third class
    a. I only
    b. II only
    c. I and III only
    d. II and III only

CHAPTER 3

Bioenergetics of Exercise and Training

Trent J. Herda, PhD, and Joel T. Cramer, PhD

 After completing this chapter, you will be able to

- explain the basic energy systems available to supply ATP during exercise;
- understand lactate accumulation, metabolic acidosis, and cellular manifestations of fatigue;
- identify patterns of substrate depletion and repletion during various exercise intensities;
- describe the bioenergetic factors that limit exercise performance;
- develop training programs that demonstrate the metabolic specificity of training;
- explain the metabolic demands of and recovery from interval training, high-intensity interval training, and combination training to optimize work-to-rest ratios.

Metabolic specificity of exercise and training is based on an understanding of the transfer of energy in biological systems. Efficient and productive training programs can be designed through an understanding of how energy is made available for specific types of exercise and how energy transfer can be modified by specific training regimens. After defining essential bioenergetics terminology and explaining the role of adenosine triphosphate (ATP), this chapter discusses the three basic energy systems that work to replenish ATP in human skeletal muscle. Then we look at substrate depletion and repletion, especially as they relate to fatigue and recovery; bioenergetic factors that limit performance; and aerobic and anaerobic contributions to oxygen uptake. Finally, the metabolic specificity of training is discussed.

Essential Terminology

Bioenergetics, or the flow of **energy** in a biological system, concerns primarily the conversion of macronutrients—carbohydrate, protein, and fats, which contain chemical energy—into biologically usable forms of energy. It is the breakdown of the chemical bonds in these macronutrients that provides the energy necessary to perform biological work.

The breakdown of large molecules into smaller molecules, associated with the release of energy, is termed **catabolism**. The synthesis of larger molecules from smaller molecules can be accomplished using the energy released from catabolic reactions; this building-up process is termed **anabolism**. The breakdown of protein into amino acids is an example of catabolism, while the formation of protein from amino acids is an anabolic process. **Exergonic reactions** are energy-releasing reactions and are generally catabolic. **Endergonic reactions** require energy and include anabolic processes and the contraction of muscle. **Metabolism** is the total of all the catabolic or exergonic and anabolic or endergonic reactions in a biological system. Energy derived from catabolic or exergonic reactions is used to drive anabolic or endergonic reactions through an intermediate molecule, **adenosine triphosphate (ATP)**. Adenosine triphosphate allows the transfer of energy from exergonic to endergonic reactions. Without an adequate supply of ATP, muscular activity and muscle growth would not be possible. Thus, it is apparent that when designing training programs, strength and conditioning professionals need to have a basic understanding of how exercise affects ATP hydrolysis and resynthesis.

Adenosine triphosphate is composed of adenosine and three phosphate groups (figure 3.1). Adenosine is the combination of adenine (a nitrogen-containing base) and ribose (a five-carbon sugar). The breakdown of one molecule of ATP to yield energy is known as **hydrolysis**, because it requires one molecule of water. The hydrolysis of ATP is catalyzed by the presence of an enzyme called **adenosine triphosphatase (ATPase)**. Specifically, **myosin ATPase** is the enzyme that catalyzes ATP hydrolysis for crossbridge recycling. Other specific enzymes hydrolyze ATP at other locations, such as **calcium ATPase** for pumping calcium into the sarcoplasmic reticulum and **sodium-potassium ATPase** for maintaining the sarcolemmal concentration gradient after depolarization (59). The following equation depicts the reactants (left), enzyme (middle), and products (right) of ATP hydrolysis:

$$ATP + H_2O \xleftrightarrow{\text{ATPase}} ADP + P_i + H^+ + \text{Energy} \quad \textbf{(3.1)}$$

where ADP represents **adenosine diphosphate** (only two phosphate groups, figure 3.1), P_i is an **inorganic phosphate** molecule, and H^+ is a hydrogen ion (proton). Further hydrolysis of ADP cleaves the second phosphate group and yields **adenosine monophosphate (AMP)**. The energy released primarily from the hydrolysis of ATP and secondarily from ADP results in biological work.

Adenosine triphosphate is classified as a high-energy molecule because it stores large amounts of energy in the chemical bonds of the two terminal phosphate groups. Because muscle cells store ATP only in limited amounts and activity requires a constant supply of ATP to provide the energy needed for muscle actions, ATP-producing processes must occur in the cell.

Biological Energy Systems

Three basic energy systems exist in mammalian muscle cells to replenish ATP (85, 122):

- Phosphagen system
- Glycolysis
- Oxidative system

In discussion of exercise-related bioenergetics, the terms *anaerobic* and *aerobic metabolism* are often used. **Anaerobic** processes do not require the presence of oxygen, whereas **aerobic** mechanisms depend on oxygen. The **phosphagen** and **glycolytic systems** are anaerobic mechanisms that occur in the sarcoplasm of a muscle cell. The **Krebs cycle**, electron transport, and the rest of the **oxidative system** are aerobic mechanisms that occur in the **mitochondria** of muscle cells and require oxygen as the terminal electron acceptor.

Of the three main macronutrients—carbohydrate, protein, and fats—only carbohydrate can be metabolized for energy without the direct involvement of oxygen

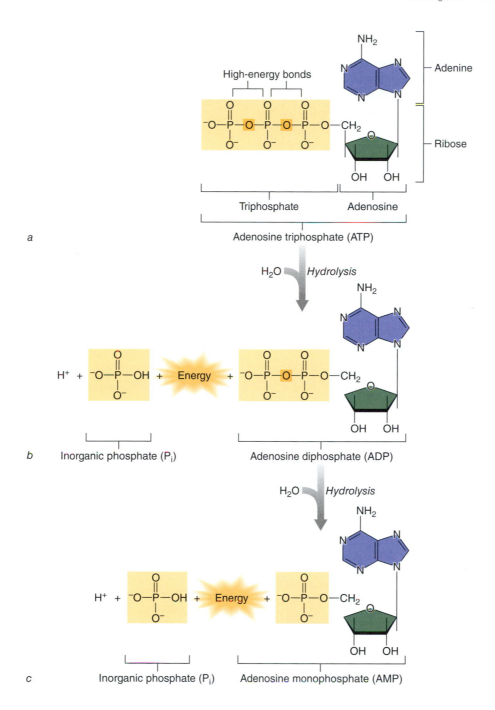

FIGURE 3.1   *(a)* The chemical structure of an ATP molecule showing adenosine (adenine + ribose), the triphosphate group, and locations of the high-energy chemical bonds. *(b)* The hydrolysis of ATP breaks the terminal phosphate bond, releases energy, and leaves ADP, an inorganic phosphate (P_i), and a hydrogen ion (H^+). *(c)* The hydrolysis of ADP breaks the terminal phosphate bond, releases energy, and leaves AMP, P_i, and H^+.

> **Energy stored in the chemical bonds of adenosine triphosphate (ATP) is used to power muscular activity. The replenishment of ATP in human skeletal muscle is accomplished by three basic energy systems: (a) phosphagen, (b) glycolytic, and (c) oxidative.**

(21). Therefore, carbohydrate is critical during anaerobic metabolism. All three energy systems are active at any given time; however, the magnitude of the contribution of each system to overall work performance is primarily dependent on the intensity of the activity and secondarily on the duration (45, 85).

Phosphagen System

The phosphagen system provides ATP primarily for short-term, high-intensity activities (e.g., resistance training and sprinting) and is highly active at the start of all exercise regardless of intensity (62, 70, 153). This energy system relies on the hydrolysis of ATP (equation 3.1) and breakdown of another high-energy phosphate molecule called **creatine phosphate (CP)**, also called **phosphocreatine (PCr)**. **Creatine kinase** is the enzyme that catalyzes the synthesis of ATP from CP and ADP in the following reaction:

$$\text{ADP} + \text{CP} \xleftrightarrow{\text{Creatine kinase}} \text{ATP} + \text{Creatine} \qquad (3.2)$$

Creatine phosphate supplies a phosphate group that combines with ADP to replenish ATP. The creatine kinase reaction provides energy at a high rate; however, because CP is stored in relatively small amounts, the phosphagen system cannot be the primary supplier of energy for continuous, long-duration activities (30).

ATP Stores

The body stores approximately 80 to 100 g (about 3 ounces) of ATP at any given time, which does not represent a significant energy reserve for exercise (107). In addition, ATP stores cannot be completely depleted due to the necessity for basic cellular function. In fact, ATP concentrations may decrease by up to 50% to 60% (34, 71, 100, 143) of the preexercise levels during experimentally induced muscle fatigue. Therefore, the phosphagen system uses the creatine kinase reaction (equation 3.2) to maintain the concentration of ATP. Under normal circumstances, skeletal muscle concentrations of CP are four to six times higher than ATP concentrations (107). Therefore, the phosphagen system, through CP and the creatine kinase reaction, serves as an energy reserve for rapidly replenishing ATP. In addition, Type II (fast-twitch) muscle fibers contain higher concentrations of CP than Type I (slow-twitch) fibers (95, 132); thus, individuals with higher percentages of Type II fibers may be able to replenish ATP faster through the phosphagen system during anaerobic, explosive exercise.

Another important single-enzyme reaction that can rapidly replenish ATP is the **adenylate kinase** (also called **myokinase**) **reaction**:

$$2\text{ADP} \xleftrightarrow{\text{Adenylate kinase}} \text{ATP} + \text{AMP} \qquad (3.3)$$

This reaction is particularly important because AMP, a product of the adenylate kinase (myokinase) reaction, is a powerful stimulant of **glycolysis** (22, 28).

Control of the Phosphagen System

The reactions of the phosphagen system (often represented by equations 3.1, 3.2, and 3.3) are largely controlled by the **law of mass action** or the **mass action effect** (107). The law of mass action states that the concentrations of reactants or products (or both) in solution will drive the direction of the reactions. With enzyme-mediated reactions, such as the reactions of the phosphagen system, the rate of product formation is greatly influenced by the concentrations of the reactants. This is denoted in equations 3.1, 3.2, and 3.3 by the two-way arrow between reactants and products. For example, as ATP is hydrolyzed to yield the energy necessary for exercise (equation 3.1), there is a transient increase in ADP concentrations (as well as P_i) in the sarcolemma. This will increase the rate of the creatine kinase and adenylate kinase reaction (equations 3.2 and 3.3) to replenish the ATP supply. The process will continue until (a) the exercise ceases or (b) the intensity is low enough that it does not deplete CP stores and it allows glycolysis or the oxidative system to become the primary supplier of ATP and rephosphorylate the free creatine (equation 3.2) (37). At this point, the sarcoplasmic concentration of ATP will remain steady or increase, which will slow down or reverse the directions of the creatine kinase and adenylate kinase reactions. As a result, equations 3.1, 3.2, and 3.3 are often referred to as **near-equilibrium reactions** that proceed in a direction dictated by the concentrations of the reactants due to the law of mass action.

Glycolysis

Glycolysis is the breakdown of carbohydrate—either glycogen stored in the muscle or glucose delivered in the blood—to resynthesize ATP (22, 143). The process of glycolysis involves multiple enzymatically catalyzed reactions (figure 3.2). As a result, the ATP resynthesis rate during glycolysis is not as rapid as with the single-step phosphagen system; however, the capacity to produce ATP is much higher due to a larger supply of glycogen and glucose compared to CP. As with the phosphagen system, glycolysis occurs in the sarcoplasm.

As depicted in figure 3.2, **pyruvate**, the end result of glycolysis, may proceed in one of two directions:

1. Pyruvate can be converted to **lactate** in the sarcoplasm.
2. Pyruvate can be shuttled into the mitochondria.

When pyruvate is converted to lactate, ATP resynthesis occurs at a faster rate via the rapid regeneration of NAD^+, but is limited in duration due to the subsequent H^+ production and resulting decrease in cytosolic pH. This process is sometimes called **anaerobic glycolysis** (or **fast glycolysis**). However, when pyruvate is shuttled into the mitochondria to undergo the Krebs cycle, the ATP resynthesis rate is slower because of the numerous reactions, but can occur for a longer duration if the

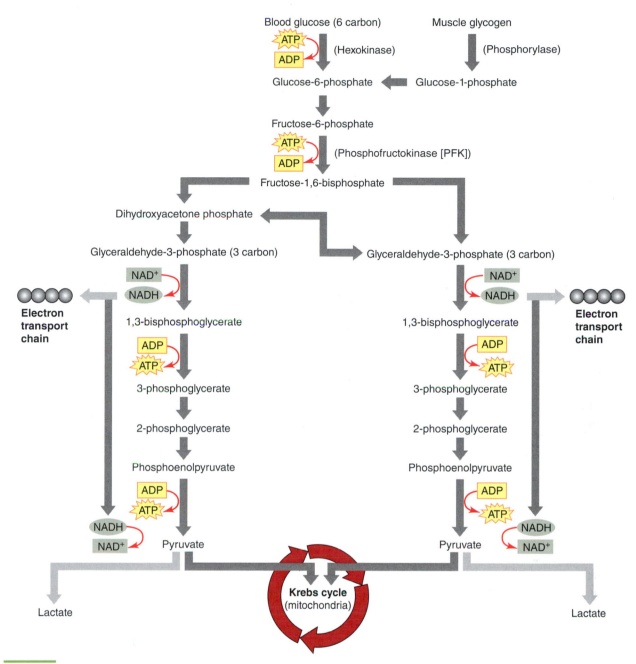

FIGURE 3.2   Glycolysis. ADP = adenosine diphosphate; ATP = adenosine triphosphate; NAD+, NADH = nicotinamide adenine dinucleotide.

exercise intensity is low enough. This process is often referred to as **aerobic glycolysis** (or **slow glycolysis**). At higher exercise intensities, pyruvate and NADH will increase above what can be handled by pyruvate dehydrogenase and will then be converted into lactate and NAD+. Unfortunately, because glycolysis itself does not depend on oxygen, the terms *anaerobic* and *aerobic* (or *fast* and *slow*, respectively) *glycolysis* are probably not practical for describing the processes. Nevertheless, the fate of pyruvate is ultimately controlled by the energy demands within the cell. If energy demand is high and

must be transferred quickly, as during resistance training, pyruvate is primarily converted to lactate for further support of anaerobic glycolysis. If energy demand is not as high and oxygen is present in sufficient quantities in the cell, pyruvate can be further oxidized in the mitochondria.

Glycolysis and the Formation of Lactate

The formation of lactate from pyruvate is catalyzed by the enzyme lactate dehydrogenase. Sometimes, mistakenly, the end result of this reaction is said to be the formation of **lactic acid**. However, due to the physiological pH (i.e., near 7) and earlier steps in glycolysis that consume protons (123), lactate—rather than lactic acid—is the product of the lactate dehydrogenase reaction. Although the muscular fatigue experienced during exercise often correlates with high tissue concentrations of lactate, lactate is not the cause of fatigue (22, 27, 123). Proton (H^+) accumulation during fatigue reduces the intracellular pH, inhibits glycolytic reactions, and directly interferes with muscle's excitation–contraction coupling—possibly by inhibiting calcium binding to troponin (57, 113) or by interfering with crossbridge recycling (51, 57, 78, 113, 144). Also, the decrease in pH inhibits the enzymatic turnover rate of the cell's energy systems (9, 78). Overall, this process of an exercise-induced decrease in pH is referred to as **metabolic acidosis** (123), and may be responsible for much of the peripheral fatigue that occurs during exercise (42, 154). More recently, the role of metabolic acidosis in peripheral fatigue has been questioned (128); and other factors have been reported to play a prominent role in peripheral fatigue, such as an increased interstitial K^+ concentration and P_i that impairs Ca^{++} release (118, 137). However, evidence suggests that other mechanisms, such as the simple hydrolysis of ATP (equation 3.1), are responsible for most of the H^+ accumulation and that lactate itself actually works to decrease metabolic acidosis rather than accelerate it (27, 123). See the sidebar titled "Lactic Acid Does Not Cause Metabolic Acidosis!" In fact, lactate is often used as an **energy substrate**, especially in Type I and cardiac muscle fibers (10, 106, 160). It is also used in **gluconeogenesis**—the formation of glucose from noncarbohydrate sources—during extended exercise and recovery (19, 106).

Normally there is a low concentration of lactate in blood and muscle. The reported normal range of lactate concentration in blood is 0.5 to 2.2 mmol/L at rest (67) and 0.5 to 2.2 mmol for each kilogram of **wet muscle** (muscle that has not been desiccated) (67). Lactate production increases with exercise intensity (67, 127) and appears to depend on muscle fiber type. Researchers have reported that the maximal rate of lactate production for Type II muscle fibers is 0.5 mmol·g⁻¹·s⁻¹ (46, 105) and for Type I muscle is 0.25 mmol·g⁻¹·s⁻¹ (111). The higher rate of lactate production by Type II muscle fibers may reflect a higher concentration or activity of glycolytic enzymes than in Type I muscle fibers (10, 120). Although the highest possible concentration of lactate accumulation is not known, severe fatigue may occur at blood concentrations between 20 and 25 mmol/L (105); one study, however, showed blood lactate concentrations greater than 30 mmol/L following multiple bouts of dynamic exercise (79). Along with exercise intensity and muscle fiber type, exercise duration (67), state of

training (66), and initial glycogen levels (67) can also influence lactate accumulation.

Blood lactate concentrations reflect the net balance of lactate production and clearance as a result of bicarbonate (HCO_3^-) buffering. HCO_3^- minimizes the disrupting influence of the H^+ on pH by accepting the proton (H_2CO_3). The clearance and buffering of lactate from the blood reflect a return to homeostatic range. Lactate can be cleared by oxidation within the muscle fiber in which it was produced, or it can be transported in the blood to other muscle fibers to be oxidized (106). Lactate can also be transported in the blood to the liver, where it is converted to glucose. This process is referred to as the **Cori cycle** and is depicted in figure 3.3.

Gollnick and colleagues (67) and others (8, 72, 116) have reported that blood lactate concentrations normally return to preexercise values within an hour after activity, depending on the duration and intensity of exercise, training status, and type of recovery (i.e., passive versus active). Light activity during the postexercise period has been shown to increase lactate clearance rates (55, 67, 72, 79, 116). For example, an active recovery following a 200-yard (182.9 m) maximal-effort swim resulted in the greatest lactate clearance in comparison to a passive recovery in competitive swimmers (72). In addition, both aerobically trained (67) and anaerobically trained (62) athletes have faster lactate clearance rates than untrained people. Peak blood lactate concentrations occur approximately 5 minutes after the cessation of exercise (67), a delay frequently attributed to the time required to buffer and transport lactate from the tissue to the blood (93).

Blood lactate accumulation is greater following high-intensity, intermittent exercise (e.g., resistance training and sprints) than following lower-intensity, continuous exercise (79, 101, 150). However, trained people experience lower blood lactate concentrations

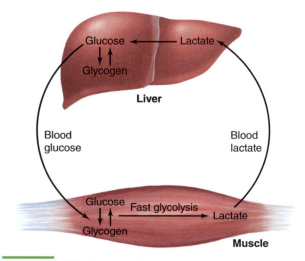

FIGURE 3.3   The Cori cycle.

Lactic Acid Does Not Cause Metabolic Acidosis!

Lactic acidosis is a common misnomer, as lactic acid is inaccurately believed to cause the burning sensations experienced with muscle fatigue during high-intensity exercise. This is based on the assumption that there is an immediate dissociation of lactic acid into lactate and H⁺ when produced by glycolysis in skeletal muscle (1, 60, 123). However, the phosphoglycerate kinase reaction of glycolysis involves the transfer of a phosphate leaving a carboxylate (COO⁻) group (103). Thus, as shown in figure 3.4, no proton (H⁺) exists to dissociate from lactate (60, 123).

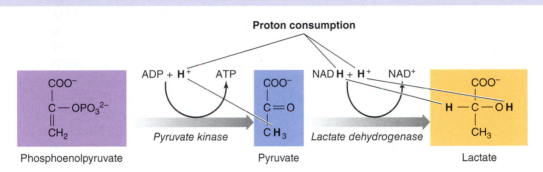

FIGURE 3.4   The phosphoglycerate kinase reaction of glycolysis, illustrating that there is no proton (H⁺) to dissociate from lactate.

Furthermore, the lactate dehydrogenase reaction itself consumes protons, which alkalizes the cell (60, 123)—quite the opposite of acidosis. In fact, Busa and Nuccitelli (27) stated, "ATP hydrolysis, not lactate accumulation, is the dominant source of the intracellular acid load . . ." (p. 430). The take-home message from Robergs and colleagues (123) is that the hydrolysis of ATP outside the mitochondria is primarily responsible for the proton (H⁺) accumulation during exercise-induced metabolic acidosis—not the conversion of pyruvate to lactate as is commonly believed. Consequently, the term *lactic acidosis* is indeed a misnomer, and the term *metabolic acidosis* is recommended to describe the reduced pH within skeletal muscle during high-intensity, fatiguing exercise.

than untrained people when exercising at an absolute workload (same resistance) (66, 89, 141). This indicates that resistance training results in alterations in lactate response similar to those from aerobic endurance training (67, 89, 141). These alterations include a lower blood lactate concentration at a given workload in trained individuals and higher blood lactate concentrations in trained individuals during maximal exercise (67, 89, 141).

The net reaction for glycolysis when pyruvate is converted to lactate may be summarized as follows:

$$\text{Glucose} + 2P_i + 2\text{ADP} \rightarrow 2\text{Lactate} + 2\text{ATP} + H_2O \quad \textbf{(3.4)}$$

Glycolysis Leading to the Krebs Cycle

If oxygen is present in sufficient quantities in the mitochondria (specialized cellular organelles where the reactions of aerobic metabolism occur), the end product of glycolysis, pyruvate, is not converted to lactate but is transported into the mitochondria. Also transported are two molecules of reduced **nicotinamide adenine dinucleotide (NADH)** produced during glycolytic reactions (*reduced* refers to the added hydrogen). When pyruvate enters the mitochondria, it is converted to acetyl-CoA

(CoA stands for coenzyme A) by the pyruvate dehydrogenase complex, resulting in the loss of a carbon as CO_2. Acetyl-CoA can then enter the Krebs cycle for further ATP resynthesis. The NADH molecules enter the electron transport system, where they can also be used to resynthesize ATP.

The net reaction for glycolysis when pyruvate is shuttled to the mitochondria may be summarized as follows:

$$\text{Glucose} + 2P_i + 2\text{ADP} + 2\text{NAD}^+ \rightarrow$$
$$2\text{Pyruvate} + 2\text{ATP} + 2\text{NADH} + 2H_2O \quad \textbf{(3.5)}$$

Energy Yield of Glycolysis

There are two primary mechanisms for resynthesizing ATP during metabolism:

1. Substrate-level phosphorylation
2. Oxidative phosphorylation

Phosphorylation is the process of adding an inorganic phosphate (P_i) to another molecule. For example, $\text{ADP} + P_i \rightarrow \text{ATP}$ is the phosphorylation of ADP to ATP. **Oxidative phosphorylation** refers to the resynthesis of

ATP in the **electron transport chain (ETC)**. In contrast, **substrate-level phosphorylation** refers to the direct resynthesis of ATP from ADP during a single reaction in the metabolic pathways. To illustrate, in glycolysis there are two steps that result in substrate-level phosphorylation of ADP to ATP (42):

$$\text{1,3-bisphosphoglycerate} + \text{ADP} + \text{P}_i$$
$$\xrightarrow{\text{Phosphoglycerate kinase}} \text{3-phosphoglycerate} + \text{ATP} \quad \textbf{(3.6)}$$

$$\text{Phosphoenolpyruvate} + \text{ADP}$$
$$+ \text{P}_i \xrightarrow{\text{Pyruvate kinase}} \text{Pyruvate} + \text{ATP} \quad \textbf{(3.7)}$$

The gross number of ATP molecules that are resynthesized as a result of substrate-level phosphorylation during glycolysis is four (figure 3.2). However, the reaction that converts fructose-6-phosphate to fructose-1,6-bisphosphate (catalyzed by the enzyme **phosphofructokinase [PFK]**) in glycolysis requires the hydrolysis of one ATP molecule. In addition, there are two possible sources of glucose: blood glucose and muscle glycogen. When blood glucose enters the muscle cell, it must be phosphorylated to remain in the cell and to maintain the glucose concentration gradient (67). The phosphorylation of one molecule of blood glucose, which is catalyzed by hexokinase, also requires the hydrolysis of one ATP. In contrast, when muscle glycogen is broken down (i.e., **glycogenolysis**) to glucose with the help of the enzyme glycogen phosphorylase, the glucose is already phosphorylated, and it does not require the hydrolysis of ATP. Therefore, when glycolysis begins with one molecule of blood glucose, two ATP molecules are used and four ATP are resynthesized, which results in a net resynthesis of two ATP molecules. When glycolysis begins from muscle glycogen, only one ATP is used and four ATP are resynthesized, which yields a net resynthesis of three ATP molecules.

Control of Glycolysis

In general, the rate of glycolysis is stimulated to increase during intense muscle actions by high concentrations of ADP, P_i, and ammonia and by a slight decrease in pH and AMP (22, 61, 140), all of which are signs of increased ATP hydrolysis and a need for energy. In contrast, glycolysis is inhibited by markedly lower pH, ATP, CP, citrate, and free fatty acids (22), which are usually present at rest. (Note that a slight decrease in pH increases glycolysis, but if pH continues to decrease significantly it will inhibit the rate of glycolysis.) However, there are more specific factors that contribute to the regulation of glycolysis (107), such as the concentrations and turnover rates of three important glycolytic enzymes: hexokinase, PFK, and pyruvate kinase. All three of these are regulatory enzymes in glycolysis, because each has important allosteric (meaning "other site") binding sites. Allosteric regulation occurs when the end product of a reaction or series of reactions feeds back to regulate the turnover rate of key enzymes in the metabolic pathways. Consequently, this process is also called *end product regulation* (85) or *feedback regulation* (61). **Allosteric inhibition** occurs when an end product binds to the regulatory enzyme and decreases its turnover rate and slows product formation. In contrast, **allosteric activation** occurs when an "activator" binds with the enzyme and increases its turnover rate.

Hexokinase, which catalyzes the phosphorylation of glucose to glucose-6-phosphate, is allosterically inhibited by the concentration of glucose-6-phosphate in the sarcoplasm (61). Thus, the higher the concentration of glucose-6-phosphate, the more hexokinase will be inhibited. In addition, the phosphorylation of glucose commits it to the cell so that it cannot leave. Similarly, the PFK reaction (fructose-6-phosphate → fructose 1,6-bisphosphate) commits the cell to metabolizing glucose rather than storing it as glycogen. Phosphofructokinase is the most important regulator of glycolysis because it is the **rate-limiting step.** Adenosine triphosphate is an allosteric inhibitor of PFK; therefore, as intracellular ATP concentrations rise, PFK activity decreases and reduces the conversion of fructose-6-phosphate to fructose 1,6-bisphosphate and, subsequently, decreases activity of the glycolytic pathway. However, AMP is an allosteric activator of PFK and a powerful stimulator of glycolysis. Moreover, the ammonia produced during high-intensity exercise as a result of AMP or amino acid deamination (removing the amine group from the amino acid molecule) can also stimulate PFK. Pyruvate kinase catalyzes the conversion of phosphoenolpyruvate to pyruvate and is the final regulatory enzyme. Pyruvate kinase is allosterically inhibited by ATP and acetyl-CoA (the latter is a Krebs cycle intermediate) and activated by high concentrations of AMP and fructose-1,6-bisphosphate (61).

Lactate Threshold and Onset of Blood Lactate Accumulation

Recent evidence suggests that there are specific break points in the lactate accumulation curve (figure 3.5) as exercise intensity increases (39, 98). The exercise intensity or relative intensity at which blood lactate begins an abrupt increase above the baseline concentration has been termed the **lactate threshold (LT)** (161). The *LT* represents a significantly increased reliance on anaerobic mechanisms for energy production to meet demand. The LT corresponds well with the ventilatory threshold (breaking point in the relationship between ventilation and $\dot{V}O_2$) and is often used as a marker of the anaerobic threshold.

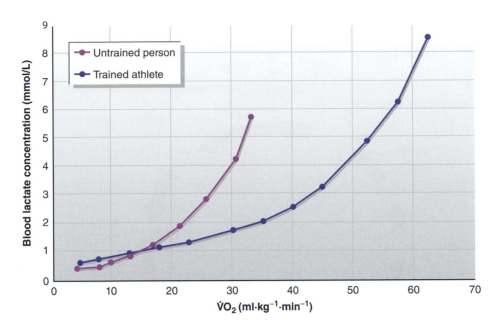

FIGURE 3.5 Lactate threshold (LT) and onset of blood lactate accumulation (OBLA).

The LT typically begins at 50% to 60% of maximal **oxygen uptake** in untrained individuals and at 70% to 80% in aerobically trained athletes (29, 52). A second increase in the rate of lactate accumulation has been noted at higher relative intensities of exercise. This second point of inflection has been termed the **onset of blood lactate accumulation (OBLA)** and occurs when the concentration of blood lactate reaches 4 mmol/L (83, 136, 142). The breaks in the lactate accumulation curve may correspond to the points at which intermediate and large motor units are recruited during increasing exercise intensities (92). The muscle cells associated with large motor units are typically Type II fibers, which are particularly suited for anaerobic metabolism and lactate production.

Some studies suggest that training at intensities near or above the LT or OBLA pushes the LT and OBLA to the right (i.e., lactate accumulation occurs later at a higher exercise intensity) (39, 43). This shift probably occurs as a result of changes in hormone release, particularly reduced catecholamine release at high exercise intensities, and increased mitochondrial content that allows for greater production of ATP through aerobic mechanisms. The shift allows the athlete to perform at higher percentages of maximal oxygen uptake without as much lactate accumulation in the blood (22, 41).

The Oxidative (Aerobic) System

The oxidative system, the primary source of ATP at rest and during low-intensity activities, uses primarily carbohydrate and fats as substrates (62). Protein does not provide a significant contribution to total energy; however, the use of protein does significantly increase during long-term starvation and long bouts (>90 minutes) of exercise (41, 102). At rest, approximately 70% of the ATP produced is derived from fats and 30% from carbohydrate. Following the onset of activity, as the intensity of the exercise increases, there is a shift in substrate preference from fats to carbohydrate. During high-intensity aerobic exercise, almost 100% of the energy is derived from carbohydrate if an adequate supply is available, with only minimal contributions from fats and protein. However, during prolonged, submaximal, steady-state work, there is a gradual shift from carbohydrate back to fats, and to a very small extent protein, as energy substrates (22).

Glucose and Glycogen Oxidation

The oxidative metabolism of blood glucose and muscle glycogen begins with glycolysis. If oxygen is present in sufficient quantities, the end product of glycolysis, pyruvate, is not converted to lactate but is transported to the mitochondria, where it is converted to acetyl-CoA (a two-carbon molecule), which enters the Krebs cycle, also known as the citric acid cycle or tricarboxylic acid cycle (7, 61). The Krebs cycle is a series of reactions that continues the oxidation of the substrate from glycolysis and produces two ATP indirectly from guanine triphosphate (GTP), via substrate-level phosphorylation, for each molecule of glucose (figure 3.6).

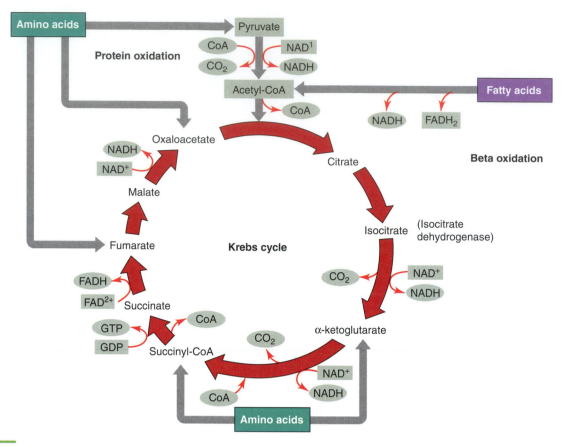

FIGURE 3.6   The Krebs cycle. CoA = coenzyme A; FAD^{2+}, FADH, $FADH_2$ = flavin adenine dinucleotide; GDP = guanine diphosphate; GTP = guanine triphosphate; NAD^+, NADH = nicotinamide adenine dinucleotide.

Also produced from the two pyruvate molecules subsequent to the production of one molecule of glucose are six molecules of NADH and two molecules of reduced **flavin adenine dinucleotide (FADH$_2$)**. These molecules transport hydrogen atoms to the ETC to be used to produce ATP from ADP (22, 107). The ETC uses the NADH and FADH$_2$ molecules to rephosphorylate ADP to ATP (figure 3.7).

The hydrogen atoms are passed down the chain (a series of electron carriers known as **cytochromes**) to form a proton concentration gradient, which provides the energy for ATP production, with oxygen serving as the final electron acceptor (resulting in the formation of water). Because NADH and FADH$_2$ enter the ETC at different sites, they differ in their ability to produce ATP. One molecule of NADH can produce three molecules of ATP, whereas one molecule of FADH$_2$ can produce only two molecules of ATP. The production of ATP during this process is referred to as *oxidative phosphorylation*. The oxidative system, beginning with glycolysis and including the Krebs cycle and ETC, results in the production of approximately 38 ATP from the degradation of one molecule of blood glucose (22, 85). However, if the initiation of glycolysis is muscle glycogen, the net ATP production is 39, since the hexokinase reaction is not necessary with muscle glycogenolysis. Nevertheless, oxidative phosphorylation accounts for over 90% of ATP synthesis compared to substrate-level phosphorylation,

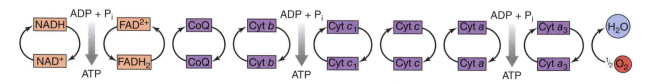

FIGURE 3.7   The electron transport chain. CoQ = coenzyme Q; Cyt = cytochrome.

which demonstrates the capacity of energy transfer by the oxidative system. See table 3.1 for a summary of these processes.

Fat Oxidation

Fats can also be used by the oxidative energy system. Triglycerides stored in fat cells can be broken down by an enzyme, hormone-sensitive lipase, to produce free fatty acids and glycerol. This releases a portion of the total free fatty acids from the fat cells into the blood, where they can circulate and enter muscle fibers and undergo oxidation (88, 121). Additionally, limited quantities of triglycerides are stored within the muscle along with a form of hormone-sensitive lipase to produce an intramuscular source of free fatty acids (22, 47). Free fatty acids enter the mitochondria, where they undergo **beta oxidation**, a series of reactions in which the free fatty acids are broken down, resulting in the formation of acetyl-CoA and hydrogen protons (figure 3.6). The acetyl-CoA enters the Krebs cycle directly, and the hydrogen atoms are carried by NADH and FADH$_2$ to the ETC (22). The result is hundreds of ATP molecules supplied by beta oxidation. For example, the breakdown of a single triglyceride molecule containing three 16-carbon chain free fatty acids (palmitic acid) can be metabolized by beta oxidation to yield over 300 ATP molecules (>100 ATP per palmitic acid). The overarching concept is that

TABLE 3.1   Total Energy Yield From the Oxidation of One Glucose Molecule

Process	ATP production
Slow glycolysis:	
Substrate-level phosphorylation	4
Oxidative phosphorylation: 2 NADH (3 ATP each)	6
Krebs cycle (2 rotations through the Krebs cycle per glucose):	
Substrate-level phosphorylation	2
Oxidative phosphorylation: 8 NADH (3 ATP each)	24
Via GTP: 2 FADH$_2$ (2 ATP each)	4
Total	40*

*Glycolysis consumes 2 ATP (if starting with blood glucose), so net ATP production is 40 − 2 = 38. This figure may also be reported as 36 ATP depending on which shuttle system is used to transport the NADH to the mitochondria. ATP = adenosine triphosphate; FADH$_2$ = flavin adenine dinucleotide; GTP = guanine triphosphate; NADH = nicotinamide adenine dinucleotide.

fat oxidation is capable of a tremendous capacity for ATP synthesis compared to carbohydrate and protein oxidation.

Protein Oxidation

Although not a significant source of energy for most activities, protein can be broken down into its constituent amino acids by various metabolic processes. Most of these amino acids can then be converted into glucose (in a process known as *gluconeogenesis*), pyruvate, or various Krebs cycle intermediates to produce ATP (figure 3.6). The contribution of amino acids to the production of ATP has been estimated to be minimal during short-term exercise but may contribute 3% to 18% of the energy requirements during prolonged activity (20, 138). The major amino acids that are oxidized in skeletal muscle are believed to be the **branched-chain amino acids** (leucine, isoleucine, and valine), although alanine, aspartate, and glutamate may also be used (69). The nitrogenous waste products of amino acid degradation are eliminated through the formation of urea and small amounts of ammonia (22). The elimination through formation of ammonia is significant because ammonia is toxic and is associated with fatigue.

Control of the Oxidative (Aerobic) System

The rate-limiting step in the Krebs cycle (see figure 3.6) is the conversion of isocitrate to α-ketoglutarate, a reaction catalyzed by the enzyme isocitrate dehydrogenase. Isocitrate dehydrogenase is stimulated by ADP and allosterically inhibited by ATP. The reactions that produce NADH or FADH$_2$ also influence the regulation of the Krebs cycle. If NAD$^+$ and FAD^{2+} are not available in sufficient quantities to accept hydrogen, the rate of the Krebs cycle is reduced. Also, when GTP accumulates, the concentration of succinyl CoA increases, which inhibits the initial reaction (oxaloacetate + acetyl-CoA → citrate + CoA) of the Krebs cycle. The ETC is inhibited by ATP and stimulated by ADP (22). A simplified overview of the metabolism of fat, carbohydrate, and protein is presented in figure 3.8.

Energy Production and Capacity

The phosphagen, glycolytic, and oxidative energy systems differ in their ability to supply energy for activities of various intensities and durations (tables 3.2 and 3.3). Exercise intensity is defined as a level of muscular activity that can be quantified in terms of power (work performed per unit of time) output (99). Activities such as resistance training performed at a high power output require a rapid rate of energy supply and rely almost entirely on the energy provided by the

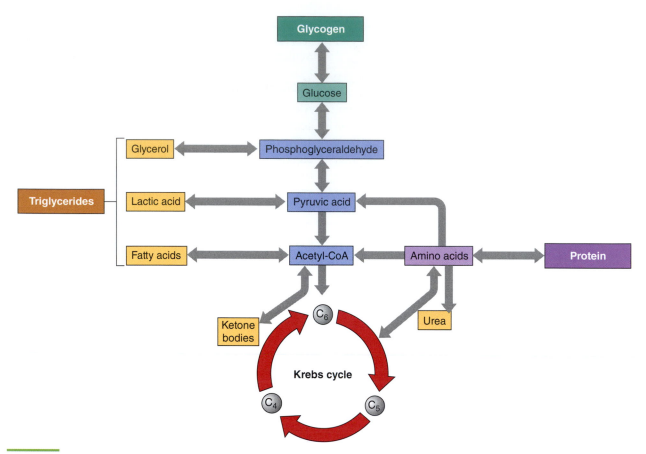

FIGURE 3.8   The metabolism of fat and that of carbohydrate and protein share some common pathways. Note that many are oxidized to acetyl-CoA and enter the Krebs cycle.

TABLE 3.2   Effect of Event Duration and Intensity on Primary Energy System Used

Duration of event	Intensity of event	Primary energy system
0-6 s	Extremely high	Phosphagen
6-30 s	Very high	Phosphagen and fast glycolysis
30 s to 2 min	High	Fast glycolysis
2-3 min	Moderate	Fast glycolysis and oxidative system
>3 min	Low	Oxidative system

The relationships between duration, intensity, and primary energy systems used assume that the athlete strives to attain the best possible performance for a given event.

TABLE 3.3   Rankings of Rate and Capacity of ATP Production

System	Rate of ATP production	Capacity of ATP production
Phosphagen	1	5
Fast glycolysis	2	4
Slow glycolysis	3	3
Oxidation of carbohydrates	4	2
Oxidation of fats and proteins	5	1

Note: 1 = fastest/greatest; 5 = slowest/least.

phosphagen system. Activities that are of low intensity but long duration, such as marathon running, require a prolonged energy supply and rely predominantly on the energy supplied by the oxidative energy system. The primary source of energy for activities between these two extremes shifts, depending on the intensity and duration of the event (table 3.2). In general, short, high-intensity activities (e.g., high-intensity resistance training and sprinting) rely largely on the phosphagen energy system and fast glycolysis. As the intensity decreases and duration increases, the emphasis gradually shifts to slow glycolysis and the oxidative energy system (45, 129).

> In general, there is an inverse relationship between a given energy system's maximum rate of ATP production (i.e., ATP produced per unit of time) and its capacity (i.e., the total amount of ATP produced over time). The phosphagen system is capable of achieving the highest rate of ATP production, while fat oxidation has the greatest capacity of ATP production. As a result, the phosphagen energy system primarily supplies ATP for high-intensity activities of short duration (e.g., 100 m dash), the glycolytic system for moderate- to high-intensity activities of short to medium duration (e.g., 400 m dash), and the oxidative system for low-intensity activities of long duration (e.g., marathon).

The duration of the activity also influences which energy system is used. Athletic events range in duration from 1 to 3 seconds (e.g., snatch and shot put) to more than 4 hours (e.g., long-distance triathlons and ultramarathons). If an athlete makes a best effort (an effort that results in the best possible performance for a given event), the time considerations shown in table 3.2 are reasonable (48, 78, 124, 144, 147).

At no time, during either exercise or rest, does any single energy system provide the complete supply of energy. During exercise, the degree to which anaerobic and oxidative systems contribute to the energy being produced is determined primarily by the exercise intensity and secondarily by exercise duration (22, 45, 48).

> The extent to which each of the three energy systems contributes to ATP production depends primarily on the intensity of muscular activity and secondarily on the duration. At no time, during either exercise or rest, does any single energy system provide the complete supply of energy.

Substrate Depletion and Repletion

Energy substrates—molecules that provide starting materials for bioenergetic reactions, including phosphagens (ATP and CP), glucose, glycogen, lactate, free fatty acids, and amino acids—can be selectively depleted during the performance of activities of various intensities and durations. Subsequently, the energy that can be produced by the bioenergetic systems is reduced. Fatigue experienced during many activities is frequently associated with the depletion of phosphagens (66, 87) and glycogen (21, 78, 90, 131); the depletion of substrates such as free fatty acids, lactate, and amino acids typically does not occur to the extent that performance

is limited. Consequently, the **depletion** and **repletion** pattern of phosphagens and glycogen following physical activity is important in exercise and sport bioenergetics.

Phosphagens

Fatigue during exercise appears to be at least partially related to the decrease in phosphagens (i.e., ATP and CP). Phosphagen concentrations in muscle are more rapidly depleted as a result of high-intensity anaerobic exercise compared to aerobic exercise (66, 87). Creatine phosphate can decrease markedly (50-70%) during the first stage of high-intensity exercise of short and moderate duration (5-30 seconds) and can be almost completely depleted as a result of very intense exercise to exhaustion (84, 91, 96, 108). Muscle ATP concentrations may decrease only slightly (34) or may decrease up to 50% to 60% (143) of the preexercise levels during experimentally induced fatigue. It should also be noted that dynamic muscle actions that produce external work use more metabolic energy and typically deplete phosphagens to a greater extent than do isometric muscle actions (18).

The intramuscular ATP concentration is largely sustained during exercise as a consequence of CP depletion and the contribution of additional ATP from the myokinase reaction and oxidation of other energy sources, such as glycogen and free fatty acids. Postexercise phosphagen repletion can occur in a relatively short period; complete resynthesis of ATP appears to occur within 3 to 5 minutes, and complete CP resynthesis can occur within 8 minutes (75, 87). Repletion of phosphagens is largely accomplished as a result of aerobic metabolism (75), although glycolysis can contribute to recovery after high-intensity exercise (29, 40).

The effects of training on concentrations of phosphagens are not well studied or understood. Aerobic endurance training may increase resting concentrations of phosphagens (49, 97) and decrease their rate of depletion at a given absolute submaximal power output (33, 97) but not at a relative (percentage of maximum) submaximal power output (33). Although researchers have noted indications of increased resting concentrations of phosphagens (12, 125), short-term (eight weeks) studies of sprint and six months of resistance or explosive training have not shown alterations in resting concentrations of phosphagens (11, 16, 145, 148). However, total phosphagen content can be larger following sprint training due to increases in muscle mass (148). Resistance training has been shown to increase the resting concentrations of phosphagens in the triceps brachii after five weeks of training (104). The increases in phosphagen concentration may have occurred due to selective hypertrophy of Type II fibers, which can contain a higher phosphagen concentration than Type I fibers (103).

Glycogen

Limited stores of glycogen are available for exercise. Approximately 300 to 400 g of glycogen are stored in the body's total muscle and about 70 to 100 g in the liver (135). Resting concentrations of liver and muscle glycogen can be influenced by training and dietary manipulations (56, 135). Research suggests that both anaerobic training, including sprinting and resistance training (16, 104), and stereotypical aerobic endurance training (64, 65) can increase resting muscle glycogen concentration with concomitantly appropriate nutrition.

The rate of glycogen depletion is related to exercise intensity (135). Muscle glycogen is a more important energy source than liver glycogen during moderate- and high-intensity exercise. Liver glycogen appears to be more important during low-intensity exercise, and its contribution to metabolic processes increases with duration of exercise. Increases in relative exercise intensity of 50%, 75%, and 100% of maximal oxygen uptake result in increases in the rate of muscle glycogenolysis (the breakdown of glycogen) of 0.7, 1.4, and 3.4 mmol $\cdot kg^{-1} \cdot min^{-1}$, respectively (131). At relative intensities of exercise above 60% of maximal oxygen uptake, muscle glycogen becomes an increasingly important energy substrate; the entire glycogen content of some muscle cells can become depleted during exercise (130).

Relatively constant blood glucose concentrations are maintained at very low exercise intensities (below 50% of maximal oxygen uptake) as a result of low muscle glucose uptake; as duration increases beyond 90 minutes, blood glucose concentrations fall, but rarely below 2.8 mmol/L (2). Long-term exercise (over 90 minutes) at higher intensities (above 50% of maximal oxygen uptake) may result in substantially decreased blood glucose concentrations as a result of liver glycogen depletion. Hypoglycemic reactions may occur in some people with exercise-induced blood glucose values less than 2.5 mmol/L (3, 35). A decline in blood glucose to around 2.5 to 3.0 mmol/L results from reduced liver carbohydrate stores and causes decreased carbohydrate oxidation and eventual exhaustion (32, 35, 135).

Very high-intensity, intermittent exercise, such as high-intensity resistance training, can cause substantial depletion of muscle glycogen (decreases of 20% to 60%) with relatively few sets (low total workloads) (99, 124, 144, 146). Although phosphagens may be the primary limiting factor during resistance exercise with high resistance and few repetitions or few sets, muscle glycogen may become the limiting factor for resistance training with many total sets and larger total amounts of work (124). This type of exercise could cause selective muscle fiber glycogen depletion (more depletion in Type II fibers), which can also limit performance (50, 124). As with other types of dynamic exercise, the rate of muscle glycogenolysis during resistance exercise depends on intensity (i.e., the greater the intensity, the faster the rate of glycogenolysis). However, it appears that when the total work performed is equal, the absolute amount of glycogen depletion is the same, regardless of the intensity of the resistance training session (69, 124).

Repletion of muscle glycogen during recovery is related to postexercise carbohydrate ingestion. Repletion appears to be optimal if 0.7 to 3.0 g of carbohydrate per kilogram of body weight is ingested every 2 hours following exercise (56, 135). This level of carbohydrate consumption can maximize muscle glycogen repletion at 5 to 6 mmol/g of wet muscle mass per hour during the first 4 to 6 hours following exercise. Muscle glycogen may be completely replenished within 24 hours, provided that sufficient carbohydrate is ingested (56, 135). However, if the exercise has a high eccentric component (associated with exercise-induced muscle damage), more time may be required to completely replenish muscle glycogen (119, 162).

Bioenergetic Limiting Factors in Exercise Performance

Factors limiting maximal performance (22, 49, 78, 86, 102, 154) must be considered in the mechanisms of fatigue experienced during exercise and training. Understanding the possible limiting factors associated

Differences in Phosphocreatine Depletion and Resynthesis in Children Versus Adults

Kappenstein and colleagues (94) tested the hypothesis that a greater oxidative capacity in children results in lower CP depletion, faster CP resynthesis, and lower metabolic acidosis than in adults during high-intensity intermittent exercise. Sixteen children (mean age = 9 years) and 16 adults (mean age = 26 years) completed 10 bouts of 30-second dynamic, plantar flexion contractions at 25% of 1-repetition maximum (1RM). Creatine phosphate, ATP, inorganic phosphate (P_i), and phosphomonoesters were measured during and after exercise. Creatine phosphate breakdown was significantly lower in children during the first exercise bout, and average CP levels were higher in children at the end of exercise and during the recovery periods. In addition, muscle pH was significantly higher in children at the end of exercise. The results suggested that children are better able to meet energy demands with oxidative metabolism during high-intensity intermittent exercise.

with a particular athletic event is required when one is designing training programs and attempting to delay fatigue and possibly enhance performance. Table 3.4 depicts examples of various limiting factors based on depletion of energy sources and increases in muscle hydrogen ions, although other potential factors have been postulated.

Glycogen depletion can be a limiting factor both for long-duration, low-intensity exercise supported primarily by aerobic metabolism and for repeated, high-intensity exercise supported primarily by anaerobic mechanisms. Of importance to resistance training, sprinting, and other primarily anaerobic activities is the effect of metabolic acidosis on limiting contractile force (53, 78, 114, 115, 123). Several other factors have been implicated in the development of muscle fatigue and may limit exercise performance, including increased intracellular inorganic phosphate, ammonia accumulation, increased ADP, and impaired calcium release from the sarcoplasmic reticulum (4, 5, 129, 154, 158). Further research is needed to delineate the causes of muscular fatigue and the limiting factors in exercise performance.

Oxygen Uptake and the Aerobic and Anaerobic Contributions to Exercise

Oxygen uptake (or consumption) is a measure of a person's ability to take in oxygen via the respiratory system and deliver it to the working tissues via the cardiovascular system, and the ability of working tissues (predominantly skeletal muscle) to use oxygen. During low-intensity exercise with a constant power output,

oxygen uptake increases for the first few minutes until a steady state of uptake (oxygen demand equals oxygen consumption) is reached (figure 3.9) (7, 83).

At the start of an exercise bout, however, some of the energy must be supplied through anaerobic mechanisms because the aerobic system responds slowly to the initial increase in the demand for energy (62, 153). This anaerobic contribution to the total energy cost of exercise is termed the **oxygen deficit** (83, 107). After exercise, oxygen uptake remains above preexercise levels for a period of time that varies according to the intensity and length of the exercise. Postexercise oxygen uptake has been termed the **oxygen debt** (83, 107), recovery O_2 (107), or the **excess postexercise oxygen consumption**

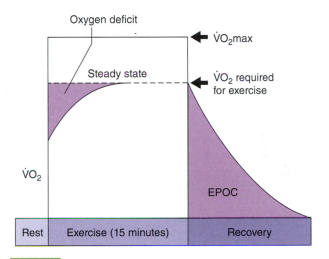

FIGURE 3.9 Low-intensity, steady-state exercise metabolism: 75% of maximal oxygen uptake ($\dot{V}O_2$max). EPOC = excess postexercise oxygen consumption; $\dot{V}O_2$ = oxygen uptake.

TABLE 3.4   Ranking of Bioenergetic Limiting Factors

Exercise	ATP and creatine phosphate	Muscle glycogen	Liver glycogen	Fat stores	Lower pH
Marathon	1	5	4-5	2-3	1
Triathlon	1-2	5	4-5	1-2	1-2
5,000 m run	1-2	3	3	1-2	1
1,500 m run	2-3	3-4	2	1-2	2-3
400 m swim	2-3	3-4	3	1	1-2
400 m run	3	3	1	1	4-5
100 m run	5	1-2	1	1	1-2
Discus	2-3	1	1	1	1
Repeated snatch exercise at 60% of 1RM (10 sets)	4-5	4-5	1-2	1-2	4-5

Note: 1 = least probable limiting factor; 5 = most probable limiting factor.

(EPOC) (22). The EPOC is the oxygen uptake above resting values used to restore the body to the preexercise condition (139). Only small to moderate relationships between the oxygen deficit and the EPOC have been observed (13, 77); the oxygen deficit may influence the size of the EPOC, but the two are not equal. The possible factors affecting the EPOC are listed in the sidebar (17, 21, 22, 58, 107).

Anaerobic mechanisms provide much of the energy for work if the exercise intensity is above the maximal oxygen uptake that a person can attain (figure 3.10). Generally, as the contribution of anaerobic mechanisms supporting the exercise increases, the exercise duration decreases (7, 68, 156, 157).

The approximate contribution of anaerobic and aerobic mechanisms to maximal sustained efforts on a cycle ergometer is shown in table 3.5 (110, 149, 159). Contributions from anaerobic mechanisms are primary up to 60 seconds, after which aerobic metabolism becomes the primary energy-supplying mechanism. The contribution of anaerobic mechanisms to this type of exercise represents the maximal anaerobic capacity (109, 149).

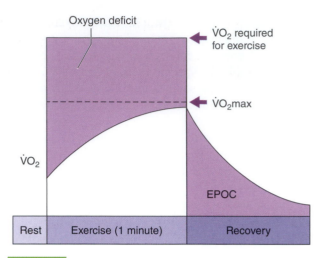

FIGURE 3.10 High-intensity, non–steady-state exercise metabolism (80% of maximum power output). The required $\dot{V}O_2$ here is the oxygen uptake that would be required to sustain the exercise if such an uptake were possible to attain. Because it is not, the oxygen deficit lasts for the duration of the exercise. EPOC = excess postexercise oxygen consumption; $\dot{V}O_2$max = maximal oxygen uptake.

Excess Postexercise Oxygen Consumption Is Intensity, Duration, and Mode Dependent

Excess postexercise oxygen consumption (EPOC) refers to the prolonged increase in $\dot{V}O_2$ that may be observed for hours after exercise (58).

Aerobic Exercise and EPOC (17)

- Intensity has the greatest effect on EPOC.
- The greatest EPOC values are found when both exercise intensity (i.e., >50-60% $\dot{V}O_2$max) and durations (i.e., >40 minutes) are high.
- Performing brief, intermittent bouts of supramaximal exercise (i.e., >100% $\dot{V}O_2$max) may induce the greatest EPOC with lower total work.
- There is interindividual variability for EPOC in response to a given relative exercise stimulus.
- The effects of aerobic exercise modes on EPOC are unclear.

Resistance Exercise and EPOC (17)

- Heavy resistance exercise (i.e., three sets, eight exercises to exhaustion, 80-90% 1RM) produces greater EPOCs than circuit weight training (i.e., four sets, eight exercises, 15 repetitions, 50% 1RM).
- Thus, EPOC is also intensity dependent in response to resistance training.

Factors Responsible for EPOC (17)

- Replenishment of oxygen in blood and muscle
- ATP/CP resynthesis
- Increased body temperature, circulation, and ventilation
- Increased rate of triglyceride–fatty acid cycling
- Increased protein turnover
- Changes in energy efficiency during recovery

TABLE 3.5   Contributions of Anaerobic and Aerobic Mechanisms to Maximal Sustained Efforts in Bicycle Ergometry

	0-5 s	30 s	60 s	90 s	150 s	200 s
Exercise intensity (% of maximum power output)	100	55	35	31	Not available	Not available
Contribution of anaerobic mechanisms (%)	96	75	50	35	30	22
Contribution of aerobic mechanisms (%)	4	25	50	65	70	78

Metabolic Specificity of Training

Appropriate exercise intensities and rest intervals can permit the "selection" of specific primary energy systems during training for specific athletic events (22, 107, 155). Few sports or physical activities require maximal sustained effort to exhaustion or near exhaustion, such as competitive middle-distance sprints (400 m to 1,600 m). Most sports and training activities produce metabolic profiles that are very similar to those of a series of high-intensity, constant- or near-constant-effort exercise bouts interspersed with rest periods, such as American football, basketball, and hockey. In this type of exercise, the required exercise intensity (power output) that must be met during each exercise bout is much greater than the maximal power output that can be sustained using aerobic energy sources alone. Increasing aerobic power through primarily aerobic endurance training while simultaneously compromising or neglecting anaerobic power and anaerobic capacity training is of little benefit to athletes in these sports (82, 109). For example, it would be of little benefit for a baseball player to run miles during training rather than focusing on exercises that improve anaerobic power and capacity.

> The use of appropriate exercise intensities and rest intervals allows for the "selection" of specific primary energy systems during training and, because this is more reflective of the actual metabolic demands of the sport, results in more efficient and productive regimens for specific athletic events with various metabolic demands.

Interval Training

Interval training is a method that emphasizes bioenergetic adaptations for a more efficient energy transfer within the metabolic pathways by using predetermined intervals of exercise and rest periods (i.e., **work-to-rest ratios**). Theoretically, properly spaced work-to-rest intervals allow more work to be accomplished at higher exercise intensities with the same or less fatigue than during continuous training at the same relative intensity. An early paper by Christensen and colleagues (31) compared the total running distance, average oxygen uptake, and blood lactate concentration during continuous running for 5 minutes and interval running totaling 30 minutes with 2:1, 1:1, and 1:2 work-to-rest ratios. Subjects were assigned a continuous running intensity (speed) that would result in fatigue within 5 minutes. At that fast pace during the continuous run, the subjects were able to complete 0.81 miles (1.30 km) before exhaustion. Using 2:1, 1:1, and 1:2 work-to-rest ratios and the same running intensity for a total duration of 30 minutes, however, the subjects were able to complete 4.14 miles (6.66 km), 3.11 miles (5.00 km), and 2.07 miles (3.33 km), respectively, all while working aerobic capacity in a manner similar to that in the continuous running condition. Therefore, much more training can be accomplished at higher intensities with interval training; this concept has been established for over 45 years (31).

A series of short-term (two-week) interval training studies used six sessions of four to seven 30-second maximum cycling efforts interspaced with 4 minutes of recovery (1:8 work-to-rest ratio). These studies demonstrated improvements in muscle oxidative potential (26, 63), muscle buffering capacity (26, 63), muscle glycogen content (25, 26), and time-trial performance (25), as well as doubled aerobic endurance capacity (26). In addition, a similar four-week interval training program exhibited increases in muscle activation and total work output (38) in trained cyclists. Thus, even the results of recent studies support the use of interval training for metabolic adaptations.

Few studies provide results that can be used to generate definitive guidelines for choosing specific work-to-rest ratios. One such study, however, reported aerobic and anaerobic metabolic variables, total work, and time to exhaustion differences between two different work-to-rest ratios in elite cyclists (117). The cyclists performed two intermittent protocols that included either a 40:20-second or a 30:30-second work-to-rest interval to exhaustion at a fixed work rate. The 40:20-second work-to-rest ratio resulted in significantly reduced total work and time to exhaustion while producing higher metabolic values ($\dot{V}O_2$max, lactate concentration, ETC). In contrast, the 30:30-second work-to-rest ratio provided sustained but slightly lower metabolic values for a considerably longer period of time. Another study manipulated the work variable via intensity and duration of the work-to-rest ratios. Wakefield and Glaister (152) reported a greater amount of time above 95% $\dot{V}O_2$max during running at an intensity of 105% of $\dot{V}O_2$max rather than 115% of $\dot{V}O_2$max with a work duration of 30 seconds rather than 20 and 25 seconds (rest = 20 seconds). When one is determining the proper work-to-rest ratio for athletes, knowledge of the time intervals, intensity of work, and recovery periods for each of the energy systems is critical to maximizing the amount of work that can be accomplished for a given exercise intensity. For example, after a bout of maximal exercise that depletes CP stores, the complete resynthesis of CP may take up to 8 minutes (75), which suggests that short-duration, high-intensity exercise requires greater work-to-rest ratios due to the aerobic mechanisms that replete phosphagen stores (75).

In contrast, as the goals of training change to longer-duration, lower-intensity tasks, the durations of the work intervals can be longer; this will lengthen the rest periods and decrease the work-to-rest ratios. Table 3.6 provides some general guidelines for work-to-rest ratios that are designed to emphasize the development of specific energy systems based on the theoretical time course for metabolic system involvement and substrate recovery. However, it should be noted that more research is necessary to provide evidence-based recommendations for optimal work-to-rest ratios.

High-Intensity Interval Training

High-intensity interval training (HIIT) involves brief repeated bouts of high-intensity exercise with intermittent recovery periods. High-intensity interval training typically incorporates either running- or cycling-based modes of exercise and is an efficient exercise regimen for eliciting cardiopulmonary (23) and metabolic and neuromuscular (24) adaptations. In fact, Buchheit and

Laursen (23) stated that HIIT "is today considered one of the most effective forms of exercise for improving physical performance in athletes" (p. 314). High-intensity interval training is often discussed in terms of duty cycles involving a high-intensity work phase followed by a lower-intensity recovery phase. It has been suggested that nine different HIIT variables can be manipulated to achieve the most precise metabolic specificity (23), including

- intensity of the active portion of each duty cycle,
- duration of the active portion of each duty cycle,
- intensity of the recovery portion of each duty cycle,
- duration of the recovery portion of each duty cycle,
- number of duty cycles performed in each set,
- number of sets,
- rest time between sets,
- recovery intensity between sets, and
- mode of exercise for HIIT.

The authors (24) indicate, however, that the intensities and durations of the active and recovery portions of each duty cycle are the most important factors to consider. To optimize HIIT training adaptations for athletes, HIIT sessions should maximize the time spent at or near $\dot{V}O_2$max. More specifically, the cumulative duration and intensity of the active portions of the duty cycles should equate to several minutes above 90% of $\dot{V}O_2$max (24).

The benefits of a HIIT protocol designed to repeatedly elicit a very high percentage of $\dot{V}O_2$max are primarily the result of the concurrent recruitment of large motor units and near-maximal cardiac output (6). Thus, HIIT provides a stimulus for both oxidative muscle fiber adaptation and myocardial hypertrophy. Additional HIIT adaptations include increases in $\dot{V}O_2$max, proton buffering, glycogen content, anaerobic thresholds, time to exhaustion, and time-trial performance. For example, Gibala and coworkers (63) reported equivalent improvements in muscle buffering capacity and glycogen content for HIIT at 250% of $\dot{V}O_2$peak during four

TABLE 3.6 Using Interval Training to Train Specific Energy Systems

% of maximum power	Primary system stressed	Typical exercise time	Range of work-to-rest period ratios
90-100	Phosphagen	5-10 s	1:12 to 1:20
75-90	Fast glycolysis	15-30 s	1:3 to 1:5
30-75	Fast glycolysis and oxidative	1-3 min	1:3 to 1:4
20-30	Oxidative	>3 min	1:1 to 1:3

to six 30-second cycling sprints compared to continuous cycling for 90 to 120 minutes at 65% of $\dot{V}O_2$peak over six total training sessions. In addition, 750 kJ cycling time trials decreased in both groups by 10.1% and 7.5% in the HIIT and long, slow endurance training groups, respectively. Thus, HIIT provided performance and physiological adaptations equivalent to those of long, slow endurance training, but in a time-efficient manner.

The strength and conditioning professional should consider a number of factors when designing a HIIT program. For example, a 400 m sprinter would need a HIIT program geared toward anaerobic-based durations and intensities more than a 2-mile (3,200 m) runner. Other considerations for the desired training adaptations are periodization, similar to that for resistance training, and the number of exercise sessions per day and week. Periodization allows for the general development of aerobic and anaerobic systems during the preseason with transitioning to sport-specific HIIT sessions during the competitive season. In addition, HIIT sessions in conjunction with other training sessions (i.e., team practices) may result in greater stress and risk for injury as a result of overtraining. Therefore, careful consideration is warranted in determining the appropriate number of HIIT sessions when concurrent with other sport-related activities.

Combination Training

Some suggest that aerobic endurance training should be added to the training of anaerobic athletes (a process that can be termed **combination training** or cross-training) to enhance recovery, because it is postulated that recovery relies primarily on aerobic mechanisms. Several studies have demonstrated that recovery in power output is related to endurance fitness (14, 15, 74). Bogdanis and colleagues (14) reported relationships in power recovery in the first 10 seconds of a cycling sprint, the resynthesis of PCr, and endurance fitness ($\dot{V}O_2$max). However, aerobic endurance training may reduce anaerobic performance capabilities, particularly for high-strength, high-power performance (80). Aerobic endurance training has been shown to reduce anaerobic energy production capabilities in rats (151). Additionally, combined anaerobic and aerobic endurance training can reduce the gain in muscle girth (36, 126), maximum strength (36, 76, 126), and speed- and power-related performance (44, 73).

Even though the exact mechanism for this phenomenon is not known, it has been suggested that combination training may increase training volume to a level that may result in overtraining in comparison to aerobic and anaerobic training alone. Hickson and colleagues

(82) provide evidence that combination training that includes progressive endurance running and cycling and resistance training may produce a plateau effect and, ultimately, a decrease in strength gains. Specifically, it was reported that heavy resistance training combined with an endurance program provided significant improvements in squat strength during the first seven weeks of the program, followed by a plateau period (two weeks) and then a decrease in squat strength during the remaining weeks of the program (two weeks). The results provided evidence that the upper limits of strength may be inhibited with progressive endurance training such as running and cycling. Other mechanisms that have been suggested to hinder the development of strength when in combination with endurance training are (a) decreasing rapid voluntary activation, (b) chronically lower muscle glycogen levels that can limit intracellular signaling responses during resistance training, and (c) and fiber type transition to slow-twitch fibers (112).

On the other hand, some studies and reviews indicate that the opposite holds true; these suggest that anaerobic training (strength training) can improve low- and high-intensity exercise endurance (54, 81, 82, 134). Sedano and colleagues (134) reported improvements in performance of highly trained runners as a result of concurrent endurance, resistance, and plyometric training. There was no reduction in $\dot{V}O_2$max over the 12 weeks in runners who participated in resistance and plyometric training. Furthermore, the combination training improved performance measures such as maximal strength, peak running velocity, and 3 km time trial compared to endurance training alone. Thus in highly trained runners it would appear that strength training would improve performance while not hindering metabolic parameters ($\dot{V}O_2$max).

Although oxidative metabolism is important for increased postexercise $\dot{V}O_2$, lactate removal, and PCr restoration from heavy anaerobic exercise (e.g., resistance training and sprint training) (133), care must be used in prescribing aerobic endurance training for anaerobic sports. In this context, it should be noted that specific anaerobic training can stimulate increases in aerobic power and enhance markers of recovery (54). Thus, it appears that extensive aerobic endurance training to enhance recovery from anaerobic events is not necessary and may be counterproductive in most strength and power sports.

Conclusion

Training programs with increased productivity can be designed through an understanding of how energy is produced during various types of exercise and how energy production can be modified by specific training regimens. Which energy system is used to supply energy for muscular contraction is determined primarily by the intensity of exercise and secondarily by the duration of exercise. Metabolic responses and training adaptations are largely regulated by exercise characteristics (e.g., intensity, duration, and recovery intervals). How these responses and adaptations occur following physical activity forms the basis for metabolic specificity of exercise and training. This principle allows for enhanced athletic performance through the implementation of improved training programs.

KEY TERMS

adenosine diphosphate (ADP)
adenosine monophosphate (AMP)
adenosine triphosphatase (ATPase)
adenosine triphosphate (ATP)
adenylate kinase reaction
aerobic
aerobic glycolysis
allosteric activation
allosteric inhibition
anabolism
anaerobic
anaerobic glycolysis
beta oxidation
bioenergetics
branched-chain amino acid
calcium ATPase
catabolism
combination training
Cori cycle
creatine kinase
creatine phosphate (CP)
cytochrome
depletion
electron transport chain (ETC)
endergonic reaction
energy

energy substrate
excess postexercise oxygen consumption (EPOC)
exergonic reaction
fast glycolysis
flavin adenine dinucleotide (FADH$_2$)
gluconeogenesis
glycogenolysis
glycolysis
glycolytic
high-intensity interval training (HIIT)
hydrolysis
inorganic phosphate
interval training
Krebs cycle
lactate
lactate threshold (LT)
lactic acid
law of mass action
mass action effect
metabolic acidosis
metabolic specificity
metabolism

mitochondria
myokinase reaction
myosin ATPase
near-equilibrium reactions
nicotinamide adenine dinucleotide (NADH)
onset of blood lactate accumulation (OBLA)
oxidative phosphorylation
oxidative system
oxygen debt
oxygen deficit
oxygen uptake
phosphagen system
phosphocreatine (PCr)
phosphofructokinase (PFK)
phosphorylation
pyruvate
rate-limiting step
repletion
slow glycolysis
sodium-potassium ATPase
substrate-level phosphorylation
wet muscle
work-to-rest ratio

1. Which of the following substances can be metabolized anaerobically?
   a. glycerol
   b. glucose
   c. amino acids
   d. free fatty acids

2. Which of the following reactions is the primary cause of metabolic acidosis (i.e., the decrease in intramuscular pH during high-intensity, fatiguing exercise)?
   a. $ATP \rightarrow ADP + P_i + H^+$
   b. $pyruvate + NADH \rightarrow lactate + NAD^+$
   c. $ADP + creatine\ phosphate \rightarrow ATP + creatine$
   d. $fructose\text{-}6\text{-}phosphate \rightarrow fructose\text{-}1,6\text{-}bisphosphate$

3. Which of the following energy systems produces ATP at the quickest rate?
   a. phosphagen
   b. aerobic glycolysis
   c. fat oxidation
   d. fast glycolysis

4. Approximately how many net ATP are produced via the oxidative energy system from the metabolism of one glucose molecule?
   a. 27
   b. 34
   c. 38
   d. 41

5. Which of the following energy substrates cannot be depleted during extreme exercise intensities or durations?
   a. creatine phosphate
   b. glycogen
   c. water
   d. ATP

CHAPTER 4

Endocrine Responses to Resistance Exercise

William J. Kraemer, PhD, Jakob L. Vingren, PhD, and Barry A. Spiering, PhD

 After completing this chapter, you will be able to

- understand basic concepts of endocrinology, including what hormones are and how they interact with each other and target tissues;
- explain the physiological roles of anabolic hormones;
- describe hormonal responses to resistance exercise; and
- develop training programs that demonstrate an understanding of human endocrine responses.

The endocrine system supports the normal homeostatic function of the body and helps it respond to external stimuli. It is part of a complex signaling system in the human body to effect changes and support exercise demands and recovery. The importance of the endocrine system in the field of strength and conditioning is reflected by the critical role this system played in the theoretical development of periodization of training (43). Hans Selye, a Canadian endocrinologist, unknowingly provided the theoretical basis for periodization with his work on the adrenal gland and the role of stress hormones in the adaptation to stress, distress, and illness.

Former Eastern Bloc sport scientists and physicians found similarities between the pattern of the training responses in athletes and the stress patterns observed by Selye. Hans Selye coined the term **General Adaptation Syndrome** to refer to how the adrenal gland responds to a noxious stimulus (stressor) (164, 165). This response begins with an initial alarm reaction that includes a reduction of function but is followed by an increase in resistance to the stress above the previous baseline function. This increase in resistance to the stress is referred to as *adaptation*; when the stressor is exercise, it is called *training adaptation*. The key to continued beneficial adaptation to the stress is the timely removal of the stimulus (e.g., exercise) so that function can recover, and then reapplication of an often-increased stress (progressive overload).

It is important for strength and conditioning professionals to have a basic understanding of the hormonal responses to resistance exercise. Hormonal signals play roles in a variety of mechanisms from anabolic (to build) to permissive (to allow) and catabolic (to break down). It is important to understand that the changes in the circulatory responses in the blood are but one observable change that some resistance training programs produce due to the metabolic challenges. One can also see anabolic responses with heavy programs that upregulate androgen receptors to use available anabolic hormones without any change in the blood concentrations (e.g., two or three sets with 1-repetition maximum [1RM] intensity and 5 to 7 minutes of rest between sets); and while endocrine signals are involved with signaling, the changes in the circulatory blood concentrations are much more subtle and must be observed at the level of the receptor. Gaining such insights and knowledge into how the endocrine system interacts with an exercise prescription can enable strength and conditioning professionals to better understand the details of how hormones help to mediate optimal adaptations to resistance training (93, 96). Although resistance training is the only natural stimulus that causes dramatic increases in lean tissue mass (i.e., muscle hypertrophy), significant differences in resistance training programs' ability to produce increases in muscle and connective tissue size

exist (44, 128, 189). The selection from among the acute program variables (intensity, sets, order of exercise, rest period duration, and exercise selection) for a resistance exercise session dictates in large part the appearance and magnitude of hormonal responses (105, 113-115, 117, 166, 169, 189). Importantly, tissue adaptations are influenced by the changes in circulating hormonal concentrations following exercise (10, 12, 14, 47, 62, 98, 171), and manipulating the endocrine system naturally through the proper selection for each acute program variable can enhance the development of target tissues and improve performance (78, 158). Thus, understanding this natural anabolic activity that occurs in the athlete's body during and following exercise is fundamental to successful recovery, adaptation, program design, training progression, and ultimately athletic performance (42-44, 93, 94, 101, 103).

Synthesis, Storage, and Secretion of Hormones

Hormones are chemical messengers or signal molecules that are synthesized, stored, and released into the blood by **endocrine glands**—body structures specialized for this function—and certain other cells (figure 4.1, table 4.1). Similarly, neurons synthesize, store, and secrete

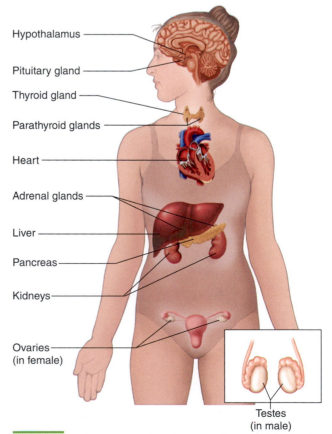

Hypothalamus

Pituitary gland

Thyroid gland

Parathyroid glands

Heart

Adrenal glands

Liver

Pancreas

Kidneys

Ovaries (in female)

Testes (in male)

FIGURE 4.1   The principal endocrine glands of the body along with other glands that secrete hormones.

TABLE 4.1   Endocrine Glands and Selected Hormones

Endocrine gland	Hormone	Selected physiological actions
Anterior pituitary gland	Growth hormone(s)	Stimulates insulin-like growth factor I secretion from the liver, protein synthesis, growth, and metabolism; other aggregates of the growth hormone (GH) also have biological function and make up the more complex super family of GH.
	Adrenocorticotropic hormone	Stimulates glucocorticoid secretion from the adrenal cortex
	Beta-endorphin	Stimulates analgesia
	Thyroid-stimulating hormone	Stimulates thyroid hormone secretion from the thyroid gland
	Follicle-stimulating hormone	Stimulates growth of follicles in ovary and seminiferous tubules in testes; stimulates ovum and sperm production
	Luteinizing hormone	Stimulates ovulation as well as secretion of sex hormones in the gonads (ovaries and testes)
	Prolactin	Stimulates milk production in mammary glands; maintains corpora lutea and secretion of progesterone
Posterior pituitary gland	Antidiuretic hormone	Increases contraction of smooth muscle and reabsorption of water by kidneys
	Oxytocin	Stimulates uterine contractions and release of milk by mammary glands
Thyroid gland	Thyroxine	Stimulates oxidative metabolism in mitochondria and cell growth
	Calcitonin	Reduces calcium phosphate levels in blood
Parathyroid glands	Parathyroid hormone	Increases blood calcium; decreases blood phosphate; stimulates bone formation
Pancreas	Insulin	Reduces blood glucose concentrations via promotion of glucose uptake by cells; promotes glycogen storage; suppresses fat oxidation and gluconeogenesis; is involved in protein synthesis
	Glucagon	Increases blood glucose levels
Adrenal cortex	Glucocorticoids (cortisol, cortisone, and so on)	Catabolic and anti-anabolic: promote protein breakdown and inhibit amino acid incorporation into proteins; conserve blood glucose concentrations via stimulation of conversion of proteins into carbohydrates (gluconeogenesis); suppress immune cell function; promote fat oxidation
	Mineralocorticoids (aldosterone, deoxycorticosterone, and so on)	Increase body fluids via sodium–potassium retention
Liver	Insulin-like growth factors	Increase protein synthesis in cells
Adrenal medulla	Epinephrine	Increases cardiac output; increases blood sugar and glycogen breakdown and fat metabolism
	Norepinephrine	Has properties of epinephrine; also constricts blood vessels
	Proenkephalin fragments (e.g., peptide F)	Enhance immune cell function, have analgesia effects
Ovaries	Estradiol	Stimulate development of female sex characteristics
	Progesterone	Stimulates development of female sex characteristics and mammary glands; maintains pregnancy
Testes	Testosterone	Anabolic and anticatabolic: promotes amino acid incorporation into proteins and inhibits protein breakdown; stimulates growth and development and maintenance of male sex characteristics
Heart (atrium)	Atrial peptide	Regulates sodium, potassium, and fluid volume
Kidney	Renin	Regulates kidney function, permeability, solute

neurotransmitters, which may have hormonal functions. The relatively new term **neuroendocrinology** refers to the study of the interactions between the nervous system and the endocrine system. Typically, endocrine glands are stimulated to release hormones by a chemical signal received by receptors on the gland or by direct neural stimulation. For example, the adrenal medulla (the internal part of the adrenal gland) releases the hormone epinephrine upon neural stimulation from the brain (91, 104, 112, 182). The adrenal cortex (the outer part of the adrenal gland) synthesizes and secretes the hormone cortisol after stimulation by another hormone, adrenocorticotropic hormone, released from the pituitary gland (110, 111, 116). Following stimulation, endocrine glands release hormones into the blood, which carries the hormones (and thereby the signal) to hormone-specific receptors located on the surface (peptide hormones) or in the cytosol (**steroid hormones** and **thyroid hormones**) of the **target tissue cells** (6-8, 11, 37, 61).

In addition to endocrine function via release into blood circulation, hormones can be secreted to function via intracrine, autocrine, and paracrine mechanisms. Intracrine and autocrine secretion of a hormone means that the cell releases the hormone to act upon the cell itself, via binding to intracellular and membrane receptors, respectively. It may be stimulated to do so via an external stimulus (e.g., another hormone), but the secreted hormone never enters the blood circulation. For example, insulin-like growth factor I (IGF-I) can be produced inside the muscle fiber when stimulated by mechanical force production or growth hormone(s) interactions with the muscle cell. Paracrine secretion of hormones involves the release of a hormone to interact with adjacent cells, without moving into the blood circulation. These mechanisms demonstrate the multiple roles that hormones can play in their interactions with a target cell.

A variety of binding proteins that carry hormones are found in the blood (6, 8). These many binding proteins carry both peptide hormones and steroid hormones. In a sense, these binding proteins act as storage sites within the circulation, help to fight degradation of the hormone, and extend its half-life. Most hormones are not active unless they are separated (free) from their specific binding protein. However, some hormone-binding proteins may actually have biological actions themselves. For instance, sex hormone–binding globulin (SHBG), the binding protein from testosterone and estrogen, can bind to specific membrane receptors and initiate activation of a cyclic adenosine monophosphate (cAMP) pathway (50). Thus, binding proteins, whether circulating in the blood or bound to a cell receptor, are major players in endocrine function and regulation. The interactions of bound hormones with receptors are just beginning to become appreciated in the field of endocrinology, and recent research has suggested the existence of even more complex regulation of hormones and target tissues (135).

Many hormones affect multiple tissues in the body (1, 3, 82, 84-86). Testosterone or one of its derivatives, for example, interacts with almost every tissue in the body. In this chapter we focus on skeletal muscle tissue as the primary target of hormonal interactions; but many other tissues, such as bone, connective tissue, kidney, and liver, are just as important to the adaptive changes observed with resistance training. It must be remembered that the whole cascade of physiological events, including hormonal signaling, is a result of the activation of motor units to create movement (i.e., size principle). The demands and magnitude of any physiological response are related to this need created by activated motor units. The amount of muscle tissue activated by the exercise dictates which physiological system is needed and how involved it is to meet the homeostatic demands of force/power production during the exercise and for the demands of recovery. For example, heart rate will be much higher to support an 80% of 1 RM squat exercise performed for 3 sets of 10 repetitions with 2 minutes rest between sets than the same protocol done for bicep curls. While similar systems will be involved with both, exercise protocol differences will exist based on the amount of muscle tissue mass affected by the protocol. Hormonal systems are also involved with other target tissues and glands that were stressed in a particular workout, but again, their needs are also dictated by the specific neural recruitment demands and their involvement to support movement. Thus, a five-set 5RM workout has different demands than a one-set 25-RM workout in its motor unit activation and its need for physiological support and recovery.

Most hormones play multiple physiological roles. These roles include regulation of reproduction; maintenance of the internal environment (homeostasis); energy production, utilization, and storage; and growth and development. In addition, hormones interact with each other in complex ways. A particular hormone may function in either an independent or a dependent manner, depending on its role in a given physiological mechanism. Such complexity and flexibility allow the endocrine system to respond in the proper magnitude to a physiological challenge and to interact differently with various physiological systems or target tissues at the same time.

Muscle as the Target for Hormone Interactions

Hormonal mechanisms are a part of an integrated signaling system that mediates change in the metabolic and cellular processes of muscle as a result of resistance exercise and training. Muscle remodeling involves the disruption and damage of muscle fibers, an inflammatory response, degradation of damaged proteins, hormonal and other signal (e.g., growth factors, cytokines) interactions, and ultimately the synthesis of new proteins and their orderly incorporation into existing or new sarcomeres (2, 20). The inflammatory process involves the immune system and various immune cells (e.g., T and B cells), which are influenced by the endocrine system (51). The study of the connection between the neural, endocrine, and immune systems is called **neuroendocrine immunology**. This term demonstrates the interdependence of these systems and the integrative nature of the remodeling process in muscle. We cannot limit our thinking about biological processes to one system.

Hormones are intimately involved with protein synthesis and degradation mechanisms that are part of muscle adaptations to resistance exercise. The production of the contractile proteins, actin and myosin, as well as structural proteins (e.g., desmin and titin), and the ultimate incorporation of all these proteins into the sarcomere complete the process at the molecular level. A multitude of hormones—including **anabolic hormones** (hormones that promote tissue building) such as insulin, insulin-like growth factors (IGFs), testosterone, and growth hormone—all contribute to various aspects of this process. Thyroid hormones act as important permissive hormones that allow the actions of other hormones to take place. As another important action in the building of tissue, anabolic hormones also block the negative effects on protein metabolism of **catabolic hormones**, such as cortisol and progesterone, which can degrade cell proteins. The negative effects of cortisol on skeletal muscle can also be seen in its roles to inactivate immune cells or block other signaling pathways such as the Akt/mechanistic target of rapamycin (mTOR) pathway involved in mRNA translation initiation. The interrelatedness of hormones, muscle fibers, and the subsequent changes in functional capabilities of muscle fibers provides the basis for the adaptive influence of hormones in hypertrophy. Yet again, the effect of hormones represents only one of the possible mechanisms for skeletal muscle adaptation to resistance training.

Role of Receptors in Mediating Hormonal Changes

The signal from a hormone (and thereby its biological effect) is relayed only to cells that express the receptor for that specific hormone. This ensures that the hormonal signal affects only the target tissue and not all cells in the body. Typically, the hormone is trying to influence cellular metabolism or affect DNA transcription in the nucleus (remember that muscle cells are multinucleated). Because many hormones cannot cross the cell membrane, their signal has to be transmitted throughout the cell via secondary messengers (often in the form of a cascade of reactions that ultimately interact and mediate the signal to the DNA machinery in the multiple nuclei of the muscle cell or single nuclei of typical cells). Receptors are generally either integrated into the cell membrane (polypeptide hormone receptors) or in the cytosol (steroid and thyroid hormone receptors). Every cell, from muscle fibers to immune cells to brain cells, has receptors to mediate the message or the signal from some hormone. One of the basic principles in endocrinology is that a given hormone interacts with a specific receptor. This principle is generally referred to as the **lock-and-key theory** (41) (in which the receptor is the lock and the hormone is the key; figure 4.2); however, it is now known that the hormone–receptor interaction is much more complex than this simple lock-and-key theory conveys. Although only one hormone has exactly the right characteristics to bind to and fully induce a signal via a specific receptor, in cases of **cross-reactivity** a given receptor partially interacts with other hormones (i.e., allosteric binding or blocking of the primary binding site). Similarly, receptors can have **allosteric binding sites** at which substances other than hormones can enhance or reduce the cellular response to the primary hormone. Finally, some hormones may need to be in an aggregated form (several hormones linked together) to produce the optimal signal via the receptor; this is believed to be the case for growth hormone, where one sees that the high molecular weight molecules do not have immune binding but do bind to bioactive receptors in the tibial line assay (65).

When an adaptation is no longer possible (e.g., the maximal amount of protein has been added to the muscle fiber) (54) or "overstimulation" by a hormone has occurred (e.g., insulin resistance), receptors can become less responsive or even nonresponsive to a specific hormone, preventing it from stimulating further actions in

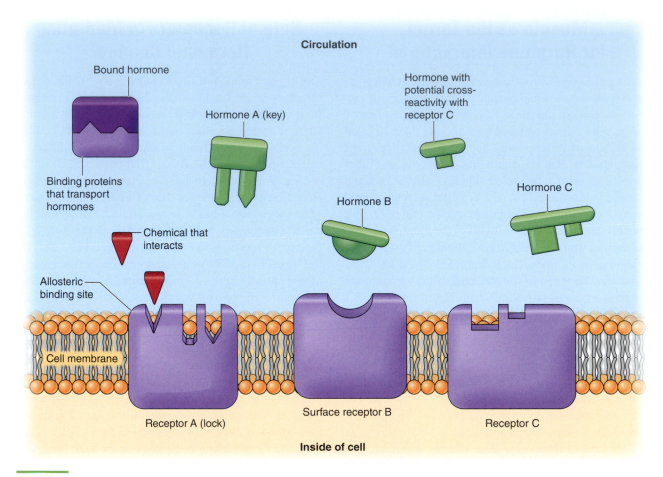

FIGURE 4.2   A schematic representation of the classic lock-and-key theory for hormonal action at the cell receptor level.

the cell. This inability of a hormone to interact with a receptor is called **downregulation** of receptor function. Receptors have the ability to increase or decrease their binding sensitivity, and the actual number of receptors present for binding can also be altered. Alterations in the receptor's binding characteristics or the number of receptors can be as dramatic an adaptation as the release of increased amounts of hormone from an endocrine gland. Obviously, if a receptor is not responsive to the hormone, little or no alteration in cell metabolism will result from that hormone. For example, it has been shown for the hormone testosterone that exercise training affects only the maximal number of receptors, not the binding sensitivity of the receptor (31). Scientists are just starting to study and understand the role that changes in receptors play in muscle adaptions to exercise training.

Categories of Hormones

In terms of molecular structure, there are three main categories of hormones: steroid, polypeptide (or simply peptide), and amine hormones. Each category of hormones interacts with muscle cells in different ways. In this chapter we focus primarily on the first two categories, as well as the most prominent amine hormones involved with exercise, the catecholamines.

Steroid Hormone Interactions

Steroid hormones, which include hormones from the adrenal cortex (e.g., cortisol) and the gonads (e.g., testosterone and estradiol), are fat soluble and passively diffuse across the cell membrane, although possible transport mechanisms have been described. The basic series of events leading to the biological effect is the same for any steroid hormone. After diffusing across the sarcolemma, the hormone binds with its receptor to form a **hormone–receptor complex (H-RC)**, causing a conformational shift in the receptor and thus activating it. The H-RC then binds to another H-RC and moves to the nucleus, where it arrives at the DNA. The H-RC "opens" the double-stranded DNA in order to expose transcriptional units that code for the synthesis of specific proteins. The H-RC recognizes specific enhancers, or upstream regulatory elements of the specific gene promoted by the given hormone, and that specific part of the DNA is transcribed. The resultant messenger RNA

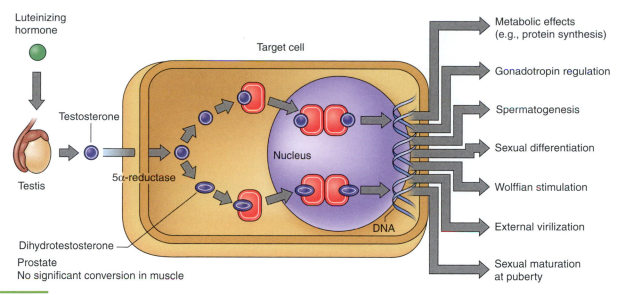

FIGURE 4.3 Typical steroid migration into a target cell by either testosterone in skeletal muscle or dihydrotestosterone in sex-linked tissues. Only one hormone pathway (testosterone or dihydrotestosterone) is targeted for one cell, but the two are shown together in this diagram. Each has different physiological outcomes.

(mRNA) then moves into the sarcoplasm of the cell, where it is translated by the ribosome into the specific protein promoted by the steroid hormone. Figure 4.3 shows a typical steroid hormone (testosterone) migrating into and through the cell. With its interaction at the genetic level of the cell, the action of the steroid hormone is completed (31, 155). However, the fact that mRNA is produced for a specific protein (e.g., actin) does not necessarily mean that that protein is produced by the ribosome and incorporated into the sarcomere. The hormone message to produce a specific mRNA is only the first part of the entire process of protein synthesis.

Polypeptide Hormone Interactions

Polypeptide hormones are made up of chains of amino acids; examples are growth hormone and insulin. Because polypeptide hormones are not fat soluble and thus cannot cross the cell membrane, **secondary messengers** inside the cell are activated by the conformational change in the receptor induced by hormone binding. In this way, the membrane receptors transmit the hormonal signal to the inside of the cell where it propagates through a cascade of signaling events inside the cell. In general, the signaling cascades initiated by polypeptide hormones affect metabolic processes, DNA transcription, or mRNA translation initiation at the ribosome. One of the signals from insulin, for example, induces a translocation of specific glucose transporters (GLUT4) from the cytosol to the cell membrane, allowing for increased glucose uptake (69). Figure 4.4 shows a typical polypeptide hormone interaction with the cell nucleus via the cytokine-activated Janus kinase (JAK)/

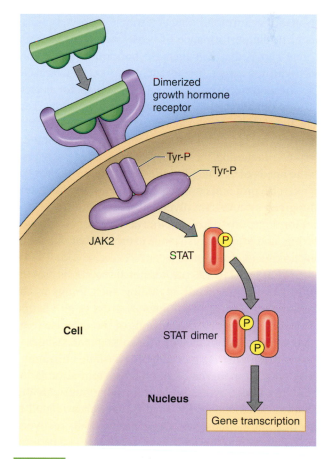

FIGURE 4.4 Typical polypeptide hormone (growth hormone in this example) interaction with a receptor via the cytokine-activated JAK/STAT signaling pathway. Although the hormone binds to an external receptor, a secondary messenger (STAT) is activated that can enter the cell nucleus. Tyr-P = tyrosinase-related protein.

signal transducer and activator of transcription (STAT) signaling pathway. The JAK/STAT pathway is used in many different interactions with various hormones and is a topic of continued investigation (21).

Amine Hormone Interactions

Amine hormones are synthesized from the amino acid tyrosine (e.g., epinephrine, norepinephrine, and dopamine) or tryptophan (e.g., serotonin). Similarly to peptide hormones, they bind to membrane receptors and act via secondary messengers. However, in contrast to peptide hormones, amine hormones are not regulated directly via negative feedback.

Heavy Resistance Exercise and Hormonal Increases

Long-term (months to years) consistent heavy resistance training brings about significant adaptive responses that result in enhanced size, strength, and power of trained musculature (71, 72, 92, 93, 102, 108, 119). The increase in anabolic hormone concentrations observed consequent to the performance of heavy resistance exercise is one signal that can increase hormonal interactions with various target tissues including skeletal muscle. On stimulation of a motor unit by the motor cortex, various signals (electrical, chemical, and hormonal) are sent from the brain and activated muscles to a number of endocrine glands. A key concept is that physiological systems, including the endocrine system, are sensitive to the needs of activated muscle, and therefore the type of exercise protocol conducted will determine the extent of a given system's involvement.

Hormones are secreted before (anticipatory response), during, and after the resistance exercise bout due to the physiological stress of resistance exercise (35, 38, 48, 53, 56, 73, 114-116). Acute hormonal secretions provide information to the body regarding such things as the amount and type of physiological stress (e.g., via epinephrine), the metabolic demands of the exercise (e.g., via insulin), and thus the need for subsequent changes in resting metabolism (e.g., change in substrate utilization). With specific patterns of nervous system stimulation from resistance exercise, certain hormonal changes occur simultaneously for specific purposes related to meeting the demands of the exercise bout, recovery, and adaptation to the acute exercise stress. The patterns of stress and hormonal responses combine to shape the tissues' adaptive response to a specific training program.

Hormonal increases in response to resistance exercise take place in a physiological environment that is unique to this type of exercise stress. The heavy external loads being lifted and resultant large muscle force requirement necessitate the activation of high-threshold motor units not typically stimulated by other types of exercise such as aerobic endurance exercise. Among the many different responses to this large force production stress are alterations in the sarcolemma's ability to import nutrients and in the sensitivity and number of hormone receptors in the muscle cells. As few as one or two heavy resistance exercise sessions can increase the number of androgen receptors, the receptor for testosterone, in the muscle (126, 192). In addition, local inflammatory processes related to tissue damage and repair mechanisms are activated by stress and run their time course with recovery (20). Combined, these alterations lead to muscle growth and strength increases in the intact muscle.

> ▶ **The specific force produced in activated fibers stimulates receptor and membrane sensitivities to anabolic factors, including hormones, which lead to muscle growth and strength changes.**

Following a resistance exercise session, remodeling of the muscle tissue takes place in the environment of hormonal secretions and other molecular signaling mechanisms that provide for anabolic actions. However, if the stress is too great, catabolic actions in the muscle may exceed anabolic actions as a result of, among other factors, the inability of anabolic hormones to bind to their receptors or the downregulation of receptors in the muscle tissue (31, 129). Thus, hormonal actions are important both during and after an exercise session to respond to the demands of the exercise stress (45-47). As noted before, the magnitude of the hormonal response (i.e., anabolic or catabolic) depends on the amount of tissue stimulated, the amount of tissue remodeling, and the amount of tissue repair required consequent to the exercise stress (51, 143). Thus, again, the characteristics of the exercise stimulus (i.e., selection among the acute program variables) are paramount to the hormonal response to the exercise protocol (94, 96).

Mechanisms of Hormonal Interactions

The mechanisms of hormonal interaction with muscle tissue depend on several factors. First, when exercise acutely increases the blood concentrations of hormones, the probability of interaction with receptors might be greater. However, if the physiological function to be affected is already close to a genetic maximum (i.e., with little adaptive potential left), the receptor is not as sensitive to the increased hormonal exposure. For example, a muscle cell that has already reached its maximum size with long-term training may not be sensitive to endogenous hormonal signals to stimulate further protein accretion. Similar receptor desensitization (decreased affinity) to a hormone can develop when resting hormone levels are chronically elevated due to disease (e.g., type 2 diabetes mellitus) or exogenous drug use. How and when this reduction in receptor sensitivity to hormonal increases occurs in human muscle has not been fully established; however, genetic predisposition ultimately limits increases in muscle size. Second, because adaptations to heavy resistance exercise typically are anabolic, the recovery mechanisms involved are related to increases in the size of muscle cells. Third, errors in exercise prescriptions can result in a greater catabolic effect or a lack of an anabolic effect (ineffective exercise program). As a result, hormonal mechanisms can adversely affect cellular development or minimally activate mechanisms that augment hypertrophy.

The combination of many different mechanisms is thought to stimulate exercise-induced hypertrophy, and molecular signaling including hormones is involved with this process. This signaling is influenced by neural factors that provide important signals to the skeletal muscle and thus can augment anabolic processes. For instance, neural activation of muscle fibers increases hormone binding affinity of receptors in muscle. The integration of the nervous system and the various hormonal mechanisms is different in trained and untrained people (73, 161). In addition, certain hormonal mechanisms for exercise-induced hypertrophy, such as those mediated by testosterone, are not fully operational in both sexes or at all ages (38, 100, 115). A wide array of hormonal mechanisms with differential effects (based on program design, training level, sex, age, genetic predisposition, and adaptation potential) provides myriad possible adaptation strategies for the maintenance or improvement of muscle size and strength (99).

Hormonal Changes in Peripheral Blood

We learn a lot about the physical stress of a workout on the human body by monitoring various measures, including the changes in hormone concentrations in the blood. This is just one biocompartment that can be monitored, and it must be viewed in the context of all of the other processes stimulating muscle and protein synthesis (e.g., neural factors, the branched-chain amino acid leucine). Hormone concentrations can be determined from blood samples drawn from athletes at various stages of exercise and training. One can also measure hormones in the fluid surrounding the muscle or within the muscle itself (151). Although interpretation of blood concentrations of hormones can be tricky, as this is only one part of the whole hormonal response puzzle, such data provide an indication of the status or responses of the glands or of the functional status of the mechanisms controlled by the hormone. It should be noted that peripheral concentrations of hormones in the blood do not indicate the status of the various receptor populations or the effects of a hormone within the cell. It is typically assumed, however, that large increases in hormone concentration indicate higher probabilities for interactions with receptors. There is little doubt that an increase in circulatory concentrations, in the absence of a plasma volume reduction, means that there was an increase in release from the endocrine glands. The physiological outcome from this increase now depends on the "status" of the receptor in the target tissue—that is, can the hormonal signal be realized in the cell by the binding to the receptor and the translation of the signal to the DNA machinery or other intracellular targets (e.g., mTOR pathway)? More difficult to interpret are decreases in hormonal concentrations that might indicate several possible fates for the hormone, including higher uptake into the target tissue receptors, greater degradation of the hormone, decreased secretion of the hormone, or some combination of these. In addition to these direct effects on hormones, many different physiological mechanisms contribute in varying degrees to the observed changes in peripheral blood concentrations of hormones with exercise, including circadian pattern, fluid volume shifts (exercise tends to push fluid from the blood to the intercellular compartment), tissue clearance rates (time spent in a tissue), venous pooling of blood, and hormone interactions with binding proteins (18, 24, 25, 89). These mechanisms interact to produce a certain concentration of a hormone in the blood, which influences the potential for interaction with the receptors in target tissue and their subsequent secondary effects, leading to the final effect of the hormone on a cell. Thus, when one is determining the specific effects of exercise on hormones, one must consider many different interpretations. An increase in hormonal concentrations in the blood is not a prerequisite for seeing gains in muscle size or strength but does represent an increased activation for hormonal release of the endocrine gland involved.

> Hormone responses are tightly linked to the characteristics of the resistance exercise protocol.

Adaptations in the Endocrine System

Although organs such as muscle and connective tissue are the ultimate targets of most resistance training programs, many adaptations occur within the endocrine system as well. In other words, when one trains muscles, endocrine glands are also being trained. As noted before, the involvement of any endocrine gland is dependent on how much support is needed by that gland's secretions to support the activated motor units. If one just does wrist curls for sets of 15, it is doubtful that any endocrine gland will be stimulated to increase release of hormones, as the normal homeostatic concentration of hormones going though circulation would be able to meet the needs of such a minor muscle group exercise. However, local receptors would be upregulated in the muscle tissue involved to meet the needs for the motor units used for that exercise. Adaptations are related to changes in the target organs and the toleration of exercise stress. The potential for adaptation in the endocrine system, with so many different sites and mechanisms that can be affected, is great. The following are examples of the potential types of adaptation that are possible:

- Amount of synthesis and storage of hormones
- Transport of hormones via binding proteins
- Time needed for the clearance of hormones through liver and other tissues
- Amount of hormonal degradation that takes place over a given period of time
- How much blood-to-tissue fluid shift occurs with exercise stress
- How tightly the hormone binds to its receptor (receptor affinity); this is an uncommon response to exercise training
- How many receptors are in the tissue
- The change in the content and in some cases the size of the secretory cells in the gland
- The magnitude of the signal sent to the cell nucleus by the H-RC or secondary messenger
- The degree of interaction with the cell nucleus (which dictates how much muscle protein to produce)

Hormones are secreted in response to a need for homeostatic control in the body; the endocrine system is part of an overall strategy to bring physiological functions back into normal range (60). These homeostatic mechanisms controlled by the endocrine system can be activated in response to an acute (immediate) resistance exercise stress or can be altered by chronic (over longer periods of time) resistance training (32, 55, 57, 64, 73, 81, 172, 173, 184). The mechanism that mediates acute homeostatic changes to acute resistance exercise stress is typically a sharp increase or decrease in hormonal concentrations to regulate a physiological variable, such as glucose level. A more subtle increase or decrease usually occurs in chronic resting hormonal concentrations in response to resistance training (172).

Primary Anabolic Hormones

The primary anabolic hormones involved in muscle tissue growth and remodeling are testosterone, growth hormone, and IGFs, which are discussed here, as well as insulin and the thyroid hormones, which are examined in greater detail in other sources (45-48, 60).

Testosterone

Testosterone is the primary androgen that interacts with skeletal muscle tissue; dihydrotestosterone is the primary androgen that interacts with sex-linked tissues (e.g., prostate in men). Although circulating testosterone concentration is important for the anabolic signal, it is the binding of testosterone to its receptor that is the key to stimulating anabolic functions. Therefore, an increase in circulating testosterone (free, bound, or both) concentration is not an absolute marker of this event. However, increased testosterone concentration does provide an indirect marker of motor unit activation and metabolic demands beyond hemostatic conditions and typically is associated with increased receptor binding. Heavy resistance training using one or two repetitions in low volume, which may not cause any changes in testosterone concentrations after a workout, could potentially still increase the absolute number of receptors and thus binding sites available to testosterone; however, this effect on receptors has yet to be fully elucidated (171, 188). Nevertheless, change in testosterone concentrations is a dramatic anabolic signal for target tissues throughout the body.

Circulating testosterone was proposed as a physiological marker for both men and women for evaluating the anabolic status of the body (70, 129). The hormonal control of testosterone release has been reviewed in detail (31, 61, 97, 106, 189). Testosterone has both direct and indirect effects on muscle tissue. It can promote growth hormone release from the pituitary, which can influence protein synthesis in muscle; and in turn growth hormone appears to have a permissive or synergistic effect on testosterone's promotion of protein synthesis (138). The potential interactions with other hormones and other signaling systems demonstrate the highly interdependent nature of the neuroendocrine–immune system in influencing the strength and size of skeletal muscles. The effects of testosterone on the development of strength and muscle size are also related to the influence of testosterone on the nervous system (12, 90). For example, testosterone can interact with receptors on neurons, increase the amounts of neurotransmitters, and influence structural protein changes. Each of these interactions can enhance the force production potential and mass of the innervated muscle.

Following secretion in the blood circulation from the testes in men and the ovaries and adrenal glands in women, testosterone is transported to target tissues by a binding protein (largely sex hormone–binding globulin and albumin). At the target tissue, testosterone disassociates from the binding protein and crosses the cell membrane in order to bind to the intracellular androgen receptor. Research studies have shown that testosterone also binds to cell membrane receptors. This binding allows a rapid intracellular effect of testosterone, such as calcium release, to occur (36, 186). The knowledge of hormone receptors and their cellular effects is rapidly growing, and the future promises to bring new discoveries that will further elucidate this content area.

Increases in peripheral blood concentrations of testosterone have been observed in men during and following many types of high-intensity aerobic endurance exercise (119) as well as resistance exercise (60). Although not a consistent finding, some data show small testosterone, especially for free testosterone, increases in women after resistance exercise (188). Variations in testosterone's cellular actions consequent to resistance exercise thus may be attributed to differences in the cell membrane, perhaps because of the forces placed on membranes with resistance exercise, or to different feedback mechanisms sending signals to the higher brain centers (e.g., higher levels of testosterone feeding back on the brain to decrease luteinizing hormone secretion). Furthermore, receptor interactions may be quite different under different exercise conditions due to the differential force on the membrane (31). High-intensity aerobic endurance exercise can cause a dramatic catabolic tissue response, and increases in testosterone may be related to the need for protein synthesis to keep up with protein loss (179, 180). Despite increased testosterone, hypertrophy does not typically take place with aerobic endurance training (119). In fact, oxidative stress may actually promote a decrease in muscle fiber size in order to optimize oxygen transport into the cell (119). Without the proper exercise stimulus, the cellular mechanisms that mediate muscle fiber growth are not activated to the extent that hypertrophy occurs.

In boys and younger men (<18 years), several factors appear to influence acute serum testosterone concentrations and might affect whether significant increases occur during or following exercise. Key among these factors is the onset of puberty. Since testosterone production in prepubescent boys is very low, these boys lack sufficient quantities to induce noteworthy hypertrophy. Independently or in various combinations, several

exercise variables can increase serum testosterone concentrations in boys and younger men (38, 57, 100, 115):

- Large muscle group exercises (e.g., deadlift, power clean, squats)
- Heavy resistance (85-95% of 1RM)
- Moderate to high volume of exercise, achieved with multiple sets, multiple exercises, or both
- Short rest intervals (30 seconds to 1 minute)
- Two years or more of resistance training experience

Increases in serum total testosterone in men are evident when blood is sampled before and immediately after exercise protocols that use very large muscle groups: deadlifts, for example, but not bench presses (38, 68, 74, 114, 190). When blood is sampled 4 or more hours after exercise and not immediately following it, other factors, such as **diurnal variations** (normal fluctuations in hormone levels throughout the day) or recovery phenomena, can affect the magnitude or direction of the acute stress response (32). Additionally, possible rebounds or decreases in testosterone blood values over time may reflect augmentation or depression of diurnal variations (103), making interpretation of late blood samples yet more difficult. Recent evidence demonstrates that acute resistance exercise does not appear to affect the diurnal changes in testosterone (122, 163). In men, testosterone concentrations are typically highest in the morning and drop with time through the day, but increases can occur at any point in the circadian pattern with exercise. However, the magnitude of change is smaller when resting concentrations are smaller, thus leading to lower absolute concentrations with exercise despite the fact that increases do occur. To date, time of day of strength training (e.g., morning or afternoon) has not been shown to have significant effects on the resting total testosterone concentrations, its diurnal pattern, or the absolute increase in maximum strength (163). Women have much lower concentrations of serum testosterone and little variation in concentrations during the day (although there are limited data to support the latter contention). However, the response of their androgen receptors is very dynamic with a much faster upregulation than in men, likely to better use the amount of testosterone present with a resistance exercise stimulus (188). Thus, an elevation in testosterone in the blood in women following resistance exercise might have an impact as it is

> **Large muscle group exercises using an adequate volume of total work result in acute increased total testosterone concentrations in men.**

more quickly responded to with receptor changes to use the newly available testosterone in the blood.

Free Testosterone and Sex Hormone–Binding Globulin

The acute exercise responses of free testosterone (testosterone not bound to a binding protein, such as sex hormone–binding globulin for transport) are beginning to be better understood. Free testosterone accounts for only 0.5% to 2% of total testosterone; thus higher total testosterone concentration allows for more free testosterone. Heavy resistance exercise (e.g., six sets of 10 repetitions at 80% of 1RM) can acutely increase free testosterone in men and women, although the increase is much smaller for women (188). For men, Kraemer and colleagues (120) showed that age appears to affect free testosterone responses to resistance exercise. In other words, younger (i.e., 30-year-old) men had higher concentrations of free testosterone after a workout than older (i.e., 62-year-old) men. This might indicate greater biological potential for testosterone to interact with the target tissues in younger men. The so-called free hormone hypothesis states that it is only the free hormone that interacts with target tissues. Nevertheless, the bound hormone could significantly influence the rate of hormone delivery to a target tissue, such as muscle, and this may be an advantage that younger men have over older men after a workout (34). That is, younger men have more absolute values for total testosterone and thus more free testosterone on a percentage value of total than older men.

The role, regulation, and interaction of binding proteins and their interactions with cells also present interesting possibilities for force production improvements, especially for women, whose total amount of testosterone is very low in comparison with that of men. Muscle

cell stimulation of growth keeps testosterone around longer in a bound state. In fact, the binding protein itself may act as a hormone with biological activity (159). The biological role of various binding proteins appears to be an important factor in tissue interactions (71, 72, 75, 159). Studies by Kvorning and colleagues (130, 131) have demonstrated that for younger men, testosterone is a major player in the anabolic responses to resistance training. When subjects were given luteinizing hormone blockers, which resulted in very low testosterone concentrations but did not affect other anabolic signaling systems, gains in muscle strength and lean tissue mass were reduced when compared to those of normally functioning men with normal testosterone concentrations. These classic studies demonstrate how important endogenous testosterone is in the adaptive mechanisms for resistance training adaptations.

Testosterone Responses in Women

Testosterone is the primary male sex hormone. Women have about 15- to 20-fold lower concentrations of circulating testosterone than men do. Most studies have not been able to demonstrate an acute increase in testosterone following a resistance exercise workout for women; data show that if increases do occur, they are relatively small (26, 38, 76, 81, 114, 190) and are sometimes observed only for free testosterone (188). Yet in younger women, a small but significant increase in serum testosterone in response to six sets of 10RM squats has been observed (144). In addition, Vingren and colleagues (188) observed acute increases in free testosterone in men and women who were trained in response to a heavy resistance exercise protocol, but the concentrations in women were dramatically lower than in men (see figure 4.5). The testosterone concentration can vary substantially between individual women, as

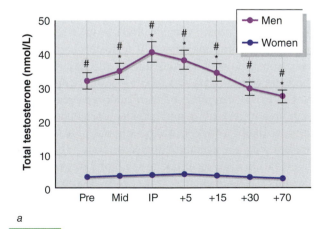

a

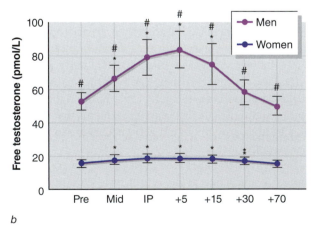

b

FIGURE 4.5 Responses of *(a)* total testosterone and *(b)* free testosterone in response to six sets of squats at 80% of 1RM with 2 minutes rest between sets. The midpoint (Mid) sample is after three sets; * indicates a significant increase from preexercise values; # indicates a significant difference from women at the corresponding time point.

some women secrete higher concentrations of adrenal androgens. In one report, changes were observed in baseline concentrations of testosterone in women who exercised regularly compared with inactive controls (26). Still, other studies have been unable to demonstrate changes in serum concentrations of testosterone with training (38, 76, 81, 114, 190). However, again, the use of testosterone by the upregulation of skeletal muscle androgen receptors in a rapid manner, in about an hour, shows the great sensitivity that women have to increases in testosterone and the importance of its use (188).

Training Adaptations of Testosterone

We are still learning about the responses of testosterone to resistance training (73, 119, 173, 188, 191). Importantly, one has to realize that testosterone increases in response to the demands of an exercise protocol; then the receptors either increase binding to use the elevated testosterone or they do not due to a lack of need for the signal to increase muscle-related metabolism. It may well be that other receptors on other target tissues (e.g., nervous, satellite cells) are more affected at certain time points in training depending on the window of adaptation available in the target tissues. So expecting increases in resting concentrations may be an outmoded concept; but one might expect an increase in the exercise-induced concentrations due to improved functional capacity and the ability to do more work in an exercise protocol. It appears that training time and experience may be very important factors in altering the resting and exercise-induced concentrations of this hormone. Its role in skeletal muscle might change, however, as upper limits of muscle cell size increases are achieved. In adult men, acute increases in testosterone are observed if the exercise stimulus is adequate (i.e., multiple sets, 5-10RM, adequate muscle mass used). In a classic study, Häkkinen and colleagues (73) demonstrated that over the course of two years of training, even in elite weightlifters, small increases in resting serum testosterone concentrations do occur, concomitant with increases in follicle-stimulating hormone and luteinizing hormone, which are involved in regulation of testosterone production and are released and secreted from the anterior pituitary in response to signals from the brain via the hypothalamus. Testosterone might have a role in nervous system development in long-term training by augmenting the neural adaptations that occur for strength gain in highly trained strength and power athletes (75, 76). Furthermore, some studies have shown greater resistance training adaptation when the training program sessions induced acutely elevated testosterone concentrations (78, 158).

Research on the effect of resistance exercise and training on the androgen receptor (the receptor for testosterone) is limited; however, recently several studies have been published underscoring the current interest in this topic (126, 156, 187, 188, 192). The findings vary, showing both increases and decreases in androgen receptor content; however, these differences might stem from variations in exercise protocols as well as the time point for tissue sampling. Despite these varying findings, it appears that resistance exercise and training ultimately increase the muscle androgen receptor content. With the increase in androgen receptor binding, the use of testosterone is enhanced. Additionally, nutritional intakes before a workout can cause upregulated skeletal muscle androgen content and are a reason why ingesting protein and some carbohydrate before a workout appears to be important (126).

Growth Hormone

There is a great amount of confusion about what GH is and what it is responsible for in the human body. Growth hormone in recent years has taken on a new complexity in both exercise and medicine. The primary hormone that arises from the DNA machinery is the 191 amino acid polypeptide (called a monomer with molecular weight of 22 kDa) that is produced in the somatotroph of the anterior pituitary gland: in two types of somatotrophs, band 1 (containing smaller molecular weight forms, e.g., 22 kDa) and band 2 (containing large molecular weight forms such as aggregates). Due to the advances of the radioimmunoassay in the 1960s and 1970s, the 22 kDa has been the primary form that has been assessed in the blood; this has blinded our view of what is going on with the other larger concentrations of aggregate forms until recent years. It is now clear that the world of pituitary GH endocrinology is much more complex than previously appreciated when only the 22 kDa variant was investigated. The blood is filled with GH splice variants and, more importantly, its many aggregates (i.e., multiple disulfide bonds linking together GH monomers) in different molecular weight combinations. Additionally, making the scenario more complex is the presence of two types of GH binding proteins that also make higher molecular weight forms (e.g., GH monomer bound with a GH binding protein). At present, scientists are just starting to unravel the complex regulatory roles this superfamily plays. Interestingly, there is a much higher concentration of bioactive GH (i.e., aggregates) when compared to just the 22 kDa GH monomer. This leads one to believe that we have gotten only a small glimpse of what GHs are doing in the body. Demonstrating that we are not completely clear as to the physiological role of the 22 kDa monomer, in medicine it has been implicated in cancer involving its interactions with liver IGF-I release (154). Thus, the aggregate forms of GH might be the important biologically functional relevant GH involved in adaptation to exercise (128).

Again, the majority of studies in exercise endocrinology have examined the 22 kDa isoform due to the ease and popularity of immunoassays (often termed radioimmunoassay [RIA], enzyme-linked immunosorbent assay [ELISA], or enzyme immunoassay [EIA]). These techniques depend on antibody interactions to determine the amount present in the blood. The antibodies used are generally specific to the 22 kDa GH variant, and thus many other forms remain undetected or underdetected with such assay techniques. Nevertheless, the current model for the regulation and targets of various forms of GH is as shown in figure 4.6. The multitude of physiological mechanisms and target tissues that have been linked to GH mediation have indicated for some time a need for a superfamily of hormones to achieve such diversity of effects.

Growth hormone is important for the normal development of a child, but it also appears to play a vital role in adapting to the stress of resistance training. A study by McCall and colleagues (139) found a positive correlation between GH responses and muscle fiber hypertrophy following 20 weeks of resistance training, yet it is possible that other GH variants followed a pattern of increase similar to that of the 22 kDa form and could also explain the relationship. This highlights the problems with using simple regression to determine a hormone's effects; and since "cause and effect" is not dictated by simple regression, great caution is needed with such interpretations for any hormone. The target tissues for GH are highly variable, and different molecular weight variants have different target tissues, which include bone, immune cells, skeletal muscle, fat cells, and liver tissue. The main physiological roles of GH and its superfamily are the following (albeit clarity is lacking as to which molecular form of the GH superfamily is directly responsible for the given role):

- Decreases glucose utilization
- Decreases glycogen synthesis
- Increases amino acid transport across cell membranes
- Increases protein synthesis
- Increases utilization of fatty acids
- Increases lipolysis (fat breakdown)
- Increases availability of glucose and amino acids
- Increases collagen synthesis
- Stimulates cartilage growth
- Increases retention of nitrogen, sodium, potassium, and phosphorus
- Increases renal plasma flow and filtration
- Promotes compensatory renal hypertrophy
- Enhances immune cell function

The secretion of GHs is regulated by a complex system of neuroendocrine feedback mechanisms (23, 39, 128, 136, 157, 170, 193). Many of the hormone's actions might be mediated by a secondary set of hormones or even be the result of other GH forms, but GH in its many forms interacts directly with target tissues. The 22 kDa GH form both stimulates the release of IGFs at the autocrine level of the cell, contributing to the overall changes in IGFs in the body, and increases the availability of amino acids for protein synthesis. This results in conditions that promote tissue repair in general and perhaps in recovery following resistance exercise. Insulin-like growth factor may be released from nonhepatic tissues (e.g., fat, white blood cells), including muscle itself, which may not produce as much endogenous IGF as other body tissues (28, 45, 77). Nevertheless, GH plays a crucial role in direct cellular interactions as one of the most potent anabolic hormones (139). The secretion of the 22 kDa GH, and thus the amount in the blood, varies according to time of day, with the highest levels observed at night during sleep (40, 98, 170). However, the higher amounts of bioactive GH have not been shown to have a circadian pattern. The 22 kDa form of release of GH is pulsatile, or burst-like; these pulses also have different amplitudes throughout the day, and exercise appears to increase their amplitude and number. It has been hypothesized that nocturnal increases are involved in various tissue repair mechanisms in the body. Thus, it is possible that GH secretion and release may directly

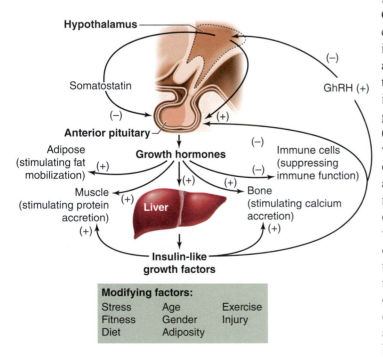

FIGURE 4.6   Diagram of growth hormone cybernetics and interactions.

influence adaptations of the contractile unit of muscle and subsequent expression of strength (139). Various external factors, such as age, male versus female sex, sleep, nutrition, alcohol consumption, and exercise, all alter GH release patterns (16, 17, 19, 152, 185). Growth hormone is released into the peripheral circulation, where it attaches to specific binding proteins, which represent the extracellular domain of the GH receptor. In general, GH acts by binding to plasma membrane–bound receptors on the target cells. The interactions with bioactive GH or its aggregates and splice variants remain a topic of current research as we now look at GH as having more than one molecular form (65, 125, 181).

Growth Hormone Responses to Stress

Pituitary hormones (e.g., proopiomelanocortin [POMC], GHs, and prolactin) respond to a variety of exercise stressors, including resistance exercise (26, 29, 56, 60, 113, 116, 132, 134). Growth hormone (22 kDa) concentrations increase in response to breath holding and hyperventilation alone (33), as well as to hypoxia (177). It appears that a substantial stimulus for 22 kDa GH release is increased hydrogen ion (drop in pH) and lactate concentrations (64). Not all resistance exercise protocols demonstrate increased serum GH concentration. Vanhelder and colleagues (184) observed that when a light load (28% of 7RM) was used with a high number of repetitions in each set, no changes in the serum concentration of the 22 kDa GH occurred. It appears that an intensity threshold must be reached in order to elicit a significant 22 kDa GH response to resistance exercise, especially when longer rest periods (>3 minutes) are used (113). This may be due to the metabolic connection with glycolytic metabolism (at least for the 22 kDa variant).

Depending on the load, rest, exercise volume, and exercise selection of a resistance exercise protocol, different 22 kDa GH responses occur (5, 43, 44, 139, 143, 166, 167, 174). In a study designed to determine the different variables related to GH increases, Kraemer and colleagues (113) found that serum increases in the 22 kDa GH are differentially sensitive to the volume of exercise, the amount of rest between sets (less rest, higher 22 kDa GH), and the resistance used (10RM produces higher lactate values and higher 22 kDa GH responses). When the intensity used was 10RM (heavy resistance) with three sets of each exercise (high total work, approximately 60,000 J) and short (1-minute) rest periods, large increases were observed in serum 22 kDa GH concentrations. The most dramatic increases occurred in response to a 1-minute rest period when the duration of exercise was longer (10RM vs. 5RM). Because such differences are related to the configuration of the exercise session (e.g., rest period length), it appears that greater attention needs to be given to pro-

gram design variables when physiological adaptations to resistance training are being evaluated.

> **Growth hormone release is affected by the type of resistance training protocol used including the duration of rest period. Short rest period types of workouts result in greater serum concentrations compared to long rest protocols of similar total work; however, at present it is not clear how the various molecular forms (e.g., aggregates and splice variants) or types of GH are affected by rest period duration.**

Growth Hormone Responses in Women

Throughout the menstrual cycle, women have higher blood concentrations of the 22 kDa GH than men due to greater frequency and amplitude of secretion. Hormone concentrations and hormone responses to exercise vary with menstrual phase (29), although the mechanisms of this variation are unclear. Kraemer and colleagues (114, 117) found that during the early follicular phase of the menstrual cycle, women had significantly higher 22 kDa GH concentrations at rest compared with men. Furthermore, with use of a heavy resistance exercise protocol characterized by long rest periods (3 minutes) and heavy loads (5RM), 22 kDa GH concentrations did not increase above resting concentrations. However, when a short-rest (1 minute) and moderate-resistance (10RM) exercise protocol was used, significant increases in serum 22 kDa GH values were observed. Hormonal response patterns to different resistance exercise routines may vary over the course of the menstrual cycle owing to alterations in resting levels (114, 117); furthermore, the use of hormonal contraception (e.g., estrogen-containing birth control pills) appears to increase the 22 kDa GH response to resistance exercise (127). However, the response patterns of men and women to the same resistance exercise protocol are similar when workouts (e.g., short rest results in a higher 22 kDa GH elevation compared to long rest period workouts) are compared (114).

Studies show that the bioactive GH is also made of many different molecular sizes based on what molecular sizes bind together (e.g., two monomers bound together results in a dimer or a 44 kDa form, and so on as GH monomers are added together) (128). Interestingly, in women, bioactive GH has been shown to be altered by resistance training. It appears that the resting concentrations are increased while little change occurs in the 22 kDa form (125). In addition, concentrations of bioactive GH are not as high in older women as in younger women, and resistance exercise is a more potent stimulus to bioactive GH than endurance exercise (65). Initial research showed that contraceptives also have minimal effects on bioactive GH forms. Furthermore, higher concentrations of bioactive GH are observed in women who have greater strength, also suggesting the importance of the higher aggregated forms of GH (123). These new insights on the GH hormone again demonstrate the potential complexity of the endocrine system and show that we have much more to learn about these important signals to tissues.

The effects of periodizing resistance training over the course of the menstrual cycle remain to be examined, and more research is needed to elucidate any sex-related neuroendocrine adaptation mechanism (43). At present, women's reduced concentrations of testosterone and different resting hormonal concentrations over the course of the menstrual cycle appear to be their most striking neuroendocrine differences from men.

Training Adaptations of Growth Hormone

It appears that GH concentrations need to be measured over longer time periods (2-24 hours) to show whether changes occur with resistance training. The area under the time curve, which includes an array of pulsatile effects, tells whether changes in release have occurred. The responses of GH to resistance training have not been extensively studied, but observations of normal, single measurements of resting 22 kDa GH concentrations in elite lifters suggest little change. It is likely that differences in feedback mechanisms, changes in receptor sensitivities, IGF potentiation, diurnal variations, and maximal exercise concentrations may mediate GH adaptations with resistance training. The typical trends for training-related changes in GH appear to be a reduction in 22 kDa GH response to an absolute exercise stress and alterations in 22 kDa GH pulsatility characteristics. The reduction in the 22 kDa GH exercise-induced responses with training perhaps indicates potential interactions with other molecular weight forms. Individual responses over a nine-month period were highly variable, with no significant group changes over time in a group of elite weightlifters (unpublished observations). This likely means that higher amounts of aggregate GH were being produced; the 22 kDa form is becoming less important as the study of the pituitary gland continues due to the majority of GH being held in aggregate or bound form. This is a hot area of current and future research. As already noted, initial data indicate that resting concentrations and some molecular weight forms of GH are also influenced by long-term resistance training in women (125). At present it would appear that the exercise-induced responses of the 22 kDa GH are what change with training with little change in the resting concentrations, except for small menstrual phase increases and decreases. For the bioactive GH

in contrast to the 22 kDa monomere GH form, it is the resting concentrations that may see the most changes with subtle alterations in some bioactive fractions of higher than 22 kDa molecular weight (125). Still, we are far from understanding how GH changes with long-term resistance training.

Insulin-Like Growth Factors

Some of the effects of 22 kDa GH are mediated through small polypeptides called *insulin-like growth factors (IGFs)* or *somatomedins* (27, 37, 45). It has been postulated that an IGF superfamily might be important as a biomarker for health and performance (145, 150). Insulin-like growth factor I is a 70 amino acid polypeptide, and IGF-II is a 67 amino acid polypeptide; the function of the latter is less clear. Again, a superfamily of peptides exists along with binding proteins. The liver secretes IGFs after 22 kDa GH stimulates liver cells to synthesize IGFs. Besides GH, factors such as thyroid hormone and testosterone are also involved in the regulation of IGF synthesis (193-196). Typical of many polypeptide hormones, both growth factors are synthesized as larger precursor molecules, which then undergo processing to form the other variants of the active hormones themselves. Insulin-like growth factors travel in the blood bound to binding proteins; in the target tissue, IGFs disassociate from the binding protein and interact with the receptors (1, 175, 176). Blood levels of IGFs are usually measured as either total levels (bound plus free) or free IGF concentrations.

At least six different circulating binding proteins that regulate the amount of IGF available for receptor interaction have been identified: IGF-I binding proteins 1 to 6, with binding protein-1 and binding protein-3 the most extensively studied in terms of their response to exercise. Each binding protein responds to exercise stress independently and has its own biological actions.

Binding proteins are important factors in the transport and physiological mechanisms of IGF (22, 23, 49). Insulin-like growth factor has been shown to stimulate the secretion of its own binding proteins from within the muscle cell itself, thus modulating the cell's responsiveness to IGF (140). The circulating IGF binding proteins play an important role in restricting access of the IGF peptides to receptors and are influenced by 22 kDa GH concentrations. Other factors, such as nutritional status and insulin levels, also have been shown to be important signal mechanisms for IGF release. The nutritional influence on IGF transport, production, and regulatory control is a dramatic variable affecting its cellular interactions. Acute changes in nitrogen balance and protein intake and nutritional status affect a variety of mechanisms (22, 121, 139). It also appears that binding proteins act as a reservoir of IGF, and release from the binding proteins is signaled by the availability of a receptor on the cell (13). This allows IGF to be viable for a longer period of time and could theoretically reduce the amount of degradation of IGF.

In strength training, many of these mechanisms are influenced by the exercise stress; by acute hormonal responses; and by the need for muscle, nerve, and bone tissue remodeling at the cellular level (20, 79, 83, 168). The dramatic interactions of multiple hormones and receptors provide powerful adaptive mechanisms in response to resistance training and can contribute to the subsequent changes in muscular strength and size.

Exercise Responses of Insulin-Like Growth Factors

Insulin-like growth factor I has been the primary IGF studied in the context of exercise because of its prolific role in protein anabolism (146, 150). It too is a superfamily of polypeptides and binding proteins with dramatic implications for health and performance (148). The exact reasons for acute increases in blood levels of IGF-I are unknown but are probably related to the disruption of various cells, including fat and muscle cells, because these cells manufacture and store IGF (183). Insulin-like growth factor I exists across different biocompartments (blood, interstitial fluid [ISF], and muscle), and whether circulating IGF-I responses to exercise reflect what is going on in local fluids surrounding the muscle has been examined. In that study of men and women, it was shown that the increase in circulating total and free IGF-I was not correlated with increases in interstitial fluid IGF-I concentrations or muscle IGF-I protein content (151). Such data indicated that exercise-induced increases in circulating IGF-I are not reflective of local IGF-I signaling that is taking place, showing that circulating concentrations are but one view of the endocrine response patterns. It takes 8 to 24 hours for IGF to be produced and released from the liver following stimulation by GH (9, 30). This seems to indicate that IGF is released from storage sources other than the liver, that release is due to cellular disruption of cells that already contain IGF, or that GH-mediated release of IGF with certain types of exercise has a different time course from that in injection–response studies. Systematic alterations in circulatory concentrations of IGF in response to various types of exercise protocols appear to be closely related to regulatory factors of IGF release and transport (13). Evaluation of serum changes over longer periods is necessary for assessment of specific effects and relationships to GH in the serum (46). In women and men, IGF-I has remained stable despite improvements in strength and power over a two-month training program (147). Exercise-related increases seem to occur more readily if resting concentrations are of a lower value (e.g., 10 to 20 nmol/L). Thus, the stability of resting concentrations may be affected by the absolute amounts of IGF-I in circulation. With training, higher resting concentrations (e.g., 35-45 nmol/L) can make acute exercise-induced increases less probable. Importantly, free forms that are not bound to any binding protein may be the effective elements that influence target tissues (66, 149, 160), especially skeletal muscle.

The autocrine and perhaps paracrine release mechanisms of IGF-I may be paramount in the IGF-I influence on muscle. At rest, fat cells contain relatively high concentrations of IGF, and skeletal muscle has very little of its own. However, mechanical stimulation, overload, and stretch of muscle cells, as in resistance exercise, cause them to substantially increase their production of IGF-I. Insulin-like growth factor I produced in muscle is often referred to as mechano growth factor, and it exerts autocrine functions (63, 141). It has been suggested that autocrine actions of mechano growth factor are the primary actions of IGF-I in muscle. It has also been proposed that IGF-I splice variants may regulate myoblast differentiation through the actions of mature IGF-I and not the E peptides, so examination of this topic remains of great interest (137). It is possible that IGF may be released from nonhepatic cells without the mediation of GH (1, 2, 45, 77, 82, 83). In addition, cells may produce and keep IGFs so that the IGFs exert their effect without entering the peripheral circulation.

Although IGF-I has been shown to be responsive to exercise in some studies, this does not follow a classic endocrine response (i.e., stimulus of gland by exercise resulting in hormone release into the blood) in all cases. It was shown that IGF-I was responsive to resistance exercise in men and women, but in those studies the starting concentrations were lower (113, 114). In another study the concentrations were higher and, despite increases in immunoreactive (22 kDa) GH, no increase in IGF-I was observed (118). From these studies it has been theorized that the starting level of IGF-I may be a factor in determining whether an increase is observed with exercise (i.e., no increases if starting concentrations are high, an increase if starting concentrations are low). A study by Kraemer and colleagues (121) supported this theory, but it was also shown that the IGF-I concentrations were more sensitive to acute caloric loads, which included carbohydrate and protein supplementation before and after a workout (figure 4.7).

Training Adaptations of Insulin-Like Growth Factors

Responses of IGF-I to heavy resistance training remain variable, but studies demonstrate that changes are based on the starting concentrations before training (i.e., if basal concentrations are low, IGF-I increases; if

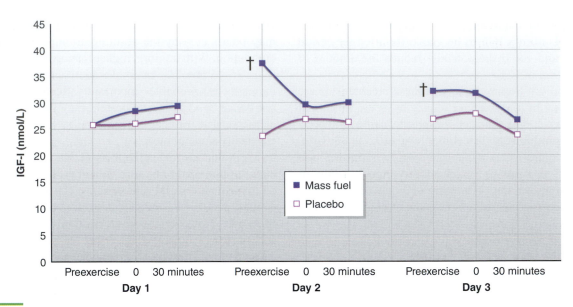

FIGURE 4.7   Responses of insulin-like growth factor I to a multiple-set, heavy resistance exercise protocol on three consecutive days with and without nutritional supplementation of protein-carbohydrate (i.e., Mass fuel) before and during the 1-hour recovery period.

† $p < 0.05$ from corresponding placebo value.

Adapted, by permission, from Kraemer et al. 1998 (121).

high, there is no change or it decreases) (W.J. Kraemer, unpublished data). Additionally, the intake of food or the level of caloric restriction (or both) influences the resting and exercise-induced concentrations in the blood (80, 109). In women, resistance training was shown to increase total IGF-I and reduced IGF binding protein-1 concentrations during acute resistance exercise, indicating that exercise mode-specific adaptations in the circulating IGF-I system can occur (67). The effects of training are still an ongoing story as to the many different aspects of the IGF superfamily response patterns (149). As with GH, training-induced adaptations in IGF-I are probably reflected in a variety of mechanisms related to type of IGFs, release, transport, and receptor interaction. Furthermore, the interaction with other anabolic hormones cannot be ignored, as these often target the same outcome (e.g., protein synthesis). Adaptations to heavy resistance training of IGF-I in the various tissues still requires further investigation.

Adrenal Hormones

The adrenal gland plays a crucial role in the fight-or-flight response phenomenon and has two major divisions: the medulla (center) and the cortex (shell). Both divisions respond to exercise stress. The adrenal medulla is stimulated directly by the nervous system and thus provides a fast and almost immediate response; the cortex is stimulated by adrenocorticotropic hormone (ACTH) released from the anterior pituitary. The adrenal

hormones most important to training and conditioning are cortisol, a glucocorticoid from the adrenal cortex, and the catecholamines (epinephrine, norepinephrine, and dopamine) and enkephalin-containing polypeptides (e.g., peptide F) from the adrenal medulla (95, 104, 109, 116, 182). Peptide F, a proenkephalin fragment, plays an important role in enhancing immune cell functions (182). Thus, the adrenal medulla secretes hormones involved in both the immediate reaction to stress and the subsequent recovery from that stress.

Cortisol

Classically, glucocorticoids, and more specifically cortisol in humans, have been viewed as catabolic hormones in skeletal muscle (45, 47, 129). In reality, however, cortisol is a primary signal hormone for carbohydrate metabolism and is related to the glycogen stores in the muscle. When glycogen concentrations are low, other substrates (proteins) must be catabolized to produce energy and to support maintenance of blood glucose concentrations. Cortisol concentrations display a strong circadian pattern; concentration is greatest in the early morning and drops throughout the day. Thus the time of day is an important consideration when one is examining or comparing results for cortisol.

Role of Cortisol

Cortisol exerts its major catabolic effects by stimulating the conversion of amino acids to carbohydrates, increasing the level of **proteolytic enzymes** (enzymes that break down proteins), inhibiting protein synthesis, and suppressing many glucose-dependent processes such as glycogenesis and immune cell function (51). Cortisol has greater catabolic effects on Type II fibers, which might, at least in part, be because they have more protein than Type I fibers; but cortisol might still be involved with the control of degradation in Type I fibers. (162). Type I fibers rely more on reducing degradation to develop muscle hypertrophy, in contrast to the dramatic increases in synthesis used by Type II fibers to develop hypertrophy.

In situations of disease, joint immobilization, or injury, an elevation in cortisol mediates a nitrogen-wasting effect with a net loss of contractile protein. This results in muscle atrophy, with associated reductions in force production capability (45, 133). In the muscle, the anabolic effects of testosterone and insulin counter cortisol's catabolic effects. If a greater number of receptors are bound with testosterone and this receptor complex then blocks the genetic element on the DNA to which cortisol and its receptor complex can bind, protein is conserved or enhanced. Conversely, if a greater number of receptors are bound to cortisol, protein is degraded and lost. The balance of anabolic and catabolic activities in the muscle affects the protein contractile unit, directly influencing strength. The acute increases in circulating cortisol following exercise also implicate acute inflammatory response mechanisms in tissue remodeling (51).

Resistance Exercise Responses of Cortisol

As with 22 kDa GH, it appears that cortisol increases with resistance exercise, most dramatically when rest periods are short or the total volume of work is high (116, 178). Increases in cortisol might not have negative effects in men after a period of training to which the body has adapted; adaptation "disinhibits" cortisol at the level of the testis, thereby maintaining testosterone's primary influence on its nuclear receptors.

Cortisol responds to resistance exercise protocols that create a dramatic stimulus to anaerobic metabolism. It is interesting that selection among the acute program variables that produce the highest catabolic responses in the body also produces the greatest GH response (116, 166, 178). Thus, though chronic high levels of cortisol have adverse effects, acute increases may be a part of a larger remodeling process in muscle tissue. Muscle must be disrupted to a certain extent (below injury levels) to remodel itself and enlarge; acute elevations in cortisol would help in this remodeling process by helping to remove damaged proteins.

Because of the catabolic role of cortisol, athletes and strength and conditioning professionals have much interest in its potential as a whole-body marker of tissue breakdown. To a certain extent, cortisol is such a marker,

but the magnitude of increase may need to be greater than 800 nmol/L to indicate potential overtraining problems (55, 56, 58, 59). The testosterone-to-cortisol ratio also has been used in the attempt to determine the anabolic–catabolic status of the body (70). Although such markers are attractive conceptually, serum cortisol measurements and the testosterone-to-cortisol ratio have met with only limited success in predicting or monitoring changes in strength and power capabilities (124). Problems with these tests probably have to do with the multiple roles of cortisol and other hormones.

Few studies have investigated the effect of resistance exercise on glucocorticoid receptors in muscle tissue, but recent data indicate that in trained men, significantly lower concentrations of receptors are found at rest and over a recovery period of 70 minutes after exercise when compared to those in women (188). Concomitantly, women with the same exercise protocol decreased and then increased their androgen binding capacity over the 70 minutes following exercise, whereas men saw only a continual downregulation. This indicates that women dealing with a lower concentration of testosterone more rapidly upregulated androgen receptors whereas glucocorticoid receptors were already upregulated before the workout.

Interestingly, for B lymphocytes, glucocorticoid receptor upregulation for men and women was observed before exercise (anticipatory), during, and after exercise for 1 hour (52). Yet with a heavy 5RM protocol, women did not exhibit an increase in cortisol concentrations in the blood, whereas men did. This indicates a differential stimulus between the sexes, yet the receptor responses of immune cells to cortisol are similar. Such data indicate that different target tissues might respond differentially to cortisol as well as to other hormone signals.

It is probable that vast differences are observed in the physiological role of cortisol in acute versus chronic exercise responses to resistance exercise. Acute cortisol responses may reflect the metabolic stress of the exercise, and chronic aspects may be primarily involved with tissue homeostasis entailing protein metabolism (45, 51). Thus, cortisol's role in overtraining, detraining, or injury may be critical when muscle tissue atrophy and decreases in force production capabilities are observed (133). Such roles remain to be demonstrated; however, cortisol's role in suppressing function of cells of the immune system (e.g., B and T cells) has a direct impact on the recovery and remodeling of skeletal muscle tissue. This impact of cortisol on immune cells can be dramatic, with the main effect one of "inactivating" immune cell functions, which partially contributes to the immune suppression observed after intense exercise stress (51). With heavy resistance exercise, glucocorticoid receptor expression in B cells decreased with exercise and increased during recovery, demonstrating a greater binding, which in turn would reduce B cell activity during recovery (52). The effects were somewhat attenuated in women compared to men of similar training levels, indicating a sex difference in the magnitude of the responses.

> **Resistance exercise protocols that use high volume, large muscle groups, and short rest periods result in increased serum cortisol values (119). Though chronic high concentrations of cortisol may have adverse catabolic effects, acute increases still contribute to the remodeling of muscle tissue and maintenance of blood glucose.**

Catecholamines

The catecholamines—primarily epinephrine but also norepinephrine and dopamine—are secreted by the adrenal medulla and are important for the acute expression of strength and power because the hormones act as central motor stimulators and peripheral vascular dilators and enhance enzyme systems and calcium release in muscle (95). Thus, the resistance exercise–induced stress leads to events similar to the classic fight-or-flight response. The importance of catecholamines during resistance exercise was highlighted by the finding that men who had a higher catecholamine release immediately before and during a heavy resistance exercise session were able to better maintain force output throughout the session (53). The role of catecholamines in growth-promoting actions in muscle tissue is less clear, but they act to stimulate other anabolic hormones.

Role of Catecholamines

The physiological functions of epinephrine and norepinephrine in muscle are these:

- Increase force production via central mechanisms and increased metabolic enzyme activity
- Increase muscle contraction rate
- Increase blood pressure
- Increase energy availability
- Increase muscle blood flow (via vasodilation)
- Augment secretion rates of other hormones, such as testosterone

Catecholamines appear to reflect the acute demands and physical stress of resistance exercise protocols (105). A high-intensity (10RM), short-rest (10-60 seconds between sets and exercises), heavy resistance exercise routine (10 exercises, three sets) typically used by bodybuilders for development of strength and

hypertrophy was shown to maintain increased plasma norepinephrine, epinephrine, and dopamine levels for 5 minutes into recovery (105). In addition, epinephrine has been correlated to lactate concentrations with exercise stress. Adrenal responses are not involved in the recovery responses until the stress is removed. Some specific endogenous opioid peptides (i.e., proenkephalins) are secreted by the adrenal medulla and affect the immune system, which is critical in recovery from exercise stress (182). If training is not varied, continued stress keeps the adrenal gland engaged, and recovery is delayed due to the secondary responses of cortisol and its negative effects on immune system cells and protein structures. Long-term continued high stress can even lead to adrenal exhaustion, at which point the ability of the adrenal medulla to release catecholamines is diminished.

Training Adaptations of Catecholamines

Heavy resistance training has been shown to increase the ability of an athlete to secrete greater amounts of epinephrine during maximal exercise (104). It has also been suggested that training reduces epinephrine responses to a single bench press workout (68). Because epinephrine is involved in metabolic control, force production, and the response mechanisms of other hormones (such as testosterone, GHs, and IGFs), stimulation of catecholamines is probably one of the first endocrine mechanisms to occur in response to resistance exercise.

> **Training protocols must be varied to allow the adrenal gland to engage in recovery processes and to prevent the secondary responses of cortisol, which can have negative effects on the immune system and protein structures.**

Other Hormonal Considerations

A host of different hormones are involved in the maintenance of normal body function and in adaptive responses of the body to resistance training (26, 45, 46, 76, 87, 97, 107). Although we might focus on one or two hormones for their roles in a particular physiological function, other hormones must create an optimal environment in which the primary hormonal actions can take place. Hormones such as insulin, thyroid hormones, and beta-endorphin have been implicated in growth, repair, pain analgesia, and exercise stress mechanisms; unfortunately, few data are available concerning their responses and adaptations to resistance exercise or training (48, 116, 120). Owing to the relatively tight homeostatic control of both insulin and thyroid hormone secretion in healthy individuals, chronic training adaptations in circulating resting con-

How Can Athletes Manipulate the Endocrine System With Resistance Training?

General Concepts

- The more muscle fibers recruited for an exercise, the greater the extent of potential remodeling process in the whole muscle.
- Only muscle fibers activated by resistance training are subject to adaptation, including hormonal adaptations to stress.

To Increase Serum Testosterone Concentrations

Serum testosterone concentrations have been shown to increase acutely with use of these methods independently or in various combinations:

- Large muscle group exercises (e.g., deadlift, power clean, squats)
- Heavy resistance (85% to 95% of 1RM)
- Moderate to high volume of exercise, achieved with multiple sets or multiple exercises
- Short rest intervals (30-60 seconds)

To Increase 22 kDa Growth Hormone Concentrations

Growth hormone levels have been shown to increase acutely with use of either of these methods or both in combination:

- Use workouts with higher lactate concentrations and associated acid–base disruptions; that is, use high intensity (10RM, or heavy resistance) with three sets of each exercise (high total work) and short (1-minute) rest periods.
- Supplement diet with carbohydrate and protein before and after workouts.

To Optimize Responses of Adrenal Hormones

- Use high volume, large muscle groups, and short rest periods to expose the body to an adrenergic stress. But be careful to vary the training protocol and the rest period length from short to long over time, provide days of complete rest, and use lower-volume workouts to allow the adrenal gland to engage in recovery processes, to reduce stress on the adrenal medulla so as not to experience adrenergic exhaustion, and to reduce stress on the adrenal cortex and prevent chronic cortisol secretions from the adrenal cortex. This way, the stress of the exercises will not result in a nonfunctional overreaching or overtraining.

centrations of these hormones would not be expected in that population. Although improvements in insulin resistance have been observed in healthy individuals following resistance training, these changes may reflect only an acute effect from the most recent exercise session (15). It is more likely that longer-term changes such as 24-hour secretion rates, sensitivity of the receptors, and binding interactions would be affected. The effect of resistance exercise and training on thyroid hormones in healthy individuals has received little attention in the literature. McMurray and colleagues (142) found that although the concentration of the thyroid hormone triiodothyronine (T3) was not affected acutely by a bout of resistance exercise, the concentration of thyroxine (T4), a precursor to T3, was elevated acutely and reduced during the subsequent night's sleep. A more recent study did not find changes to T3 or T4 concentrations at 24, 48, or 72 hours after a bout of resistance exercise (88). This suggests that any acute resistance exercise effects on thyroid hormones are brief. Transient reductions in T3 and T4 concentrations with long-term resistance training have been found after six months (4) and three and five months (4, 153), respectively, but they returned to baseline concentrations after nine months of training. Although little change occurs for these hormones, they are very important for physiological adaptations to resistance training as they have permissive effects in metabolic control, amino acid synthesis, and augmentation of other hormonal release mechanisms.

Conclusion

As we continue to study the endocrine system and its interactions with the nervous system, the immune system, and the musculoskeletal system, we find that the functions of these systems are truly integrated and very complex. Signaling communication among systems is accomplished with hormones and other signaling molecules (e.g., cytokines, chemokines, molecular signal molecules). For years, strength and conditioning professionals and athletes have appreciated the importance of anabolic hormones for mediating changes in the body and helping with the adaptive response to heavy resistance training. Whether trying to optimize a workout or avoid overtraining, the strength and conditioning professional must remember that the endocrine system plays an important role. The goal of this chapter has been to provide an initial glimpse into this complex but also highly organized system that helps to mediate changes in the body with resistance exercise training.

KEY TERMS

allosteric binding site
anabolic hormone
catabolic hormone
cross-reactivity
diurnal variation
downregulation
endocrine gland

General Adaptation Syndrome
hormone
hormone–receptor complex (H-RC)
lock-and-key theory
neuroendocrine immunology
neuroendocrinology

polypeptide hormone
proteolytic enzyme
secondary messenger
steroid hormone
target tissue cell
thyroid hormone

STUDY QUESTIONS

1. After a bout of resistance training, acute hormonal secretions provide all of the following information to the body EXCEPT
    a. amount of physiological stress
    b. metabolic demands of exercise
    c. type of physiological stress
    d. energy expended

2. Which of the following hormones enhance(s) muscle tissue growth?
    I. growth hormone
    II. cortisol
    III. IGF-I
    IV. progesterone
    a. I and III only
    b. II and IV only
    c. I, II, and III only
    d. II, III, and IV only

3. Which of the following is NOT a function of growth hormone?
    a. increase lipolysis
    b. decrease collagen synthesis
    c. increase amino acid transport
    d. decrease glucose utilization

4. Which of the following hormones has the greatest influence on neural changes?
    a. growth hormone
    b. testosterone
    c. cortisol
    d. IGF

5. What type of resistance training workout promotes the highest growth hormone increases following the exercise session?

Rest	Volume	Sets
a. 30 seconds	High	3
b. 30 seconds	Low	1
c. 3 minutes	High	1
d. 3 minutes	Low	3

CHAPTER 5

Adaptations to Anaerobic Training Programs

Duncan French, PhD

> **After completing this chapter, you will be able to**
>
> - differentiate between aerobic training adaptations and the anatomical, physiological, and performance adaptations following anaerobic training;
> - discuss the central and peripheral neural adaptations to anaerobic training;
> - understand how manipulating the acute training variables of a periodized program can alter bone, muscle, and connective tissue;
> - explain the acute and chronic effects of anaerobic training on the endocrine system;
> - elucidate the acute and chronic effects of anaerobic training on the cardiovascular system;
> - recognize the causes, signs, symptoms, and effects of anaerobic overtraining and detraining; and
> - discuss how anaerobic training programs have the potential to enhance muscular strength, muscular endurance, power, flexibility, and motor performance.

The author would like to acknowledge the significant contributions of Nicholas A. Ratamess to this chapter.

Characterized by high-intensity, intermittent bouts of exercise, **anaerobic training** requires adenosine triphosphate (ATP) to be regenerated at a faster rate than the aerobic energy system is capable of. Consequently, the difference in energy requirement is made up by the anaerobic energy system, which works in the absence of oxygen and includes the **anaerobic alactic system** (also known as the phosphagen or creatine phosphate system) and the **anaerobic lactic system** (also known as the glycolytic system). Long-term adaptations that occur in response to anaerobic training are specifically related to the characteristics of the training program. For example, improvements in muscular strength, power, hypertrophy, muscular endurance, motor skills, and coordination are all recognized as beneficial adaptations following anaerobic training modalities. These include resistance training; plyometric drills; and speed, agility, and interval training. The aerobic system ultimately has limited involvement in high-intensity anaerobic activities, but does play an important role in the recovery of energy stores during periods of low-intensity exercise or rest (45).

Exercises such as sprints and plyometric drills primarily stress the phosphagen system; they are usually less than 10 seconds in duration and minimize fatigue by allowing almost complete recovery between sets (e.g., 5-7 minutes). Longer-duration interval-type anaerobic training predominantly uses energy production from the glycolytic system, in which shorter rest intervals (e.g., 20-60 seconds) are adopted during high-intensity exercise. The integration of high-intensity exercise with short rest periods is considered an important aspect of anaerobic training, as athletes are often required to perform near-maximally under fatigued conditions during competition. It is, however, critical that appropriate anaerobic training be programmed and prescribed in such a way as to optimize the physiological adaptations that determine performance. Competitive sport requires the complex interaction of all the energy systems and demonstrates how each of them contributes to a varying extent in order to fulfill the global metabolic demands of competition (table 5.1).

A wide variety of physical and physiological adaptations are reported following anaerobic training, and these changes enable individuals to improve athletic performance standards (see table 5.2). Adaptations include changes to the nervous, muscular, connective tissue, endocrine, and cardiovascular systems. They range from changes that take place in the early phase of training (e.g., one to four weeks) to those that take place following many years of consistent training. The majority of research has typically dealt with adaptations in the early to intermediate stages of training (i.e., 4 to 24 weeks). Understanding how the individual systems of the human body respond to physical activity using anaerobic metabolism provides a knowledge base from which the strength and conditioning professional can plan and predict the outcome of a specific training program to then focus on effectively influencing individual strengths and weaknesses.

Neural Adaptations

Many anaerobic training modalities emphasize the expression of muscular speed and power and depend greatly on optimal neural recruitment for maximal performance (and high quality of training). Anaerobic training has the potential to elicit long-term adaptations throughout the neuromuscular system, beginning in the higher brain centers and continuing down to the level of individual muscle fibers (figure 5.1). Neural adaptations are fundamental to optimizing athletic performance, and increased neural drive is critical to maximizing the expression of muscular strength and power. Augmented neural drive is thought to occur via increased agonist (i.e., the major muscles involved in a specific movement or exercise) muscle recruitment, improved neuronal firing rates, and greater synchronization in the timing of neural discharge during high-intensity muscular contractions (4, 69, 166, 167, 174). In addition, a reduction in inhibitory mechanisms (i.e., from Golgi tendon organs) is also thought to occur with long-term training (1, 63). While it is not fully understood how these complex responses coexist, it is apparent that neural adaptations typically occur before any structural changes in skeletal muscle are apparent (167).

Central Adaptations

Increased motor unit activation begins in the higher brain centers, where the intent to produce maximal levels of muscular force and power causes motor cortex activity to increase (41). As the level of force developed rises, or when a new exercise or movement is being learned, primary motor cortex activity is elevated in an effort to support the enhanced need for neuromuscular function. Adaptations to anaerobic training methods are then reflected by substantial neural changes in the spinal cord, particularly along the descending corticospinal tracts (3). Indeed, after use of anaerobic training methods, the recruitment of fast-twitch motor units has been shown to be elevated as a means to support heightened levels of force expression (151). This is in comparison to what is seen in untrained individuals (4), in whom the ability to maximally recruit motor units is limited, especially fast-twitch motor units. In untrained individuals or in those rehabilitating from injury, electrical stimulation has been shown to be more effective than voluntary

TABLE 5.1   Primary Metabolic Demands of Various Sports

Sport	Phosphagen system	Glycolytic system	Aerobic system
American football	High	Moderate	Low
Archery	High	Low	—
Baseball	High	Low	—
Basketball	High	Moderate to high	Low
Boxing	High	High	Moderate
Diving	High	Low	—
Fencing	High	Moderate	—
Field events (athletics)	High	—	—
Field hockey	High	Moderate	Moderate
Golf	High	—	Moderate
Gymnastics	High	Moderate	—
Ice hockey	High	Moderate	Moderate
Lacrosse	High	Moderate	Moderate
Marathon running	Low	Low	High
Mixed martial arts	High	High	Moderate
Powerlifting	High	Low	—
Rowing	Low	Moderate	High
Skiing:			
Cross-country	Low	Low	High
Downhill	High	High	Moderate
Soccer (football)	High	Moderate	Moderate
Strongman	High	Moderate to high	Low
Swimming:			
Short distance	High	Moderate	—
Long distance	Low	Moderate	High
Tennis	High	Moderate	Low
Track (athletics):			
Sprints	High	Moderate	—
Middle distance	High	High	Moderate
Long distance	—	Moderate	High
Ultra-endurance	—	—	High
Volleyball	High	Moderate	—
Weightlifting	High	Moderate	Low
Wrestling	High	High	Moderate

Note: All types of metabolism are involved to some extent in all activities.

activations in eliciting beneficial gains. This response further indicates the potential inability of these populations to successfully activate all available muscle fibers. Indeed, research has shown that only 71% of muscle tissue is activated during maximal efforts in untrained populations (7).

Adaptations of Motor Units

The functional unit of the neuromuscular system is the **motor unit**. Consisting of the alpha motor neuron and the muscle fibers that it activates, a motor unit may innervate <10 muscle fibers for small, intricate muscles or >100

TABLE 5.2 Physiological Adaptations to Resistance Training

Variable	Resistance training adaptation
Performance	
Muscular strength	Increases
Muscular endurance	Increases for high power output
Aerobic power	No change or increases slightly
Anaerobic power	Increases
Rate of force production	Increases
Vertical jump	Improved ability
Sprint speed	Improves
Muscle fibers	
Fiber cross-sectional area	Increases
Capillary density	No change or decreases
Mitochondrial density	Decreases
Myofibrillar density	No change
Myofibrillar volume	Increases
Cytoplasmic density	Increases
Myosin heavy chain protein	Increases
Enzyme activity	
Creatine phosphokinase	Increases
Myokinase	Increases
Phosphofructokinase	Increases
Lactate dehydrogenase	No change or variable
Sodium–potassium ATPase	Increases
Metabolic energy stores	
Stored ATP	Increases
Stored creatine phosphate	Increases
Stored glycogen	Increases
Stored triglycerides	May increase
Connective tissue	
Ligament strength	May increase
Tendon strength	May increase
Collagen content	May increase
Bone density	No change or increases
Body composition	
% body fat	Decreases
Fat-free mass	Increases

ATP = adenosine triphosphate; ATPase = adenosine triphosphatase.

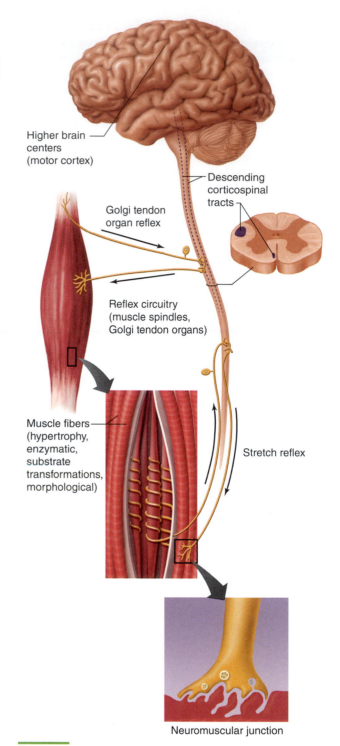

FIGURE 5.1 Potential sites of adaptation within the neuromuscular system.

fibers for large, powerful trunk and limb muscles. When expression of maximal force is desired, all the available motor units must be activated within a muscle. Change in the firing rate or frequency of the motor unit also affects the ability to generate force. Increased force with greater firing rates reflects the summation of successive muscle contractions, whereby action potentials temporarily overlap. With increased motor unit firing rates, the muscle fibers are continually activated by subsequent action potentials before they have time to completely relax following a prior action potential. The summation of overlapping action potentials is expressed as augmented contractile strength (1). These firing rates represent an adaptive mechanism shown to improve following heavy resistance training (166). Gains in maximal strength and power of agonist muscles are generally associated with (a) an increase in recruitment; (b) an increased rate of firing; (c) greater synchronization of neural discharge, which acts to coordinate the activity of multiple muscles in synergy (173); or (d) a combination of all these factors.

The recruitment or decruitment of motor units in an orderly manner is governed by the **size principle** (figure 5.2), which represents the relationship between motor unit twitch force and recruitment threshold (166, 167). According to this principle, motor units are recruited in an ascending order according to their recruitment thresholds and firing rates. This represents a continuum of voluntary force in the agonist muscle. Because most muscles contain a range of Type I and Type II muscle fibers, force production can range from very low to maximal levels. Those motor units high in the recruitment order are used primarily for high force, speed, or power production. As the demands of force expression increase, motor units are recruited in a sequential fashion from low- to high-threshold motor units. Thus, with heavy resistance training, all muscle fibers get larger (77, 183, 184) because for the most part they are all recruited to

some extent in order to produce the higher levels of force required to lift progressively heavier loads. Maximal force production not only requires the recruitment of a maximum percentage of available motor units, including the high-threshold motor units, but also relies on the recruitment occurring at very high firing frequencies, which promotes the summation of activated motor units and as a consequence augments the magnitude of contractile activity. Once a motor unit is recruited, less activation is needed in order for it to be rerecruited (69). This phenomenon may have important ramifications for strength and power training, as the high-threshold motor units may be more readily reactivated subsequent to prior recruitment.

Exceptions to the size principle do exist. Under certain circumstances, an athlete is able to inhibit the lower-threshold motor units and in their place activate higher-threshold motor units (148, 189). This **selective recruitment** is critical when force production is required at very high speeds for the expression of muscular power. Indeed, both rapid changes in the direction of force production and ballistic muscular contractions—as found in the movement patterns of Olympic weightlifting, plyometrics, speed, power, and agility training—have been shown to lead to preferential recruitment of fast-twitch motor units (148, 189). This variation in recruitment order benefits high-velocity training modalities in which rate of force production is vital to success. For example, it would be very difficult for athletes to generate enough angular velocity and power to attain maximal height for the vertical jump if they had to recruit the entire slow-twitch motor unit pool before activation of the fast-twitch units. As the time between the countermovement and the subsequent jump takeoff is often less than 0.4 seconds, there simply is insufficient time to recruit all of the motor units in order and still perform an explosive jump (4, 113). Instead, selective recruitment appears to be a beneficial intrinsic neural mechanism favoring explosive exercise. In addition, using specific training methods may enhance selective recruitment, which in turn may improve sport performance (149).

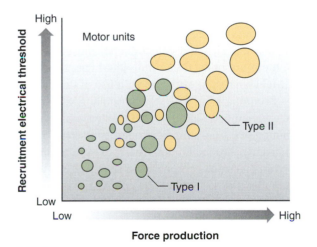

FIGURE 5.2 Graphic representation of the size principle, according to which motor units that contain Type I (slow-twitch) and Type II (fast-twitch) fibers are organized based on some "size" factor. Low-threshold motor units are recruited first and have lower force capabilities than higher-threshold motor units. Typically, to get to the high-threshold motor units, the body must first recruit the lower-threshold motor units. Exceptions exist, especially with respect to explosive, ballistic contractions that can selectively recruit high-threshold units to rapidly achieve more force and power.

> With heavy resistance training, all muscle fibers get larger (i.e., hypertrophy) because motor units are recruited in a sequential order by their size to produce high levels of force. In advanced lifters, the central nervous system may adapt by allowing well-trained athletes to recruit some motor units in a nonconsecutive order, by recruiting larger ones first to promote greater production of power or speed in a movement.

Another critical element of adaptation in neural recruitment is the level of tissue activation that results from chronic resistance training for muscular hypertrophy. Research has shown that as muscle size increases it does not require as much neural activation to lift a given load. Ploutz and colleagues (157) reported that fewer quadriceps muscle fibers were activated when subjects lifted a set load following nine weeks of resistance training that resulted in a 5% increase in muscle size. Such results demonstrate the importance of progressive overloading during resistance training and how it promotes the continual recruitment of an optimal amount of muscle tissue.

Other motor unit adaptations include changes in the rate and sequence of firing. A positive relationship exists between the magnitude of force produced and the rate of motor unit firing; high firing rates from the onset of ballistic muscle contraction are especially critical to increased rates of force development (1). The increase in firing rate (vs. recruitment) appears to be dependent on muscle size, such that smaller muscles rely more on an increased firing rate to enhance force production whereas larger muscles depend more on recruitment (48, 63). Evidence suggests that anaerobic training can play a role in enhancing firing rates of recruited motor units (4). For example, resistance training may result in a more synchronized pattern (i.e., the firing of two or more motor units at a fixed interval) of activation during the exertion of large forces, rather than the customary asynchronous pattern usually common to motor function (50, 174). Although the specific role of motor unit synchronization during anaerobic training remains to be fully elucidated, synchronization is potentially more critical to the *timing* of force production and less significant with regard to the overall level of force developed.

Neuromuscular Junction

The **neuromuscular junction (NMJ)** is the interface between the nerve and the skeletal muscle fibers, and it represents another potential site for neural adaptation following anaerobic training (38, 39). Because of the difficulty in investigating this structure, most studies examining the NMJ have used animal models to demonstrate its adaptation to exercise. Deschenes and colleagues (40) examined the impact of high-intensity versus low-intensity treadmill exercise training on NMJ in the soleus muscle of rats. Following both high- and low-intensity running, the NMJ was found to increase in its total area. High-intensity training, however, resulted in more dispersed, irregular-shaped synapses and a greater total length of nerve terminal branching compared to low-intensity training. In another study, greater end-plate perimeter length and area, as well as greater dispersion of acetylcholine receptors within the end-plate region, were also found after seven weeks of resistance training (39). These adaptations suggest that anaerobic training appears to induce beneficial morphological changes in the NMJ that are conducive to enhanced neural transmission capabilities.

Neuromuscular Reflex Potentiation

Anaerobic training causes positive changes in the reflex (i.e., muscle spindle or stretch reflex) response of the neuromuscular system and enhances the magnitude and rate of force development via this reflex. This **myotatic reflex** harnesses the involuntary elastic properties of the muscle and connective tissue and acts to positively increase force production without any additional energy requirement. Resistance training in particular has been shown to increase reflex potentiation by between 19% and 55% (5). Furthermore, resistance-trained athletes (weightlifters, bodybuilders) are found to have greater reflex potentiation in the soleus muscle compared to untrained individuals (170).

Anaerobic Training and Electromyography Studies

Electromyography (EMG) is a common research tool used to examine the magnitude of neural activation within skeletal muscle. Two kinds of EMG are commonly used in research and applied settings: surface EMG and intramuscular (needle or fine wire) EMG. Surface EMG requires placement of adhesive electrodes on the surface of the skin where they are able to monitor a large area of underlying muscle (152). Surface EMG is often more effective for monitoring superficial muscle, as it is unable to bypass the action potentials of superficial muscles and detect deeper muscle activity. Also, the more body fat an individual has, the weaker the EMG signal is likely to be with use of this methodology. In comparison, with intramuscular EMG, the skin surface is numbed, and a needle electrode, or a needle containing two fine-wire electrodes, is inserted through the skin and positioned into the belly of the muscle itself. Fine-wire electrodes emphasize a specificity of assessment in that they are located in a muscle of interest and accurately record localized motor unit action potentials (85). Because of its invasiveness, intramuscular EMG is primarily adopted in research settings or under clinical conditions. While it is often difficult to determine the specific underpinning mechanism(s) (i.e., increased recruitment, discharge rate, or synchronization; Golgi tendon organ inhibition) affecting EMG output, an increase in EMG signal indicates greater neuromuscular activity.

An important consideration when examining the neuromuscular system is the training status of an individual. Neural adaptations (improved motor learning and coordination) predominate in the early phase of training without any concomitant increases in muscle hypertrophy (73, 75-77). In addition, the onset of hypertrophy is associated with a decline in EMG activity (145). It appears that as an individual's training status advances, there exists an interplay between neural and hypertrophic mechanisms that contribute to further gains in strength and power.

Sale (166, 167) reported that dramatic increases in neural adaptation take place in the early part of a training program (6 to 10 weeks). As the duration of training increases (>10 weeks), muscle hypertrophy then occurs, and it is these structural changes that contribute to strength and power gains more than neural adaptations. Eventually muscle hypertrophy plateaus as *accommodation* to the training load occurs. However, at that time, if an athlete incorporates new variation or progressive overload into the training plan, neural adaptations will once again contribute to the performance improvements by acting to tolerate the "new" physical insult from training. This pattern is replicated with every stepwise change in the training demand, and as athletes progress in training, the type of program used may be one of the most important factors to consider (77, 80, 161). Neural factors are especially important for strength gains in programs that use very high training intensities (>85% of 1-repetition maximum [1RM]) (145). Training programs designed to elicit muscular power also provide a potent stimulus to the nervous system and result in higher posttraining EMG activity (149).

Electromyography studies have also yielded some interesting findings regarding neural adaptations to anaerobic training:

- Exercising muscle undergoing unilateral resistance training produces increased strength and neural activity in the contralateral resting muscle, a phenomenon known as **cross-education** (89). A review of the literature has shown that strength in the untrained limb may increase up to 22%, with an average strength increase of approximately 8% (147). The increase in strength of the untrained limb is accompanied by greater EMG activity in that limb (176), thereby suggesting that a central neural adaptation accounts for the majority of strength gains.

- In untrained individuals, a **bilateral deficit** is evident. The force produced when both limbs contract together is lower than the sum of the forces they produce when contracting unilaterally. Research has shown that the corresponding EMG activity is lower during bilateral contractions (63), suggesting that neural mechanisms are, at least in part, a contributing factor. With longitudinal bilateral training, the magnitude of the bilateral deficit

is reduced. In fact, trained or stronger individuals often show a **bilateral facilitation** effect in which an increase in voluntary activation of the agonist muscle groups occurs (15, 171).

- The EMG activity of antagonist muscle groups has been shown to change in response to anaerobic training during agonist movements. In most instances, cocontraction of antagonist muscles serves as a protective mechanism to increase joint stability and reduce the risk of injury (96). However, when too much antagonist activity opposes agonist movement, it creates a resistance to maximal force production. A number of studies have shown reduced antagonist cocontraction following resistance training, resulting in an increase in net force without an increase in agonist motor unit recruitment (26, 76, 151). Elsewhere, sprint and plyometric training have also been shown to alter the timing of cocontractor activation (96). The specific role of altering antagonist cocontraction patterns remains unclear. Greater antagonist activity may be observed during ballistic movements that require high levels of joint stability, or when people are unfamiliar with a task and require more inherent stability (48).

Muscular Adaptations

Skeletal muscle adaptations following anaerobic training occur in both structure and function, with reported changes encompassing increases in size, fiber type transitions, and enhanced biochemical and ultrastructural components (i.e., muscle architecture, enzyme activity, and substrate concentrations). Collectively, these adaptations result in enhanced performance characteristics that include strength, power, and muscular endurance, all of which are critical to athletic success.

Muscular Growth

Muscle **hypertrophy** is the term given to the enlargement of muscle fiber cross-sectional area (CSA) following training. A positive relationship exists between hypertrophy and the expression of muscular strength. Biologically, the process of hypertrophy involves an increase in the net accretion (i.e., an increase in synthesis, reduction in degradation, or both) of the contractile proteins **actin** and **myosin** within the myofibril, as well as an increase in the number of myofibrils within a muscle fiber. In addition to these contractile proteins, other structural proteins such as **titin** and **nebulin** are also synthesized proportionately to the myofilament changes. The new myofilaments are added to the periphery of the myofibril and result in an increase in its diameter. The cumulative effect of these additions is an enlargement of the fiber and, collectively, the size of the muscle or muscle group itself. During exposure to mechanical loading (e.g., resistance training), a series of intracellular processes regulate gene expression and subsequently promote increased protein synthesis (165).

Mechanical deformation of muscle stimulates various proteins independent of hormone concentrations, and these proteins have been shown to increase in activity before evidence of muscle hypertrophy appears. In particular, mechanical tissue deformation activates the protein kinase B (Akt)–mammalian target of rapamycin (mTOR) pathway, the adenosine monophosphate–activated protein kinase (AMPK) pathway, and the mitogen-activated protein kinase (MAPK) pathway. Of these, the Akt/mTOR pathway in particular is important in directly regulating adaptations to resistance training (179). When muscle fibers contract, Akt/mTOR signaling increases dramatically, and this response is critical for increasing muscle protein synthesis and subsequent growth (a process known as **myogenesis**). At the same time, the downregulation of inhibitory growth factors (e.g., myostatin) suggests that resistance exercise significantly affects a plethora of growth-signaling and breakdown pathways (18, 98, 101). Protein synthetic rates are elevated after acute resistance exercise and remain elevated for up to 48 hours (130, 156). The magnitude of increased protein synthesis depends on a variety of factors including carbohydrate and protein intake, amino acid availability, timing of nutrient intake, mechanical stress of the weight training workout, muscle cell hydration levels, and the anabolic hormonal and subsequent receptor response (19, 115, 162).

> ▶ **The process of hypertrophy involves both an increase in the synthesis of the contractile proteins actin and myosin within the myofibril and an increase in the number of myofibrils within the muscle fiber itself. The new myofilaments are added to the external layers of the myofibril, resulting in an increase in its diameter.**

Exercise-induced muscle damage (EIMD) and disruption of myofibrils and the uniform structure of muscle fiber sarcomeres following high-intensity anaerobic training (e.g., resistance training) also have a marked effect on muscle growth. The theoretical basis for this suggests that structural changes associated with EIMD influence gene expression in an effort to strengthen muscle tissue and protect it from further damage. The repair and remodeling process itself may involve a host of regulatory mechanisms (e.g., hormonal, immune, and metabolic) that interact with the training status of the individual (105, 193). However, it is understood that

both the inflammatory responses and increased protein turnover (i.e., increased net protein synthesis) ultimately contribute to long-term hypertrophic adaptations (179). The sequence of protein synthesis involves (a) water uptake, (b) noncontractile protein synthesis, and (c) contractile protein synthesis (192). At the same time, reduced degradation acts to maintain the size of fibers by reducing net protein loss.

After the initiation of a heavy resistance training program, changes in the type of muscle proteins (e.g., fast myosin heavy chains) start to take place within several appropriately timed workouts (113, 183). However, muscle fiber hypertrophy requires a longer period of training (>16 workouts) before significant changes in CSA actually become apparent (185). As with initial gains in performance variables (e.g., strength, power), hypertrophic responses are at their greatest in the early stages, after which the rate of muscle growth diminishes over time (113). Athletes studied across two years of heavy resistance training showed increases in strength that paralleled optimal training intensities, although muscle fiber hypertrophy contributed little to increased lifting performance (80).

The magnitude of hypertrophy ultimately depends on the training stimulus and the manner in which the acute training variables are prescribed. In order to optimize muscle growth, appropriate training periodization is essential for maximizing the combination of mechanical and metabolic stimuli. Mechanical factors include the lifting of heavy loads, the inclusion of eccentric muscle actions, and moderate to high training volumes (114), all of which are characteristic of strength training. An increasing amount of evidence is also supporting the use of novel training modalities (e.g., occlusion training [177]) as alternative methods of inducing appropriate mechanical or metabolic stress. Metabolic factors center on low- to moderate-intensity or moderately high-intensity training with high volumes and short rest intervals (characteristic of bodybuilding training) (114). Collectively, mechanical factors result in optimal recruitment of muscle fibers (as muscle fibers need to be recruited before growth), growth factor expression, and potential disruption to the sarcomeres, all of which increase muscle CSA (67, 161). The metabolic factors stress the glycolytic energy system and result in increased metabolites that may be involved in muscle growth. These programs also elicit the most potent anabolic hormone response (115).

Also proposed as a mechanism for increasing muscle size, and something that has been debated by exercise scientists for years, is hyperplasia. **Hyperplasia** is the term given to an increase in the number of muscle fibers via longitudinal fiber splitting in response to high-intensity resistance training. Hyperplasia has been shown to occur in animals (68, 87), but the findings are controversial in humans, with some studies providing support (129, 132, 191) and others rejecting its occurrence in humans (131). Part of the reason for this confusion may arise from cross-sectional studies comparing resistance-trained athletes to untrained individuals, showing a greater number of fibers in the trained population. In this scenario it is difficult to determine if the difference is due to genetics or hyperplasia. One must also consider that the procedures scientists perform on animals simply cannot be done on humans for ethical and logistical reasons. Consequently, some of the more convincing data supporting skeletal muscle hyperplasia emerge from animal studies (68, 87). When examining hyperplasia in animal models, researchers remove whole muscle and strip back the fascia in order to analyze muscle fiber numbers longitudinally under a microscope. In humans, removal of whole muscle is not feasible. Instead, needle biopsies techniques are used to harvest a small sample of muscle tissue, which is then examined in cross section, and a prediction of hyperplasia is made indirectly from extrapolation mathematics. While hyperplasia cannot be completely ruled out, it does not appear to be a major strategy for muscle tissue adaptation to resistance training; and, if it occurs at all, it involves only a small amount of the stimulated tissue (maybe less than 10%) if the conditions are optimal. It may be hypothesized that if hyperplasia occurs, it may be in response to muscle fibers reaching a theoretical upper limit in size, which may occur in athletes using anabolic steroids and other growth agents or undergoing long-term training that produces large to extreme levels of hypertrophy. This remains to be fully elucidated and continues to be an area of contention among scientific researchers.

Fiber Size Changes

The magnitude of muscle hypertrophy experienced following anaerobic training is intimately associated with muscle fiber type. Muscle fibers, in particular those within the high-threshold motor units governed by the size principle, must be activated in order to promote significant hypertrophy (36). During resistance training, both Type I and Type II muscle fibers have the potential to be recruited, with the frequency at which they are recruited ultimately determining the extent of their adaptive processes. According to the size principle, only following hierarchical activation do Type I or Type II fibers receive a signaling mechanism that initiates the cascade of regulatory processes promoting protein synthesis. Collectively, however, following muscle fiber activation these hypertrophic responses translate into enlarged CSA of the intact muscle after several months of training. Typically, Type II fibers manifest greater increases in size than Type I fibers; thus the magnitude

of hypertrophy is not uniform between the two major fiber types (83). In fact, it has been argued that the ultimate potential for hypertrophy may reside in the relative proportion of Type II fibers within a given athlete's muscles (131, 191). That is, athletes who genetically possess a relatively large proportion of fast-twitch fibers may have a greater potential for increasing muscle mass than individuals possessing predominately slow-twitch fibers.

Fiber Type Transitions

The pattern of neural stimulation dictates the extent to which fiber type adaptations occur following anaerobic training. Muscle fibers are theoretically positioned on a continuum from the least oxidative to the most oxidative type (see figure 5.3 and the description of muscle fiber types in chapter 1). The continuum is as follows: IIx, IIax, IIa, IIac, IIc, Ic, and I, with a concomitant myosin heavy chain (MHC) expression (i.e., MHC IIx, IIa, and I) (181). Although the proportions of Type I and Ix fibers are genetically determined (154), changes within each subtype can occur following anaerobic training. With training and activation of the high-threshold motor units, there is a transition from Type IIx to IIa fiber type (25). In other words, Type IIx muscle fibers change their myosin adenosine triphosphatase (ATPase) isoform content and progressively become more oxidative IIa fibers. In fact, research has shown nearly full transitions from Type IIx to IIa fiber profiles following the combination of high-intensity resistance and aerobic endurance training (112). The changes in fast-twitch fiber types have typically not been linked to the rate at which changes in the muscle fiber CSA take place.

Type IIx fibers represent a "reservoir" that, upon consistent activation, changes into a more oxidative form along the continuum (i.e., to an intermediate fiber Type IIax and then to a IIa) (25). Any change in the muscle fiber type continuum and associated MHCs occurs in the early stages of a resistance training program. In an early study, Staron and colleagues (183) examined the

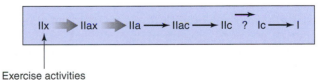

Exercise activities

FIGURE 5.3 Muscle fiber transitions occur during training. This means that a shift of the type of myosin adenosine triphosphatase (ATPase) and heavy chains takes place during training. Transformations from IIx to IIax to IIa can be seen, and then small percentages change to IIac and IIc. Exercise activities that recruit motor units with Type IIx muscle fibers initiate a shift toward IIa fibers.

effects of a high-intensity resistance training protocol (multiple sets of squat, leg press, and knee extension exercises using 6- to 12RM loads and 2-minute rest periods) performed by men and women two times per week for eight weeks. They reported a significant decrease in the Type IIx percentage in women after just two weeks of training (four workouts) and in the men after four weeks of training (eight workouts). Over the eight-week training program, Type IIx fiber types decreased from ~18% to about 7% of the total muscle fibers in both men and women. Analysis of the MHCs showed that in this early phase of training, IIx MHCs were replaced with IIa MHCs. In addition, this study demonstrated that changes in hormonal factors (testosterone and cortisol interactions) correlated with changes in muscle fiber type. Interestingly, detraining has the opposite effect, resulting in an increase in Type IIx fibers and a reduction in Type IIa fibers (153), with a possible overshoot of Type IIx fibers (i.e., higher IIx percentages than observed pretraining ([10]). While transformation within muscle fiber subtypes appears typical, transformation from Type I to Type II or vice versa appears less probable, most likely due to differing MHC isoforms and relative oxidative enzyme content (155). Whether these transformations are possible remains doubtful at this point, as insufficient evidence is currently available. These possibilities need to be explored in future studies; it is intriguing to consider whether or not the continuum of adaptations extends beyond Type I and II subpopulations, especially in extreme cases in which a marathon runner (high percentage of Type I fibers) follows a high-intensity resistance training program or a powerlifter (high percentage of Type II fibers) begins an extensive aerobic endurance training program.

Structural and Architectural Changes

Pennate muscle has fascicles that attach obliquely (in a slanted position) to its tendon. **Pennation angle** affects the force production capabilities as well as the range of motion of a muscle. Larger pennation angles can also accommodate greater protein deposition and allow for greater increases in CSA (2). In pennate muscle, resistance training has been shown to increase the angle of pennation, with strength-trained athletes displaying larger pennation angles in the triceps brachii and vastus lateralis muscles compared to untrained individuals (2). In addition, fascicle length has been shown to be greater in strength-trained athletes (94), and fascicle length of the gastrocnemius and vastus lateralis has been found to be greater in sprinters compared to distance runners (6). The combination of resistance, sprint, and jump training has been shown to increase rectus femoris fascicle length; and sprint and jump training have been shown to increase vastus lateralis fascicle length (20).

These architectural changes have a positive effect on the manner in which force is ultimately transmitted to tendons and bones.

Other Muscular Adaptations

Resistance training has been shown to increase myofibrillar volume (128), cytoplasmic density (132), sarcoplasmic reticulum and T-tubule density (9), and sodium–potassium ATPase activity (71). Collectively, these changes act to facilitate hypertrophy and enable greater expression of muscular strength. Sprint training has been shown to enhance calcium release (150), which assists in increasing speed and power production by promoting actin and myosin crossbridge formation.

Heavy resistance training has also been shown to reduce mitochondrial density (133). While the number of mitochondria actually remains constant or can slightly increase throughout a training phase, mitochondrial density is expressed relative to muscle area. Increases in muscle CSA occur disproportionately to mitochondrial proliferation, and consequently the density of mitochondria per unit volume is actually found to decrease with hypertrophy. Muscle hypertrophy also results in decreased capillary density by similar mechanisms, again with the number of capillaries per fiber actually increasing somewhat (184). Powerlifters and weightlifters show significantly lower capillary densities than control subjects, whereas bodybuilders have capillary densities similar to those of nonathletes (107). Bodybuilding workouts produce large hydrogen ion concentrations, but having more capillaries per fiber may assist in the clearance of metabolites from exercising muscle (111, 190).

Anaerobic exercise results in substantial reductions in muscle and blood pH (33), with several mechanisms regulating a change in acid–base balance during exercise. With adaptations to consistent acute changes in pH during training (i.e., increased H^+ concentration), buffering capacity can improve. This increased capacity then allows an athlete to better tolerate the accumulation of H^+ within the working muscle, resulting in delayed fatigue and greater muscular endurance (175). By its nature, high-intensity interval training (sprints, cycling) performed above the lactate threshold has been shown to significantly increase buffering capacity by 16% to 38% (17, 175). Elsewhere, athletes competing in anaerobic team sports have been shown to have higher buffering capacity than endurance athletes and untrained control subjects (47).

Within skeletal muscle, substrate content and enzyme activity represent further areas of adaptation in response to anaerobic training. Most notably, when ATP and creatine phosphate (CP) concentrations are repeatedly exhausted following bouts of intermittent high-intensity muscular contraction, the storage capacity of these high-energy compounds is increased via a "supercompensation" effect. MacDougall and colleagues (135) reported a 28% increase in resting CP and an 18% increase in ATP concentrations following five months of resistance training (i.e., three to five sets of 8-10 repetitions with 2-minute rest periods). In addition, it appears that bodybuilding-style programs such as this, which stress anaerobic glycolysis, may also be a potent stimulus for enhancement of glycogen content, as this was found to increase up to 112%.

Connective Tissue Adaptations

Bone, tendons, ligaments, fascia, and cartilage are examples of connective tissue. Anaerobic exercise imparts mechanical forces that cause deformation of specific regions of the skeleton. These forces, created by muscular actions on the tendinous insertion into bone, can be bending, compressive, or torsional. In response to

mechanical loading, **osteoblasts** migrate to the bone surface and begin bone modeling (figure 5.4). Osteoblasts manufacture and secrete proteins—primarily collagen molecules—that are deposited in the spaces between bone cells to increase strength. These proteins form the **bone matrix** and eventually become mineralized as calcium phosphate crystals (**hydroxyapatite**). New bone formation occurs predominantly on the outer surface of the bone (**periosteum**), increasing diameter and strength.

General Bone Physiology

The rate of bone adaptation occurs differently in the axial (skull-cranium, vertebral column, ribs, and sternum) and appendicular (shoulder girdle, pelvis, and bones of the upper and lower extremities) skeleton, owing to differing amounts of **trabecular** (spongy) **bone** and **cortical** (compact) **bone**. Cortical bone is dense and forms a compact outer shell surrounding the trabecular bone, with the two types of bone linked by interlocking narrow and delicate plates of trabecular bone. The

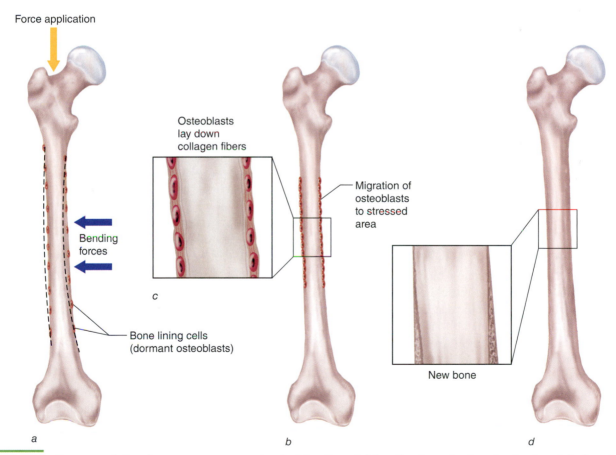

FIGURE 5.4   Bone modeling in response to mechanical loading. *(a)* Application of a longitudinal weight-bearing force causes the bone to bend (as depicted by the dotted line), creating a stimulus for new bone formation at the regions experiencing the greatest deformation. *(b)* Osteoblasts lay down additional collagen fibers at the site. *(c)* Previously dormant osteoblasts migrate to the area experiencing the strain. *(d)* The collagen fibers become mineralized, and the bone diameter effectively increases.

spaces between the trabecular plates are occupied by bone marrow that consists of adipose tissue and blood products such as immature red blood cells. Blood vessels from the marrow cavity extend into the dense cortical bone through a network of vertical and horizontal canals. Because it is less dense and has a greater surface area–to–mass ratio, trabecular bone is able to respond more rapidly to stimuli than cortical bone as it is softer, weaker, and more flexible and therefore more inclined to adaptive change.

The term **minimal essential strain (MES)** refers to the threshold stimulus that initiates new bone formation. Consistently exceeding these thresholds signals osteoblasts to migrate to the region experiencing the stress and to form bone, while forces that fall below the MES do not present an appropriate stimulus for new bone formation. Bone cells work to regulate the formation of new bone tissue such that forces experienced on a regular basis do not exceed the MES, thereby establishing a margin of safety against fracture. Strain registered by bone is a function of the force per unit area of bone (stress). The MES is thought to be approximately 1/10 of the force required to fracture bone. Increasing the diameter of bone allows the force to be distributed over a larger surface area, thereby decreasing the amount of mechanical stress. Following bone growth, a force that previously exceeded the MES will now be below the MES threshold. Progressive weight-bearing physical activities that generate forces exceeding the MES are therefore the most effective at increasing bone size and strength.

> Forces that reach or exceed a threshold stimulus initiate new bone formation in the area experiencing the mechanical strain.

Anaerobic Training and Bone Growth

As muscular strength and hypertrophy increase in response to anaerobic training modalities, the forces generated by the increased muscle contractions subsequently increase the mechanical stress on bone, and the bone itself must increase in mass and strength to provide an adequate support structure. Any increase in muscle strength or mass may therefore result in a corresponding increase in **bone mineral density (BMD)**, or the quantity of mineral deposited in a given area of the bone (93). Interestingly, inactivity or immobilization has the opposite effect and results in a more rapid rate of loss of bone matrix and BMD (178). Numerous studies have shown a positive correlation between BMD and muscle strength and mass (158, 198). Researchers have reported that resistance-trained athletes have higher BMD than age-matched sedentary control subjects (28, 29, 164). In some individuals (e.g., professional soccer players),

physical activity seems to influence bone mass, area, and width more than BMD (198). Thus, exercise that stimulates muscle hypertrophy and strength gains also appears to stimulate bone growth.

Quantitatively, the time course for bone adaptations is rather long—approximately six months or longer (27)—and depends intimately on the structure of the program. However, the process of adaptation begins within the first few workouts. The process of osteogenesis involves secretion of substances into the blood (substances specific to bone only) that can be measured. Therefore, any elevation in an osteogenic marker can be recognized as an early indicator of bone formation and presumably a precursor to increased BMD, provided that the stimulus is maintained over a long training period.

Principles of Training to Increase Bone Strength

Anaerobic training programs that have the objective to stimulate bone growth need to incorporate specificity of loading, speed and direction of loading, sufficient volume, appropriate exercise selection, progressive overload, and variation (30). **Specificity of loading** demands the use of exercises that directly load the particular region of interest of the skeleton. If the body interprets these forces as new or novel, they will stimulate bone growth in the area that is receiving the strain. For example, running may be a good stimulus for increased BMD in the femur but the wrong choice for promoting mineral deposits when one is trying to strengthen the wrist. The concept of specificity of loading becomes particularly important when a strength and conditioning professional prescribes exercises to increase bone mass in regions of the skeleton most commonly affected by **osteoporosis**—a disease in which BMD and bone mass become reduced to critically low levels. Research indicates that high-impact cyclical loading exercises for the lower body, such as gymnastics (187), volleyball, or basketball (42), selectively increase BMD at clinically relevant sites such as the hip and spine more than lower-impact activities do. Additionally, increases in BMD may be seen in highly trained college athletes already possessing high levels of BMD. These changes in BMD are independent of reproductive hormonal status if the stimulus is sufficient (187).

Exercise selection is critical when one is trying to elicit maximal **osteogenic stimuli** (factors that stimulate new bone formation). In essence, exercises should involve multiple joints, should direct the force vectors primarily through the spine and hip (i.e., **structural exercises**), and should apply external loads heavier than those with single-joint assistance exercises. Cussler and colleagues (35) showed a positive linear relationship between the amounts of weight lifted over the course of a training year and associated increases in BMD. In addition, the findings of this research highlighted the importance of exercise specificity in that the squat, compared to seated leg press, was more effective for increasing BMD in the trochanter of the femur (35). The use of single-joint, machine-based exercises should be limited, as these exercises isolate a single muscle group by using equipment as support to stabilize the body rather than promoting skeletal support. Therefore, exercises such as the back squat, power clean, deadlift, snatch, and push jerk (for the axial skeleton and lower body) and the shoulder press (for the upper body) are recommended as more effective methods for increasing bone strength.

Because bone responds favorably to mechanical forces, the principle of **progressive overload**—progressively placing greater than normal demands on the exercising musculature—applies when one is training to increase bone mass (70, 196). Although the maximal strength of bone is maintained well above the voluntary force capabilities of the associated musculature, bone responds to higher forces (e.g., 1- to 10RM loads) that are repetitively applied over time. The adaptive response of bone ensures that forces do not exceed a critical level that increases the risk of **stress fractures** (microfractures in bone due to structural fatigue). Support for progressive overload comes from studies that have compared BMD of various groups of athletes to that of nonathletes (42, 198). In fact, elite adolescent weightlifters have been found to possess levels of bone mineralization that far exceed values found in untrained adults (29, 91). This observation is interesting because it indicates that young bone may be more responsive to osteogenic stimuli than mature bone. Evidence indicates that physical activity during growth modulates the external geometry and trabecular architecture of bone, potentially enhancing skeletal strength (84). Recent evidence shows that physical activity–associated bone loading during skel-etal growth (i.e., adolescence) and after skeletal growth (i.e., early adulthood) elevates **peak bone mass** and is positively associated with adult bone mass in later life (186).

Another important consideration in the design of programs to stimulate new bone formation is training variation. The internal architecture of the human skeleton has a mechanism through which it compensates for new strain patterns experienced by the bone. To optimally dissipate the imposed forces, the direction of the collagen fibers within the bone matrix may change to conform to the lines of stress experienced by the bone. Thus, changing the distribution (and direction) of the force vectors by using a variety of exercises continually presents a unique stimulus for new bone formation within a given region of bone. Subsequently, collagen formation occurs in multiple directions, increasing bone strength in various directions. Overall, if the magnitude of the load or the rate of force application is sufficient, it is not typically necessary to perform more than a total of 30 to 35 repetitions, as a greater volume of loading is not likely to provide any additional stimulus for bone growth (57, 178).

> ▶ The components of mechanical load that stimulate bone growth are the magnitude of the load (intensity), rate (speed) of loading, direction of the forces, and the volume of loading (number of repetitions).

Adaptations of Tendons, Ligaments, and Fascia to Anaerobic Training

Tendons, ligaments, fascia, and cartilage are complex and dynamic structures that are the critical link between muscles and bones. The primary structural component of all connective tissue is the **collagen** fiber (Type I for bone, tendon, and ligaments and Type II for cartilage;

How Can Athletes Stimulate Bone Formation?

In order to promote bone formation, athletes should use specific programming of acute training variables in order to maximize optimal adaptations.

- Select multijoint, structural exercises that involve many muscle groups at once. Avoid isolated, single-joint movements.
- Select exercises that direct axial force vectors through the spine and hip and apply heavier loads than single-joint assistance exercises.
- Use the principle of progressive overload to stress the musculoskeletal system, and continue to progressively increase load as the tissues become accustomed to the stimulus.
- Use both heavy-load exercises and ballistic or high-impact exercises to expose the bone to different intensities of force.
- By varying exercise selection, it is possible to change the distribution of force insults and present a unique stimulus for new bone formation.

figure 5.5). The parent protein, **procollagen**, is synthesized and secreted by fibroblasts, which are the most common cells found in the connective tissue of animals and act as stem cells in the synthesis of the extracellular matrix, as well as playing a critical role in wound healing. Procollagen molecules consist of three protein strands twisted around each other in a triple helix. Procollagen leaves the cell with protective extensions on the ends to prevent premature collagen formation. Cleavage of the extensions via enzymes results in the formation of active collagen that aligns with other collagen molecules to form a long filament. Measurement of these enzymes provides an indication of collagen metabolism. In fact, enzyme levels increase in response to training, thereby showing increased net Type I collagen synthesis (125). The parallel arrangement of filaments is called a **microfibril**. Collagen has a striated (striped) appearance under a light microscope, somewhat like skeletal muscle, owing to the orderly alignment of the gaps between the collagen molecules within a microfibril. As bone grows, microfibrils become arranged into fibers, and the fibers into larger bundles. The true strength of collagen comes from the strong chemical bonds (**cross-linking**) that form between adjacent collagen molecules throughout the collagen bundles. Collagen bundles are bunched together longitudinally to form tendons or ligaments, or

are arranged in sheets with the layers oriented in different directions, as found in bone, cartilage, and fascia.

Tendons and ligaments are composed primarily of tightly packed, parallel arrangements of collagen bundles. Mature tendons and ligaments contain relatively few cells. The small number of metabolically active cells in tendons and ligaments makes the requirement for oxygen and nutrients in these tissues relatively low. Ligaments contain elastic fibers (**elastin**) in addition to collagen, as a certain amount of stretch is needed within a ligament to allow normal joint motion. Tendons and ligaments attach to bone with great strength, allowing the maximal transmission of forces. The fibrous connective tissues that surround and separate the different organizational levels within skeletal muscle are referred to as fascia. Fascia has sheets of fibrocollagenous support tissue, containing bundles of collagen fibers arranged in different planes, to provide resistance to forces from different directions. Fascia within muscles converges near the end of the muscle to form a tendon through which the force of muscle contraction is transmitted to bone. Compared with that of muscle tissue, tendon metabolism is much slower due to poorer vascularity and circulation (92). In fact, the increase in blood flow to skeletal muscle via exercise is not paralleled by the same flow perfusion in tendons (99). This limited

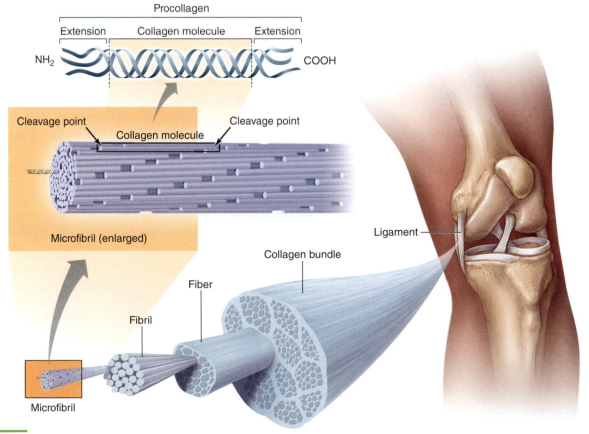

FIGURE 5.5 Formation of a collagen fiber.

vascularity has implications for regeneration and is the reason tendons can take significant amounts of time to heal following injury.

The primary stimulus for growth of tendons, ligaments, and fascia is the insult from mechanical forces created during high-intensity exercise. The degree of tissue adaptation appears to be proportional to the intensity of exercise (99). Consistent anaerobic exercise that exceeds the threshold of strain has a positive effect on stimulating connective tissue changes (92).

Empirical evidence suggests that connective tissues must increase their functional capabilities in response to increased muscle strength and hypertrophy. The sites where connective tissues can increase strength and load-bearing capacity are

- the junctions between the tendon (and ligament) and bone surface,
- within the body of the tendon or ligament, and
- in the network of fascia within skeletal muscle (99).

As muscles become stronger, they pull on their bony attachments with greater force and cause an increase in bone mass at the tendon–bone junction and along the line over which the forces are distributed.

High-intensity anaerobic training results in connective tissue growth and other ultrastructural changes that enhance force transmission. Specific changes within a tendon that contribute to its increase in size and strength include the following:

- An increase in collagen fibril diameter
- A greater number of covalent cross-links within the hypertrophied fiber
- An increase in the number of collagen fibrils
- An increase in the packing density of collagen fibrils

Collectively, these adaptations increase the tendon's ability to withstand greater tensional forces (143).

Muscle hypertrophy in animals relates to an increase in the number and size of fibroblasts, thereby resulting in a greater supply of total collagen. Activation of fibroblasts and subsequent growth of the connective tissue network are prerequisites for hypertrophy of active muscle (142). This may explain why biopsies of trained athletes have shown that hypertrophied muscle contains greater total collagen than in untrained individuals but that the collagen content remains proportional to the existing muscle mass (143). Recent studies indicate that **tendon stiffness** (force transmission per unit of strain, or tendon elongation) increases as a result of resistance training (123). In fact, Kubo and colleagues (121) reported a 15% to 19% increase in Achilles tendon stiffness following eight weeks of resistance training. The intensity of exercise is critical, as heavy loads (80% of 1RM) increase tendon stiffness but light loads (20% of 1RM) do not (122).

Adaptations of Cartilage to Anaerobic Training

Cartilage is a dense connective tissue capable of withstanding considerable force without damage to its structure. The main functions of cartilage are to

- provide a smooth joint articulating surface,
- act as a shock absorber for forces directed through the joint, and
- aid in the attachment of connective tissue to the skeleton.

How Can Athletes Stimulate Connective Tissue Adaptations?

Tendons, Ligaments, Fascia

- Long-term adaptations in tendons, ligaments, and fascia are stimulated through progressive high-intensity loading patterns using external resistances.
- High-intensity loads should be used, as low to moderate intensities do not markedly change the collagen content of connective tissue.
- Forces should be exerted throughout the full range of motion of a joint, and wherever possible multiple-joint exercises should be used.

Cartilage

- Moderate-intensity anaerobic exercise seems to be adequate for increasing cartilage thickness. Strenuous exercise does not appear to cause any degenerative joint disease when progressively overloaded appropriately.
- Tissue viability can be maintained by adopting a variety of exercise modalities and ensuring that load is applied throughout the range of motion.

A feature unique to cartilage is that it lacks its own blood supply and must depend on diffusion of oxygen and nutrients from synovial fluid (which is why cartilage does not easily repair itself following injury). Two primary types of cartilage are significant in relation to physical activity. **Hyaline cartilage** (articular cartilage) is found on the articulating surfaces of bones. **Fibrous cartilage** is a very tough form of cartilage found in the intervertebral disks of the spine and at the junctions where tendons attach to bone.

The fact that articular cartilage gets its nutrient supply via diffusion from synovial fluid provides a link for joint mobility to joint health. Movement about a joint creates changes in pressure in the joint capsule that drive nutrients from the synovial fluid toward the articular cartilage of the joint (180). Immobilization of a joint prevents proper diffusion of oxygen and essential nutrients throughout the joint. This results in the death of the healthy cells within cartilage, called chondrocytes, and a resorption of the cartilage matrix (195). Current understanding indicates that human cartilage undergoes atrophy, or thinning, when external loading is removed (e.g., postoperative immobilization and paraplegia). However, the effect that increased external loading has on average cartilage thickness remains to be fully elucidated (46). In any case, it is likely that genetic contribution plays a greater role in determining cartilage morphology.

Endocrine Responses and Adaptations to Anaerobic Training

Hormones have a variety of regulatory roles during anaerobic training and affect homeostatic mechanisms dedicated to keeping the body's functions within normal range during rest and exercise (60, 61, 102, 106, 109). These include the development of muscle, bone, and connective tissue through both anabolic and catabolic processes. As discussed in chapter 4, endocrine responses to anaerobic training can include (a) acute changes during and after exercise, (b) chronic changes in the acute response to a workout, (c) chronic changes in resting concentrations, and (d) changes in hormone receptor content.

Acute Anabolic Hormone Responses

Following anaerobic exercise (in particular resistance training), elevated concentrations of testosterone, molecular variants of growth hormone, and cortisol have been found for up to 30 minutes in men (104, 105, 115, 117). These fluctuations occur quickly and then rapidly stabilize in response to homeostatic challenges from the initial demands of acute exercise (119, 183) and longer-term training (136). The magnitude of elevation is greatest when large muscle mass exercises are performed, or during workouts with moderate to high intensity and volume combined with shorter rest intervals (111, 115) For example, high correlations exist between blood lactate (i.e., from high-intensity anaerobic exercise), growth hormone, and cortisol (78), and thus it is thought that hydrogen ion accumulation may be a primary factor influencing growth hormone and cortisol release. Elsewhere, elevations in free testosterone have been shown to be greater in resistance-trained men compared to aerobic-trained men (82, 193), with some studies reporting slight testosterone elevations in women following anaerobic exercise (149).

> The acute anabolic hormone response to anaerobic exercise is critical for exercise performance and subsequent training adaptations. Upregulation of anabolic hormone receptors is important for mediating the hormonal effects.

Insulin-like growth factor I (IGF-I) is a primary mediator of growth hormone; it acts as a hormonal messenger that stimulates growth-promoting effects in almost every cell of the body, especially skeletal muscle, cartilage, and bone. Insulin-like growth factor I has a delayed response to exercise and is dependent upon the acute growth hormone response. However, alternative *mechano growth factors* are upregulated in skeletal muscle in response to mechanical loading and act independently of growth hormone (66). Insulin secretion in comparison parallels blood glucose and amino acid changes, with insulin mostly affected by supplementation before, during, or after exercise and not by the anaerobic exercise stimulus (13). Catecholamines (epinephrine, norepinephrine, dopamine) reflect the acute demands of anaerobic exercise (22, 56, 105, 111), with increasing concentrations important for regulating force production, muscle contraction rate, energy availability, and augmentation of other hormones (e.g., testosterone).

Chronic Changes in the Acute Hormonal Response

Adherence to a long-term resistance training program results in an increased ability to exert greater levels of muscular force (80), with relative training intensities increasing over time as the body adapts to tolerate progressively heavier loads. As a consequence, acute endocrine responses to anaerobic training will likely mirror these improvements, as has been predominantly shown with growth hormone (34). The longitudinal changes in endocrine function reflect the increased exercise "stress" being tolerated by the body in response to incremental external loading. It is thus hypothesized that any chronic adaptations in acute hormonal response patterns potentially augment the ability to better tolerate and sustain prolonged higher exercise intensities.

Chronic Changes in Resting Hormonal Concentrations

Chronic changes in resting hormone concentrations following anaerobic exercise are unlikely, with research providing inconclusive changes in testosterone, growth hormone, IGF-I, and cortisol over time (115). Instead, resting concentrations likely reflect the current state of the muscle tissue in response to substantial changes to the training program (i.e., volume or intensity) and nutritional factors. It appears that the elevation during and immediately following a workout may present receptors with enough of a stimulus to affect tissue remodeling without the need for chronic elevations in basal concentrations (162). It is important to note that chronic elevations in an anabolic hormone may be counterproductive over the long term. Receptors tend to downregulate over time when exposed consistently to high levels of hormones. For example, in type 2 diabetes mellitus, sensitivity of skeletal muscle to insulin is reduced due to chronic elevated blood insulin. This is why anabolic steroid users repeatedly cycle drug use rather than maintaining consistently high doses.

Hormone Receptor Changes

Receptor content is important for mediating the adaptations elicited by any hormonal response. Androgen receptors (AR) have received much attention in the literature, and their content (i.e., number of receptors per area on the target tissue) depends on several factors including muscle fiber type, contractile activity, and the concentrations of testosterone. Resistance training has been shown to upregulate AR content within 48 to 72 hours after the workout (15). The resistance exercise stimulus appears to mediate the magnitude of acute AR modifications. Ratamess and colleagues (162) compared one set versus six sets of 10 repetitions of squats and reported no differences in AR content following the single-set protocol; however, the higher-volume protocol elicited significant downregulation of AR content 1 hour after the workout. This study also demonstrated that when sufficient volume is reached, AR protein content may initially downregulate, before the upregulation that has been shown in other studies. However, Kraemer and colleagues (118) have shown that consumption of a protein-carbohydrate supplement before and after the workout attenuates this AR downregulation.

Cardiovascular and Respiratory Responses to Anaerobic Exercise

Both acute bouts of anaerobic exercise and long-term anaerobic training have a significant impact on cardiovascular and respiratory function. This is reflected in both anaerobic athletes (51) and sedentary individuals (97), where enhanced cardiac function and dimensions are apparent. Heavy-load resistance training can benefit the cardiovascular system, but differently from resistance training with more repetitions of light loads and less rest or conventional aerobic endurance training (52). Improved ability of the heart, lungs, and circulatory system to function under conditions of high pressure and force production can prepare the athlete's body for the extreme demands of sporting competition.

Acute Cardiovascular Responses to Anaerobic Exercise

An acute bout of anaerobic exercise significantly increases cardiovascular responses. Heart rate, stroke volume, cardiac output, and blood pressure all increase significantly during resistance exercise. Peak blood pressures of 320/250 mmHg and a heart rate of 170 beats/min have been reported during a high-intensity (i.e., 95% of 1RM) leg press exercise (134). Generally, the blood pressure response increases nonlinearly with the magnitude of active muscle mass and is higher during the concentric phase of each repetition than during the eccentric phase, especially at the "sticking point" of an exercise. Although large elevations in blood pressure have been reported, there are limited data to indicate that resistance training has any negative effects on resting blood pressure (31). In addition, intrathoracic pressure increases, and plasma volume reductions of up to 22% have been reported (157, 162).

> **Acute anaerobic exercise results in increased cardiac output, stroke volume, heart rate, oxygen uptake, systolic blood pressure, and blood flow to active muscles.**

During a set of resistance exercise, stroke volume and cardiac output increase mostly during the eccentric phase of each repetition, especially when the Valsalva technique is used (see chapter 2) (49). Because the concentric phase of a repetition is much more difficult and elevations in intrathoracic and intra-abdominal pressures are more prominent (via the Valsalva maneuver), limiting venous return and reducing end-diastolic volume, the hemodynamic response of resistance exercise is delayed such that cardiac output increases more during the eccentric phase or during the rest period between sets. This is especially true for an individual's heart rate response; during the first 5 seconds after completion of a set, heart rate is higher than during the set itself (160).

The degree to which blood flow is increased in the working muscles during anaerobic training is dependent on a number of factors, including (a) the intensity of resistance, (b) the length of time of the effort (i.e., the number of repetitions performed), and (c) the size of the muscle mass activated. When lower resistances are lifted for many repetitions, the responses are relatively similar to those observed during aerobic exercise (64). However, heavy resistance exercise decreases blood flow to the working muscles as a result of contracted muscle tissue's clamping down on capillaries and creating a localized occlusion. Muscular contractions greater than 20% of maximal voluntary contraction impede peripheral blood flow within the muscle during a set, but blood flow increases during the subsequent rest period (**reactive hyperemia**) (116). Interestingly, the lack of blood flow (and subsequent increase in metabolites such as hydrogen ions and reduction in pH) during heavy external loading is a potent stimulus for muscle growth (188). Overall, the magnitude of the acute cardiovascular responses depends on the intensity and volume of exercise, muscle mass involvement, rest period length, and contraction velocity (113, 160).

Chronic Cardiovascular Adaptations at Rest

The effect of anaerobic training modalities on resting heart rate remains to be fully elucidated. Short-term resistance training has been shown to decrease resting heart rate between 5% and 12% (53, 57). However, when this effect is studied longitudinally over time, mixed responses are reported, with either no change in resting heart rate or reductions of 4% to 13% (53, 57). In chronically resistance-trained athletes (e.g., bodybuilders, powerlifters, weightlifters), both average and lower than average resting heart rates (60-78 beats/min) have been reported compared to those in untrained individuals.

A meta-analysis of resting blood pressure indicated that both systolic and diastolic blood pressure decreased by 2% to 4% as an adaptation to resistance training (95). It appears that the response is greatest in those individuals who initially have a slightly elevated blood pressure. Similarly, the **rate–pressure product** (heart rate $\times$ systolic blood pressure; a measure of myocardial work) has been shown to either remain constant or decrease following resistance training (52, 53). Stroke volume has been shown to increase in absolute magnitude, but not relative to body surface area or lean body mass (53). That is, stroke volume will increase as lean tissue mass

increases during long-term resistance training. Lastly, resistance training may either not change or slightly decrease total cholesterol and low-density lipoproteins and increase high-density lipoproteins (90). Therefore, heavy resistance training does little to enhance resting cardiac function, but greater improvements may result from adaptations to a high-volume program with short rest periods (i.e., bodybuilding, circuit training) in which the overall continuity of the exercise stress in a workout is much higher.

Chronic resistance training also alters cardiac dimensions. Increased left ventricular wall thickness and mass have been reported, but the increase disappears when expressed relative to body surface area or lean body mass (52, 53). It is thought that this increase may result from exposure to intermittently elevated blood pressures and increases in intrathoracic pressure in addition to accommodating changes from increases in lean body mass and body size. Highly resistance-trained athletes have greater than normal absolute posterior left ventricular and intraventricular septum wall thickness (55). Little or no change in left ventricular chamber size or volume is observed with resistance training; this is a major difference between resistance exercise and aerobic exercise. Greater than normal absolute left and right ventricular end-diastolic and end-systolic volumes have been reported in bodybuilders but not weightlifters (55), which indicates that high-volume training may be more conducive to increasing absolute left ventricular volumes. It is important to note that bodybuilders frequently incorporate aerobic exercise into their training programs in an effort to metabolize body fat and promote a lean body composition; therefore, it is possible that some of these adaptations have been brought about, in part, by aerobic endurance training. Bodybuilders as well as weightlifters have greater than normal absolute and relative (to lean body mass and body surface) left atrial internal dimensions, with the bodybuilders showing a significantly greater dimension (37).

Chronic Adaptations of the Acute Cardiovascular Response to Anaerobic Exercise

Chronic resistance training reduces the cardiovascular response to an acute bout of resistance exercise of a given absolute intensity or workload. Short-term studies have shown that resistance training results in adaptations that blunt the acute increases in heart rate, blood pressure, and double product caused by the resistance training workout (139, 169). In addition, male bodybuilders have been found to have lower systolic and diastolic blood pressure and heart rates during sets of 50% to 100% of 1RM performed to momentary muscular failure compared to both sedentary and lesser-trained men (54). Interestingly, bodybuilders' peak cardiac output and stroke volume are significantly greater than those of powerlifters (49), demonstrating that stroke volume and cardiac output may be greater per absolute workload as a result of training. It is thought that these adaptations result from a decreased afterload on the left ventricle, which in turn increases cardiac output and decreases myocardial oxygen consumption (49). Lastly, oxygen extraction is generally not improved with resistance training using heavy loads and low volume. It is enhanced to a greater extent with continuous aerobic exercise or perhaps slightly with a resistance training program using high volume and short rest periods (116).

Ventilatory Response to Anaerobic Exercise

Ventilation rate generally does not limit resistance exercise and is either unaffected or only moderately improved by anaerobic training. With resistance exercise, ventilation is significantly elevated during each set, but the elevation is even greater during the first minute of recovery (160). Ventilations in excess of 60 L/min have been reported (160), and the rest interval length had a large effect such that short rest intervals (30 seconds to 1 minute) produced the most substantial elevation. Training adaptations include increased tidal volume and breathing frequency with maximal exercise. With submaximal activity, however, breathing frequency is often reduced while tidal volume is increased. It appears that such ventilatory adaptations result from local, neural, or chemical adaptations in the specific muscles trained through exercise (14). Additionally, improved ventilation efficiency, as characterized by reduced **ventilatory equivalent** for oxygen (the ratio of air ventilated to oxygen used by the tissues, $\dot{V}_E/\dot{V}O_2$), is observed in trained versus untrained individuals (14).

Compatibility of Aerobic and Anaerobic Modes of Training

Strength/power training and work capacity–endurance training have divergent physiology that presents a programming challenge to the strength and conditioning professional working to optimize concurrent gains in both these physical and physiological characteristics. Combining resistance and aerobic endurance training may interfere with strength and power gains, primarily if the aerobic endurance training is high in intensity, volume, or frequency (44, 86, 112). Callister and colleagues (24) showed that simultaneous sprint and aerobic endurance training decreased sprint speed and jump power. Possible explanations for this less-than-optimal

power development include adverse neural changes and the alterations of muscle proteins in muscle fibers. In contrast, most studies have shown no adverse effects on aerobic power resulting from heavy resistance exercise despite the expected cellular changes caused by this type of exercise (112). Few studies have shown that resistance training can hinder $\dot{V}O_2$max improvements (65). Interestingly, Kraemer and colleagues (120) reported that women who performed both resistance exercise and aerobic endurance training had greater aerobic development than those who performed the aerobic endurance training alone. Such data have encouraged some athletes (e.g., distance runners) to add supplemental sport-specific resistance training to their total training regimen. Indeed, the majority of research indicates that heavy resistance training has very limited, if any, negative effects on aerobic power (197) but instead can serve to actually enhance performance in endurance sports (172).

In a study examining the potential incompatibility of strength and endurance exercise, Kraemer and colleagues (112) used three months of simultaneous high-intensity strength and aerobic endurance training under five conditions:

1. A combination group (C) that performed both resistance and aerobic endurance training
2. A group (UC) that performed upper body resistance and aerobic endurance training
3. A resistance training–only group (S)
4. An aerobic endurance training–only group (E)
5. A control group

The S group increased 1RM strength and rate of strength development more than did the C group. In addition, maximal oxygen consumption improvements were not affected by the simultaneous training (i.e., almost identical improvements in 2-mile [3.2 km] run times). Thus, no overtraining state for aerobic endurance was apparent.

A fascinating finding of the research by Kraemer and colleagues (112) was change in the muscle fiber size of the thigh musculature. Previous studies have shown decreases in muscle fiber size during aerobic endurance training (15, 65). Kraemer's group (112), however, indicated that the transformation of Type IIx to Type IIa fibers was almost complete in the S group (19.1±7.9% Type IIx pretraining to 1.9±0.8% posttraining) and C group (14.11±7.2% pre to 1.6±0.8% post). Interestingly, the UC and E groups (who performed only interval training) also had significant Type IIx fiber transformation after training (22.6±4.9% pre to 11.6±5.3% post for UC, and 19.2±3.6% pre to 8.8±4.4% post for E). This indicates that heavy resistance training recruits more of the Type IIx fibers than high-intensity aerobic endurance interval training. In addition, a small number (<3%) of

Type IIa fibers were converted to Type IIc fibers in the aerobic training group. The combined group increased muscle size only in Type IIa fibers, while the S group demonstrated increases in Type I, IIc, and IIa fibers. The lack of change in Type I fiber area and increase in Type IIa fiber area in the C group appear to represent a cellular adaptation that shows the antagonism of simultaneous strength and aerobic endurance stimuli, since strength training alone produced increases in both Type I and II muscle fiber areas. The E group showed decreased size in Type I and IIc fibers, presumably due to higher observed cortisol levels (and reduced testosterone) and their physiological need for shorter distances between capillary and cell to enhance oxygen kinetics.

The majority of studies use untrained subjects to examine the effects of simultaneous high-intensity resistance training and aerobic endurance training (65, 74, 127, 138). Few studies have looked at concurrent

What Performance Improvements Occur Following Anaerobic Exercise?

Muscular Strength

- A review of more than 100 studies has shown that mean strength can increase approximately 40% in "untrained," 20% in "moderately trained," 16% in "trained," 10% in "advanced," and 2% in "elite" participants over periods ranging from four weeks to two years (103).
- With training, a positive shift in muscle fiber types reflects an augmented recruitment of higher-order motor units. Type IIx fibers transition to Type IIa fibers and reflect a greater fatigue resistance at similar absolute force output.

Power

- The optimal load for maximizing absolute peak power output in the jump squat is 0% of 1RM (i.e., body weight [31]). However, it has been reported that peak power output is maximized in trained power athletes with higher loads corresponding to 30% to 60% of squat 1RM (12).
- Peak power in the squat is maximized at 56% of 1RM and in the power clean at 80% of 1RM (31).
- For the upper body, peak power output can be maximized during the ballistic bench press throw using loads corresponding to 46% to 62% of 1RM bench press (11).

Local Muscular Endurance

- Cross-sectional data in anaerobic athletes have shown enhanced muscular endurance and subsequent muscular adaptations consistent with improved oxidative and buffering capacity (100).
- Skeletal muscle adaptations to anaerobic muscular endurance training include fiber type transitions from Type IIx to Type IIb, as well as increases in mitochondrial and capillary numbers, buffering capacity, resistance to fatigue, and metabolic enzyme activity (64, 116).

Body Composition

- Resistance training can increase fat-free mass and reduce body fat by up to 9% (116).
- Increases in lean tissue mass, daily metabolic rate, and energy expenditure during exercise are outcomes of resistance training (53).

Flexibility

- Anaerobic training potentially can have a positive impact on flexibility, and a combination of resistance training and stretching appears to be the most effective method to improve flexibility with increasing muscle mass (116).

Aerobic Capacity

- In untrained people, heavy resistance training can increase $\dot{V}O_2max$ from 5% to 8%. In trained individuals, resistance training does not significantly affect aerobic capacity (52).
- Circuit training and programs using high volume and short rest periods (i.e., 30 seconds or less) have been shown to improve $\dot{V}O_2max$ (64).

Motor Performance

- Resistance training has been shown to increase running economy, vertical jump, sprint speed, tennis serve velocity, swinging and throwing velocity, and kicking performance (116).

training in elite athlete populations (172). Several studies have shown an incompatibility using three days a week of resistance training alternating with three days a week of aerobic endurance training (i.e., training on six consecutive days), or four to six days a week of combined high-intensity resistance and aerobic endurance training (16, 44, 112), thereby lending credibility to the suggestion that the onset of overtraining mechanisms could have played a role. When both modalities are performed during the same workout (yielding a frequency of three days a week with at least one day off between workouts), the incompatibility has not been shown as frequently (127, 137, 138). An exception was a study by Sale and colleagues (168), who showed that training four days (two days of resistance training and two days of aerobic endurance training) per week was better than training two days (combined resistance training and aerobic endurance training) per week for increasing leg press 1RM (25% vs. 13%). These studies show that increasing the recovery period between workouts may decrease the incompatibility, a principle supported by a recent meta-analysis of concurrent training by Wilson and colleagues (197).

Power development appears to be negatively affected more than strength during concurrent high-intensity resistance and aerobic endurance training. Häkkinen and colleagues (74) reported similar dynamic and isometric strength increases following 21 weeks of concurrent training or resistance training only; however, the resistance training–only group showed improvements in the rate of force development whereas the concurrent training group did not match this increase. Kraemer and colleagues (112) also showed that a resistance training–only group increased muscle power whereas a combined group did not. The resistance training–only group also increased peak power in upper and lower body tests while the combined group did not. It appears that power development is much more susceptible to the antagonistic effects of combined strength and aerobic endurance training than is slow-velocity strength (112). Lastly, the sequence may play a role in the magnitude of adaptation. Leveritt and Abernethy (126) examined lifting performance 30 minutes following a 25-minute aerobic exercise workout and found that the number of repetitions performed during the squat was reduced by 13% to 36% over three sets.

Overtraining

The goal of training is to provide incremental overload on the body so that physiological adaptations can subsequently contribute to improved performance. Successful training must not only involve overload, but must also avoid the combination of excessive overload with inadequate recovery (140). When training frequency, volume, or intensity (or some combination of these) is excessive without sufficient rest, recovery, and nutrient intake, conditions of extreme fatigue, illness, or injury (or more than one of these) can occur (110, 124, 185). This accumulation of training stress can result in *long-term* decrements in performance with or without associated physiological and psychological signs and symptoms of maladaptation, and is referred to as **overtraining**. Depending on the extent to which an athlete is overtrained, restoration of performance can take several weeks or months (81, 140).

When an athlete undertakes excessive training that leads to *short-term* decrements in performance, this temporary response has been termed **overreaching** or **functional overreaching (FOR)** (58, 163). Recovery from this condition is normally achieved within a few days or weeks of rest; consequently, overreaching can be prescribed as a planned phase in many training programs. The rationale is to overwork (to suppress performance and build up tolerance) and then taper in order to allow for a "supercompensation" in performance. In fact, it has been shown that short-term overreaching followed by an appropriate tapering period can result in beneficial strength and power gains (163). When mismanaged, however, it can lead to detrimental effects (144).

When the intensification of a training stimulus continues without adequate recovery and regeneration, an athlete can evolve into a state of extreme overreaching, or **nonfunctional overreaching (NFOR)**. This NFOR leads to stagnation and a decrease in performance that will continue for several weeks or months. When an athlete does not fully respect the balance between training and recovery, the first signs and symptoms of prolonged training distress are decreased performance, increased fatigue, decreased vigor, and hormonal disturbances. When those occur, it becomes difficult to differentiate between NFOR and what has been termed **overtraining syndrome (OTS)**. Central to the definition of OTS is a "prolonged maladaptation" not only of the athlete, but also of several biological, neurochemical, and hormonal regulation mechanisms. Many alternative terms have been suggested for OTS, including *burnout, chronic overwork, staleness, unexplained underperformance syndrome,* and *overfatigue* (21, 23). Figure 5.6 illustrates the progression that composes the overtraining continuum.

Overtraining syndrome can last as long as six months or beyond; and in the worst-case scenario, OTS can ruin an athletic career. Two distinct types of OTS have been proposed: sympathetic and parasympathetic. The **sympathetic overtraining syndrome** includes increased sympathetic activity at rest, whereas the **parasympathetic overtraining syndrome** involves increased

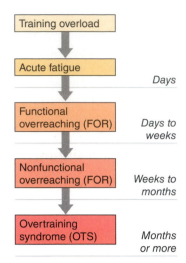

FIGURE 5.6   The overtraining continuum.

parasympathetic activity at rest and with exercise (140). The sympathetic syndrome is thought to develop before the parasympathetic syndrome and predominates in younger athletes who train for speed or power (58). Eventually all states of overtraining culminate in the parasympathetic syndrome and the chronic suppression of most physiological systems throughout the body (140). Because rebounds are possible, it is difficult to determine exactly when overtraining becomes chronic. In addition, some athletes respond positively to overreaching strategies (163) whereas for others, overreaching can be the catalyst for OTS.

A predominant feature of OTS is the inability to sustain high-intensity exercise when training load is maintained or increased (141). In many cases OTS is a consequence of prolonged NFOR, which in itself can result from mistakes in the prescription of training load and a mismanagement of the acute training variables (e.g., intensity, volume, rest). A common mistake in overtrained athletes is a rate of progressive overload that is too high. That is, increasing either the volume or intensity (or both) too rapidly over a period of several weeks or months with insufficient recovery can result in greater structural damage over time and, potentially, overtraining. A theoretical overview of anaerobic overtraining is presented in table 5.3.

For the purpose of investigating overtraining, deliberately causing OTS is not easy in a laboratory setting. What is more, while the symptoms of OTS are generally thought of as more severe than those of NFOR, there is no scientific evidence to confirm or refute this suggestion (140), making it hard to confirm that OTS has occurred. Instead, longitudinal monitoring of athletes has been the most practical way of documenting the physiological responses and performance effects of overtraining. The majority of this research has been conducted in endurance-type sports, where it is perhaps more prevalent. However, a survey of overtrained athletes showed that 77% were also involved in sports requiring high levels of strength, speed, or coordination (58). The symptoms of overtraining found in anaerobic activities (sympathetic) were also different from those in aerobic–endurance activities (parasympathetic) (23, 58).

TABLE 5.3   Theoretical Development of Anaerobic Overtraining

Stages of overtraining	Day(s)	Anaerobic performance							
		Performance	Neural	Skeletal muscle	Metabolic	Cardiovascular	Immune	Endocrine	Psychological
Acute fatigue	Day(s)	No effect or **increase**	Altered neuron function	—	—	—	—	—	—
Functional overreaching (FOR)	Days to weeks	**Temporary** decrease, returns to baseline	Altered motor unit recruitment	—	—	—	—	Altered sympathetic activity and hypothalamic control	—
Nonfunctional overreaching (NFOR)	Weeks to months	**Stagnation** or decrease	Decreased motor coordination	Altered excitation–contraction coupling	Decreased muscle glycogen	Increased resting heart rate and blood pressure	Altered immune function	Altered hormonal concentrations	Mood disturbances
Overtraining syndrome (OTS)	Many months to years	**Decrease**	—	Decreased force production	Decreased glycolytic capacity	—	Sickness and infection	—	Emotional and sleep disturbances

Reprinted, by permission, from Fry et al., 1993 (62); Meeusen et al., 2013 (140).

Sympathetic-type overtraining is a little more difficult to characterize than parasympathetic overtraining. It can be speculated that increased neural activity consequent to excessive motor unit activation may bring about this type of overtraining; however, there are many other factors that could potentially contribute. Adopting a short-term NFOR model (eight sets of machine squats with a 95% 1RM load for six consecutive days), Fry and colleagues (59) examined intensity-specific responses and reported nonspecific performance decreases in isokinetic torque production, longer sprint times, and longer agility times. They did, however, find that 1RM strength was preserved. In a subsequent study by Fry and associates (62), subjects performed 10 sets of 1RM over seven days with a day's rest. This resulted in a significant decrease (>9.9 pounds [4.5 kg]) in the 1RM in 73% of the subjects. Interestingly, some subjects made progress and did not reach a NFOR state. This demonstrates that the time course for the onset of overreaching or overtraining symptoms is greatly dependent on individual responses, training status, and genetic endowment.

Mistakes That Can Lead to Anaerobic Overtraining

The overtraining state is associated with damage to or negative physiological alterations in the neuromuscular system. As with any form of training, the structure of an anaerobic training program ultimately dictates the nature of the physical and physiological adaptations

---

What Are the Markers of Anaerobic Overtraining?

Although the knowledge of central pathological mechanisms of OTS has increased significantly, there remains a strong demand for relevant tools for the early identification of OTS. Until a definitive evaluative tool is developed, coaches and athletes need to use performance decrements as verification that overtraining is evident. The following criteria may be considered:

1. Is the athlete experiencing any of the following symptoms?
   - Unexplained underperformance
   - Persistent fatigue
   - Increased sense of effort during training
   - Disordered sleep patterns
   - Loss of appetite

2. Are the athlete's scores in maximal exercise tests, sport-specific performance tests, or vital signs assessments (heart rate, blood pressure) poorer than on previous tests or what would be considered normal or baseline?

3. Are there errors in the design of the athlete's training program?
   - Training volume increased significantly (<5%)
   - Training intensity increased significantly
   - Training monotony present
   - High number or frequency of competitions

4. Are there other confounding factors?
   - Psychological signs and symptoms (disturbed Profile of Mood States [POMS], higher than normal rating of perceived exertion [RPE])
   - Social factors (family, relationships, finances, work, coach, team)
   - Recent or multiple time zone travel

5. Does the athlete have any common exclusion criteria?
   - Confounding illnesses
   - Anemia
   - Infectious diseases
   - Muscle damage (high creatine kinase levels)
   - Endocrine disorders (diabetes, catecholamines, adrenal, thyroid)
   - Major eating disorders
   - Biological abnormalities (C-reactive protein, creatinine, decreased ferritin)
   - Musculoskeletal injury
   - Cardiologic symptoms
   - Adult-onset asthma
   - Allergies

It should be noted that no single marker can be taken as an indicator of impending OTS. A plethora of research (140, 185, 194) suggests that OTS is multifactorial in its nature and that regular monitoring of a combination of performance, physiological, biochemical, immunological, and psychological variables should be considered.

that take place in response to the training stimulus. A mistake in the prescription of any acute program variable could theoretically contribute to OTS if it is consistently repeated over time. This can often occur when highly motivated athletes use a high volume of heavy training loads with high training frequency and take limited rest to recover between workouts. Training volume has been shown to be important for augmenting continued gains in performance. Conversely, however, an excessively high volume of exercise can create a stimulus that exceeds the athlete's ability to recover from the stress and may result in excessive soreness and residual fatigue. Training periodization should therefore consist of careful planning to avoid overtraining.

Hormonal Markers of Anaerobic Overtraining

Regular monitoring of performance standards is central in any attempt to avoid the onset of NFOT or OTS, but some researchers have used biological markers to try to characterize anaerobic overtraining. Indeed, it has long been hypothesized that endocrine factors mediate the central dysfunction that occurs during the pathogenesis of OTS (140).

The resting plasma testosterone/cortisol ratio has long been considered an indicator of an overtraining state. This ratio decreases in relation to the intensity and duration of exercise; however, it is now evident that it indicates only the actual physiological strain of training and cannot be used for diagnostic purposes (43). A blunted rise in pituitary hormones (adrenocorticotropic hormone [ACTH], growth hormone, luteinizing hormone, follicle-stimulating hormone [FSH]) in response to a stressful stimulus has been reported (194). However, despite this seemingly uniform acute hormonal response following exercise, explaining the disturbance in the neuroendocrine system caused by OTS is not simple. Indeed, whether peripheral metabolic hormones can be used as accurate markers of OTS remains a topic of ongoing discussion. In efforts to predict overtraining responses from FOR, decreased resting concentrations of testosterone and IGF-I have been observed (159); but in response to resistance exercise, augmented acute testosterone responses are found in trained individuals with previous exposure to overreaching (61). *Volume-related overtraining* has been shown to increase cortisol and to decrease resting luteinizing hormone and total and free testosterone concentrations (58). In addition, the exercise-induced elevation in total testosterone can potentially be blunted (79).

Intensity-related overtraining does not appear to alter resting concentrations of hormones (58). Fry and colleagues (60) reported no changes in circulating testos-

terone, free testosterone, cortisol, and growth hormone concentrations during high-intensity anaerobic overtraining (e.g., 10 1RM sets of the squat exercise each day for two weeks). Interestingly, Meeusen and colleagues (141) have reported that the *training status* of an athlete has an impact on hypothalamic–pituitary reactivity, with differing neuroendocrine responses exhibited in response to NFOR. Initially, highly trained athletes are likely to experience a large, hypersensitive sympathetic hormone response, following which a suppression of circulating hormone concentrations will occur that reflects a down-regulation of pituitary sensitivity and long-term pituitary exhaustion (141). Collectively, endocrine responses appear to require longer than one week of monitoring in order to serve as adequate markers. What remains clear, however, is that the most effective biological markers are perhaps those that allow for early detection of NFOR, and it is this early recognition that will support the prevention of OTS.

Psychological Factors in Overtraining

Mood disturbances and psychological symptoms, as determined from the Profile of Mood States (POMS), have been associated with OTS in athletes for many years. Heavy resistance training is accompanied by decreased vigor, motivation, and confidence; raised levels of tension, depression, anger, fatigue, confusion, anxiety, and irritability; and impaired concentration (110). Altered psychological characteristics are also related to changing endocrine profiles (141). Many athletes sense overtraining by the associated psychological alterations that are often observed before actual decrements in performance occur. Monitoring the mood and mental state of an athlete is very important to gain insights into overtraining (111, 140).

Detraining

Detraining is the term given to a decrement in performance and loss of the accumulated physiological adaptations following the cessation of anaerobic training or when there is a substantial reduction in frequency, volume, intensity, or any combination of these variables. According to the principles of *reversibility,* training-induced adaptations are transient and thus can disappear when the training load is insufficient or removed completely. The result is a partial or complete loss of the anatomical, physiological, and performance adaptations that have been made. The magnitude of these losses is dependent on the length of the detraining period as well as the initial training status of the individual.

Following the removal of a training stimulus is a lag time before the effects of detraining are fully observed.

Strength performance in general is readily maintained for up to four weeks of inactivity; but in highly trained athletes, eccentric force and sport-specific power may decline significantly faster (146). In trained weightlifters, removing the training stimulus for 14 days did not significantly affect 1RM strength performance in the bench press (−1.7%) and squat (−0.9%), isometric (−7%) and isokinetic concentric knee extension force (−2.3%), or vertical jump performance (1.2%) (88). In recreationally trained men, very little change is seen during the first six weeks of detraining (108). Longer periods of training cessation are accompanied by significantly pronounced declines in the strength performance of strength-trained athletes (146), but this loss is still limited to 7% to 12% during periods of inactivity ranging from 8 to 12 weeks. This strength loss is coupled with decreased average maximal bilateral and unilateral intramuscular EMG. Indeed, strength reductions appear related to neural mechanisms initially, with atrophy predominating as the detraining period extends. Interestingly, the amount of muscle strength retained is rarely lower than pretraining values, indicating that resistance training has a residual effect when the stimulus is removed. However, when the athlete returns to training, the rate of strength reattainment is high, supporting the paradigm of "muscle memory."

With respect to muscle fiber characteristics following the cessation of training, it appears that fiber disruption remains unchanged during the initial weeks of inactivity, but oxidative fibers may increase in strength-trained athletes (decrease in endurance athletes) within eight weeks of stopping training (146). In strength-trained athletes, 14 days of inactivity has been reported to have no effect on muscle fiber type distribution (88). In comparison, muscle fiber cross-sectional area declines rapidly in strength and sprint athletes (146). In 12 trained weightlifters, Hortobagyi and colleagues (88) observed a decline of 6.4% in fast-twitch fiber cross-sectional area in 14 days. These changes specifically targeted fast-twitch fibers initially, with no significant change immediately found in the slow-twitch fiber population. Longer periods of stoppage bring about declines in both fast- and slow-twitch fiber cross-sectional area and muscle mass in anaerobically trained athletes. In professional rugby league players, cross-sectional area of fast-twitch fibers decreased more than that of slow-twitch fibers, with the former being 23% larger at the end of a competitive season but only 9% larger after six weeks without training (8). After seven months with no training, an average of 37.1% atrophy was observed in all fiber types of a powerlifter (182); in elite body builders after 13.5 months without training, fat-free mass, thigh and arm girth, and average fiber area decreased by 9.3%, 0.5%, 11.5%, and 8.3%, respectively (72).

Conclusion

Anaerobic exercise represents a specific type of training stress to the anatomy and various systems of the body, and adaptations consequent to anaerobic training are specific to the nature of the exercise performed. It is also apparent that an individual's age, nutrition, prior fitness level, and training motivation can affect adaptations. Integration of a training program that has many components requires careful planning and monitoring in order to minimize the occurrence of incompatibilities or overtraining. Explosive training evokes marked increases in muscular power, whereas more conventional heavy resistance training mainly increases muscle size and strength. Anaerobic training (resistance, sprint, plyometric, agility, high-intensity interval training) in general elicits specific adaptations in the nervous system leading to greater recruitment, rate of firing, synchronization, and enhanced muscle function that enable increases in strength and power.

Anaerobic training also has positive effects on bone, muscle, and the associated connective tissue; the entire musculoskeletal system undergoes a coordinated adaptation to exercise. Athletes undertaking strenuous exercise training experience changes in the force-generating capabilities of muscle, resulting in a coordinated and proportional increase in the load-bearing capacity of bone and other connective tissue. Anaerobic training can increase skeletal muscle mass, force-generating capability, and metabolic capacity and may lead to subtle alterations of the endocrine system that enhance the tissue remodeling process.

Anaerobic training generally results in fewer acute and chronic responses in the cardiovascular and respiratory systems, although low-intensity, high-volume resistance exercise produces some responses that are similar to those with aerobic exercise. Collectively, improved neuromuscular, musculoskeletal, endocrine, and cardiovascular function contribute to enhanced muscle strength, power, hypertrophy, muscular endurance, and motor performance—all of which contribute to increased athletic performance. The adaptations observed in athletes are directly related to the quality of the exercise stimulus and accordingly to the levels of progressive overload, specificity, and variation incorporated into program design. The scientific basis of program design is ultimately seen in the effectiveness with which the athlete improves performance.

KEY TERMS

actin
anaerobic alactic system
anaerobic lactic system
anaerobic training
bilateral deficit
bilateral facilitation
bone matrix
bone mineral density (BMD)
collagen
cortical bone
cross-education
cross-linking
detraining
elastin
electromyography (EMG)
fibrous cartilage
functional overreaching (FOR)
hyaline cartilage
hydroxyapatite
hyperplasia

hypertrophy
mechanical loading
microfibril
minimal essential strain (MES)
motor unit
myogenesis
myosin
myotatic reflex
nebulin
neuromuscular junction (NMJ)
nonfunctional overreaching
 (NFOR)
osteoblasts
osteogenic stimuli
osteoporosis
overreaching
overtraining
overtraining syndrome (OTS)
parasympathetic overtraining
 syndrome

peak bone mass
pennation angle
periosteum
procollagen
progressive overload
rate–pressure product
reactive hyperemia
selective recruitment
size principle
specificity of loading
stress fractures
structural exercises
sympathetic overtraining
 syndrome
tendon stiffness
titin
trabecular bone
ventilatory equivalent

STUDY QUESTIONS

1. Following resistance training, augmented neural drive to the working musculature is the result of
   I. increased agonist muscle recruitment
   II. muscle hypertrophy
   III. improved firing rate
   IV. greater synchronization
   a. all of the above
   b. I and IV only
   c. I, II, and III only
   d. I, III, and IV only

2. When one is performing a box-to-box plyometric drop jump, in order to generate sufficient force in a limited amount of time (<200 ms), which muscle fibers are bypassed through the principle of selective recruitment?
   a. I
   b. IIa
   c. IIx
   d. IIc

3. Which of the following performance or physiological characteristics is NOT usually observed in a state of nonfunctional overreaching (NFOR) within athlete populations?
   a. stagnation and a decrease in performance
   b. hormonal disturbances
   c. sleep disturbances
   d. increased levels of fatigue

4. Following prolonged periods of detraining in elite strength/power athletes, which of the following physical characteristics will likely show the largest reduction as a consequence of the removal of an anaerobic training stimulus?
    a. total fat mass
    b. fast-twitch fiber cross-sectional area
    c. slow-twitch fiber cross-sectional area
    d. total Type I muscle fiber content

5. Following a period of chronic high-intensity resistance training, a variety of physiological adaptations take place in a number of systems within the body that promote improved athletic performance in strength/power activities. If an elite athlete were to undergo 12 weeks of heavy strength training, which of the following adaptations would NOT be expected consequent to this type of anaerobic exercise?
    a. a transition from Type IIx to Type IIa muscle fiber
    b. increased pennation angle in certain muscle groups
    c. reduced sarcoplasmic reticulum and T-tubule density
    d. elevated sodium–potassium ATPase activity

6. In which of the following athletes might you expect limited bone mineral density (BMD) levels as a consequence of the force vectors and the physical demands associated with the given sport?
    a. a 16-year-old gymnast with a seven-year training history in her sport
    b. a 23-year-old offensive lineman who has lifted weights for eight years
    c. a 33-year-old track cyclist who has a 1RM squat of 352 pounds
    d. a 19-year-old 800 m freestyle swimmer with one year of dryland training

CHAPTER 6

Adaptations to Aerobic Endurance Training Programs

Ann Swank, PhD, and Carwyn Sharp, PhD

 After completing this chapter, you will be able to

- identify and describe the acute responses of the cardiovascular and respiratory systems to aerobic exercise;

- identify and describe the impact of chronic aerobic endurance training on the physiological characteristics of the cardiovascular, respiratory, nervous, muscular, bone and connective tissue, and endocrine systems;

- recognize the interaction between aerobic endurance training and optimizing physiological responses of all body systems;

- identify and describe external factors that influence adaptations to acute and chronic aerobic exercise including altitude, sex, blood doping, and detraining; and

- recognize the causes, signs, symptoms, and effects of overtraining.

An understanding of responses of body systems to both acute and chronic aerobic exercise is crucial to the strength and conditioning professional for providing effective exercise training. This chapter describes the acute responses of the cardiovascular and respiratory systems to aerobic exercise and the associated physiological variables used to measure these responses. Also presented are chronic adaptations that occur with aerobic endurance training. The chapter concludes with discussions of external factors, such as altitude, detraining, and blood doping, that influence responses to aerobic endurance training, as well as the deleterious impact of overtraining.

Acute Responses to Aerobic Exercise

A single bout of aerobic exercise places a significant metabolic demand on the body (see table 5.1 in chapter 5), especially the cardiovascular, respiratory, and muscular systems. Repeated exposure to the acute stress of exercise that occurs with chronic exercise training results in many changes in the function and responses of all body systems. A basic knowledge of the acute effects of aerobic exercise provides the foundation for an understanding of the chronic adaptations that are discussed in the next section.

Cardiovascular Responses

The primary functions of the cardiovascular system during aerobic exercise are to deliver oxygen and other nutrients to the working muscles and remove metabolites and waste products. This section describes the cardiovascular mechanisms of these acute responses.

Cardiac Output

Cardiac output is the amount of blood pumped by the heart in liters per minute and is determined by the quantity of blood ejected with each beat (**stroke volume**) and the heart's rate of pumping (**heart rate**):

$$\dot{Q} = \text{Stroke volume} \times \text{Heart rate} \qquad (6.1)$$

where $\dot{Q}$ is the cardiac output. Stroke volume is measured in milliliters of blood per beat, and heart rate is measured in beats (contractions) per minute (46).

In the progression from rest to steady-state aerobic exercise, cardiac output initially increases rapidly, then more gradually, and subsequently reaches a plateau. With maximal exercise, cardiac output may increase to four times the resting level of about 5 L/min to a maximum of 20 to 22 L/min (4). Stroke volume (see next section) begins to increase at the onset of exercise and continues to rise until the individual's oxygen consumption is at

approximately 40% to 50% of maximal oxygen uptake (4). At that point, stroke volume begins to plateau. Sedentary college-aged men have maximal stroke volumes averaging between 100 and 120 ml of blood per beat; maximal stroke volumes for college-aged women are approximately 25% less, due to a smaller average body size as well as a smaller heart muscle (99). The effect of training on the responses to exercise is marked, and we see an increase in maximal stroke volume for college-aged men up to 150 to 160 ml per beat and approximately 100 to 110 for college-aged women (99).

Stroke Volume

Two physiological mechanisms are responsible for the regulation of stroke volume. The first is a result of the **end-diastolic volume**, the volume of blood available to be pumped by the left ventricle at the end of the filling phase, or diastole. The second is due to the action of catecholamines including epinephrine and norepinephrine, which are hormones of the sympathetic nervous system that produce a more forceful ventricular contraction and greater systolic emptying of the heart.

With aerobic exercise, the amount of blood returning to the heart (also called **venous return**) is increased due to a combination of venoconstriction (induced via increased sympathetic nervous system activation) (6), the skeletal muscle pump (muscular contractions combine with one-way venous valves to "push" more blood to the heart during exercise [44]), and the respiratory pump (increased respiratory frequency and tidal volume) (93). All of these result in alterations in the pressure on the chambers of the heart and thoracic vena cava, which promote increased venous return (93), and thus end-diastolic volume is significantly increased. With the increased volume, the myocardial fibers become more stretched than at rest, resulting in a more forceful contraction (this is analogous to greater stretch on a rubber band resulting in greater elastic recoil) and an increase in force of systolic ejection and greater cardiac emptying (46). This principle, called the **Frank-Starling mechanism**, is related to the concept that the force of contraction is a function of the length of the fibers of the muscle wall. This increase in cardiac emptying is characterized by an increase in the **ejection fraction**, the fraction of the end-diastolic volume ejected from the heart (32, 46). At the onset of exercise, or even with the anticipation of exercise, sympathetic stimulation increases myocardial contractility and consequently increases stroke volume (32, 91).

Heart Rate

Just before and at the beginning of an exercise session, a reflex or anticipatory stimulation of the sympathetic nervous system results in an increase in heart rate. Heart

How Can Athletes Estimate Maximal Heart Rate?

A simple estimate of **maximal heart rate** is to subtract one's age from 220; for example, the estimated maximal heart rate for a 47-year-old person is

$$220 - 47 \text{ (age in years)} = 173 \text{ beats/min.}$$

The variance, or standard deviation, around this estimate is ±10 to 12 beats/min; thus the actual maximal heart rate for this individual could be expected to fall within the range of 161 to 185 beats/min. See chapter 20 for more exercise heart rate calculations. More recently a meta-analysis determined that the equation 208 − 0.7 × age could be used in healthy adults to more accurately predict maximal heart rate (123).

rate increases linearly with increases in intensity during aerobic exercise (32). The rate of increase in heart rate, the actual heart rate response, and the maximal heart rate achieved relate to a variety of individual characteristics of the human system, including fitness and age, in addition to exercise workload.

Oxygen Uptake

Oxygen uptake is the amount of oxygen consumed by the body's tissues. The oxygen demand of working muscles increases during an acute bout of aerobic exercise and is directly related to the mass of exercising muscle, metabolic efficiency, and exercise intensity. Aerobic exercise involving a larger mass of muscle or a greater level of work is likely to be associated with a higher total oxygen uptake. Increased metabolic efficiency allows for an increase in oxygen uptake, especially at maximal exercise.

Maximal oxygen uptake is the greatest amount of oxygen that can be used at the cellular level for the entire body. Maximal oxygen uptake has been found to correlate well with the degree of physical conditioning and is recognized as the most widely accepted measure of cardiorespiratory fitness (32). The capacity to use oxygen is related primarily to the ability of the heart and circulatory system to transport oxygen and the ability of body tissues to use it. Resting oxygen uptake is estimated at 3.5 ml of oxygen per kilogram of body weight per minute ($ml \cdot kg^{-1} \cdot min^{-1}$) for an average person; this value is defined as 1 **metabolic equivalent (MET)**. Maximal oxygen uptake values in normal, healthy individuals generally range from 25 to 80 $ml \cdot kg^{-1} \cdot min^{-1}$, or 7.1 to 22.9 METs, and depend on a variety of physiological parameters, including age and conditioning level (46).

Oxygen uptake ($\dot{V}O_2$) can be calculated with the **Fick equation**, which expresses the relationship of cardiac output, oxygen uptake, and arteriovenous oxygen difference:

$$\dot{V}O_2 = \dot{Q} \times \text{a-}\bar{v} O_2 \text{ difference} \qquad (6.2)$$

where $\dot{Q}$ is the cardiac output in milliliters per minute and a-$\bar{v}$ O_2 difference is the **arteriovenous oxygen dif-**

ference (the difference in the oxygen content between arterial and venous blood) in milliliters of oxygen per 100 ml of blood. Recalling equation 6.1, we can calculate oxygen uptake as shown in the following example:

$$\dot{V}O_2 = \text{Heart rate} \times \text{Stroke volume} \times \text{a-}\bar{v} O_2 \text{ difference}$$

$$\dot{V}O_2 = 72 \text{ beats/min} \times 65 \text{ ml blood/beat} \times 6 \text{ ml } O_2/100 \text{ ml blood} = 281 \text{ ml } O_2/\text{min}$$

To express oxygen uptake in its common unit (i.e., $ml \cdot kg^{-1} \cdot min^{-1}$), we would then divide the result by the person's weight in kilograms. This is an example for an 80 kg (176-pound) athlete:

$$\dot{V}O_2 = 281 \text{ ml } O_2/\text{min} \div 80 \text{ kg}$$

$$\dot{V}O_2 = 3.5 \text{ ml} \cdot kg^{-1} \cdot min^{-1}$$

Blood Pressure

Systolic blood pressure estimates the pressure exerted against the arterial walls as blood is forcefully ejected during ventricular contraction (**systole**) and, when combined with heart rate, can be used to describe the myocardial oxygen consumption (work) of the heart. This estimate of the work of the heart is obtained according to the following equation and is referred to as the **rate–pressure product**, or **double product**:

Rate–pressure product =
Heart rate × Systolic blood pressure   **(6.3)**

Diastolic blood pressure is used to estimate the pressure exerted against the arterial walls when no blood is being forcefully ejected through the vessels (**diastole**). Diastolic blood pressure provides an indication of peripheral resistance and can decrease with aerobic exercise due to vasodilation. In systemic circulation, pressure is highest in the aorta and arteries and rapidly falls off within the venous circulation. Also, because pumping by the heart is pulsatile, resting arterial pressure on average fluctuates between a systolic level of 120 mmHg and a diastolic level of 80 mmHg (approximate values). As the blood flow continues through the systemic circulation, its pressure falls progressively to nearly 0 mmHg (venous pressure) by the time it reaches the termination of the vena cava in the right atrium (46).

The **mean arterial pressure** is the average blood pressure throughout the cardiac cycle (equation 6.4). Mean arterial pressure is not the average of systolic and diastolic pressures, because the arterial pressure usually remains nearer the diastolic level than the systolic level during a greater portion of the cardiac cycle. Thus, the mean arterial pressure is usually less than the average of the systolic and diastolic pressures.

Mean arterial blood pressure =
[(Systolic blood pressure − Diastolic blood
pressure) ÷ 3] + Diastolic blood pressure   **(6.4)**

Normal resting blood pressure generally ranges from 110 to 139 mmHg systolic and from 60 to 89 mmHg diastolic. With maximal aerobic exercise, systolic pressure can normally rise to as much as 220 to 260 mmHg, while diastolic pressure remains at the resting level or decreases slightly (46, 91).

Control of Local Circulation

Resistance to blood flow is also increased with increasing viscosity of the blood and the length of the vessel. However, these factors remain relatively constant under most circumstances. Thus, **vasoconstriction** and **vasodilation** of blood vessels are the primary mechanisms for regulating regional blood flow.

During aerobic exercise, blood flow to active muscles is considerably increased by the dilation of local arterioles; at the same time, blood flow to other organ systems is reduced by constriction of the arterioles. At rest, 15% to 20% of cardiac output is distributed to skeletal muscle, whereas with vigorous exercise this value may rise to 90% of cardiac output (32, 91).

> Acute aerobic exercise results in increased cardiac output, stroke volume, heart rate, oxygen uptake, systolic blood pressure, and blood flow to active muscles and a decrease in diastolic blood pressure.

Respiratory Responses

Aerobic exercise provides for the greatest impact on both oxygen uptake and carbon dioxide production as compared to other types of exercise, such as anaerobic resistance training. Significant increases in oxygen delivered to the tissue, carbon dioxide returned to the lungs, and **minute ventilation** (the volume of air breathed per minute) provide for appropriate levels of alveolar gas concentrations during aerobic exercise (91).

With aerobic exercise, increased minute ventilation occurs as a result of increases in the depth of breathing, frequency of breathing, or both. During strenuous exercise, the breathing frequency of healthy young adults usually increases from 12 to 15 breaths per minute at rest to 35 to 45 breaths per minute, while **tidal volume** (TV), the amount of air inhaled and exhaled with each breath, increases from resting values (of 0.4 to 1 L) to as much as 3 L or greater. Consequently, the minute ventilation can increase to 15 to 25 times the resting value, or to values of 90 to 150 L of air per minute (32, 46, 91).

During low- to moderate-intensity aerobic exercise, there is an increase in ventilation directly associated with both increased oxygen uptake and carbon dioxide production. In this instance, the increase in ventilation is primarily due to increased tidal volume. The ratio of minute ventilation to oxygen uptake is termed the **ventilatory equivalent** and ranges between 20 and 25 L of air per liter of oxygen consumed. In more intense exercise (generally above 45% to 65% of maximal oxygen uptake in untrained individuals and 70% to 90% in trained athletes), breathing frequency takes on a greater role. At these levels, minute ventilation rises disproportionately to the increases in oxygen uptake and begins to parallel the abrupt rise in blood lactate. At this point, the ventilatory equivalent may increase to 35 or 40 L of air per liter of oxygen consumed with this high-intensity activity (32, 91).

With inspiration, air enters the **alveoli**, the functional unit of the pulmonary system where gas exchange occurs. However, with inspiration, air also occupies areas of the respiratory passages: the nose, mouth, trachea, bronchi, and bronchioles. This area is not functional for gas exchange and is called the **anatomical dead space**. The normal volume of this air space is approximately 150 ml in young adults and increases with age. Because the respiratory passages stretch with deep breathing, the anatomical dead space increases as tidal volume increases (figure 6.1). Nevertheless, the increase in tidal volume with deep breathing is proportionately greater than any increase in anatomical dead space. Thus, increasing tidal volume (deeper breathing) provides for more efficient ventilation than increasing frequency of breathing alone (46, 91).

Physiological dead space refers to alveoli in which poor blood flow, poor ventilation, or other problems with the alveolar surface impair gas exchange. The physiological dead space in the lungs of healthy people is usually negligible because all or nearly all alveoli are functional. Certain types of lung disease such as chronic obstructive lung disease or pneumonia can significantly reduce alveolar function, increasing physiological dead space by as much as 10 times the volume of anatomical dead space (46, 91).

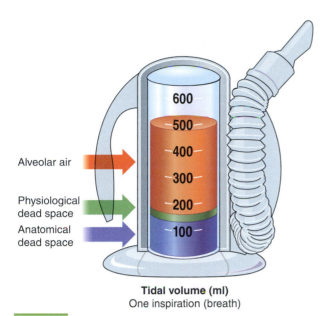

Alveolar air

Physiological
dead space

Anatomical
dead space

Tidal volume (ml)
One inspiration (breath)

FIGURE 6.1 Distribution of tidal volume in a healthy athlete at rest. The tidal volume comprises about 350 ml of room air that mixes with alveolar air, about 150 ml of air in the larger passages (anatomical dead space), and a small portion of air distributed to either poorly ventilated or incompletely filled alveoli (physiological dead space).

During aerobic exercise, large amounts of oxygen diffuse from the capillaries into the tissues; increased levels of carbon dioxide move from the blood into the alveoli; and minute ventilation increases to maintain appropriate alveolar concentrations of these gases.

Gas Responses

Diffusion is the movement of oxygen and carbon dioxide across a cell membrane and is a function of the concentration of each gas and the resulting partial pressure exerted by the molecular motion of each gas. Diffusion results from the movement of gas from high concentration to low concentration. At the tissue level, where oxygen is used in metabolism and carbon dioxide is produced, the partial pressures of these gases in some instances differ considerably from those in arterial blood (figure 6.2). At rest, the partial pressure of oxygen in the interstitial fluid (fluid immediately outside a muscle cell) rapidly drops from 100 mmHg in arterial blood to as low as 40 mmHg, while the partial pressure of carbon dioxide is elevated above that of arterial blood to about

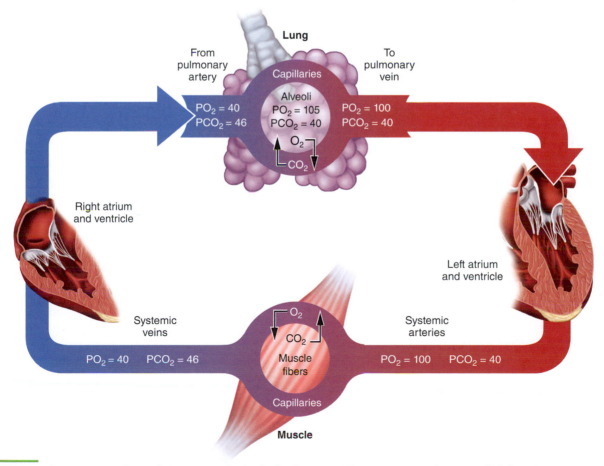

FIGURE 6.2 Pressure gradients for gas transfer in the body at rest. The pressures of oxygen (PO_2) and carbon dioxide (PCO_2) in alveolar air, venous and arterial blood, and muscle tissue are shown.

46 mmHg. During high-intensity aerobic exercise, the partial pressures of these gases are approximately 3 mmHg for oxygen and 90 mmHg for carbon dioxide. Consequently, these pressure gradients cause the movement of gases across cell membranes. In addition, the diffusing capacities of oxygen and, in particular, carbon dioxide increase dramatically with exercise, which facilitates their exchange (32, 46, 91).

Blood Transport of Gases and Metabolic By-Products

Oxygen is carried in blood either dissolved in the plasma or combined with hemoglobin. Because oxygen is not readily soluble in fluids, only about 3 ml of oxygen can be carried per liter of plasma. Nonetheless, this limited amount of oxygen transported in plasma contributes to the partial pressure of oxygen in blood and other body fluids, thus playing a role in the mechanisms that regulate breathing and in the diffusion of oxygen into alveolar blood and the cells of body tissues (46, 91).

Given the limited capacity of plasma to carry oxygen, the majority of oxygen in blood is carried by the hemoglobin. Men have about 15 to 16 g of hemoglobin per 100 ml of blood, and women have about 14 g of hemoglobin per 100 ml of blood. One gram of hemoglobin can carry 1.34 ml of oxygen; thus, the oxygen-carrying capacity of 100 ml of blood is about 20 ml of oxygen in men and a little less in women (91).

The way in which carbon dioxide is removed from the system has some similarities to oxygen transport, but the vast amount of carbon dioxide is removed by a more complex process. After carbon dioxide is formed in the cell, it easily diffuses across the cell membranes and is subsequently transported to the lungs. As with oxygen, only a limited quantity of carbon dioxide—about 5% of that produced during metabolism—is carried in the plasma; similar to the situation with oxygen, this limited amount of carbon dioxide contributes to establishing the partial pressure of carbon dioxide in the blood. Some carbon dioxide is also transported via hemoglobin, but this amount is limited (91).

The greatest amount of carbon dioxide removal (approximately 70%) is from the combination with water and delivery to the lungs in the form of bicarbonate (HCO_3^-). The initial step in this reversible reaction is the combination of carbon dioxide in solution with water in the red blood cells to form carbonic acid. The reaction would normally be quite slow except for the impact of the enzyme carbonic anhydrase, which significantly speeds up this process. Once carbonic acid is formed, it is broken down to hydrogen ions and bicarbonate ions. Because hemoglobin is a significant acid–base buffer, hydrogen ions combine with hemoglobin. This process

helps to maintain the pH of the blood. Bicarbonate ions diffuse from the red blood cells to the plasma while chloride ions diffuse into the blood cells to replace them (46, 91).

Lactic acid is another important metabolic by-product of exercise. During low- to moderate-intensity exercise, sufficient oxygen is available to the working muscles and lactic acid does not accumulate, as the removal rate is greater than or equal to the production rate. This removal of lactate includes the Cori cycle, in which muscle-derived lactate is transported via the blood to the liver, where it undergoes gluconeogenesis. If, at higher work intensities, aerobic metabolism is not sufficient to keep up with the formation of lactic acid, then the lactic acid level in the blood begins to rise. The aerobic exercise level at which lactic acid (converted to blood lactate at this point) begins to show an increase is termed the onset of blood lactate accumulation or OBLA (see chapter 3).

Chronic Adaptations to Aerobic Exercise

Understanding the effects of aerobic endurance training on the body systems is important for assessing physical or athletic performance and determining the impact of training programs. This section deals with the effects of aerobic endurance training on the cardiovascular, respiratory, nervous, muscular, bone and connective tissue, and endocrine systems of the body (see table 6.1).

Cardiovascular Adaptations

Aerobic endurance training results in several changes in cardiovascular function, including increased maximal cardiac output, increased stroke volume, and reduced heart rate at rest and during submaximal exercise. In addition, muscle fiber capillary density increases as a result of aerobic endurance training, supporting delivery of oxygen and removal of carbon dioxide.

For optimal aerobic exercise performance, increasing maximal oxygen uptake is of paramount importance. One of the primary mechanisms for increasing maximal oxygen uptake is the enhancement of central cardiovascular function (cardiac output). The normal discharge rate of the sinoatrial (SA) node ranges from 60 to 80 times per minute. Aerobic endurance training results in a significantly slower discharge rate due to an increase in parasympathetic tone. Increased stroke volume also affects the resting heart rate—more blood is pumped per contraction, so the heart needs to contract less frequently to meet the same cardiac output. Aerobic endurance training can increase the heart's ability to pump blood per contraction at rest and thus may account for some of the significant **bradycardia** (slower heart rate) observed

TABLE 6.1   Physiological Adaptations to Aerobic Endurance Training

Variable	Aerobic endurance training adaptations
Performance	
Muscular strength	No change
Muscular endurance	Increases for low power output
Aerobic power	Increases
Maximal rate of force production	No change or decreases
Vertical jump	Ability unchanged
Anaerobic power	No change
Sprint speed	No change
Muscle fibers	
Fiber size	No change or increases slightly
Capillary density	Increases
Mitochondrial density	Increases
Myofibrillar	
Packing density	No change
Volume	No change
Cytoplasmic density	No change
Myosin heavy chain protein	No change or decreases in amount
Enzyme activity	
Creatine phosphokinase	Increases
Myokinase	Increases
Phosphofructokinase	Variable
Lactate dehydrogenase	Variable
Sodium–potassium ATPase	May slightly increase
Metabolic energy stores	
Stored ATP	Increases
Stored creatine phosphate	Increases
Stored glycogen	Increases
Stored triglycerides	Increase
Connective tissue	
Ligament strength	Increases
Tendon strength	Increases
Collagen content	Variable
Bone density	No change or increases
Body composition	
% body fat	Decreases
Fat-free mass	No change

ATP = adenosine triphosphate; ATPase = adenosine triphosphatase.

in highly conditioned aerobic endurance athletes, whose resting heart rates commonly range from 40 to 60 beats/min (46, 91).

The most significant change in cardiovascular function with long-term (6-12 months) aerobic endurance training is the increase in maximal cardiac output, resulting primarily from improved stroke volume. A significantly lower heart rate in response to a standardized submaximal level of work is another hallmark of aerobic endurance training. Furthermore, heart rate increases more slowly in trained athletes than in sedentary people for a given workload (33, 91). Because maximal heart rate may actually decrease slightly with prolonged training (83), perhaps as a result of increased parasympathetic tone (11), the size of the left ventricle (both chamber volume and wall thickness) and the strength of contractions (increased contractility) are key to increasing stroke volume with submaximal as well as maximal exercise.

In addition to delivering oxygen, nutrients, and hormones, the capillary circulation provides the means for removing heat and metabolic by-products. Increased muscle fiber capillary density has been observed in response to the increased density of muscle associated with aerobic endurance training and is a function of volume and intensity of training. This increase in capillary density decreases the diffusion distance for oxygen and metabolic substrates (76).

Respiratory Adaptations

Ventilation generally does not limit aerobic exercise and is either unaffected or only moderately affected by training (7, 24). Furthermore, the ventilatory adaptations observed appear to be highly specific to activities that involve the type of exercise used in training; that is, adaptations observed during lower extremity exercise primarily occur as a result of lower extremity training. If exercise training focuses on the lower extremities, one will not likely observe ventilatory adaptation during upper extremity activities. Training adaptations include increased tidal volume and breathing frequency with maximal exercise. With submaximal activity, breathing frequency is often reduced and tidal volume is increased. Ventilatory adaptations result from local, neural, or chemical adaptations in the specific muscles trained through exercise (7, 24).

Neural Adaptations

Nervous system adaptations play a significant role in the early stages of aerobic endurance training (108). At the outset, efficiency is increased and fatigue of the contractile mechanisms is delayed. Additionally, improved aerobic performance may result in a rotation of neural activity among synergists (i.e., rather than maintaining a constant state of activation, synergistic muscles alternate between active and inactive to maintain low-level muscular force production [122]) and among motor units within a muscle. Thus, the athlete produces more efficient locomotion during the activity with lower energy expenditure.

Muscular Adaptations

One of the fundamental adaptive responses to aerobic endurance training is an increase in the aerobic capacity of the trained musculature. This adaptation allows the athlete to perform a given absolute intensity of exercise with greater ease. More impressively, after training, an athlete can exercise at a greater relative intensity of a now-higher maximal aerobic power. Thus, measuring an athlete's maximal oxygen uptake only before and after aerobic endurance training may not accurately portray his or her ability to perform during competition. For example, an athlete who can run the marathon at a pace equal to 75% of maximal oxygen uptake may, after training, be able to maintain a pace that is 80% of maximal aerobic power. This adaptation occurs as a result of glycogen sparing (less glycogen use during exercise) and increased fat utilization within the muscle, which prolongs performance at the same intensity (59). Consequently, the OBLA occurs at a higher percentage (up to 80-90%) of the trained athlete's aerobic capacity. This advantageous response may be due to the aerobic endurance athlete's muscle fiber type, specific local adaptations resulting from aerobic endurance training that reduce the production of lactic acid, changes in hormone release (particularly catecholamine release at high-intensity exercise), and a more rapid rate of lactic acid removal (91).

The muscular component of an aerobic endurance training program involves submaximal muscle contractions extended over a large number of repetitions with little recovery. Therefore, the relative intensity is very low, and the overall volume is very high. This manner of training encourages relative increases in aerobic potential that are similar in Type I and Type II fibers (134). Compared to Type II fibers, Type I fibers have a higher preexisting initial aerobic capacity, to which the increase in aerobic potential from training is added (43). Thus, Type I fibers possess an oxidative capacity greater than that of Type II fibers both before and after training. However, if the intensity is sufficient, as in running repeated 800 m intervals, fast-twitch fibers (especially Type IIx fibers) also make a significant contribution to the effort. Under such conditions, their aerobic capacity also increases with training, but chronic aerobic endurance training reduces the concentration of glycolytic enzymes and can reduce the overall muscle mass of these fibers (82).

Conversely, selective hypertrophy of Type I muscle fibers occurs (19) due to their increased recruitment during aerobic activities, although the resulting cross-sectional diameter is not as great as that seen in Type II fibers adapted to resistance exercise. Also, the change is smaller than the hypertrophy of Type I fibers from a bodybuilding-style resistance training program.

There is little evidence to show that Type II fibers change into Type I fibers as a result of aerobic endurance training, but there may be a gradual conversion within the two major Type II fiber subgroups—of Type IIx fibers to Type IIa fibers (2, 134). This adaptation is significant, in that Type IIa fibers possess a greater oxidative capacity than Type IIx fibers and have functional characteristics more similar to those of Type I fibers. The result of this conversion is a greater number of muscle fibers that can contribute to aerobic endurance performance.

At the cellular level, muscular adaptations to aerobic exercise include an increase in the size and number of mitochondria (56) and increased myoglobin content (21, 52). **Myoglobin** is a protein that transports oxygen within the cell. **Mitochondria** are the organelles in cells that are responsible for aerobically producing adenosine triphosphate (ATP) via oxidation of glycogen and free fatty acids. When the larger and more numerous mitochondria are combined with an increase in the quantity of oxygen that can be delivered to mitochondria by the greater concentration of myoglobin, the capacity of the muscle tissue to extract and use oxygen is enhanced. This adaptation is further augmented by increases in the level and activity of the enzymes involved in the aerobic metabolism of glucose (61) and a parallel increase in glycogen (41, 43) and triglyceride (94) stores.

Bone and Connective Tissue Adaptations

The selection of different forms of aerobic exercise has met with some success in bringing about improvements in bone mass. Aerobic programs that are the most successful in stimulating bone growth involve the more intense physical activities such as running and high-intensity aerobics (10, 15). The key to the success of aerobic exercise in stimulating new bone formation is that the activity must be significantly more intense than the daily activities the person normally engages in, so as to exceed the minimum threshold intensity, as well as at a cyclical strain to exceed the minimum and strain frequency for bone growth (10). The intensity of the activity must systematically increase in order to continually overload the bone. Eventually, it may become difficult to overload bone through aerobic exercise when the oxygen transport system rather than limitations of the musculoskeletal system restricts the progression to new exercise intensity. Bone responds to the magnitude and rate of external loading. Therefore, to enhance the stimulus to the musculoskeletal system, it is also necessary to increase the rate of limb movement. Using high-intensity interval training techniques is one method of providing a greater osteogenic stimulus while still providing the benefits associated with aerobic exercise (12, 34).

In mature adults, the extent to which tendons, ligaments, and cartilage grow and become stronger is proportional to the intensity of the exercise stimulus, especially from weight-bearing activities (98). As with bone and muscle, exercise intensity that consistently exceeds the strain placed on the connective tissues during normal daily activities is needed to create connective tissue changes (see chapter 5 for more information).

An example of the positive effects of weight-bearing activity on cartilage is evidenced in a typical knee joint, where the surfaces of the joint that experience the greatest degree of weight bearing are thicker than the non–weight-bearing surfaces (98). Complete movement through a full range of motion during weight bearing is likely essential to maintain tissue viability (119).

Animal studies evaluating the potential negative effects of aerobic exercise on cartilage have shown encouraging results. Although studies have found that strenuous running (12.5 miles [20 km] per session) decreases cartilage thickness (66), other studies using dogs as subjects demonstrated that a moderate running program (1 hour per day, five days per week for 15 weeks) increased cartilage thickness and stimulated positive remodeling of bone tissue (67). And running 25 miles (40 km) per session for one year, or weighted running (using jackets weighing 130% of the animals' weight) 2.5 miles (4 km) five days per week for 550 weeks, did not cause degenerative joint disease (15).

Endocrine Adaptations

While the significance of endocrine responses to resistance training is well accepted (75), the changes in hormone production that contribute to the body's adaptation to aerobic exercise are equally important (38, 39, 69, 91, 94). Testosterone, insulin, insulin-like growth factors (IGF-I), and growth hormone affect the integrity of muscle, bone, and connective tissue as well as assist in maintaining metabolism within a normal range (35, 36, 71, 72, 127). Increases in hormonal circulation and changes at the receptor level (both number of receptors and turnover rate) are specific responses to aerobic exercise.

High-intensity aerobic training augments the absolute secretion rates of many hormones in response to maximal exercise, although trained athletes have attenuated hormonal responses to submaximal exercise (87). The hormone concentrations of a trained athlete equal those of their untrained counterparts at the same relative submaximal exercise intensity (115). The greater hormonal response patterns to maximal exercise appear to augment the athlete's ability to tolerate and sustain prolonged high aerobic exercise intensities (138). When exercise intensity is very high and exercise duration is very short (from 5 to 10 seconds), only "fight-or-flight" changes in peripheral blood hormone concentrations occur (e.g., epinephrine and norepinephrine concentrations increase) (74).

Aerobic training, especially running, is often associated with an increase in net protein breakdown from the muscle (124), brought about in part by stress-induced cortisol secretion (115, 116) that the body attempts to offset by increasing hormonal anabolic responses in testosterone and IGF-1 (128). However, recent evidence suggests that net protein synthesis in skeletal muscle of endurance-trained athletes does occur and may lead to muscle hypertrophy (68), but most likely is due to mitochondrial rather than contractile proteins (131, 133).

Adaptations to Aerobic Endurance Training

Much research has been done on training adaptations associated with aerobic endurance exercise (5, 13, 17, 26, 37, 53, 54, 131). Aerobic metabolism plays a vital role in human performance and is basic to all sports, if for no other reason than recovery (125). Metabolically, the Krebs cycle and electron transport chain are the main pathways in aerobic energy production. Aerobic metabolism produces far more ATP energy than anaerobic metabolism and uses fats, carbohydrates, and proteins as fuel sources for generating ATP. Many sports involve interactions between the aerobic and anaerobic metabolic systems and thus require appropriate training. For example, soccer, lacrosse, basketball, field hockey, and ice hockey involve continuous movement (and thus constant aerobic demand) mixed with bursts of sprint and power activities. Proper conditioning of the aerobic system is vital to the ability of the player to sustain such activity and adequately recover within and between exercise sessions.

Every athlete needs a basic level of cardiovascular endurance—if not for performance, for health reasons—that can be achieved using a wide variety of training modalities and programs. Apart from the stereotypical submaximal aerobic training methods, another method that can produce significant gains in aerobic fitness (e.g., increased $\dot{V}O_2max$, lactate threshold) is interval training (14, 37, 80).

One of the most commonly measured adaptations to aerobic endurance training is an increase in maximal oxygen uptake associated with an increase in maximal cardiac output (13, 23, 53, 131). As the intensity of exercise increases, oxygen consumption rises to maximal levels. When oxygen consumption can no longer increase to meet the demands, maximal oxygen uptake has been achieved even in the presence of continuing oxygen availability. Aerobic endurance training can improve an athlete's aerobic power by 5% to 30%, depending, in part, on the starting fitness level as well as the genetic potential of the individual (5). Most adaptations in maximal oxygen consumption can be achieved within a 6- to 12-month training period. After that, further changes in aerobic endurance performance consist of increases in running efficiency and increased lactate threshold (62). Metabolic changes include increased respiratory capacity, lower blood lactate concentrations at a given submaximal exercise intensity, increased mitochondrial and capillary densities, and improved enzyme activity. It may be that experienced runners do not experience further increases in their $\dot{V}O_2max$ through chronic endurance training but that their performance improves due to enhanced running economy (13, 54).

The intensity of training is one of the most important factors in improving and maintaining aerobic power. Short, high-intensity bouts of interval sprints can improve maximal oxygen uptake if the interim rest period is also short. Callister and colleagues (17) showed that long rest periods used with sprints improve sprint speed without significant increases in maximal aerobic power. Therefore, longer training sessions with higher amounts of rest between exercise bouts result in less improvement in aerobic capacity. The use of shorter recovery periods between high-intensity training intervals has been shown in various studies to improve various skeletal muscle metabolic processes, resulting in improved endurance performance (40).

Aerobic endurance training is generally associated with alterations in body composition, assuming appropriate nutritional intake. Aerobic endurance training usually decreases the relative percentage of body fat but has little or no significant effect on fat-free mass. Longer-term programs can result in greater decreases in the percentage of body fat (13, 26, 61). Excessive training may lead to a predominance of catabolic activity in the body and cause an imbalance between catabolic and anabolic processes (114).

> **Aerobic endurance training results in reduced body fat, increased maximal oxygen uptake, increased running economy, increased respiratory capacity, lower blood lactate concentrations at submaximal exercise, increased mitochondrial and capillary densities, and improved enzyme activity.**

Table 6.2 lists the physiological changes that occur with short-term (three- to six-month) aerobic endurance training and compares the results for previously untrained and elite aerobic endurance athletes.

External and Individual Factors Influencing Adaptations to Aerobic Endurance Training

A variety of external and individual factors can influence both the acute responses and the chronic adaptations of

TABLE 6.2   Physiological Variables in Aerobic Endurance Training

	Previously untrained subjects		Highly trained or elite subjects
	Pre	Post	
Heart rate (beats/min)			
Resting (104, 109)	76.4	57.0	45
Maximal (104, 109)	192.8	190.8	196
Stroke volume (ml)			
Resting (109, 137)	79	76	94
Maximal (109, 137)	104	120	187
Cardiac output (L/min)			
Resting (109, 137)	5.7	4.4	4.2
Maximal (109, 137)	20.0	22.8	33.8
Heart volume (ml) (104, 109)	860	895	938
Blood pressure (mm Hg) (104, 109)			
Resting (104, 109)	131/75	144/78	112/75
Maximal (104, 109)	204/81	201/74	188/77
Pulmonary ventilation (body temperature [37 °C] and pressure [ambient], saturated [47 mmHg]) (L/min)			
Resting (104, 109)	10.9	12.0	11.8
Maximal (104, 109)	128.7	156.4	163.4
Arteriovenous oxygen difference (ml/100 ml)			
Resting	5.8	7.5	—
Maximal (109, 137)	16.2	17.1	15.9
Maximal oxygen uptake ($ml \cdot kg^{-1} \cdot min^{-1}$) (104, 109)	36.0	48.0	74.1
% Type I fibers (1)	48	51	72
Fiber area (μm^2)			
Type I (27)	4,947*	6,284*	6,485
Type II (27)	5,460*	6,378*	8,342
Capillary density			
Number/mm² (1, 51)	289	356	640
Number/fiber (1)	1.39	1.95	2.15
Skeletal muscle enzymes			
Citrate synthase ($\mu mol \cdot min^{-1} \cdot g^{-1}$ wet weight) (132)	35.9	45.1	—
Lactate dehydrogenase ($\mu mol \cdot g^{-1} \cdot min^{-1}$) (27)	843*	788*	746
Succinate dehydrogenase ($\mu mol \cdot g^{-1} \cdot min^{-1}$) (27)	6.4*	17.7*	21.6
Phosphofructokinase ($\mu mol \cdot g^{-1} \cdot min^{-1}$) (42, 43)	27.13	58.82	20.1
Maximal fiber shortening velocity (fiber lengths/s)			
Type I (48, 126)	0.99	1.27	1.65
Type II (48, 126)	3.18	3.38	3.72

*Data not from training study; subjects were untrained or "good distance runners."

Data compiled by Carwyn Sharp. Unless otherwise indicated, data is from Saltin, B, Blomqvist, G, et al. Response to exercise after bed rest and after training. Circulation 38(Suppl. 7):1-78, 1968.

the cardiovascular and respiratory systems to exercise. The effects of altitude, hyperoxic breathing, smoking, and blood doping (external factors), as well as genetic potential, age, and sex (individual factors), are briefly described in this section.

Altitude

At elevations greater than 3,900 feet (1,200 m), acute physiological adjustments begin to occur to compensate for the reduced partial pressure of oxygen in the

What Are the Improvements in Performance From Aerobic Exercise?

The body systems affected by aerobic exercise include musculoskeletal, cardiovascular, and respiratory. Adaptations include the following:

Respiratory system: Decreased submaximal respiration rate (31).

Cardiovascular system: Decreased heart rate for fixed submaximal workloads (106) associated with increased stroke volume and cardiac output. Blood volume is also increased, supporting increased stroke volume and cardiac output (45).

Musculoskeletal system: Increased arterial–venous O_2 difference associated with increased capillarization in muscle (110, 123), increased oxidative enzyme concentrations, and increased mitochondrial size and density (58).

Aerobic power (maximal oxygen uptake): Arguably the most significant change in physiological variables with aerobic exercise training is an increase in maximal oxygen uptake ($\dot{V}O_2max$), often used as the criterion variable for cardiovascular fitness. The $\dot{V}O_2max$ is determined in part by genetics and by the training program undertaken by the athlete. Elite athletes may show minor changes in $\dot{V}O_2max$ with training (5-10%), while untrained individuals may increase $\dot{V}O_2max$ by as much as 20% (55, 62). A high $\dot{V}O_2max$ coupled with increased lactate threshold allows enhanced performance for running sports as well as sports requiring intermittent sprinting (soccer, basketball, and other team sports).

Lactate threshold: Aerobic training increases the absolute lactate threshold, allowing the highly trained individual to work at both a higher relative and absolute percentage of their $\dot{V}O_2max$ than an individual less well trained. This increased tolerance of lactate translates into a variety of performance outcomes; these include running at a higher percentage of $\dot{V}O_2max$ for a race (resulting in reduced time), covering more distance during a game, enhanced recovery for second-half performance, and working at higher exercise intensities throughout an event. The importance of having a high lactate threshold can be seen in the following example. Two individuals can have the same $\dot{V}O_2max$, perhaps 50 ml·kg^{-1}·min^{-1}; however, if one has a lactate threshold of 80% of $\dot{V}O_2max$ (i.e., threshold occurs at 40 ml·kg^{-1}·min^{-1}) whereas the other's occurs at 70% (i.e., 35 ml·kg^{-1}·min^{-1}), the first individual will be able to maintain a power output equivalent to 5 ml·kg^{-1}·min^{-1} higher than the second individual. All other things being equal, such as movement economy, this would result in a greater speed of movement and thus superior performance.

Effective utilization of substrate: Carbohydrates are the preferred source of fuel for high-intensity intermittent exercise in many team sports. Aerobic exercise training results in a greater use of fat as a substrate for exercise with a relative sparing of carbohydrate. With a sparing of carbohydrate, an endurance-trained individual can maintain higher-intensity exercise for longer periods of time. Aerobic exercise may be further improved through various carbohydrate loading manipulations to increase endogenous glycogen stores (16).

Muscle fiber adaptations: When muscle fibers are examined from a cross-sectional point of view, elite distance runners have a higher proportion (percentage) of Type I fibers, and the available Type I fibers are functionally very efficient for aerobic metabolism (increased mitochondrial density and oxidative enzyme capacity [57] and capillary network for oxygen delivery). Aerobic exercise training, especially long-distance and high-intensity intermittent exercise, results in an increase in the oxidative capacity of Type I fibers. Research indicates that skeletal muscle fibers can alter their myosin heavy chain and internal characteristics, leading to alterations in the classification of fibers and the observation that Type IIx fibers are increased in endurance trained athletes (8, 102). From a performance standpoint, these metabolic and fiber changes result in a more efficient use of aerobic energy production.

Exercise efficiency: The economy of exercise is mostly a function of biomechanics and technique. Two aerobic endurance athletes may have the same maximal oxygen uptake and lactate threshold yet not show the same performance outcomes. The athlete with the more efficient exercise (i.e., requiring less energy to maintain the same power output) would be able to sustain the same power output for a longer duration even though the two athletes have the same $\dot{V}O_2max$ and lactate threshold.

atmosphere (49). Table 6.3 presents the adjustments to altitude hypoxia that are immediate and longer-term. Two adjustments that occur early in the acclimatization process are particularly important. First, there is an increase in pulmonary ventilation (**hyperventilation**) at rest and during exercise. This increase in ventilation is primarily the result of increased breathing frequency. With longer stays at high elevation, however, increased tidal volume also contributes to augmented ventilation. Stabilization of ventilation is dependent on the level of altitude and the duration at altitude (64). Second, in the early stages of altitude exposure, there is an increase

TABLE 6.3   Adjustments to Altitude Hypoxia

System	Immediate adjustments	Longer-term adjustments
Pulmonary	Hyperventilation	Increase in ventilation rate stabilizers
Acid-base	Body fluids become more alkaline due to reduction in CO_2 with hyperventilation.	Excretion of HCO_3^- by the kidneys with concomitant reduction in alkaline reserve
Cardiovascular	Cardiac output increases at rest and during submaximal exercise. Submaximal heart rate increases. Stroke volume remains the same or is slightly lowered. Maximal heart rate remains the same or is slightly lowered. Maximal cardiac output remains the same or is slightly lowered.	Continued elevation in submaximal heart rate Decreased stroke volume at rest and with submaximal and maximal exercise Lowered maximal heart rate Lowered maximal cardiac output
Hematologic		Increased red cell production (polycythemia) Increased viscosity Increased hematocrit Decreased plasma volume
Local tissue		Increased capillary density of skeletal muscle Increased number of mitochondria Increased use of free fatty acids, sparing muscle glycogen

in cardiac output at rest and during submaximal exercise, due primarily to increases in heart rate (49, 91). Submaximal heart rate and cardiac output can increase 30% to 50% above sea level values, and stroke volume is constant or slightly reduced. Increased submaximal cardiac output reflects the need for increased blood flow at a time when arterial blood oxygen content is reduced in order to maintain adequate oxygen delivery to the tissues.

Within 10 to 14 days at a given altitude, heart rate and cardiac output begin to return to normal values because of the longer-term acclimatization response of increased red blood cell production. Thus, with acute exposure to altitude, hyperventilation and increased submaximal cardiac output are rapid and relatively effective responses to offset the challenges of the reduced partial pressure of oxygen. However, despite these adjustments, during this acute period, arterial oxygen saturation decreases and results in decreases in maximal oxygen uptake and aerobic performance at altitudes above 3,900 feet (1,200 m). Acclimatization changes revert in about one month after return to sea level. As indicated in table 6.3, chronic physiological and metabolic adjustments that occur during a prolonged altitude exposure include

- increased formation of hemoglobin (generally 5-15% increase, although higher values have been reported) and red blood cells (30-50% increase),

- increased diffusing capacity of oxygen through the pulmonary membranes,

- maintenance of the acid–base balance of body fluids by renal excretion of HCO_3^- and through hyperventilation, and

- increased capillarization.

All these adaptations generally improve tolerance of the relative hypoxia at medium and high altitudes (46, 49, 91) and may result in nearly sea level exercise capacities with adequate acclimatization. A minimum of three to six weeks is needed to adapt at moderate altitude (2,200 to 3,000 m). However, reduced performance, compared to sea level, is generally expected with altitude exposure regardless of the period of acclimatization. Strength and conditioning professionals are encouraged to inform athletes of both expected acute responses and chronic adaptations to altitude so that they can maintain appropriately adjusted training regimens and a positive mental approach to the impact of altitude.

Hyperoxic Breathing

Breathing oxygen-enriched gas mixtures (**hyperoxic breathing**) during rest periods or following exercise has been proposed to positively affect some aspects of exercise performance, although the mechanisms for these results are not well understood and the procedure remains controversial and the research divided (117, 118). Hyperoxic breathing may increase the amount of oxygen carried by the blood and therefore increase the supply of oxygen to working muscles. However, the breathing of ambient air at sea level by healthy people results in arterial hemoglobin oxygen saturation between 95% to 98%. Thus, the potential for hyperoxic breathing during rest periods or following exercise has yet to be fully elucidated (46, 103).

Smoking

Relatively little research is available regarding smoking and exercise performance, possibly because athletes and active individuals may tend to avoid smoking for fear of impairing performance or increasing disease risk (85, 101). Smokers experience impairments in lung function and are at increased risk for chronic obstructive pulmonary diseases (88, 120) including chronic bronchitis (65) and emphysema (86). Decrements in exercise tolerance and cardiopulmonary function have been observed in teenagers (85), demonstrating that the harmful effects of smoking occur in even young smokers within a relatively short period of time. The detrimental effects of smoking include

- increased airway resistance due to nicotine-related bronchiole constriction or increased fluid secretion and swelling in the bronchial tree due to the irritation of smoke; and
- paralysis of the cilia on the surfaces of the respiratory tract by nicotine, which limits the ability to remove excess fluids and foreign particles, causing debris to accumulate in the respiratory passageways and adding to the difficulty of breathing.

Thus, even the light smoker may feel respiratory strain during exercise and experience a reduction in the level of performance (46, 91).

Carbon monoxide, a component of cigarette smoke, is associated with an impaired hemodynamic response to exercise and increased catecholamine release. Carbon monoxide has a higher affinity for hemoglobin than does oxygen. The resulting carboxyhemoglobin (carbon monoxide and hemoglobin) reduces the amount of oxygen that can be carried by hemoglobin and thus reduces the oxygen that can be provided to the working muscles. The reduction in oxygen-carrying capacity may reduce maximal exercise capacity, and submaximal cardiovascular responses may increase in an effort to provide adequate oxygenated blood to the working muscles. The increased catecholamine release increases heart rate and blood pressure.

Blood Doping

The practice of artificially increasing red blood cell mass (**blood doping**) as a means to improve athletic performance has been criticized as unethical and as one that poses serious health risks to the athlete (100). Nonetheless, research has suggested that this practice can improve aerobic exercise performance and may enhance tolerance of certain environmental conditions (112).

Blood doping can be accomplished through infusion of an individual's own red blood cells or those from someone else, or through administration of **erythropoietin (EPO)**, which stimulates red blood cell production. Infusion of red blood cells rapidly increases red blood cell mass, but for just a few weeks (97), whereas the effects of the drug EPO produce changes over weeks and last as long as EPO continues to be administered (112). In either case, it is theorized that increasing red blood cell mass increases the blood's ability to carry oxygen and thus increases oxygen availability to working muscles. Maximal oxygen uptake has been demonstrated to increase by up to 11% with either red blood cell infusion or EPO administration (112, 113). At standardized submaximal workloads, blood doping has also been associated with decreased heart rate and blood lactate as well as higher pH values (112).

The effects of blood doping suggest the potential for diminishing the impact of various environmental conditions. The effects of altitude appear to be lessened with blood doping, although as altitude increases, the positive influence of blood doping is reduced (107). Environmental stressors such as heat and cold exposure may also be affected by blood doping. During heat exposure, a blood-doped athlete will be able to tolerate submaximal exercise stress more easily (63, 111-113). The increased blood volume associated with increased red blood cell mass allows the body to shunt more blood to the skin for improved thermoregulation while still providing sufficient blood to transport oxygen to the working muscles. However, blood doping appears to confer these benefits primarily to individuals who are already acclimatized to heat and provides very little aid relating to the response to heat of those who are not acclimatized (112). Much less is known about blood doping with respect to cold stress, and although some theoretical benefit has been suggested, this practice could conceivably increase health risks (112).

The health risks associated with blood doping further complicate the controversy surrounding this practice. Theoretically, high hematocrit levels may increase risks for embolic events such as stroke, myocardial infarction, deep vein thrombosis, or pulmonary embolism. Increased arterial blood pressure, flu-like symptoms, and increased plasma potassium levels may present themselves with EPO use (113). Finally, there is risk associated with infusion or transfusion, although in most cases the risk is relatively small (113).

Genetic Potential

The upper limit of an individual's genetic potential contributes significantly to the absolute magnitude of the training adaptations. The magnitude of change also depends on the current training status of the individual. Each biological system adaptation, such as that of the cardiovascular system, has an upper limit, and as the athlete gets closer to that upper limit, smaller and smaller gains are observed. For example, in some elite competitions (e.g., swimming), small gains in performance may be the difference between the gold medal and 26th place. Thus, in an event in which tenths or hundredths of a second make a big difference, it may be worth the extra training time to gain that 0.05% improvement in performance. Because of the small gains possible with training in elite athletes, careful program design and monitoring become even more critical (26, 70, 77, 135).

Age and Sex

Physiological adaptations to aerobic endurance training vary according to age and sex (3, 131). Maximal aerobic power decreases with age in adults as a consequence of various physiological changes that accompany aging—for example, reduced muscle mass and strength (also called sarcopenia) (79) and increased fat mass (3, 78). On the average, when women and men are matched by age, the aerobic power values of women range from 73% to 85% of the values of men (131). However, the general physiological response to training is similar in men and women (84). The differences in aerobic power may be caused by several factors, including women's higher percentage of body fat and lower blood hemoglobin values and men's larger heart size and blood volume (13, 18).

Overtraining: Definition, Prevalence, Diagnosis, and Potential Markers

Improving sport performance for competitive athletes through appropriately designed training programs is crucial to success. Equally important to the success of an athlete in any sport is adequate recovery from intense training. When there is an imbalance between training loads and recovery, the potential for **overtraining** and development of the **overtraining syndrome (OTS)** exists (28). While considerable research exists on OTS,

controversy remains regarding how to define, evaluate, and remedy this syndrome (73, 121).

Recently, the European and American Colleges of Sports Medicine published a joint consensus statement about OTS (92). This section of the chapter presents some of the findings of this consensus statement, particularly with regard to definitions, potential markers, and prevention.

For effectively studying OTS, consistent terminology is needed. The recommendations of the consensus statement are from the work of Halson (47) and Urhausen (130). In these definitions, overtraining is considered a process (expressed as a verb) that can result in **overreaching** in the short term (**functional overreaching**) or extreme overreaching (**nonfunctional overreaching [NFOR]**) or OTS in the long term. Each of these conditions results in a sport performance decrement that is a hallmark of overtraining. In the case of functional overreaching, training is purposely intensified to cause a brief decrement in performance followed by a few days or weeks of recovery. The result is a supercompensative improvement in performance. An example is a final maximal training session (which causes functional overreaching) a few weeks before a competition, followed by a gradual tapering period leading up to an enhanced performance. Nonfunctional overreaching is characterized by a stagnation or decrease in sport performance, with recovery requiring weeks to months in order for the athlete to return to the previous level of performance. If intensified training continues without adequate recovery, an athlete can progress to OTS, in which performance is decreased and for which months of recovery would be required to return the athlete to prior levels of performance. These definitions for overtraining assume a continuum for which the common trigger for the progression from functional overreaching to OTS is continued intensified training with insufficient rest. While it is difficult to measure the prevalence of OTS, a recent study (105) indicated that about 10% (7% to 21%) of collegiate swimmers and other aerobic endurance athletes experienced either NFOR or OTS.

> Overtraining syndrome can lead to dramatic performance decreases in all athletes; the most common cause is intensified training without adequate recovery.

Cardiovascular Responses

Greater volumes of training associated with OTS can affect heart rate. Interestingly, resting heart rate can be either decreased or increased in association with OTS (136). Heart rate variability can decrease with onset of OTS, indicating reduced parasympathetic input or excessive sympathetic stimulation. Exercise-induced maximum heart rates decrease from overtraining, as have heart rates at absolute submaximal exercise intensities (50). Increased training volumes, within a given time period, associated with overtraining do not generally affect resting blood pressures. However, increased training intensity can produce increased resting diastolic blood pressures without affecting resting systolic pressures.

Biochemical Responses

Unusually high training volume can result in increased levels of creatine kinase (CK), indicating muscle damage (30). Lactate concentrations, on the other hand, either decrease or stay the same when training volumes increase. Blood lipids and lipoproteins are not altered by volume overtraining. Muscle glycogen decreases with prolonged periods of overtraining, although this may be largely due to dietary considerations. Decreased glycogen levels may contribute to the lowered lactate responses.

Endocrine Responses

In men, total testosterone decreases after an initial increase in response to the exercise stimuli; however, this should be viewed as a response to a stressful stimulus rather than an indication of overtraining (92). Concentrations of free testosterone also decrease in some cases. These changes do not appear to be regulated by the pituitary, since luteinizing hormone levels are not affected (129). The changes in free testosterone appear to be independent of protein-binding capacity, because concentrations of sex hormone–binding globulin are not altered (129). Therefore, the decreased ratio of total testosterone to sex hormone–binding globulin that can accompany increased volumes of training seems to be due to altered total testosterone levels.

The anabolic–catabolic state of an athlete may be quantified by the testosterone-to-cortisol ratio, which decreases or stays the same with greater training volumes. The free testosterone component may be more influential physiologically. Decreases of 5% to 50% in the ratio of free testosterone to cortisol have also been reported with increased training volumes. A possible marker of OTS is a decrease of 30% or more in this ratio.

Decreased pituitary secretion of growth hormone occurs with overtraining. This and other endocrine responses to an overtraining stimulus appear to be due primarily to impaired hypothalamic function, not pituitary function. Whether these endocrine alterations are responsible for performance decrements is open to debate. Levels of free testosterone, total testosterone, cortisol, and creatine kinase seem to simply reflect training volumes. Actual physical performance is occasionally related to total testosterone concentrations, but not in all cases.

Catecholamines appear very responsive to an overtraining stimulus. Alterations in basal levels of epinephrine, norepinephrine, and dopamine are reported to be significantly related to the severity of self-reported complaints in overtrained runners. Changes in catecholamine and cortisol concentrations may mirror each other during overtraining, although cortisol is not as sensitive to increased training volume as catecholamines are. Severely increased volumes of training can result in decreased nocturnal levels of epinephrine, which indicate basal levels. Preexercise or resting levels of epinephrine and norepinephrine are either unchanged or increased. A given absolute load of exercise results in increased epinephrine and norepinephrine levels in the presence of overtraining compared with before overtraining, although maximum levels of epinephrine and norepinephrine are unchanged. Basal levels of dopamine decrease with volume overtraining, as do dopamine concentrations at the same absolute workload. With submaximal exercise, dopamine responses vary, but they appear to counter norepinephrine patterns. Although often difficult to document, severe volume overtraining of aerobic endurance athletes produces characteristics of the parasympathetic OTS, including reduced sensitivity to catecholamines, and may result in advanced cases of severe OTS.

Strategies for Prevention of Overtraining Syndrome

The overtraining syndrome represents a cumulative sum of stressors with the primary cause of intensified training without adequate recovery (92). However other contributors include lack of sleep, environmental considerations (heat, cold, altitude, pollution), interpersonal difficulties, and traveling, among others. While the definitive identification of OTS remains somewhat controversial, there are still some strategies that athletes and coaches can follow to prevent OTS.

An effective tactic includes making sure the athlete is following good nutrition guidelines as well as getting sufficient sleep and recovery time. Coaches should track an athlete's training program, and the program should provide variety in intensity and volume. Keeping an accurate record of an athlete's performance can also help "catch" a marker of OTS early in the process so that training can be adjusted. Most importantly, athletes should have access to a multidisciplinary health team (coach, physician, nutritionist, and psychologist) to discuss any issues related to their lives; this access may lead to early information that would assist in avoiding OTS (92).

What Are the Markers of Aerobic Overtraining?

Several criteria characterize a variable as a reliable marker for the onset of overtraining syndrome:

- The marker should be sensitive to the training load.
- It should not be affected by other factors.
- Changes in the marker should precede development of overtraining syndrome.
- The marker should be easy to measure accurately.
- Measurement should not be profoundly invasive.
- The marker should not be expensive to use or measure.

The following variables have been identified as potential markers, but none satisfy all of the criteria listed (92).

- Decreased performance
- Decreased percentage of body fat
- Decreased maximal oxygen uptake
- Altered blood pressure
- Increased muscle soreness
- Decreased muscle glycogen
- Altered resting heart rate and decreased heart rate variability
- Increased submaximal exercise heart rate
- Decreased lactate
- Increased creatine kinase
- Altered cortisol concentration
- Decreased total testosterone concentration
- Decreased ratio of total testosterone to cortisol
- Decreased ratio of free testosterone to cortisol
- Decreased ratio of total testosterone to sex hormone–binding globulin
- Decreased sympathetic tone (decreased nocturnal and resting catecholamines)
- Increased sympathetic stress response
- Change in mood states
- Decreased performance in psychomotor speed tests

Detraining

Detraining is defined as the partial or complete loss of training-induced adaptations in response to an insufficient training stimulus (95, 96). Detraining is governed by the principle of training reversibility, which states that whereas physical training results in several physiological adaptations that enhance athletic performance, stopping or markedly reducing training induces a partial or complete reversal of these adaptations, compromising athletic performance. A distinction needs to be made with regard to cessation of training that results in a reversal of adaptations and tapering. **Tapering** is the planned reduction of volume of training (usually in duration and frequency but not intensity) that occurs before an athletic competition or a planned recovery microcycle. This type of reduction in training is designed to enhance athletic performance and adaptations.

Aerobic endurance adaptations are most sensitive to periods of inactivity because of their enzymatic basis.

The exact cellular mechanisms that dictate detraining changes are unknown, and further research is needed to clarify the underlying physiological alterations. Two review articles (95, 96) address the factors that contribute to aerobic performance, most importantly $\dot{V}O_2max$ and the factors determining $\dot{V}O_2max$ (cardiac output and arteriovenous oxygen difference) and the impact of detraining. The authors discuss the impact of short-term (four weeks) (95) and long-term (more than four weeks) (96) detraining. In highly trained athletes, maximal oxygen uptake is reduced 4% to 14% with short-term (22, 90) and 6% to 20% with long-term detraining (21, 25, 90). The reduction in $\dot{V}O_2max$ is primarily a result of decreased blood volume (20), decreased stroke volume (20, 21), decreased maximal cardiac output (20, 21), and increased submaximal heart rate (20, 23, 25, 89). The decrease in $\dot{V}O_2max$ supports the loss of aerobic-related endurance performance (20, 21, 23, 25, 60, 89).

> ▶ **Proper exercise variation, intensity, maintenance programs, and active recovery periods can adequately protect against serious detraining effects (29).**

Conclusion

Aerobic endurance exercise produces many acute cardiovascular and respiratory responses, and aerobic endurance training produces many chronic adaptations. This information can be of particular value for developing the goals of a conditioning program and can provide a basis for clinical evaluation and the selection of parameters to be included in such an evaluation process. Knowledge of cardiovascular, respiratory, nervous, muscular, bone and connective tissue, and endocrine system responses to aerobic endurance training can help the strength and conditioning professional understand the scientific basis for aerobic conditioning and the adaptations to expect and monitor during training. Adaptations to specific types of exercise stimuli take place in the body. Optimal adaptations reflect careful design, implementation, and performance of strength and conditioning programs.

KEY TERMS

alveoli
anatomical dead space
arteriovenous oxygen difference
blood doping
bradycardia
cardiac output
detraining
diastole
diastolic blood pressure
diffusion
double product
ejection fraction
end-diastolic volume
erythropoietin (EPO)
Fick equation

Frank-Starling mechanism
functional overreaching
heart rate
hyperoxic breathing
hyperventilation
maximal heart rate
maximal oxygen uptake
mean arterial pressure
metabolic equivalent (MET)
minute ventilation
mitochondria
myoglobin
nonfunctional overreaching
overreaching

overtraining
overtraining syndrome (OTS)
oxygen uptake
physiological dead space
rate–pressure product
stroke volume
systole
systolic blood pressure
tapering
tidal volume
vasoconstriction
vasodilation
venous return
ventilatory equivalent

STUDY QUESTIONS

1. A 17-year-old high school cross-country runner has been training aerobically for six months in preparation for the upcoming season. Which of the following adaptations will occur in the muscles during that time?
   a. increased concentration of glycolytic enzymes
   b. hyperplasia of Type II fibers
   c. transformation from Type I to Type II fibers
   d. hypertrophy of Type I fibers

2. The amount of blood ejected from the left ventricle during each beat is the
   a. cardiac output
   b. a-$\bar{v}$O$_2$ difference
   c. heart rate
   d. stroke volume

3. Which of the following does NOT normally increase during an aerobic exercise session?
   a. end-diastolic volume
   b. cardiac contractility
   c. cardiac output
   d. diastolic blood pressure

4. The mean arterial pressure is defined as the
   a. average blood pressure throughout the cardiac cycle
   b. average of the systolic and diastolic blood pressures
   c. average systolic blood pressure during exercise
   d. average of blood pressure and heart rate

5. Primary training adaptations of elite aerobically trained athletes include which of the following?
   I. increased maximal oxygen uptake
   II. decreased blood lactate concentration
   III. increased running economy
   IV. decreased capillary density
   a. I and III only
   b. II and IV only
   c. I, II, and III only
   d. II, III, and IV only

CHAPTER 7

Age- and Sex-Related Differences and Their Implications for Resistance Exercise

Rhodri S. Lloyd, PhD, and Avery D. Faigenbaum, EdD

▶ **After completing this chapter, you will be able to**

- evaluate the evidence regarding the safety, effectiveness, and importance of resistance exercise for children;
- discuss sex-related differences in muscular function and their implications for females;
- describe the effects of aging on musculoskeletal health and comment on the trainability of older adults; and
- explain why adaptations to resistance exercise can vary greatly among these three distinct populations.

Resistance exercise has proven to be a safe and effective method of conditioning for individuals with various needs, goals, and abilities. Though much of what we understand about the stimulus of resistance exercise has been gained through examination of the acute and chronic responses of adult men to various training protocols, resistance exercise for children, women, and older people has received increasing public and medical attention. When designing and evaluating resistance training programs, strength and conditioning professionals need to understand age- and sex-related differences in body composition, muscular performance, and trainability and their implications for each individual.

For the purposes of this chapter, **resistance exercise** is defined as a specialized method of conditioning whereby an individual is working against a wide range of resistive loads to enhance health, fitness, and performance. This term should be distinguished from the sport of weightlifting, in which individuals attempt to lift maximal amounts of weight in competition, specifically in the clean and jerk and snatch exercises. The term **childhood** refers to a period of life before the development of secondary sex characteristics (e.g., pubic hair and reproductive organs), and the term **adolescence** refers to the period between childhood and **adulthood**. For ease of discussion, the term **youth** or **young athlete** refers to both children and adolescents. The terms **older** and **senior** have been arbitrarily defined to include men and women over 65 years of age. In this chapter, muscular strength is expressed on an absolute basis (i.e., total force measured in pounds or kilograms) or on a relative basis (i.e., ratio of absolute strength to total body mass, fat-free mass, or muscle cross-sectional area).

Children

With the growing interest in youth resistance training, it is important for strength and conditioning professionals to understand the fundamental principles of growth, maturation, and development. An understanding of these principles and an appreciation for how they can influence training adaptations and confound interpretation of research data are essential to the development and evaluation of safe and effective resistance training programs. Because the training of young athletes is becoming more intense and complex, anatomical, physiological, and psychosocial factors that may be associated with acute and chronic injury also need to be considered.

The Growing Child

In this section, the terms **growth**, **development**, and **maturation** are used to describe changes that occur in the body throughout life. The term *growth* refers to an increase in body size or a particular body part; *development* describes the natural progression from prenatal life to adulthood; and *maturation* refers to the process of becoming mature and fully functional. **Puberty** refers to a period of time in which secondary sex characteristics develop and a child transitions to young adulthood. During puberty, changes also occur in body composition and the performance of physical skills, with such changes varying markedly between individuals.

Chronological Age Versus Biological Age

Because of considerable variation in the rates of growth and development, it is not particularly accurate to define a stage of maturation or development by age in months or years, which is known as **chronological age**. Children do not grow at a constant rate, and there are substantial interindividual differences in physical development at any given chronological age. A group of 14-year-old children can have a height difference as great as 9 inches (23 cm) and a weight difference up to 40 pounds (18 kg). Furthermore, an 11-year-old girl may be taller and more physically skilled than an 11-year-old boy. These differences correspond to variations in the timing, tempo, and magnitude of growth during puberty (131). The onset of puberty can vary from 8 to 13 years in girls and from 9 to 15 years in boys, with girls typically beginning puberty approximately two years before boys.

Stages of maturation, or pubertal development, can be better assessed by **biological age**, which can be measured in terms of skeletal age, somatic (physique) maturity, or sexual maturation. For example, two girls on a team may have the same chronological age but differ by several years in their biological age. One girl may be sexually mature, whereas the other may not begin the process of sexual maturation for several years. In girls the onset of menstruation (**menarche**) is a marker of sexual maturation, whereas in boys the closest indicators of sexual maturity include the appearance of pubic hair, facial hair, and deepening of the voice. The assessment of maturation in children is important for several reasons. Maturity assessment can be used to evaluate growth and development patterns in children. In addition, since the degree of maturation is related to measures of fitness, including muscular strength and motor skill performance (114), techniques used to assess maturation can help ensure that children are more fairly matched for fitness testing and athletic competition, as opposed to grouped according to chronological age. In adequately nourished children there is no scientific evidence that physical training delays or accelerates growth or maturation in boys and girls (72, 135). Further, the osteogenic benefits of physical activity, specifically weight-bearing activities that generate compressive forces, are essential for skeletal remodeling and growth (215).

The gold standard for determining biological maturation is skeletal age assessment. This technique involves trained radiographers comparing x-rays or radiographs of a child against standard reference radiographs to determine the extent of ossification of the bones of the left wrist (89, 186, 205-207). Ossification refers to the process of laying down new bone material by cells called osteoblasts. While skeletal age provides the most accurate and reliable form of assessing maturity, concerns with cost, specialist equipment, time constraints, and the need for specific radiography expertise make the method unrealistic for most practitioners working with youth.

An alternative method of evaluating biological age, devised by Tanner (206), involves visually assessing the development of identifiable secondary sex characteristics: breast development in girls, genital development in boys, and pubic hair development in both sexes. The Tanner classification has five stages: Stage 1 represents the immature, preadolescent state, and stage 5 represents full sexual maturation. While certain methodological limitations are apparent with Tanner staging (131), its greatest constraint surrounds the invasive nature of the procedure and the inherent concerns for both the child and the parents. Consequently, this technique should not be used by strength and conditioning professionals and should be performed only when necessary by suitably qualified clinicians. For most practitioners, the most realistic and feasible means of estimating biological age is from somatic assessments (131). Somatic age reflects the degree of growth in overall stature or smaller, subdimensions of the body (e.g., limb length). Techniques available to the practitioner include longitudinal growth curve analysis, percentages and predictions of final adult height, and the prediction of age from **peak height velocity (PHV)**, which is defined as the age at maximum rate of growth during the pubertal growth spurt. Measures of growth are relatively easy to collect, are noninvasive, and require minimal equipment. In some cases, it may be appropriate to measure somatic growth every three months (131).

Sensitivity to individual differences in ability, technical competency, and past experience is especially important for children in the weight room. An early-maturing 14-year-old girl may be ready to train for a sport such as weightlifting, whereas a late-maturing 14-year-old boy may not be ready for the demands of heavy resistance exercise. In addition, a child's **training age** (i.e., the length of time the child has consistently followed a formalized and supervised resistance training program) can influence adaptations to resistance training; the magnitude of gain in any strength-related measure is affected by the amount of adaptation that has already occurred. For example, a 12-year-old with two years of resistance training experience (i.e., a training age of 2

years) may not achieve the same strength gains in a given period of time as a 10-year-old who has no experience of resistance training (i.e., a training age of zero). It is also important for practitioners to evaluate and monitor technical competency in youth, as two children with the same training age may present with different standards of technical competency and may develop competency at different rates. Strength and conditioning professionals must recognize all of these variables and should individualize training program design based on each child's technical competency, training age, and maturity level. When creating any youth resistance training program, strength and conditioning professionals should also take into consideration the unique psychosocial needs of each individual child and then design, implement, and revise programs according to these needs. For example, a strength and conditioning professional needs to use different interpersonal skills to coach an inexperienced child with a low training age and low levels of self-confidence versus an experienced and highly competent adolescent who simply lacks motivation.

During the period of peak height velocity, young athletes may be at an increased risk of injury (143). Peak height velocity usually occurs around age 12 in females and age 14 in males. Alterations in center of mass, muscle imbalances, and the relative tightening of the muscle–tendon units spanning rapidly growing bones are potential risk factors for overuse injuries in children during the pubertal growth spurt (154, 213). Strength and conditioning professionals may need to modify training programs (i.e., reinforce high-quality movement patterns, target flexibility restrictions, correct muscle imbalances, or decrease the volume or intensity of training or both) during periods of rapid growth. If a young athlete complains of pain or discomfort during a growth spurt, the strength and conditioning professional should consider the possibility of an overuse injury rather than labeling these complaints "growing pains" and, in consultation with the child's parents or guardians, should refer the child to a medical practitioner.

Muscle and Bone Growth

As children grow, muscle mass steadily increases throughout the developing years. At birth, approximately 25% of a child's body weight is muscle mass, and by adulthood this percentage increases to about 40% (136). During puberty, marked increases in hormonal concentrations (e.g., testosterone, growth hormone, and insulin-like growth factor) in boys result in a marked increase in muscle mass and widening of the shoulders, whereas in girls an increase in estrogen production causes increased body fat deposition, breast development, and widening of the hips. Although muscle mass in girls continues to increase during adolescence, the increase occurs at a slower rate than in boys due to hormonal differences (136). Throughout this time period the increase in muscle mass in both sexes is due to the hypertrophy of individual muscle fibers and not hyperplasia (136). Peak muscle mass occurs between the ages of 16 and 20 years in females and between 18 and 25 years in males unless affected by resistance exercise, diet, or both (136).

The majority of bone formation occurs in the **diaphysis** (primary ossification center), which is the central shaft of a long bone, and in the **growth cartilage** (secondary ossification center), which is located at three sites in the child: the epiphyseal (growth) plate, the joint surface, and the **apophyseal** insertions of muscle–tendon units. When the epiphyseal plate becomes completely ossified, the long bones stop growing (figure 7.1). Although bones typically begin to fuse during early adolescence, girls generally achieve full bone maturity about two to three years before boys. The actual age varies considerably, but most bones are fused by the early 20s.

A particular concern in children is the vulnerability of the growth cartilage to trauma and overuse (103). Injuries to the growth cartilage may disrupt the bone's blood and nutrient supply and result in permanent growth disturbances (e.g., skeletal undergrowth, skeletal overgrowth, or malalignment of bone). Trauma from falls or excessive repetitive stress that may result in a ligament tear in an adult may produce an epiphyseal plate fracture in a child. Because the peak incidence of epiphyseal plate fractures in children occurs at about the time of peak height velocity, it seems that a preadolescent child may be at less risk for an epiphyseal plate fracture than an adolescent child experiencing the growth spurt (145). It has been suggested that the epiphyseal plates of younger children may be stronger and more resistant to shearing-type forces, which may be the cause of injuries to the growth cartilage (145). The potential for injury to the epiphyseal plate during resistance training is discussed later in this chapter.

> ▶ Growth cartilage in children is located at the epiphyseal plate, the joint surface, and the apophyseal insertions. Damage to the growth cartilage may impair the growth and development of the affected bone. However, the risk of such damage can be reduced with appropriate exercise technique, sensible progression of training loads, and instruction by qualified strength and conditioning professionals.

Developmental Changes in Muscular Strength

As muscle mass increases throughout preadolescence and adolescence, there is an increase in muscular strength. In fact, the growth curves for strength are similar to those for body mass. In boys, peak gains in strength typically occur about 1.2 years after peak height velocity and 0.8 years after peak weight velocity, with body weight being the clearer indicator (136). This pattern suggests that during periods of rapid growth, muscle increases first in mass and later in its ability to express and attenuate high levels of force (23). This is reflected by a recent meta-analysis showing that adolescents were able to attain increases in muscular strength that were nearly 50% greater than children (14). In girls, peak gains in strength also typically occur after peak height velocity, although there is more individual variation in the relationship of strength to height and body weight

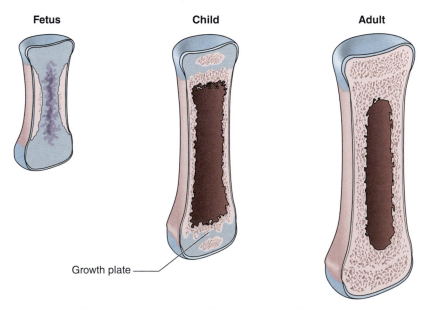

Fetus   **Child**   **Adult**

Growth plate ————

FIGURE 7.1   Bone formation, which takes place as a result of growth and development.

for girls than for boys (136). Although the strength of boys and girls is essentially equal during preadolescence, hormonal differences during puberty are responsible for acceleration in the strength gains of boys and a general plateau in the strength development of girls during adolescence (129, 136). On average, peak strength is usually attained by age 20 in untrained women and between the ages of 20 and 30 in untrained men (136).

An important factor related to the expression of muscular strength in children is the development of the nervous system. If myelination of nerve fibers (motor neurons) is absent or incomplete, fast reactions and skilled movements cannot be successfully performed, and high levels of strength and power are impossible. As the nervous system continues to develop with age, children improve their performance in skills that require balance, agility, strength, and power. Since the myelination of many motor neurons is incomplete until sexual maturation, children should not be expected to respond to training in the same way or to reach the same skill level as adults until they reach full neural maturity (121).

Because physiological functions are more closely related to biological age than to chronological age, at any given time an early-maturing child probably has an advantage in measures of absolute strength when compared with a later-maturing child of the same sex who has less muscle mass. Toward the end of adolescence the body type of early-maturing youngsters tends to be **mesomorphic** (muscular and broader shoulders) or **endomorphic** (rounder and broader hips), whereas late maturers tend to be **ectomorphic** (slender and tall) (136). Clearly, physical differences in body proportions can affect the execution of resistance exercises. For example, short arms and a large chest cavity are a biomechanical advantage in upper body pressing exercises, whereas long legs and a long torso are a disadvantage in squatting movements. These factors have implications for strength and conditioning professionals who are attempting to standardize fitness tests or develop a resistance training program for a group of boys and girls who vary greatly in physical size. It should be noted that whether in a testing or training environment, the practitioner should use child-size resistance machines or exercises using body weight, medicine balls, elastic bands, dumbbells, or barbells. The reasons for individualized training programs should be explained to all participants, and special encouragement should be offered to late maturers who may be smaller and weaker than chronological-age peers with more advanced biological maturity. Although late maturers tend to eventually catch up to the early maturers as they proceed through adolescence, young athletes should realize that many factors including motivation, coaching, and innate ability contribute to success in sport.

Youth Resistance Training

Clinicians, coaches, and exercise scientists now agree that resistance exercise can be a safe and effective method of conditioning for children (12, 19, 54, 57, 64, 66, 74, 121, 129, 130). An increasing number of boys and girls are participating in resistance training activities, and major sports medicine organizations support children's participation in a range of resistance exercise modes, provided that the programs are appropriately designed and supervised by qualified professionals (2, 3, 7, 22, 57, 129). National standards and grade-level outcomes for physical education include guidelines and recommendations that recognize the importance of fitness activities that enhance muscle and bone strength (199).

It is imperative that strength and conditioning professionals remember that children are not miniature adults. No matter how big or strong a child is, children are physically less mature and are often experiencing training activities for the very first time. Children should begin resistance training at a level that is commensurate with their maturity level, physical abilities, and individual goals. Adult programs and training philosophies should not be superimposed on younger populations. In such instances, the intensity and volume of training are often too severe, and the recovery between training sessions is inadequate to enable training adaptation to take place. When introducing children to resistance training activities, it is always better to underestimate their physical abilities and gradually increase the volume and intensity of training than to exceed their abilities and risk injury or long-term negative health outcomes.

Responsiveness to Resistance Training in Children

Much of the controversy surrounding youth resistance training stemmed from the issue of children's trainability, that is, children's responsiveness to the stimulus of resistance exercise. Early studies failed to demonstrate a strength increase in preadolescents who participated in a resistance training program (50, 99). Although the lack of significant findings in these studies could be explained by methodological shortcomings, such as short study duration or inadequate training volume or intensity, the results from these reports are sometimes cited as proof that resistance training is ineffective for children. As previously discussed, muscular strength normally increases from childhood and throughout the teenage years; thus a more appropriate conclusion from these reports may be that training-induced gains from a short-duration, low-volume and low-intensity training program are not distinguishable from gains attributable to normal growth and maturation.

Other investigations have clearly demonstrated that boys and girls can increase muscular strength above and beyond that accompanying growth and maturation alone, provided that the intensity and volume of training are adequate (62, 63, 71, 127, 175, 184, 220). Children as young as age 5 have benefited from resistance training (8, 115), and a variety of training modalities have proven to be effective (129). While gains in a maximum strength range of approximately 10% to 90% have been reported in the literature (14), strength gains of roughly 30% to 40% are typically observed in untrained preadolescent children following short-term (8 to 20 weeks) resistance training programs (57, 129). However, following the initial adaptation period, the rate of change in strength gains will be attenuated as youth adapt to the training program, thus highlighting the need for continued, progressive training. The variability in strength gain may be due to several factors, including the biological age of the child, program design, quality of instruction, and background level of physical activity.

Children who participate in resistance training programs are likely to undergo periods of reduced training or inactivity due to program design factors, extended travel plans, busy schedules, injury, involvement in multiple sports, or decreased motivation. This temporary reduction or withdrawal of the training stimulus is called *detraining*. In children, unlike adults, the evaluation of strength changes during the detraining phase is complicated by the growth-related strength increases during the same period of time. Nevertheless, data suggest that training-induced strength gains in children are impermanent and tend to return to untrained control group values during the detraining period (56, 70, 108, 211). In one report, participation in physical education classes and organized sports throughout a detraining period did not maintain the preadolescents' training-induced strength gains (70). In another study comparing the effects on children of one and two days per week of resistance training, participants who resistance trained only once per week averaged 67% of the strength gains of participants who resistance trained twice per week (63). While a recent review suggested that increased training frequency is related to a greater strength training effect in youth (14), this finding must be considered in light of the many other commitments that youth or young athletes may have (e.g., competitive playing schedule, schoolwork, time to interact with peers). Collectively, these findings underscore the importance of continuous training to maintain the strength advantage of exercise-induced adaptations in children. Though the precise mechanisms responsible for the detraining response remain unclear, it seems likely that changes in neuromuscular functioning are at least partly responsible. Interestingly, recent research suggests that the detraining effect may not be homogenous, with different neuromuscular qualities in young children showing different responses following the cessation of a training program (56).

Changes in muscle hypertrophy can significantly contribute to training-induced strength gains in adolescents and adults, yet it is unlikely that muscle hypertrophy is primarily responsible for training-induced strength gains (at least up to 20 weeks) in preadolescents (172, 184). Although some findings do not agree with this suggestion (81), preadolescents appear to experience more difficulty increasing their muscle mass through a resistance training program due to inadequate levels of circulating hormones (testosterone, growth hormone, insulin-like growth factor). In preadolescent boys and girls, testosterone concentration is between 20 and 60 ng/100 ml; in contrast, during adolescence, testosterone levels in males increase to about 600 ng/100 ml while the levels in females remain unchanged (136).

It appears that preadolescents have more potential for an increase in strength owing to neural factors, such as increases in motor unit activation and synchronization, as well as enhanced motor unit recruitment and firing frequency (87, 129, 172, 184). It has also been suggested that intrinsic muscle adaptations, improvements in motor skill performance, and the coordination of the involved muscle groups could be partly responsible for training-induced strength gains in preadolescents (184). One cannot state without qualification, however, that resistance training does not result in muscle hypertrophy in preadolescents, because it is possible that longer study durations, higher training volumes, and more precise measuring techniques (e.g., computerized imaging) may be needed to uncover potential training-induced muscle hypertrophy in youth who are following a resistance training program. Additionally, as muscle fiber pennation angle increases with age (16), whether resistance training can change the architectural properties of the muscle without making substantial changes in overall muscle cross-sectional area remains unclear.

During and after puberty, however, training-induced gains in strength are typically associated with gains in muscle hypertrophy due to hormonal influences. Although lower levels of testosterone in adolescent females limit the magnitude of training-induced increases in muscle hypertrophy, other hormone and growth factors (e.g., growth hormone and insulin-like growth factor) may be at least partly responsible for their muscle development (119). Figure 7.2 highlights the factors that contribute to the development of muscular strength, namely fat-free mass, testosterone concentrations, nervous system development, and the differentiation of fast-twitch and slow-twitch muscle fibers.

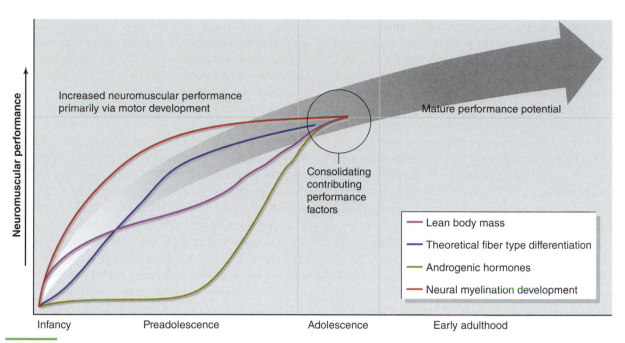

FIGURE 7.2   Theoretical interactive model for the integration of developmental factors related to the potential for muscular strength adaptations and performance.

Reprinted, by permission, from Faigenbaum et al., 2013 (58).

> ▶ **Preadolescent boys and girls can significantly improve their strength above and beyond growth and maturation with resistance training. Neurological factors, as opposed to hypertrophic factors, are primarily responsible for these gains.**

Potential Benefits

In addition to increasing muscular strength, power, and muscular endurance, regular participation in a youth resistance training program has the potential to influence many other health- and fitness-related measures (129, 198). Resistance exercise may favorably alter selected anatomic and psychosocial parameters, reduce injuries in sport and recreational activities (212), and improve motor skills and sport performance (13, 68, 203).

From a clinical perspective, it has been reported that regular participation in a resistance training program can result in a decrease in body fat, improvements in insulin sensitivity, and enhanced cardiac function among obese children and adolescents (15, 139, 162, 193, 218, 219). The grades for indicators of youth physical activity around the world are low, which suggests that there is widespread evidence of a physical inactivity crisis (210). Children who are obese or those who lead sedentary lives (e.g., who take a bus to school and watch television or play computer games after school and on weekends) are not ready for 1 to 2 hours of sport training four or five days a week. Current global findings based on data from

183 countries indicate that between 1980 and 2013, the prevalence of children with a body mass index ≥ 25 kg/m^2 increased substantially in both developed and developing countries (165). Specifically to the United States, data from 2011 and 2012 show that 16.9% (95% confidence interval [CI], 14.9-19.2%) of American youth aged 2 through 19 years were obese (168); and while childhood prevalence data appear to be plateauing, the number of young children who are currently obese or overweight remains high (168). Although the treatment of childhood obesity is complex, it seems that obese youth enjoy resistance training because it is not aerobically taxing and provides an opportunity for all participants to experience success and feel good about their performance.

In addition to the high prevalence of childhood obesity, other secular trends in muscular fitness in youth are of concern regarding those engaging in organized sport or recreational activity. For example, research indicates that within various cohorts of school-aged children, a range of muscular strength measures (e.g., bent-arm hang, handgrip strength) (36, 152, 189) and motor skill competencies (96, 189) have shown a decrease in recent times. Therefore, while all aspiring young athletes will likely benefit from preparatory conditioning inclusive of resistance training, it seems that those who might benefit the most are the ones who are less fit to begin with.

While resistance training does not affect the genotypic maximum, it probably has a favorable influence on growth at any stage of development, as long as appropriate guidelines are followed (10, 72). In fact, regular participation in an exercise program that includes resistance training and weight-bearing physical activities has been shown to enhance bone mineral density in children and adolescents (139, 153, 166). In support of these observations, it has been reported that elite adolescent weightlifters who regularly train with heavy weights while performing multijoint exercises display levels of bone density well above values of age-matched controls (40, 216). These findings may be especially important for girls who are at an increased risk for developing **osteoporosis** later in life, a clinical condition characterized by low bone mass and an increased susceptibility to fractures.

It has also been suggested that regular participation in a preseason conditioning program that includes resistance training may increase a young athlete's resistance to injury (52, 103). Every year, millions of injuries occur during sport participation among children and adolescents in the United States (146), and it has been estimated that more than 50% of overuse injuries sustained by children could be prevented with simple approaches including coaching education, preparatory conditioning, and delayed specialization (144, 212). Strength and conditioning professionals can play a pivotal role in preparing young athletes for sport and thereby minimize or offset the incidence and severity of sport-related injuries common to young athletes. In many cases, modern-day youth who enroll in organized sport programs are unfit and ill prepared to handle the demands of their chosen sport.

Even though some coaches argue that early sport specialization is the key to success, youth who participate in a single sport or specialize in a single position at an early age are likely to be at an increased risk of developing muscle imbalances, overuse injuries, overtraining, and potential burnout (2, 21, 49, 212). Additionally, it seems that late specialization and involvement in a variety of sports and activities during the younger years may be better related to sporting success at a later age (2, 79, 134, 151). Although the total elimination of youth sport injuries is an unrealistic goal, the addition of resistance training to a youth preseason fitness program may better prepare the young athlete to handle the duration and magnitude of unanticipated forces that develop in practice and game situations (35, 66, 103). Because of individual differences in stress tolerance, resistance training intensity, volume, and rate of progression need to be carefully prescribed since this form of training adds to the chronic repetitive stress placed on the young musculoskeletal system. Proper progression and program variation will optimize gains, prevent boredom, and reduce the stress that can lead to overtraining. In addition, well-planned recovery strategies (e.g., proper cool-down, postexercise meal or snack, and adequate sleep) can help to maximize training adaptations. For example, research shows that youth athletes responded more favorably to a combination of active recovery and cold-water therapy in comparison to passive postcompetition regimens including stretching and raising of the legs (117).

Because many sports have a significant strength or power component, it is attractive to assume that resistance training will enhance athletic performance. Though comments from parents and children support this contention, scientific reports on this issue are limited. Improvements in selected motor performance skills, such as the long jump, vertical jump, 30 m dash, and agility run, have been observed in children who participated in a resistance training program of between 8 and 20 weeks (13, 55, 73, 127, 167, 220). Although only a few reports have provided direct evaluations of the effects of youth resistance training on sport performance (18, 24, 78), a progressive resistance training program will in all likelihood result in some degree of improvement in sport performance in young athletes (85, 86, 97, 180).

Potential Risks and Concerns

Appropriately prescribed youth resistance training programs are relatively safe when compared with other sports and activities in which children and adolescents regularly participate (95). Paradoxically, it seems that the forces placed on the joints of young athletes during sport participation may be far greater, and more difficult to anticipate, than those generated from resistance training programs (66). The belief that resistance training is dangerous for children is not consistent with the needs of children and the documented risks associated with this type of training. Children have been injured in the weight room; however, such injuries are more likely to be accidental in children (158) and typically occur in cases in which the levels of supervision and instruction, technical competency, and training loads are inappropriate (66). This highlights the need for strength and conditioning professionals to heed safety guidelines when working with younger populations. Although epiphyseal plate fractures have been reported in adolescents who were following a resistance training program, these reports were case studies and typically involved the performance of heavy overhead lifts in unsupervised settings (90, 187, 189). An epiphyseal plate fracture has not been reported in any prospective youth resistance training study that adhered to established training guidelines (66). Of note, 1-repetition maximum (1RM) testing in children and adolescents has proven to be safe, provided that appropriate testing guidelines are followed (i.e., adequate warm-up periods, individual progression of loads, and close supervision) (61, 65, 100, 123, 192). If children and adolescents are taught how to resistance train properly and understand resistance training guidelines and procedures, the risk of an epiphyseal plate fracture is minimal.

Program Design Considerations for Children

It is important to view resistance training as part of a well-rounded exercise program for a child that also addresses other fitness goals. Although there is no minimal age requirement for participation in a youth resistance training program, children should have the emotional maturity to receive and follow directions and should want to try this type of activity (129, 157). A pretraining medical examination is not mandatory for apparently healthy children; however, all participants should be screened for any injury or illness that may limit or prevent safe participation in a resistance training program (2). The goals of youth resistance training programs should not be limited to increasing muscular strength but should also include teaching children about their bodies, promoting an interest in physical activity, teaching weight room etiquette, and having fun. It seems likely that children who enjoy participating in physical activities and sport are more likely to be active later in life (208).

Two important areas of concern in the development of youth resistance training programs are the quality of instruction and rate of progression. Strength and condi-

tioning professionals must have a thorough understanding of youth resistance training guidelines, a willingness to demonstrate proper exercise technique, and the requisite pedagogical skills to speak with children at a level they understand (59, 129). Professionals should play down competition between participants and focus on proper technique instead of the amount of weight lifted. The use of individualized workout logs can help each child understand the concept of individual progression. Although increasing the resistance or the number of sets is necessary to make continual gains, this does not mean that every session needs to be more intense or higher in volume than the previous one. While it is important to keep the program fresh and challenging, children should be given an opportunity to develop proper form and technique. When working with youth it is important to focus on intrinsic factors such as skill improvement, personal successes, and having fun.

Although only limited data are available regarding the relationship between repetitions and selected percentages of the 1RM in children, it appears that the number of repetitions that can be performed at a given percentage of the 1RM is specific to the given exercise (69). Thus, the minimal strength threshold, when expressed as a percentage of 1RM, may vary between muscle groups, possibly due to the amount of muscle mass involved with each exercise. While practitioners have safely used

How Can We Reduce the Risk of Overuse Injuries in Youth?

- Before organized or recreational sport participation, children and adolescents should be evaluated by a sports medicine physician to identify the existence of any medical problems.
- Parents should be educated about the benefits and risks of competitive sport and should understand the importance of preparatory conditioning for aspiring young athletes.
- Children and adolescents should be encouraged to participate in long-term training programs with adequate time for recovery between sport seasons to suitably prepare them for the demands of sport and physical activities.
- Training programs should be multidimensional, incorporating elements of resistance training, fundamental movement skills, speed, plyometric and agility development, and dynamic stabilization. Additionally, these programs should vary in type, volume, and intensity throughout the year and meet the specific needs of each individual child.
- Youth coaches should implement well-planned recovery strategies between hard workouts and competitions in order to maximize recovery and enable growth and maturational processes to occur. This approach should help reduce the chances of overtraining and burnout in youth.
- All youth should follow healthy lifestyle habits (e.g., appropriate nutrition, hydration, and sleep quality).
- Youth sport coaches should participate in continued professional development programs to learn more about conditioning, sport skills, safety rules, equipment, the psychosocial needs of children, and the physiology of growth and development.
- Coaches should support and encourage all children and adolescents to participate but should not excessively pressure them to perform at a level beyond their capabilities. Child welfare and well-being should at all times remain the priority.
- Children in most sports should be encouraged to participate in a variety of sports and activities and delay early sport specialization until adolescence if possible.

1RM testing to determine strength levels in youth within research settings and sport environments, where this is not possible (perhaps owing to time limitations, class size, or a lack of coach expertise), alternative means of assessing strength are available. Strength and conditioning professionals can use predictive equations that estimate 1RM loads from multiple submaximal repetitions (e.g., 5RM or 10RM) (129). However, strength and conditioning professionals should recognize that such approaches might place the child at heightened risk due to the cumulative fatiguing effects of multiple repetitions on technical form. In order to obtain a surrogate measure of muscular strength without the use of repetition maximum schemes, practitioners could use field-based measures of different jump protocols (e.g., vertical jump or long jump) or handgrip strength, as these measures have been significantly correlated to 1RM values in youth (30, 149). Irrespective of the strength testing protocol used, the child or adolescent must be able to demonstrate and maintain correct technical competency throughout the entire test under the watchful eye of a qualified professional.

Advanced multijoint exercises such as the snatch and clean and jerk can be incorporated into a child's program at the appropriate time (i.e., after foundational strength and technique progressions have been completed), but the primary focus must be on developing proper form and technique (25, 67). Poor technique can put abnormal stress on musculoskeletal tissues and lead to injury. The resistance must be lowered if proper exercise technique cannot be maintained. When learning new exercises, children should start with an unloaded barbell, a long wooden stick, or PVC piping to learn the correct technique. The importance of correct feedback, delivered at the correct time and in the correct manner, cannot be overestimated during this stage of development to ensure the facilitation of skill development. Youth training should involve the regular grading and evaluation of the technical performance of different exercises by a trained observer, as opposed to simply assessing performance measures (e.g., load lifted or the velocity of movement) (60). Such an approach can be used to continually educate young lifters about proper exercise technique, raise awareness about common technical flaws, and provide coaches and teachers with a tool for assessing learning during practice or physical education. A summary of youth resistance training guidelines is presented in the sidebar.

Female Athletes

Women who regularly participate in resistance training activities can improve their health, reduce their risk of degenerative diseases (e.g., osteoporosis) and their injury

---

Youth Resistance Training Guidelines

- Each child should understand the benefits and risks associated with resistance training.
- Competent and caring strength and conditioning professionals should design and supervise training sessions.
- The exercise environment should be safe and free of hazards, and the equipment should be appropriately sized to fit each child.
- Dynamic warm-up exercises should be performed before resistance training.
- When appropriate, static stretching exercises should be performed after resistance training.
- Carefully monitor each child's tolerance to the exercise stress.
- Begin with light loads to allow appropriate adjustments to be made.
- Increase the resistance gradually (e.g., 5% to 10%) as technique and strength improve.
- Depending on individual needs and goals, one to three sets of 6 to 15 repetitions on a variety of single- and multijoint exercises can be performed.
- Advanced multijoint exercises, such as the snatch and clean and jerk, may be incorporated into the program, provided that appropriate loads are used and technical proficiency remains a key outcome.
- Two or three nonconsecutive training sessions per week are recommended; however, youth with higher training ages may participate in more frequent resistance training sessions per week.
- When necessary, adult spotters should be nearby to actively assist the child in the event of a failed repetition.
- The resistance training program should be systematically periodized throughout the year to ensure that the child or adolescent is exposed to a sequential and varied training stimulus with adequate rest and recovery between training cycles.

Adapted, by permission, from A. Faigenbaum et al., 1996, "Youth resistance training position statement paper and literature review," *Strength and Conditioning* 16(6): 71.

rates, and enhance their overall sporting performance. Whereas in the past women may have questioned the value of resistance training or even avoided this type of exercise due to social stigma, evidence clearly indicates that women are capable of tolerating and adapting to the stresses of resistance exercise and that the benefits are substantial (122, 161). Furthermore, to enhance health and fitness and reduce injury rates, it is now suggested that resistance training be an essential component of any training program that females follow (155, 159, 204).

Sex Differences

Strength and conditioning professionals need to understand sex-related differences in physique, body composition, and physiological responses to resistance exercise when designing and evaluating resistance training programs for females. An understanding of these differences and the areas of concern that are unique to female athletes can help to optimize performance and decrease the risk of sport-related injuries.

Body Size and Composition

Before puberty there are essentially no differences in height, weight, and body size between boys and girls. As puberty begins and progresses, sex-related anthropometric discrepancies become more evident, primarily because of hormonal changes. During puberty the production of estrogen in girls increases fat deposition and breast development, whereas testosterone production in boys increases bone formation and protein synthesis. Though estrogen also stimulates bone growth, boys have a longer growth period and commence puberty at a later stage, and therefore adult men tend to achieve greater overall stature than adult women. On average, adult women tend to have more body fat, less muscle, and lower bone mineral density than adult males. Furthermore, women tend to be lighter in total body weight than men. Although some female athletes have lower fat percentages than untrained men, extremely low fat percentages in women may be associated with adverse health consequences (171, 221). Anthropometric measurements of adults indicate that men tend to have broader shoulders relative to their hips and women tend to have broader hips relative to their waist and shoulders. The broader shoulders in men can support more muscle tissue and can also provide a mechanical advantage for muscles acting at the shoulder.

Strength and Power Output

When comparing training-induced changes in muscular strength between sexes, it is important to distinguish between absolute and relative measures. In terms of absolute strength, women generally have about two-thirds the strength of men (124). The absolute lower body strength of women is generally closer to male values as compared to the absolute values for upper body strength. Sex-related differences in body composition, anthropometric characteristics, and fat-free mass distribution (women tend to have less muscle mass above the waist) can partly explain these sex-related differences, which are apparent in recreationally trained individuals as well as highly trained athletes (17).

When considered on a relative basis, sex-related differences in muscular strength are greatly reduced. Because the average man and woman differ considerably in body size, it is useful to compare sex differences in strength relative to body weight, fat-free mass, and muscle cross-sectional area. When expressed relative to body weight, the lower body strength of women is similar to that of men, while the upper body strength of women is still somewhat less (105). If comparisons are made relative to fat-free mass, differences in strength between men and women tend to disappear (105). Of note, limited data suggest that eccentric strength may be more similar between men and women than concentric strength when compared relative to fat-free mass (37, 196).

When strength is expressed relative to muscle cross-sectional area, no significant difference exists between sexes, which indicates that muscle quality (peak force per cross-sectional area) is not sex specific (29, 148). Even though the muscle fibers in men and women are also similar in fiber type distribution and histochemical characteristics, men tend to have a larger muscle fiber cross-sectional area than women. Notwithstanding the importance of these observations, strength and conditioning professionals need to remember that there is a wide range of strength abilities and that in some cases differences between two women (or two men) may in fact be greater than differences between a man and a woman.

> ▶ In terms of absolute strength, women are generally weaker than men because of their lower quantity of muscle. Relative to muscle cross-sectional area, differences in strength are reduced between the sexes, which indicates that muscle quality is not sex specific.

Sex-related differences in power output are similar to those for muscular strength. Measurements comparing power outputs of competitive lifters revealed that during the entire snatch or clean pulling movements, women's power output relative to total body weight was about 63% of men's (83). Similar findings regarding power output were obtained in presumably untrained women (118). Maximal vertical jump and standing long jump scores also tend to be lower in women than in men (38, 45, 137), although when expressed relative to fat-free mass, the gap between sexes tends to narrow. Though men still perform better in general than women, it appears that differences in fat-free mass are not entirely responsible for differences in power output. Although the data are equivocal, sex-related differences in the rate of force development (182, 183) and the recruitment strategy of muscle activation (173) could partly explain these findings (191).

Resistance Training for Female Athletes

Despite sex-related differences, men and women respond to resistance exercise from their pretraining baseline levels in similar ways. Although the magnitudes of change in selected variables may differ somewhat, the overall trends suggest that the value of resistance exercise for women extends far beyond an increase in muscular strength and includes favorable changes in other important measures of health and fitness (122).

Responsiveness to Resistance Training in Women

Through participation in a resistance training program, women can apparently increase their strength at the same rate as men or faster. Although absolute gains in strength are often greater for men, relative (percentage) increases are about the same or greater in women (156). However, this may reflect that baseline neuromuscular levels are lower on average in females (156). Even though nervous system adaptations clearly contribute to the development of strength, the influence of hypertrophic factors in women should not be overlooked. When sophisticated techniques (e.g., computed tomography) are used to accurately measure changes in muscle cross-sectional area, relative short-term gains (up to 16 weeks) in muscle hypertrophy are similar between sexes (43, 93).

Judging by the muscular development of female weightlifters, bodybuilders, and track and field athletes who have not used anabolic steroids, it is obvious that muscle hypertrophy is possible in women who regularly participate in high-volume or high-intensity training programs, even though these gains may be less than in males. Although further study is warranted, it is possible that testosterone concentrations in women vary with training and that women with relatively high levels of testosterone may have more potential for an increase in muscle size and strength (42, 94). Furthermore, it is possible that the complexity of the exercise movement used during training may influence the degree of muscle hypertrophy (33). More complex, multijoint movements, such as the squat, clean and jerk, and snatch (as compared with single-joint exercises such as the biceps curl),

may require a relatively longer neural adaptation period, thereby delaying muscle hypertrophy in the trunk and legs (33). A genetic disposition to develop a large muscle mass may also be a contributing factor (201).

Female Athlete Triad

Strength and conditioning professionals working with female athletes should be aware of the potential negative health outcomes associated with the **female athlete triad** (6). The triad, which refers to the interrelationships between energy availability, menstrual function, and bone mineral density, is a health risk for female athletes who train for prolonged periods of time with insufficient caloric intake to meet the high energy expenditure of training and adaptations (6, 47). In instances in which female athletes have low energy availability (due to high training volumes or intensities, or both, and inadequate dietary intake), osteoporosis is more likely (47). In addition to the heightened risk of osteoporosis, low energy can also lead to subclinical menstrual disorders. **Amenorrhea** is defined as the absence of a menstrual cycle for more than three months (6) and is caused by a reduced secretion frequency of luteinizing hormone by the pituitary gland. Amenorrhea can negatively affect the health and well-being of females, with bone stress fractures, endocrine and gastrointestinal complications, and sporting performance decrements more common in women experiencing prolonged reproductive suppression (47).

Resistance training offers a multitude of benefits for females, including the attenuation of age-related declines in bone mineral density (116). Specifically, the stress from the mechanical loading applied via resistance training directly increases the magnitude of skeletal remodeling and therefore bone mass. Data show that in females, resistance training increases bone mineral density in various skeletal regions of the body (116). It is also known that higher intensities of resistance training promote greater degrees of osteogenesis (133), and that preadolescence is an opportune time to participate in weight-bearing activities in order to enhance bone mineral density (91, 104).

However, when prescribing resistance training programs for females, strength and conditioning professionals must ensure that nutritional intake supports the training prescription in order to stimulate adaptation and facilitate recovery. For example, a female middle-distance runner who fails to consume sufficient levels of calcium, vitamin D, and protein may be at risk of increasing the likelihood of entering into a negative energy balance and experiencing the early onset of female athlete triad. Athletes considered to be at risk for nutritional deficiencies should receive a nutritional assessment by a fully qualified registered sport dietician

(47). It should be noted that insufficient energy intake may simply reflect an inadvertent lack of a biological drive to match activity-induced energy expenditure, or it could be attributable to clinical eating disorders or disordered eating behaviors that are more prevalent in female athletes (6). Females at high risk of eating disorders are likely to be those involved in sports or activities that use subjective scoring based on aesthetics (e.g., dance or gymnastics); and in such cases individuals should be referred to trained medical and dietary professionals.

Program Design Considerations for Women

Since the physiological characteristics of muscle in the sexes are the same, there is no sensible reason why resistance training programs for women need to be different from those of men. In fact, because the muscle groups involved in a particular sport or physical activity are obviously the same for men and women, resistance training programs should be designed to improve the performance of the muscles needed for successful sport performance and everyday activities, regardless of sex. The only real difference between training programs for men and women is generally the amount of absolute resistance used for a given exercise, which is based on the individual's strength capabilities. It is particularly important for young female athletes to perform some type of resistance exercise regularly if they are to approach their genetic potential in musculoskeletal strength and power during adulthood. Observations that elite female gymnasts are able to perform 40 pull-ups and that competitive female weightlifters can clean and jerk over two times their body weight demonstrate what is possible.

Upper Body Strength Development

Two areas of concern regarding the prescription of resistance training programs for women relate to the development of upper body strength and the prevention of sport-related injuries, in particular those that involve the knee. Since the upper body absolute strength of women tends to be less than that of men (122), emphasizing development of the upper body is especially worthwhile for female athletes who play sports that require upper body strength and power. The addition of one or two upper body exercises or one or two extra sets may be beneficial for women who have difficulty performing multijoint free weight exercises (e.g., various full and partial snatching and cleaning movements) because of limitations in upper body strength. Female athletes can benefit by incorporating various snatches, cleans, and derivative weightlifting movements into their training programs, because adaptations resulting from these large

muscle mass, multijoint exercises transfer well to performance in recreational and sport activities. Furthermore, the caloric cost of performing these lifts can be relatively high (84), which may aid in the maintenance of healthy body composition.

Anterior Cruciate Ligament Injury in Females

It is important for strength and conditioning professionals to be aware of the increased incidence of knee injuries in female athletes, particularly in sports such as soccer and basketball (6, 34, 73). According to a number of reports, female athletes are six times more likely to incur an **anterior cruciate ligament (ACL)** tear than male players (39, 102, 111, 147, 160). On the basis of these findings, some observers suggest that over 15,000 debilitating knee injuries can be expected to occur in female intercollegiate athletes during any given year (103). Although it is possible that the increasing number of knee injuries simply reflects an increase in participation by women in organized sport, others have suggested causative factors. It is possible that joint laxity, limb alignment, notch dimensions, ligament size, body movement, shoe–surface interaction, skill level, hormonal changes, use of ankle braces, and training deficiencies contribute to the observed difference in the number of knee injuries between male and female athletes (9, 101, 150, 194, 224). While anatomical and hormonal factors may contribute to heightened ACL injury risk in females, it is believed that the most significant contributing factor is a neuromuscular deficiency, which ultimately leads to abnormal biomechanics (increased dynamic knee valgus upon contact with the ground) (159). Evidence suggests that in order to reduce the risk of ACL injury, youth should participate in preparatory conditioning before puberty to optimize training adaptations (159). Engaging in a well-balanced conditioning program (including resistance training, plyometrics, and agility and balance training) that is designed and delivered by a qualified professional, in order to strengthen muscle and connective tissues as well as enhancing neuromuscular control of the knee joint before sport participation, is merited in order to reduce injury risk (1). Since most ACL injuries in female athletes occur from noncontact mechanisms (e.g., deceleration, lateral pivoting or landing [20]), regular participation in a conditioning program that is designed to enhance the strength of supporting structures and increase neuromuscular control of the knee joint may reduce the risk of sport-related injuries (52, 103). Furthermore, it is important that female athletes consume adequate energy and emphasize quality protein and healthy fat consumption within a well-rounded diet to optimize training adaptations (47). Although additional clinical trials are needed to determine the best method for reducing the incidence of ACL injuries in female athletes

How Can Female Athletes Reduce Their Risk of ACL Injury?

To help female athletes reduce their risk of ACL injury, strength and conditioning professionals should do to the following:

- Recommend preparticipation screening by a sports medicine physician. This should include identification of risk factors for injury along with musculoskeletal testing.

- Encourage female athletes to participate in a year-round conditioning program that includes resistance, plyometric, speed and agility, and flexibility training. The conditioning program should meet the specific needs of each athlete and should progress in a periodized fashion that allows for training adaptations to continually manifest.

- Ensure that females learn, and can repeatedly demonstrate, correct movement mechanics (e.g., jumping, landing, twisting, and cutting) within a variety of environments.

- Precede every exercise session with a general dynamic warm-up and a specific warm-up using movements that resemble those involved in the activity and that target the activation of key muscle groups (e.g., posterior chain muscle groups).

- Provide augmented feedback within training sessions to optimize skill transfer and enhance biomechanics related to ACL injury.

- Encourage children to participate in injury prevention programs (which include progressive resistance training to develop both skill- and health-related fitness components); early intervention appears to benefit the effectiveness of such programs (159).

- Recommend that athletes wear appropriate clothing and footwear during practice and games.

and improving adherence to these training protocols, the strategies listed in the sidebar will likely be effective.

Older Adults

The number of men and women over the age of 65 is growing, and it seems that more opportunities for participation in sports ranging from marathon running to weightlifting are available to older athletes. While the cardiovascular endurance and muscular strength of older competitors or masters athletes are truly exceptional, even the most highly trained athletes experience some decline in performance after age 30. For example, competitive weightlifting ability has been shown to decline with age at a rate of approximately 1% to 1.5% per year until approximately age 70, after which a more dramatic decrease occurs (140). Older athletes who do not engage in physical activity typically see greater decrements in a number of physical performance measures and increase their risk of debilitating injury (174). Strength and conditioning professionals should understand the physiological changes that occur with aging and the trainability of older individuals. In addition, the potential health risks associated with physical activity for older individuals need to be considered.

Age-Related Changes in Musculoskeletal Health

Significant changes in body composition with advancing age can lead to the development of physical functional impairments and injury. The well-documented loss of bone and muscle with age not only makes activities of daily life such as getting out of a chair and opening a window more difficult, but also increases the risk for falls, fractures, and long-term disability (34, 105, 106). Bones become fragile with age because of a decrease in bone mineral content that causes an increase in bone porosity. The bone mineral content and microarchitecture of bone can deteriorate to such an extent that the risk of bone fracture, particularly of the hip, spine, or wrist during a fall, is increased (5). **Osteopenia** is defined by a bone mineral density between −1 and −2.5 standard deviations (SD) of the young adult mean; osteoporosis is defined by a bone mineral density below −2.5 SD of the young adult mean (112). These conditions, which result in bones with less density and strength, are serious concerns for older people (particularly women) as they heighten the risk of skeletal fracture and poor bone health (5). The slow but progressive loss of bone with age has been linked to physical inactivity and to hormonal, nutritional, mechanical, and genetic factors (51). Figure 7.3 shows the structural difference between normal, healthy bone and low mineral density osteporotic bone.

Advancing age is also associated with a loss of muscle mass and strength, which has been termed **sarcopenia** (5). Computed tomography has revealed that after age 30 there is a decrease in the cross-sectional areas of individual muscles, along with a decrease in muscle density, reductions in tendon compliance, and an increase in intramuscular fat (5, 107). These changes seem to be a predictable consequence of advancing age and seem to be most pronounced in women (107). The observed muscle atrophy with aging appears to result from physi-

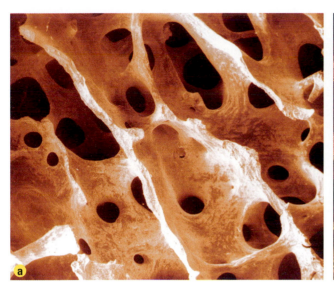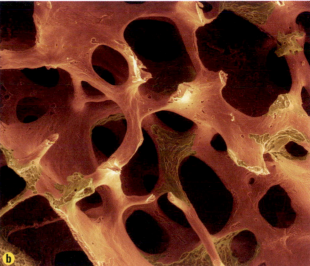

FIGURE 7.3 Differences between *(a)* healthy bone and *(b)* bone showing increased porosity resulting from osteoporosis.

cal inactivity and a gradual and selective denervation of muscle fibers (126, 181, 213). Decreased muscle mass results in a loss of muscle strength. In one report, 40% of women aged 55 to 64 years, 45% of women aged 65 to 74 years, and 65% of women aged 75 to 84 years were unable to lift about 10 pounds (4.5 kg) (110). The reduction in the size and number and the gradual denervation of muscle fibers also lead to a decrease in the ability of a muscle to generate power (i.e., exert force rapidly) (11, 92, 181); in fact, power recedes at a faster rate than muscle strength with aging (142). Since everyday activities require a certain degree of power production, a decrease in the ability of muscles to produce force rapidly may adversely affect the ability of older adults to safely perform activities such as stair climbing and walking. Factors that may contribute to the age-related decline in muscle strength and power include reductions in muscle mass, nervous system changes, hormonal changes, poor nutrition, and physical inactivity (48, 98, 170). The functional consequences of these age-related changes are significant because the magnitude and rate of change influence the age at which a person may become functionally dependent (e.g., unable to perform household tasks or rise from a chair) or reach a threshold of disability. A summary of adaptations to aging and resistance training is presented in table 7.1.

> ▶ **Advancing age is associated with a loss of muscle mass, which is largely attributable to physical inactivity. A direct result of the reduction in muscle mass is a loss of muscular strength and power.**

TABLE 7.1   Summary of the Effects of Aging and Resistance Training

Physical or physiological variable	Effect of aging	Effect of resistance training
Muscular strength	Decreases	Increases
Muscular power	Decreases	Increases
Muscular endurance	Decreases	Increases
Muscle mass	Decreases	Increases
Muscle fiber size	Decreases	Increases
Muscular metabolic capacity	Decreases	Increases
Resting metabolic rate	Decreases	Increases
Body fat	Increases	Decreases
Bone mineral density	Decreases	Increases
Physical function	Decreases	Increases

Age-Related Changes in Neuromotor Function

Seniors are at an increased risk of falling, which can lead to serious health, psychosocial, and economic consequences that negatively affect overall quality of life. Specifically, falls can result in pain syndromes, joint dislocations, skeletal fractures, limitations on daily functional activities, and a reduction in self-confidence (113). Falls can also lead to permanent disability, institutionalization, and fatalities (26). Intrinsic factors that lead to increased risk of falls in seniors include decrements in muscle strength and power (177), reaction time (5), and impaired balance and postural stability (188). Muscle activity before (**preactivation**), and immediately following (**cocontraction**) contact with the ground is an important mediator of braking and dynamic stabilization in both young and old individuals. Increased preactivation helps increase stiffness of the limb using fast stretch reflexes to better prepare the limb for ground contact. Cocontraction is a motor control strategy that dynamically stabilizes the joint; however, due to the simultaneous activation of both the agonist and antagonist muscle groups crossing the same joint, net joint moments and agonistic force outputs are reduced (223). Research shows that seniors rely on increased levels of muscle cocontraction as a compensatory mechanism to offset their increased balance difficulties and to minimize postural sway (164). Intuitively, this literature would suggest that older adults should use a variety of training modes specifically designed to offset these natural reductions in preactivation. Such methods would include low-intensity plyometrics, balance and dynamic stabilization exercises, and proprioception training to develop the ability to react more efficiently with the ground (88, 176).

Research shows that physical activity interventions can be effective in improving neuromotor function and preventing falls in seniors (209). However, it would appear that simply increasing physical activity per se will not prevent falls on its own. Rather, seniors must engage with, and adhere to, multidimensional programs that incorporate elements of both resistance and balance training (209). Furthermore, guidelines suggest that as with any population, training programs for seniors should overload progressively to promote a challenging training environment, and that training should be completed on a frequent basis to provide individuals with a sufficient training dosage (209). Of note, resistance training as a stand-alone training method does not seem to prevent the risk of falls (197), and it would appear that balance and flexibility training must accompany resistance training in order to provide the requisite training stimulus to reduce fall risk. However, the relative importance and potency of resistance training in increasing muscular strength, muscular power, and bone mineral density, in addition to its many other health benefits for seniors, cannot be overlooked.

Resistance Training for Older Adults

Aging does not appear to enhance or reduce the ability of the musculoskeletal system to adapt to resistance exercise. Significant improvements in muscular strength, muscular power, muscle mass, bone mineral density, and functional capabilities (e.g., gait speed) have been observed in older people who participated in progressive resistance training programs (5, 34, 106, 132). For older adults, such improvements enhance exercise performance, decrease the risk for injury, promote independent living, and improve quality of life. Because of the age-related changes in musculoskeletal health, resistance exercise is a beneficial mode of training for older populations who need to enhance musculoskeletal strength and power and resist decrements in muscle mass, bone mineral density, and functional abilities. Data also show that muscular strength is an important factor for reducing mortality risk in seniors (41, 128).

Responsiveness to Resistance Training in Older Adults

A great deal of attention has focused on strategies to improve the musculoskeletal health of older men and women. Because of the deconditioned state of many seniors, desirable changes in muscle strength and function can result from a variety of resistance training protocols, particularly during the first few weeks of training (82). Previously sedentary older men have more than doubled knee extensor strength and tripled knee flexor strength following a 12-week resistance training program (80), and similar observations have been made in older women after 12 weeks of resistance training (32). In one study, the ability of very old men and women (87 to 96 years old) to improve muscular strength was demonstrated following only eight weeks of resistance training (75). Improvements in gait speed, stair climbing ability, balance, and overall spontaneous activity have also been associated with training-induced strength gains in older populations (34, 76, 132). Evidence also suggests that resistance training specific to power development may help optimize functional abilities in older adults (5, 88, 98, 170), and that power training may be as effective as traditional resistance training in developing muscle architecture and neuromuscular activation properties of the lower limb (217). In some instances, it has been suggested that high-velocity power training has a greater influence on the ability to produce explosive force than traditional progressive resistance training (88, 179). For example, Fielding and colleagues (77) showed that older adults who completed high-velocity resistance training made greater gains in peak power and similar gains in maximum strength compared to seniors who trained at slower velocities over a 16-week training period. Similar results were reported by Reid and colleagues (185); in that study, older adults who completed a high-velocity, high-power resistance training program made significantly greater gains in leg press peak power than individuals who followed a slow-velocity, progressive resistance training program. While the optimal training protocol for improving muscular strength and power in seniors is not known, it appears there is a dose–response relationship between training intensity and improvements in muscular strength and power (48), with higher-intensity resistance training being more effective in developing maximal muscle strength than moderate- or low-intensity training (200).

Regular participation in a resistance training program also seems to have profound anabolic effects in older populations (32, 75, 80). Computed tomography and muscle biopsy analysis showed evidence of muscle hypertrophy in older men who participated in a high-intensity resistance training program (80); and other investigations involving older adults have shown that resistance training can improve nitrogen retention, which can have a positive effect on muscle protein metabolism (28, 225). Resistance training has also been shown to have an important effect on energy balance in older adults, as evidenced by an increase in the resting metabolic rate of men and women who resistance train (27). It is noteworthy that dietary modifications (a change in total food intake or selected nutrients) in addition to resistance training promotes a greater hypertrophic response than resistance training alone in elderly men (141).

Although the response of bone to resistance exercise is influenced by a complex interaction of many variables (e.g., hormonal status, activity history, and nutrition), it has been reported that resistance exercise has a positive effect on bone health in older men and women (44, 125, 163). Regularly performed resistance training can offset the age-related declines in bone health by maintaining or increasing bone mineral density. Resistance training may also reduce the risk of osteoporotic fractures by improving dynamic balance, muscle mass, and overall level of physical activity (5). While there is no doubt that resistance exercise can improve bone health in older adults, the interaction of exercise with hormonal and nutritional factors influences the degree of benefit of the exercise program. Furthermore, bones retain the beneficial effects of exercise only as long as training is continued. During periods of inactivity, bone density tends to revert to preexercise levels (109).

> ▶ **Though aging is associated with a number of undesirable changes in body composition, older men and women maintain their ability to make significant improvements in strength and functional ability. Aerobic, resistance, and balance exercise are beneficial for older adults, but only resistance training can increase muscular strength, muscular power, and muscle mass.**

Program Design Considerations for Older Adults

Whereas aerobic exercise has been recommended for many years as a means of increasing cardiovascular fitness, resistance training is currently recognized as an important component of a well-rounded fitness program for older adults (5, 34, 82, 120, 222). Because age-related losses of musculoskeletal strength, power, and mass may be almost universal, programs designed to maintain or improve musculoskeletal health in older adults should be implemented. Not only can regular participation in a resistance training program offset some of these age-related losses, but it can help older people maintain an active, high-quality lifestyle.

The fundamental principles of designing a resistance training program for an older person and a younger person are basically the same, but there are several concerns that strength and conditioning professionals need to be aware of when working with seniors. Attention should be given to preexisting medical ailments, prior training history, and nutritional status before the beginning of a resistance training program that may predispose seniors to increased risk of exercise-induced injury or illness. Even though older populations retain the capacity to adapt to increased levels of physical activity, safe and effective exercise guidelines must be followed.

Before participation in an exercise program, seniors should complete a medical history and risk factor questionnaire (4). Potential limitations and possible restrictions for physical activity can be ascertained from this information. In some cases physician clearance is required before the initiation of a moderate or vigorous exercise program (4), for example, in cardiac rehabilitation patients or cancer survivors. Any questions regarding a participant's medical status (e.g., heart disease, hypertension, arthritis, osteoporosis, or diabetes mellitus) should be answered by a health professional. After this information has been obtained, a preprogram evaluation to document baseline measurements and assess responses to specific exercise modalities should be performed. Although a treadmill exercise test is often used to evaluate cardiovascular responses to aerobic exercise, a strength test (preferably on the equipment used in training) should be performed to assess responses to resistance exercise and aid in the exercise prescription. Of note, while resistance machines may be used in the early stages of a training program with older adults due to balance and flexibility limitations, where appropriate, older adults should use free weight, multijoint resistance training exercises, which provide a greater overall training stimulus and place a greater demand on postural stability. Various methods of assessing muscular strength, including repetition maximum testing, can be used in senior populations, provided that appropriate testing guidelines are followed (195). Strength and conditioning professionals should be aware of the potential risks of breath holding (Valsalva maneuver) for older adults. While the Valsalva maneuver assists in stabilizing the trunk and vertebral column during performance of various resistance training exercises, owing to the sudden rise in systolic and diastolic blood pressure that the technique creates, this technique is generally discouraged in seniors (4, 178). This is especially true for adults with a history of cardiovascular disease (heart arrhythmias, angina) or cerebral conditions (i.e., stroke, dizziness).

Evidence suggests that resistance training can be safe for seniors when individuals adhere to appropriate training guidelines (53, 138, 222). On the other hand, poorly designed programs can be potentially hazardous. For example, failing to provide sufficient rest periods between sets and between different exercises, programming exercises that are technically too challenging, or increasing the intensity of exercise (typically the external load against which the individual is working) all increase the likelihood of resistance training–related injury. Similar to the situation with youth and females, the resistance training stimulus should never be increased at the expense of technical competency.

Untrained seniors who begin resistance training should start at a relatively low exercise intensity and volume, and the exercise prescription should be individualized. Although higher intensities and volumes can be tolerated by some older men and women who have resistance training experience, the early phase of the training program should be directed toward learning proper exercise technique while minimizing the potential for muscle soreness and injury. Less intense training during the first few weeks of an exercise program may also be beneficial for seniors who are apprehensive about participating in a resistance training program. Following the initial adaptation period, the training program can gradually progress, provided that it continues to meet the needs and medical concerns of each person. In training older men and women, it is particularly important to focus on the interaction of major muscle groups used in everyday activities, such as load carrying and climbing stairs.

Once participants master the performance of basic resistance exercises, more advanced and demanding exercises such as standing postures with free weights (barbells and dumbbells), multidirectional medicine ball exercises, and advanced balance training (e.g., one-legged stands and circle turns) can be incorporated into the program. Seniors should gradually progress from one set of 8 to 12 repetitions at a relatively low intensity (e.g., 40% to 50% 1RM) to higher training volumes and intensities (e.g., three sets per exercise with 60% to 80% of 1RM), depending on individual needs, goals, and abilities (82, 120). In addition, high-velocity power exercises can be gradually incorporated into the overall training regimen, provided that seniors have successfully completed a general resistance training program. Current recommendations for increasing power in healthy older adults include the performance of one to three sets per exercise with a light to moderate load (40% to 60% 1RM) for 6 to 10 repetitions with high repetition velocity (120).

A resistance training program for older men and women should vary in volume and intensity throughout the year to lessen the likelihood of overtraining and ensure that progress is made throughout the training period. Because recovery from a training session may take longer in older populations, a training frequency of twice per week is recommended, at least during the initial adaptation period. Strength and conditioning

What Are the Safety Recommendations for Resistance Training for Older Adults?

- Older adult participants should be prescreened, since many older people suffer from a variety of age-related medical conditions. If necessary, medical advice should be sought concerning the most appropriate type of activity.
- Participants should warm up for 5 to 10 minutes before each exercise session. An acceptable warm-up includes low- to moderate-intensity aerobic activity and calisthenics.
- Older adults should perform static stretching exercises either before or after—or both before and after—each resistance training session.
- Older adults should use a resistance that does not overtax the musculoskeletal system.
- Participants should avoid performing the Valsalva maneuver during resistance training to avoid an abnormal increase in blood pressure.
- Older adults should be allowed 48 to 72 hours of recovery between exercise sessions.
- They should perform all exercises within a range of motion that is pain free.
- As with any individual engaging with resistance training, older adults should receive exercise instruction from qualified instructors.

professionals should be sensitive to the concerns of individuals and be able to modify a training program based on the person's health history and individual goals. With competent instruction and support from friends, older men and women can gain confidence in their ability to resistance train, which may be enough to ensure good adherence to the program. However, since a majority of older adults do not currently engage in resistance training activities (31, 202), professionals may initially need to increase awareness of the fitness benefits associated with resistance exercise and address the concerns that seniors may have about participating in a resistance training program.

An additional consideration related to resistance training in older men and women is appropriate nutrition. The quality and quantity of a person's food intake (or perhaps selected nutrients) may mean the difference between losing and gaining muscle mass. In particular, it seems that adequate amounts of protein are essential for muscle hypertrophy in older people (169). Furthermore, inadequate intakes of macronutrients (fat, protein, and carbohydrate) and micronutrients (vitamins and minerals) are associated with potential negative health consequences, including fatigue, compromised immune function, and delayed recovery from injury. Improving an older person's food intake not only improves health but may also optimize adaptations to resistance training.

Conclusion

Research shows that resistance exercise can be a safe and effective method of conditioning for males and females of all ages and abilities. The potential benefits are multifactorial, including positive effects on a variety of physical performance variables (e.g., strength and power), health markers (e.g., body composition and cardiac function), and psychosocial development (e.g., self-image and confidence). Moreover, regular participation in a resistance training program can reduce the risk of sport- and physical activity–related injuries in athletes and promote independent living in seniors. Though the fundamental principles of resistance training are similar for people of both sexes and all ages, there are unique concerns specific to each population. Knowledge of age- and sex-related differences is essential to the development and evaluation of safe and effective resistance training programs. Strength and conditioning professionals should be aware that individual responses to resistance exercise may vary greatly and should be sensitive to the individual needs of all participants.

Over the past few decades, coaches, clinicians, and exercise scientists have added to our understanding of age- and sex-related differences and their implications for resistance exercise. Their work has quantified the impact of resistance training on males and females of all ages and has provided the foundation for recommendations about the design of strength and conditioning programs. The information in this chapter and other chapters should help strength and conditioning professionals understand and appreciate age- and sex-related differences and enhance their ability to develop safe and effective resistance training programs for children, women, and older adults alike.

KEY TERMS

adolescence	ectomorphic	osteoporosis
adulthood	endomorphic	peak height velocity (PHV)
amenorrhea	female athlete triad	preactivation
anterior cruciate ligament (ACL)	growth	puberty
apophyseal	growth cartilage	resistance exercise
biological age	maturation	sarcopenia
childhood	menarche	senior
chronological age	mesomorphic	training age
cocontraction	older	youth
development	osteopenia	young athlete
diaphysis		

STUDY QUESTIONS

1. An 8-year-old boy dramatically increased his upper body strength after following a six-month resistance training program. Which of the following is MOST likely responsible for this gain?
   a. increased number of muscle fibers
   b. enhanced cross-sectional area
   c. greater muscle density
   d. improved neuromuscular functioning

2. Growth cartilage in children is located at all of the following EXCEPT the
   a. diaphysis
   b. epiphyseal plate
   c. joint surface
   d. apophyseal insertion

3. The condition characterized by a bone mineral density more than 2.5 SD below the young adult mean is called
   a. sarcopenia
   b. osteopenia
   c. osteoporosis
   d. scoliosis

4. Which of the following should be evaluated FIRST when one is designing a training program for a 68-year-old competitive female tennis player?
   a. cardiovascular fitness
   b. lower body strength
   c. balance and agility
   d. medical history

5. Deconditioned female college athletes who participate in sports such as basketball and soccer appear to be at increased risk for developing injuries to the
   a. back
   b. knee
   c. wrist
   d. neck

Psychology of Athletic Preparation and Performance

Traci A. Statler, PhD, and Andrea M. DuBois, MS

> **After completing this chapter, you will be able to**
>
> - understand the psychological constructs of arousal, motivation, focus, and confidence and be able to ascertain their impact on physical performance;
> - comprehend terms relevant to psychological areas of concern, such as anxiety, attention, the ideal performance state, self-efficacy, imagery, and goal setting;
> - understand varying ways to manipulate practice schedules including whole–part, random, and variable practice, and how to use these schedules to facilitate skill acquisition and learning;
> - understand different types of instructions and feedback and their application in a practice and performance setting.

The authors would like to acknowledge the significant contributions of Bradley D. Hatfield and Evan B. Brody to this chapter.

Excellence in athletic performance is the result of sound skill and physical training accompanied by optimal rest and recovery cycles and appropriate diet. At any particular stage of biological maturity, the phenotypic development of the athlete's genetic potential represents a relatively stable ceiling for performance, but the expression of that skilled performance can vary tremendously from contest to contest and even from moment to moment. The role of sport psychology is to help athletes achieve more consistent levels of performance at or near their physical potential by carefully managing their physical resources through appropriate psychological strategies and techniques. By understanding these strategies and techniques, strength and conditioning professionals can design sport-specific and even position-specific training programs that have the ultimate goal of maximizing performance.

After introducing foundational concepts, we address how one's mind, through cognitions, can influence physical performance, and then we describe the **ideal performance state**—the ultimate goal of every athlete. In part, this state is marked by psychological and **physiological efficiency** (i.e., employing only the amount of mental and physical energy required to perform the task). We discuss the primary psychological influences—motivation, attention, and arousal—on skill acquisition and performance, citing several theories of how these phenomena can change psychomotor learning and athletic performance. Finally, we discuss techniques, including goal setting, energy management and relaxation, imagery, and confidence development, that can be employed to enhance overall performance in strength and conditioning environments, as well as other performance venues.

Role of Sport Psychology

An athlete is someone who engages in a social comparison (i.e., competition) involving psychomotor skill or physical prowess (or both) in an institutionalized setting, typically under public scrutiny or evaluation. The essence of athletic competition involves comparing oneself to others and putting ego and self-esteem on the line in a setting that is bound by rules and regulations. The psychologically well-prepared athlete is characterized by efficiency of thought and behavior. Efficiency is typically associated with skilled performance, when actions are fluid and graceful. The concept can also be extended to psychological activity; an efficient athlete adopts a task-relevant focus, not wasting attention on task-irrelevant processing such as worrying, catastrophizing, or thinking about other things such as a critical audience or coach.

Sport psychology is a multifaceted discipline, drawing on constructs of exercise science and psychological principles, that seeks to understand the influence of behavioral processes and cognitions on movement. Sport psychology is typically classified as a scientific field of study within sports medicine, and has three major goals:

- Measuring psychological phenomena
- Investigating the relationships between psychological variables and performance
- Applying theoretical knowledge to improve athletic performance

By applying the information gained through an awareness of sport psychology principles, athletes can better manage their physical resources, thereby producing more effective performances. In reality, many athletes come to the training environment with some solid mental skills already in their repertoire, but this often seems to "just happen," with little understanding of how these skills evolved, or even how to best use them for effective performance. Throughout this chapter we introduce a structure for understanding the interrelationships not only between the mental skills themselves, but between the mental skills and the physical, technical, and tactical skills being developed in the weight room and on the practice field. Note, however, that these skills can be truly effective only if they are understood, practiced, and applied to the performance setting. Like the physical, technical, and tactical constructs described throughout the rest of this book, mental skills too need to be taught, practiced, integrated into performance, and evaluated for effectiveness.

Ideal Performance State

The ideal performance state has been studied from a number of perspectives. Williams and Krane (42) listed the following characteristics that athletes typically report about this state:

- Absence of fear—no fear of failure
- No thinking about or analysis of performance (related to the motor stage of automaticity)
- A narrow focus of attention concentrated on the activity itself
- A sense of effortlessness—an involuntary experience
- A sense of personal control
- A distortion of time and space, in which time seems to slow

In a sense, this ideal performance state seems to represent everything that applied sport psychology programs attempt to promote. There is an absence of negative self-talk, a strong feeling of efficacy, and an adaptive focus on task-relevant cues. An important aspect is that the athletes trust in their skill and conditioning levels and just "let it happen," without interference from negative associative processes in the cerebral cortex.

Kobe Bryant, one of the premier players in the National Basketball Association, describes being in this state, saying,

> When you get in that zone it's just a supreme confidence that you know it's going in. It's not a matter of if or this [or] that. It's going in. Things just slow down. Everything slows down and you just have supreme confidence. When that happens, you really do not try to focus on what's going on because . . . you could lose it in a second. Everything becomes one noise—you don't hear this or that; everything's just one noise—you're not paying attention to one or the other. . . . You just really try to stay in the present and not let anything break that rhythm. Again, as long as you just kind of stay there, you become oblivious to everything that's going on. You don't think about your surroundings or what's going on with the crowd or the team. You're kind of locked in. . . . You have to really try to stay in the present and not let anything break that rhythm. (see YouTube at https://www.youtube.com/watch?v=wl49zc8g3DY)

Bryant's comments richly reinforce many of the concepts discussed throughout this chapter. It is important to remember that his mental state rests largely on a sound physical training program and on a history of performance success. Bryant exhibits phenomenal physical prowess, arduously running sprints, training on the court, and lifting weights in the off-season. Combined with superior performance on the basketball court, such preparatory physical effort contributes greatly to his focused, confident psychological state.

Energy Management: Arousal, Anxiety, and Stress

In order for athletes to perform effectively, they need to learn how to best manage their mental and physical energy levels. Athletes who deplete energy through worry, anger, frustration, or anxiety experience a greater likelihood of distraction and decreased self-confidence, and they have less physical energy for when they really need to perform (11). Thus, the ability to maintain self-control and manage energy in a performance environment is a critical skill for any performer.

Mental energy is generated, maintained, depleted, and refreshed via our emotions. **Emotions** are temporary feeling states that occur in response to events and that have both physiological and psychological components (10). These emotions affect mental and physical energy and therefore can have both beneficial and detrimental effects on human performance, often depending on how they get interpreted. Emotions can be beneficial to performance when they get us excited, cause us to feel motivated, elevate confidence in ourselves, and reinforce our commitment levels. However, emotion can be detrimental when there is either too much or too little (a performer being too "amped up" or "too flat") or when we lose control of our emotions and cease to function effectively in a performance environment (e.g., an athlete who cannot control his or her anger or frustration). Training athletes to tap into their emotions to generate or elevate energy, while maintaining a sense of control over those emotions so as not to let them interfere with performance, is a key toward generating that ideal performance state (40).

By arming athletes with the mental tools to combat inappropriate thoughts, enhance confidence, and reinforce motivation and commitment, coaches are providing many of the skills necessary to allow the athlete to maintain composure as well.

Arousal

The training environment provides a host of new and unfamiliar experiences that create multiple opportunities to test oneself and be evaluated for effectiveness. Because of this, athletic performance is frequently affected by arousal, anxiety, and stress. These terms are often used interchangeably; however, in reality, they are different elements within the same construct.

Arousal is simply a blend of physiological and psychological activation in an individual and refers to the intensity of motivation at any given moment (40). For example, a "psyched-up" athlete may experience tremendous mental activation characterized by positive thoughts and a strong sense of control, whereas a "flat" athlete could experience minimal activation characterized by wandering thoughts and feelings of boredom. Arousal is always present in an individual to some degree, on a continuum ranging from being deeply asleep, or comatose, to highly excited; but in and of itself it is not automatically associated with pleasant or unpleasant events. It is simply a measurement of activation, and as such can be indexed by such metrics as heart rate, blood pressure, electroencephalography (EEG), electromyography (EMG), and catecholamine levels, or with self-report instruments such as the activation–deactivation checklist (39). The optimal arousal required for efficient performance depends on several factors that are discussed later in the chapter.

Anxiety

Anxiety is a subcategory of arousal in that it is a negatively perceived emotional state characterized by nervousness, worry, apprehension, or fear and is associated with a physiological activation of the body (40). Because anxiety requires the individual's negative perception of a situation, it incorporates a cognitive component, called **cognitive anxiety**, as well as the physical reaction, or **somatic anxiety**, evidenced through physical symptoms such as tense muscles, tachycardia (fast heart rate), and upset stomach.

The term *anxiety* is often confusingly used to refer to both a stable, enduring personality construct and a more short-term, changeable mood state. These are, in fact, different constructs within the emotional state of anxiety. **State anxiety** refers to a subjective experience of apprehension and uncertainty accompanied by elevated autonomic and voluntary neural outflow and increased endocrine activity (36). State anxiety is a generally negative experience, but its effects on athletic performance can be positive, negative, or indifferent, depending on such factors as the athlete's skill level and personality and the complexity of the task to be performed.

State anxiety is distinct from but related to **trait anxiety**, a personality variable or disposition relating to the probability that one will perceive an environment as threatening. In essence, trait anxiety acts as a primer for the athlete to experience state anxiety (37). Trait anxiety also affects the appropriate level of arousal for a given individual. People with high levels of trait anxiety tend to flood attentional capacity with task-irrelevant cognitions, such as thoughts of failure, catastrophe, or ego-oriented concerns. During a complex decision-making task, these attentionally demanding cues could compromise a player's selective attention. The athlete with low trait anxiety can handle higher levels of pressure because of the decreased probability of engaging in such personal catastrophizing.

> State anxiety is the actual experience of apprehension and uncontrolled arousal. Trait anxiety is a personality characteristic, which represents a latent disposition to perceive situations as threatening.

In a nonanxious state, arousal is under the control of the athlete; it can be elevated or lowered as needed. The athlete who is psychologically well prepared knows the appropriate zone for optimal performance and can manage it accordingly. In an anxious state, arousal is relatively uncontrolled. Typically, arousal is too high

during periods of ineffective state anxiety; the skeletal muscles are tense, the heart is racing, and negative thoughts intrude. This lack of physical and **psychological efficiency** is typically initiated by uncertainty about a present or anticipated event. At least three important factors are usually present:

- A high degree of ego involvement, in which the athlete may perceive a threat to self-esteem
- A perceived discrepancy between one's ability and the demands for athletic success
- A fear of the consequences of failure (such as a loss of approval from teammates, coach, family, or peers)

Because these constructs of anxiety and arousal are complex and interrelated, figure 8.1 provides a summary of the interrelationships of arousal, state anxiety, and trait anxiety, and anxiety cognitive and somatic components.

Stress

Stress is defined as a substantial imbalance between demand (physical, psychological, or both) and response capability, under conditions in which failure to meet that demand has important consequences (31). A **stressor** is an environmental or cognitive event that precipitates stress (i.e., the stress response). Stress can be described as a negative (**distress**) or a positive (**eustress**) state. Both of these generate arousal, but only when the perception of the stressor is negative—distress—does it also generate anxiety. Therefore, distress comprises cognitive and somatic anxiety, whereas eustress comprises positive mental energy and physiological arousal.

Influence of Arousal and Anxiety on Performance

Once an understanding of the general concepts of arousal, anxiety, and stress is attained, the next step lies in deconstructing how these emotional elements influence performance. Why does arousal affect one athlete beneficially and another detrimentally? This section examines a number of theories and models that attempt to explain this relationship between arousal and performance. It begins with the simplest construct—Hull's (35) drive theory—and builds on it with Yerkes and Dodson's (50) inverted-U theory, describing the mediating influences of skill level, task complexity, and personality. Other related theories that further explain this relationship are outlined, including Hanin's (12) individual zones of optimal functioning (IZOF), Fazey and Hardy's (13) catastrophe theory, and finally, Kerr's (17) reversal theory.

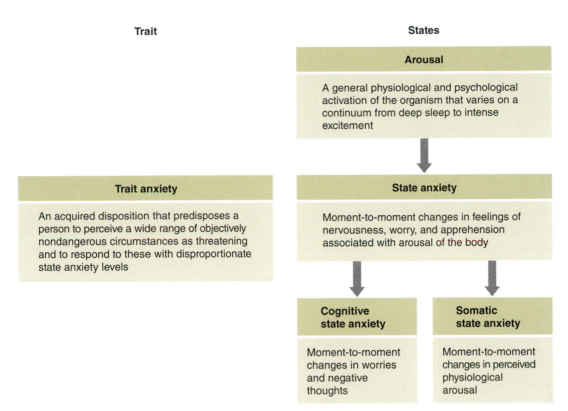

Trait

States

Arousal

A general physiological and psychological activation of the organism that varies on a continuum from deep sleep to intense excitement

Trait anxiety

An acquired disposition that predisposes a person to perceive a wide range of objectively nondangerous circumstances as threatening and to respond to these with disproportionate state anxiety levels

State anxiety

Moment-to-moment changes in feelings of nervousness, worry, and apprehension associated with arousal of the body

Cognitive state anxiety

Moment-to-moment changes in worries and negative thoughts

Somatic state anxiety

Moment-to-moment changes in perceived physiological arousal

FIGURE 8.1   The interrelationships of arousal, trait anxiety, and state anxiety.

Reprinted, by permission, from Weinberg and Gould, 2015 (40).

Drive Theory

When researchers first started examining the relationship between arousal and performance, it was thought to follow a direct and linear progression. Hull's **drive theory** (35) proposes that as an individual's arousal or state anxiety increases, so too does performance. Thus, the more psyched up athletes become, the better they perform. This may hold true as an athlete progresses from relatively low levels of arousal to somewhat higher amounts; but most would recognize that more arousal is not always better, as performers can clearly be too "pumped up" to perform well. Depending on the skill and experience levels of the performer, the complexity of the activity, or both, more arousal may be beneficial, but it can in fact also be detrimental. When people perform well-learned or simple skills, a higher level of arousal can benefit performance. However, the more complex a given skill becomes, or the less experience an athlete has with that skill, the more arousal can produce catastrophic performance outcomes (40).

Skill Level

An athlete's skill level can increase the latitude of optimal arousal; that is, the more skill an athlete has developed, the better he or she can perform during states of less-than or greater-than-optimal arousal (40). In the

beginning stages of learning a skill, the athlete is in a stage of analysis or cognition (9). This means that he or she has to think about actions. For example, a novice basketball player has to be conscious of the ball while dribbling and needs to devote some attention to the task. At a given level of arousal, worrisome thoughts compete with an attentional capacity already filled by details of motor performance (i.e., dribbling). If a new situation suddenly develops, the novice's mind is already occupied, and he or she may not see it.

The optimal arousal point is lower for less skilled athletes than for more advanced players. Therefore, coaches should lower arousal and decrease the decision-making responsibilities of developing or unseasoned athletes (players who are skilled but lack competitive experience) and have them focus on simple assignments to prevent attentional overload. In coaching Olympic-style lifters during an important meet, instructions to novice competitors should be simple, clear, and direct. When they experience success, the derived self-confidence may reduce negative self-talk and the sense of uncertainty that typically characterizes such performers.

Task Complexity

A second factor that influences the appropriate level of arousal to achieve optimal performance is task complexity (26). Most athletic skills are exceedingly complex from a biomechanical perspective, but the more concerning complexity relates to conscious decision making. For example, running is a very complex task in terms of motor control and functional anatomy, but athletes fortunately do not have to devote much conscious attention to the coordinated action. In fact, the action can become altered and inefficient if they think about it too much, because they change the neural sequences for movement initiation. From an attentional perspective, simple or well-learned skills are less affected by a high degree of arousal because they have few task-relevant cues to monitor (40). Fortunately, then, physiological arousal, which typically accompanies emotional arousal, may be beneficial. However, the situation is dramatically reversed for skills that necessitate conscious decision-making effort, such as those required by a goalie in

soccer or a baseball catcher who is facing a critical, bases-loaded pitch. In these instances, arousal must be kept relatively low because of the need to maintain a wider focus so as to recognize relevant attentional cues.

Inverted-U Theory

Building on the basic relationship outlined in drive theory, Yerkes and Dodson (50) proposed one of the major tenets of the arousal–performance relationship—the **inverted-U theory**. Basically, this theory states that arousal facilitates performance up to an optimal level, beyond which further increases in arousal are associated with reduced performance. Figure 8.2 graphically shows this relationship. Most coaches and athletes intuitively accept this hypothesis, as they have all experienced poor performance when feeling flat or underaroused, as well as when they feel too "amped up" or "out of

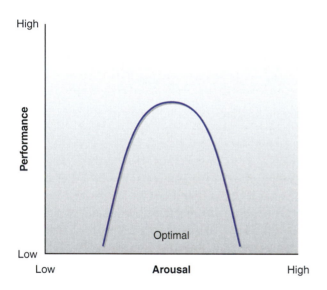

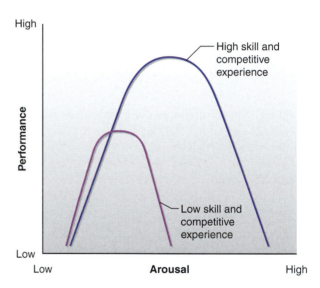

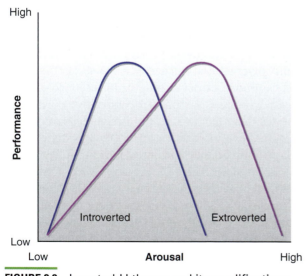

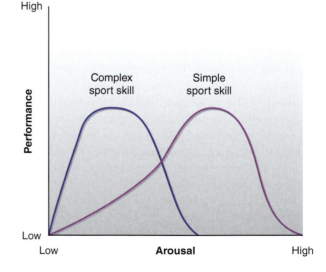

FIGURE 8.2   Inverted-U theory and its modifications.

Reprinted, by permission, from Hatfield and Walford, 1987 (14).

control." The inverted-U concept helps coaches and athletes understand why arousal affects performance and enables them to gain greater control over the appropriate level of arousal for a given athlete within a given sport. It should be noted, however, that the generic shape of the curve in this relationship has been criticized, given our understanding of the individual influences of skill, ability, experience, and task complexity as described previously (11).

Individual Zones of Optimal Functioning Theory

Hanin (12) noted the interactions of individual factors that affect optimal arousal for performance and developed the **individual zones of optimal functioning** theory. Dr. Hanin holds that different people, in different types of performances, perform best with very different levels of arousal. This theory differs from the inverted-U hypothesis in two ways: (1) Ideal performance does not seem to always occur at the midpoint of the arousal continuum, and (2) rather than there being a single defined arousal point at which optimal performance occurs, this best performance can occur within a small range, or bandwidth, of arousal level. Further, Hanin proposed that there are positive and negative emotions (e.g., excited, nervous) that can generate enhanced performance, just as there are positive and negative emotions (e.g., comfortable, annoyed) that can debilitate performance. This proposal is important because it recognizes that any specific emotion can be positively perceived by one athlete but negatively perceived by another. In practice, then, athletes can retrospectively recall the arousal associated with several of their performances that differed in quality. They can then monitor emotions and arousal levels before an important match and make adjustments to increase the chances of falling into this individual ideal zone.

Catastrophe Theory

According to Hardy (13), assessment of the cognitive and somatic dimensions of arousal can sharpen the ability to predict (and therefore control) their impact on performance. Earlier assumptions associated with the inverted-U theory held that increases in arousal beyond the optimal level resulted in gradual, proportionate declines in performance. However, common observation tells us that this is not always the case—an athlete may suffer a severe and catastrophic decline rather than a gradual quadratic or curvilinear decline in performance, and restoring a degree of calm does not necessarily bring a return to the level of performance exhibited before the decline. In this model, the **catastrophe theory**, somatic arousal has a curvilinear, inverted-U relationship to athletic performance, whereas cognitive anxiety shows a steady negative relationship to performance. When increases in physiological arousal occur in the presence of cognitive anxiety, a sudden drop—rather than a gradual decline—in performance occurs. The practical implication of this theory is that the arousal constructs need to be more clearly delineated as cognitive anxiety, physiological arousal, somatic anxiety, or some combination of these.

Reversal Theory

Kerr's (17) interpretation of **reversal theory** posits that the way in which arousal and anxiety affect performance depends on the individual's interpretation of that arousal. Essentially, one athlete might interpret high levels of arousal as excitement and indicative of performance readiness, while another athlete, experiencing the same emotion at the same arousal level, would interpret that feeling as unpleasant and reflective of a lack of confidence. This idea implies that athletes have within their power the ability to reverse their interpretation of their own arousal; instead of perceiving high arousal as scary and worrisome, they can choose to reverse their perception and interpret the arousal as reflecting excitement and anticipation. This theory is important because it emphasizes that one's interpretation of arousal, and not just its amount, is significant. Further, it shows that the way in which arousal and anxiety influence performance—whether they are beneficial or detrimental to performance—is within the control of the individual.

Motivation

As mentioned earlier in this chapter, motivation is a primary psychological factor in the acquisition and effective performance of motor skills. **Motivation** can be defined as the intensity and direction of effort (40). Selected aspects of motivational phenomena are highlighted in the following sections. We first discuss intrinsic and extrinsic motivation, which greatly influence the athlete's desire to train and compete. Then we discuss achievement motivation, which helps to explain individual differences in competitiveness. Finally, positive and negative reinforcement are explained as they apply to skill learning and performance.

Intrinsic and Extrinsic Motivation

Intrinsic motivation is important for any athlete. Deci (7) defined this construct as a desire to be competent and self-determining. With intrinsic motivation, athletes are driven because of their love of the game and the inherent reward they feel from participation. This is motivation that comes from within the athlete and is exhibited regardless of the existence of material reward or punishment. Intrinsically motivated athletes focus on the enjoyment or fun they experience in the activity and generally desire to learn and improve because of this love for the behavior in and of itself (40). How can such a desirable state be maintained or encouraged? The answer lies in Deci's (7) definition, which stresses success (competence) and "pulling one's own strings" (self-determination). Appropriate goals, especially process or performance goals, can increase perceived competence. Additionally, giving the athlete some latitude in decision making increases perceived self-determination (7). Although authoritarian behavior is sometimes warranted in sport, in that clear directives are needed in a stressful and competitive environment, a total lack of delegated responsibilities could result in a loss of initiative and drive in athletes (40).

In opposition, **extrinsic motivation** is motivation that comes from some external as opposed to internal source. Numerous examples of this exist, as it is founded on an individualized reward construct; examples of more common extrinsic rewards in sport settings include awards, trophies, praise from coaches and teammates, social approval, and fear of punishment. It should be noted that athletes are rarely completely intrinsically or extrinsically motivated; rather, they exhibit varying degrees along this motivation continuum depending on the activity, their perceptions of competence, the level of importance the activity has, and a host of other variables (5, 7, 23, 40, 42).

Achievement Motivation

Within the general construct of motivation lies a more specifically targeted type called **achievement motivation**, which refers to a person's efforts to master a task, achieve excellence, overcome obstacles, and engage in competition or social comparison. All things being equal between two athletes, whoever is higher in achievement motivation will be the better athlete because he or she has a greater appetite for competition.

McClelland and colleagues (23) theorized that all people have opposing personality traits within themselves: the **motive to achieve success (MAS)** and the **motive to avoid failure (MAF)**. The MAS relates to the capacity to experience pride in one's accomplishments and is characterized by a desire to challenge oneself and evaluate one's abilities. On the other hand, the MAF relates to the desire to protect one's ego and self-esteem. Despite its name, however, MAF is not really about avoiding failure itself. It is more about avoiding the perception of shame that accompanies the failure.

Generally, MAS-dominated athletes are most intrigued by situations that are either uncertain or challenging, with an approximate 50% probability of success (40). This creates opportunities to assess one's abilities. On the other hand, MAF-dominated players are more comfortable in situations in which it is either very easy to achieve success (thereby avoiding shame) or so extremely difficult that there would be no expectation of winning (again, eliminating the likelihood of feeling shame) (40). At higher levels of sport involvement, it is unlikely that athletes would be dominated by MAF, but they would certainly show degrees or a range of competitiveness. Confronted by a very challenging goal, such as gaining a significant amount of lean muscle weight during the hypertrophy phase of a periodized cycle, the MAF-dominated individual might reduce effort because he or she fears failure and the threat to self-esteem (and might also claim that the goal is unrealistic), whereas the MAS-dominated individual might heighten effort in response to the challenge and not perceive any threat.

Motivational Aspects of Skill Learning (Self-Controlled Practice)

In addition to providing the individual with information for skill acquisition, practice, instructions, and feedback can also act as motivational factors for enhancing performance. Practice schedules that address the fundamental psychological needs of autonomy, competence, and social relatedness can influence motivation (47). Of recent interest in the motor learning literature is the role of **self-controlled practice** in enhancing motivation, performance, and skill learning. Self-controlled practice involves the athlete in decisions related to the practice structure, including when to receive feedback or which skill to practice; it also involves simply asking athletes how they believe they are doing (4-6, 47). This promotes a more active involvement in the practice session and can enhance feelings of competence and autonomy (5, 6). As a result of this heightened motivation, performance and learning improve (5, 6). Engaging the athletes in some decisions related to the practice schedule is an easy yet effective way to have them assist themselves in reaching their sport performance goals. The concepts of instructions, feedback, and practice schedules are discussed in greater depth later in this chapter.

Positive and Negative Reinforcement in Coaching

Coaches can also benefit from understanding the concepts of positive and negative reinforcement and positive and negative punishment as they relate to motivation (22). **Positive reinforcement** is the act of increasing the probability of occurrence of a given behavior (a target behavior, such as correct footwork in basketball, is termed an **operant**) by following it with a positive action, object, or event such as praise, decals on the helmet, or prizes and awards. **Negative reinforcement** also increases the probability of occurrence of a given operant, but it is accomplished through the removal of an act, object, or event that is typically aversive. For example, if the team showed great hustle in practice (i.e., the operant is enthusiasm and hustle), then the coach could announce that no wind sprints would be required at the session's end. This coaching reinforcement style focuses attention on what the athlete is doing correctly.

Punishment, on the other hand, is designed to decrease the occurrence of a given operant, that is, negative behaviors such as mistakes or a lack of effort. **Positive punishment** is the presentation of an act, object, or event following a behavior that could decrease the behavior's occurrence. An example is reprimanding a player after a mistake or making an athlete do push-ups or sprints after a fumble. **Negative punishment**, or the removal of something valued, could take the form of revoking privileges or playing time, as in benching. Although coaches use a mixture of both reward and punishment, reinforcement (i.e., reward), or a positive approach, is arguably better because it focuses on what athletes should do and what they did right (termed *specific positive feedback*). Reinforcement (both positive and negative) increases task-relevant focus rather than worry focus. A task-relevant focus facilitates reaction time and decision making. With reinforcement, athletes also build long-term memories of success, self-esteem, self-efficacy, and confidence. Successful experiences more likely color the athlete's view of competition as desirable and as an opportunity to perform. Of course, coaches may punish unwarranted lack of effort, but it seems ineffective to punish athletes for mistakes if they are making the effort to perform correctly.

Attention and Focus

The athlete's ability to focus can be better understood through the construct of attention. **Attention** is defined as the processing of both environmental and internal cues that come to awareness. A performer's conscious attention is continuously bombarded with a variety of external stimuli and internal thoughts to which it can be directed. The ability to inhibit awareness of some

stimuli in order to process others is termed **selective attention**, and it suppresses task-irrelevant cues (e.g., people on the sidelines, planes flying over the stadium) in order to process the task-relevant cues in the limited attentional space. For a baseball pitcher, task-relevant cues might include the hitter's tendencies and the locations of runners on base.

> ► **Selective attention, commonly referred to by athletes as their *level of focus*, is the suppression of task-irrelevant stimuli and thoughts.**

American football coaches often exploit the strategic potential of selective attention of their opponents by calling a time-out just before a field goal attempt. During the time-out, the opposing athlete might selectively attend more to task-irrelevant thoughts of self-doubt and the potential for failure, rather than the more beneficial thoughts of self-reassurance or a focus on minor instructional cues. Placekickers can deal with this anxiety and attentional challenge by adopting a ritual or a mental checklist, commonly referred to as a **routine**, that consciously directs thoughts to task-relevant and controllable concerns (e.g., breathing, checking the turf, and stretching the hamstrings).

The important underlying principle is that thinking one set of thoughts actively precludes attending to other worrisome thoughts because of the limited capacity of working memory. This human shortcoming can be used to advantage. Before a lifting performance, for example, the athlete might use key phrases to focus on the task-relevant cues associated with the lift, such as foot placement, back position, point of visual focus, and knee angle during a squat. This strategy can reduce distractions, which often deter optimal effort. Such focusing strategies can promote mental consistency during the preparatory state, which in turn can promote physical consistency—the hallmark of a skilled athlete.

It is also important to note that the ability to focus attention on task-relevant cues and to control distraction is a skill that can be learned and that improves with increased experience. According to Fitts and Posner's (9) classic theory, the athlete progresses through three

---

How Should Positive and Negative Reinforcement Be Applied?

- Coaches should generally subscribe to a reinforcement strategy to assist athletes in focusing on what they do correctly.
- Punishment should be used sparingly, as it increases the likelihood that athletes will focus on what they are doing incorrectly.
- Under conditions that promote a narrow focus of attention, positive reinforcement aids a focus on task-relevant cues, while punishment floods attentional capacity with a predominance of task-irrelevant cues.

stages when learning new motor skills. The first stage, termed the cognitive stage, is characterized by effortful and conscious regulation of the movement. That is, the athlete has to think about the details of the task. During the second stage, the associative stage, the athlete must focus on the task but is less concerned with the details of the movement. Finally, the athlete achieves the stage of automaticity, during which the mind is relaxed and the skill is executed automatically without thinking. Assuming proper instruction and coaching, the relaxed mind focuses only on what is relevant to the task at that moment and, at the same time, automatically filters out all irrelevant cues. Attaining automaticity of action and the clarity of thought that often accompanies it is a goal for many athletes.

Attentional Styles

Nideffer (25) formulated an important concept in sport psychology when he theorized that individuals tend to experience shifting categories of attentional styles during performance. These categories are characterized by two dimensions: direction (internal-external) and width (broad-narrow). The first dimension refers to an introspective versus an externally oriented perspective, whereas the second dimension refers to an integrative (expansive) versus a highly selective orientation. These dimensions each occur on overlapping continuums, creating four "quadrants" of attentional focus: (1) broad external, in which the athlete assesses the situation by looking at the environment and various elements within it; (2) broad internal, in which the athlete processes information and develops a strategy; (3) narrow internal, in which the athlete mentally rehearses the upcoming action; and (4) narrow external, in which the athlete specifically focuses on one or two external cues to generate action. These constructs and their relationships to each other can be seen in figure 8.3.

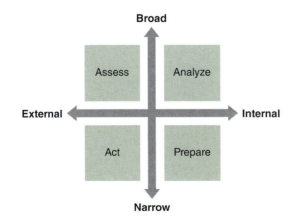

FIGURE 8.3 Four quadrants of attentional focus.
Adapted from Nideffer, 1976 (25).

Understanding attentional styles can improve coaching effectiveness. For example, a player who tends to become overloaded with external stimuli might be coached to focus on one important cue, such as an opponent's footwork. Athletes who seem to get lost in their own head could practice describing out loud, to a coach, what they are feeling during a lunge. Without such coaching, these players would likely attend to inappropriate cues and react too slowly.

Psychological Techniques for Improved Performance

Improving one's use of mental skills can enhance performance on sporting courts and in training rooms and on practice fields; it can also transfer over into better performance in all areas of life. Business or work, academic, and even general social interaction in any domain can be improved with a little attention to building up mental skills. These psychological skills are quite similar to physical, technical, and tactical skills in that they can be taught and learned and must be practiced on a regular basis if they are to generate long-term behavioral change. This next section introduces several of these psychological skills that can be integrated into training to improve overall performance.

Relaxation Techniques to Control Elevated Arousal and Anxiety

Several techniques can be used to help athletes manage their psychological processes through relaxation. Relaxation techniques are designed to reduce physiological arousal and increase task-relevant focus. These techniques are important when people are executing complex tasks or practicing new ones, when they are dealing with pressure situations, or when deliberate focus is necessary.

Diaphragmatic Breathing

One simple technique for reaching a higher level of physical and mental relaxation is **diaphragmatic breathing** (39). Referred to as belly breathing, this form of breathing is a basic stress management technique and a precursor to virtually all other mental training techniques. It focuses attention on the process of breathing to clear the mind and therefore increase concentration. During any mental training exercise, athletes should attempt to engage in deep, rhythmic breathing in a relaxed, natural manner. Physiologically, this form of breathing has a major influence on heart rate and muscle tension due to feedback mechanisms that link the respiratory and cardiac control centers in the brain stem. The relatively deep inspiration, followed by a controlled expiration, alters autonomic nervous system (ANS) balance so that increased vagal tone or parasympathetic activity can occur (28). The parasympathetic branch of the ANS promotes the effect opposite the sympathetic-mediated fight-or-flight response. Thus, rhythmic breathing can decrease neural stimulation of both the skeletal muscles and organs (e.g., heart, lungs, liver), resulting in a sense of deep relaxation.

Diaphragmatic breathing requires that attention be directed to the abdominal region. It is best to get familiar with this starting from a standing position so that breathing is not inhibited. The athlete should let the arms hang loosely and concentrate on relaxing, particularly in the neck and shoulder region, by first taking a couple of deep breaths. Next, the athlete should relax the abdominal muscles so that they appear flaccid. The initiation of each breath should occur simultaneously with the relaxed protrusion of the abdominal muscles; placing a hand on the abdomen gives feedback to ensure that the abdomen protrudes with the initiation of each breath. With each breath the abdomen should become naturally distended. When this portion of the technique is performed properly, the diaphragm (a muscle at the base of the lungs) contracts and drops, allowing a deeper breath to occur. This is the first stage of taking a maximal inhalation. The entire process of inhalation takes place in three different areas and stages: the lower abdomen, the midchest, and finally the upper chest. Diaphragmatic breathing can be combined with more dynamic muscular relaxation techniques like progressive muscular relaxation and autogenic training.

Progressive Muscular Relaxation

To achieve an appropriate level of cognitive and somatic activation before performance, athletes may employ progressive muscle relaxation (PMR) (15). **Progressive muscle relaxation** is a technique by which psychological and physical arousal are self-regulated through the control of skeletal muscle tension. In essence, by going through a series of alternating muscular tensing and relaxing phases, the athlete learns to become aware of somatic tension and thereby control it. The hope is that a relaxed body will promote a relaxed mind.

These tensing and relaxing cycles progress from one muscle group to the next until all muscle groups are optimally relaxed. Each cycle involves maximally tensing each muscle for a short period of time (10-15 seconds), followed by a conscious attempt to relax that muscle completely, before moving on to the next muscle group. With practice, an athlete learns to rapidly discern the difference between a tense muscle and a relaxed one and then actively take steps to generate the needed muscular relaxation.

In many cases, a positive side effect of the reduced muscle tension is an increase in smooth, fluid, or effi-

cient movement as well as an increased range of motion around the joint. This can be an effective self-regulation technique for some athletes before practice or competition, or even during an intense moment in a given contest. However, it should be noted that when athletes first begin using PMR, there can be a period of lethargy following use. Therefore, athletes should practice this technique in the days leading up to competition (rather than on the day of) to determine its individual impact.

Autogenic Training

For athletes who are injured or who for some reason find it uncomfortable or impractical to experience high muscular tension levels, the PMR cycle for each muscle group can be replaced with an attentional state that simply focuses on the sense of warmth and heaviness for a particular limb or muscle group. This kind of technique, referred to as **autogenic training**, consists of a series of exercises designed to produce physical sensations in the body—generally warmth and heaviness (40). Because autogenic training eliminates the need for uncomfortable levels of muscle tension in the contraction–relaxation cycles, older athletes or athletes in rehabilitation from injury may find this an attractive alternative to PMR.

> ▶ **Relaxation techniques are designed to reduce physiological arousal and increase task-relevant focus. These techniques are of extreme importance when one is executing complex or novel tasks or performing in high-pressure situations.**

Systematic Desensitization

Sometimes fears are learned by association of previously neutral stimuli with a stressful event. For example, an adult nonswimmer who experienced a threatening event in the water as a child may avoid activities around water because of a learned association. This individual may become fearful and therefore tense doing basic resistance or stretching exercises in a pool, even ones that require no swimming skill. This example illustrates the importance of understanding exercise science. For example, the aquatic environment is a great aid in enhancing flexibility. To benefit maximally from a stretching program, however, a participant must learn to fully relax. If the purpose of the pool session is to enhance flexibility, the inability of a nonswimmer to relax in the environment could easily prevent gains in flexibility.

One technique that helps an athlete initially confront or reduce fear is **systematic desensitization (SD)** (45). Systematic desensitization combines mental and physical techniques that allow an athlete to replace a fear response to various cues with a relaxation response.

Like cognitive–affective stress management training (SMT) and stress inoculation training (SIT), systematic desensitization teaches the athlete to use a specific relaxation skill-based coping response to control for cognitive arousal (40). This adaptive, learned replacement process, the principle behind SD, is called **counterconditioning**.

To practice the technique, an athlete should be reasonably skilled at both PMR and mental imagery. The athlete should construct a hierarchy, or progression, of events and situations that he or she specifically perceives as fearful. For example, a competitive gymnast who suffered a serious injury on the balance beam may list a series of fearful scenes, proceeding from warming up before the event to the actual movement that precipitated the injury.

In a relaxed setting the athlete visualizes the first scene and experiences a mild degree of anxiety. At the same time, diaphragmatic breathing, PMR, or another physical relaxation technique is instituted, and a strong relaxation response theoretically should overcome the relatively weak fight-or-flight syndrome. This technique is practiced until the athlete can hold the image clearly while maintaining a relaxed state. The athlete progresses through the hierarchy, experiencing conditioned fear in small, manageable doses that are overcome by the relaxation achieved with the relaxation technique. This procedure prevents cognitive avoidance and counterconditions a new response (relaxation) to the formerly fear-inducing stimuli (40).

Imagery

Imagery can be defined as a cognitive skill in which the athlete creates or recreates an experience in his or her mind (40). Ideally, for athletes, it uses all the senses to create a mental experience of an athletic performance. The athlete simulates reality by mentally rehearsing a movement, imagining visual, auditory, kinesthetic, olfactory, and even gustatory (taste) cues. Feltz and Landers (8) provided convincing evidence for the effectiveness of mental imagery in the **enhancement** of sport skill based on a meta-analytic review of the literature. During the initial stages of using imagery, the athlete may start with a relatively simple, somewhat familiar visual image. This helps successful practice of the technique. As with learning any skill by proceeding from simple to complex, the person starts with static images, such as visualizing a golf ball or mentally examining the visual characteristics of a tennis racket. The vividness or detail of the image should become clearer and clearer with continued practice. Some people have a natural talent for achieving image clarity, but everyone can improve with repeated practice.

The perspective of the image can be internal (first person) or external (third person). Although the research literature is unclear as to whether one is superior, it seems that an image that is more engaging and natural to the athlete would be most appropriate. Of course, the internal, first-person perspective seems more specific to skill execution, inasmuch as the actual task is performed with such an orientation. However, as many athletes are familiar with reviewing film or recordings of their performances, an external perspective may also feel natural.

After the athlete successfully visualizes a stationary object with vivid detail, he or she may start to move the object or begin to "walk around" it in the mind, viewing it from a number of different perspectives. For an image such as a basketball, the athlete may attempt to bounce the ball and feel it against the fingertips. In this manner, the athlete increases complexity by controlling the image or moving it with control (e.g., bouncing the ball) and by bringing a multisensory perspective to bear (i.e., using tactile or kinesthetic as well as visual sensation).

Rehearsing successful execution of a skill during imagined competitive conditions can provide the subconscious mind with positive memories, thus increasing the athlete's sense of confidence and preparedness for the particular sport. Of course, mental imaging is not as powerful a determinant of self-efficacy as actual success, but it does offer two potentially potent ingredients. First, successful performance is entirely under the control of the athlete during imaging, whereas a degree of uncertainty about the outcome is inherent in reality. In imagery the athlete has a great opportunity to "experience" success. We believe that athletes should be realistic in the kinds of success they imagine; that is, the mental images should be personally challenging yet within the realm of possibility. Second, the athlete can

---

How Should Athletes Use Arousal Control Techniques?

- An athlete should employ arousal reduction techniques when performing a new skill or one that is complex, or when performing in high-pressure situations.
- Athletes should employ arousal enhancement techniques when executing simple skills, ones that are well learned, or in situations of minimal pressure.
- The purpose of employing such techniques is to allow the athlete to perform with an unburdened mind while matching his or her mental and physical intensity to the demands of the task.

"experience" competition repeatedly, fostering a sense of familiarity and preparedness.

For some athletes, the months of preparation for a season of play—involving off-season, preseason, and in-season conditioning and skill development—may lead to only a few minutes of actual competitive experience. Even for the starters in team sports, actual competitive experience may be extremely small relative to physical practice time. **Mental imagery**, however, allows the athlete to get used to this uncertain environment over longer periods of time despite minimal real-world competitive opportunity.

Self-Efficacy

Of course, one of the main objectives for applied sport psychology is generating a psychological perspective that improves performance, and it has been argued that perceived self-confidence, or self-efficacy (1), is a better predictor of task execution than either arousal or anxiety. **Self-confidence** is the belief that one can successfully perform a desired behavior (40), while **self-efficacy**, a situationally specific form of self-confidence, is the perception of one's ability to perform a given task in a specific situation (1). Someone who is highly self-efficacious does not doubt his or her ability to succeed at a given task, even when failure is experienced.

According to Bandura's theory (1), a person's self-efficacy derives from a number of sources:

- Performance accomplishments—past experiences of success or failure
- Vicarious experiences—watching others (modeling)
- Verbal persuasion—encouragement from self or others
- Imaginal experience—using imagery to see oneself perform
- Physiological states—perception of arousal as facilitative or debilitative
- Emotional states—affect or mood

These sources translate well into sport and training environments and can be influenced by the coaches as well as the athlete themselves.

It is thought that if an athlete has the necessary skill set and an acceptable level of motivation, then the resulting performance is largely determined by self-efficacy (1). Skill alone is not enough to ensure effective performance—athletes have to want to perform well and need to believe they can be successful in their endeavors. Furthermore, individuals' level of self-efficacy influences the choices made—whether toward certain activities that they feel confident about, or away from those about which confidence is lacking. Similarly, this construct additionally influences level of overall effort as well as persistence in the face of obstacles, as those who believe in themselves generally work harder and are more determined to attain the desired outcome than those without the necessary levels of self-efficacy (40). Clearly, the perception of one's ability to successfully perform the tasks of sport or training has a direct impact on the actual performance.

> ▶ Self-efficacy influences people's choice of activity, their level of effort in that activity, and how much persistence they will have in the face of challenging obstacles.

Self-Talk

A technique frequently used to enhance self-efficacy, aid in directing proper focus, assist in regulating arousal levels, and reinforce motivation is **self-talk**. Self-talk, or intrapersonal communication, is the inner dialogue we have with ourselves (40). It is what we say to ourselves, either out loud or in our heads, that provides the "sound track" for our behaviors and performances.

Self-talk is generally categorized as positive, negative, or instructional and can be either spontaneously generated or more purposefully used to generate changes in mood or behaviors (38). Positive self-talk can include utterances or statements that are encouraging (e.g., "Come on!"), motivational (e.g., "I can do this!"), or reinforcing (e.g., "I am ready!") and generally reflects favorable emotions or feelings. Negative self-talk generally reflects anger, discouragement, doubt, or negative judgment (e.g., "You suck!" "You can't do this" "What were you thinking?") Instructional self-talk generally provides specific direction or focus on necessary performance cues for a particular skill or strategy (e.g., "feet shoulder-width apart," "Keep your torso erect").

Positive and instructionally focused self-talk have been found to improve performance in laboratory settings; however, significant individual and environmental differences may modify these findings in actual performance settings (38). For example, instructional self-talk can be harmful for expert performers, as relaying specific performance cues may actively interfere with the automaticity of the movement. Furthermore, some evidence exists that positive self-talk can result in decreased self-efficacy in some performers (46). Generally, however, negative self-talk is associated with poor performance, as it directs one's focus to inappropriate cues, can trigger negative emotional energy, and can decrease confidence. Therefore, in order to employ self-talk most effectively, athletes should begin by examining their current use of self-talk and its effects on performance. Then, an assessment of the most appropriate way to modify their self-talk can be made.

Goal Setting

Not surprisingly, many of the concepts discussed in this chapter can have a direct influence on one another. Self-efficacy is one of these in that it has a significant impact on the types of goals people set for themselves. Those with higher confidence and efficacy generally envision, create, and strive to accomplish more challenging goals. **Goal setting** can be characterized as a process whereby progressively challenging standards of performance are pursued with a defined criterion of task performance that increases the likelihood of perceived success (21). For example, a goal for a swimmer may be to execute a technically correct stroke throughout a sanctioned distance, such as the 50 m freestyle. In the beginning, the swimmer's skill level might be so low that such a task would seem overwhelming and produce a strong sense of failure and frustration, yet physiological testing may show the coach that the athlete has the physical resources to excel at such an event (i.e., the swimmer has a high degree of fast-twitch, or Type II, muscle fibers, exhibits superior muscular power or speed-strength in the upper and lower body, and seems to have a high capacity for anaerobic metabolism). However, the stroke mechanics are inefficient; the athlete is highly aware of this and therefore lacks confidence. First, the coach and athlete can break the skill and conditioning units down into manageable components (the traditional whole–part–whole method of learning). Then as the athlete focuses on and masters each component, a sense of progress and success is nurtured, developing more confidence and better motivating the athlete to complete the challenging goal.

Systematic goal setting can simultaneously increase the psychological development and performance of the athlete (40). A number of reasons explain why goal setting affects performance:

- Goals direct an athlete's attention by prioritizing efforts.
- Goals increase effort because of the contingency of success on goal attainment.
- Goals increase positive reinforcement through the feedback given to athletes.

It seems that the informational nature of thoughtfully derived goals, which increase effort because they are challenging yet attainable, is a powerful ingredient in behavioral change.

Process Goals

An important distinction related to setting goals is the difference between the process versus the outcome (2). **Process goals** are those over whose achievement the athlete has control. They focus on the actions the individual must engage in during performance to execute the skill well. If the effort is expended, success occurs with a relatively high degree of probability. Examples of process goals within the skill domain relate to form and technique, although an individually determined time (in the case of a swimmer or track athlete) could also be considered a process goal. An example of a process goal within strength and conditioning is to have the athlete focus on the strategy for weight reduction (e.g., what the athlete must do on a daily basis, such as aerobic activity and dietary modifications) rather than on the actual result (e.g., a loss of weight), thereby increasing a sense of control over actions. With process goals, success is strongly contingent on effort.

Outcome Goals

On the other hand, **outcome goals** are ones over which the athlete has little control; typically, winning is the primary focus. Outcome goals in sport generally focus on the competitive result of an event, so earning a medal, scoring points, and generating a high ranking would all fall in this category. The accomplishment of outcome goals is contingent not only on individual effort, but also on the efforts and abilities of others—something out of the individual's personal control. We believe that winning is a sound goal orientation that can surely generate high levels of motivation but that, ironically, an athlete can increase the likelihood of its achievement by having both a process and an outcome goal orientation as opposed to a winning-only attitude. Undue emphasis on winning alone may occupy such a proportion of fixed attentional capacity that it causes narrowing of attentional focus. As such, task-relevant cues are missed, reaction time is slowed, and coordination is diminished by forced movements and compromised automaticity, which alter neuromuscular sequencing—all inhibiting the attainment of the desired goal.

Both process and outcome goals can be applied to strength and conditioning settings as well. For example, emphasizing technique during the power clean illustrates a process orientation, whereas focusing only on completing the set illustrates an outcome orientation. An exception to the general caveat about avoiding outcome goals is the situation in which an athlete is extremely confident and undermatched in competition. He or she may want to focus solely on outcome and a personal best to maximize motivation.

Short-Term Goals

In addition to the process and outcome distinction just discussed, goals can also be categorized as short-term and long-term. **Short-term goals** are generally those that are directly related to current training or competition and are guidelines that can be attained in a relatively

Guidelines for Using Goal Setting
• Long-term goals and short-term goals are interdependent.
• Long-term goals provide a sense of meaningfulness and direction for pursuing short-term goals.
• The attainment of short-term goals provides a hierarchical sense of mastery and success that builds self-confidence.
• Athletes should define process goals to focus on elements of their performance over which they have control.

short time frame. Short-term goals also increase the likelihood of success because, although challenging, they are relatively close to the athlete's present ability level. They also increase confidence, self-efficacy, and motivation because of the likelihood of success. In this regard, short-term process and outcome goals counteract the boredom and frustration that are potential side effects of long, arduous training regimens.

Long-Term Goals

However, the full meaning of the short-term standards of success is framed by an appropriate long-term goal. **Long-term goals** are those that overarch the series of linked short-term goals. The attainment of those short-term goals should lead to the accomplishment of the related long-term goal. The athlete may see more relevance in everyday practice goals if it is apparent how they help attain the ultimate level of performance. For example, a gymnast who has a long-term goal of winning the floor routine for the national championship during her senior year may be much more intense and positive about weight room conditioning exercises when she perceives their relevance to her dream. An athlete may be more aroused psychologically and physiologically during practice by the perception that today's activity is another step on the ladder to a personal, long-term dream.

Lastly, the specificity of the goals—whether short- or long-term—is important in relation to giving the athlete feedback in effective coaching. Feedback, or the knowledge of success and failure, is more effective in the presence of specific, quantifiable goals, as opposed to vague standards of performance. Feedback is a corrective mechanism, like a thermostat or cybernetic device. Both success and failure can help the athlete stay on course toward long-term success. For example, a specific goal of 25 minutes of continuous running in a heart rate range of 160 to 170 beats/min is a much more engaging objective than "going out for a run." The vague phrasing may be fine for a recreational participant, but it is not helpful for a competitive cross-country runner, especially when the goal is to develop physiological capacity.

Optimal goal setting requires knowledge of the exercise sciences in both the biophysical and behavioral domains. The efficacy of goals for improving athletic performance lies in their relevance to the physical needs of the athlete. For example, formulating a series of appropriate goals to enable a 400 m runner to decrease his or her time in the event rests on understanding the physical profile, relevant metabolic pathways, and biomechanical technique to be developed.

Of course, some goals may be completely psychological and therefore only indirectly performance based. An example of such a goal is to adopt a positive mood state for an entire practice. Although such goals demand less biophysical knowledge, they may be profoundly useful in increasing performance because they are goals that an athlete has tremendous control over and can facilitate inhibiting habitual negative self-talk. However, the most comprehensive goal-setting programs encompass several areas of exercise science in that they might involve goals from any number of subdisciplines, including physiological, metabolic, biomechanical, nutrition, and psychological. This requirement uniquely distinguishes sport psychology from other behavioral sciences.

Enhancing Motor Skill Acquisition and Learning

A comprehensive understanding of the impact and value of sport psychology on athletic performance is not complete without a working knowledge of the overlap of motor skill acquisition and learning topics. The integration of this significantly related behavioral science will improve both the athletes' performance and the ability of those who coach them. Selected techniques to enhance motor skill learning are discussed in the next sections, including those pertaining to practice schedule, instructions, and feedback. While research demonstrates favorable outcomes for particular techniques, it is important to consider the uniqueness of the athlete, the task, and the environment. What may facilitate learning for one athlete may have a different effect on another. The following sections can thus serve as a basic guide that can be tailored to the needs of the athlete, the task, and the environment.

Learning–Performance Distinction

Before considering techniques to enhance motor skill learning, it is important to recognize the learning–

performance distinction. Learning is a process that results in a relatively permanent change in the capability for a motor skill (30). Performance is the execution of the skill in the current environment (16). As has been discussed throughout this chapter, performance can be affected by arousal, motivation, and numerous other factors and therefore may not be indicative of the skill capabilities of the individual (3). While the techniques discussed here will facilitate skill learning of the individual, some might actually lead to performance decrements during the practice session. It is imperative to recognize this possibility and not to assume that an athlete's performance during a given practice session reflects his or her learning of the given skill.

Practice Schedule

Practice is essential for motor skill learning. More importantly, challenging practice enables motor skill acquisition; mere repetitions alone are not enough to change behavior (27). One of the many ways to facilitate skill learning is through the manipulation of the practice structure and schedule.

Whole Versus Part Practice

With respect to teaching a complex motor skill, there is debate about the effectiveness of whole versus part practice. **Whole practice** addresses the skill in its entirety, whereas **part practice** separates the skill into a series of subcomponents. As a general rule, tasks that are challenging but have low interrelatedness of the subcomponents are learned better with part practice (24). For example, the snatch is a skilled power movement that can be broken down into four subcomponents: the first pull, transition, second pull, and catch. On the other hand, whole practice would tend to be favored for a task with subcomponents that are highly interrelated, as part practice can inhibit the effective regrouping of the subcomponents (24). In the instance of a lunge, it would be ineffective to separate the movements of the front leg from the movements of the lead leg, because these two components are highly interrelated. Therefore, a lunge would be better learned as a whole. Regardless of the task interrelatedness, in instances in which the skill may be dangerous or costly to learn as a whole, part practice is the favored choice.

If part practice is to be used, there are numerous ways to separate a task into subcomponents. **Segmentation** breaks down the task into a series of subcomponents that have clear breaks between them (41). For example, as mentioned previously, the snatch can be broken down into the first pull, the transition, the second pull, and the catch. **Fractionalization** breaks the tasks into subcomponents that occur simultaneously (41). In performing the push press, the athlete practices the press motion of the arms and the push motion of the legs independently. **Simplification** adjusts the difficulty of the tasks by changing task characteristics such as the execution speed or the equipment used (41). In the snatch, the athlete first practices the subcomponents with a PVC pipe. In this instance, both segmentation and fractionalization are used.

When teaching the subcomponents of the task, there are multiple methods to integrate the parts back into the whole skill. **Pure-part training** (also known as the part–whole method) has the athlete practice each subcomponent of the skill multiple times independently. After all components have been practiced, the skill is practiced in its entirety (41). In a snatch, the first pull is practiced, then the transition, followed by the second pull and ending with the catch. After all skills have been practiced multiple times, the snatch is practiced. **Progressive-part training** has the athlete practice the first two parts in isolation before practicing these parts together (41). The athlete then practices the third subcomponent before practicing all three parts together. In the snatch, the athlete first practices the first pull and then the transition, then the first pull with the transition. The athlete then practices the second pull before practicing the first pull, transition, and second pull as a combined skill. This progression continues until the whole skill has been reintegrated. **Repetitive part training** has the athlete practice only the first part in isolation; then each subsequent part is added until the whole task is reintegrated (41). The athlete in this instance would first practice the first pull; then the first pull with the transition; then the first pull, transition, and second pull; and so forth. With use of simplification, characteristics of the task can be added gradually, increasing the difficulty of the task. The choice of sequencing will be dependent on the task and the goals of the given training session.

Random Practice

Traditionally, skills are practiced in a blocked fashion, such that the athlete practices the same skill multiple times before progressing to another skill. In **random practice**, multiple skills are practiced in a random order during a given practice session. For example, during blocked practice, the athlete performs multiple squat depth jumps before progressing to another skill. In random practice, an athlete may perform a squat depth jump, a depth jump with a lateral movement, a split-squat jump, and a side-to-side push-off in a random order. The athlete continues to repeat these skills in a random order. While performance on each individual skill initially declines during random practice, learning is facilitated by this practice design (33). As applied to a sport setting, an integration of blocked and random practice (a few repetitive attempts at each skill before proceeding) maximizes the benefits of both practice schedules (18). In the instance of the jumps, the athlete would perform a few repetitions of the squat depth jump before moving on to another movement such as the side-to-side push-off.

Variable Practice

Similar to random practice, **variable practice** includes variations of the same skill within a single practice session as opposed to specific practice in which a specific skill (i.e., depth jump to second box of a specific height) is repeated multiple times. In variable practice, the athlete would practice stepping from and jumping to boxes of varying heights. Similar to random practice, variable practice can impair performance during the practice session, but can enhance performance on a novel variation of a skill (19) such as the ability to quickly jump to a second box after stepping off a box from an unpracticed height. A combination of specific and variable practice allows the athlete to develop sport-specific skills while also providing the athlete with the flexibility to perform in unfamiliar contexts (19). This flexibility is important to an athlete's success, as sport requires the athlete to perform in unfamiliar environments (travel games) and to accurately modify a practice skill in response to an opponent. As an example, training to land from and jump to varying heights will allow the athlete to respond in a game and execute the skill in an unfamiliar context.

Observational Learning

Observational practice (action observation), or practice through observation of the task or skill to be performed, has important implications for motor skill learning. Observational practice frequently uses prerecorded videos or live demonstrations. The individual executing the observed skill can be a novice or a competent or expert performer. When physical practice is combined with observational practice, learning is enhanced (32). In a strength and conditioning setting, partner work can facilitate learning. As one athlete completes a lift or a drill, the other athlete can observe during his or her rest period and vice versa. Sakadjian and colleagues (29) found that observational practice combined with physical practice facilitated improved power clean technique as compared to physical practice alone. Observational practice can assist athletes in achieving the desired technique, thus maintaining athlete safety and allowing for a more rapid progression to heavier lifting.

Instructions

A coach can facilitate learning by varying the amount of detail provided in the instruction to the athletes' strongest learning style. Instructional styles can be divided into explicit instructions, guided discovery, and discovery. **Explicit instructions** include prescriptive information that gives the athlete the "rules" for effectively executing the given task. In learning a squat, the athlete receives detailed instructions about the specific body position throughout the movement as well as the type (e.g., flexion-extension) and amount of movement at each of the joints. **Guided discovery** provides the athlete with instructions about the overall movement goal and important prompts for task accomplishment without explicitly telling the athlete how to accomplish the task. The athlete is told the goal of the squat depth jump and a few key reminders to prevent injury, such as maintaining a neutral spine. This style provides some direction while allowing the athlete to explore relationships between the executed movement patterns and the associated movement goal. Finally, **discovery** instructs the athlete on the overarching goal of the task and the athlete receives little to no direction. In this instance the athlete is just told to squat to a particular depth and is allowed to explore methods to accomplish this task. A discovery instructional style can slow the learning process while explicit instructions can impair performance in a stressful environment (34). The decreased attentional demands of discovery and guided discovery instructional styles allow athletes to increase their focus on the task-relevant cues related to task execution (49).

Feedback

Feedback plays a significant role in motor skill acquisition by providing the athlete with information about the movement pattern and the associated goal. This information can then be used to make appropriate adjustments to achieve the desired movement pattern and goal. **Intrinsic feedback** is feedback provided to the athlete by the athlete from the senses—for example, sensory information about missing a box during a squat box jump. Integration of the sensory information allows the athlete to fine-tune and adjust the movement pattern to produce the desired movement and associated task goal. **Augmented feedback** is feedback provided to the athlete by either an observer, such as a coach, or technology, such as video or laboratory equipment. After the squat box jump, a coach can tell the athlete that the hips countermovement was too slow, resulting in missing the box.

The remainder of this section focuses on augmented feedback. Augmented feedback can be broken down into knowledge of results and knowledge of performance. **Knowledge of results** provides the athlete with information about the execution of the task goal. For example, with a T-drill, the coach can tell the athlete how quickly he or she completed the drill. The athlete can also be given normative information about how this time compares with others. Both positive normative feedback and feedback without comparison augment skill learning compared to negative normative feedback (20). **Knowledge of performance** feedback provides the athlete with information about his or her movement pattern. This can be delivered in the form of video analysis or through the use of specialized laboratory equipment such as a force plate. In the instance of the T-drill, the coach gives the athlete specific information about the movement during the T-test such as body position during changes of direction. When the task goal is a movement outcome—for example, proper form on a power clean—there is an overlap between knowledge of results and knowledge of performance and thus they can become one and the same.

The timing and frequency of feedback also influence learning outcomes. Feedback that is offered concurrently with the task enhances performance while impairing learning; therefore, this feedback is beneficial in a competition setting (43). However, feedback that is provided after task execution facilitates skill learning (43). This feedback can be provided either after every trial or after a series of trials. While decreased frequency impairs performance during practice, less frequent feedback enhances skill acquisition as compared to feedback after every trial (44), except in instances in which the skill is complex (48). Therefore, in initial skill learning it would be beneficial to provide more frequent feedback that decreases as athletes progress in their skill level.

> **Feedback can be used to facilitate both learning and performance. The timing and frequency of the feedback have different influences on performance and learning. While concurrent feedback is beneficial for competition, delayed feedback that is initially frequent and decreases with time will facilitate learning of complex movement patterns.**

Conclusion

Although a scientific and motivationally sound coaching program can greatly help in the development of athletes, several other complementary psychological techniques can enhance their overall effectiveness. In reality, most athletes probably have had both adaptive and maladaptive experiences in the form of countless practices and competitions and, as a result, have developed a more or less effective mental skills repertoire. A working understanding of some of the psychological principles and tools for the generation of cognitive–behavioral change included in this chapter may help facilitate improved performance and an enhanced quality of life.

The coach and athlete can each contribute to improved performance outcomes and increase the enjoyment of competition by attending to the psychological aspects of instruction and performance. A positive, goal-oriented coaching approach is one of the most powerful contributors to psychological preparation for sport. The physical and nutritional preparation of the athlete represents the foundation on which performance potential is based, as the role of psychology is to mentally manage the developed physical resources (i.e., strength, speed, flexibility, and skill), thereby allowing the athlete to achieve his or her potential on a more consistent basis. Additionally, an adequate understanding of the mind–body relationship, as reflected in the constructs of this chapter, can facilitate communication between the strength and conditioning professional and the athlete and aid the athlete in controlling and managing emotion, arousal, focus, and motivation. Using appropriate psychological techniques can help this self-management process. The experience of success in sport may be important in and of itself, but we believe that the greater outcome of improved mental skills utilization may be the enhanced self-esteem, confidence, and positive self-concept that athletes achieve in their lives in general.

KEY TERMS

achievement motivation
anxiety
arousal
attention
augmented feedback
autogenic training
catastrophe theory
cognitive anxiety
counterconditioning
diaphragmatic breathing
discovery
distress
drive theory
emotions
enhancement
eustress
explicit instructions
extrinsic motivation
fractionalization
goal setting
guided discovery
ideal performance state
imagery
individual zones of optimal
  functioning

intrinsic feedback
intrinsic motivation
inverted-U theory
knowledge of performance
knowledge of results
long-term goals
mental imagery
motivation
motive to achieve success
  (MAS)
motive to avoid failure (MAF)
negative punishment
negative reinforcement
observational practice
operant
outcome goals
part practice
physiological efficiency
positive punishment
positive reinforcement
process goals
progressive muscle relaxation
  (PMR)
progressive-part training

psychological efficiency
pure-part training
random practice
repetitive part training
reversal theory
routine
segmentation
selective attention
self-confidence
self-controlled practice
self-efficacy
self-talk
short-term goals
simplification
somatic anxiety
sport psychology
state anxiety
stress
stressor
systematic desensitization (SD)
trait anxiety
variable practice
whole practice

STUDY QUESTIONS

1. An Olympic weightlifter attempting a personal record is able to ignore the audience to concentrate solely on her performance. Which of the following abilities is this athlete most likely using to perform the exercise?
   a. selective attention
   b. somatic anxiety
   c. guided discovery
   d. self-efficacy

2. An athlete's desire to perform to his or her potential is an example of
   a. motive to avoid failure
   b. autogenic training
   c. selective attention
   d. achievement motivation

3. For a high school American football team, if any player squats two times his body weight, his name is placed on the wall. This is an example of
   a. negative reinforcement
   b. positive reinforcement
   c. negative punishment
   d. positive punishment

4. How does an athlete's optimal level of arousal change with limited skill and ability to perform the activity?
   a. It increases.
   b. It decreases.
   c. It has no effect.
   d. It is not related to the activity.

5. In teaching the push press, which of the following is an example of segmentation with pure-part training integration?
   a. Practice the push press without any equipment, progress to practice with a PVC pipe, and end with an unloaded bar.
   b. Practice the dip, followed by the dip with the drive, and end with practice of the entire push press.
   c. Practice the dip, the drive, and the catch independently before practicing the entire push press.
   d. Practice the dip and the drive independently, followed by practice of the dip with the drive; then practice the catch independently and end with practice of the entire push press.

Basic Nutrition Factors in Health

Marie Spano, MS, RD

After completing this chapter, you will be able to

- know when to refer an athlete to the appropriate resource, a medical doctor or a sports dietitian;
- identify the protein, carbohydrate, and fat recommendations for athletes;
- list the dietary recommendations for disease prevention and overall health; and
- list hydration and electrolyte guidelines for different age groups and scenarios and help athletes develop an individualized hydration plan.

Good nutrition provides athletes with the nutrients necessary for general health, growth, development, and repairing and building muscle tissue, as well as the energy needed to train, compete, and maintain mental focus and concentration. A nutrition plan that is tailored to an athlete's specific needs can help decrease risk of injuries and illness and maximize training adaptations (improvements made from training) while helping the athlete reach his or her performance goals. This chapter focuses on the scientific rationale for performance-enhancing nutrition practices while providing suggestions that will help readers apply sports nutrition science to real-life scenarios.

Given the amount of nutrition misinformation and conflicting nutrition advice circulating on the Internet, in print, and via word of mouth, nutrition can be very confusing for athletes (185). In addition, each athlete's dietary needs differ from those of age- and sex-matched sedentary counterparts because of the physiological demands of his or her sport. Nutrition guidelines created for the general public are not necessarily applicable to athletes. Because each athlete's nutrition needs depend on many factors (age; body size and composition; sex; genetics; environmental training conditions; injuries; medical nutrition needs; and duration, frequency, and intensity of training), nutrition requirements can vary tremendously between athletes, even if they play the same position. And finally, because nutrition is a complex, constantly evolving science, it is important for strength and conditioning professionals to have some basic nutrition knowledge in addition to a list of nutrition professionals they can refer athletes to for individualized nutrition advice based on the latest science.

Role of Sports Nutrition Professionals

Sports nutrition is a complex multidisciplinary field, and athletic trainers, strength and conditioning professionals, physicians, exercise scientists, and food service providers have varying degrees of nutrition knowledge. Job responsibilities of player development staff should be outlined based on the nutrition education and knowledge of the staff member, the type of nutrition information provided, and state licensure laws regarding nutrition practice.

All sports nutrition professionals should be able to answer basic nutrition questions (for example, "What are some healthy snack ideas?"). However, athletes with complex nutrition issues should be referred to the appropriate resource, either a team physician or sports dietitian. The team physician is responsible for overseeing the athlete's medical care while the sports dietitian is responsible for providing individualized dietary advice. A **sports dietitian** is a registered dietitian (also referred to as a registered dietitian nutritionist) with specific education and experience in sports nutrition. The Academy of Nutrition and Dietetics (AND) Board Certified Specialist in Sports Dietetics (CSSD) certification distinguishes registered dietitians with expertise in sports nutrition from other registered dietitians who specialize in other areas of nutrition (see the sidebar on this topic). And though some sports dietitians have complementary skills or training and may therefore be social workers, athletic trainers, or chefs, a comprehensive sports nutrition program requires full-time attention; therefore these secondary skills should be considered a complement to the sports dietitian's knowledge rather than be used to try to fill two distinct job positions with one individual. And finally, higher-level positions generally a sports dietitian with a master's degree or PhD. A sports dietitian can help athletes make the connection between plate and performance.

At times, physicians and sports dietitians may work together to help athletes with eating disorders, nutrient deficiencies, or specific disease states such as diabetes. Because an athlete's nutrition and medical information may be shared with other members of the player development or coaching staff or family members in order to provide comprehensive care, in the United States all staff should follow Health Insurance Portability and Accountability Act (HIPAA) guidelines for handling an athlete's protected health information.

A sports nutrition coach is a professional who is not a registered dietitian but has basic training in nutrition and exercise science. For example, the strength and conditioning professional can act as a sports nutrition coach, providing basic nutrition education and suggestions. More complex situations in which food or nutrition is being used to treat or manage a medical condition (that includes a nutrient deficiency) require medical nutrition therapy and fall under the role of the sports dietitian. Sports nutrition coaches may obtain additional education by getting a sports nutrition certification. For example, the American Council on Exercise (ACE) has a Fitness Nutrition Specialist certification designed for personal trainers, health coaches, group fitness instructors, and health care professionals. Also, the International Society of Sports Nutrition (ISSN) Sports Nutrition Specialist Certification requires a high school diploma for the exam and is geared toward personal trainers or other fitness professionals who do not hold a four-year college degree. The ISSN also has a Certified Sports Nutritionist credential (CISSN), which requires a four-year undergraduate degree (or current status as a student majoring in exercise science, nutrition, or a related field) and is

Board Certified Specialist in Sports Dietetics (CSSD)

According to the Academy of Nutrition and Dietetics, a CSSD does the following (these competencies are also what strength and conditioning professionals should look for in a sports dietitian):

- Counsels individuals and groups on daily nutrition for performance and health
- Translates the latest scientific evidence into practical sports nutrition recommendations
- Tracks and documents outcomes of nutrition services, serving as a food and nutrition resource for coaches, trainers, and parents
- Assesses and analyzes dietary practices, body composition, and energy balance (intake and expenditure) of athletes in the context of athletic performance and health
- Counsels athletes on optimal nutrition for exercise training (match nutrition to training phases and goals), competition, recovery from exercise, weight management, hydration, immune health, disordered eating, travel, and supplementation
- Counsels athletes on achieving and maintaining a level of body mass, body fat, and muscle mass that is consistent with good health and good performance
- Provides personalized meal and snack plans to promote achieving short- and long-term goals for athletic performance and good health
- Develops hydration protocols that help athletes meet their own specific fluid and electrolyte needs
- Addresses nutritional challenges to performance, such as food allergies, bone mineral disturbances, gastrointestinal disturbances, iron depletion, and iron-deficiency anemia
- Provides medical nutrition therapy, as needed, to help manage or treat medical conditions, which may include diabetes, irritable bowel disease, hypertension, and more
- Counsels athletes on optimal nutrition for recovery from illness or injury
- Coordinates nutritional care as a member of multidisciplinary sports medical/sports science teams
- Is a liaison to in- and out-patient programs for conditions such as disordered eating
- Evaluates nutritional supplements, including herbal and sports supplements, for legality, safety, quality, and efficacy; monitors use of appropriate supplementation
- Collaborates with the individual's family, physician, coach, and other health professionals as appropriate while also following HIPAA guidelines
- Develops resources to support educational efforts
- Educates athletes and teams on food selection (grocery store tours) food storage, and food preparation (cooking classes)
- Documents nutrition services provided and evaluates the effectiveness of nutrition strategies towards meeting desired outcomes using the Nutrition Care Process
- Develops and oversees nutrition policies and procedures

Reprinted, by permission, from Sports, Cardiovascular and Wellness Nutrition (SCAN), 2008; Hornick, 2008 (62).

intended for health, fitness, and medical professionals who work with athletes and active individuals.

A sports nutritionist with an advanced degree is a professional who may work in the sports nutrition industry or conduct research in the area of sports nutrition and would therefore be able to discuss the literature on a particular topic. The sports nutritionist with an advanced degree may also choose to obtain a sports nutrition certification. One option is the IOC (International Olympic Committee) Diploma in Sports Nutrition. This two-year program includes coursework, seminars, tutorials, and laboratory practical work. The IOC states that students interested in this course typically have a degree in nutrition or dietetics, biological sciences (including biochemistry, physiology, or sport science), or medicine.

All sports nutrition professionals must follow state nutrition licensure laws, which vary from state to state and specify who is allowed to provide individualized nutrition counseling and medical nutrition therapy. For instance, in Louisiana, general nutrition education can be provided by various disciplines if the information is general, accurate, and not individualized (based on a specific person's dietary needs). However, only a licensed dietitian or nutritionist can provide nutrition assessment and counseling. Nutrition counseling is defined as "the provision of the individual guidance on appropriate food and nutrient intake for those with special needs, taking into consideration health, cultural, socioeconomic, functional, and psychological facts from the nutrition assessment. Nutrition counseling may include advice to increase or decrease nutrients in the diet; to change the timing and size of and composition of meals; to modify food textures, and in extreme instances, to change the route of administration" (www.lbedn.org).

Many individuals without any (or with minimal) education in nutrition and exercise science and little to no formal training refer to themselves as sports nutritionists. Regardless of the specific title of the person providing sports nutrition information or individualized dietary advice, strength and conditioning professionals should take a close look at the person's education (including the curriculum), previous work history (especially the person's day-to-day job duties), knowledge of sports nutrition, and years of experience.

> **Experienced sports dietitians help athletes make the connection between plate and performance. They have advanced knowledge, skills, and expertise in sports nutrition.**

The first step in nutrition coaching involves defining the athlete's goals and identifying the coach's goals (since the two may be different). After this, similar to the strength and conditioning professional undertaking a needs analysis, the sports dietitian will take a detailed look at the athlete's diet, individual food preferences (including cultural and religious considerations), cooking skills, access to food, financial constraints, barriers to making wise dietary choices, supplement use, weight and body composition history, medical history, training program, and injuries. The sports dietitian will then work with the athlete to develop a plan that fits his or her lifestyle and taste preferences while including (1) the appropriate calorie level; (2) macronutrients and micronutrients in recommended amounts; (3) adequate fluids and electrolytes; and (4) supplements as necessary to help correct a nutrient deficiency, make up for potential nutrient shortfalls, or meet training goals.

Standard Nutrition Guidelines

For general nutrition information, strength and conditioning professionals may want to refer their athletes to **MyPlate**, a food guidance system created by the U.S. Department of Agriculture and based on the 2010 Dietary Guidelines for Americans to help consumers make better food choices (98). MyPlate is an icon of five food groups based on a mealtime visual, the place setting (figure 9.1).

MyPlate

Information related to MyPlate can be found at www.choosemyplate.gov. Although the basic guidelines represented by the MyPlate icon and corresponding educational materials are universal, they include calorie

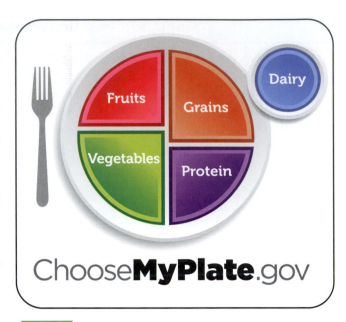

FIGURE 9.1   The MyPlate icon.

From USDA's Center for Nutrition Policy and Promotion.

guidelines and portion recommendations for fruit, grains, and protein and an allowance for oil based on age and sex for individuals who get less than 30 minutes of moderate physical activity most days, as noted in tables 9.1 and 9.2. Those who are more physically active should adjust the guidelines to meet their specific dietary needs (136). And though oils are not a food group, they contain nutrients such as essential fatty acids and vitamin E. Therefore, a daily allowance is provided for oils.

MyPlate should be considered a starting point that athletes can use to evaluate their diet. In general, if a diet provides a variety of foods from each group, it is more likely to contain an adequate amount of each vitamin and mineral. However, if the diet excludes an entire food group, specific nutrients may be lacking. For example, an athlete who excludes dairy from the diet may have a tough time meeting his or her nutrition requirements for calcium, potassium, and vitamin D (in fortified milk and fortified yogurts). Even though calcium-fortified nondairy replacement foods may help people meet their calcium needs, they are not a nutritionally equivalent substitute for dairy and may therefore be lacking in other nutrients (46). Individuals who exclude all animal foods and fish might not meet their vitamin B_{12} needs. (B_{12} is found in meat, poultry, fish, eggs, and dairy foods, though some breakfast cereals, nondairy milk alternatives, meat substitutes, and nutritional yeast are fortified with B_{12}.) Thus it is highly recommended that individuals who exclude food groups work with their sports dietitian to find suitable replacements or replacement combinations to ensure that they meet their nutrient requirements for health and performance.

TABLE 9.1　Food Group Recommendations From MyPlate

		Estimated daily calories for those who are not physically fit*	Fruit*	Vegetables**	Grains* (minimum)	Protein foods*	Dairy	Oils***
Children	2-3	1,000	1 cup	1 cup	3 oz. equivalents (1.5)	2 oz. equivalents	2 cups	3 tsp
	4-8	1,200-1,400	1-1.5 cups	1.5 cups	5 oz. equivalents (2.5)	4 oz. equivalents	2.5 cups	4 tsp
Girls	9-13	1,600	1.5 cups	2 cups	5 oz. equivalents (3)	5 oz. equivalents	3 cups	5 tsp
	14-18	1,800	1.5 cups	2.5 cups	6 oz. equivalents (3)	5 oz. equivalents	3 cups	5 tsp
Boys	9-13	1,800	1.5 cups	2.5 cups	6 oz. equivalents (3)	5 oz. equivalents	3 cups	5 tsp
	14-18	2,200	2 cups	3 cups	8 oz. equivalents (4)	6.5 oz. equivalents	3 cups	6 tsp
Females	19-30	2,000	2 cups	2.5 cups	6 oz. equivalents (3)	5.5 oz. equivalents	3 cups	6 tsp
	31-50	1,800	1.5 cups	2.5 cups	6 oz. equivalents (3)	5 oz. equivalents	3 cups	5 tsp
	51+	1,600	1.5 cups	2 cups	5 oz. equivalents (3)	5 oz. equivalents	3 cups	5 tsp
Males	19-30	2,400	2 cups	3 cups	8 oz. equivalents (4)	6.5 oz. equivalents	3 cups	7 tsp
	31-50	2,200	2 cups	3 cups	7 oz. equivalents (3.5)	6 oz. equivalents	3 cups	6 tsp
	51+	2,000	2 cups	2.5 cups	6 oz. equivalents (3)	5.5 oz. equivalents	3 cups	6 tsp

tsp = teaspoon; oz. = ounce.

The amount you need from each group depends on age, sex, and level of physical activity. Recommended daily amounts are shown in the chart.

*These amounts are appropriate for individuals who get less than 30 minutes of moderate physical activity most days. Those who are more physically active may be able to consume more while staying within calorie needs. To find your personal total calorie needs and empty calories limit, enter your information into "My Daily Food Plan": www.choosemyplate.gov/myplate/index.aspx.

**See table 9.2 for weekly vegetable subgroup recommendations.

***Oils have a recommended daily allowance versus recommended daily amount. The daily allowance is appropriate for individuals who get less than 30 minutes of moderate physical activity most days. Those who are more physically active may be able to consume more while staying within calorie needs.

Fruit. In general, 1 cup of fruit or 100% fruit juice, or 1/2 cup of dried fruit, can be considered as 1 cup from the Fruit Group.

Vegetables. Any vegetable or 100% vegetable juice counts as a member of the Vegetable Group. Vegetables may be raw or cooked; fresh, frozen, canned, or dried-dehydrated; and may be whole, cut up, or mashed.

Grains. Any food made from wheat, rice, oats, cornmeal, barley, or another cereal grain is a grain product. Bread, pasta, oatmeal, breakfast cereals, tortillas, and grits are examples of grain products.

Protein foods. All foods made from meat, poultry, seafood, beans and peas, eggs, processed soy products, nuts, and seeds are considered part of the Protein Foods Group. Beans and peas are also part of the Vegetable Group. In general, 1 ounce of meat, poultry, or fish, 1/4 cup cooked beans, 1 egg, 1 tablespoon of peanut butter, or 1/2 ounce of nuts or seeds can be considered as 1 ounce equivalent from the Protein Foods Group.

Dairy. All fluid milk products and many foods made from milk are considered part of this food group. Most Dairy Group choices should be fat free or low fat. Foods made from milk that retain their calcium content are part of the group. Foods made from milk that have little to no calcium, such as cream cheese, cream, and butter, are not. Calcium-fortified soymilk (soy beverage) is also part of the Dairy Group.

Oils. Oils are fats that are liquid at room temperature, like the vegetable oils used in cooking. Oils come from many different plants and from fish. Oils are not a food group, but they provide essential nutrients. Therefore, oils are included in USDA food patterns.

From U.S. Department of Agriculture and U.S. Department of Health and Human Services.

TABLE 9.2   MyPlate Vegetable Subgroup Recommendations

		Amount per week				
		Dark green vegetables	Red and orange vegetables	Beans and peas	Starchy vegetables	Other vegetables
Children	2-3	1/2 cup	2.5 cups	1/2 cup	2 cups	1.5 cups
	4-8	1 cup	3 cups	1/2 cup	3.5 cups	2.5 cups
Girls	9-13	1.5 cups	4 cups	1 cup	4 cups	3.5 cups
	14-18	1.5 cups	5.5 cups	1.5 cups	5 cups	4 cups
Boys	9-13	1.5 cups	5.5 cups	1.5 cups	5 cups	4 cups
	14-18	2 cups	6 cups	2 cups	6 cups	5 cups
Females	19-30	1.5 cups	5.5 cups	1.5 cups	5 cups	4 cups
	31-50	1.5 cups	5.5 cups	1.5 cups	5 cups	4 cups
	51+	1.5 cups	4 cups	1 cup	4 cups	3.5 cups
Males	19-30	2 cups	6 cups	2 cups	6 cups	5 cups
	31-50	2 cups	6 cups	2 cups	6 cups	5 cups
	51+	1.5 cups	5.5 cups	1.5 cups	5 cups	4 cups

Vegetable subgroup recommendations are given as amounts to eat WEEKLY. It is not necessary to eat vegetables from each subgroup daily. However, over a week, try to consume the amounts listed from each subgroup as a way to reach your daily intake recommendation.

These recommendations are for the general population; athletes may need different recommendations depending on their level and type of training.

From U.S. Department of Agriculture and U.S. Department of Health and Human Services.

Foods within each group share similar nutrient compositions and are considered interchangeable; however, a variety of foods should be consumed within each group. For example, eating an orange, an apple, and a pear provides a broader array of essential nutrients than is provided by three apples. A diet providing a variety of foods from each group is more likely to meet a person's **macronutrient** (carbohydrate, protein, and fat) as well as **micronutrient** (vitamins and minerals) needs.

The SuperTracker section of the MyPlate website contains sample food plans based on calorie needs, as well as information on empty calories and food labels. It also gives users the ability to calculate how much they eat and to track foods, physical activities, and weight.

Dietary Reference Intakes

Because athletes eat food, not individual nutrients, dietary recommendations should be presented in terms of specific food choices. However, it is also important to have an understanding of the athlete's nutrient requirements in order to make food recommendations. The **Dietary Reference Intakes (DRIs)**, created by the Food and Nutrition Board, Institute of Medicine, National Academies, are a complete set of nutrient intakes for use when evaluating and planning diets for healthy individuals. Dietary Reference Intakes are listed for the macronutrients as well as micronutrients, electrolytes, and water (68, 70, 72, 142, 169). The DRIs are based

on the body of literature regarding nutrient intake and the reduction of chronic disease, as opposed to simply prevention of dietary deficiencies (36). Because nutrient intake can vary considerably from day to day, the DRIs apply to a person's usual intake. Therefore, when a sports dietitian assesses a person's nutrient intake, she looks at several days in order to get an average daily intake for each nutrient. This is especially true with regard to evaluating intake of nutrients found in few foods or in very small amounts in foods (115). Fewer days' worth of food records are needed to get a good estimation of average protein intake, since this doesn't vary much from day to day (115). The DRIs include the following:

Recommended Dietary Allowance (RDA)—the average daily nutrient requirement adequate for meeting the needs of most healthy people within each life stage and sex.

Adequate Intake (AI)—the average daily nutrient intake level recommended when a RDA cannot be established.

Tolerable Upper Intake Level (UL)—the maximum average daily nutrient level not associated with any adverse health effects. Intakes above the UL increase potential risk of adverse effects. (The UL represents intake from all sources including food, water, and supplements.)

Estimated Average Requirement (EAR)—the average daily nutrient intake level considered sufficient to meet the needs of half of the healthy population within each life stage and sex.

Studies point to several nutrients of concern, nutrients that large portions of the population are not consuming in adequate amounts. All subgroups (males and females in all age groups) have a high prevalence of inadequacy of vitamin E and magnesium (71, 173). Vitamin E is found in many foods, though oils, nuts, and seeds are among the best sources of this nutrient. Magnesium is in a wide variety of foods, though often in small quantities. A few of the best sources of magnesium are nuts and seeds (particularly pumpkin seeds, almonds, and cashews) and beans, including mung beans and lima beans (175). In addition, for all individuals over the age of 2, mean usual intakes of fiber and potassium are below the DRI (175). The Scientific Report of the 2015 Dietary Guidelines Advisory Committee (176) lists fiber, potassium, calcium, and vitamin D as nutrients of concern. Dairy foods, fortified beverages (soy beverages, orange juice, and so on), and canned sardines are excellent sources of calcium while fatty fish, fortified beverages (milk, orange juice, soy beverages) and fortified yogurt are excellent sources of vitamin D (176). Also, iron is a concern for specific populations. Many women and adolescent females who are capable of becoming pregnant are deficient in iron, and many in these same groups are not meeting their dietary folate

needs. Red meat, iron-fortified cereals, and beans are excellent sources of iron. Beans, peas, peanuts, and sunflower seeds are among the best sources of dietary folate (176). And finally, though no longer considered a nutrient of concern, vitamin B_{12} absorption is affected by insufficient hydrochloric acid in the stomach, found in about 10-30% of older adults. Therefore, adults over the age of 50 are encouraged to consume foods fortified with synthetic vitamin B_{12} or take dietary supplements, because their bodies can typically absorb vitamin B_{12} from these sources (176). B_{12} is found in animal foods, fortified nutritional yeast, and fortified cereals. Beef, lamb, veal, and fish are some of the best sources of this nutrient (175).

Macronutrients

A macronutrient is a nutrient that is required in significant amounts in the diet. Three important classes of macronutrients are protein, carbohydrate, and fat.

Protein

Protein is the primary structural and functional component of every cell in the human body. Dietary proteins are used for growth and development and to build and repair cells; they also serve as enzymes, transport carriers, and hormones. Therefore dietary protein intake

---

For More Information on Nutrition

Strength and conditioning professionals can rely on the following websites for more information about nutrition:

Interactive DRI for Healthcare Professionals (based on the DRIs, this dietary planning tool calculates daily nutrient recommendations):

http://fnic.nal.usda.gov/fnic/interactiveDRI

Information on dietary supplements, including regulations; reports and warnings; macronutrient, phytonutrient, vitamin, and mineral supplementation; herbal information; ergogenic aids; and complementary and alternative medicine:

USDA's National Agricultural Library, Dietary Supplements:

http://fnic.nal.usda.gov/dietary-supplements

Weight Management, Food and Nutrition Information Center:

http://fnic.nal.usda.gov/consumers/eating-health/weight-management

Peer-reviewed journal articles:

www.pubmed.com

Collegiate and Professional Sports Dietitians Association:

www.sportsrd.org

International Society of Sports Nutrition:

www.sportsnutritionsociety.org

Sports, Cardiovascular, and Wellness Nutritionists:

www.scandpg.org

is essential for maintaining health, reproduction, and cellular structure and function (69).

Proteins are composed of carbon, hydrogen, oxygen, and nitrogen. "Amino" means "nitrogen containing," and **amino acids** are the molecules that, when joined in groups of a few dozen to hundreds, form the thousands of proteins occurring in nature. Proteins in the human body are composed of various combinations of the individual amino acids. Four amino acids can be synthesized by the human body and are therefore considered "nonessential" because they do not need to be consumed in the diet. Nine amino acids are "essential" because the body cannot manufacture them—they must be obtained through the diet. And finally, eight amino acids are considered conditionally essential. These amino acids are typically not essential though they become essential, and therefore must be obtained through the diet, during times of illness and stress (169). The amino acids are listed in table 9.3.

Amino acids are joined together by peptide bonds. Two amino acids together are referred to as a dipeptide, and several amino acids together are referred to as a **polypeptide**. Polypeptide chains bond together to form a multitude of proteins with various structures and functions. Almost half of the body's protein reserve exists as skeletal muscle, while approximately 15% makes up structural tissues including skin and blood. The rest of the body's protein reserves are in visceral tissues such as the liver and kidney and in the bones (48).

Protein Quality and Dietary Recommendations

Protein quality is determined by amino acid content and **protein digestibility**, as calculated by how much of the protein's nitrogen is absorbed during digestion and its ability to provide the amino acids necessary for growth,

maintenance, and repair. Higher-quality proteins are highly digestible and contain all of the essential amino acids. Animal-based proteins—including eggs, dairy foods, meat, fish, and poultry—contain all of the essential amino acids, while soy is the only plant-based protein that contains all nine essential amino acids. In general, plant proteins are less digestible than animal proteins, though digestibility can sometimes be improved through processing and preparation (69, 110). And though measures of protein quality, such as the **protein digestibility correct amino acid score (PDCAAS)**, take protein digestibility (or **bioavailability**) into account as well as a protein's ability to provide the essential amino acids necessary for the synthesis of body proteins and other metabolites, they do not take into account how other compounds within the food alter the bioavailability of the protein's amino acids. Foods contain antinutritional factors—compounds that reduce the digestion and absorption of a nutrient, making it less available for use by the body (159). Several antinutritional factors lead to digestive losses and structural changes of amino acids that limit amino acid bioavailability (110). For instance, during cooking, some foods will brown; this browning, called a Maillard reaction, leads to compounds that can decrease the bioavailability of certain amino acids. And though the majority of plant-based foods fall short in one or more essential amino acids, vegetarians and vegans (those who consume only plants and plant products—no meat, fish, poultry, eggs, milk, or other foods that come from animals) can meet their protein needs by consuming a variety of plant foods including legumes, vegetables, seeds, nuts, rice, and whole grains that provide different amino acids so that all essential amino acids are consumed over the course of the day (184).

While dietary recommendations are stated as protein requirements, the actual requirement is for amino acids. The need for amino acids in sedentary, healthy adults results from the constant turnover of cells and cellular proteins. During cell turnover—the constant breakdown and regeneration of cells—the body's free amino acid pool is the immediate and largest supplier of amino acids (106). The pool is replenished from dietary protein digestion, as well as the amino acids released from tissue turnover. Substantially more protein is turned over daily than is ordinarily consumed, indicating that amino acids are recycled (119). This process is not completely efficient, however, so dietary amino acid intake is required to replace losses.

The RDA for protein for men and women 19 years of age and older, based on nitrogen balance studies, is 0.80 g of good-quality protein per kilogram body weight per day (69). Children, teens, and pregnant and lactating women have higher dietary protein needs as reflected in the RDA for these groups. However, protein needs are

TABLE 9.3   Essential, Nonessential, and Conditionally Essential Amino Acids

Essential	Nonessential	Conditionally essential
Histidine	Alanine	Arginine
Isoleucine	Asparagine	Cysteine (cystine)
Leucine	Aspartic acid	Glutamine
Lysine	Glutamic acid	Glycine
Methionine		Ornithine
Phenylalanine		Proline
Threonine		Serine
Tryptophan		Tyrosine
Valine		

From Institute of Medicine (US).

inversely proportional to calorie intake because small amounts of protein can be metabolized as a source of energy when a person is in a state of negative calorie balance, when fewer calories are consumed than are expended (e.g., typically only 1-6% of total caloric expenditure in most circumstances but up to 10% during prolonged exercise in a glycogen-depleted state) (69, 95, 165). In this case, the protein cannot be used for the intended purpose of replacing the amino acid pool. When caloric intake goes down, protein requirement goes up (101). Therefore, the Institute of Medicine (IOM) established an **Acceptable Macronutrient Distribution Range (AMDR)** for protein, which covers a wide range of protein intake. The AMDR is 5% to 20% of total calories for children ages 1 to 3 years, 10% to 30% of total calories for children ages 4 to 18 years, and 10% to 35% of total calories for adults older than age 18 years. Men and women typically consume an average of 15% of their calories from protein (172). The AMDR for a nutrient includes a range of intakes associated with reduced risk of chronic disease while still providing recommended intakes of other essential nutrients (176). Though the DRI for protein fits within the AMDR, the DRI is based solely on body weight and therefore does not take low or high calorie intakes into account. Based on the AMDR, when calorie intake is lower, protein needs go up as a percentage of total calorie intake by approximately 1% for every 100-calorie decrease below 2,000 calories. When total calorie intake is higher, protein needs, expressed as a percentage of total caloric intake, go down to a certain point. In practice, sports dietitians should first establish an athlete's protein intake and then add carbohydrate and fats as determined by total calorie needs (93).

Concerns About the RDA for Protein

There is controversy surrounding the RDA for protein since some scientists suggest that adults should consume more than the RDA for bone health (54), weight management, and building and repairing muscle (121, 122). In addition, research suggests that higher-protein, lower-carbohydrate diets can favorably affect blood lipids, particularly in obese individuals, and therefore also decrease some of the risk factors for cardiovascular disease and metabolic syndrome (94).

Protein is a building block for strong bones, contributing to 50% of bone volume and 33% of bone mass (56). Protein's effect on bone may be due, in part, to its influence on insulin-like growth factor-I (IGF-I), which is produced in the liver and promotes bone and muscle formation (151). And though research suggests that supplemental, but not dietary, protein increases calcium losses through urine, in healthy individuals consuming 0.7 to 2.1 g of protein per kilogram body weight, both urinary calcium excretion and intestinal calcium absorption

increase (87). In fact, low dietary protein intake (0.7 g protein per kilogram body weight per day) suppresses intestinal calcium absorption (86).

Protein also plays a multifaceted role in weight management. First, it promotes satiety in a dose-dependent manner: Greater amounts of protein lead to a greater increase in satiety (41). However, the satiating effect of protein also depends on the timing of protein intake, form (solid vs. liquid), concurrent intake of other macronutrients, and time until the next meal (5). The type of protein may also have an effect on satiety, though research has not fully elucidated which proteins may have the greatest impact (16, 59, 101). Protein also has the greatest thermic effect of feeding—more calories are burned during the digestion of protein as compared to carbohydrate or fat. And finally, higher protein diets help spare muscle loss while a person is on a reduced-calorie diet (91, 134).

The amino acids in protein are used for growth (including muscle growth) and for repairing tissue, synthesizing enzymes and hormones, and repairing and making new cells. And though adults in a general fitness program can likely meet their protein requirements by consuming 0.8 to 1.0 g of protein per kilogram body weight per day, athletes and those who exercise intensely require more protein (21). Aerobic endurance athletes who consume a sufficient number of calories require approximately 1.0 to 1.6 g of protein per kilogram body weight per day (128, 165). Strength athletes need approximately 1.4 to 1.7 g of protein per kilogram body weight per day (96). Athletes who generally do a combination of strength and aerobic endurance or anaerobic sprint training and who are consuming adequate calories should ingest 1.4 to 1.7 g of protein per kilogram body weight. Athletes who are on a reduced-calorie diet may need more protein per day to preserve muscle tissue during weight loss.

In addition to eating the right amount of protein per day, research supports the idea of athletes consuming sufficient protein right after exercise, when muscle tissue is most receptive to amino acids. In fact, after exercise, both **muscle protein synthesis** and breakdown are increased, though net protein balance is negative when the exercise is done in a fasted state (127). Protein consumed after exercise increases muscle protein synthesis, and muscle sensitivity to amino acids is enhanced for up to 48 hours after a bout of exercise. However, this sensitivity goes down over time; therefore consuming protein sooner, rather than waiting, has a greater effect on acute muscle protein synthesis (28, 42, 97, 145). The amount of protein an athlete should consume after aerobic endurance exercise has yet to be fully elucidated. However, some suggest a 4:1 or 3:1 ratio of carbohydrate to protein as a general guideline (85). After resistance training, a wide range of protein intakes, 20 to 48 g, has proven beneficial for maximally stimulating acute muscle protein synthesis (82). The amount appears to depend, at least in part, on the leucine content of the protein (28) and is also affected by age, since sensitivity to amino acids decreases in older adults (84).

Concerns surrounding protein intakes above the RDA are unfounded for the most part in healthy individuals (105). Proteins consumed in excess of the amount needed for the synthesis of tissue are broken down (65), the nitrogen is excreted as urea in urine, and the remaining ketoacids are either used directly as sources of energy or converted to carbohydrate (**gluconeogenesis**) or body fat (60). In fact, a study examining high protein intake in athletes found that protein intakes up to 2.8 g per kilogram body weight (as assessed by a seven-day diet record) didn't impair any measures of renal function (132). The strength and conditioning professional should be aware that consistently high protein intakes, above recommended levels for building and repairing muscle, are not recommended because carbohydrate and fat intake (and the nutrients commonly found in carbohydrate- and fat-rich foods) may be compromised.

The protein content of commonly consumed foods is listed in table 9.4.

> ▶ **Athletes require more than the RDA for protein to build and repair muscle. Depending on the sport and the training program, 1.0 to 1.7 g per kilogram body weight of protein is recommended.**

Carbohydrate

Carbohydrate primarily serves as a source of energy. However, carbohydrate is not an essential nutrient, because the body can break down the carbon skeletons of certain amino acids and convert them into glucose (i.e., gluconeogenesis). Carbohydrates are composed of carbon, hydrogen, and oxygen. Carbohydrates can be classified into three groups according to the number of sugar (saccharide) units they contain: monosaccharides, disaccharides, and polysaccharides.

Monosaccharides (**glucose**, **fructose**, and **galactose**) are single-sugar molecules. In the body, glucose is present as circulating sugar in the blood, where it is used as the primary energy substrate for cells. In addition, glucose molecules make up glycogen, a polysaccharide stored in muscle and liver cells. In food, glucose is typically combined with other monosaccharides to form various sugars, such as sucrose. Isolated glucose found in candy or sport drinks is found in the form of dextrose, a chemical isomer of glucose. Fructose has the same chemical formula as glucose, but because the atoms are arranged differently, it tastes much sweeter and has different properties. Fructose accounts for the sweet taste of honey and occurs naturally in fruits and vegetables. In the body, fructose causes less insulin secretion than other sugars, which has made it a focus of much research in the area of aerobic endurance performance. Galactose, the third monosaccharide, combines with glucose to form lactose, milk sugar.

Disaccharides (**sucrose**, **lactose,** and **maltose**) are composed of two simple sugar units joined together. Sucrose (or table sugar), the most common disaccharide, is a combination of glucose and fructose. Sucrose occurs naturally in most fruits and is crystallized from the syrup of sugar cane and sugar beets to make brown, white, or powdered sugar. Lactose (glucose + galactose) is found only in mammalian milk. Maltose (glucose + glucose) occurs primarily when polysaccharides are broken down during digestion. It also occurs in the fermentation process of alcohol and is the primary carbohydrate in beer.

Polysaccharides, also known as complex carbohydrates, contain up to thousands of glucose units. Some of the most common polysaccharides of nutritional importance are starch, fiber, and glycogen. *Starch* is the storage form of glucose in plants. Grains, legumes, and vegetables are good sources of starch. Before starch can be used as a source of energy, it must be broken down into glucose components. Dietary fiber, a constituent of the plant cell wall, is also a form of carbohydrate. Cellulose, hemicellulose, beta-glucans, and pectins are fibers; these and noncarbohydrate fibrous materials (lignins) are partially resistant to human digestive enzymes. Fibers have different physiological effects in the body. Some delay gastric emptying, which may temporarily influence feelings of fullness, while other types of fiber increase bulk and water content, reducing constipation and decreasing transit time of feces. In addition, some soluble fibers decrease the absorption of cholesterol and may therefore help reduce blood cholesterol levels after ingestion (104), while prebiotic dietary fibers selectively stimulate the growth of bacteria in the gut (32, 135). Fiber-rich foods include beans, peas, bran, many fruits and vegetables, and some whole-grain foods.

Glycogen is found in small (77, 166) amounts in human liver and muscle, totaling approximately 15 g of glycogen per kilogram body weight (1), and in animal tissue as a temporary source of stored energy (20). While present in animal meats we eat such as steak, chicken breast, and fish fillets, it is not present to any large extent. When glucose enters the muscles and liver, if it is not metabolized for energy it can be synthesized to form glycogen. Three-quarters of the glycogen in the body is stored in skeletal muscle; the remaining quarter is stored in the liver (20). The process of converting glucose to glycogen is called **glycogenesis**.

TABLE 9.4   Protein Content of Common Foods

Food	Serving size in ounces	Serving size in grams	Average amount of protein (in grams) per serving
Almonds	1/4 cup	39	8
Bacon, pork	3 slices	27.3	10.5
Black beans	1/2 cup	92.5	7.5
Cashews	1/4 cup	32	5.5
Cheese slice, cheddar	1 slice	21	5.5
Cheese slice, Swiss	1 slice	28	7.5
Cheese, string, part skim	1 oz. (1 stick)	28	7
Chicken breast	3 oz.	85	25
Cottage cheese, 1%	4 oz.	113	14
Deli turkey	5 oz.	142	19
Edamame	1/2 cup	73.5	8.5
Egg	1	56	7
Garbanzo beans	1/3 cup	83.5	6
Greek yogurt, nonfat	6 oz.	170	17
Hamburger patty	3 oz.	85	22
Kidney beans	1/2 cup	88.5	7.5
Lamb chop	3 oz.	85	23.5
Lima beans	1/2 cup	94	7
Milk, 1%, low fat	8 fl. oz.	245	8
Peanut butter	2 Tbsp	32	8
Peanuts	1/4 cup	35.5	9
Pistachios	1/4 cup	30.5	6.5
Pork tenderloin	3 oz.	85	22.5
Salmon	3 oz.	85	17
Sausage links	3 links	63	10
Shrimp, large	4	22	5
Sirloin steak	3 oz.	85	26
Soy milk	8 fl. oz.	245	8
Soy nuts	1/4 cup	23	9
Tortilla, flour, 8 in.	1	51	4.5
Tuna, canned	3 oz. (1/2 can)	85	21.5
Wheat bagel, 5 in.	1 bagel	98	10
Wheat bread	1 slice	29	3
Yogurt, low fat	6 oz.	170	7

From U.S. Department of Agriculture, Agricultural Research Service.

Athletes typically consume a variety of carbohydrates in their normal diets. However, when they want to improve the quality of their diet, by consuming fewer foods that have untoward effects on overall health or performance, they may consider macronutrient ranking systems such as the glycemic index or glycemic load.

Glycemic Index and Glycemic Load

The **glycemic index (GI)** ranks carbohydrates according to how quickly they are digested and absorbed, and therefore raise blood glucose levels, in the 2-hour time period after a meal, compared to the same amount (by weight in grams) of a reference food, typically white bread or glucose, which is given a GI of 100 (76).

Glycemic index = [Incremental area under the curve for the blood glucose response after consumption of a 25 or 50g carbohydrate portion of a test food ÷ Incremental area under the curve for the blood glucose response after consumption of the same portion (in grams) of a standard food] × 100

Low-GI foods are digested and absorbed slowly, resulting in a smaller rise in blood glucose and subsequent insulin release from the pancreas compared to the reference food (45). Insulin helps lower blood glucose levels by facilitating glucose transport into cells. The fate of glucose within cells depends on where it is shuttled. For instance, muscle cells use glucose for energy while fat cells convert glucose into triglycerides (fat).

Though the GI was developed to help people better control their blood sugar levels—something that is particularly helpful for those with diabetes—some researchers hypothesized that diets composed of lower- versus higher-GI foods may also help decrease risk of obesity and other diseases (99, 100). However, the GI system has a few issues that may limit its accuracy. First, published GI values for a given type of food may vary considerably due to differences in testing and variations in ingredients used, ripeness of food, method of food processing, cooking, and storage (27, 60). Secondly, consuming carbohydrate as part of a meal or in different quantities affects the GI (45). Low-GI foods generally include vegetables, legumes, beans, and whole grains (see table 9.5).

Although some scientists have speculated that consumption of low-GI foods before exercise might spare carbohydrate by minimizing insulin secretion and therefore improve performance, there is insufficient evidence to support this hypothesis (21). The research is mixed, with some studies showing that consumption of a low-GI food as compared to a high-GI food before exercise improves exercise time to exhaustion (35, 167) and others finding that consuming a preexercise low-GI food versus a high-GI food had no effect on running performance (160, 180).

Therefore, athletes who use the GI to guide their food choices can try preexercise low- and high-GI foods in training while sticking with high-GI foods during exercise to provide immediate sources of energy (sugar) for activity (23) and immediately after exercise to more rapidly replenish glycogen stores (131).

The **glycemic load** (GL) takes the amount of carbohydrate, in grams, in a portion of food into account—a factor that also influences glycemic response. Because GL takes portion size into account, it is a more realistic gauge of glycemic response than the GI, which is based on a standard serving size. Table 9.6 shows the difference in GI and GL for specific foods. The GL is equal to the GI multiplied by the amount of carbohydrate in a portion of the food and dividing this total by 100.

$$\text{Glycemic load} = \frac{\text{GI of an individual food} \times \text{grams of carbohydrate per serving of food}}{100}$$

TABLE 9.5   Glycemic Index (GI) of Various Foods

Low GI foods (55 or less)	Medium GI foods (55-69)	High GI foods (70 or more)
Apple juice	Brown rice, boiled	Cornflakes cereal
Carrots, boiled	Couscous	Glucose
Chocolate	Honey	Potato, boiled
Corn tortilla	Pineapple, raw	Potato, instant mashed
Ice cream	Popcorn	Rice crackers, crisps
Kidney beans	Potato, French fries	Rice milk
Lentils	Rolled oats	Watermelon, raw
Orange, raw	Soft drink, soda	White bread
Milk, soy or dairy	Sucrose	White rice, boiled
Yogurt, fruit	Sweet potato, boiled	Whole wheat bread

Based on Atkinson, Foster-Powell, and Brand-Miller, 2008 (8).

TABLE 9.6   Glycemic Index and Glycemic Load

Food	Serving size (g)	Glycemic index (GI; glucose = 100)	Available carbohydrates (g/serving)	Glycemic load (GL; per serving)
Angel food cake	50	67	29	19
Apple (different varieties)	120	38± 2	15	6
Apple juice, unsweetened	(250 ml) 8 fl. oz.	40 ± 1	29	12
Bagel, white, frozen	70	72	35	25
Banana, ripe	120	51	25	13
Cheese pizza (Pillsbury Canada Ltd)	100	60	27	16
Chocolate milk (powder dissolved in milk)	250 ml (8.5 fl. oz.)	43	11	5
Chocolate pudding, instant, made from powder and whole milk	100	47 ± 4	16	7
Corn, sweet	150	53 ± 4	32	17
English muffin	30	77 ± 7	14	11
Grapes	120	46 ± 3	18	8
Ice cream	50	61 ± 7	13	8
Kidney beans, canned	150	52	17	9
Mashed potatoes, instant	150	85 ± 3	20	17
Oatmeal, prepared	50	69	35	24
Raisins	60	64 ± 11	44	28
Rice, brown (steamed, USA)	150	50	33	16
Rice, white, long grain, boiled 20-30 min	150	50	36	18
Soft drink (Coca Cola)	250 ml (8.5 fl. oz.)	63	26	16
Strawberries	120	40 ± 7	3	1
Sweet potato	150	61 ± 7	28	17
Vanilla wafers	25	77	18	14
Wheat bread, 75% cracked wheat kernels	30	53 ± 3	20	11
Yogurt, low-fat (0.9%), wild strawberry	200	31 ± 14	30	9

Adapted, by permission, from Foster-Powell, Holt, and Brand-Miller, 2002 (45).

Foods with a higher GL are expected to lead to greater increases in blood sugar and subsequent insulin release (45).

A low-GL diet, combined with exercise, has been shown to improve insulin sensitivity in older, obese adults and therefore may be a potential treatment for this population (90), while observational and intervention studies suggest that low-GI and low-GL diets are associated with lower levels of inflammatory markers. Chronic low-grade inflammation is considered a potential risk factor for chronic diseases (19). In addition, some (though not all) studies have found that diets with a lower GI or GL are associated with lower levels of fasting insulin as well as fewer cardiovascular risk factors (63, 152).

Fiber

Diets low in **fiber** have been associated with constipation, heart disease, colon cancer, and type 2 diabetes. The DRI for fiber ranges from 21 to 29 g/day for women (depending on age, pregnancy, and lactation) and 30 to 38 g/day for men based on age group. Fiber is commonly found in fruits, vegetables, nuts, seeds, legumes, and whole-grain products such as whole-grain bread, oatmeal, and popcorn.

Carbohydrate Requirements for Athletes

Numerous studies show that carbohydrates can improve time to exhaustion during aerobic endurance performance as well as work output and performance in high-intensity intermittent sports (2, 11). High glycogen levels have also been shown to spare the use of protein for fuel, thereby helping attenuate muscle breakdown (though differences in protein intake also affect muscle breakdown) (64).

Carbohydrate recommendations are largely based on type of training. Aerobic endurance athletes training 90 minutes or more per day at moderate intensity (70-80% $\dot{V}O_2max$) should aim for 8 to 10 g of carbohydrate per kilogram body weight per day (75). Athletes who benefit from this level of carbohydrate intake include those engaged in continuous aerobic activity such as distance runners, road cyclists, triathletes, and cross-country skiers. Research has shown that athletes consistently engaged in high-intensity, intermittent activities, such as soccer players, also benefit from high-carbohydrate diets (10, 163). Research on the carbohydrate needs of athletes in a wide variety of sports such as basketball players, wrestlers, and volleyball players is limited. Athletes who participate in strength, sprint, and skill activities need approximately 5 to 6 g of carbohydrate per kilogram body weight per day (153).

Within 30 minutes after aerobic endurance training, approximately 1.5 g of higher-glycemic carbohydrate per kilogram of body weight should be consumed to quickly stimulate glycogen resynthesis (74). Athletes can consume less carbohydrate in the time period immediately postexercise as long as they consume a higher-carbohydrate meal or snack at regular intervals (approximately every 2 hours) after finishing training. Athletes who do not train every day can restore their glycogen over the course of a 24-hour period if they consume enough total carbohydrate in their diet. And finally, despite the profound effect glycogen has on performance, athletes adapt to low-carbohydrate diets, which will decrease their reliance on carbohydrate as a fuel source during exercise (43). Some athletes also use this strategy to decrease their total calorie intake.

> Athletes adapt to dietary changes in carbohydrate intake. Though athletes who regularly consume carbohydrates use them as a primary source of energy during aerobic exercise, consistent intake of a low-carbohydrate diet leads to greater reliance on fat as a source of fuel.

Fat

Although the terms **fat** and *lipid* are often used interchangeably, *lipid* is a broader term. Lipids include **triglycerides** (fats and oils) as well as related fatty compounds, such as sterols and phospholipids. The lipids of greatest significance in nutrition are triglycerides, **fatty acids**, phospholipids, and cholesterol. Triglycerides are formed by the union of glycerol with three fatty acids. The majority of lipids found in foods and in the body are in the triglyceride form, and within this chapter the term *fat* refers to triglycerides.

Like carbohydrate, fat contains carbon, oxygen, and hydrogen atoms; but because the fatty acid chains have more carbon and hydrogen relative to oxygen, they provide more energy per gram. For example, fats provide approximately 9 kcal/g, while carbohydrates and protein provide approximately 4 kcal/g. Dietary fats and oils are composed of different types of fatty acids.

Saturated fatty acids have no double bonds, and their carbon molecules are saturated with hydrogen. Saturated fatty acids are used for certain physiological and structural functions, but the body can make these fatty acids; therefore there is no dietary requirement for saturated fatty acids (174). Unsaturated fatty acids contain some carbon molecules that are joined together by double bonds, making them more chemically more reactive. Fatty acids containing one double bond are **monounsaturated**. With two or more double bonds, a fatty acid is **polyunsaturated**. Two polyunsaturated fatty acids are considered essential, meaning that the body cannot make them: omega-6 and omega-3 fatty acids. These two fatty acids are necessary for the formation of healthy cell membranes, proper development and functioning of the brain and nervous system, and hormone production. Omega-6 fatty acids are abundant in the food supply and found in foods such as soybean, corn, and safflower oil and products made with these oils. Fewer foods contain omega-3 fatty acids; these include fish, particularly fatty fish such as salmon, herring, halibut, trout, and mackerel, which contain the omega-3 fatty acids **eicosapentaenoic acid (EPA)** and **docosahexaenoic acid (DHA)**. Eicosapentaenoic acid and DHA are tied to a dose-dependent decrease in triglycerides; a small, but statistically significant, decrease in blood pressure, especially in the elderly; and potential antiarrhythmic effects (107, 113).

One could also consume flaxseeds, walnuts, soybean oil, or canola oil to meet omega-3 requirements since these contain the **omega-3 fatty acid alpha-linolenic acid (ALA)**, which is converted to EPA and DHA. However, this conversion process is inefficient. According to vivo studies, approximately 5% of ALA is converted to EPA and <0.5% of ALA is converted to DHA in adults (130). Therefore, while foods that contain ALA count toward one's omega-3 intake, they do not have a substantial effect on EPA and DHA levels in the body. Foods rich in ALA may improve some risk factors for cardiovascular disease; however, it isn't clear which is responsible—ALA, the other compounds in these nutrient-rich foods, or a combination of the two (38). In addition to its physiological functions, fat is important because it is responsible for the characteristic flavor, aroma, and texture of many foods. Generally, most dietary fats and oils are a mix of all three types of fatty acids, with one type predominating. Soy, corn, sunflower, and safflower oils are relatively high in polyunsaturated fatty acids; olive, peanut, and canola oils are high in monounsaturated fatty acids; and most animal fats and tropical oils (e.g., coconut, palm kernel) are relatively high in saturated fatty acids.

When stored in the human body, fat serves many functions. Energy is stored primarily as adipose tissue in humans, but small amounts are also found in skeletal muscle, especially in aerobically trained athletes (150). Body fat insulates and protects organs, regulates hormones, and carries and stores the fat-soluble vitamins A, D, E, and K.

Relationship With Cholesterol

Cholesterol is a waxy, fat-like substance that is an important structural and functional component of all cell membranes. In addition, cholesterol is used for the production of bile salts, vitamin D, and several hormones, including the sex hormones (estrogen, androgen, and progesterone) as well as cortisol. And though cholesterol has many essential functions in the body, high levels of cholesterol may lead to atherosclerosis, hardening of the arteries due to plaque build up on artery walls, which narrows the area within arteries that blood can pass through. Therefore, having high levels of blood cholesterol is a risk factor for heart disease and stroke.

High levels of total cholesterol, **low-density lipoproteins (LDL)**, and triglycerides are all associated with increased risk of heart disease. Low-density lipoprotein is further divided into subfractions based on particle size. Smaller, more dense particles, called **very low-density lipoproteins (VLDL)**, are more atherogenic (artery clogging) than larger LDL particles (44). High levels

of saturated or trans fats, weight gain, and anorexia can all increase LDL cholesterol (162). However, VLDL levels increase with increasing intake of carbohydrate (116). High levels of **high-density lipoproteins (HDL)** are protective against heart disease, but are not a target of therapy (practitioners are told not to focus on HDL). Table 9.7 shows how LDL, total, and HDL cholesterol are classified.

High intake of refined carbohydrates, weight gain, excessive alcohol intake, and very-low-fat diets can increase triglycerides (blood fats). However, as with cholesterol, several factors affect triglycerides, including a sedentary lifestyle, overweight or obesity, smoking, genetics, and certain diseases and medications (125, 162).

The Scientific Report of the 2015 Dietary Guidelines Advisory Committee recommends avoiding partially hydrogenated oils containing trans fat and limiting saturated fat to less than 10% of total calories and replacing saturated fat with unsaturated fat, particularly polyunsaturated fat. In addition, it is advised that added sugars consumed be a maximum of 10% of total calories (176).

Fat and Performance

Both intramuscular and circulating fatty acids are potential energy sources during exercise (126). Compared with the limited capacity of the body to store carbohydrate, fat stores are large and represent a vast source of fuel

TABLE 9.7   Classification of LDL, Total, and HDL Cholesterol (mg/dl)

LDL cholesterol	
<100	Optimal
130-159	Borderline high
160-189	High
>190	Very high
Total cholesterol	
<200	Desirable
200-239	Borderline high
>240	High
HDL cholesterol	
<40	Low
>60	High

LDL = low-density lipoprotein; HDL = high-density lipoprotein.

Lipoprotein level testing should be completed after a 9- to 12-hour fast.

LDL cholesterol is the primary target of therapy.

Macronutrient Guidelines

Protein

- Choose a variety of protein foods, which include seafood, lean meat and poultry, eggs, beans and peas, soy products, nuts, and seeds.
- Increase the amount and variety of seafood consumed by choosing seafood in place of some meat and poultry.
- Replace protein foods that are higher in solid fats with choices that are lower in solid fats and calories (171).
- Young adults in a general fitness program: 0.8 to 1.0 g of protein per kilogram body weight per day.
- Aerobic endurance athletes: 1.0 to 1.6 g of protein per kilogram body weight per day.
- Strength athletes: 1.4 to 1.7 g of protein per kilogram body weight per day.
- Athletes on a reduced-calorie diet: approximately 1.8 to 2.7 g per kilogram body weight per day.

Carbohydrate

- Reduce intake of calories from added sugars.
- Increase intake of vegetables (prepared without added salt or fat) and fruit (prepared without added sugars).
- Eat a variety of vegetables, including beans; peas; and dark-green, red, and orange vegetables.
- Consume at least half of all grains as whole grains. Increase whole-grain intake by replacing refined grains with whole grains.

Fats and Alcohol

- Consume less than 10% of calories from saturated fats by replacing them with unsaturated fats, particularly polyunsaturated fats.
- Avoid partially hydrogenated oils containing trans fats.
- Reduce the intake of calories from solid fats.
- Decrease consumption of refined grains.
- If alcohol is consumed, it should be consumed in moderation—up to one drink per day for women and two drinks per day for men—and only by adults of legal drinking age (176). Pregnant women should avoid alcohol, and breastfeeding women should be cautious about their intake if they choose to drink (176). Alcohol should be avoided in the time period postexercise because it reduces muscle protein synthesis (123).

for exercise (54). For example, a lean runner who is 160 pounds (72 kg) with 4% body fat has approximately 22,400 calories stored within fat tissue (53). At rest and during low-intensity exercise, a high percentage of the energy produced is derived from fatty acid oxidation (140). When the intensity of exercise increases, there is a gradual shift from fat to carbohydrate as the preferred source of fuel. Consistent aerobic training increases the muscle's capacity to use fatty acids (79). In addition to training, the body adapts to using greater amounts of fat for energy when a higher-fat, lower-carbohydrate diet is consumed over a period of time (57, 79). And because the type of diet to which the body is adapted may influence performance (66), the effects of high-fat,

> ▶ **The human body has a sufficient amount of fat to fuel long training sessions or competition.**

low-carbohydrate diets vary, depending on the individual (129, 139, 143).

Vitamins

Vitamins are organic substances (i.e., containing carbon atoms) needed in very small amounts to perform specific metabolic functions (67, 177). Vitamins typically act as coenzymes, facilitating numerous reactions in the body. For instance, B vitamins help the body make energy from the metabolism of carbohydrates. Table 9.8 describes the functions and some food sources of individual vitamins.

Water-soluble vitamins, including the B vitamins and vitamin C, dissolve in water and are transported in the blood. With the exception of vitamin B_{12}, which is stored in the liver for years, water-soluble vitamins are not stored in appreciable amounts in the body; instead the body uses what is needed and then excretes the

TABLE 9.8 Vitamins

Vitamin	Function	Food sources (171)	DRI and UL** per day (67, 70, 71, 72)
Vitamin A	Necessary for vision, healthy skin, teeth, body tissues, and healthy mucous membranes and skin.	Animal foods including animal liver (veal, beef, goose, lamb, turkey), meat, fortified milk, cheese, herring	Males: 300-900 mcg RAE (retinal activity equivalents) (RDA) Females: 300-1,300 mcg RAE (RDA) Males: 600-3,000 mcg RAE (UL) Females: 600-3,000 mcg RAE (UL)
Beta-carotene	An antioxidant.** Converted into vitamin A in the body.	Sweet potato, carrots, pumpkin, spinach, collards, kale, winter squash, lamb quarters, beet greens, turnip greens, cabbage	No RDA or AI; however, 1 IU beta-carotene from food = 0.05 mcg RAE vitamin A UL is not determinable due to lack of data. Supplementation is advised only for individuals at risk for vitamin A deficiency.
Vitamin D	Aids calcium absorption, helps maintain blood levels of calcium and phosphorus. Necessary for building bone mass and preventing bone loss.	Fish (swordfish, salmon, tuna, sardines, mackerel, carp, eel, whitefish), fortified milk, fortified breakfast cereals, egg yolks	Males: 15-20 mcg (600-800 IU) (RDA) Females: 15-20 mcg (600-800 IU) (RDA) Males: 63-100 mcg (2,500-4,000 IU) (UL) Females: 63-100 mcg (2,500-4,000 IU) (UL)
Vitamin E	An antioxidant.* Needed for immune functioning and metabolism.	Oils (wheat germ, vegetable), fortified breakfast cereals, nuts and seeds, wheat germ, peanut butter, corn oil	Males: 6-15 mg (7.5-22.4 IU) (RDA) Females: 6-19 mg (9-28.4 IU) (RDA) Males: 200-1,000 mg (300-1,500 IU) (UL) Females: 200-1,000 mg (300-1,500 IU) (UL)
Vitamin K (phylloquinone)	Needed for blood clotting; supports tissue and bone health.	Dark green leafy vegetables (kale, Brussels sprouts, spinach, chard, turnip and mustard greens, beet greens, radicchio), broccoli, asparagus, lamb quarters	Males: 30-120 mcg (AI) Females: 30-90 mcg (AI) No UL due to lack of data
Vitamin C	Promotes healthy cell development, wound healing, and resistance to infections. Serves as an antioxidant.** Necessary for conversion of the inactive form of folic acid to the active form. Makes iron available for hemoglobin synthesis.	Sweet peppers, peaches, guava, broccoli, kiwifruit, citrus fruit (strawberries, oranges, limes, lemons, grapefruit, tangerine), papayas, cantaloupe, tomatoes, potatoes, onions	Males: 15-90 mg (RDA) Females: 15-120 mg (RDA) Males: 400-2,000 mg (UL) Females: 400-2,000 mg (UL)
Thiamin (B$_1$)	Coenzyme for carbohydrate metabolism. Needed for normal functioning of the nervous system and muscles, including the heart.	Fortified breakfast cereals, sunflower seeds, peas, pork, oranges, orange juice, lima beans, pecans, enriched rice	Males: 0.5-1.2 mg (RDA) Females: 0.5-1.4 mg (RDA) No UL due to lack of data
Riboflavin (B$_2$)	Coenzyme in red blood cell formation, nervous system functioning, and metabolism of carbohydrate, protein, and fat. Needed for vision and may help protect against cataracts.	Liver, wheat germ, brewer's yeast, almonds, cheese, fortified breakfast cereal, whey protein, milk, eggs, lamb, pork, veal, beef, broccoli, yogurt	Males: 0.5-1.3 mg (RDA) Females: 0.5-1.6 mg (RDA) No UL due to lack of data

(continued)

TABLE 9.8 *(continued)*

Vitamin	Function	Food sources (171)	DRI and UL** per day (67, 70, 71, 72)
Niacin	Coenzyme for carbohydrate, protein, and fat metabolism and proper nervous system functioning. High intakes can lower elevated cholesterol.	Soy protein, soy flour, textured vegetable protein, whey protein, beef, peanuts, peanut butter, sunflower seeds, fortified breakfast cereals	Males: 6-16 mg (RDA) Females: 6-18 mg (RDA) Males: 10-35 mg (UL) Females: 10-35 mg (UL)
Pyridoxine (B$_6$)	Coenzyme for protein metabolism and nervous and immune system function. Involved in synthesis of hormones and red blood cells.	Liver, bananas, fortified breakfast cereals, soybeans, chicken, tuna, raw carrots, beef, broccoli, spinach, potatoes, alfalfa sprouts, navy beans, peanut butter, garbanzo beans, walnuts, sunflower seeds, avocados, eggs, lima beans, cabbage, salmon	Males: 0.5-1.7 mg (RDA) Females: 0.5-2.0 mg (RDA) Males: 30-100 mg (UL) Females: 30-100 mg (UL)
Folate	Needed for normal growth and development and red blood cell formation. Reduces risk of neural tube birth defects. May reduce risk of heart disease and cervical dysplasia.	Brewer's yeast, fortified breakfast cereals, liver, black-eyed peas, beans (pinto, black, lima, white, garbanzo, soy), peanuts, peanut butter, spinach, turnip greens, asparagus, mustard greens, seaweed, eggs, enriched bread, oranges, orange juice	Males: 150-400 mcg (RDA) Females: 150-600 mcg (RDA) Males: 300-1,000 mcg (UL) Females: 300-1,000 mcg (UL)
Cobalamin (B$_{12}$)	Vital for blood formation and healthy nervous system.	Liver, oysters, lamb, eggs, beef, shellfish, fish, poultry, pork, chicken, fortified breakfast cereals	Males: 0.9-2.4 mcg (RDA) Females: 0.9-2.8 mcg (RDA) No UL due to lack of data
Biotin	Assists in the metabolism of fatty acids and utilization of B vitamins.	Nuts (peanuts, hazelnuts, almonds, cashews, macadamia), soybeans, peanut butter, black-eyed peas, liver, milk, egg yolks, yeast, cheese, cauliflower, carrots, avocados, sweet potatoes	Males: 8-30 mcg (AI) Females: 8-35 mcg (AI) No UL due to lack of data
Pantothenic acid	Aids in normal growth and development.	Liver, sunflower seeds, fortified breakfast cereals, egg yolks, whey protein, soy protein, peanuts, peanut butter, pecans, veal, enriched rice, broccoli, lima beans	Males: 2-5 mg (AI) Females: 2-7 mg (AI) No UL due to lack of data

*Antioxidants are substances that modify cell-signaling pathways and counteract oxidative stress-induced cell damage caused by reactive oxygen and nitrogen species (free radicals). Free radicals are both beneficial and harmful to human health. An overproduction of, or overexposure to, free radicals combined with a deficiency in antioxidants can result in oxidative stress and subsequent damage to cellular lipids, proteins, and DNA (67, 177).

**Dietary Reference Intake (DRI): A set of nutrient recommendations that include the values Recommended Dietary Allowance (RDA), Adequate Intake (AI), Estimated Average Requirement (EAR), and the Tolerable Upper Level Intake (UL).

Tolerable Upper Level Intake (UL): The highest daily intake of a nutrient that is likely to not pose a risk of adverse health effects in most of the general population.

DRIs and UL are listed as a range across the life span for each sex.

remaining amounts in urine (170). And though there are no known side effects from excess vitamin B$_{12}$ consumption, consuming more than the body can use will not increase energy or improve health (17, 72). Vitamins A, D, E, and K are fat soluble and therefore carried by fat in the blood and stored in fat tissue in the body (142). Excess preformed vitamin A (not beta carotene, alpha carotene, or beta cryptoxanthin, which are converted into vitamin A in the body) is toxic and associated with significant adverse effects including liver damage, intracranial pressure (pseudotumor cerebri), dizziness, nausea, headaches, skin irritation, pain in joints and bones, coma, and even death (67, 141). Excess vitamin A intake can occur through diet but typically results from high levels of vitamin A in supplements (70, 142). Toxic levels of vitamin D can lead to heart arrhythmias and increased levels of blood calcium, which can cause blood vessel and tissue calcification, as well as damage to the heart, blood vessels, and kidneys (142). Vitamin E acts as an anticoagulant and therefore thins the blood. Regular intake of excessive amounts of vitamin E can lead to high serum vitamin E levels, which is associated with increased risk of hemorrhagic stroke, particularly in individuals on blood thinners (124). Because vitamin K helps blood clot, excess intake of this vitamin can interfere with the effects of some anticlotting medications such as warfarin (Coumadin) (92).

Minerals

Minerals contribute to the structure of bone, teeth, and nails; are a component of enzymes; and perform a wide variety of metabolic functions. For example, calcium is needed for bone and tooth formation and function, nerve transmission, and muscle contraction. Iron is necessary for oxygen transport and is also a component of enzymes necessary for energy metabolism. Calcium, phosphorus, magnesium, iron, and the **electrolytes** sodium, potassium, and chloride are often called the major minerals. For the athlete, minerals are important for bone health, oxygen-carrying capacity, and fluid and electrolyte balance. The minerals, their functions, and good food sources are listed in table 9.9.

Two minerals, iron and calcium, deserve additional attention. Athletes who do not consume enough dietary iron can develop iron deficiency or iron deficiency **anemia**, both of which can impair performance.

TABLE 9.9   Minerals

Mineral	Function	Food sources (153)	DRI and UL (67, 68, 70, 71)
Calcium	Essential for developing and maintaining healthy bones and teeth. Assists with blood clotting, muscle contraction, and nerve transmission.	Fruit juices and fruit drinks fortified with calcium, cheese, sardines, milk, cottage cheese, yogurt, ice cream, calcium-set tofu, turnip greens, Chinese cabbage, mustard greens, kale, rutabaga	Males: 700-1,300 mg (RDA) Females: 700-1,300 mg (RDA) Males: 2,000-3,000 mg (UL) Females: 2,000-3,000 mg (UL)
Phosphorus	Works with calcium to develop and maintain strong bones and teeth. Enhances use of other nutrients. Essential for energy metabolism, DNA structure, and cell membranes.	Cheese, fish, beef, pork, whole-wheat products, cocoa powder, pumpkin seeds, sunflower seeds, almonds	Males: 460-1,250 mg (RDA) Females: 460-1,250 mg (RDA) Males: 3-4 g (UL) Females: 3-4 g (UL)
Magnesium	Activates nearly 100 enzymes and helps nerves and muscles function. Constituent of bones and teeth.	Bran (wheat and rice), cocoa powder, fortified breakfast cereals, seeds (pumpkin, sunflower), soybeans, nuts (almonds, pine nuts, hazelnuts, cashews, walnuts, peanuts), spinach	Males: 80-420 mg (RDA) Females: 80-400 mg (RDA) Males: 65-350 mg (UL) Females: 65-350 mg (UL)
Molybdenum	Needed for metabolism of DNA and ribonucleic acid (RNA) and production of uric acid.	Milk, milk products, peas, beans, liver, whole-grain products	Males: 17-45 mcg (RDA) Females: 17-50 mcg (RDA) Males: 300-2,000 mcg (UL) Females: 300-2,000 mcg (UL)
Manganese	Necessary for the normal development of the skeletal and connective tissues. Involved in metabolism of carbohydrates.	Wheat germ, wheat bran, rice bran, fortified breakfast cereals, rice cakes, nuts (peanuts, pecans, pine nuts, walnuts, almonds, hazelnuts), soybeans, mussels, whole-wheat products (pastas, breads, and crackers)	Males: 1.2-2.3 mg (AI) Females: 1.2-2.6 mg (AI) Males: 2-11 mg (UL) Females: 2-11 mg (UL)

(continued)

TABLE 9.9   *(continued)*

Mineral	Function	Food sources (153)	DRI and UL (67, 68, 70, 71)
Copper	Involved in iron metabolism, nervous system functioning, bone health, and synthesis of proteins. Plays a role in the pigmentation of skin, hair, and eyes.	Liver, shellfish (especially oysters), lobster, nuts (cashews, Brazil nuts, hazelnuts, walnuts, peanuts, almonds, pecans, pistachios), seeds (sunflower, pumpkin), fortified breakfast cereals, great northern beans	Males: 340-900 mcg (RDA) Females: 340-1,300 mcg (RDA) Males: 1,000-10,000 mcg (UL) Females: 1,000-10,000 mcg (UL)
Chromium	Aids in glucose metabolism and may help regulate blood sugar and insulin levels in people with diabetes.	Mushrooms (white), raw oysters, wine, apples, brewer's yeast, beer, pork, chicken	Males: 11-35 mcg (AI) Females: 11-45 mcg (AI) No UL due to lack of data.
Iodine	Part of the thyroid hormone. Helps regulate growth, development, and energy metabolism.	Iodized salt, saltwater fish and seafood	Males: 90-150 mcg (RDA) Females: 90-290 mcg (RDA) Males: 200-1,100 mcg (UL) Females: 200-1,100 mcg (UL)
Iron	Necessary for red blood cell formation and function. Constituent of myoglobin and component of enzyme systems.	Liver, beef, lamb, pork, veal, poultry, clams, oysters, fortified breakfast cereals, enriched bread products, brewer's yeast, nuts (pine nuts, cashews, almonds), beans (kidney, green, garbanzo)	Males: 7-11 mg (RDA) Females: 7-27 mg (RDA) Males: 40-45 mg (UL) Females: 40-45 mg (UL)
Selenium	Essential component of a key antioxidant enzyme. Necessary for normal growth and development and for use of iodine in thyroid function.	Tenderloin of beef, pollock, trout, tuna, oysters, mackerel, flounder, liver, sunflower seeds, wheat bran, wheat germ, some pork, fortified breakfast cereals, perch, crab, clams, cod, haddock, whole-wheat breads	Males: 20-55 mcg (RDA) Females: 20-70 mcg (RDA) Males: 90-400 mcg (UL) Females: 90-400 mcg (UL)
Zinc	Essential part of more than 100 enzymes involved in digestion, metabolism, reproduction, and wound healing.	Oysters, beef, veal, lamb, pork, chicken, lima beans, black-eyed peas, white beans	Males: 3-11 mg (RDA) Females: 3-13 mg (RDA) Males: 7-40 mg (UL) Females: 7-40 mg (UL)

Inadequate dietary calcium can contribute to low bone density and possibly future risk of developing osteopenia or osteoporosis.

Iron

Iron is essential for both the functioning and synthesis of hemoglobin, a protein that transfers oxygen throughout the body (158). In addition, iron is a component of the protein myoglobin, which transports oxygen to muscles (51). This mineral plays important roles in growth, development, cell functioning, and the synthesis and functioning of some hormones (41, 46, 85).

Iron deficiency is the most prevalent nutrition deficiency in the world (183). And though it disproportionately affects those in developing countries, it is common in industrialized countries as well. The National Nutrition and Health Examination Survey (NHANES) found that approximately 16% of teenage girls aged 16 to 19 and 12% of women aged 20 to 49 were deficient in iron. In some studies examining iron deficiency in female aerobic endurance athletes, more than one in four women tested positive for iron deficiency (102, 137). Iron deficiency occurs in three stages (in order of severity): depletion, marginal deficiency, and anemia (89, 118). Iron carries oxygen to the working muscles, and even marginal iron deficiency may impair athletic performance (18, 61). Iron deficiency anemia develops when low iron stores persist for a period of time and the body cannot make enough healthy red blood cells to deliver oxygen throughout the body (157, 161). Symptoms depend on the individual; some people are asymptomatic or get used to their symptoms and assume that they are normal. Symptoms of deficiency iron deficiency or iron deficiency anemia may include weakness, fatigue, irritability, poor concentration, headache, decreased exercise capacity, hair loss, and dry mouth (15). Other symptoms associated with iron deficiency anemia include feeling cold often, inflamed tongue (glossitis), shortness of breath during routine activities, and pica (the desire to eat nonfood substances such as laundry starch, dirt, clay, and ice) (111).

Women of childbearing age, teenage girls, pregnant women, infants, and toddlers have the greatest need for iron and therefore an increased risk of becoming deficient. In addition, distance runners, vegetarian athletes, female athletes, those who lose a significant amount of blood during their menstrual cycle, people who take excessive amounts of antacids, and people with certain digestive diseases such as celiac disease have an increased risk of developing iron deficiency anemia (70).

The two types of iron found in food are heme and nonheme iron. Heme iron, derived from hemoglobin, is found in foods that originally contained hemoglobin and myoglobin—animal foods including red meats, fish, and poultry. Heme iron is absorbed better than nonheme iron, and absorption isn't affected by anything else we eat. We absorb approximately 15% to 35% of the heme iron we eat (111).

Nonheme iron is the form of iron found in all other, non-meat foods including vegetables, grains, and iron-fortified breakfast cereal. Only 2% to 20% of nonheme iron is absorbed (165). And, while heme iron is not affected by compounds found in food eaten concurrently, many factors affect the absorption of nonheme iron. For instance, the nonheme iron in spinach is bound to a substance called phytic acid, the storage form of phosphorus in plants. Phytic acid decreases the absorption of nonheme iron. In addition, several other substances may decrease the absorption of nonheme iron, including tannins (found in tea and wine), calcium (found in dairy and multivitamins), polyphenols, phytates (found in legumes and whole grains), and some of the proteins in soy. A person can increase the amount of nonheme iron absorbed by consuming vitamin C–rich foods or beverages at the same time or consuming a nonheme source at the same time heme iron is consumed. For example, pairing spinach with meat increases iron absorption from spinach (70, 165).

There are many supplemental forms of iron; each supplies a different amount of elemental iron while also varying in bioavailability and the potential for side effects such as stomach upset (103). In addition, both calcium and supplemental magnesium may interfere with iron absorption (179). Yet many Americans are not consuming enough calcium and magnesium through diet alone. Because of the many factors affecting iron intake and absorption, including intake of other minerals the athlete may not be consuming in adequate quantities, only a medical doctor or registered dietitian should recommend iron supplements and how to take an iron supplement for maximum absorption and minimal stomach upset (24, 47, 114, 144, 179).

Calcium

Adequate calcium intake throughout childhood and adolescence is essential for the development of strong bones. Calcium helps bones grow in length and density during adolescence, with up to 90% of peak bone mineral density occurring during late adolescence (58, 154). And in adults, calcium helps maintain bone density. When dietary calcium intake falls short, calcium is pulled from its storage site in bone to meet the demands of the body and keep calcium concentrations in the blood, muscle, and intercellular fluids constant. Calcium is essential for attaining peak bone mass, and calcium deficiencies can impair the attainment of peak bone mineral density and increase risk of fracture later in life (71). Calcium also keeps teeth strong, helps regulate muscle contraction, and plays a role in nerve functioning, blood vessel expansion and contraction, and hormone and enzyme secretion (71).

The NHANES found that just 15% of 9- to 13-year-old females and less than 10% of females aged 14 to 18 and over the age of 51 met the adequate intake (AI) for calcium from diet alone (9). Therefore, athletes should be encouraged to include dairy products and other

---

Caloric Versus Nutrient-Dense Foods

Given the rise in obesity in America, some classify the American diet as calorie dense but nutrient poor. The Scientific Report of the 2015 Dietary Guidelines Advisory Committee recommends a dietary pattern including a variety of nutrient-dense foods. Though there is no standardized definition of the term **nutrient density**, in general, choosing nutrient-dense foods means looking for foods based on the nutrients such as vitamins, minerals, and fiber, as well as the healthy plant-based compounds that they provide, whereas caloric density refers to the caloric content of a food. Foods high in nutrient density include milk, vegetables, protein foods, and grains, while foods high in caloric density but low in nutrient density typically include potato chips, desserts, and candy (39). For more information on nutrient versus caloric density, the reader is referred to the work of Drewnowski (39).

calcium-rich foods in their diets. The athlete's medical doctor or registered dietitian may suggest a calcium supplement if calcium needs cannot be met through diet alone.

Fluid and Electrolytes

Water is the largest component of the body, representing 45% to 75% of a person's body weight (68). In the human body, water acts as a lubricant, shock absorber, building material, and solvent. In addition, water is essential for body temperature regulation (water loss through sweat helps cool off skin, particularly in hot environments and during exercise), nutrient transport and waste product removal, and maintaining fluid balance and therefore normal blood pressure (78). Water is so important that even under optimal temperature conditions, the body can survive only a few days without water (99).

While maintaining adequate **hydration** is important for all individuals, athletes must pay close attention to their hydration status since sweat losses that exceed fluid intake can quickly lead to a hypohydrated state with a subsequent increase in core body temperature, decrease in blood plasma volume, and increase in heart rate and perceived exertion (31, 147). When this happens, sweat output cannot keep up with increases in core body temperature unless fluids are given. Repeated exercise in hot environments helps the body adapt to heat stress (e.g., greater sweat volume, lower electrolyte concentration of sweat, and lower temperature for the onset of sweating), and therefore athletes may be more prone to **dehydration** and heat stress at the beginning of the season (50). In addition, athletes with less training may be more prone to heat stress than trained athletes (45). Due to physiological changes that alter water conservation in the body as well as age-related decline in fluid intake, the elderly have an increased risk of dehydration and **hypohydration** (45). Children may have a greater risk of dehydration as well, resulting from increased heat gain from the environment due to greater surface area–body mass ratio compared to adults, increased heat production during exercise, decreased ability to dissipate heat through sweat, and a decreased sensation of thirst compared to adults (12, 40). In addition, those with sickle cell trait, cystic fibrosis, and some other diseases have an increased risk of becoming dehydrated (12, 168). Even mild dehydration, representing 2% to 3% weight loss, can increase core body temperature and significantly affect athletic performance by increasing fatigue and decreasing motivation, neuromuscular control, accuracy, power, strength, muscular endurance, and overall performance (13, 25, 37, 55, 81, 83, 112, 149, 158). Dehydration can increase core body temperature, reduce stroke volume and cardiac output, decrease blood pressure, reduce blood flow to muscles, increase heartbeat, exacerbate symptomatic exertional rhabdomyolysis, and increase risk of heatstroke and death (31, 52, 109, 146). One's risk for dehydration is greater in hot, humid environments and at altitude (26, 109, 117).

Fluid Balance

The AI for water is 3.7 L (125.1 fluid ounces or 15.6 cups) and 2.7 L (91.3 fluid ounces or 11.4 cups) per day, respectively, for men and women. However, the AI for pregnant and lactating women is 3.0 L (101.4 fluid ounces or 12.7 cups) and 3.8 L (128.49 fluid ounces or 16.1 cups) per day, respectively. All sources of fluid, including beverages such as coffee, tea, juice, and soda, as well as the fluid in foods, contribute to meeting a person's water needs (68).

Maintaining fluid balance during training and competition can be a challenge for many athletes, particularly those who sweat profusely or train in hot, humid environments or at altitude. In addition to environmental conditions, clothing, equipment, and larger body size can increase sweat rate, while unsafe weight loss practices such frequent use or overuse of diuretics or laxatives can increase risk of dehydration (31, 34). American football players, particularly linemen, have a greater risk of becoming dehydrated because of their equipment and in many cases, larger body size (31). For example, a study in National Football League players found that backs and receivers, with an average body mass of 93 ± 6 kg (204.6 ± 13.2 pounds), lost an average of 1.4 ± 0.45 L (47.3 ± 15.2 fluid ounces; or approximately 6 ± 2 cups) of sweat per hour, while linemen, with an average body mass of 135.6 ± 17 kg (298 ± 37.4 pounds), lost an average 2.25 ± 0.68 L (75.1 ± 1.5 fluid ounces; approximately 9 cups) of sweat per hour during practice. Calculated sweat losses for both groups during a total of 4.5 hours of practice on days with two practice sessions were 6.4 ± 2.0 L (216.4 ± 67.6 fluid ounces; approximately 27 ± 8 cups) for backs and receivers and 10.1 ± 3.1 L (341.5 ± 104.8 fluid ounces; 42.7 ± 13.1 cups) for linemen (51). Multiple layers of clothing and protective equipment contribute to sweat losses and dehydration risk in hockey players (14), while intentional dehydration and other unsafe weight loss practices can increase dehydration risk in wrestlers (52, 181). In addition, it is important to note that a very wide range of fluid losses through sweat exists. For instance, National Basketball Association players lost from 1.0 to 4.6 L (33.8-155.5 fluid ounces; 4.2-19.4 cups) and had a mean loss of 2.2 ± 0.8 L (74.4 ± 27.1 fluid ounces; 9.3 ± 3.4 cups) of sweat over the course of a 40-minute game in which the average playing time was 21 ± 8 minutes (120). When people are sedentary, respiration and sweat combined contribute to water losses equal to approximately 0.3 L (20.2 fluid ounces; 2.5 cups) per hour (148).

Preventing Dehydration

Given the negative effects associated with dehydration, athletes should try to prevent water weight losses exceeding 2% of body weight while also restoring electrolytes lost through sweat (146, 147). The first step to preventing dehydration is to assess hydration status (table 9.10). Urine specific gravity (USG) can be used to access hydration status because the test is easy to use, inexpensive, and portable (178). However, USG is not a sensitive indicator of acute changes in hydration; instead it is better as a measure of chronic hydration status (120, 133). A quick and simple method for estimating hydration status involves measuring changes in body weight from pre- to postworkout. Athletes should weigh themselves in minimal, lightweight clothing, after drying off and urinating, immediately before and after their workout. Sweaty clothes should be removed before weighing. Each pound (0.45 kg) lost during practice represents 16 ounces (0.5 L) of fluid. A loss of 2% or more of body weight indicates the athlete is not adequately replacing fluid lost through sweat (146). In addition to identifying acute dehydration from one workout, assessing weight changes over time may help identify athletes who are chronically dehydrated—those who lose several pounds over the course of a few days (22).

In addition to identifying athletes who do not adequately hydrate, one can calculate sweat rate, thereby giving a better idea of fluid needs during exercise, by weighing athletes preexercise and again after an intense 1-hour practice session while also measuring fluid intake and urine volume produced. Sweat rate is equal to preexercise body weight minus postexercise body weight + fluid intake during exercise − urine produced (14, 22). Assessments of urine quantity, through USG or urine volume, may be misleading during the immediate rehydration period after dehydration. When athletes consume large quantities of hypotonic fluid, they produce copious amounts of urine long before they become adequately hydrated (156).

In addition to monitoring weight changes, athletes are sometimes advised to check their urine color. However, the relationship between urine color and hydration status is very subjective (68, 109, 146). Also, beets, blackberries, certain food colors, and medications can turn urine pink, red, or light brown (49). In addition, B vitamins, carotenoids (such as beta carotene), and some medications can turn urine dark yellow, bright yellow, or orange, while artificial food colors (such as those found in some sport drinks) may also turn urine blue or green (178).

> A very wide range of fluid losses, in the form of sweat, exists among athletes. Therefore each athlete should develop an individualized hydration plan.

Electrolytes

The major electrolytes lost in sweat include sodium chloride, and, to a lesser extent and in order, potassium, magnesium, and calcium (88). Sodium influences fluid regulation by helping retain more of the fluid consumed (108). In addition, all of the electrolytes lost through sweat are essential to muscle contraction and nerve conduction. Thus, any disturbance in the balance of electrolytes in body fluids could potentially interfere with performance. Sodium losses through sweat vary tremendously between athletes, with reported concentrations ranging from 0.2 to greater than 12.5 g/L (10 to over 544 mEq/L) (31, 146). Given the large quantity of sodium some athletes lose through sweat, replacing sodium losses may require a conscious decision to choose higher-sodium foods, salt their food, and add electrolytes to their sport drinks. Athletes who exercise intensely or for hours and hydrate excessively with only water or a no- or low-sodium beverage may dilute their

TABLE 9.10   Biomarkers of Hydration Status

Measure	Practicality	Validity (acute vs. chronic changes)	EUH cutoff
Total body water	Low	Acute and chronic	<2%
Plasma osmolality	Medium	Acute and chronic	<290 mOsmol
Urine specific gravity	High	Chronic	<1.020 g/ml
Urine osmolality	High	Chronic	<700 mOsmol
Body weight	High	Acute and chronic*	<1%

EUH = euhydration.

* = potentially confounded by changes in body composition during very prolonged assessment periods.

Reprinted, by permission, from Sawka et al., 2007 (146).

blood sodium levels to dangerously low levels—below 130 mmol/L—a condition called **hyponatremia**. This leads to intracellular swelling, and, when blood sodium levels fall below 125 mmol/L, to headaches, nausea, vomiting, muscle cramps, swollen hands and feet, restlessness, and disorientation. When blood sodium drops below 120 mmol/L, risk of developing cerebral edema, seizures, coma, brain stem herniation, respiratory arrest, and risk of death increase (4, 6, 146). To avoid hyponatremia, fluid intake shouldn't exceed sweat losses (athletes should not weigh more after they finish exercising than they did at the start of their training session), and athletes should consume sodium through either sport drinks or food (120, 146).

Sport drinks provide small amounts of potassium to replace sweat potassium losses. However, they are not a significant contributor to total potassium intake. And, because research shows that <2% of adults in the United States meet the dietary recommendations for potassium (29), athletes should focus on consuming more potassium-rich foods in their diet, such as tomatoes, citrus fruits, melons, potatoes, bananas, and milk.

> **Athletes who exercise intensely or for hours and hydrate excessively with only water or a no- or low-sodium beverage may dilute their blood sodium to dangerously low levels.**

Fluid Intake Guidelines

Ideally, athletes should start exercise or training in a hydrated state, avoid losing more than 2% of body weight (due to sweat losses) during exercise, and rehydrate completely after exercise and before the next training session. The amount of fluid necessary to fully achieve rehydration depends on the time period before the next bout of training. However, studies show that some athletes start practice or competition in a hypohydrated state, making it more difficult to consume enough fluid during the exercise session to make up for poor preexercise hydration status (120, 138). In addition, athletes with significant sweat losses may not voluntarily drink enough fluid to adequately rehydrate and prevent dehydration during training and competition. A systematic approach to fluid replacement is necessary for this reason and also because thirst may not be a reliable indicator of fluid needs for athletes who are heavy sweaters or those who are practicing intensely in hot environmental conditions (22). Though fluid and electrolyte guidelines should be individualized as much as possible, given the wide range of fluid and electrolyte losses in athletes, the general guidelines presented next are a good starting place with athletes until specific recommendations can be provided based on sweat rate (7). In addition, strength coaches should ensure that athletes are given adequate time to drink and access to cool fluids (10-15 °C [50-59 °F]) (80).

Fluid Intake Guidelines at a Glance

Before Training

- Athletes should have a USG reading <1.020. They should prehydrate, if necessary, several hours before exercise to allow for fluid absorption and urine output (146).

During a Training Session

Children and Adolescents

- Children weighing 88 pounds (40 kg) should drink 5 ounces (150 ml) of cold water or a flavored, salted beverage every 20 minutes during training.
- Adolescents weighing 132 pounds (60 kg) should drink 9 (250 ml) ounces of cold water or a flavored, salted beverage every 20 minutes (30, 182).

Adults

- Athletes should follow an individualized hydration plan. During prolonged activity in hot weather, they should consume a sport drink containing 20 to 30 mEq of sodium (460-690 mg with chloride as the anion) per liter, 2 to 5 mEq of potassium (78-195 mg) per liter, and carbohydrate in a concentration of 5% to 10%.

After Training

- Athletes should consume adequate food and fluids, as well as sodium, to restore hydration. If dehydration is significant or the athlete has <12 hours before the next exercise bout, a more aggressive approach is warranted and the athlete should consume approximately 1.5 L (50 ounces) of fluid (with sufficient electrolytes) for each kilogram of body weight lost (0.7 L or 24 ounces for each pound of body weight).

Before Activity

Prehydrate, if necessary, several hours before exercise to allow for fluid absorption and urine output (146).

During Activity

Due to large variations in sweat rates and electrolyte concentrations, athletes should measure weight changes during training and competition in specific weather conditions and develop individualized hydration strategies based on this information (146). During prolonged activity in hot weather, the IOM recommends sport drinks containing 20 to 30 mEq of sodium (460-690 mg with chloride as the anion) per liter, 2 to 5 mEq of potassium (78-195 mg) per liter, and carbohydrate in a concentration of 5% to 10% (73). In addition, when a sport drink is ingested at high rates during intense or prolonged exercise, athletes may want to choose one that contains multiple types of carbohydrates with different intestinal transport mechanisms, such as glucose, fructose, and maltodextrin. Ingestion of multiple types of carbohydrate versus a single carbohydrate will lead to greater gastric emptying, carbohydrate absorption, oxidation, and possibly better performance (33, 80). All beverages provided should be cool—10-15 °C (50-59 °F)—but not cold (22).

The American Academy of Pediatrics recommends periodic drinking be enforced in children. These guidelines suggest that children weighing 88 pounds (40 kg) drink 5 ounces (148 ml) of cold water or a flavored salted beverage every 20 minutes during practice and that adolescents weighing 132 pounds (60 kg) drink 9 ounces (266 ml) even if they do not feel thirsty. Another recommendation is a sodium chloride concentration of 15 to 20 mmol/L (1 g per 2 pints), which has been shown to increase voluntary hydration by 90% when compared to unflavored water (30, 182).

After Activity

After exercise, athletes should replace fluid and electrolyte losses. If time permits, normal meals, snacks (provided that they contain some sodium), and water will restore fluid and electrolyte losses. Additional salt can be added to foods when sweat sodium losses are substantial (68, 146). If dehydration is significant, or the athlete has a short recovery period before the next bout of exercise (<12 hours), then a more aggressive approach is warranted: Athletes should consume approximately 1.5 L (50 ounces) of fluid (with sufficient electrolytes) for each kilogram of body weight loss (0.7 L or 24 ounces for each pound of body weight). This amount of fluid helps account for increased urine production stemming from the consumption of a large volume of fluid (146, 155).

Conclusion

Nutrition plays an important role in strength and conditioning. Adequate hydration and electrolytes, appropriate energy intake, and adequate protein, carbohydrate, fat, vitamin, and mineral intakes allow athletes to reap maximal benefits from training. A general understanding of nutrition principles and applications is essential for strength and conditioning professionals so that they can help athletes sort through nutrition misinformation and provide sound guidelines that athletes can use to improve their diets.

KEY WORDS

Acceptable Macronutrient Distribution Range (AMDR)
Adequate Intake (AI)
amino acids
anemia
bioavailability
carbohydrate
cholesterol
dehydration
Dietary Reference Intakes (DRIs)
disaccharides
docosahexaenoic acid (DHA)
eicosapentaenoic acid (EPA)
electrolytes
Estimated Average Requirement (EAR)
fat
fatty acids
fiber
fructose
galactose
gluconeogenesis
glycemic index (GI)
glycemic load
glycogen
glycogenesis
glucose
high-density lipoprotein (HDL)
hydration
hypohydration
hyponatremia
lactose
low-density lipoprotein (LDL)
macronutrient
maltose
micronutrient
minerals
monosaccharides
monounsaturated
muscle protein synthesis
MyPlate
nutrient density
omega-3 fatty acid alpha-linolenic acid (ALA)
polypeptide
polysaccharides
polyunsaturated
protein
protein digestibility
protein digestibility correct amino acid score (PDCAAS)
Recommended Dietary Allowances (RDA)
saturated
sports dietitian
sucrose
Tolerable Upper Intake Level (UL)
triglycerides
very low-density lipoproteins (VLDL)
vitamins

STUDY QUESTIONS

1. Maintaining adequate glycogen stores
    a. spares the use of protein for energy
    b. improves maximum power
    c. decreases endurance performance
    d. helps athletes gain weight

2. The following is the most likely contributor to fatigue and poor performance:
    a. low protein intake
    b. iron deficiency
    c. low calcium intake
    d. omega-3 fatty acid deficiency

3. Which of the following is a recommendation for lowering undesirably high levels of blood lipids?
    a. reduce complex carbohydrate intake
    b. limit saturated fatty acid intake to 30% of total calories
    c. consume a minimum of 500 mg of dietary cholesterol per day
    d. replace saturated fatty acids with monounsaturated or polyunsaturated fatty acids

4. Which of the following protein sources does not contain all essential amino acids in appreciable quantities?
    a. poultry
    b. eggs
    c. lentils
    d. beef

CHAPTER 10

Nutrition Strategies
for Maximizing Performance

Marie Spano, MS, RD

 After completing this chapter, you will be able to

- list pre-, during- and postcompetition nutrition recommendations for different sports;
- provide guidelines for weight gain and weight loss;
- recognize signs and symptoms of eating disorders;
- understand the importance of having an intervention and referral system in place for athletes suspected of having an eating disorder;
- recognize the prevalence and etiologies of obesity; and
- assist in the assessment process for obese individuals.

What athletes eat and drink before and during competition can affect their performance, while their postevent meal has a greater impact on their recovery, and, if the time period between events is less than 24 hours, performance in the next event or game. Therefore this chapter focuses on pre-, during-, and postcompetition nutrition while also providing guidelines for athletes who want to lose or gain weight. In addition, no talk about weight is complete unless it includes information on **disordered eating** and **eating disorders**. It is imperative that the strength and conditioning professional recognize when an athlete may have signs and symptoms of an eating disorder and be an active member of the treatment team.

Precompetition, During-Event, and Postcompetition Nutrition

Athletes' dietary practices over time will influence their overall health and performance. In addition, what athletes eat before and during competition can have both physiological and psychological effects on performance, while their postcompetition meal affects recovery and may therefore influence how they perform during their next bout of training or competition.

Precompetition Nutrition

The **precompetition meal** helps provide fluid to maintain adequate hydration and carbohydrate to maximize blood glucose and stored glycogen levels (5, 25) while also keeping hunger pangs at bay. Glycogen is the main form of energy used during high-intensity (>70% $\dot{V}O_2max$) exercise; once these stores become depleted, the athlete will experience muscular fatigue (56). Small quantities of glycogen are stored in liver and muscle, totaling approximately 15 g of glycogen per kilogram body weight (1). For example, an 80 kg man can store approximately 1,200 grams of glycogen. Glycogen stored in the liver is used for the whole body, while glycogen stored in muscle tissue is used by muscle (56).

Despite the vital roles that both hydration and glycogen play in athletic performance, studies examining the importance of the precompetition meal and its effect on performance are equivocal due to differences in study subjects and methods used. Some show that a high-carbohydrate preexercise meal enhances aerobic time to exhaustion (24, 93, 113) as well as anaerobic performance in adolescent males (71), while other studies found no effect on time-trial performance (100). Despite these differences and the fact that studies simulating performance can't take into account several factors that distinguish the competitive environment from a lab setting, such as precompetition nerves, temperature, humidity, and altitude, athletes can adapt general precompetition

guidelines based on the literature to fit their own unique needs and the competitive environment they are in.

All precompetition meals should take timing, meal and fluid composition, event or sport, and individual athlete preferences into account. In order to minimize the potential for stomach upset, smaller quantities of fluids and food should be consumed when the precompetition meal is consumed closer in temporal proximity to competition. Precompetition foods and beverages should be familiar to the athlete (tried in practice), low in fat and fiber so that they empty rapidly from the stomach and minimize any potential for gastrointestinal distress, and moderate in protein (protein promotes longer-lasting satiety) (5).

Athletes can choose from either high or low glycemic index (124) carbohydrates before competition, since the research does not indicate that one is more advantageous than the other (12). Even though consuming carbohydrates that rapidly increase insulin, such as glucose, will lead to an initial drop in blood sugar at the beginning of exercise, blood sugar levels typically return to normal within approximately 20 minutes, and the initial drop has no negative effect on performance (78).

Aerobic Endurance Sports

The precompetition meal may be most important for aerobic endurance athletes who compete in long-duration activity (>2 hours) in the morning after an overnight fast. Upon waking in the morning, blood sugar levels are low and liver glycogen stores are substantially reduced. Both conditions decrease the amount of carbohydrate available for use as energy. Carbohydrates at the precompetition meal can significantly enhance glycogen stores and improve exercise time to exhaustion in those who regularly include carbohydrate in their diets, when consumed 3 or more hours before competition (27, 137).

A crossover study examined whether a precompetition high-carbohydrate meal combined with a carbohydrate-electrolyte sports drink consumed during exercise improved aerobic endurance running capacity (70% $\dot{V}O_2max$ until exhaustion) more than the sports drink alone (23). The scientists had men perform three treadmill runs, each separated by one week, after an overnight fast followed by (1) a carbohydrate meal 3 hours before exercise in addition to a carbohydrate-electrolyte sports drink during running; (2) a carbohydrate meal 3 hours before exercise and water during running; or (3) a low-calorie placebo drink (same flavor as the sports drink) 3 hours before exercise and water during running. In the two-day period before the first main trial, subjects weighed and recorded their food intake. They replicated the same diet for the two-day period before each trial. No differences were noted in average daily caloric intake between the three trials. Consumption of

Minimizing Gastrointestinal Issues

To minimize the likelihood of stomach discomfort during competition, athletes should do the following:

- Try food in practice first. Always try new foods during several practice sessions before competition (5).
- When the meal is closer in time to the start of the game or event, consume smaller amounts of food and liquids.
- Avoid high-fat and high-fiber foods. Both fat and fiber slow down the rate of digestion. When food is still being digesting as you are exercising, you may experience stomach cramps (5).
- Avoid sugar alcohols. Despite their name, sugar alcohols contain no alcohol. But their chemical structure resembles that of both sugar and alcohol. Sugar alcohols are a type of carbohydrate that is not completely absorbed in the gut. Consequently, consumption can cause gas, bloating, and cramping and may have a laxative effect. Sugar alcohols are found in some low-carbohydrate and sugar-free products, including sugar-free gum, toothpaste, and mouthwashes. The two sugar alcohols most likely to cause gastrointestinal issues are sorbitol and mannitol (131). Any product that could result in consumption of 20 g of mannitol must carry this warning on the label: "Excess consumption may have a laxative effect." Individual responses to sugar alcohol vary. Sugar alcohols include xylitol (the most common one found in dental products), erythritol, sorbitol, mannitol, maltitol, isomalt, lactitol, hydrogenated starch hydrolysates, and hydrogenated glucose syrups (131).

the high-carbohydrate meal preexercise improved endurance running capacity by 9% compared to the placebo drink before exercise and water during the run. However, the high-carbohydrate meal plus sports drink during the run improved endurance capacity by 22% compared to the placebo beforehand and sports drink during the run. These results indicate that a high-carbohydrate preexercise or precompetition meal can help improve aerobic endurance running capacity (23).

Endurance athletes who are not chronically adapted to a low-carbohydrate diet and start exercise with depleted glycogen stores will break down muscle to use protein for energy and may acutely suppress immune and central nervous system functioning. Therefore, a high-carbohydrate preexercise meal can help attenuate the breakdown of skeletal muscle while also providing carbohydrate for immune and nervous system functioning (20, 72). Over time, adaptation to chronic consumption of a low-carbohydrate diet increases the body's reliance on its vast storage of fat as a fuel source during exercise, though training with low glycogen stores may suppress immune and central nervous system functioning (20, 45). In a study examining protein catabolism, six subjects rode a cycle ergometer for 1 hour at 61% $\dot{V}O_2$max after a **carbohydrate loading** protocol or carbohydrate depletion. In the carbohydrate-depleted state, protein breakdown was calculated at 13.7 g per hour, which represented 10.7% of the calories used during exercise (72).

It is clear that a preexercise meal consumed hours before competition can help improve aerobic endurance performance. However, extremely early morning start times can complicate the desire to feed with a concurrent desire for maximum sleep. For instance, a runner who must be at the starting line of a race at 7 a.m. may find

that waking up at 3 or 4 a.m. to eat isn't practical. Athletes who find themselves in this scenario should practice eating small amounts of food 1 to 2 hours before they start while also ensuring that they consume an adequate amount of carbohydrate during competition.

The following are general recommendations that can be adapted to meet each athlete's individual needs. More research needs to be done to examine the needs of athletes in a variety of sports and to determine the effects of varying amounts of each macronutrient on performance (95). Until this is done, the guidelines for aerobic endurance athletes are adapted to other sports.

- Athletes should prehydrate, if necessary, several hours before exercise to allow for fluid absorption and urine output. Their urine specific gravity (USG) reading should be <1.020 (112).
- Athletes who tend to get nauseated easily, who have experienced diarrhea during competition, who get anxious or experience precompetition jitters, or who compete in high-intensity sports (jarring movements can increase the likelihood of stomach upset), as well as those who are competing in the heat, may want to consider eating at least 4 hours before competition. Aerobic endurance athletes who eat at least 4 hours before competition should include approximately 1 to 4 g of carbohydrate per kilogram body weight and 0.15 to 0.25 g of protein per kilogram body weight (124).
- If the precompetition meal is consumed 2 hours before exercise, athletes should aim for approximately 1 g of carbohydrate per kilogram body weight. Athletes should follow an individualized

hydration plan. During prolonged activity in hot weather, they should consume a sports drink containing 20 to 30 mEq of sodium (460-690 mg with chloride as the anion) per liter, 2 to 5 mEq of potassium (78-195 mg) per liter, and carbohydrate in a concentration of 5% to 10% (112).

- When consumed closer to the start of competition, the preexercise meal should be smaller. In addition, liquid sources of carbohydrate may be preferable when the preexercise meal is 1 hour before the event because they are emptied from the stomach faster than solid food (5). Gels, gummies, and similar sources of carbohydrate are also digested very quickly. Table 10.1 summarizes these recommendations while providing sample food options.

Athletes may want to keep a record of their food intake, including the time each meal or snack was consumed and how they felt while training. By recording the types and amounts of food consumed and when these are consumed in relation to training, they may be able to identify any issues they are having with performance or stomach upset and develop a better precompetition plan.

> ▶ **The primary purpose of the precompetition meal is to provide sufficient fluid to maintain hydration and carbohydrate to maximize blood glucose and stored glycogen while also satisfying hunger.**

Carbohydrate Loading

Depletion of muscle and liver glycogen leads to fatigue during long-term aerobic endurance exercise (109, 123, 133). Therefore, a technique called carbohydrate loading has been used for decades to enhance muscle glycogen before aerobic endurance events. And though there are many different variations of carbohydrate loading, all include high carbohydrate intake in the days leading up to an event to maximize glycogen stores and therefore carbohydrate availability in the later stages of the event

TABLE 10.1   Precompetition Food and Fluid Recommendations for Aerobic Endurance Athletes*

Time before competition	Food recommendations	Fluid recommendations	Sample precompetition meals for a 68.2 kg (150 lb) athlete	Sample meals based on food and fluid recommendations	
≥1 hour	0.5 g carbohydrate per kilogram body weight		34 g carbohydrate	1 small banana 8 oz. sports drink	37 g carbohydrate 8 oz. fluid
2 hours	1 g carbohydrate per kilogram body weight	If not adequately hydrated, sip on 3-5 ml (0.10-0.17 oz.) of fluid per kilogram body weight (112)	68 g carbohydrate 7-12 oz. fluid	2.5 cups boiled, plain potato, flesh only 2 mini bagels with 1 Tbsp jam + 8 oz. sports drink	66 g carbohydrate 72 g carbohydrate 8 g protein 8 oz. fluid
4 hours or more	1-4 g carbohydrate per kilogram body weight and 0.15-0.25 g protein per kilogram body weight (100)	Should consume approximately 5-7 ml of water or a sports drink per kilogram body weight (112)	68-272.8 g carbohydrate 10-17 g protein Minimal fat	Bowl of cereal and fruit: 8 oz. skim milk + 2 cups of Cheerios + 1/4 cup (measured unpacked) raisins	74 g carbohydrate 11 g protein 14 oz. water
				Egg white sandwich: 2 egg whites on 2 pieces of white bread (skip high-fiber breads preworkout)	72 g carbohydrate (based on 1 slice = 64 g weight) 17 g protein 14 oz. water

*These recommendations are for aerobic endurance athletes and can be adapted for other types of athletes.

(25). Carbohydrate loading offers potential benefits for distance runners, road cyclists, cross-country skiers, and other aerobic endurance athletes who risk depleting glycogen stores, and it may conceivably benefit other athletes as well (105).

A commonly used carbohydrate loading regimen includes three days of a high-carbohydrate diet in concert with tapering exercise the week before competition and complete rest the day before the event. The diet should provide adequate calories and carbohydrate per day: 8 to 10 g of carbohydrate per kilogram body weight. This regimen should increase muscle glycogen stores 20% to 40% above normal (25). However, higher intakes, 10 to 12 g of carbohydrate per kilogram body weight, have been suggested for runners during the 36 to 48 hours before a marathon (19).

Studies show that carbohydrate loading is effective in men (123, 139). However, the studies in women have been mixed. One study examined the effects of carbohydrate loading on aerobic endurance performance and substrate utilization in eight 20- to 40-year-old weight-stable, eumenorrheic female runners with an average running history of 53 km (24 miles) per week for at least 12 months before the study and a typical carbohydrate intake below 65% of total caloric intake (7). Each female completed three different 24.2 km (15-mile) self-paced treadmill performance runs after four days on each experimental diet regimen: (1) carbohydrate supplementation (50% of calories from carbohydrate), (2) carbohydrate loading and supplementation (75% of calories from carbohydrate), and (3) placebo (50% of calories from carbohydrate). Both the carbohydrate-supplemented and carbohydrate loading plus supplementation groups consumed a 6% carbohydrate-electrolyte solution before exercise (6 ml/kg) and every 20 minutes during exercise (3 ml/kg). And though the carbohydrate-supplemented and carbohydrate loading plus supplementation groups used a greater portion of energy from carbohydrate during their runs, there was no significant difference in running performance between the groups. However, both total calories and grams of carbohydrate per day were not reported; therefore, it is possible that total calorie or carbohydrate intakes (or both) were not adequate for the runners. In addition, given the small number of subjects included in this study, differences in performance may have been noted if more subjects had been included (7).

In another study, researchers found that males increased glycogen content significantly while female athletes did not after increasing carbohydrate intake from 58% to 74% of calories for four days before a submaximal aerobic endurance exercise test, due to either inadequate carbohydrate or calorie intake (or both) or sex differences in glycogen storage (123). In a follow-up study, the same researchers examined glycogen storage capacity in six well-trained men and six well-trained women (125). Subjects were randomly assigned to one of three diets for four days: a high-carbohydrate diet (75% of total calorie intake), a high-carbohydrate diet plus extra calories (75% of calories from carbohydrate and a 34% increase in total calories), or their habitual daily diet. In men, both the higher-carbohydrate diet and higher-carbohydrate plus extra calories diet led to significantly greater levels of glycogen than the habitual diet. However, in women, only the higher-carbohydrate plus extra calories diet resulted in significant increases in glycogen storage compared to the habitual diet. In the high-carbohydrate conditions, men increased their total carbohydrate intake to 7.9 g of carbohydrate per kilogram body weight whereas women reached just 6.4 g of carbohydrate per kilogram body weight. No differences were noted between men and women in their ability to use glycogen as measured by enzymatic activity. Therefore, the failure of previous studies to show improved performance from carbohydrate loading in women was likely due to inadequate overall carbohydrate intake (125). This theory (that women were not consuming enough total carbohydrate in many of the protocols) was backed up in a study examining female cyclists. In trained female cyclists, three or four days on a moderate-carbohydrate diet (48% of calories from carbohydrates) followed by three or four days consuming 78% of calories from carbohydrates (8.14 g of carbohydrate per kilogram body weight) led to significant increases in glycogen stores and greater cycling time to exhaustion compared to seven days on the moderate-carbohydrate diet (133). Researchers have found that glycogen storage capacity in the 4-hour time period after exercise did not differ between men and women when they consumed the same amount of carbohydrate per unit body weight (1 g of carbohydrate per kilogram body weight immediately and 1 hour after the completion of exercise) (122). And while glycogen storage capacity is greater during the luteal phase of the menstrual cycle in women as compared to the early follicular phase due to hormonal differences, carbohydrate loading can make up for this difference (94).

The main challenge with carbohydrate loading in females appears to be their overall daily calorie intake. Women who habitually consume less than 2,400 calories per day may find it difficult to consume greater amounts of carbohydrate. Therefore, female athletes may need to increase their total energy intake above 2,400 calories, in addition to consuming a higher-carbohydrate diet, in order to increase glycogen stores (123, 133).

Though the majority of studies on carbohydrate loading have been done in aerobic endurance athletes, some research has attempted to examine carbohydrate loading for athletes in high-intensity sports as well. In a randomized, crossover design, seven professional soccer players who consumed an average of 46% of calories from carbohydrates ate either a 39% or a 65% carbohydrate diet two days before being testing. Each test consisted of 6,856 m of field work (completed at 65%, 57%, and 81% $\dot{V}O_2$max) followed by a treadmill run to exhaustion in an attempt to mimic a soccer game. After the high-carbohydrate diet, the players ran 17.1 km total, which was 0.9 km longer (a significant difference) than the distance run while on the lower-carbohydrate diet. However, three of the athletes ran less than 420 m longer, indicating significant variability in the athletes' responses to a higher-carbohydrate regimen (11). The results of this study may or may not be applicable to soccer players, since the average distance covered in a soccer match is considerably shorter (10.3 km with a range of 9.7 to 11.3 km, as reported in one study), and it is covered in an intermittent manner and at varying levels of intensity (68).

In a study examining the effect of carbohydrate loading on resistance exercise performance, eight healthy young men were randomly assigned to either a higher-carbohydrate (6.5 g of carbohydrate per kilogram body weight) or a moderate-carbohydrate diet (4.4 g of carbohydrate per kilogram body weight) for four days. After this period, they participated in a resistance exercise test including four sets of 12 repetitions of maximal-effort jump squats with a load of 30% of 1-repetition maximum (1RM) and a 2-minute rest period between sets (44). There was no significant difference in power performance between subjects on the high-carbohydrate and the moderate-carbohydrate diets. Therefore, in this study a higher-carbohydrate diet did not enhance power performance during a four-set resistance exercise test. However, it is unclear whether the carbohydrate loading regimen could have affected power performance if more sets were performed or if the carbohydrate loading regimen more closely resembled that of an endurance athlete, providing 8-10 g carbohydrate per kilogram bodyweight (44).

The degree of benefit derived from carbohydrate loading varies among individuals, even among aerobic endurance athletes, and therefore athletes should determine the value of this regimen while weighing any negative side effects, such as temporary weight gain, in practice before competition. Athletes who use carbohydrate loading as a means to maximize glycogen storage should also know how different types of carbohydrates affect them. For instance, oligosaccharides, which are found in dry beans and peas, onions, and foods with added inulin or other oligosaccharides (such as some nutrition bars and shakes), are rapidly fermented by bacteria in the gut, which can lead to excessive intestinal

gas and bloating. Dietary fiber is found in vegetables, fruits, whole grains, dry beans and peas, nuts, and seeds (130). Table 10.2 provides a sample daily meal plan for a 68 kg (150-pound) athlete following research-based carbohydrate recommendations for aerobic endurance athletes.

> ▶ **Carbohydrate loading is an effective strategy to maximize glycogen storage. However, athletes must consume 8 to 10 g of carbohydrate per kilogram body weight per day during the loading period to notice any benefit from carbohydrate loading.**

During-Event Nutrition

Nutrition is an important factor during aerobic endurance events lasting greater than 45 minutes, intermittent-activity sports, or when an athlete has multiple events in one day. Fluids and carbohydrates can affect performance, while the provision of amino acids may minimize muscle damage.

Proper hydration during competition is essential for performance while also helping to prevent overheating, dehydration, and heat illness. Athletes should hydrate themselves several hours before exercise to allow for fluid absorption and urine output before competing. In addition, they should consume enough fluid during exercise to prevent water weight losses exceeding 2% of body weight (112). The optimal sports drink contains 20 to 30 mEq of sodium (460-690 mg with chloride as the anion) per liter, 2 to 5 mEq of potassium (78-195 mg) per liter, and carbohydrate in a concentration of 5% to 10% (53). Sports drinks with a higher concentration of carbohydrate—those that contain more than 8%—delay gastric emptying (how quickly the drink is emptied from the stomach), which could lead to stomach discomfort (82). Therefore a carbohydrate concentration of 6% to 8% may be ideal (112).

Fluid intake guidelines are different for children. According to the American Academy of Pediatrics, children weighing 40 kg (88 pounds) should drink 5 ounces (148 ml) of cold water or a flavored salted beverage every 20 minutes during practice, while adolescents weighing 60 kg (132 pounds) should drink 9 ounces (256 ml) every 20 minutes even if they do not feel thirsty. They also recommend a sodium chloride concentration of 15 to 20 mmol/L (1 g per 2 pints), which has been shown to increase voluntary hydration by 90% when compared to unflavored water (4, 13, 138). Despite these recommendations, keep in mind that 9 ounces of fluid at one time is a considerable amount for an adolescent and may cause stomach distress. Therefore these guidelines may need to be adjusted for individual athletes.

TABLE 10.2 Carbohydrate Loading Regimens and Sample Daily Meal Plans for Aerobic Endurance Athletes*

Amount of carbohydrate	Sample meal plan for a 68 kg (150 lb) athlete	Nutrition breakdown

8-10 g carbohydrate per kilogram body weight consumed on day 3 before an event (25)	**Breakfast:**
	3 eggs
	4 slices 15-grain toast
	1 cup mixed chopped fruit
	1 170 g fruit-on-the-bottom yogurt
	Snack:
	40 mini pretzels
	Lunch:
	Chicken stir fry including
	  2 cups brown rice
	  6 oz. cooked chicken breast
	  1 cup mixed stir fry vegetables cooked in 2 Tbsp sesame oil
	Early afternoon snack:
	1 bagel with 2 Tbsp 100% fruit jam
	Post taper run:
	8 oz. 100% juice
	2 cups whole-grain cereal
	8 oz. skim milk
	Dinner:
	3 cups pasta
	1 cup pasta sauce
	Green salad with a variety of colorful vegetables and 2 oz. cheese
	1 Tbsp salad dressing
		91 g fat
		576 g carbohydrate
		141 g protein
		8.5 g carbohydrate per kilogram body weight

10-12 g carbohydrate per kilogram body weight consumed on each of the two days before an event (19)	**Breakfast:** 3 eggs 4 slices 15-grain toast 1 cup mixed chopped fruit 1 170 g fruit-on-the-bottom yogurt **Snack:** 40 mini pretzels 1 glass 100% juice **Lunch:** Chicken stir fry including 2 cups brown rice 4 oz. cooked chicken breast 1 cup mixed stir fry vegetables all cooked in 2 Tbsp sesame oil **Early afternoon snack:** 1 bagel with 2 Tbsp 100% fruit jam **Post taper run:** 8 oz. 100% juice 2 cups whole-grain cereal 1/3 cup packed raisins added 8 oz. skim milk **Dinner:** 3 cups pasta 1 cup pasta sauce Green salad with a variety of colorful vegetables and 2 oz. cheese 1 Tbsp salad dressing	91 g fat 689 g carbohydrate 128 g protein 10.1 g carbohydrate per kilogram body weight

*These recommendations are for aerobic endurance athletes and can be adapted for other types of athletes.

Aerobic Endurance Sports

Consuming carbohydrates during prolonged aerobic endurance exercise can improve performance while also reducing exercise-induced stress and suppression of immune system functioning (90). And though sports drinks provide carbohydrates, they cannot keep up with an athlete's carbohydrate utilization during prolonged, intense activity (unless an excessive amount of fluid is consumed). In fact, athletes who train intensely may burn 600 to 1,200 calories or more per hour (66). Several studies show that a carbohydrate intake ranging from 28 to 144 g per hour (with higher amounts studied during cycling) during aerobic endurance activity can decrease reliance on limited glycogen stores, extend time to exhaustion, and improve performance by providing a steady stream of carbohydrate that can be used for energy (26, 62, 85, 128).

Despite greater intakes per hour, as noted earlier, exogenous (external; that which is consumed) carbohydrate oxidation rates do not exceed 1.0 to 1.1 g per minute, likely due to the rate of glucose absorption and possibly also the limited delivery rate of 1 g per minute of glucose into the bloodstream (61). However, each carbohydrate has a different rate of oxidation. Glucose, sucrose, maltose, maltodextrins, and amylopectin are oxidized quickly; the oxidation rates of fructose, galactose, and amylose are 25% to 50% slower (61). In addition, each type of carbohydrate has a different intestinal transport system. If an athlete consumes one type of carbohydrate, fructose for instance, carbohydrate digestion will be limited when the intestinal transporter for fructose becomes saturated. Therefore, consuming multiple types of carbohydrates together, such as sucrose, fructose, and glucose or maltodextrin, increases the rate of carbohydrate absorption and exogenous carbohydrate oxidation compared to consuming an **isocaloric** amount of just one sugar (58). In addition to improving the rate of carbohydrate utilization by the body, consuming multiple types of carbohydrate during exercise was found to improve cycling time-trial performance after 120 minutes of cycling (the study design simulated the last few stages of an aerobic endurance race when an athlete must provide maximum effort) when subjects were provided glucose combined with fructose versus glucose only at a rate of 1.8 g per minute (108 g of carbohydrate per hour) (28). In addition, athletes given 36 g of glucose and fructose every 15 minutes had a better 100 km cycling time than cyclists given only glucose every 15 minutes (128).

In addition to actually ingesting carbohydrates, simply rinsing carbohydrates through the mouth (without actually ingesting them) seems to improve performance lasting approximately 1 hour by 2% to 3%, presumably by affecting the central nervous system (60).

In addition to providing carbohydrates during aerobic endurance activity, adding protein to a carbohydrate gel led to increased time until exhaustion during a bout of cycling while also attenuating the rise in creatine kinase (a marker of muscle damage) during cycling, due either to the protein itself or to the additional calories provided by the protein (111). A meta-analysis and review of the research examining how the addition of protein to carbohydrate affects aerobic endurance performance revealed mixed findings (111). Only time-to-exhaustion studies showed that the addition of protein made a significant difference. However, these studies were not controlled for calorie intake during the trial; therefore, it is unclear if any benefit was due to protein or the added calories provided by the protein. The three time-trial studies showed no difference between carbohydrate only and carbohydrate plus protein (120).

Intermittent High-Intensity Sports

Many team sports, such as soccer, tennis, basketball, and American football, include repeated bouts of short-duration, high-intensity activity in addition to involving a wide range of skills. Fatigue during play could stem from a number of factors, including decreased or depleted glycogen stores and dehydration. The provision of both fluids and carbohydrate is essential for performance during prolonged intermittent sports. For instance, a long tennis match may last 4 hours—considerably longer than many aerobic endurance events. Because tennis players cannot drink continuously during a match and can lose

---

Fructose and Gastrointestinal Symptoms

Fructose, a sugar found naturally in fruit and also added to a number of foods and beverages, including many sports nutrition products, is often blamed for symptoms of stomach upset during exercise. Though some people do not completely absorb fructose and may therefore experience bloating, gas, abdominal discomfort, and alterations in bowel functioning after consuming this sugar (116), studies have not examined gastrointestinal symptoms related to fructose ingestion alone in athletes. Thus athletes need to test, in practice, whether changing their sports drinks or other products they consume during training (and testing fructose-free conditions) helps alleviate any gastrointestinal symptoms they may be having (119). Athletes with irritable bowel syndrome are more likely to have a problem absorbing fructose and therefore experience side effects (116).

more than 2.5 L of fluid per hour, a recommendation of 200 to 400 ml (6.8-13.5 ounces) per changeover (switching sides) has been put forth for these athletes (65). In addition to maintaining hydration status, research shows that carbohydrate supplementation may not affect ratings of perceived exertion (38) but improves stroke quality (which includes measures of velocity, precision, and error rate) during prolonged play (132).

In soccer players, 5 ml per kilogram body weight of a 6.9% glucose-polymer drink, consumed 15 minutes before each match and at halftime, made no difference in several measures of performance such as successful tackles, heading, dribbling, or shooting ability (142). Yet another soccer study, this one with professional soccer players, found that the group consuming a carbohydrate-electrolyte beverage improved some parameters of performance during match play. In this study, 22 professional male soccer players consumed the same diet for seven days (55% of the calories were derived from carbohydrate, 25% from fat, and 20% from protein), refrained from exercise for three days before the match, and consumed a standardized breakfast 4 hours before the match on game day. They were divided into two groups, receiving either (a) a carbohydrate-electrolyte drink (7% carbohydrates, sodium 24 mmol/L, chloride 12 mmol/L, potassium 3 mmol/L) or (b) placebo. Each group drank 5 ml (0.17 ounces) per kilogram body weight before the match and 2 ml (0.7 ounces) per kilogram body weight every 15 minutes during the 90-minute game. The group receiving the carbohydrate-electrolyte drink finished the specific dribble test faster than those receiving the placebo. In addition, ratings of precision were higher in the carbohydrate-electrolyte trial versus placebo. However, there were no differences in the coordination or power tests between groups. In this particular study, supplementation with a carbohydrate-electrolyte drink

improved soccer-specific skill performance compared with a placebo (96).

In another study that found that during-play carbohydrate consumption was beneficial, a randomized, double-blind protocol was used. Seventeen male soccer players received 8 ml (0.27 ounces) of a 6.4% carbohydrate-electrolyte beverage per kilogram body weight before exercise plus 3 ml (0.10 ounces) per kilogram body weight after every 15 minutes (for a total of 52 g of carbohydrate per hour) during a 90-minute intermittent shuttle test (3). Consuming the carbohydrate-electrolyte beverage attenuated a significant decrease in skill reduction from before exercise until the last 15 to 30 minutes of exercise compared to placebo. In the carbohydrate trial, there was a 3% reduction in skill performance during this time period, while in the placebo trial a 15% decline in skill performance was noted. However, this trial was performed after carbohydrate-depleting exercise followed by a low-carbohydrate meal and then an overnight fast; therefore, the effect of carbohydrates on performance may depend not only on the amount consumed during intermittent activities but also on whether the athlete is competing in a fed or fasted and glycogen-depleted state (3).

In another study, which used four 15-minute quarters of intermittent high-intensity shuttles at various intensities (walking, jogging, running, sprinting, and jumping), separated by a 20-minute rest at halftime and followed by a shuttle run to fatigue (designed to mimic a competitive soccer or basketball game), subjects who consumed a carbohydrate-electrolyte (carbohydrate) drink before exercise (5 ml of a 6% solution per kilogram body weight) and at halftime (5 ml of a 18% solution per kilogram body weight) ran 37% longer in the run to fatigue than those receiving a placebo and were significantly faster in a 20 m sprint during the fourth

During-Competition Food and Fluid Recommendations

Due to large variations in sweat rates and electrolyte concentrations, athletes should measure weight changes during training and competition in specific weather conditions and develop individualized hydration strategies based on this information (112). During prolonged activity in hot weather, the Institute of Medicine recommends sports drinks containing 20 to 30 mEq of sodium (460-690 mg with chloride as the anion) per liter, 2 to 5 mEq of potassium (78-195 mg) per liter, and carbohydrate in a concentration of 5% to 10% (53).

- Children weighing 40 kg (88 pounds) should drink 5 ounces (148 ml) of cold water or a flavored salted beverage every 20 minutes during practice.
- Adolescents weighing 60 kg (132 pounds) should drink 9 ounces (256 ml) every 20 minutes even if they do not feel thirsty (4, 13).
- Aerobic endurance athletes should consume 28 to 144 g of multiple types of carbohydrates together, such as sucrose, fructose, and glucose, or maltodextrin, each hour during prolonged aerobic endurance activity (26, 28, 62, 85, 128).
- Tennis players should aim for approximately 200 to 400 ml fluid per changeover and have some of this fluid from a carbohydrate-electrolyte sports drink (65).

quarter. In addition, the carbohydrate-supplemented group performed better on a whole-body motor skill test during the later stages of exercise and reported decreased perceptions of fatigue, indicating that the consumption of a carbohydrate-electrolyte beverage during intermittent sports is advantageous (136).

Strength and Power Sports

Carbohydrates are also an essential source of energy used during resistance training and therefore in strength and power sports. Research studies using a series of different weightlifting protocols found that participants used a significant amount of muscle glycogen (74). Most of these studies had participants perform just a few sets of exercises. Therefore, athletes who perform in strength and power competitions or sports, or in positions that rely on muscle strength and power (hammer throwers, offensive linemen in American football), could deplete their muscle glycogen stores. Furthermore, starting with already low carbohydrate stores will increase muscle breakdown (72). Strength and power athletes can maintain their glycogen stores, which may decrease muscular fatigue in slow-twitch fibers and possibly lead to better performance, by supplementing with carbohydrate before and during competition (39, 54).

Postcompetition Nutrition

The postcompetition meal helps athletes rehydrate, replenish glycogen stores, and repair muscle tissue. Therefore, what they consume in the time period soon after training or competition helps prepare their body for the next bout of activity. Each athlete's postcompetition needs vary based on the sport he or she plays, intensity during play, amount of time played, the individual's weight and age, and probably the person's sex. However, much more research has been conducted with male subjects as opposed to females; therefore, recommendations are not broken out based on sex due to a lack of sufficient data in females.

After competition, athletes should replace fluid and electrolyte losses. If time permits, normal meals, snacks (provided they contain some sodium), and water will restore fluid and electrolyte losses. More salt can be added to foods when sweat sodium losses are substantial (51, 112). Athletes can choose a carbohydrate-electrolyte sports drink or plain water alongside foods that contain sodium chloride (or they can salt their foods) since sodium is essential for helping the body retain fluid (79, 112, 118). Rehydration strategies should be individualized as much as possible. Athletes competing in weight-class sports such as wrestling and mixed martial arts may deliberately dehydrate themselves to make weight and attempt to rehydrate before competition, though short time periods between weighing and competing may mean starting competition in a dehydrated state, leading to poor performance and health risks.

Aerobic Endurance Events

After prolonged aerobic endurance events, it is important to replenish carbohydrate stores before the next training session or competition (whichever comes first) and consume enough protein to build and repair muscle. Glycogen synthesis occurs in two distinct phases. The first phase is independent of insulin and lasts 30 to 60 minutes, and glycogen synthesis occurs rapidly. The second phase lasts several hours, and glycogen synthesis occurs at a much slower pace. Glycogen synthesis occurs at a rapid rate when large amounts of carbohydrate, 1.0 to 1.85 g per kilogram body weight per hour, are consumed immediately after exercise or competition and at regular intervals every 15 to 60 minutes thereafter for up to 5 hours (57). Though athletes may be able to fully replenish their glycogen stores right away or over the course of a 24-hour period after a long training session, this isn't necessarily the case after competition. Strenuous aerobic endurance events that result in measurable muscle damage, such as the marathon, lead to delayed glycogen resynthesis even if an athlete consumes a higher-carbohydrate diet, possibly due to either metabolic disturbance or mechanical damage to muscle cells (9, 117, 134).

Though athletes are often told that they need to eat carbohydrate immediately after they finish competing, research shows that this isn't always necessary; they may be able to wait 2 hours after finishing a glycogen-depleting event before eating carbohydrate. In a study examining the rate of glycogen resynthesis, five high-glycemic meals were given to athletes over the course of a 24-hour period after a 2-hour-long glycogen-depleting bout of cycling. One group received the first three meals over the 4-hour period after exercise, while the second group received the first three meals at regular 2-hour intervals starting 2 hours after they finished over the first 6 hours after exercise. The rate of glycogen resynthesis was the same between groups after 8 hours and after 24 hours (98). Therefore, athletes who have more than 24 hours to recover can likely wait before eating after exercise and replace their glycogen over the 24-hour time period after exercise as long as they consume an adequate amount of carbohydrate. However, athletes who train two or three times a day or have less than 24 hours to recover may want to consider eating or drinking a high-carbohydrate meal immediately after finishing their event and at regular intervals thereafter to quickly replenish glycogen stores.

Because prolonged aerobic endurance exercise breaks down muscle tissue, protein should be included in the aerobic endurance athlete's posttraining meal to help start muscle building and repair, which may attenuate posttraining and post-event muscle soreness (80). Consuming protein after training has another benefit: it increases the rate of glycogen storage if carbohydrate intake is inadequate (i.e., <1.2 g of carbohydrate per kilogram body weight per hour) (57). In a randomized, controlled trial, 18 elite orienteers participated in 13 exercise sessions during one week. Half of the orienteers (the PRO-CON group) ingested a protein drink before (0.3 g per kilogram body weight) and a protein-carbohydrate drink after (0.3 g protein per kilogram body weight + 1 g carbohydrate per kilogram body weight) training. The other half of participants consumed an isocaloric carbohydrate-only beverage before and after exercise (CHO). Diet was kept consistent throughout the study (15/63/22% protein/carbohydrate/fat) except for the addition of the supplements. The basic diet + supplements provided 3.0 g of protein per kilogram body weight/day and 8.3 to 9.3 g of carbohydrate per kilogram body weight/day in the PRO-CON group; the CHO group consumed 1.8 g of protein per kilogram body weight/day and 8.8 to 10.8 g carbohydrate per kilogram body weight/day. A 4 km run test was performed at the beginning and end of the study and 2 hours after participants consumed a standardized breakfast. PRO-CON significantly improved performance and reduced markers of muscle breakdown, while CHO did not improve performance. However, it isn't clear from this study if the timing of protein made the difference or the increased total daily intake of protein in the PRO-CON as compared to the CHO group (40).

Other research does suggest that protein is important after endurance exercise. For instance, a single-blind, randomized, triple-crossover design was used to assess how different doses of a protein–leucine blend affected myofibrillar protein fractional synthetic rate (FSR; muscle protein synthesis) in 12 endurance-trained men after 100 minutes of high-intensity cycling (performed 3 hours after a standardized breakfast; diet the day before the test was standardized based on calorie needs and provided the same percentage of carbohydrate, protein, and fat for each subject). Cyclists consumed 70/15/180/30 g protein/leucine/carbohydrate/fat, or 23/5/180/30 g, or 0/0/274/30 g (Control) in four servings during the first 90 minutes of a 240-minute (4-hour) recovery period. The lower-protein, lower-leucine supplement (23/5/180/30 g) increased FSR by 33% ± 12% compared to Control, while additional protein and leucine (70/15/180/30 g) increased FSR by 51% ± 12% compared to Control. Though no significant differences were noted between the two protein and leucine groups, both fared better than placebo, indicating that protein is important after a long, tough workout (110). Given different workouts, exercise completed in a fasted or unfasted state,

and different doses of protein (10-96 g) used in other studies, the precise minimum dose of protein needed to maximize FSR after endurance exercise isn't clear (18, 49). In addition, it isn't clear if maximizing FSR in the time period immediately after endurance exercise will translate to improved performance over time. And finally, the ideal time period after endurance training during which protein should be consumed is not clear and may depend on whether training was completed in a fasted or unfasted state as well as on total daily protein intake. However, one study found that delaying protein intake after endurance exercise by as little as 3 hours blunts its anabolic effects (73).

High-Intensity Intermittent Sports

Because athletes who participate in intermittent high-intensity sports—such as basketball, hockey, and soccer—may play more than one game per day, sometimes with just a few hours in between tournament games, immediate recovery after a game is imperative for performance in their next game. And when competing in sports that involve prolonged high-intensity intermittent activity, such as soccer, American football, field and ice hockey, rugby, and tennis, athletes may significantly reduce their muscle glycogen stores, leading to muscular fatigue (10, 55). Fully replacing muscle glycogen before a subsequent bout of exercise or competition may prolong time until fatigue and improve performance. In a study designed to mimic a soccer game, Nicholas and colleagues had six males complete the same exercise test separated by 22 hours on two consecutive days—75 minutes of a prolonged, intermittent, high-intensity shuttle run test after which they completed as many 20 m shuttles as possible (each shuttle alternated between jogging and sprinting). Subjects were assigned to one of two diets for the 22-hour recovery period: a recovery diet including 10 g of carbohydrate per kilogram body weight or an isocaloric diet with more protein and fat than their normal daily diet. Intermittent running capacity improved after the higher-carbohydrate diet as compared to the higher-calorie condition with more protein and fat (89). Also, Balsom and colleagues found that male study subjects performed significantly more work in both short-term (<10 minutes) and prolonged (>30 minutes) high-intensity intermittent exercise sessions after consuming a high- versus low-carbohydrate diet for the 48-hour period before the exercise sessions (10).

High-intensity intermittent sports can lead to some degree of muscle damage depending on many factors including the time and intensity of play and body size. Studies show that consuming protein postexercise helps decrease some markers of muscle damage (34). The ideal amount of protein an athlete should consume immediately after play in a game such as American football or soccer remains unclear at this time. And though postexercise carbohydrate intake can affect performance in a subsequent event or training session, particularly when sessions are close together in time, the addition of protein will not affect performance in a subsequent bout of exercise during the 4-hour recovery period following the initial event or exercise session (80).

Strength and Power Sports

Athletes in strength and power sports rely on both blood glucose and glycogen for energy during competition. Because a single bout of resistance training can lead to significant reductions in glycogen (74) and decreases in glycogen can impair force production and isometric strength while accentuating muscle weakness, it is imperative that these athletes restore glycogen levels before their next bout of exercise (39, 54). During the recovery period after strength and power competitions, athletes should focus on consuming higher-glycemic carbohydrates immediately postexercise if they must compete or train again over the course of the 24-hour period after the initial training session or competition. The amount of carbohydrate they need to fully replenish glycogen stores depends on many factors, including intensity and the time spent competing, their overall body weight and muscle mass, their preexercise meal (and state of glycogen stores before competition), and whether or not they consumed carbohydrate during the competition. In a crossover study, after an overnight fast, eight men who completed six sets of single-leg knee extensions at 70% of 1RM, until 50% of full knee extension was no longer possible, depleted glycogen levels to 71%. They replaced glycogen stores to 91% of preexercise levels by six hours after training after consuming 1.5 g of carbohydrate per kilogram body weight immediately after the resistance training session and again one hour later. However, when study subjects consumed water only immediately after training and again one hour later, they barely increased muscle glycogen content above depletion levels to 75% (99).

Net protein balance depends on both muscle protein synthesis and breakdown. And though carbohydrates have no effect on muscle protein synthesis, they help attenuate acute protein breakdown resulting from resistance exercise. The increase in protein breakdown likely depends on the resistance stimulus, the person's overall nutrition intake, and dietary intake before and during training or competition. One study in untrained young men found that acute protein breakdown increased by 51% ± 17% after a bout of resistance training (14). In another study, the rate of both mixed muscle protein fractional synthesis rate (muscle protein synthesis) and fractional breakdown rate (breakdown) were measured after a bout of either concentric or eccentric exercise in

four untrained men and four untrained women. The rate of synthesis increased significantly above resting levels by 112% in the 3-hour period after exercise, 65% over the 24-hour period after exercise, and 34% over the 48-hour period after exercise. Muscle breakdown also increased by 31% and 18% in the 3- and 24-hour periods after exercise yet returned to baseline by 48 hours after exercise (104). Relatively small amounts of carbohydrate, somewhere between 30 and 100 g, can sufficiently reduce muscle protein breakdown (16, 35). And though muscle protein breakdown has a role in overall protein balance, muscle protein synthesis plays a much bigger role in overall protein balance (35).

Supplementing with protein after a muscle-damaging bout of resistance training increases acute muscle protein synthesis. Varying amounts of protein have been used after resistance training to stimulate muscle protein synthesis, though maximal stimulation occurs with 20 to 25 g (providing about 8.5 to 10 g of essential amino acids) of a high-quality, high-leucine, fast protein (one that leads to a rapid rise in amino acids in the bloodstream) in younger individuals, while 40 g or more may be necessary in older adults (103). Rice is an intermediate-speed leucine-poor protein (though the rise in leucine in the bloodstream appears quickly after consumption of rice protein); larger doses of rice effectively stimulated muscle protein synthesis to the same extent as a higher-quality protein when matched for leucine content (63). Therefore the leucine content of the protein, and possibly the speed of leucine delivery, appears to be the determining factor for acute changes in maximal stimulation of muscle protein synthesis. A protein dose that contains 2 to 3 g of leucine or 0.05 g of leucine per kilogram body weight will maximally stimulate muscle protein synthesis in younger adults (91, 97, 127).

In addition to the acute increase in muscle protein synthesis, consistently supplementing with protein after resistance training led to small to moderate increases in muscle hypertrophy over time compared to conditions in which subjects were not given protein supplements (22, 115). Only one study to date has directly examined the relationship between acute measures of muscle protein synthesis and hypertrophy due to resistance training. In this study 23 young men who were recreationally active but had not participated in a resistance training exercise program in at least a year were tested for initial strength and resting and postexercise rates of muscle protein synthesis. Then they participated in a 16-week linear resistance training program consisting of two days of lower body (leg press, leg extension, leg curl, and calf press) and two days of upper body (chest press, shoulder press, seated row, lat pulldown, biceps curl, triceps extension) exercises performed first thing in the morning after an overnight fast. After exercise each day and at breakfast on nontraining days they consumed a nutrition drink containing 30 g of milk protein, 25.9 g of carbohydrate, and 3.4 g of fat. The study authors found no relationship between the acute rise (6 hours posttraining) in muscle protein synthesis due to exercise training and the nutrition drink provided and muscle hypertrophy. However, the authors also noted that changes in muscle protein synthesis with training were not uniform among study subjects; therefore, though acute changes in muscle protein synthesis are important for muscle hypertrophy, they are not the sole determining factor that predicts a person's potential to increase muscle growth (81). Thirty grams of milk protein, as used in this study, provides an estimated 24 g of casein, 6 g of whey protein, and a total of 2.8 g of leucine (129).

Concurrent Training

Exercise interference is a concept suggesting that endurance exercise, when combined with strength training (back-to-back sessions), blunts gains in strength compared to strength training alone but results in improvements in endurance performance (140). While interest in concurrent training-based research has increased recently, nutrition recommendations for concurrent training are often based on isolated studies examining the impact of nutrition interventions on endurance or resistance training alone. The consumption of carbohydrate after endurance exercise and prelift can help suppress skeletal muscle breakdown. Also, given the impact of protein intake after endurance exercise on muscle protein synthesis, as well as the research suggesting that protein intake during prolonged (>2 hours) resistance training supports greater rates of muscle protein synthesis during exercise compared to a carbohydrate control, athletes should consider consuming protein after endurance exercise and prelift or during their lifting session (101).

Protein at Mealtime

In addition to consuming protein right after working out, adults should also focus on their protein intake at each main meal, especially since resistance training can increase muscle sensitivity to amino acids for 24 to 48 hours after exercise whereas the anabolic effect of a meal lasts approximately 3-5 hours. For optimal muscle remodeling, experts suggest consuming at least 20 to 30 g of protein per meal and eating meals every 3 to 4 hours (77, 101).

The amount of data on muscle protein synthesis in children is limited because invasive measurement procedures are required (15), and no studies have examined muscle protein synthesis after training and postworkout protein ingestion in healthy children. However, one thing is clear with regard to children: They do not need to follow the same per-meal protein guidelines as adults because the drive for protein synthesis is regulated by insulin and calorie intake as opposed to leucine. Children can therefore consume protein in smaller amounts spread throughout their day to meet their protein needs (75). For more information about protein needs by sport, see table 10.3.

TABLE 10.3   Sport-Specific Protein Needs

Sport	Daily protein needs in grams per kilogram body weight	Sample daily intake for a 200 lb man or woman (grams of protein)	Postexercise protein needs	Postexercise protein examples
Low to moderate endurance activity (e.g., jogging, triathlon)	1.0-1.1	1 cup Greek yogurt (22 g) Grilled chicken sandwich (28 g) 1 higher-protein nutrition bar (20 g) Spaghetti with meatballs (4 oz. meatballs) (20 g)	0.2-0.5 g per kilogram body weight	1 higher-protein nutrition bar (20 g) 1 cup higher-protein Greek yogurt with 2 Tbsp. peanut butter mixed in 25 g whey protein
Elite endurance athlete or one who trains intensely	>1.6	1 cup Greek yogurt (22 g) Grilled chicken sandwich (28 g) 2 oz. cheese with whole-grain crackers (20 g) Spaghetti with meatballs (6 oz. meatballs) (30 g) 8 oz. glass of milk (8 g) 1/2 cup cottage cheese (15 g)	0.2-0.5 g per kilogram body weight	20 oz. milk or higher-protein soy milk (20 g)

(continued)

TABLE 10.3 *(continued)*

Sport	Daily protein needs in grams per kilogram body weight	Sample daily intake for a 200 lb man or woman (grams of protein)	Postexercise protein needs	Postexercise protein examples
American football	1.0-2.0, though likely at the upper end of this range for those playing at an intense level	2 g protein per kilogram body weight: 5 large egg whites or whole eggs, cooked with 1 oz. cheese (38 g) Grilled chicken sandwich (28 g) 1 glass of milk (or high-protein soy milk) (8 g) 2 Tbsp peanut butter mixed in 1/2 cup oatmeal (made with milk) (about 20 g) 6 oz. grilled salmon (48 g) 12 oz. glass of milk + 1 scoop whey protein (37 g)	Not clarified by research; therefore, players may want to follow the guidelines for resistance training and consume a minimum of 20-25 g of a fast, high-quality, leucine-rich (2-3 g leucine) protein	Whey protein shake + fruit Other examples (though not fast proteins): ≥1 cup higher-protein Greek yogurt Grilled cheese sandwich with turkey or chicken
Gymnastics	Dietary restriction increases protein needs (if they restrict calories); no studies conducted on gymnasts' protein needs		Not yet clarified by research	
Team sports	Likely 1.0-2.0 g per kilogram body weight, depending on the sport and intensity of exercise	2.0 g per kilogram body weight; follow the same sample daily meal plan as noted above for American football	Not clarified by research	
Weightlifting	1.5-2.0	2.0 g per kilogram body weight; follow the same sample daily meal plan as noted above for American football	20 g egg protein or 25 g whey protein pre- or postexercise or both; studies have used 20-70 g protein in close temporal proximity to resistance exercise, though a protein containing approximately 2-3 g leucine per serving of protein is recommended	Whey protein shake
Wrestling	Not known, though dietary restriction increases protein needs		No studies have been conducted that specifically outline protein needs for wrestling pre- or postexercise	

Nutrition for Aerobic Endurance Performance and Recovery

- Aerobic endurance athletes need to consume 8 to 10 g of carbohydrate and 1.0 to 1.6 g of protein per kilogram body weight per day, especially if training for 90 or more minutes.

- Athletes who eat at least 4 hours before competition should include approximately 1 to 4 g of carbohydrate per kilogram body weight and 0.15 to 0.25 g of protein per kilogram body weight (124). If the precompetition meal is consumed 2 hours before exercise, athletes should aim for approximately 1 g of carbohydrate per kilogram body weight (112).

- Athletes should consume 28 to 144 g of multiple types of carbohydrate (such as sucrose, fructose, and glucose or maltodextrin) per hour during prolonged aerobic endurance exercise to extend time until exhaustion and improve performance (26, 28, 62, 85, 128).

- During prolonged activity in hot weather, athletes should consume sports drinks containing 20 to 30 mEq of sodium (460-690 mg with chloride as the anion) per liter, 2 to 5 mEq of potassium (78-195 mg) per liter, and carbohydrate in a concentration of 5% to 10% (53).

- Postexercise, approximately 1.5 g of carbohydrate per kilogram body weight should be consumed within 30 minutes after stopping the exercise. Some, though not all, studies show that the addition of protein to carbohydrate postworkout may attenuate muscle breakdown and soreness and increase muscle protein synthesis. The ideal amount of protein and the time period after exercise in which it should be consumed are not clear based on the current body of literature and may depend on whether the exercise was performed in the fed versus fasted state and on total calories consumed postworkout (36, 49, 80). However, as a general guideline, at least 10 g of protein should also be consumed within a 3-hour time period after endurance exercise (sooner may be better, though the exact time period has yet to be elucidated in the research) (73).

- Glycogen stores should be replenished after exercise and before the next bout of training. A regular diet with sufficient carbohydrate intake can restore glycogen over the course of a 24-hour period. For faster glycogen synthesis, athletes should eat or drink a high-carbohydrate meal immediately after exercise and at regular intervals thereafter. This is especially important for athletes who train again less than 24 hours after their initial training session (57).

Nutrition for Strength

- Athletes should consider supplementing with carbohydrate before and during competition to maintain strength and minimize muscle breakdown (39, 54). In general, strength/speed athletes should consume 5 to 6 g of carbohydrate per kilogram body weight per day. As little as 30 g of carbohydrate after training may reduce muscle breakdown. The ideal time period for carbohydrate consumption postresistance training has yet to be fully clarified; however, consuming carbohydrate sooner (rather than waiting) may be more beneficial, particularly if training was carried out in a fasted state (35).

- Because low glycogen can impair muscle force, athletes should consume higher-glycemic carbohydrates immediately following weightlifting or strength and power competitions if they must compete or train again over the course of the 24-hour period after their initial competition. Otherwise, they can consume enough carbohydrate over the course of the day to restore glycogen levels before the next bout of training or competition (39, 54, 99).

- In general, strength/speed athletes should consume 1.4 to 1.7 g of protein per kilogram body weight per day, even if their sport or training includes an aerobic endurance component. After resistance training, younger individuals should consume at least 20 to 25 g (providing about 8.5 to 10 g of essential amino acids) of a high-quality, high-leucine protein (2-3 g), while older adults should consume 40 g or more to maximally stimulate muscle protein synthesis in the acute time period after training (103). If the exercise was performed in a fasted state (first thing in the morning or more than 3 hours after the last protein-rich meal), the protein should be consumed within 30 minutes after the end of the session; but if the exercise was performed in a fed state (preexercise protein-rich meal or supplement), this postexercise time window may be considerably longer (8).

- Between 30 and 100 g of high-glycemic carbohydrates should be consumed after muscle-damaging exercise to reduce muscle protein breakdown (16, 35).

- Adult athletes should eat meals containing at least 20 to 30 g of a higher-leucine protein.

(continued)

(continued)

Nutrition for Hypertrophy

- Between 30 and 100 g of high-glycemic carbohydrates should be consumed after muscle-damaging exercise to reduce muscle protein breakdown (16, 35).
- After resistance training, younger individuals should consume at least 20 to 25 g (providing about 8.5 to 10 g of essential amino acids) of a high-quality, high-leucine protein (2-3 g), while older adults should consume 40 g or more to maximally stimulate muscle protein synthesis in the acute time period after training (103).
- Adult athletes should eat meals containing at least 20 to 30 g of a higher-leucine protein every 3 to 4 hours.

Nutrition for Muscular Endurance

- Maintain adequate hydration by preventing water weight losses exceeding 2% of body weight.
- During prolonged training or competition, consider a carbohydrate-electrolyte beverage to delay fatigue and improve performance, particularly if performing after an overnight fast (136) (3).
- Fully replace glycogen stores before the next training session or competition.
- Consume protein after training or games to minimize muscle damage and soreness (34).

Nutrition Strategies for Altering Body Composition

Athletes who want to alter their body composition typically need to gain muscle, lose body fat, or both. Although there are some scenarios (typically in those with eating disorders) in which an athlete may need to gain both muscle and fat, this section focuses on gaining muscle and losing body fat.

The first step toward altering body composition involves estimating calorie needs (though *calorie* is the common term, the technical term is *kilocalorie*). The number of calories an athlete needs each day depends on a number of factors including genetics, body weight, body composition, training program, and age. Children and adolescents also need calories for growth and development.

Basal metabolic rate (BMR) is by far the largest contributor to total energy expenditure, accounting for approximately 65% to 70% of daily energy expenditure (59, 107). It is a measure of the calories required for maintaining normal body functions such as respiration, blood circulation, and gastrointestinal and renal processing. *Basal metabolic rate* and *resting metabolic rate* (RMR) are often used interchangeably, though they are slightly different. Basal metabolic rate is measured after an overnight fast (12 to 14 hours without food) with the subject resting supine and motionless but awake (32, 52). Resting metabolic rate is often used instead of BMR due to the ease of measurement (an overnight fast is not required), yet it is 10% to 20% higher than BMR due to increased energy expenditure resulting from recent food intake or physical activity completed earlier in the day. Several factors influence BMR and RMR, particularly

fat-free mass, which explains approximately 70% to 80% of the difference in RMR among individuals (52, 88, 108). Other factors include age, nutrition status, genetics, and differences in endocrine functioning (such as hypo- or hyperthyroidism).

The second-largest component of an individual's energy requirement is the energy expended in physical activity. Of all the components, it is the most variable among individuals. The number of calories expended through physical activity increases with the frequency, intensity, and duration of the training program, as well as nontraining daily activity (washing a car, doing housework, and so on). Typically, 20% to 30% of total daily energy expenditure is from physical activity, though this figure may be considerably higher in athletes (59, 107). The highest energy costs are seen in aerobic activities performed by large athletes for long periods of time, whereas lowest energy costs are associated with skill and power sports performed by smaller athletes.

The thermic effect of food, also known as **diet-induced thermogenesis**, is the increase in energy expenditure above the RMR that can be measured for several hours following a meal. The thermic effect of food includes the energy cost of digestion, absorption, metabolism, and storage of food in the body. The thermic effect of food accounts for approximately 10% to 15% of total calories burned each day (59, 107).

Many different equations can be used to calculate calorie needs, including the Cunningham equation and Harris-Benedict equation, which are prediction equations. Harris-Benedict takes sex, body weight, height, and age into account to predict RMR. Resting metabolic rate can then be multiplied by an activity factor from 1.2 (sedentary) to 1.9 (heavy physical activity) to predict energy requirements (42). However, the Harris-Benedict does not take into account how muscle mass affects RMR (83). The Cunningham equation takes the same variables into account as Harris-Benedict but also includes fat-free mass, making it more applicable to athletes (126).

$$RMR = 500 + 22(LBM \text{ in kg})$$

After using the Cunningham equation to estimate RMR based on lean body mass (LBM), an activity factor can be used to estimate total daily energy expenditure. Instead of using a basic activity factor, the strength and conditioning coach may choose to use metabolic equivalents (MET values)—an estimate of caloric expenditure during activity. One MET is the energy equivalent of sitting quietly; therefore, the greater the intensity of exercise, the higher the MET value (2).

Another, more laborious method that can be used by very motivated athletes is to record dietary intake for a minimum of three consecutive, representative days during a period of stable body weight. The individual's daily energy requirement is assumed to equal the average number of calories consumed each day. The pitfall of this method is that recording food intake usually alters normal eating habits and people do not always accurately record their food intake (47, 114). Finally, a very simple method for quickly assessing calorie needs is presented in table 10.4.

Weight Gain

An athlete's ability to gain weight depends on numerous factors; the ones that can be controlled include diet and training. The off-season should be used as a time to make dietary changes that focus on weight gain since athletes do not have the pressures of competition on their mind.

If athletes increase their calorie intake dramatically and consistently, they could gain more fat than they would like. A general guideline, which should be adjusted based on the athlete, is to consume approximately 500 additional calories per day in order to gain weight (106). Eating larger portion sizes, increasing meal frequency, and focusing on choosing calorie-dense foods are all strategies that can help an athlete gain weight. In addition to increasing total calorie intake, athletes should ensure that they are eating enough protein to maximize gains in lean body mass: 1.5 to 2.0 g per kilogram body weight per day. Increasing an athlete's protein intake may make weight gain tough, given the profound effect that protein has on satiety, as well as the increased thermic effect of feeding associated with higher-protein diets. However, overfeeding protein is advantageous if the athlete can sustain the diet. In a randomized, controlled overfeeding study, 16 healthy adults lived in a metabolic ward for eight weeks and were overfed a diet containing low (5% of total calories), normal (15% of total calories), or high (25% of total calories) protein. The subjects who consumed the normal- and high-protein diet stored approximately 45% of the excess calories as lean body mass, whereas those on the low-protein diet stored 95% of the excess calories consumed as body fat (31). In addition to making dietary changes, athletes who want to gain weight should consider supplementing with creatine monohydrate, a supplement that safely and effectively increases lean body weight (69).

Finally, though athletes may know their energy and protein needs, putting this knowledge into practice can be perplexing. Therefore, regular nutrition counseling (or coaching) by a sports dietitian or sports nutritionist with an advanced degree is a recommended strategy for facilitating greater weight gain. A study in 21 elite athletes with heavy training loads, who were randomized to receive nutrition counseling or to eat ad libitum, showed that over the course of the 8- to 12-week weight gain period, the group receiving dietary counseling had greater total and lean body mass gains during the intervention and after 12 months; this means that the group receiving nutrition counseling continued to benefit from the nutrition guidance for several months after counseling ended (33).

TABLE 10.4   Estimated Daily Calorie Needs of Male and Female Athletes by Activity Level

Activity level	Male		Female	
	kcal/lb	kcal/kg	kcal/lb	kcal/kg
Light	17	38	16	35
Moderate	19	41	17	37
Heavy	23	50	20	44

Light activity level: Walking on a level surface at 2.5 to 3.0 miles per hour (4.0 to 4.8 km/h), garage work, electrical trades, carpentry, restaurant trades, housecleaning, child care, golf, sailing, table tennis.

Moderate activity level: Walking 3.5 to 4.0 miles per hour (5.6 to 6.4 km/h), weeding and hoeing, cycling, skiing, tennis, dancing.

Heavy activity level: Walking with load uphill, heavy manual digging, basketball, climbing, American football, soccer.

Weight (Fat) Loss

Athletes participating in a variety of sports may need to lose body fat to improve aspects of performance such as speed or endurance. Plus, regulating body weight may give certain athletes a mental advantage going into competition (102). In addition, maintaining or making weight is a recurring aspect of sports that include weight classes, weight limitations, or judging based on appearance such as weightlifting, wrestling, boxing, lightweight crew, and gymnastics.

Despite diet books on the bestseller lists, there is no ideal diet that works for everyone. Instead, studies show that a variety of types of diets, including low-carbohydrate and low-fat diets, result in weight loss as long as the people following them are consuming fewer calories than needed to maintain weight. In addition, there appears to be no difference between the amount of weight loss on a low-carbohydrate as compared to a low-fat (and therefore higher-carbohydrate) diet (17, 30). Total calorie intake and dietary adherence, the ability to stick with a diet over time, are the two most important factors that predict successful weight loss. However, a good portion of weight loss during dieting may come from muscle (135). And because muscle protein synthesis is an energy-expensive process, during times of dieting, caloric restriction may decrease muscle protein synthesis. Athletes who want to maintain muscle and lose body fat while dieting should consume about 1.8

> There is no one ideal diet. Instead, athletes need to choose a dietary approach based on whether it is safe for them, contains enough protein to meet their needs, and fits their lifestyle so that they can easily adhere to it.

to 2.7 g protein per kilogram body weight per day (or approximately 2.3-3.1 g protein per kilogram fat-free mass per day) in addition to maintaining a moderate energy deficit of approximately 500 calories/day (84).

In order to be sustainable in the long term, diets should be individualized, be easy to adhere to, and take into account lifestyle habits, medical history (including diabetes, insulin resistance, other diseases and medical concerns), diet history, and food preferences while providing all of the nutrients an athlete needs to train and perform optimally. And finally, research shows that ongoing behavior therapy and support can improve long-lasting results (76).

Overweight and Obesity

Overweight and **obesity**, defined as a **body mass index (BMI)** of 25 to 29.9 kg/m^2 and $\geq$30 kg/m^2, respectively, increase a person's risk of morbidity from hypertension; dyslipidemia; coronary heart disease; gallbladder disease; stroke; type 2 diabetes; sleep apnea; osteoarthritis; respiratory problems; and endometrial, breast, prostate, and colon cancers (86). Obesity is categorized as a disease and affects 34.9% of adults and 17% of children in the United States (92).

The causes of obesity are complex and include an interaction of genes and environment, involving social, behavioral, cultural, metabolic, physiological, and genetic factors. However, many treatment options are effective, including dietary therapy, altering physical activity patterns, behavior therapy techniques, pharmacotherapy, and surgery. Some patients and clinicians employ a combination of these treatments. The initial goal for weight loss in overweight and obese individuals should be 10% of initial weight within six months (86).

Low-Carbohydrate Diets

The popularity and effectiveness of low-carbohydrate diets may have less to do with cutting carbohydrates (in healthy individuals) and more to do with a temporary decrease in water weight, cutting calories, and increasing protein intake. When people significantly reduce their carbohydrate intake, they deplete their glycogen stores (carbohydrate stored with three to four parts water) and therefore quickly drop pounds from water weight. Once carbohydrates are reintroduced into the diet, they can rapidly gain the weight back (67).

Over time, however, low-carbohydrate diets may work for some people because of increased levels of protein. Protein increases feelings of fullness (satiety) in a dose-dependent manner—the more protein consumed at one sitting, the greater its effect on satiety. However, at this time the "optimal dose" for maximum satiety remains unclear. Protein also increases the thermic effect of feeding. More calories are burned during digesting and processing protein than carbohydrate or fat. And finally, protein helps spare metabolically active lean muscle tissue during weight loss. This is important because muscle burns a few more calories at rest than fat does, and over time this can affect body weight. Plus, more muscle may mean that a person can train harder and therefore burn more calories during training (84).

Though cutting carbohydrates may be detrimental for a number of competitive athletes, particularly during precompetition and competition phases, it is a very effective approach for someone with insulin resistance (a condition that leads to the buildup of glucose in the blood because the body doesn't use insulin effectively), as well as type 2 diabetes. It may also be a very effective approach for overweight and obese individuals (43, 46, 141).

Body mass index is considered a measure of body fat calculated from height and weight. Body mass index is often used to assess risk for diseases associated with more body fat; however, in reality, it is a measure of excess weight as opposed to excess body fat (86) because BMI cannot distinguish between excess fat and muscle or bone mass (21). Lastly, age, sex, ethnicity, and muscle mass affect the association between BMI and body fat. Therefore, BMI can overestimate body fat in athletes and others with muscular builds and underestimate body fat in older persons or those who have lost muscle (86). The same factors that affect the relationship between BMI and body fat in adults are applicable to children. In addition, height and sexual maturation influence a child's BMI. The same calculation is used for children, but BMI interpretations for children take into account age and sex.

Body mass index should not be used as a diagnostic tool but instead as an initial screening tool to identify potential weight issues in individuals and to track population-based rates of overweight and obesity. In addition, no single body fat measure should be used to assess health, disease, or disease risk (21). Overweight and obesity combined with other risk factors, including high blood pressure, high low-density lipoprotein cho-

lesterol, low high-density lipoprotein cholesterol, high triglycerides, high blood glucose, physical inactivity, family history of premature heart disease, or cigarette smoking, increase a person's risk for heart disease (86).

> **Body mass index should not be used as a diagnostic tool but instead as an initial screening tool to identify potential weight issues in individuals and to track population-based rates of overweight and obesity.**

Waist circumference is another measure commonly used to assess disease risk. Men have an increased relative risk for disease if they have a waist circumference greater than 40 inches (102 cm), while women have an increased relative risk if they have a waist circumference greater than 35 inches (88 cm) (86).

Table 10.5 describes the various classifications of overweight and obesity. For reference, table 10.6 provides the weights and heights that correspond to BMIs of 25, 27, and 30. Table 10.7 lists BMI categories for corresponding percentile rankings for children. For more information about the screening process and risk assessment, refer to Clinical Guidelines on the Identification, Evaluation, and Treatment of Overweight and Obesity in

---

Calculating BMI

To estimate BMI using kilograms and meters, use this equation:

$$\text{Weight (kilograms) / Height (meters)}^2$$

To estimate BMI using pounds and inches, use this equation:

$$[\text{Weight (pounds) / Height (inches)}^2] \times 703$$

Overweight is defined as a BMI of 25 to 29.9 kg/m² and obesity as a BMI of 30 kg/m² or more.

TABLE 10.5   Classification of Adult Weight by Body Mass Index (BMI) and Associated Disease Risk (86)

Classification	Obesity class	*BMI (kg/m²)	Disease risk** relative to normal weight and waist circumference	
			Men <102 cm (<40 in.) Women <88 cm (<35 in.)	Men >102 cm (>40 in.) Women >88 cm (>35 in.)
Underweight		<18.5		
Normal		18.5-24.9		
Overweight		25.0-29.9	Increased	High
Obesity	I	30.0-34.9	High	Very high
	II	35.0-39.9	Very high	Very high
Extreme obesity	III	≥40	Extremely high	Extremely high

Increased waist circumference can also be a marker for increased risk even in persons of normal weight.

*BMI may overestimate fat in athletes and others with muscular builds and underestimate fat in older persons and others who have lost muscle.

**Disease risk for type 2 diabetes, hypertension, and cardiovascular disease.

Reprinted, by permission, from National Heart, Lung, and Blood Institute, 1998 (86).

Adults on the National Heart, Lung, and Blood Institute's website. Strength and conditioning professionals should use other, more accurate measures of body composition such as skinfolds or dual-energy X-ray absorptiometry (DEXA) in athletes with more muscle than their age- and

TABLE 10.6   Selected BMI Units Categorized by Height and Weight

Height in inches (cm)	Body weight in pounds (kg)		
	BMI = 25	BMI = 27	BMI = 30
58 (147.32)	119 (53.98)	129 (58.51)	143 (64.86)
59 (149.86)	124 (56.25)	133 (60.33)	148 (67.13)
60 (152.40)	128 (58.06)	138 (62.60)	153 (69.40)
61 (154.94)	132 (59.87)	143 (64.86)	158 (71.67)
62 (157.48)	136 (61.69)	147 (66.68)	164 (74.39)
63 (160.02)	141 (63.96)	152 (68.95)	169 (76.66)
64 (162.56)	145 (65.77)	157 (71.21)	174 (78.93)
65 (165.10)	150 (68.04)	162 (73.48)	180 (81.65)
66 (167.64)	155 (70.31)	167 (75.75)	186 (84.37)
67 (170.18)	159 (72.12)	172 (78.02)	191 (86.64)
68 (172.72)	164 (74.39)	177 (80.29)	197 (89.36)
69 (175.26)	169 (76.66)	182 (82.56)	203 (92.08)
70 (177.80)	174 (78.93)	188 (85.28)	207 (93.89)
71 (180.34)	179 (81.19)	193 (87.54)	215 (97.52)
72 (182.88)	184 (83.46)	199 (90.27)	221 (100.25)
73 (185.42)	189 (85.73)	204 (92.53)	227 (102.97)
74 (187.96)	194 (88.00)	210 (95.26)	233 (105.69)
75 (190.50)	200 (90.72)	216 (97.98)	240 (108.86)
76 (193.04)	205 (92.99)	221 (100.25)	246 (111.58)

BMI = body mass index.

Metric conversion formula: weight/height^2 (kg/m^2).

Example of BMI calculation: A person who weighs 78.93 kg and is 177 cm tall has a BMI of 25: weight/height^2 = 78.93 kg/(1.77 m)^2 = 25.

Reprinted, by permission, from National Heart, Lung, and Blood Institute, 1998 (86).

sex-matched counterparts since BMI is more likely to overestimate overweight and obesity (70).

Although all obese individuals share the trait of excess body fat, they cannot be treated homogeneously. They must be screened for coexisting illnesses such as diabetes, orthopedic problems, cardiac disease, psychological disorders such as **binge-eating disorder** or depression, social and cultural influences, and readiness for change. Obese athletes who are mandated to lose weight (e.g., by a physician) pose a special challenge because losing weight is dictated by an external source and is not an internalized goal. Weight loss takes a great deal of dedication from within the individual, and these athletes may need to work closely with a mental health professional or registered dietitian to help them meet their goal.

Rapid Weight Loss

Though there is no uniform definition in the literature, *rapid weight loss* generally refers to quick weight loss, faster than can be achieved by lowering calorie intake and increasing exercise, in a short period of time (29). Athletes may use any variety of techniques to cut weight quickly in order to compete in a desired weight class, meet a weight goal set by their coach, or improve performance. Potentially dangerous weight loss techniques may include fasting, fad diets, **voluntary dehydration** (diuretics, sauna, water and salt manipulation, wearing multiple layers of clothing), excessive spitting, self-induced vomiting, laxative abuse, and inappropriate or excessive use of thermogenic aids (29).

Athletes who attempt to lose too much weight too quickly may lose lean body mass, feel fatigued, experience headaches or mood swings, put their training and performance in jeopardy, and suffer from several potentially serious side effects. These include dehydration, heat illness, muscle cramping, fatigue, dizziness, suppressed immune system functioning, hormone imbalances, hyperthermia, reduced muscle strength, decreased plasma and blood volume, low blood pressure, electrolyte imbalances, kidney failure (diuretic abuse), fainting, and death (extreme cases) (29).

The strength and conditioning professional should be able to recognize the signs and symptoms associated

TABLE 10.7   BMI-for-Age Categories and Corresponding Percentiles for Children

Percentile ranking	Weight status
Less than 5th percentile	Underweight
5th percentile to less than 85th percentile	Healthy weight
85th percentile to less than 95th percentile	Overweight
Equal to or greater than the 95th percentile	Obese

Reprinted from Centers for Disease Control.

with rapid weight loss techniques and refer athletes to the appropriate professional while also communicating concerns to the rest of the coaching staff. In addition, the strength and conditioning professional may want to consider documenting the steps he or she has taken to assist the athlete (for good record keeping and to prevent liability) while also working with a medical doctor or registered dietitian to set appropriate weight goals after body composition, dieting, medical, and eating disorder history have been taken into account. Some athletes may need to reconsider which weight class they are competing in if they cannot make weight without putting their health or performance in jeopardy.

Feeding and Eating Disorders

Eating disorders, including binge-eating disorder, **anorexia nervosa**, and **bulimia nervosa**, are serious mental health disorders that can affect both men and women, appear at any point in life, and increase risk of mortality. Those with eating disorders have a high prevalence of other psychiatric disorders, including anxiety disorders, mood disorders such as depression, impulse-control disorders, and substance abuse disorders (41, 50).

Studies show an increased prevalence of both disordered eating and eating disorders in athletes compared to controls (37, 121, 143). In particular, athletes in sports with weight classes such as wrestling, those in sports that emphasize leanness such as cross-country running, and aesthetic sports such as gymnastics may be more prone to disordered eating and eating disorders (37, 121, 143). Signs of disordered eating may include restrictive eating, fasting, skipping meals, and taking diet pills, laxatives, or diuretics. However, those with disordered eating do not meet the full diagnostic criteria for an eating disorder (37).

Eating disorders are multifactorial diseases and, as such, require a multidisciplinary team approach. The strength and conditioning professional must be aware of signs and symptoms of an eating disorder and have a referral network in place so athletes can get the psychological, medical, and nutrition help they need from experts who work with eating disorders.

Anorexia Nervosa

Anorexia nervosa is characterized by a distorted body image and an intense fear of gaining weight or becoming fat, leading those with this disease to excessive calorie restriction and severe weight loss (6). Those with anorexia nervosa also put a great deal of emphasis on their weight or shape yet do not recognize the seriousness of their illness. Also, people with anorexia nervosa typically engage in ritualistic behaviors including repeated weighing, cutting food into small pieces, and carefully portioning their food (87).

Two subtypes fall under anorexia nervosa. The restricting type does not regularly binge eat or purge, while the binge-eating or purging type regularly engages in binge eating or purging.

The average age of onset is 19 years old, and the lifetime prevalence in females and males is 0.9% and 0.3%, respectively. Just 33.8% of those with anorexia nervosa are in treatment (50). However, these statistics are based on older criteria for anorexia nervosa; prevalence rates may go up with the 2013 revised diagnostic criteria (48). It is important to note that among all mental health disorders, anorexia nervosa has the highest mortality rate

---

Symptoms of Anorexia Nervosa

- Thinning of the bones (osteopenia or osteoporosis)
- Brittle hair and nails
- Dry and yellowish skin
- Growth of fine hair all over the body (lanugo)
- Mild anemia and muscle wasting and weakness
- Severe constipation
- Low blood pressure, slowed breathing and pulse
- Damage to the structure and function of the heart
- Brain damage
- Multiorgan failure
- Drop in internal body temperature, causing a person to feel cold all the time
- Lethargy, sluggishness, or feeling tired all the time
- Infertility

Reprinted from National Institute of Mental Health.

(41). For more information about anorexia nervosa, the reader is encouraged to read the American Psychiatric Association's *Diagnostic and Statistical Manual of Mental Disorders, Fifth Edition* (2013).

Binge-Eating Disorder

Previously categorized under "eating disorder not otherwise specified," binge-eating disorder has its own category in the *Diagnostic and Statistical Manual of Mental Disorders, Fifth Edition* (6). Binge-eating disorder is characterized by repeated episodes, occurring at least once a week for a period of three weeks, of uncontrolled binge eating (eating significantly more food in a short period of time than most people would eat under the same circumstances) (6). The binge-eating episodes are associated with three or more of the following:

- Eating much more rapidly than normal
- Eating until feeling uncomfortably full
- Eating large amounts of food when not feeling physically hungry
- Eating alone because of feeling embarrassed by how much one is eating
- Feeling disgusted with oneself, depressed, or very guilty afterward (6)

Because binge-eating episodes are not followed by purging, as is the case with bulimia nervosa, people with binge-eating disorder are often overweight or obese. The lifetime prevalence for men and women is 2.0% and 3.5%, respectively, and average age of onset is 25 years old. A lifetime prevalence of binge-eating disorder is associated with morbid obesity (BMI >40). Over the course of a lifetime, only 43.6% of people with binge-eating disorder are receiving treatment (50). However, these statistics are based on older criteria for binge-eating disorder, before its inclusion as a specific eating disorder in 2013. Prevalence rates may go up with the revised criteria (48). Binge eating is associated with significant physical and psychological problems. In addition, people with binge-eating disorder may feel embarrassed, guilty, or disgusted with their behavior and may attempt to hide their behavior by eating alone (6).

Bulimia Nervosa

Bulimia nervosa is characterized by recurrent consumption of food in amounts significantly greater than would customarily be consumed in a discrete period of time—for example, an entire pizza and a half-gallon of ice cream, plus a package of cookies. Purging follows episodes of binge eating and may include one or more of the following: self-induced vomiting, intense exercise, laxative use, or diuretic use. The binging and purging occur at least once a week for a period of three months (6). People with bulimia nervosa feel a lack of control over their eating during binge episodes and are more likely to be normal weight as opposed to underweight, are unhappy with their weight and body, and fear weight gain. Average age of onset for bulimia nervosa is 20 years old, and the lifetime prevalence is 0.6%. Only 43.2% of those with bulimia nervosa are receiving treatment (50). However, these statistics are also based on older criteria for bulimia nervosa, and prevalence rates may go up with the revised criteria in the *Diagnostic and Statistical Manual of Mental Disorders, Fifth Edition* (48). For more information about bulimia, the reader is encouraged to read this source.

Avoidant/Restrictive Food Intake Disorder

Avoidant/restrictive food intake disorder (ARFID) is an eating or feeding disturbance, including apparent lack of interest in eating or food; avoidance based on the sensory

---

Symptoms of Bulimia Nervosa

- Chronically inflamed and sore throat
- Swollen salivary glands in the neck and jaw area
- Worn tooth enamel, increasingly sensitive and decaying teeth as a result of exposure to stomach acid
- Acid reflux disorder and other gastrointestinal problems
- Intestinal distress and irritation from laxative abuse
- Severe dehydration from purging of fluids
- Electrolyte imbalance (too low or too high levels of sodium, calcium, potassium, and other minerals), which can lead to heart attack.

Reprinted from National Institute of Mental Health.

characteristics of food; or concern about aversive consequences of eating. This disorder is manifested by persistent failure to meet appropriate nutritional or energy needs associated with one (or more) of the following (6):

- Significant weight loss (or failure to achieve expected weight gain or faltering growth in children)
- Significant nutritional deficiency
- Dependence on enteral feeding or oral nutritional supplements
- Marked interference with psychosocial functioning

The disturbance is not better explained by lack of available food or by associated culturally sanctioned practice.

The eating disturbance does not occur exclusively during the course of anorexia nervosa or bulimia nervosa, and there is no evidence of a disturbance in the way in which one's body weight or shape is experienced.

The eating disturbance is not attributable to a concurrent medical condition or not better explained by another mental disorder. When the eating disturbance occurs in the context of another condition or disorder, the severity of the eating disturbance exceeds that routinely associated with the condition or disorder and warrants additional clinical attention (6).

Pica

People with pica eat nonnutritive substances for a period of at least one month. Common nonnutritive substances include clay, laundry starch, ice, cigarette butts, hair, or chalk (64). Those with pica may have electrolyte and metabolic disorders, intestinal obstruction, wearing away of tooth enamel, and gastrointestinal problems, among other issues. Testing for anemia is recommended since pica is associated with iron deficiency (64).

Rumination Disorder

Rumination involves chewing, reswallowing, or spitting of regurgitated food. To be classified as having this disorder, one must display this behavior, unrelated to any medical condition, for at least one month.

Rumination disorder can occur alongside other eating issues or disorders (6).

Eating Disorders: Management and Care

It is not the responsibility of the strength and conditioning professional to treat or diagnose an eating disorder. It is his or her ethical responsibility to assist the athlete in attaining the proper diagnosis from a qualified physician and treatment from a qualified treatment team. Therefore, strength and conditioning professionals should be mindful of the symptoms of each eating disorder as well as signs of disordered eating. Keep in mind that abnormal eating patterns and amenorrhea alone are not indicative of an eating disorder. A professional who is experienced and qualified in diagnosing and treating eating disorders should be contacted when an athlete's behavior is concerning.

> The strength and conditioning professional is not responsible for treating eating disorders but instead should be aware of the symptoms associated with an eating disorder and refer athletes to the appropriate professional.

Eating Disorder Resources

National Eating Disorders Association
www.nationaleatingdisorders.org

International Association of Eating Disorders Professionals
www.iaedp.com

The Renfrew Center Foundation
www.renfrewcenter.com

National Association of Anorexia Nervosa and Associated Disorders, Inc.
www.anad.org

Remuda Ranch
www.remudaranch.com

Conclusion

The primary role of nutrition in strength and conditioning is to support athletic performance. A general understanding of nutrition principles and applications is essential for strength and conditioning professionals so that they can provide consistent, accurate informa-tion to their athletes while also being able to identify the potential signs and symptoms of an eating disorder. And though pre-, during-, and postcompetition nutrition can lead to better performance, a nutritionally sound daily diet should be emphasized as well, for overall health, greater training adaptations, and performance.

KEY TERMS

anorexia nervosa
binge-eating disorder
body mass index (BMI)
bulimia nervosa

carbohydrate loading
diet-induced thermogenesis
disordered eating
eating disorders

isocaloric
obesity
precompetition meal
voluntary dehydration

STUDY QUESTIONS

1. The primary macronutrient that is addressed in the precompetition meal is
   a. fat
   b. carbohydrate
   c. protein
   d. vitamin

2. Which of the following makes the GREATEST contribution to total energy expenditure?
   a. resting metabolic rate
   b. physical activity energy expenditure
   c. thermic effect of food
   d. resting blood sugar levels

3. Which of the following is characteristic of anorexia nervosa?
   a. normal body weight
   b. very low dietary fat intake
   c. preoccupation with food
   d. secretive eating

4. When an eating disorder is suspected, the strength and conditioning professional should
   a. monitor the athlete's daily food intake
   b. require frequent weigh-ins
   c. encourage further assessment by an eating disorder specialist
   d. provide nutritional information

Performance-Enhancing Substances and Methods

Bill Campbell, PhD

> **After completing this chapter, you will be able to**
>
> - provide reliable and up-to-date information to athletes on the risks and benefits of performance-enhancing substances, including anabolic steroids;
> - understand the efficacy and adverse effects of over-the-counter dietary supplements marketed to athletes for enhancing sport and exercise performance;
> - determine which performance-enhancing supplements are beneficial for strength/power performance, endurance performance, or both; and
> - distinguish between those performance-enhancing supplements that mimic the effects of hormones in the body and those that improve performance through some other means.

The author would like to acknowledge the significant contributions of Jay R. Hoffman and Jeffrey R. Stout to this chapter.

Athletes who choose to use performance-enhancing substances do so with the hope that they will augment their training adaptations and ultimately improve their sport performance (198). Ideally, performance-enhancing substances also support the health of the athlete and are within the ethical and stated guidelines of the athlete's sport. Because of the ethical considerations relating to unfair advantage during competition and the potential for adverse events, most athletic governing bodies have generated a list of substances that are banned from national and international competition. Athletes caught using such substances can be suspended or forced to forfeit their medals or both. In situations in which the athlete tests positive for a banned substance on repeated occasions, he or she risks a lifetime ban on participation in the given sport. However, numerous nutritional supplements and ergogenic aids are permissible and are frequently used by athletes to maximize performance enhancement. Often the use of these substances is promoted on the basis of unfounded claims (198). Thus, it is imperative that the athlete become informed about the legality of these substances, understand the potential risks associated with consumption, and know whether scientific research supports the claims (i.e., the efficacy of the product). The strength and conditioning professional can greatly assist athletes in this regard by giving them relevant information related to these issues, as well as by referring them to nutrition specialists. Although an **ergogenic aid** can be any substance, mechanical aid, or training method that improves sport performance, for the purposes of this chapter the term refers specifically to pharmacologic aids.

Athletes may try to gain a competitive advantage by using supplements that are reputed to be ergogenic but are not banned, or they may knowingly use banned substances in the belief that they can stay ahead of the drug testers (198). A consequence may be that athletes who would normally refrain from using these substances may feel pressured to use them just to stay abreast of their competitors. However, athletes who are well informed can confidently ignore useless and possibly harmful products despite what their fellow athletes claim. It may also be possible to steer athletes away from the use of banned drugs if they are aware of the risks to their health and safety and are aware that competitors who cheat run a high risk of being detected.

Athletes should focus on using appropriately periodized strength and conditioning methods and sound nutritional practices designed to enhance performance. If these two factors are addressed, at that point the athlete can consider using sport supplements or ergogenic aids. It is important that athletes seek guidance from appropriate professionals in order to make sure that what they are considering is both legal and efficacious.

▶ **An athlete's first priority should be to apply sound principles of training, including adequate nutrition, before using any nutritional supplement or ergogenic aid. Before purchasing or consuming a product, an athlete should seek guidance from qualified professionals to make sure the choice is both legal and effective.**

Types of Performance-Enhancing Substances

This chapter discusses two categories of performance-enhancing substances: (1) hormones and the drugs that mimic their effects and (2) dietary supplements. Certain hormones, such as testosterone, play an integral role in the adaptive response to strength and conditioning activities; others, such as epinephrine, are important for energy mobilization during training. These and several other types of hormones are covered more extensively in the next part of this chapter. The distinction between a drug and a dietary supplement is not intuitively obvious. For example, caffeine, which is found in many beverages such as coffee, is categorized as a drug. The distinction between a drug and a dietary supplement affects whether or not a product meets United States Food and Drug Administration (FDA) approval for safety and effectiveness. If a product is not classified as a drug or advertised as having therapeutic value, FDA regulations concerning its sale are relatively relaxed. This means that any manufacturer can introduce a new dietary supplement to the market without special approval and that the FDA will not investigate its safety or effectiveness unless a health risk is brought to the agency's attention (87). The FDA's definition of a drug encompasses substances that change the body's structure or function. This includes substances that stimulate hormone secretion. In addition, if a compound is administered differently from the way in which foods would be consumed, it may be classified as a drug.

▶ **The distinction between a drug and a dietary supplement is linked to FDA approval for safety and effectiveness.**

Generally, **dietary supplements** are highly refined products that would not be confused with a food. They may not have any positive nutritional value; hence they are not referred to as nutritional supplements. Carbohydrate loading to bolster glycogen stores before an athletic competition is considered sport nutrition, as is a tablet of a single purified amino acid (not promoted for medicinal properties); however, the tablet is considered a dietary supplement.

Definition of Products That Can Be Sold as Dietary Supplements

The following points define which products can be sold as dietary supplements in the United States:

1. A product (other than tobacco) intended to supplement the diet that contains one or more of the following dietary ingredients:
   a. A vitamin
   b. A mineral
   c. An herb or other botanical
   d. An amino acid
   e. A dietary substance for use by humans to supplement the diet by increasing the total dietary intake
   f. A concentrate, metabolite, constituent, extract, or combination of any ingredient identified in *a* through *e*
2. The product must also be intended for ingestion and cannot be advertised for use as a conventional food or as the sole item within a meal or diet.

The FDA regulates both finished dietary supplement products and dietary ingredients. The FDA regulates dietary supplements under a different set of regulations than those covering conventional foods and drugs (see FDA website at www.fda.gov/Food/Dietarysupplements/default.htm). In 1994, the U.S. Congress passed a seminal piece of legislation known as the Dietary Supplement Health and Education Act (DSHEA). Under DSHEA, manufacturers and distributors of dietary supplements are prohibited from marketing products that are adulterated or misbranded. This means that these firms are responsible for evaluating the safety and labeling of their products before marketing to ensure that they meet all the requirements of DSHEA and FDA regulations. Companies can, however, make claims about effects on the body's structure and function as long as the manufacturers can show that the statements are truthful and not misleading; this is a much less stringent requirement than for effectiveness claims made for drugs.

Ergogenic substances are usually banned from athletic competition when a consensus is reached that they may provide an unfair competitive edge or pose a significant health risk. This prohibition does not need to be based on conclusive proof that a substance does anything advantageous; it simply represents an agreement among administrators or clinicians that this may be the case. As mentioned previously, every sport's governing body publishes its own list of banned substances. Probably the most widely recognized international organization regulating doping worldwide is the World Anti-Doping Agency (WADA), which oversees the doping controls and establishes the banned substances list for the International Olympic Committee (69). Each country has an affiliated agency (e.g., United States Anti-Doping Agency [USADA], Australian Anti-Doping Agency [ASADA]). ASADA not only polices doping in Olympic sports but also oversees doping controls for professional sports in Australia. The prohibited substances list is standardized and updated by WADA each year. While the WADA list is the international standard, other organizations, such as collegiate and professional sports in the United States, have different prohibited substances lists as well as penalties for doping. Regardless of which organization regulates doping controls, it is incumbent upon the athlete, sport coach, strength and conditioning professional, and all support staff to ensure that they are compliant with their respective organizations. Figure 11.1

Major Sport Organizations' Lists of Banned Substances

Major League Baseball

http://mlbplayers.mlb.com/pa/info/cba.jsp

National Collegiate Athletic Association

www.ncaa.org/health-and-safety/policy/2013-14-ncaa-banned-drugs

National Football League

www.nflplayers.com/About-us/Rules--Regulations/Player-Policies/Banned-Substances

National Hockey League (uses the WADA banned substances list)

www.nhl.com/ice/page.htm?id=26397

World Anti-Doping Agency (WADA)

https://www.wada-ama.org/en

2013-2014 National Collegiate Athletic Association Banned Drug Classes

A. Stimulants

Amphetamine (Adderall), caffeine (guarana), cocaine, ephedrine, fenfluramine (Fen), methamphetamine, methylphenidate (Ritalin), phentermine (Phen), synephrine (bitter orange), methylhexaneamine, "bath salts" (mephedrone), and so on
> The following stimulants are not banned: phenylephrine and pseudoephedrine.

B. Anabolic Agents

(Sometimes listed as a chemical formula, such as 3,6,17-androstenetrione), androstenedione, boldenone, clenbuterol, dehydroepiandrosterone (DHEA), epi-trenbolone, etiocholanolone, methasterone, methandienone, nandrolone, norandrostenedione, stanozolol, stenbolone, testosterone, trenbolone, and so on

C. Alcohol and Beta-Blockers (Banned for Rifle Only)

Alcohol, atenolol, metoprolol, nadolol, pindolol, propranolol, timolol, and so on

D. Diuretics (Water Pills) and Other Masking Agents

Bumetanide, chlorothiazide, furosemide, hydrochlorothiazide, probenecid, spironolactone (canrenone), triamterene, trichlormethiazide, and so on

E. Street Drugs

Heroin, marijuana, tetrahydrocannabinol (THC), synthetic cannabinoids (e.g., spice, K2, JWH-018, JWH-073)

F. Peptide Hormones and Analogues

Growth hormone (hGH), human chorionic gonadotropin (hCG), erythropoietin (EPO), and so on

G. Anti-Estrogens

Anastrozole, tamoxifen, formestane, 3,17-dioxo-etiochol-1,4,6-triene (ATD), and so on

H. Beta-2 Agonists

Bambuterol, formoterol, salbutamol, salmeterol, and so on

FIGURE 11.1   The National Collegiate Athletic Association's list of substances banned for athletes at colleges and universities in the United States. Check with your institution or governing body for the list specific to your situation.

lists the 2013-2014 National Collegiate Athletic Association banned drug classes. This list is used by many universities in the United States and is subject to change on a yearly basis.

Some of the substances are illegal under governmental statute as well. Anabolic steroids are a Class III substance, which makes their possession, for other than medical use, punishable with a maximum penalty of one year in prison and a minimum US$1,000 fine if this is the individual's first drug offense. The maximum penalty for trafficking (to deal or trade in something illegal) is five years in prison and a fine of US$250,000 if this is the individual's first felony drug offense. If this is the second felony drug offense, the maximum period of imprisonment and the maximum fine both double. While these penalties are for federal offenses, individual states have also implemented fines and penalties for illegal use of anabolic steroids.

Hormones

A variety of endogenously produced hormones are used to enhance athletic performance. The most commonly used hormone is **testosterone**, along with its synthetic derivatives (121). Testosterone is the primary androgen hormone that interacts with skeletal muscle tissue. In addition to testosterone, a variety of other hormones produced by the body have been employed by athletes as ergogenic aids to stimulate the testes to produce testosterone, or they have anabolic properties in themselves; growth hormone is an example. Erythropoietin, which is secreted by the kidneys, is used to stimulate red cell production for enhancement of aerobic endurance performance; and catecholamines such as adrenaline (or epinephrine), which have metabolic and nervous system effects, are often used to enhance weight loss and to provide greater arousal for performance.

Anabolic Steroids

Anabolic steroids are the synthetic (human-made) derivatives of the male sex hormone testosterone. Physiologically, elevations in testosterone concentrations stimulate protein synthesis, resulting in improvements in muscle size, body mass, and strength (27). In addition, testosterone and its synthetic derivatives are responsible for the development and maturation of male secondary sex characteristics (i.e., increase in body hair; masculine voice; development of male pattern baldness, libido, sperm production, and aggressiveness). These androgenic properties include the full development of the primary sexual characteristics of the male. Thus it is more accurate to refer to synthetic derivatives of testosterone as anabolic-androgenic steroids. However, they are also referred to as androgens, androgenic steroids, or anabolic steroids.

Secretion of testosterone occurs primarily in the interstitial Leydig cells in the testes. Although several other steroid hormones with anabolic-androgenic properties are produced in the testes (e.g., dihydrotestosterone and androstenedione), testosterone is produced in far greater quantities. Testosterone and these other male sex hormones are also secreted in significantly smaller amounts from the adrenal glands (in men and women) and ovaries (in women). Many of the ergogenic aids on the market today are precursors for testosterone (i.e., androstenedione) and are discussed in more detail later in this chapter.

It was not until the 1930s that testosterone was isolated, synthesized, and subsequently investigated for its effects in humans (61). The physiological changes that testosterone regulates have made it one of the drugs of choice for strength and power athletes or other athletes interested in increasing muscle mass (121). However, testosterone itself is a very poor ergogenic aid. Rapid degradation occurs when testosterone is given either orally or through injectable administration (256). Thus, chemical modification of testosterone was necessary to retard the degradation process in order to achieve androgenic and anabolic effects at lower concentrations and to provide effective blood concentrations for longer periods of time (256). Many derivatives of testosterone were developed from 1940 to 1960 (207); once these modifications occurred, anabolic steroid use through either oral or injectable administration became possible. In recent years, anabolic steroid administration via creams and gels for topical applications and skin patches has increased in popularity, primarily for medical reasons. However, the most commonly used forms for administration in athletes are oral and injectable forms (121). Examples of oral and injectable anabolic steroids are listed in table 11.1.

TABLE 11.1 Types of Anabolic Steroids Used by Athletes

Generic name or category	Examples of trade names
Orally active steroids	
Methandrostenolone	Dianabol
Oxandrolone	Anavar
Stanozolol	Winstrol
Oxymetholone	Anadrol 50
Fluoxymesterone	Halotestin
Methyltestosterone	Metandren
Mesterolone	Proviron
Injectable steroids	
Testosterone esters*	Depo-Testosterone
Nandrolone esters*	Deca-Durabolin
Stanozolol	Winstrol
Methenolone enanthate	Primobolan Depot
Boldenone undecylenate	Equipoise
Trenbolone acetate	Finaject

*These are generic categories of substances; many different preparations of each are available.

Dosing

Athletes typically use anabolic steroids in a "**stacking**" regimen, in which they administer several different drugs simultaneously (187). The rationale for stacking is to increase the potency of each drug via an additive effect. That is, the potency of one anabolic agent may be enhanced when it is consumed simultaneously with another anabolic agent. Research in this area is limited, and the efficacy of stacking has not been proven one way or the other. Individuals use both oral and injectable compounds. Most users take anabolic steroids in a cyclic pattern, meaning they use the drugs for several weeks or months and alternate these cycles with periods of discontinued use (187). Often users administer the drugs in a pyramid (step-up) pattern in which dosages are steadily increased over several weeks (121). Toward the end of the cycle, the athlete "steps down" to reduce the likelihood of negative side effects. At this point, some athletes discontinue the drug use or perhaps initiate another cycle of different drugs (e.g., drugs that may increase endogenous testosterone production, taken to prevent the undesirable drop in testosterone concentrations that follows the removal of the pharmaceutical agents). One study showed that the typical steroid regimen involved an average of 3.1 agents, with a typical cycle ranging from 5 to 10 weeks (187). The dose that the athlete administered was reported to vary from between 5 and 29 times greater than physiological replacement doses (187). These higher pharmacologic dosages appear necessary to elicit the gains that the athletes desire. In a classic study on the dose–response curve of anabolic steroids, Forbes (81) demonstrated that the total dose of anabolic steroids has a logarithmic relationship to increases in lean body mass; low doses produce only slight effects, but there is a progressive augmentation of lean body mass with increasingly larger doses. These results reinforce the athlete's philosophy that if a low dose is effective, then more must be better.

Athletes typically use higher doses of the substances than are prescribed for men with low testosterone levels. Methandrostenolone (Dianabol), for example, maintains normal secondary sexual characteristics in hypogonadal men at a replacement dose of approximately 15 mg/day; athletes have reported using up to 300 mg/day (88). This orally active drug has not been available for medical use in the United States for more than a decade but is still available through black market sources. Testosterone enanthate is a testosterone ester and is an injectable steroid that is readily available in the United States and is used clinically for some rare diseases and for replacement treatment. A replacement dose is approximately 75 to 100 mg/week administered every one to two weeks. Injectable steroids are administered intramuscularly, typically by deep gluteal injections. They are also more potent than oral steroids because of their route of delivery, and perhaps as well because they do not require additional modification to protect them from immediate metabolism by the liver. The injectable compounds have a wide range of half-lives. Among the testosterone esters, testosterone propionate remains in the circulation for approximately 1.5 days, whereas testosterone buciclate lasts for three months after a single injection (18).

Who Uses Anabolic Steroids?

It is believed that athletes (particularly strength athletes) whose goals are to improve athletic performance are the primary users of anabolic steroids. George J. Mitchell, a former United States senator, in the famous 2007 "Mitchell Report" stated that use of androgenic–anabolic steroids by Major League Baseball players in the United States was pervasive (49). Before this revelation of anabolic steroid use in athletes, earlier reports date back to the 1952 and 1956 Olympics, in which there were accounts of systematic use of androgens by the Soviet weightlifting team (49). State-sponsored anabolic steroid use in other countries has also been documented. In the former German Democratic Republic after the fall of the communist government in 1990, classified documents revealed a secret state program beginning

in 1966 to improve national athletic performance using androgens (49, 86). In the United States, widespread use has also been reported in powerlifters (59), National Football League players (125), and collegiate athletes (167). Although results of several surveys suggest that anabolic steroid use appears to have been declining over the last few decades (133, 238), anabolic steroids are among the top sport issues today because of accusations of widespread use in many sports during the past few years (84).

Strength athletes are not the only users of anabolic steroids. People outside organized sport use steroids to enhance appearance rather than performance (66). National surveys of male American high school seniors showed that approximately 7% were using, or had used, anabolic steroids (14, 39). One-third of the admitted steroid users were not involved in school-sponsored sports, and more than one-fourth stated that their main reason for using steroids was to improve appearance, as opposed to athletic performance. Pope and his colleagues (191, 193) described a subset of bodybuilders with an altered self-image who believed that they looked small and weak even though they were large and muscular. These individuals used ergogenic substances and weight training to increase their body size. Pope calls this condition "reverse anorexia nervosa"; it is also known as **muscle dysmorphia**. These bodybuilders appear to be substantially different from competitive athletes in terms of their objectives, the substantial health risks that some of them are willing to take, and their strategies of using extremely large doses of anabolic steroids. This phenomenon may suggest why the most serious illnesses associated with steroid use have occurred almost exclusively in bodybuilders and not in other steroid-using athletes (88).

Efficacy

The purported ergogenic benefits commonly attributed to anabolic steroid use are increased muscle mass, strength, and athletic performance, particularly in sports requiring maximal strength levels. When anabolic steroids are taken at supraphysiologic doses, these ergogenic benefits are realized (27, 240). The degree and incidence of these changes are variable, depending greatly on, among other factors, the training status of the individual (27).

Muscle Mass and Strength   One of the primary reasons athletes and nonathletes take anabolic steroids is to increase lean muscle mass and maximal strength. If such improvements do occur, this will lead to better performance on the field, with all other variables of athleticism held constant. When anabolic steroids are given in doses similar to those used by recreationally trained and competitive athletes, increases in muscle protein synthesis are seen (106). These increases in protein synthesis are likely responsible for the increases observed in lean body mass in both recreationally trained and competitive athletes taking anabolic steroids (111, 113, 153, 240, 250). Even when anabolic steroids are administered to normal adult men not engaged in intensive resistance training, increases in body mass, including the nonfat component, are observed (27, 82, 88, 252). The extent to which gains in lean body mass and maximal strength occur with anabolic steroid use has been reported in the scientific literature as a case study (2). In this study, an adult male international-level bodybuilder self-injected androgenic hormones (at a dosage of 53 mg/day) for a training period of one year that included only a four-week abstinence from drugs in the middle of the year. During this time, the bodybuilder was able to gain about 7 kg (15 pounds) of fat-free weight, increase the mean fiber area of the vastus lateralis muscle by approximately 11% in six months' time, and significantly increase maximal strength. Despite these improvements in muscle mass and strength, the individual's health status was negatively affected. Specifically, after drug withdrawal, the subject experienced atrophic testicles and low luteinizing hormone, follicle-stimulating hormone, and testosterone levels. High-density lipoprotein (HDL) cholesterol was also significantly lowered, which indicates a higher risk for atherogenesis. See more information on the health consequences of anabolic steroid use in the "Adverse Effects" section.

For some time it was postulated that increases in body mass with androgen use came from an increase in body water (113). An increase in total body water is expected with an increase in muscle mass, since water constitutes a majority of the cellular weight; however, it has been postulated that anabolic steroids may increase water retention as well by increasing interstitial and extracellular volume. Although water retention may explain why not all of the weight gain is sustained after cessation of anabolic steroid use, this issue is still not well understood. In a study of experienced male bodybuilders, an eight-week cycle of nandrolone decanoate (200 mg/week, intramuscularly) resulted in a significant 2.2 kg (4.8-pound) increase in body mass, a 2.6 kg (5.7-pound) increase in fat-free mass, and a 0.4 kg (0.88-pound) decrease in fat mass, with no change in hydration of fat-free mass (240). In addition, the extracellular and intracellular water ratio was unaltered. Even after six weeks of discontinued androgen use, the body mass of the bodybuilders was still significantly greater than baseline levels (1.6 kg [3.5 pounds] greater), yet no hydration changes were seen. The increase in fat-free mass and possible reduction in fat mass may last for several months after cessation of use (82) (figure 11.2). Thus, athletes may derive a benefit from steroid use

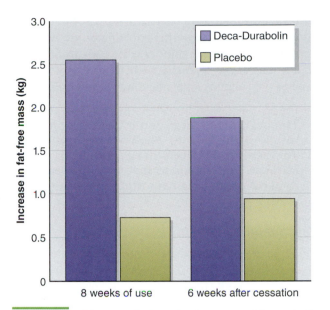

FIGURE 11.2 Changes in lean body mass with anabolic steroid administration and following drug cessation.
Data from Forbes, Porta, Herr, and Griggs, 1992 (82).

even if they stop taking the drugs long enough before competition to obtain a negative drug test. This is why unannounced, year-round drug testing of some elite athletes is important for the prevention of unfair drug use.

Athletic Performance   Initially, researchers examining the ergogenicity of exogenously administered anabolic steroids were unable to see any significant performance effects (75, 85, 161, 223). Consequently, the scientific and medical community suggested that anabolic steroids had little influence on athletic performance. This, however, was contrary to anecdotal reports emanating from gyms and training centers that showed large strength improvements in the athletes. Upon further examination of the initial studies, several methodological flaws became apparent. Several of these studies used physiological doses, in contrast to the suprapharmacologic doses that are typically taken by athletes self-administering androgens. In essence, these subjects were shutting down their own endogenous production and replacing it with an exogenous anabolic steroid. Another flaw in some of these investigations was the method of strength assessment. In several studies, strength performance was evaluated using a mode of exercise that was different from the training stimulus. This lack of specificity likely masked any possible training effect. In addition, several studies used subjects who had only minimal resistance training experience (85, 223). When exogenous androgens have been administered to experienced resistance-trained athletes, significant strength gains have been consistently reported (3, 113, 217, 250). Strength gains in experienced strength-trained athletes are generally quite small relative to those seen in novice lifters; but when strength-trained athletes use anabolic steroids, their strength gains may be two- to threefold higher than those typically seen in similarly trained athletes who are not supplementing (113, 240, 250).

> The purported ergogenic benefits commonly attributed to anabolic steroid use are increased muscle mass, strength, and athletic performance, but these changes depend on the training status of the individual.

Psychological Effects

Anabolic steroid use is also associated with changes in aggression, arousal, and irritability (174). The East Germans reportedly used anabolic steroids for this effect, delivering high doses to the central nervous system by taking steroids through the nose. The issue has not been well studied, but anecdotal reports suggest that this practice markedly increased aggressiveness and enhanced performance among athletes (65). Elevations in arousal and self-esteem may be a positive side effect for the anabolic steroid user. Increases in aggressiveness may also be perceived as a benefit, especially for athletes participating in contact sports.

Increased aggressiveness may not be confined to athletic performance, however. Anabolic steroid users experiencing increased aggressiveness may pose a threat both to themselves and to those they come in contact with (183, 192). Anabolic steroids are also associated with mood swings and psychotic episodes. Studies have shown that nearly 60% of anabolic steroid users experience increases in irritability and aggressiveness (192). Pope and colleagues (194) reported significant elevations in aggressiveness and manic scores following 12 weeks of testosterone cypionate injections in a controlled double-blind crossover study. Interestingly, the results of this study were not uniform across the subjects. Most subjects showed little psychological effect, and few developed prominent effects. A cause-and-effect relationship has yet to be identified in anabolic steroid users, but it does appear that individuals who experience psychological or behavioral changes recover when steroid use is discontinued (91).

Adverse Effects

Adverse effects associated with anabolic steroid use are listed in table 11.2. It is important to note that there are differences between the side effects of anabolic steroid use under medical supervision and those associated with abuse (i.e., consumption of many drugs at high doses). Most of the information concerning adverse medical events associated with anabolic steroid use

TABLE 11.2 Signs and Symptoms of Ergogenic Aid Abuse

Affected system	Adverse effects
Cardiovascular	Lipid profile changes Elevated blood pressure Decreased myocardial function
Endocrine	Gynecomastia Decreased sperm count Testicular atrophy Impotence and transient infertility

Genitourinary	Males
	  Decreased sperm count
	  Decreased testicular size
	Females
	  Menstrual cycle irregularities
	  Clitoromegaly
	  Deepening of voice
	  Masculinization
	Males and females
	  Gynecomastia
	  Libido changes

Dermatological	Acne Male pattern baldness
Hepatic	Increased risk of liver tumors and liver damage
Musculoskeletal	Premature epiphyseal plate closure Increased risk of tendon tears Intramuscular abscess
Psychological	Mania Depression Aggression Hostility Mood Swings

has been acquired from athletes self-administering the drugs. In conjunction, some of the scientific literature has suggested that the medical problems related to anabolic steroids may be somewhat overstated (26, 258), considering that many of the side effects linked to abuse are reversible upon cessation. Anecdotally, it appears that a disproportionate magnitude of use and incidence of adverse events are evident in bodybuilders (who are also known for consuming several other drugs—such as diuretics, thyroid hormones, insulin, and anti-estrogens—that relieve some side effects but potentiate other risk factors as well) compared to strength and power athletes.

Testosterone Precursors (Prohormones)

Prohormones are precursors to the synthesis of other hormones and are theorized to increase the body's ability to produce a given specific hormone. The basis for the use of prohormones as an ergogenic aid evolved from a study showing a threefold increase in testosterone in healthy women who were given 100 mg of either androstenedione or dehydroepiandrosterone (163). Athletes who have continued to supplement with these testosterone precursors (androstenedione, androstenediol, and dehydroepiandrosterone [DHEA]) likely do so on the premise that they will increase testosterone concentrations, strength, muscle size, and willingness to train, as well as providing overall athletic performance enhancements similar to those experienced by people taking anabolic steroids. However, these precursors have only relatively weak androgenic properties in themselves; androstenedione and DHEA have only 1/5th and 1/10th the biological activity of testosterone, respectively (175). Nevertheless, testosterone precursors were officially listed as controlled substances in the 2004 Anabolic Steroid Control Act passed by the U.S. Congress, which mandated a physician's prescription for these substances.

Studies examining the efficacy of testosterone precursors have produced varying results. No significant differences in strength or body composition were seen in middle-aged men performing a resistance training program while supplementing with either DHEA, androstenedione (100 mg), or a placebo for three months (248). When DHEA supplementation (150 mg) was examined in a group of younger males (19-29 years) on a two-weeks-on, one-week-off cycle for eight weeks, there were no gains in strength or lean tissue (37). In addition, the investigators were unable to see any changes in serum testosterone, estrone, estradiol, or lipid concentrations with supplementation. Even in studies using higher dosages (300 mg) of androstenedione for eight weeks, in a similar two-weeks-on, one-week-off protocol, no significant effect was observed in strength, muscle size, or testosterone concentrations (144). However, androstenedione supplementation did cause an increase in serum concentrations of estradiol and estrone and was associated with lower high-density lipoprotein (HDL) levels. These results suggest that although performance changes may not occur in athletes taking this supplement,

they may be at higher risk for some of the negative side effects associated with anabolic steroid use. Broeder and colleagues (34), in the conclusion to their Andro Project study in which they investigated the physiological and hormonal influences of androstenedione in conjunction with a high-intensity resistance training program, made the following statement:

> Testosterone precursors do not enhance adaptations to resistance training when consumed in dosages recommended by manufacturers. Testosterone precursor supplementation does result in significant increases in estrogen-related compounds, dehydroepiandrosterone sulfate concentrations, down-regulation in testosterone synthesis, and unfavorable alterations in blood lipid and coronary heart disease risk profiles of men aged 35 to 65 years. (p. 3093)

Based on the scientific evidence, it appears as if prohormones fall far short of providing the anabolic effects generally associated with androgens (36). However, scientific research has focused almost exclusively on only a few prohormone supplements—DHEA, androstenediol, 19-nor-androstenedione, and 19-nor-androstenediol. There are many other prohormone supplements available that have not been clinically tested. Also, use of prohormones has not been studied in highly trained athletes. In addition, oral administration has been the primary method of taking prohormones. The oral use of prohormones may not be as effective as other means of intake (e.g., injection). All of this suggests that continued study of the efficacy of the testosterone precursors for performance enhancement is still needed; specifically warranted is examination of other routes of ingestion in a trained competitive athletic population.

HCG (Human Chorionic Gonadotropin)

Human chorionic gonadotropin (HCG) is a hormone obtained from the placenta of pregnant women and is very closely related in structure and function to luteinizing hormone. In fact, it is the pregnancy indicator used by

Examples of Banned Prohormone Supplements

This list contains some examples of prohormones that have been banned as part of the Anabolic Steroid Control Act of 2004, but it is not a comprehensive list.

- Androstanediol
- Androstanedione
- Bolasterone
- Methyltestosterone
- Norandrostenediol
- Norandrostenedione
- 19-nor-4-androstenediol
- 19-nor-5-androstenediol
- 1-testosterone

over-the-counter pregnancy test kits, since it is generally not found in the body at any other time. In the general population, HCG is sometimes injected into overweight females under medical supervision in conjunction with low-calorie diets for the purposes of weight loss (99). Research suggests that when used for this purpose, HCG is not effective for inducing weight loss. The caloric restriction that accompanies the HCG injections appears to be the main contributing factor to associated weight loss (99).

Efficacy

While HCG offers females no performance-enhancing ability, it is cited anecdotally as useful for males who take anabolic steroids. When injected into men, HCG can increase testicular testosterone production; testosterone levels can nearly double within four days after a large intramuscular injection (54). The activity of HCG in the male body is due to its ability to mimic luteinizing hormone, a pituitary hormone that stimulates the Leydig cells in the testicles to manufacture testosterone (160). The reason males would want to be injected with HCG to increase endogenous testosterone levels is that endogenous testosterone production is suppressed at the end of a steroid cycle (173, 176). For that reason, if HCG is used by athletes, it is likely used by those who are finishing a cycle of anabolic steroids and are looking to activate their own endogenous testosterone production.

Adverse Effects

Human chorionic gonadotropin is given as an injection under the skin or into a muscle; the side effects that are common to such administration are pain, swelling, and tenderness around the injection site. There is very little research on the side effects of HCG injections. In one investigation in which HCG was injected into obese women, no adverse effects were reported in relation to blood pressure or routine blood work (218).

Insulin

Insulin is a potent anabolic hormone. It is secreted by the pancreas in response to elevations in blood glucose or specific amino acid (e.g., leucine) concentrations. Its role is to facilitate the uptake of glucose and amino acids into the cell. Since insulin increases protein synthesis, it is considered an anabolic hormone.

Efficacy

When insulin concentrations are elevated naturally (i.e., endogenously from the pancreas following carbohydrate ingestion), there are no safety concerns in otherwise healthy individuals. Additionally, several reports indicate that postworkout carbohydrate ingestion suppresses muscle protein breakdown via the anticatabolic effects of insulin (32, 201). Theoretically, if protein breakdown is suppressed over several weeks to months, gains in lean muscle mass could be realized.

Adverse Effects

Because of insulin's anabolic properties and its rumored ability to potentiate the effects of growth hormone and insulin-like growth factors, some individuals (primarily bodybuilders) take insulin by injection. The use of insulin in this manner comes with serious consequences. Possible outcomes in a previously healthy athlete include immediate death, coma, or the development of insulin-dependent diabetes (160).

Human Growth Hormone

Human growth hormone (HGH), a protein secreted from the anterior pituitary gland, has several important physiological functions that enhance its ergogenic effect. It is anabolic due to its stimulation of bone and skeletal muscle growth, but it also has important metabolic functions such as maintaining blood glucose levels, increasing the uptake of glucose and amino acids into muscle cells (80), and stimulating release of fatty acids from the fat cells.

The primary source of pharmacologic growth hormone is a relatively complicated molecule from which it is synthetically derived using recombinant DNA technology. However, until 1986, the only source of the hormone was the pituitaries of human cadavers. Because HGH receptors are unable to cross-react with growth hormone from animal sources, the financial cost of HGH was very high before 1986. Although the use of cadaver growth hormone did not come without significant health risks, these consequences did not prevent athletes from taking the supplement but instead only substantially restricted use (121). The development of recombinant HGH provided clinicians with a relatively low-risk drug at a lower cost (as compared to cadaver growth hormone) with greater availability. Clinicians can now prescribe recombinant HGH to increase stature in short children with growth hormone deficiency and alter body composition in adults. The use of HGH as a performance-enhancing substance is believed to be widespread among professional athletes; it is either taken alone or stacked with anabolic steroids (17). Even though recombinant technology has increased the availability of HGH, its cost, especially on the black market, is extremely high—between several hundred and a few thousand dollars per month. Humatrope, Nutropin, Norditropin, Genotropin, Serostim, Saizen, and Protropin are brand names of HGH commonly used in the United States.

Efficacy

There appear to be no studies on the efficacy of HGH in professional athletes. Most investigations of HGH have focused on HGH as replacement therapy in growth hormone–deficient adults and children or in healthy elderly individuals. These studies have consistently shown positive alterations in body composition (increases in lean body tissue with decreases in body fat) (79, 120, 204, 228). In men with established growth hormone deficiencies, nightly injections of recombinant HGH for six months resulted in an average increase of 12 pounds (5.4 kg) in lean body mass and a similar amount of fat loss (204). Most studies have not addressed the effect of HGH therapy on muscle strength and performance. One study showed no changes in isokinetic strength following 12 months of therapy (120). However, the subjects in that study did not perform any resistance training during the course of treatment. A study involving trained adults given growth hormone (three days per week for six weeks) showed modest changes in body composition, but no strength assessment was performed (58). Although the scientific literature does not provide support for the efficacy of HGH use in athletic populations, it is likely that the inability to perform such studies (due to ethical constraints) will limit much of our understanding of HGH and human performance. In years past, the use of HGH by athletes may have been prevalent in some professional sports because of its perceived efficacy and the fact that it could not be detected in **random drug tests**. Currently, HGH cannot be detected in the urine via a drug test, and it may be postulated that athletes opt to use it for this reason. However, a blood test for HGH was first introduced at the 2004 Summer Olympic Games in Athens, Greece.

Growth hormone is a protein molecule. Injection is necessary in order to avoid its complete metabolism and maintain its effectiveness. Oral ingestion does not result in any benefit. Many of the actions of growth hormone are mediated through insulin-like growth factor I (IGF-I), another peptide hormone, which is produced and secreted from the liver in response to growth hormone stimulation. Insulin-like growth factor I is now being synthesized using recombinant DNA technology and will likely produce the same effects as HGH.

Adverse Effects

The use of HGH does, however, present some potential significant health risks. Excessive secretion of growth hormone during childhood causes gigantism, a condition in which a person becomes abnormally tall. After puberty, once linear growth has stopped, excess secretion of growth hormone causes **acromegaly**, a disfiguring disease characterized by a widening of the bones, arthri-

tis, organ enlargement, and metabolic abnormalities. This is a potential risk for athletes who use HGH as an ergogenic aid. In addition, these side effects may provide some indication that the athlete could be using this drug. In clinical studies in growth hormone–deficient adults, side effects appear to be minimal for even up to two years of replacement therapy (1, 120, 237). However, athletes who supplement with HGH generally use dosages that far exceed the doses commonly administered in replacement treatment (17). Thus, one should not assume that HGH use is benign with regard to adverse medical events in doses commonly used by an athletic population. Adverse side effects for HGH abuse are diabetes in prone individuals; cardiovascular dysfunction; muscle, joint, and bone pain; hypertension; abnormal growth of organs; and accelerated osteoarthritis (17).

> ▶ Although growth hormone used as replacement therapy for people with growth hormone or IGF-I deficiency can be effective and can have minimal adverse consequences, the dosages that are likely used by athletes may pose a significant risk for acromegaly.

Erythropoietin

One of the limiting factors for endurance performance is the athlete's ability to deliver oxygen to the contracting skeletal muscle. Over the years, several methods have been developed to increase the body's ability to deliver oxygen. Some methods include novel training programs that may naturally elevate red blood cell and hemoglobin levels (i.e., altitude training), while other methods involve synthetic means to elevate the oxygen-carrying capacity of the blood (i.e., blood doping). Blood doping increases one's red blood cell mass and is typically conducted using blood transfusions or taking a hormone known as erythropoietin. There are two forms of blood doping via blood transfusions: autologous and homologous. Autologous blood doping is the transfusion of one's own blood, which has been stored (refrigerated or frozen) until needed. Homologous blood doping is the transfusion of blood that has been taken from another person with the same blood type. Since the late 1980s, blood doping via autologous blood transfusion has taken a back seat to the more popular method, administration of recombinant human erythropoietin (47).

Erythropoietin (EPO) is produced in the kidneys and stimulates the production of new red blood cells. It is also a protein hormone that can be produced by recombinant DNA techniques and is reportedly being abused by athletes (72). Erythropoietin use was one of the methods of doping that Lance Armstrong admitted to over the course of his cycling career. The EPO level in the blood increases in response to chronic aerobic endurance exercise. In certain types of anemia, especially in kidney patients with inadequate EPO production, recombinant human EPO can improve the quality of life of the individual.

Efficacy

Injections of EPO are generally associated with elevations in both hematocrit and hemoglobin. When EPO was given to normal men during six weeks of treatment, hematocrit levels increased from 44.5% to 50%; hemoglobin concentrations increased by 10%; aerobic capacity increased between 6% and 8%; and the time to exhaustion improved by up to 17% (25, 73). The enhanced oxygen-carrying capacity of the blood makes EPO an effective ergogenic aid for the aerobic endurance athlete.

Adverse Effects

While medically supervised use of EPO provides therapeutic benefit in the treatment of anemia related to kidney disease, its misuse can lead to serious health risks for athletes who use this substance simply to gain a competitive edge. The increase in hematocrit resulting from EPO injection presents a significant health risk. Increases in red blood cell number increase blood viscosity (the thickening of the blood). This poses several problems that include increased risk of blood clotting, elevations in systolic blood pressure, stroke, and cerebral or pulmonary embolism (95). During aerobic endurance events, the additional problem of dehydration could compound cardiovascular risks by eliminating any safety margin in the balance between performance advantages from artificially increased hematocrit and decrements from increased blood viscosity. The deaths of a number of competitive cyclists have been related to EPO administration (95). The primary risk associated with EPO is its lack of predictability compared to red blood cell infusion. Once EPO is injected into the body, the stimulus for producing red blood cells is no longer under control. Consequently, aerobic endurance athletes should avoid this drug because of the significant cardiovascular risk, leading to possible death, associated with its administration.

β-Adrenergic Agonists

Synthetic β-adrenergic agonists, or **β-agonists**, are substances chemically related to epinephrine, a hormone produced in the adrenal medulla that regulates physiological effects, such as **lipolysis** (the breakdown of fat) and **thermogenesis** (increased energy expenditure resulting in the production of heat). β-Agonists were originally developed for the treatment of asthma and other life-threatening medical conditions. Some of these compounds have been found to have specific effects on body composition, such as increases in lean mass and decreases in stored fat (195); because of this, these drugs are sometimes referred to as *partitioning agents* (24). One of the more popular β-agonists used by athletes is the drug clenbuterol (195).

Efficacy

Clenbuterol is a β_2-agonist and is a widely used bronchodilator (used to reverse bronchial restriction) in many parts of the world. Athletes use clenbuterol as an ergogenic aid to increase lean muscle tissue and reduce subcutaneous fat (195). Data on the effectiveness of clenbuterol have typically been based not on healthy athletes, but rather subjects with heart failure (138), patients experiencing muscle-wasting conditions (165), and animal models (162, 164). Though studies in humans are limited, several findings have indicated an ergogenic potential of β_2-agonists for strength improvements (164, 166). Athletes generally use clenbuterol in doses twice the recommended amounts administered for clinical purposes, in a cyclic fashion (three weeks on alternated with three weeks off, with a two-days-on, two-days-off cycle during the "on" week) (195). It is believed that this cycling regimen avoids β_2-receptor downregulation (160).

Adverse Effects

Athletes consume clenbuterol in a capsule form, in contrast to the inhalation route that is often used for relieving bronchial constriction. Although a number of potential side effects have been suggested (i.e., transient tachycardia, hyperthermia, tremors, dizziness, palpitations, and insomnia), actual documented events are quite limited (160). In addition, the scarcity of data on the ergogenic potential of clenbuterol in humans makes determining its efficacy difficult.

β-Blockers

β-Blockers are a class of drugs that block the β-adrenergic receptors, preventing the catecholamines (i.e., norepinephrine and epinephrine) from binding. β-Blockers are generally prescribed by cardiologists for the treatment of a wide variety of cardiovascular diseases, including hypertension. The ergogenic benefit of these drugs may reside in their ability to reduce anxiety and tremors during performance (155). Thus, athletes who rely on steady, controlled movements during performance (i.e., archers or marksmen) would appear to benefit from these drugs. Also, β-blockers may improve physiological adaptations from aerobic endurance training by causing an upregulation of β-receptors.

If this is true, it would result in an exaggerated response to sympathetic discharge during intense exercise upon cessation of supplementation.

Efficacy

Several studies have shown that β-blockers can improve both slow and fast shooting accuracy (7, 152). In addition, the dose taken appears to have significant effects on the magnitude of improvement. In shooters who administered β-blockers in two different doses (80 mg vs. 40 mg of oxprenolol), the group taking the higher dose shot with greater accuracy (7). In certain sports, however, some degree of anxiety may be important. Tesch (229) reported that bowlers whose performance was improved during blockade with oxprenolol had significantly greater heart rates before, during, and after competition than subjects whose performance did not improve while on β-blockers.

Adverse Effects

β-Blockers may also have an **ergolytic** effect (reduce performance). Studies have shown that β-blockers impair the cardiovascular response to exercise by reducing maximal heart rate, oxygen consumption, and 10 km race time performance (6). Also, β-blockers are associated with an increased rate of perceived exertion (229). Risks associated with these drugs include bronchospasm, heart failure, prolonged hypoglycemia, bradycardia, heart block, and intermittent claudication (89).

Dietary Supplements

The sport supplement industry throughout the world continues to increase, with the global sport nutrition market valued at US$20.7 billion in 2012 and having an expected value of over US$37 billion by 2019 (235). Some sport nutrition companies make unsubstantiated claims concerning the efficacy of their products. At times, unscrupulous companies have knowingly placed analogues of banned substances in their products to enhance their effects (50). As a result, much confusion has been created among athletes regarding appropriate supplements and the ethics of companies. This section describes dietary supplements that are commonly used by athletes and presents scientific examination of their efficacy.

Essential Amino Acids, Branched-Chain Amino Acids

Essential amino acids (EAAs) are not produced in the body and must be obtained through the diet. They include histidine, isoleucine, leucine, valine, lysine, methionine, phenylalanine, threonine, and tryptophan. High levels of the EAAs can be found in any number of animal-based proteins or as supplements sold over the counter. Leucine can also be found in plants such as spinach and broccoli, but the amount of leucine is minimal when compared to that in animal-based sources.

Efficacy

Scientists have been able to delineate certain categories of amino acids as well as individual amino acids and their role in stimulating muscle protein synthesis. For example, Tipton and colleagues (230, 231) reported that nonessential amino acids were not necessary to stimulate muscle protein synthesis; rather, only the presence of EAAs is needed. In this research (230), six healthy adults (three males and three females) participated in resistance exercise (eight sets of eight repetitions at 80% of 1-repetition maximum [1RM]) and then consumed either 40 g of mixed amino acids (composed of both nonessential and essential amino acids), 40 g of EAA, or a placebo. While the mixed amino acids and the EAA induced an anabolic response that was significantly greater than with the placebo treatment, there was no difference between the amino acid treatments. Since there was no difference, it was concluded that nonessential amino acids are not needed to stimulate muscle protein synthesis. In a follow-up study, using the same protocol (but with only 6 g EAA and 35 g sugar), Rasmussen and colleagues (197) demonstrated significantly greater anabolic drive—that is, the building of new muscle tissue—with the EAA supplement (when given shortly after resistance exercise) versus the placebo.

Subsequently, Tipton and colleagues (232) examined the effects of consuming 6 g EAA plus 36 g of sugar, before or after resistance training, on muscle protein metabolism. They reported that when the EAA plus sugar was consumed 30 minutes before resistance training, the acute (3 hours postexercise) anabolic response was 158% greater than when the EAA and sugar supplement were consumed posttraining. As a result of these acute findings, Tipton and colleagues (232) and Rasmussen and colleagues (197) theorized that a person who consumed EAA before or after (or both before and after) every resistance training session over a period of weeks would experience greater changes in muscle mass than with training only. It is important to note that although the nonessential amino acids are not required to stimulate muscle protein synthesis, this does not mean that they are not important for maximizing training adaptations in the athlete. The conditionally essential and nonessential amino acids serve as the substrates that are incorporated into the newly formed muscle proteins; further, they also spare the conversion of these amino acids from the essential ones, thus effectively increasing the levels of EAAs.

Prior work in animal models further identified that of the eight EAAs, it is the **branched-chain amino acids** (BCAAs)—isoleucine, leucine, and valine—that are responsible for increasing muscle protein synthesis (96). Of the BCAAs, it appears that leucine is the key amino acid for stimulating muscle protein synthesis (42, 139, 199) via the Akt/mechanistic target of rapamycin (mTOR) pathway (figure 11.3). Norton and coworkers (180) demonstrated in rodent models that a leucine threshold for stimulating muscle protein synthesis exists. Based on this pioneering research, many nutrition researchers now believe that the leucine content in any given protein intake is the rate-limiting factor in terms of maximizing muscle protein synthesis within the capacity of skeletal muscle, rather than simply the total amount of protein ingested. To support this theory of the importance of the content of a protein meal, Pasiakos and colleagues (185) reported that a leucine-enriched EAA beverage resulted in a significant elevation of muscle protein synthesis compared to a normal leucine-containing EAA beverage. In this study, trained males ingested one of two different 10 g EAA beverages during cycling exercise—one containing 3.5 g of leucine (46 mg/kg body mass) and the other containing 1.87 g of leucine (~25 mg/kg body mass). After the exercise bout (during a 3-hour assessment period), muscle protein synthesis was 33% greater in the leucine-enriched EAA beverage. The importance of leucine intake and its role in the anabolic response of skeletal muscle following resistance training is a popular topic in sport nutrition research today.

Adverse Effects

No known reports or scientific studies have investigated the adverse effects of branched-chain amino acid or EAA supplementation.

> The branched-chain amino acid leucine is a key regulator in stimulating muscle protein synthesis. Leucine directly activates the Akt/mTOR pathway in skeletal muscle, which is a key pathway in skeletal muscle protein synthesis.

Arginine

Arginine is a conditionally essential amino acid and has crucial roles in nutrition and metabolism. Arginine is required for the synthesis of protein and creatine, and its metabolism results in the production of nitric oxide. The claims often attributed to arginine supplementation are its ability to elevate nitric oxide levels, increase muscle blood flow, and improve exercise performance. Each of these claims is directed at athletes or physically active individuals, as these are all outcomes that would be beneficial for enhancing sport performance or maximizing training adaptations. Unfortunately, there is very little scientific evidence supporting these claims regarding arginine supplementation in the populations that these outcomes would benefit.

Efficacy

Oral arginine supplementation is most often marketed for its potential to elevate nitric oxide levels. Nitric oxide possesses many physiological roles in the human body, but its effects on **vasodilation** (i.e., the widening of blood vessels) are what make it important during exercising conditions. During exercise, nitric oxide levels are naturally increased so that more blood can flow through the arteries and arterioles for the purpose of delivering oxygen and fuel substrates to the working skeletal muscles (30). While nitric oxide is essential for vasodilation, the overwhelming majority of the scientific literature does not support the claim that oral arginine supplementation increases nitric oxide production to levels that are greater than the effects of exercise alone in healthy individuals (5, 159, 208). In contrast to healthy individuals, those with risk factors for cardiovascular disease or people who have diabetes may benefit from increased nitric oxide production resulting from oral arginine supplementation (135, 136).

A natural outcome of nitric oxide production is an increased muscle blood flow. Therefore, increasing muscle blood flow is also a popular claim that is made regarding arginine's effectiveness. Despite the common perception among athletes and consumers

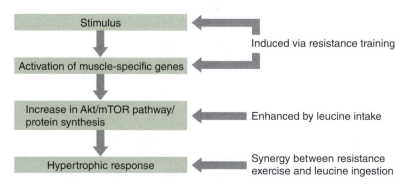

FIGURE 11.3   Role of leucine in muscle protein synthesis.

of dietary supplements that arginine supplementation does increase muscle blood flow, nearly all scientific investigations into this area are in agreement that muscle blood flow is not increased in healthy individuals following arginine supplementation (76, 77, 226). Oral arginine supplementation has also been purported to improve endurance exercise performance. However, in research investigating arginine's effectiveness in healthy populations, it was reported that time to exhaustion, local muscular endurance, and intermittent anaerobic exercise performance were not improved as a result of supplementation (104, 159, 239). Due to its inability to increase nitric oxide production, enhance muscle blood flow, or improve several modes of endurance exercise, oral arginine supplementation is not recommended for healthy athletes.

Adverse Effects

A majority of the scientific investigations in which arginine was given to participants to improve exercise performance used a 6 g dose. While this dose of arginine was not effective in improving endurance performance, this amount was well tolerated and posed no adverse side effects. Oral supplementation at doses up to 13 g is generally well tolerated. The most common adverse reactions to higher doses (13 to 30 g) include gastrointestinal distress consistent with nausea, abdominal cramps, and diarrhea (51).

> **Due to its inability to increase nitric oxide production, enhance muscle blood flow, or improve endurance exercise performance, oral arginine supplementation is not recommended for healthy athletes.**

β-Hydroxy-β-Methylbutyrate

β-Hydroxy-β-methylbutyrate (HMB) is a derivative of the EAA leucine and its metabolite α-ketoisocaproic acid. Evidence shows that HMB stimulates protein synthesis (74) and decreases protein breakdown by inhibiting the ubiquitin–proteasome pathway (211). Due to HMB's role in the regulation of protein breakdown, it may be an effective supplement for minimizing losses of lean muscle mass in situations that promote a catabolic state. β-Hydroxy-β-methylbutyrate is not currently banned or restricted by sport organizations.

Efficacy

The initial research study that highlighted HMB's anti-catabolic potential was conducted by Nissen and colleagues (179). In this study, untrained subjects ingested one of three levels of HMB (0, 1.5, or 3.0 g per day) and two protein levels (117 or 175 g per day) and resistance

trained three days per week for three weeks. As a measure of myofibrillar protein breakdown, urinary 3-methyl-histidine levels were measured (higher levels of urinary 3-methyl-histidine mean that more muscle protein is catabolized, or broken down). After the first week of the resistance training protocol, urinary 3-methyl-histidine was increased by 94% in the control group and by 85% and 50% in those individuals ingesting 1.5 and 3 g of HMB per day, respectively. During the second week of the study, urinary 3-methyl-histidine levels were still elevated by 27% in the control group but were 4% and 15% below basal levels for the 1.5 and 3 g of HMB per day groups. At the end of the third week of resistance training, urinary 3-methyl-histidine levels were not significantly different between the groups (179).

Research in other catabolic-inducing environments has also demonstrated the effectiveness of HMB supplementation. For example, when older adults were confined to complete bed rest (a catabolic state) for 10 days, it was reported that the subjects who were supplemented with 3 g of HMB per day lost significantly less lean body mass (lost only 0.37 pounds [0.17 kg]) as compared to those subjects who were supplemented with a placebo (lost 4.5 pounds [2.05 kg]) (64). Other research findings are in agreement with these observations and have shown that HMB exerts an anticatabolic effect and suppresses muscle damage (146, 241).

In previously untrained individuals initiating a resistance training program lasting four to eight weeks, HMB has been shown to exert significantly greater improvements in strength and lean body mass as compared to a placebo (94, 179, 184). The muscle damage and soreness that result from resistance training are predictably greater in those who have little training experience as compared to individuals who have engaged in resistance training for longer periods of time. Given HMB's ability to suppress muscle damage and muscle protein breakdown, it is not surprising that HMB is effective for people beginning a new training program.

The ergogenic effects of HMB in trained individuals are less conclusive. Studies using resistance-trained or competitive athletes were unable to duplicate the results seen in a recreationally trained population using similar supplementation schedules (150, 181, 196). However, many of the studies investigating the effects of HMB on strength and lean body mass in trained individuals were of short duration (less than five weeks) and lacked the presence of a periodized, high-intensity training program. In order for HMB to be effective, it may be essential to provide novel stimuli to individuals to induce either muscle damage or stimulate elevated protein breakdown.

Research suggests that trained individuals instructed not to change their programs do not benefit from HMB

(150). In a recent investigation, it was reported that highly resistance-trained males undergoing a periodized resistance training program and ingesting supplemental HMB realized significant improvements in total strength and lean body mass as compared to a placebo group that participated in an identical training program (257). Other investigations that have provided an adequate training stimulus in trained individuals have also reported increases in maximal strength and lean body mass as compared to placebo treatments (179, 184).

Adverse Effects

The duration, dosage, and timing of HMB supplementation have notably varied in the scientific literature. In nearly every published investigation related to HMB supplementation, 3 to 6 g per day was ingested. Three grams per day (often divided into several doses) is the most common dosage used in published studies. The majority of studies investigating HMB have used the calcium salt of HMB—HMB-Ca. Recently, another form of HMB, HMB-free acid, has been investigated as well (257). The safety of HMB supplementation has been widely studied and to date there is a consensus that HMB presents no known adverse effects.

> ▶ β-Hydroxy-β-methylbutyrate is most effective when an adequate training stimulus is provided. For untrained individuals, this does not likely require high-volume training. For trained individuals, a high-intensity, high-volume resistance training program is likely needed in order for benefits to be realized with HMB supplementation.

Nutritional Muscle Buffers

During high-intensity anaerobic exercise, a significant accumulation of hydrogen ions (H^+) is coupled with a reduction of pH within skeletal muscle and has been shown to adversely affect performance (200). The ability to regulate H^+ concentration in skeletal muscle during high-intensity exercise has been termed **muscle buffering capacity (MBC)** (22, 178). There is a strong positive relationship between MBC and exercise performance (repeated-sprint ability, high-intensity exercise capacity, anaerobic threshold, and training volume) (70, 71). In fact, researchers have demonstrated a positive relationship between exercise performance and MBC in athletes who participate in sports like basketball, soccer, hockey, cycling, crew (rowing), triathlons, and sprinting (29, 70, 71). In theory, improving MBC by training or nutritional means (β-alanine, sodium bicarbonate, or citrate) would improve performance in sports and activities that may be limited by H^+ buildup. Therefore a brief review of β-alanine, sodium bicarbonate, and sodium citrate and their effects on high-intensity exercise performance follows.

β-Alanine

β-Alanine is a nonessential amino acid that is common in many foods that we eat, such as chicken. By itself, β-alanine has limited ergogenic properties. However, in muscle cells, it is the rate-limiting substrate for carnosine synthesis (68). Harris and colleagues (110) reported that four weeks of supplementing with β-alanine (4 to 6 g/day) resulted in a mean increase of 64% in skeletal muscle β-alanine concentrations. In humans, carnosine is found primarily in fast-twitch (Type II) skeletal muscle and is estimated to contribute up to 40% of the skeletal MBC of H^+ produced during intense anaerobic exercise, thus encouraging a drop in pH (110, 114). Theoretically, increasing skeletal muscle carnosine levels through chronic training or β-alanine supplementation (or both) would improve MBC and most likely improve anaerobic performance. Interestingly, carnosine concentrations in athletes such as sprinters and bodybuilders appear to be significantly higher than those in marathoners, untrained individuals, and people who are elderly (110, 224).

Suzuki and colleagues (224) examined the relationship between skeletal muscle carnosine levels and high-intensity exercise performance in trained cyclists. The authors reported a significant and positive relationship between carnosine concentration and mean power in a 30-second maximal sprint on a cycle ergometer. This finding supported the theory that skeletal muscle carnosine levels have a positive correlation with anaerobic performance because of the relationship between carnosine and MBC.

Efficacy β-Alanine has been studied for its effects on strength, aerobic power, and high-intensity short-term exercises interspersed with short recovery intervals. In contrast to creatine, β-alanine does not seem to improve maximal strength (140, 122, 123). Similarly, aerobic power does not appear to be improved with β-alanine supplementation (123, 140). Even though aerobic power is not improved, supporting data indicate that anaerobic threshold is improved with β-alanine supplementation (221, 259). Practically, improving anaerobic threshold (as measured by the lactate and ventilatory thresholds) means that endurance activities can be performed at relatively higher intensities for longer periods. Hill and colleagues (114) examined the effect of β-alanine supplementation on muscle carnosine levels and exercise performance in untrained subjects. In a double-blind fashion, 25 male subjects (19-31 years) supplemented with either 4.0 g β-alanine or sugar placebo for the first week, then with up to 6.4 g for an additional nine weeks. Muscle carnosine levels (via muscle biopsy) and total work done (kilojoules) were measured at weeks 0, 4, and 10 during cycling to exhaustion at maximal power established from a graded exercise cycle ergometry test. Mean carnosine levels increased by 58% at week 4 and an additional 15% at week 10. Additionally, 13% and 16% increases in total work done during cycle ergometry were seen at weeks 4 and 10, respectively.

In a comprehensive review summarizing the effects of β-alanine supplementation on high-intensity performance, Artioli and colleagues (9) stated that β-alanine ingestion is capable of improving performance in exercises resulting in an extreme intramuscular acidotic environment, such as multiple bouts of high-intensity exercises lasting more than 60 seconds, as well as single bouts undertaken when fatigue is already present. High-intensity exercises performed with a lower level of acidosis are unlikely to benefit from β-alanine supplementation.

Adverse Effects   In the published literature, β-alanine ingestion has ranged from 2.4 to 6.4 g per day. In many β-alanine trials, the total daily amount of β-alanine ingestion was divided into two to four smaller doses. The reason for the smaller dosing strategies is to prevent the only reported adverse effect of β-alanine supplementation, which is the symptom of paresthesia (tingling, pricking, or numbness of a person's skin) (9). Symptoms of paresthesia are triggered by a high and acute single dose and disappear within approximately 1 hour after the ingestion (9, 110).

Sodium Bicarbonate

Sodium bicarbonate is an antacid (alkalinizing agent), meaning that it counteracts or neutralizes acid (low pH). Sodium bicarbonate is naturally formed in the body and is also found in baking soda. Supplementation with sodium bicarbonate has been shown to increase the pH of blood (219). A pH difference is created between the inside and outside of muscle cells that causes an accelerated movement of H^+ out of the contracting muscle, helping to regulate intramuscular pH. Supplementing with sodium bicarbonate has been shown to improve MBC and in turn high-intensity exercise performance.

Efficacy   Most research investigating the efficacy of sodium bicarbonate for enhancing sport performance has focused on short bouts of high-intensity exercise lasting 60 seconds to 6 minutes (172). McNaughton and colleagues (169, 171) and Coombes and McNaughton (55) have demonstrated improved total work capacity, peak power, peak torque, and strength from acute sodium bicarbonate supplementation in men and women. Recently, Hobson and coworkers (117) examined the effects of sodium bicarbonate ingestion during a 2,000 m rowing ergometer time trial in experienced male

rowers. The rowers were supplemented before exercise with 0.3 g/kg body mass of sodium bicarbonate or a placebo. Time to complete the 2,000 m and time taken for each 500 m split were recorded. While there were no significant differences in the overall 2,000 m time trial, the sodium bicarbonate did result in significant improvements in the third and final 500 m time splits. Some investigations (28, 157), but not all (10), have reported similar improvements in high-intensity exercise following 0.3 g/kg body mass sodium bicarbonate supplementation. The timing of the sodium bicarbonate ingestion used in many scientific investigations is typically 60 to 90 minutes before the bout of exercise.

Adverse Effects   It appears that a dosage of 0.3 g/kg body mass (136 mg/pound of body mass) sodium bicarbonate ingested approximately 60 to 90 minutes before activity improves short-duration, high-intensity exercise performance (117, 172). Dosages above this amount have been associated with unpleasant side effects such as diarrhea, cramping, nausea, and vomiting. A more tolerable dose (0.2 g/kg [90 mg/pound] of body weight) has been shown to reduce these side effects; however, research has revealed that this dose does not improve exercise performance (156). It appears that a minimum sodium bicarbonate dose of 0.3 g/kg body mass, 60 to 90 minutes before exercise, is needed to improve performance (126, 251). Due to the severity of the side effects (which may be experienced by some athletes even when ingesting 0.3 g/kg body mass), many sport scientists recommend that athletes try sodium bicarbonate supplementation during practice before using it as a precompetition aid.

Sodium Citrate

Although sodium citrate is not actually a base, it can increase blood pH without the gastrointestinal distress that is commonly seen with sodium bicarbonate supplementation (242). It is believed that once in the blood, sodium citrate actually breaks down into bicarbonate, thus increasing the extracellular pH (233). As a result, sodium citrate would help regulate intramuscular pH during high-intensity exercise by the same mechanism as sodium bicarbonate.

Efficacy   The data are equivocal in terms of the effectiveness of sodium citrate's ergogenic potential during short-duration, high-intensity exercise, with some investigations reporting no benefit (15, 57, 203, 242) and others having observed an ergogenic effect (158, 170). For example, a dose of 200 mg per pound of body weight (0.44 g per kilogram of weight) given 60 to 90 minutes before exercise led to significant improvement (about 20% greater) in leg muscular endurance during maximal isometric knee extensions (112). More research, however, is needed before sodium citrate can be recommended before a workout or competition for performance enhancement.

Adverse Effects   Sodium citrate may possess MBC and has been used without the typical gastrointestinal discomfort usually associated with sodium bicarbonate ingestion (15, 158). Even though it appears that the adverse effects of sodium citrate supplementation are lower than those of sodium bicarbonate, ingestion of 0.4 to 0.6 g/kg body mass sodium citrate has the potential to cause gastrointestinal distress (182, 205). The gastrointestinal response seems to vary among individuals; therefore athletes should individually test sodium citrate supplementation before using it in competition.

L-Carnitine

L-carnitine is synthesized from the amino acids lysine and methionine and is responsible for the transport of fatty acids from the cytosol into the mitochondria to be oxidized for energy (142). Carnitine's role in lipid oxidation has generated interest in its efficacy as a dietary supplement, primarily to enhance exercise performance by increasing fat utilization and sparing muscle glycogen. However, studies examining L-carnitine's role as an ergogenic aid for increasing lipid oxidation have not shown clear efficacy in either human or rat models (8, 33). Although Bacurau and colleagues (13) showed enhanced fatty acid oxidation following three weeks of L-carnitine supplementation, which was attributed to a greater carnitine content in the muscle, most studies have been unable to demonstrate elevated muscle carnitine levels following supplementation (16, 247). This may be related to limits in the amount of carnitine that can be absorbed through oral supplementation (131), or potentially related to limits in the amount of fat that can be transported into the mitochondria through the carnitine system due to feedback regulators within the muscle, such as malonyl–coenzyme A, which is a product of metabolism.

Efficacy

Interestingly, several studies have suggested that L-carnitine may enhance recovery from exercise (116, 129, 245). Decreases in pain and muscle damage (97), decreases in markers of metabolic stress (214), and enhanced recovery (245) have also been demonstrated following high-intensity resistance exercise in untrained or recreationally trained individuals who supplemented with L-carnitine. The mechanisms that have been proposed involve enhancing blood flow regulation through an enhanced vasodilatory effect that reduces the magnitude of exercise-induced hypoxia (130). In addition, Kraemer and colleagues indicated that L-carnitine

supplementation (2 g/day for three weeks) upregulates androgen receptors (147) and increases IGF binding proteins that preserve IGF-I concentrations (148). These endocrine adaptations from the supplement may have an important role in the enhanced recovery seen following high-intensity exercise.

Adverse Effects

Up to 3 g of daily L-carnitine supplementation (for three weeks) appears to be well tolerated in healthy volunteers, with no adverse subjective, hematological, or metabolic events reported (202). Yet as with most supplements, this information should not be extrapolated to suggest the safety of greater dosing or of use for prolonged supplementation periods.

Creatine

Creatine is a nitrogenous organic compound that is synthesized naturally in the body, primarily in the liver, and helps to supply energy to all cells in the body. It can also be synthesized in smaller amounts in both the kidneys and pancreas. The amino acids arginine, glycine, and methionine are the precursors for the synthesis of creatine in those organs. Creatine can also be obtained though dietary sources. It is found in relative abundance in both meat and fish. Approximately 98% of creatine is stored within skeletal muscle in either its free form (40%) or its phosphorylated form (60%). Smaller amounts of creatine are also stored in the heart, brain, and testes. Creatine is transported from its site of synthesis to the skeletal muscle via circulation.

Importance of Creatine to Exercise

Creatine, in the form of creatine phosphate (CP; also called phosphocreatine [PCr]), has an essential role in energy metabolism as a substrate for the formation of adenosine triphosphate (ATP) by rephosphorylating adenosine diphosphate (ADP), especially during short-duration, high-intensity exercise. The ability to rapidly rephosphorylate ADP is dependent on the enzyme creatine kinase and the availability of CP within the muscle. As CP stores become depleted, the ability to perform high-intensity exercise declines. In short-duration sprints (e.g., 100 m sprint), the energy for fueling the activity is derived primarily through the hydrolysis of CP (93). However, as high-intensity exercise increases in duration, the ability of CP to serve as an energy source is drastically reduced.

Depletion of muscle CP during high-intensity exercise is the primary mechanism leading to fatigue in such events. During a 6-second bout of maximal exercise, CP levels within the muscle are reduced 35% to 57% from resting levels (93). As the duration of high-intensity exercise increases to 30 seconds, CP levels in the muscle are further reduced by approximately 64% to 80% from resting levels (31, 48); during bouts of repeated high-intensity exercise, CP levels in the muscle are almost completely depleted (168). As muscle CP concentrations decrease, the ability to perform maximal exercise is reduced. Hirvonen and colleagues (115) demonstrated that sprint times were slower as CP concentrations were reduced. It stands to reason that if muscle CP concentrations could be maintained, the ability to sustain high-intensity exercise would be improved. This is the basis for creatine supplementation in athletes.

Creatine Supplementation

Reports suggest that 37.2% of collegiate athletes use, or have used, creatine during their preparation for competition (90). However, the prevalence of use among strength/power athletes may approach more than 80% in certain sports (154). Creatine use has also gained popularity among high school athletes; 90% of athletes who supplement choose creatine (225). As a result of their widespread use, creatine supplements may be the most extensively studied ergogenic aid in recent history. Creatine supplementation is reported to increase the creatine content of muscles by approximately 20% (40, 78, 132). However, it appears that a saturation limit for creatine exists within muscle. Once creatine concentrations in skeletal muscle reach 150 to 160 mmol/kg dry weight, additional supplementation appears to be unable to further increase muscle creatine concentrations (102). This has important implications for the "more is better" philosophy that governs the thinking of some athletes, and may affect the development of proper and realistic dosing schemes.

A typical creatine supplementation regimen involves a loading dose of 20 to 25 g daily for five days, or 0.3 g/kg body mass if an individual wishes to dose relative to body weight, followed by a maintenance dose of 2 g/day (132). If one ingests creatine without an initial loading dose, muscle creatine content will reach levels similar to those seen in people who do initially use a loading dose, but reaching that muscle creatine concentration will take longer (~30 days vs. 5 days). Muscle creatine levels will remain elevated as long as the maintenance dose is maintained (2 g/day or 0.03 g/kg body mass per day) (132). Once creatine supplementation is stopped, muscle creatine levels will return to baseline levels in approximately four weeks (78, 132).

Efficacy

Most studies examining the effect of creatine supplementation on strength performance have been fairly consistent in showing significant ergogenic benefits (23, 141, 186, 243, 246) (refer to figure 11.4). Strength increases in the bench press, squat, and power clean may be two- to threefold higher in trained athletes supplementing with creatine compared to placebo (122, 186). These results may highlight the benefit of creatine supplementation in experienced resistance-trained athletes whose potential to improve strength may be limited. In experienced strength athletes, supplementing with creatine may also

> **Creatine supplementation has been shown to increase maximal strength, power, and lean body mass in both trained and untrained populations. Additionally, creatine supplementation is safe and relatively inexpensive.**

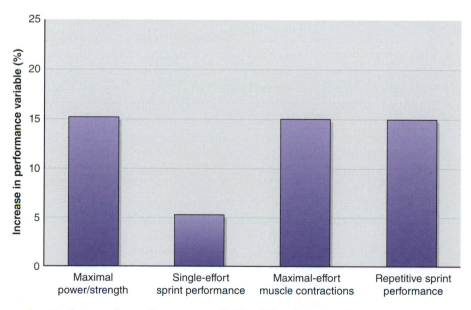

FIGURE 11.4 Approximate changes in performance variables following creatine supplementation (149).

enhance the quality of workouts (less fatigue, enhanced recovery), which may be crucial for providing a greater training stimulus to the muscle.

Most studies examining the effects of creatine supplementation on a single bout of explosive exercise (sprint performance) have not shown any significant performance improvements (62, 145, 177, 212). However, in many of these studies, subjects were supplemented with a loading dose for only five days (145, 177, 212). While ingesting creatine with a loading dose for five days will significantly increase intramuscular creatine stores, this is likely not enough time for training adaptations to occur and to be manifested in explosive exercise performance improvements. When subjects have supplemented for an extended period of time (28-84 days), significant improvements in jump and power performance have been seen (108, 243). It appears that creatine is more effective as a training supplement than as a direct performance enhancer.

Body Mass Changes

Prolonged creatine supplementation has been generally associated with increases in body weight. These increases appear to primarily relate to increases in fat-free mass. The increase in body mass is believed to be partly related to an increase in total body water. An increase in creatine content within the muscle is thought to enhance the intracellular osmotic gradient, causing water to fill the cell (244). In addition, increasing the creatine content of muscle appears to be coupled with an increased rate of muscle contractile protein synthesis (246, 255). In general, creatine supplementation during training is typically associated with a 1- to 4.5-pound (0.5-2 kg) greater increase in body mass or fat-free mass (151) over a period of several weeks to several months.

Adverse Effects

Increase in body mass has at times been referred to as a potential unwanted side effect of creatine supplementation (206), particularly in relation to strength-to-mass or power-to-mass ratio. However, in athletes supplementing with creatine, weight gain is often a desired outcome. When people talk about side effects from a drug or supplement, they are generally referring to a potentially debilitating effect. There have been many anecdotal reports of gastrointestinal, cardiovascular, and muscular problems, including muscle cramps, in association with creatine ingestion. However, controlled studies have been unable to document any significant side effects from creatine supplementation. Even during prolonged supplementation (several weeks up to many months), no increases in reported side effects were noted in subjects supplementing with creatine—either competitive athletes or recreationally trained individuals (60, 103, 151).

Another concern with any supplement is the long-term health effects. A retrospective study on health variables in 26 former or current competitive athletes who had used creatine for up to four years indicated only occasional gastrointestinal upset during the loading phase (206). These disturbances ranged from gas to mild diarrhea. Other hypothesized major concerns during creatine supplementation include a strain on the kidneys due to the high nitrogen content of creatine and increased creatine excretion during short-term ingestion. However, no renal dysfunction has been reported with either short-term (five days) or long-term (up to five years) creatine use (189, 190).

> ▶ Despite certain media and anecdotal reports linking creatine supplementation to dehydration and cramping, there is no reason to believe that creatine enhances the risk for these side effects.

Stimulants

There is little question about the usefulness of stimulants to many types of athletic endeavors; the effects of stimulants include reduced fatigue, increased alertness, increased confidence, and even euphoria. Because stimulants have to be used at the time of competition to confer an ergogenic advantage, drug testing performed immediately after the competition can effectively reduce their abuse (128). However, many stimulants (e.g., caffeine) are also available in food items, while others (e.g., ephedrine) may be found in decongestants and other medications.

Caffeine

Caffeine is a multifaceted supplement used in athletics and is popular among both endurance and resistance training athletes. It is found in coffee, tea, soft drinks, chocolate, and various other foods. It is a central nervous system stimulant, and its effects are similar to, yet weaker than, those associated with amphetamines. Caffeine has been used as a performance enhancer for more than 40 years and is one of the few ergogenic aids that may be used comparably by aerobic and anaerobic athletes.

The mechanism to explain endurance improvements is unclear. One of the mechanisms that has been proposed involves an increase in fat oxidation through the mobilization of free fatty acids from adipose tissue or intramuscular fat stores (215). The greater use of fat as a primary energy source slows glycogen depletion and delays fatigue. Alterations in muscle metabolism alone cannot fully explain the ergogenic effect of caffeine. During short-duration, high-intensity exercise, the primary ergogenic effect attributed to caffeine supplementation is enhanced power production. This is thought to be the result of an enhanced excitation–contraction coupling, affecting neuromuscular transmission and mobilization of intracellular calcium ions from the sarcoplasmic reticulum (227). In addition, caffeine ingestion is thought to enhance the kinetics of glycolytic regulatory enzymes such as phosphorylase (215).

Efficacy   For the aerobic athlete, caffeine is thought to prolong aerobic endurance exercise (56). Initial studies dealing with the effect of caffeine supplementation on aerobic endurance performance indicated a 21-minute improvement in the time to exhaustion (from 75 minutes in a placebo trial to 96 minutes in the caffeine trial) during cycling at 80% of $\dot{V}O_2$max (56). These results were confirmed by a number of additional studies demonstrating the ergogenic effect of caffeine during prolonged aerobic endurance activity (101, 216). These studies showed that caffeine in doses ranging from 3 to 9 mg/kg (equivalent to approximately 1.5 to 3.5 cups of automatic drip coffee in a 70 kg [154-pound] person) produced a significant ergogenic effect. Similar performance effects from caffeine have also been demonstrated during short-duration, high-intensity exercise (38, 67).

When the effects of caffeine ingestion on sprint or power performance are examined, however, the ergogenic benefits become less clear. Several studies have shown that caffeine ingestion does not improve power performance (52, 105), but those studies used recreational athletes. In elite Judo athletes ingesting caffeine (5 mg/kg), it was reported that peak power was significantly improved in comparison with a placebo treatment (213).

Similarly, in competitive swimmers, caffeine ingestion (250 mg) was shown to improve sprint times during repeated 100 m sprints by an average of 3% (53). The number of studies on caffeine ingestion and sprint and power performance is limited compared to the number that measured caffeine's effect on aerobic endurance performance. Thus, the results of the studies on the ergogenic benefit of caffeine for power performance are inconclusive. If there is any performance benefit, it likely occurs in the trained athlete.

Caffeine from a food source (coffee consumption) and anhydrous caffeine have both shown significant performance effects; however, the extent of performance improvements appears to be greater when caffeine is ingested in tablet form (101). When caffeine is provided as a pure caffeine supplement, the ergogenic benefit with respect to improved aerobic endurance performance has been reported to range between 28% and 43% (101). However, when it is provided in a food source such as coffee (either caffeinated coffee or decaffeinated coffee with added caffeine), the ergogenic benefit for aerobic endurance exercise may not be seen (46, 101)

or may be seen only at a reduced level (56, 236, 253). Graham and colleagues (101) suggested that although the bioavailability of caffeine is the same whether it is consumed in a food source or in an anhydrous form, some compound in coffee antagonizes the action of caffeine.

> **In doses of 3 to 9 mg/kg body weight consumed ~60 minutes before exercise or during prolonged exercise, caffeine is ergogenic. There is no further benefit when it is consumed at higher dosages (≥9 mg/kg). It can decrease feelings of perceived exertion, improve work capacity, and increase mental alertness. The scientific literature does not support caffeine-induced diuresis during exercise or any harmful change in fluid balance that would negatively affect performance.**

Adverse Effects   The side effects associated with caffeine include anxiety, gastrointestinal disturbances, restlessness, insomnia, tremors, and heart arrhythmias. Caffeine is also physically addicting, and discontinuation can result in some withdrawal symptoms, such as headache, fatigue, dysphoric mood, difficulty concentrating, and flu-like somatic symptoms (222). Caffeine intakes greater than 9 mg/kg appear to result in a greater risk for side effects (98). Caffeine overdose is an issue that can have potentially fatal consequences. A lethal dose of caffeine is typically in excess of 5 g, which equates to about 42 cups of coffee at 120 mg of caffeine per cup (143) or twenty-five 200 mg tablets of caffeine.

Preworkout Energy Drinks

Consumption of preworkout caffeine-containing liquid beverages (i.e., energy drinks) has gained in popularity over the past several years. Research has demonstrated that energy drinks are among the most popular dietary supplements consumed by young people in the United States (90). The primary reasons for ingesting energy drinks include enhancing workouts, improving sport performance, and facilitating faster training adaptations (188). The ingredients most common to commercially available energy drinks are caffeine, carbohydrates, B vitamins, tyrosine, and gingko biloba, among others. Of these ingredients, caffeine and carbohydrate are the primary ergogenic nutrients in energy drinks (43).

Efficacy   Preworkout energy drinks have been investigated for their effectiveness on several modes of exercise, including resistance exercise, anaerobic exercise, and aerobic endurance exercise. In relation to resistance exercise performance, Forbes and colleagues (83) gave 15 physically active college-aged students a commercially available energy drink or an isocaloric noncaffeinated placebo 60 minutes before exercise. The energy drink was standardized with 2 mg of caffeine/kg body mass. The exercise bout consisted of three sets of 70% 1RM bench press conducted to failure on each set with 1 minute of rest between each set. The energy drink significantly increased bench press performance as compared to the placebo treatment. Other studies investigating the effects of preworkout energy drink consumption have also reported improvements in upper and lower body total lifting volume (63, 100). While it appears that preworkout energy drink ingestion is effective for increasing resistance training volume performance, other types of anaerobic exercise (including Wingate tests and speed/agility performance) are not as responsive to energy drink consumption (11, 83, 118). In terms of endurance exercise performance, most investigations (4, 134, 249), but not all (44), have reported that energy drinks containing approximately 2 mg of caffeine/kg body mass, consumed within an hour before exercise, improve cycling and running performance in trained cyclists and recreationally active individuals (43). Interestingly, the amount of caffeine (2 mg/kg body mass) in the energy drinks is less than the amount recommended for an enhancement of exercise performance (3-9 mg/kg body mass). This contributes to the hypothesis that the synergistic effects of the various ingredients in energy drinks may be responsible for the reported improvements in exercise performance (43).

Adverse Effects   The safety issues surrounding energy drink consumption appear related to excessive caffeine intake (209) and the detrimental effects of mixing energy drinks with alcohol (127). The mixing of energy drinks with alcohol is more prevalent in certain social contexts and is not a common practice for those consuming energy drinks before a workout to enhance work capacity or to facilitate faster training adaptations. Due to the presence of caffeine in most energy drinks, the same potential adverse effects that exist for caffeine also exist for energy drinks. However, most energy drinks contain only moderate amounts of caffeine, typically less than 300 mg (234). Even though energy drinks typically contain low to moderate doses of caffeine, one should recognize that it is possible to overdose on caffeine through the consumption of energy drinks (124). While there is some information related to the side effects of excess caffeine ingestion, energy drinks contain other ingredients and stimulants. Currently, it is unknown whether inclusion of other stimulants in energy drinks may increase or decrease the threshold for experiencing side effects. Therefore, more research is needed to determine the long-term effects of habitual intake of energy drinks before definitive conclusions can be drawn.

Ephedrine

Another stimulant, ephedrine, has been widely used throughout the world for temporary relief from the symptoms of bronchial asthma, bronchitis, allergies, shortness of breath, cold and flu symptoms, and other ailments. Ephedrine is also very popular among bodybuilders due to its strong thermogenic quality (41). A thermogenic supplement or drug works by elevating basal metabolic rate, thereby increasing energy expenditure and ultimately resulting in fat loss. It often is used as a stacking agent with caffeine to enhance the thermogenic effect.

Efficacy   Studies examining the ergogenic effect of ephedrine have shown it to be effective only when it is taken in combination with caffeine (21). These results have been quite consistent with regard to improving aerobic endurance performance (19, 20). In terms of anaerobic exercise performance, the scientific literature investigating the combination of ephedrine and caffeine is equivocal (137, 254). However, side effects (vomiting and nausea) following exercise have been reported in 25% of the subjects ingesting a mixture of 5 mg/kg caffeine and 1 mg/kg ephedrine (19). A subsequent study performed by the same investigators showed that at a lower dose (4 mg/kg caffeine and 0.8 mg/kg ephedrine), similar ergogenic benefits were realized with no side effects (20). The caffeine–ephedrine mixture appears to have a greater benefit than either supplement taken alone (12).

Adverse Effects   Ephedra, also called ma huang, is a plant that contains ephedrine. In the United States before 2004, most over-the-counter sport and weight loss products contained ephedra. However, in April 2004, the FDA banned all products containing ephedra after determining that it posed an unreasonable risk to those who used it. The FDA ban was based on a report published by the Rand Institute (210) indicating that 16,000 adverse events were linked to the use of ephedra-containing dietary supplements. Further, Shekelle and colleagues (210) reported that the use of ephedra-containing dietary supplements or ephedrine plus caffeine was associated with an increased incidence of nausea, vomiting, psychiatric symptoms such as anxiety and change in mood, autonomic hyperactivity, palpitations, and in a few cases death. As a result of the many adverse effects, ephedrine use has been banned by most sport governing bodies, including the International Olympic Committee.

Citrus Aurantium

Citrus aurantium is from a fruit commonly known as "bitter orange" and is often used as an Asian herbal medicine to treat digestive problems (92, 107). However,

Summary of Ergogenic and Non-Ergogenic Dietary Supplements and Their Application

- *Essential amino acids and branched-chain amino acids*—Ability to stimulate muscle protein synthesis, particularly via the anabolic effects of the amino acid leucine.
- *Arginine*—Not effective for inducing nitric oxide or muscle blood flow in healthy individuals. Also, does not appear to have any effect on improving endurance performance in healthy populations.
- *β-Hydroxy-β-methylbutyrate (HMB)*—Most effective for trained individuals participating in a high-intensity, high-volume resistance training program.
- *β-Alanine*—Effective as a performance-enhancing substance in exercises inducing a high level of lactic acid, such as multiple bouts of high-intensity exercises lasting more than 60 seconds.
- *Sodium bicarbonate*—Has been shown to improve high-intensity exercise performance and training, but is associated with unpleasant side effects consistent with gastrointestinal discomfort.
- *Sodium citrate*—The scientific data are not conclusive in relation to sodium citrate's ergogenic potential during short-duration, high-intensity exercise.
- *L-carnitine*—May enhance recovery following high-intensity resistance exercise.
- *Creatine*—Effective for increasing maximal strength, power, and lean body mass in both trained and untrained populations.
- *Caffeine*—Effective for prolonging endurance exercise, but its effects on sprint or power performance are less clear.
- *Preworkout energy drinks*—Effective for increasing resistance training volume performance and endurance performance, but not ergogenic in their ability to improve anaerobic exercise (high-intensity cycling and speed/agility performance).
- *Ephedrine*—When combined with caffeine, is able to improve aerobic endurance performance. Not as effective in improving anaerobic exercise performance.
- *Citrus aurantium*—When combined with caffeine and other herbal products, improvements in exercise time to fatigue (a measure of endurance performance) have been reported.

it is also a mild stimulant and is thought to contribute to appetite suppression and increased metabolic rate and lipolysis (92, 107).

Efficacy

When citrus aurantium is combined with caffeine and other herbal products, significant improvements in time to fatigue have been reported (220). Citrus aurantium contains synephrine, a sympathomimetic agent, which some have suggested stimulates specific beta adrenergic receptors (β-3, but not β-1 or β-2) that in turn stimulate fat metabolism without any of the negative side effects generally associated with compounds that stimulate the other adrenergic receptors (45). Synephrine, a known active component of citrus aurantium, is thought to interact with β-3 receptors to increase lipolysis (i.e., the breakdown of body fat) and minimize the cardiovascular effect typical of adrenergic amines (45). Currently, there are not enough published data on citrus aurantium alone to recommend its use as a performance-enhancing supplement.

Adverse Effects

Synephrine has been shown to stimulate peripheral α-1 receptors, resulting in vasoconstriction and elevations in blood pressure (35). However, other research has shown that when citrus aurantium is ingested alone, no effect on blood pressure is seen (109), but in combination with other herbal products it may cause significant elevations in systolic blood pressure (109, 119). It should be noted that synephrine is currently on the National Collegiate Athletic Association's banned list of performance-enhancing drugs.

Conclusion

Athletes are frequently exposed to information about ergogenic aids. Strength and conditioning professionals play an integral part in the decision-making process regarding which ergogenic aids athletes choose to take. Therefore, it is imperative that strength and conditioning professions stay up to date on the latest scientific findings in relation to what ergogenic aids are safe, effective, and legal. If strength and conditioning professionals fail in this area, the athletes they serve will be more susceptible to hyped marketing, potentially false advertising, and influence by others who may not have the athlete's best interests in mind. The information contained in this chapter serves the strength and conditioning professional by providing fundamental information on performance-enhancing substances, including which substances are banned, effective or noneffective, and safe.

acromegaly

anabolic steroid

β-agonists

branched-chain amino acids

dietary supplement

ergogenic aid

ergolytic

erythropoietin (EPO)

essential amino acids

human growth hormone (HGH)

lipolysis

muscle buffering capacity (MBC)

muscle dysmorphia

random drug tests

stacking

testosterone

thermogenesis

vasodilation

STUDY QUESTIONS

1. Which of the following dietary supplements is (are) considered a stimulant?
   I. creatine
   II. caffeine
   III. HMB
   IV. citrus aurantium
   a. I and II
   b. II and IV
   c. III and IV
   d. I and III

2. Which of the following is NOT part of caffeine's role in improving athletic performance?
   a. increased power production
   b. decreased glycogen depletion
   c. increased fat oxidation
   d. decreased urine production

3. Which of the following is the BEST reason for aerobic endurance athletes to avoid erythropoietin use?
   a. Hematocrit and hemoglobin levels may decrease.
   b. It may cause an unregulated increase in red blood cell production
   c. Resistance to infectious disease may be impaired.
   d. It may reduce the ability of the blood to carry oxygen.

4. Creatine supplementation improves all of the following variables EXCEPT
   a. lean body mass
   b. maximal strength
   c. endurance performance
   d. power

5. Which of the following performance-enhancing substances is most likely to increase lean body mass?
   a. anabolic steroids
   b. arginine
   c. ephedrine
   d. β-alanine

CHAPTER 12

Principles of Test Selection and Administration

Michael McGuigan, PhD

The author would like to acknowledge the significant contribution of Everett Harman to this chapter.

> **After completing this chapter, you will be able to**
>
> - identify and explain reasons for performing tests,
> - understand testing terminology to communicate clearly with athletes and colleagues,
> - evaluate a test's validity and reliability,
> - select appropriate tests, and
> - administer test protocols properly and safely.

The strength and conditioning professional with a broad understanding of exercise science can effectively use tests and measurements to make training decisions that help athletes achieve their goals and maximize their potential. Tests and measurements form the objective core of the evaluation process. This chapter covers the reasons for testing, testing terminology, evaluation of test quality, the selection of appropriate tests, and aspects of proper test administration.

Reasons for Testing

Testing helps athletes and coaches assess athletic talent and identify physical abilities and areas in need of improvement. In addition, test scores can be used in goal setting. Baseline measurements can be used to establish starting points against which achievable goals can be set, and testing at regular intervals can help track an athlete's progress in reaching those goals. Using tests as a basis for goal setting allows coaches to set specific goals for individual athletes that, when taken together, help to accomplish group or team objectives (see chapter 8 for more information about goal setting).

Assessment of Athletic Talent

It is important for a coach to determine whether an individual has the physical potential to play a sport at the competitive level of the team. That judgment is not difficult if the candidate has already excelled at the sport elsewhere and is of adequate body size. However, in many cases, candidates have not clearly demonstrated their competitive abilities or may lack experience in the sport. The coach then needs some way of determining whether the candidate has the necessary basic physical abilities that, in combination with technique training and practice, could produce a competitive player. Field tests serve as tools for such assessment.

Identification of Physical Abilities in Need of Improvement

While some physical abilities are innate and not amenable to change, other physical abilities can be improved through physical training. By using appropriate testing methods and analysis, the strength and conditioning professional can determine which physical qualities of the athletes can be targeted by participation in prescribed exercise programs (25, 28).

> Testing can be used to assess athletic talent, identify physical abilities and areas in need of improvement, set goals, and evaluate progress.

Testing Terminology

To communicate clearly with athletes and colleagues, strength and conditioning professionals should use consistent terminology. The following terms and definitions are widely accepted and are used in this text:

test—A procedure for assessing ability in a particular endeavor.

field test—A test used to assess ability that is performed away from the laboratory and does not require extensive training or expensive equipment (8).

measurement—The process of collecting test data (14).

evaluation—The process of analyzing test results for the purpose of making decisions. For example, a coach examines the results of physical performance tests to determine whether the athlete's training program is effective in helping achieve the training goals or whether modifications in the program are needed.

pretest—A test administered before the beginning of training to determine the athlete's initial basic ability levels. A pretest allows the coach to design the training program in keeping with the athlete's initial training level and the overall program objectives.

midtest—A test administered one or more times during the training period to assess progress and modify the program as needed to maximize benefit.

formative evaluation—Periodic reevaluation based on midtests administered during the training, usually at regular intervals (2). It enables monitoring of the athlete's progress and adjustment of the training program according to the athlete's individual needs. It also allows evaluation of different training methods and collection of normative data. Regular modification of the training program based on formative evaluation keeps the training program fresh and interesting and helps avoid physical and mental staleness.

posttest—Test administered after the training period to determine the success of the training program in achieving the training objectives.

Evaluation of Test Quality

Test results are useful only if the test actually measures what it is supposed to measure (validity) and if the measurement is repeatable (reliability). These two characteristics are the key factors in evaluating test quality and must be present in order for the test to be beneficial.

Validity

Validity refers to the degree to which a test or test item measures what it is supposed to measure, and is one of the most important characteristics of testing (2, 22). For tests of physical properties such as height and weight, validity is easy to establish. For example, close correspondence between the readings on a spring scale and the readings on a calibrated balance scale indicates validity of weighing with the spring scale. The validity of tests of basic athletic abilities or capacities is more difficult to establish. There are several types of validity, including construct validity, face validity, content validity, and criterion-referenced validity.

> **Validity is the degree to which a test or test item measures what it is supposed to measure; this is one of the most important characteristics of testing.**

Construct Validity

Construct validity is the ability of a test to represent the underlying construct (the theory developed to organize and explain some aspects of existing knowledge and observations). Construct validity refers to overall validity, or the extent to which the test actually measures what it was designed to measure (21). Face validity, content validity, and criterion-referenced validity, defined next, are secondary to and provide evidence for construct validity.

To be valid, physical performance tests should measure abilities important in the sport, produce repeatable results (see the later section on reliability), measure the performance of one athlete at a time (unless otherwise specified in the protocol), appear meaningful, be of suitable difficulty, be able to differentiate between various levels of ability, permit accurate scoring, include a sufficient number of trials, and withstand the test of statistical evaluation. Given the choice between two valid tests, consideration should be given to simplicity and economy of test administration.

Face Validity

Face validity is the appearance to the athlete and other casual observers that the test measures what it is purported to measure. If a test or test item has face validity, the athlete is more likely to respond to it positively (1). The assessment of face validity is generally informal and nonquantitative. In other fields, such as psychology, tests may be deliberately constructed to have poor face validity because if examinees realize what a test or test item is supposed to measure, they can answer deceptively to manipulate their scores. For tests of basic athletic abilities, however, face validity is desirable based on the assumption that anyone taking a test of physical ability wants to do well and is thus motivated by a test that appears to measure a relevant capability.

Content Validity

Content validity is the assessment by experts that the testing covers all relevant subtopics or component abilities in appropriate proportions (1). For athletic testing, these include all the component abilities needed for a particular sport or sport position. Examples of component abilities in athletics are jumping ability, sprinting ability, and lower body strength (34). For example, a test battery for potential soccer players should include, at minimum, tests of sprinting speed, agility, endurance, and kicking power. To ensure content validity, the test developer should list the ability components to be assessed and make sure they are all represented on the test. In addition, the proportion of the total score attributable to a particular component ability should be proportional to the importance of that component to total performance. While the terms *face validity* and *content validity* are sometimes used interchangeably, the latter relates to actual validity while the former relates to the appearance of validity to nonexperts (1).

Criterion-Referenced Validity

Criterion-referenced validity is the extent to which test scores are associated with some other measure of the same ability. There are three types of criterion-referenced validity: concurrent, predictive, and discriminant.

Concurrent validity is the extent to which test scores are associated with those of other accepted tests that measure the same ability. Criterion-referenced validity is often estimated statistically. For example, a Pearson product–moment correlation coefficient based on the scores on a new body fat assessment device and those from dual-energy x-ray absorptiometry would provide a measure of the concurrent validity of the new test.

Convergent validity is evidenced by high positive correlation between results of the test being assessed and those of the recognized measure of the construct (the "gold standard"). Convergent validity is the type of concurrent validity that field tests used by strength and conditioning professionals should exhibit. A test may be preferable to the gold standard if it exhibits convergent validity with the standard but is less demanding in terms of time, equipment, expense, or expertise.

Predictive validity is the extent to which the test score corresponds with future behavior or performance. This can be measured through comparison of a test score with some measure of success in the sport itself. For example, one could calculate the statistical correlation between the overall score on a battery of tests used to assess potential for basketball and a measurement of actual basketball performance as indicated by a composite of such quantities as points scored, rebounds, assists, blocked shots, forced turnovers, and steals.

Discriminant validity is the ability of a test to distinguish between two different constructs and is evidenced by a low correlation between the results of the test and those of tests of a different construct (2). It is best if tests in a battery measure relatively independent ability components (e.g., flexibility, speed, aerobic endurance). Good discriminant validity of tests in a battery avoids unnecessary expenditures of time, energy, and resources in administering tests that correlate very highly with each other.

Reliability

Reliability is a measure of the degree of consistency or repeatability of a test (2, 15). If an athlete whose ability does not change is measured two times with a perfectly reliable test, the same score is obtained both times. On an unreliable test, an individual could obtain a high score on one day and a low score on another. A test must be reliable to be valid, because highly variable results have little meaning. However, even a reliable test may not be valid, because the test may not measure what it is supposed to measure. For example, both the 60 m (66-yard) dash and the 1.5-mile (2.4 km) run are reliable field tests, but only the 1.5-mile run is considered a valid field test for aerobic fitness. It is also possible for a test to be highly reliable for one group (e.g., college tennis players) but only moderately reliable for another group (e.g., high school tennis players) because of differences in physical or emotional maturity and skill level, which can affect test performance.

There are several ways to determine the reliability of a test; the most obvious one is to administer the same test several times to the same group of athletes. Statistical correlation of the scores from two administrations provides a measure of **test–retest reliability**. Any difference between the two sets of scores represents measurement error. Another statistic that can be calculated is the **typical error of measurement** (TE), which includes both the equipment error and biological variation of athletes (15). The difference between two sets of scores can arise from a number of different factors (2):

- Intrasubject (within subjects) variability
- Lack of interrater (between raters) reliability or agreement
- Intrarater (within raters) variability
- Failure of the test itself to provide consistent results

> **Reliability is a measure of the degree of consistency or repeatability of a test. A test must be reliable to be valid, because highly variable results have little meaning.**

Intrasubject variability is a lack of consistent performance by the person being tested. **Interrater reliability**, also referred to as **objectivity** or **interrater agreement** (2), is the degree to which different raters agree in their test results over time or on repeated occasions; it is a measure of consistency. A clearly defined scoring system and competent scorers who are trained and experienced with the test are essential to enhance interrater reliability. For example, even a test that appears simple, such as timing a 40-yard (37 m) dash with a stopwatch, can exhibit both random and systematic error if the timer is not trained and experienced. Sprint times obtained using handheld stopwatches are typically shorter than those obtained using automatic timers, because raters using stopwatches exhibit reaction-time delay when pressing the start button in response to the gun but do not delay in pressing the button at the finish line because they can see the athlete approaching. Interrater reliability is particularly important if different scorers administer tests to different subgroups of athletes. A subgroup with a relatively lenient scorer will have artificially inflated scores. To get an accurate measure of improvement, the same scorer should test a group at the beginning and the end of the training period. If there are two scorers and the scorer at the beginning is more or less lenient than the scorer at the end, the resulting measurements may be worthless for comparative purposes. Consider a situation in which an athlete is tested in the squat. If the pretest scorer is more lenient (requiring less depth on the squat) than the posttest scorer, the athlete may achieve a lower test score on the posttest despite having made a significant improvement in strength.

Sources of interrater differences include variations in calibrating testing devices, preparing athletes, and running the test. Different testers may motivate athletes to different degrees, based on factors such as personality, status, physical appearance, demeanor, and sex. A common scenario that increases interrater variability occurs when the coach tests some of the athletes while an assistant tests others. The athletes may be inspired to do better on the tests administered by the coach.

Intrarater variability is the lack of consistent scores by a given tester. This differs from interrater reliability, which refers to the degree of agreement between different testers. For example, a coach eager to see improvement may unintentionally be more lenient on a posttest than on a pretest. Other causes of intrarater variability include inadequate training; inattentiveness; lack of concentration; or failure to follow standardized procedures for device calibration, athlete preparation, test administration, or test scoring. To avoid such problems, accurate and consistent athletic testing should be a priority for all strength and conditioning professionals.

Finally, sometimes the test itself might fail to provide consistent results. This may occur if a physical performance test requires a technique in which the athlete has not developed consistency. More technique-intensive tests generally exhibit greater variability in results and require more pretest practice to produce consistency.

Test Selection

When evaluating tests for high levels of validity and reliability, the strength and conditioning professional must rely on her or his knowledge base and practical experience with the sport. The strength and conditioning professional must consider sport specificity (e.g., metabolic energy systems, biomechanical movement patterns), athlete experience, training status, age, and environmental factors when selecting tests.

Metabolic Energy System Specificity

A valid test must emulate the energy requirements of the sport for which ability is being assessed. Thus, the strength and conditioning professional should have a thorough understanding of the basic energy systems (phosphagen, glycolytic, and oxidative) and their interrelationships in order to apply the principle of specificity when choosing or designing valid tests to measure athletic ability for specific sports (7, 10, 16, 33). For example, in choosing an appropriate test for running ability in basketball, the strength and conditioning professional must understand that basketball is predominantly an anaerobic running sport (3, 23) and also be familiar with the distances and directions of sprints in a basketball game. It is best for the tests to simulate the physical movements and energy demands of a real game.

Biomechanical Movement Pattern Specificity

All else being equal, the more similar the test is to an important movement in the sport, the better. Sports differ in their physical demands. For example, the vertical jump test is very specific to basketball and volleyball, both of which involve vertical jumping during play, but less relevant to hockey, which does not involve vertical jumping. Positions within a sport differ as well. An American football defensive lineman needs pushing strength to move opposing linemen out of the way and 5- to 15-yard (5 to 14 m) sprint speed to reach the opposing quarterback, while a wide receiver depends less on pushing strength but must be able to sprint 30 to 100 yards (27-91 m) quickly. Thus, the bench press and 10-yard (9 m) sprint test would be more relevant to the lineman, while sprint tests of 30 to 100 yards (27-91 m) would be more relevant to the wide receiver.

> For a test to be valid, it must emulate the energy requirements and important movements of the sport for which ability is being tested.

Experience and Training Status

For a well-trained, experienced athlete, a technique-intensive test may be appropriate because it can be very sport specific, and one can assume that poor technique will not impair performance of the test. However, this assumption cannot be made for an athlete just learning or trying out for a sport. The number of one-leg hops needed to travel 27 yards (25 m) may represent a valid and reliable test of plyometric strength for an experienced long jumper but not for a novice (8).

Testers must also consider the training status of the athletes being tested. It would not be ideal, for example, to ask a baseball player to perform a 3-mile (4.8 km) run test a week before the beginning of fall practice, because the player has probably been doing interval training and relatively short runs (29). A lower body strength test using the parallel squat would not be an ideal test for an athlete who has trained using the leg press exclusively.

Age and Sex

Both age and sex can affect the validity and reliability of a test. For example, the 1.5-mile (2.4 km) run may be a valid and reliable field test of aerobic power for college-aged men and women (18) but may not be appropriate for preadolescents because of their probable lack of experience and interest in sustained running (27). A test of the maximum number of chin-ups that can be performed may be a valid test of elbow flexion muscular endurance for male wrestlers, but it may not be as valid for females due to differences in upper body pulling strength (24). The test may not be capable of differentiating muscular endurance levels in females. Therefore using a modified prone pull-up with the feet supported may be a more valid test.

Environmental Factors

It is necessary to consider the environment when selecting and administering tests of basic athletic ability. High ambient temperature, especially in combination with high humidity, can impair endurance exercise performance, pose health risks, and lower the validity of an aerobic endurance exercise test. Aerobic endurance performance (26, 32) and intermittent sprint performance (13) may be impaired when the temperature approaches 80 °F, especially if the humidity exceeds 50% (17). The effects of temperature and humidity on testing performance can create problems for comparing the results of tests administered at different times of year, on different days, and even at different times of day. For example, the maximal oxygen uptake of an athlete impaired by the heat is underestimated by the 1.5-mile (2.4 km) run test. Run times can also be impaired by cold temperatures. Thus, outdoor aerobic endurance tests may be inappropriate at locations characterized by wide fluctuations in temperature. In such places, aerobic endurance tests can be administered on an indoor track, if available, or with a treadmill or stationary cycle.

Altitude can also impair performance on aerobic endurance tests, although not on tests of strength and power (11). Norms on aerobic endurance tests should be adjusted when testing at altitudes exceeding 1,900 feet (580 m). Up to about 9,000 feet (2,740 m), maximal oxygen uptake declines by approximately 5% for each 3,000 feet (910 m) of elevation. At even higher altitudes, maximal oxygen uptake declines more sharply. Athletes who arrive at a relatively high altitude after living near sea level for an extended period of time should be given at least 10 days to acclimatize before undergoing aerobic endurance tests (31). For all testing, it is good practice to measure and document the environmental conditions and then to consider these factors when interpreting the results.

> **Athletes' experience, training status, age, and sex can affect test performance, so these factors should be considered in test selection. Environmental factors such as temperature, humidity, and altitude can also influence test performance, so testers should try to standardize environmental conditions as much as possible.**

Test Administration

To achieve accurate test results, tests must be administered safely, correctly, and in an organized manner. Strength and conditioning professionals should ensure the health and safety of athletes; testers should be carefully selected and trained; tests should be well organized and administered efficiently; and athletes should be properly prepared and instructed.

Health and Safety Considerations

Even though all athletes should be medically cleared before being permitted to physically train and compete, the strength and conditioning professional must be aware of testing conditions that can threaten the health of athletes and be observant of signs and symptoms of health problems that warrant exclusion from testing (4). The strength and conditioning professional must remain attentive to the health status of athletes, especially

before, during, and after maximal exertions that occur during training, testing, and competition. Strenuous exercise, such as maximal runs or 1-repetition maximum (1RM) tests, can uncover or worsen existing heart problems, such as impaired blood flow to the heart muscle and irregular heartbeats. Standard medical screening cannot always reveal hidden heart problems, which occasionally result in fatality among young athletes (27). Heat injury is also a risk during heavy physical exertion in hot environments, especially when humidity is high. Athletes should wear light clothing in warm weather and drink water ad libitum according to the dictates of thirst before and during heavy physical exertion in the heat (refer to chapters 9 and 10 for more detailed hydration guidelines). Musculoskeletal injuries can also be a problem. If symptoms are ignored, recovery can be greatly delayed.

Medical referral may be warranted for an athlete who persistently has any of the following symptoms: chest pressure, pain, or discomfort; listlessness; light-headedness; dizziness; confusion; headache; deeply reddened or cold and clammy skin; irregular pulse; bone or joint pain; blurred vision; nausea; or shortness of breath, rapid pulse, or weakness either not commensurate with the level of exertion or unresponsive to rest. Such symptoms can occur long after exercise is terminated. Even symptoms that occur only once, if severe (such as loss of consciousness), call for immediate medical attention.

When aerobic endurance exercise tests are being administered in a hot environment, caution must be observed to protect both the health and safety of the athlete and the validity of the test. Figure 12.1 lists temperature limits at various ranges of relative humidity for strenuous exercise testing, and the sidebar lists guidelines for aerobic endurance testing in the heat.

Selection and Training of Testers

Test administrators should be well trained and should have a thorough understanding of all testing procedures and protocols. The testing supervisor should make sure that all novice personnel perform and score all tests correctly, as in timing sprint speed with a stopwatch or determining a 1RM back squat. It is essential that all testers have sufficient practice so that the scores they obtain correlate closely with those produced by experienced and reliable personnel. The testers should be trained to explain and administer the tests as consistently as possible. Test reliability is impaired, for example, if one test administrator provides considerable verbal encouragement to a group of athletes while another tester provides no verbal encouragement to another group. Administrators should have a checklist of materials needed for testing and written test protocols to refer to if questions arise during the testing process.

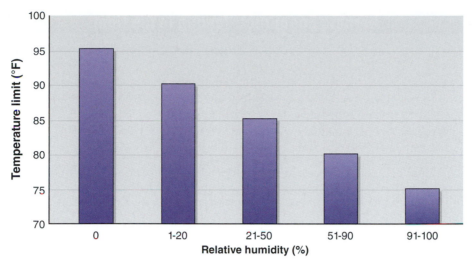

FIGURE 12.1   Temperature limits at various ranges of relative humidity for strenuous exercise testing.

Data from McArdle, Katch, and Katch (20).

Recording Forms

Scoring forms should be developed before the testing session and should have space for all test results and comments. Factors such as environmental conditions should be documented. The specific details of setup for the testing should also be noted. For example, for a 1RM squat, the tester can note the pin height that was used for the barbell. This allows test time to be used more efficiently and reduces the incidence of recording errors.

Test Format

A well-organized testing session, in which the athletes are aware of the purpose and procedures of the testing, will enhance the reliability of test measures. Reliable measures obtained from valid tests are a great asset in assessing fitness levels and evaluating changes over a period of time.

Test planning must address such issues as whether athletes will be tested all at once or in groups and whether the same person will administer a given test to all athletes. The main consideration here is the number of athletes that are being tested. It is preferable to have the same person administer a given test if time and schedules permit, because this eliminates the issue of interrater reliability. If this is not feasible, the test supervisor can allow simple, well-defined tests (such as counting correct push-ups) to be administered by different testers and tests requiring schooled judgment (as of proper form in the squat) to be scored by the most skilled and experienced personnel. As a rule, each tester should administer only one test at a time, especially when the tests require complex judgments. It is permissible to have one tester alternate between two testing stations to avoid wasting time as athletes get ready. However, the tester must focus on only one test at a time. Planning and practicing the testing sessions beforehand will go a long way toward ensuring an efficiently run testing session.

Testing Batteries and Multiple Testing Trials

When time is limited and the group of athletes is large, duplicate test setups may be employed to make efficient use of testing time. For example, when one is conducting the 300-yard (274 m) shuttle, two test courses can be set up (12). A tester can administer up to two nonfatiguing tests in sequence to an athlete as long as test reliability can be maintained. For example, at a two-test lower body power station staffed by only one tester, the athlete can perform the vertical jump test and the static jump test immediately afterward.

When multiple trials of a test (e.g., the repeated trials it takes to find a 1RM) or a battery of tests is performed, allow complete recovery between trials (28). There should be at least 2 minutes of rest between attempts that are not close to the athlete's maximum and 3 minutes between attempts that are close to the maximum, as judged by the relative difficulty of the previous trial or testing set (19). When administering a **test battery** (e.g., one in which wrestlers perform maximal repetition pull-up and push-up tests for assessment of local muscular endurance), tests should be separated by at least 5 minutes to prevent the effects of fatigue from confounding test results (also see the following section, "Sequence of Tests").

Sequence of Tests

Knowledge of exercise science can help determine the proper order of tests and the duration of rest periods

Aerobic Endurance Testing in the Heat

Follow these guidelines to minimize health risks and obtain accurate results when testing athletes in hot environments (6, 20, 27):

1. During the weeks before the test, athletes should engage in enough training to establish a baseline of fitness in the activity being tested. Strength and conditioning professionals should be aware that responses to exercise in the heat are highly individual.

2. Avoid testing under extreme combinations of heat and humidity. Figure 12.1 lists the combinations of temperature and humidity at which heat injury risk is present. Using temperature limits at least 5 °F (3 °C) below those listed is recommended, especially on sunny days, to provide a safety margin and enable better test performance. On days when the temperature has exceeded or is expected to exceed the recommended limits, indoor facilities should be used if available; or testing should be conducted during morning or early evening hours when temperatures are acceptable.

3. The athletes, especially those coming from cool climates, should be acclimatized to the heat and humidity for at least one week before testing. Start with short workouts and progress to workouts of longer duration.

4. Athletes should make sure they are well hydrated in the 24-hour period preceding aerobic endurance testing in the heat. A good indication of adequate hydration is a plentiful volume of clear urine (refer to chapter 9 for more detailed preexercise hydration guidelines). Salt tablets should generally be avoided.

5. Athletes should be encouraged to drink during exercise in the heat. Plain water is most appropriate for exercise up to 1 hour in duration. Snack breaks during longer durations of training can help replenish fluids and be important in replacing electrolytes. The amount and rate of fluid replacement depend on individual sweat rates, duration of exercise, and environment. Refer to chapter 9 for specific guidelines and how to calculate sweat rate if needed.

6. Athletes should wear a light-colored, loose-fitting tank top and shorts that are breathable (i.e., synthetic porous, moisture-wicking material). Male athletes may be allowed to go shirtless.

7. Heart rate may be monitored to detect reactions to the heat.

8. Be attentive to possible symptoms of heatstroke or heat exhaustion: cramps, nausea, dizziness, difficulty in walking or standing, faintness, garbled speech, lack of sweat, red or ashen skin, and goose bumps.

9. Be aware of the symptoms of hyponatremia or water intoxication, a potentially fatal condition in which excess water intake reduces blood sodium to dangerously low levels. Symptoms may include extremely dilute urine in combination with bloated skin, altered consciousness, or loss of consciousness, with no increase in body temperature. A victim of hyponatremia should never be given fluid and should be treated by a physician.

10. Proficient medical coverage should be readily available so that an athlete encountering a test-related health problem can be very rapidly treated or evacuated (or both).

between tests to ensure test reliability. The fundamental principle with test sequencing should be that one test should not affect the performance of a subsequent test. This should allow for optimal performance in each test and also allows for valid comparisons with previous testing results. For example, a test that maximally taxes the phosphagen energy system requires 3 to 5 minutes of rest for complete recovery (5, 9), whereas a maximal test of the anaerobic glycolytic energy system requires at least 1 hour for complete recovery (7). Therefore, tests requiring high-skill movements, such as agility tests, should be administered before tests that are likely to produce fatigue and confound the results of subsequent tests. A logical sequence, although there are some variations, is to administer tests in this order:

1. Nonfatiguing tests (e.g., height, weight, flexibility, skinfold and girth measurements, vertical jump)

2. Agility tests (e.g., T-test, pro agility test)

3. Maximum power and strength tests (e.g., 1RM power clean, 1RM squat)

4. Sprint tests (e.g., 40 m sprint with split times at 10 m and 20 m)

5. Local muscular endurance tests (e.g., push-up test)

6. Fatiguing anaerobic capacity tests (e.g., 300-yard [275 m] shuttle)

7. Aerobic capacity tests (e.g., 1.5-mile [2.4 km] run or Yo-Yo intermittent recovery test)

The test order should also be designed to require minimal recovery time between tests, allowing for a more efficient testing session. An effort should be made to administer fatiguing anaerobic capacity tests and aerobic tests on a different day than the other tests. However, if performed on the same day, these tests should be performed last, after an extended rest period.

It is important that test sessions be conducted at the same time of day to avoid fluctuations in physiological responses due to differences in circadian rhythm (30). It is also recommended that tests be conducted indoors, which will allow for climate and testing surfaces to remain more consistent.

> ▶ **The order of tests should be designed in such a way that the completion of one test does not adversely affect performance in subsequent tests.**

Preparing Athletes for Testing

The date, time, and purpose of a test battery should be announced in advance to allow athletes to prepare physically and mentally. To maximize test reliability, athletes should be familiar with test content and procedures. A short, supervised pretest practice or familiarization session one to three days before the test, in which the athletes exert themselves at somewhat less than full intensity, is often beneficial. If this is done, it should be repeated at all future testing sessions. One strategy could be to incorporate familiarization of the tests into training sessions.

The instructions should cover the purpose of the test, how it is to be performed, the amount of warm-up recommended, the number of practice attempts allowed, the number of trials, test scoring, criteria for disallowing attempts, and recommendations for maximizing performance. The instructions that are given to the athletes need to be clear and concise as this will increase the reliability and objectivity of the test (22).

As an important supplement to reading test instructions aloud, the test administrator or a competent assistant should demonstrate proper test performance when possible. The athletes should be given opportunities to ask questions before and after the demonstration. The test administrator should anticipate questions and have answers prepared. It is important to motivate all athletes equally rather than giving special encouragement to only some. Whenever possible, tell athletes their test scores immediately after each trial to motivate them to perform better on subsequent trials (2).

Reliability of testing improves with pretest warm-up (2). An appropriately organized warm-up consists of a general warm-up followed by a specific warm-up. Both types of warm-ups include body movements similar to those involved in the test. An organized, instructor-led general warm-up ensures uniformity. It is acceptable to allow two or three activity-specific warm-up trials, depending on the test protocol, and have subsequent trials actually count toward the score. Depending on the test protocol, the score can be the best or the average of the post-warm-up trials (2).

> ▶ **General and specific warm-ups performed before a test can increase the test's reliability.**

Administer a supervised cool-down period to athletes following tests that dramatically increase heart rate and at the completion of the test battery. For example, after the 300-yard (274 m) shuttle, the athlete should not sit or lie down; active recovery using low-intensity movement and light stretching will enhance the recovery process (7).

Conclusion

Tests and measurements can be used to assess athletic talent, identify physical capacities in need of improvement, provide reference values to evaluate the effectiveness of a training program, and set realistic training goals. To optimize test quality, testers must understand and consider validity and reliability. Test selection involves consideration of the physiological energy systems required by the sport; movement specificity; and the athletes' experience, training status, age, and sex. Testers must also consider environmental factors such as temperature, humidity, and altitude before administering tests. Strength and conditioning professionals must always remain conscious of potential health risks during testing and attentive to signs and symptoms of possible health problems that require medical referral. Testers must be carefully selected and well trained, and the testing session must be well planned and organized using the appropriate testing sequence. Consistent and effective preparation of athletes for testing is essential.

KEY TERMS

concurrent validity
construct validity
content validity
convergent validity
criterion-referenced validity
discriminant validity
evaluation
face validity
field test

formative evaluation
interrater agreement
interrater reliability
intrarater variability
intrasubject variability
measurement
midtest
objectivity
posttest

predictive validity
pretest
reliability
test
test battery
test–retest reliability
typical error of measurement
validity

STUDY QUESTIONS

1. A college basketball coach would like to know which one of her players has the most muscular power. Which of the following is the MOST valid test for measuring muscular power?
   a. vertical jump
   b. 1RM bench press
   c. 5RM squat
   d. 100 m (109-yard) sprint

2. When measuring maximal strength of a soccer player, which of the following could potentially adversely affect the test–retest reliability of the results?
   I. using multiple testers
   II. retesting at a different time of day
   III. an athlete's inexperience with the tested exercise
   IV. using an established testing protocol
   a. I and III only
   b. II and IV only
   c. I, II, and III only
   d. II, III, and IV only

3. All of the following procedures should be followed when testing an athlete's cardiovascular fitness in the heat EXCEPT
   a. performing the test in an indoor facility
   b. using salt tablets to retain water
   c. scheduling the test in the morning
   d. drinking fluids during the test

4. The bench press, vertical jump, and 10 m (11-yard) sprint are the MOST valid tests for which of the following American football positions?
   a. quarterback
   b. defensive back
   c. wide receiver
   d. defensive lineman

5. Which of the following sequences will produce the MOST reliable results?
   a. 1RM power clean, T-test, 1.5 mile (2.4 km) run, 1RM bench press
   b. T-test, 1RM power clean, 1RM bench press, 1.5 mile (2.4 km) run
   c. 1.5 mile (2.4 km) run, 1RM bench press, T-test, 1RM power clean
   d. 1RM bench press, 1RM power clean, T-test, 1.5 mile (2.4 km) run

CHAPTER 13

Administration, Scoring, and Interpretation of Selected Tests

Michael McGuigan, PhD

 After completing this chapter, you will be able to

- discern the best ways to measure selected parameters related to athletic performance,
- administer field tests appropriately,
- evaluate and analyze test data and make normative comparisons,
- understand appropriate statistics, and
- combine the results of selected tests to generate an athletic profile.

The author would like to acknowledge the significant contributions of Everett Harman and John Garhammer to this chapter.

As discussed in chapter 12, the strength and conditioning professional—often referred to as *tester* in this chapter—who has a broad understanding of exercise science can effectively choose and use tests and measurements to make training program decisions that help athletes optimize their physical preparation and maximize their potential. To do this effectively, the tester must administer tests correctly, analyze test data accurately, and then combine the results of selected tests to generate an athletic profile. This chapter covers these basic aspects of testing performance-related parameters and provides comprehensive age- and sport-specific descriptive and normative data for selected tests.

Measuring Parameters of Athletic Performance

Athleticism incorporates many physical abilities, some of which are much more amenable to training than others. Such abilities may be called components of **athletic performance**, that is, the ability to respond effectively to the various physical demands of the specific sport or event. This section focuses on how each component can be tested and highlights relevant issues.

Maximum Muscular Strength (Low-Speed Strength)

Maximal strength tests usually involve relatively low movement speeds and therefore reflect **low-speed muscular strength**. In this case, muscular strength is related to the force a muscle or muscle group can exert in one maximal effort while maintaining proper form, and it can be quantified by the maximum weight that can be lifted once (the 1-repetition maximum [1RM]) in exercises such as the bench press or back squat, the maximum force exerted isometrically (against an immovable object) as measured with a transducer, or the maximum force that can be exerted at a particular isokinetic speed (5, 6, 31, 48, 70, 71, 73, 77, 90). As 1RM tests do not require expensive equipment and reflect the kind of dynamic ability necessary in sport, they are the maximal strength tests of choice for most strength and conditioning professionals.

In general, 1RM tests are administered after the athlete has warmed up by performing a few sets of the test exercise with submaximal loads, beginning with a relatively light load. The first attempt is usually with approximately 50% of the athlete's estimated 1RM weight. After the athlete has rested enough to feel recovered from the previous attempt (1-5 minutes, depending on the difficulty of the attempt), the strength and conditioning professional increases the weight somewhat, based on the ease with which the previous trial was performed.

A skilled strength and conditioning professional should, within three to five attempts following warm-up, be able to find the athlete's 1RM load to within a few percentage points of the true value.

Anaerobic or Maximum Muscular Power (High-Speed Strength)

High-speed muscular strength or **maximal anaerobic muscular power** (or **anaerobic power**) is related to the ability of muscle tissue to exert high force while contracting at a high speed. Tests of such strength and power are of very short duration, are performed at maximal movement speeds, and produce very high power outputs. High-speed maximal muscular power tests are often called (maximal) anaerobic power tests. Scores on high-speed muscular strength tests include the 1RM of explosive exercises (e.g., the power clean, snatch, push jerk), the height of a vertical jump, and the time to sprint up a staircase (45, 70, 77, 90, 93). As explosive exercise tests take about 1 second while low-speed maximal strength tests generally require 2 to 4 seconds to complete, phosphocreatine and adenosine triphosphate (ATP) stored in the active muscle(s) are the primary energy sources for both types of tests. Maintaining correct technique or form is also important when measuring anaerobic power for both performance validity and safety reasons.

> ▶ Most maximal muscular strength tests use relatively slow movement speeds and therefore reflect low-speed strength. Assessment of high-speed muscular strength can involve measuring the 1RM of explosive resistance training exercises or the height of a vertical jump.

Power output reflects both force and velocity. The height of a jump is a function of the force put into the ground and the velocity at which the athlete leaves the ground. An athlete may not improve in jump height after gaining body weight during a resistance training cycle, making it appear that power output is unchanged. However, because the athlete is heavier and propels the body to the same height, indicating the same takeoff velocity, an increase in power output is evident. This applies to any test in which body weight is manipulated (e.g., running up stairs). Moving a heavier body at the same speed requires a higher power output.

An alternative class of anaerobic power tests involves the use of a cycle ergometer. This type of test can be advantageous for the strength and conditioning professional in some injury situations in which running is restricted or when the athlete participates in a non-body-weight-support sport such as rowing or cycling. The most commonly used test of this type is the Wingate anaerobic test. A field test protocol involves use of a cycle ergometer with mechanical means of adjusting resistance and measuring pedal revolutions and rate (rpm). In a laboratory setting, an electronically instrumented ergometer can simplify parameter measurement and improve accuracy. Typical protocols involve a basic warm-up followed by a 30-second test interval (27). In this test, resistance is applied quickly after the individual reaches a near-maximal pedaling rate (typically 90 to 110 rpm). The resistance applied is proportional to body weight; the percentage is greater for trained athletes than for individuals with less training. Work performed is determined from the resistance value and number of pedal revolutions. Power is generally calculated as work divided by time for each 5-second time interval during the 30-second test. Parameters typically calculated include peak power, average power, and a fatigue index such as a ratio of maximum to minimum interval power. Norms for cycle ergometer tests are available (47, 73).

Anaerobic Capacity

Anaerobic capacity is the maximal rate of energy production by the combined phosphagen and anaerobic glycolytic energy systems for moderate-duration activities. It is typically quantified as the maximal power output during muscular activity between 30 and 90 seconds using a variety of tests for the upper and lower body (27, 73, 90, 115), as opposed to maximal anaerobic power tests, which last no longer than a few seconds.

Local Muscular Endurance

Local muscular endurance is the ability of certain muscles or muscle groups to perform repeated contractions against a submaximal resistance (11, 73). A test of local muscular endurance should be performed in a continuous manner for several seconds to several minutes without the advantage of rest periods and without extraneous body movements. Examples include performing a maximal number of repetitions in the chin-up, parallel bar dip, or push-up exercises or a resistance training exercise using a fixed load (e.g., a percentage of an athlete's 1RM or body weight) (26, 64, 70, 73).

Aerobic Capacity

Aerobic capacity, also called **aerobic power**, is the maximum rate at which an athlete can produce energy through oxidation of energy sources (carbohydrates, fats, and proteins) and is usually expressed as a volume of oxygen consumed per kilogram of body weight per minute (i.e., ml·kg^{-1}·min^{-1}) (65). Few strength and conditioning professionals have the equipment to measure oxygen consumption directly, so aerobic capacity is generally estimated by performance in aerobic endurance activities such as running 1 mile (1.6 km) or more (45, 79, 88). It can also be estimated using other field tests such as the maximal aerobic speed (MAS) test (60) and the Yo-Yo intermittent recovery test (9, 13, 58, 59).

Agility

Agility has traditionally been considered the ability to stop, start, and change the direction of the whole body rapidly (101, 108). Agility consists of two main components: speed in changing direction and cognitive factors (101). More recently the definition of agility has been revised to take into account the perceptual qualities, and it is now considered "a rapid, whole-body, change of direction or speed in response to a sports-specific stimulus" (101, 108). Agility testing is generally confined to physical capacity tests such as change-of-direction speed or cognitive components such as anticipation. Tests such as the T-test, 505 agility, and pro agility test are used to assess change of direction.

Speed

Speed is movement distance per unit time and is typically quantified as the time taken to cover a fixed distance. The time taken to sprint from a stationary start over a short distance such as 10 yards (9.3 m) reflects acceleration, whereas longer sprints such as 40 yards (37.1 m) would measure maximum speed (126). Tests of speed are not usually conducted over distances greater than 100 m (109.4 yards) because longer distances reflect anaerobic or aerobic capacity more than absolute ability to move the body at maximal speed (73, 90, 126).

Electronic timing devices are becoming more accessible to strength and conditioning professionals due to increased ease of use and lower prices. However, many tests of speed and agility are administered using hand timing with a stopwatch, which can be a major source of measurement error, especially if the tester is not sufficiently trained. Even under ideal conditions, stopwatch-measured sprint times are up to 0.24 seconds faster than electronically measured times because of the tester's reaction-time delay in pressing the stopwatch button at the gun and the tendency to anticipate and press the button early as the athlete approaches the finish line (31, 44, 91). Therefore strength and conditioning professionals are encouraged to use electronic timing devices for tests of speed and agility when they are available. It is also more informative to measure split times, as this can provide the strength and conditioning professional with insight into the speed and acceleration capacities of the athletes. For example, times for 10 yards (9.1 m), 20 yards (18.3 m), and 40 yards (36.6 m) can be recorded and used to calculate split times and maximal velocity.

Finally, tests of speed and agility require proper footwear and a nonslip surface.

Flexibility

Flexibility can be defined as the range of motion about a body joint (11). Typical devices for measuring flexibility include manual and electric goniometers, which measure joint angle, and the sit-and-reach box, which is used to evaluate the combined flexibility of the lower back and hips. Flexibility measurements are more reliable when standardized warm-up and static stretching precede the flexibility assessment. During a flexibility test, the athlete should move slowly into the fully stretched position and hold this position. Ballistic stretching, characterized by bouncing to increase range of motion, cannot be allowed during any flexibility testing (45, 79).

A number of physical competency screens are available for strength and conditioning professionals and can be used to assess overall flexibility, mobility, and general movement competency of athletes. However there is no current consensus on which screen to use or a clearly established link between results of screening and injury (68, 84). Good strength and conditioning professionals perform postural and performance screening routinely by viewing the athletes' performance in training. For example, the overhead squat is a common exercise that is used as a part of movement screens as it is able to assess bilateral mobility of hips, knees, and ankles along with shoulder and thoracic spine (3, 16, 93).

Balance and Stability

Balance is the ability to maintain static and dynamic equilibrium or the ability to maintain the body's center of gravity over its base of support (73, 90). **Stability** is a measure of the ability to return to a desired position following a disturbance to the system (73). Athletes with poor balance are at a greater risk of lower limb injuries (52, 53). Athletes have also been shown to have greater balance compared to nonathletes (23). Balance testing can be used to assess stability increases with training and in a number of different ways (73). Commonly used tests include timed static standing tests (eyes closed and standing on one or both legs) (14, 66), balance tests using unstable surfaces (66), and tests using specialized balance testing equipment (NeuroCom, Biodex Balance System) (90). These include a large number of tests that can evaluate different aspects of balance and stability (73). The balance error scoring system (BESS) and star excursion balance test (SEBT) have very good reliability and a substantial body of literature supporting their use (14, 41, 43, 73, 83, 111).

Body Composition

Body composition usually refers to the relative proportions by weight of fat and lean tissue. Although there are sophisticated and expensive devices capable of partitioning the lean component into bone and nonbone lean tissue, the body composition procedures typically performed by strength and conditioning professionals use the basic two-compartment (fat and lean) model. With a trained and competent tester, the skinfold measurement technique is the most valid and reliable ($r = 0.99$) means for assessing body fatness that is generally available to the strength and conditioning professional and is preferable to body circumference methods (65), although dual x-ray absorptiometry (DEXA) and underwater (hydrostatic) weighing are often labeled as the "gold standards." The skinfold method uses calipers that measure the thickness of a double layer of finger-pinched skin and subcutaneous fat. A good skinfold measurement device should squeeze the fold of skin and fat with constant pressure regardless of the amount of tissue being measured (28, 45, 88). Circumference methods may be added, as they are relatively quick and simple and can yield important chronic disease risk information. For example, waist circumference can assess abdominal fat, and a high waist circumference is associated with an increased risk for type 2 diabetes, high cholesterol, high blood pressure, and certain types of cardiac disease (45).

Anthropometry

Anthropometry, which is the science of measurement applied to the human body, generally includes measurements of height, weight, and selected body girths (45). Ideally, height should be measured with a stadiometer. If a stadiometer is not available, measurement of height requires a flat wall against which the athlete stands, with a measuring tape attached or unattached to the wall. Height is usually measured without shoes to the nearest quarter-inch or half-centimeter (73).

The most accurate body mass or body weight measurement is performed with a certified balance scale, which is generally more reliable than a spring scale and should be calibrated on a regular basis (73). A calibrated electronic scale is an acceptable alternative. Athletes should be weighed while wearing minimal dry clothing (e.g., gym shorts and T-shirt, no shoes). For comparison measurements at a later date, they should dress similarly and be weighed at the same time of day. The most reliable body mass measurements are made in the morning upon rising, after elimination and before ingestion of food or fluids. Level of hydration can result in variability of body mass (weight). Thus, athletes should be encouraged to avoid eating salty food (which increases water retention) the day before weighing and to go to bed normally hydrated.

The most reliable girth measurements are usually obtained with the aid of a flexible measuring tape equipped with a spring-loaded attachment at the end that, when pulled out to a specified mark, exerts a fixed amount of tension on the tape. Girth measurements should be made at the beginning of a training period for comparison with subsequent measurements (45, 73).

Testing Conditions

As discussed in detail in chapter 12, in order to maximize the reliability of tests, it is essential that testing conditions be as similar as possible for all the athletes tested and from test to retest of the same athlete. The environmental conditions should not differ from test to test. For any particular test conducted on the ground, the surface should always be the same and should not be wet for one test and dry for another. Maximum strength tests should use the same type of racks with the supports set at the same height for a given athlete. For jumping tests, the type of equipment used should be consistent.

Athletes should never be tested after fatiguing sport activities or workouts. They should arrive for testing normally hydrated and with standard nutrition before commencing the testing. Standardization of testing also includes not taking supplements before performing the test (e.g., creatine monohydrate can enhance performance on some tests) (119). It is best to perform tests and retests at approximately the same time of day (92). Warm-up for the tests should be standardized and should include both a general dynamic warm-up such as jogging or light calisthenics and a specific warm-up that involves movements like those required by the test, such as practice of the test at submaximal intensity. Familiarization and practice of the tests to be performed by the athletes are also critical aspects. Stretching is appropriate for any test requiring flexibility.

SELECTED TEST PROTOCOLS AND SCORING DATA

13.1　1RM BENCH PRESS

Equipment

- A barbell, weight plates, and two safety locks; enough total weight to accommodate the maximum load of the strongest athlete; and a variety of plate sizes to allow for 5-pound (2.5 kg) gradations in weight
- A sturdy bench press bench with integral bar rack (preferably of adjustable height)

Personnel

- One spotter, one recorder

Procedure

1. Instruct the athlete in proper technique for the flat barbell bench press as described in chapter 15.
2. The spotter stands at the head end of the bench throughout the test to help in raising the bar on a failed attempt and to help the athlete place the bar back on the rack.
3. As with any maximal strength test, the athlete first does a specific warm-up of 5 to 10 repetitions with a light to moderate load.
4. Usually, at least two heavier warm-up sets of two to five repetitions each are completed before the first actual 1RM attempt.
5. Generally, it is desirable to measure the 1RM within three to five attempts after the warm-up; otherwise fatigue may detract from the final result.
6. A more detailed step-by-step method for the 1RM protocol is shown in figure 17.1.

Note: Normative and descriptive data for the 1RM bench press are presented in tables 13.1 and 13.4 near the end of the chapter.

13.2　1RM BENCH PULL

Equipment

- A barbell, weight plates, and two safety locks; enough total weight to accommodate the maximum load of the strongest athlete; and a variety of plate sizes to allow for 5-pound (2.5 kg) gradations in weight
- A sturdy bench

Personnel

- One spotter, one recorder

Procedure

1. Instruct the athlete in proper technique for the bench pull (figure 13.1).
2. The athlete grasps the bar with a closed pronated grip, wider than shoulder-width.
3. Bench height is set so the athlete can use a comfortable grip while the weight is off the ground in the hang position.
4. The athlete starts the lift from the hang position, and the grip should be consistent from test to test.
5. The bar is pulled up toward the lower chest or upper abdomen with the elbows pointed up.
6. The head position can remain either down or to the side but must remain in contact with the bench throughout the test.
7. A valid repetition is one in which the bar touches the underside of the bench and the bar is lowered in a controlled manner to the hang position with full elbow extension without touching the ground.
8. The feet should remain off the ground throughout the test and in the same position throughout.
9. A more detailed step-by-step method for the 1RM protocol is shown in figure 17.1.

Note: Descriptive data for the 1RM bench pull are presented in table 13.4 near the end of the chapter.

(continued)

13.2 *(continued)*

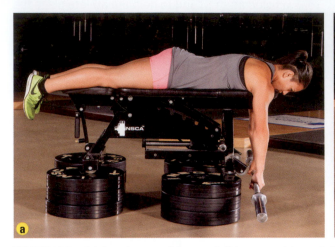 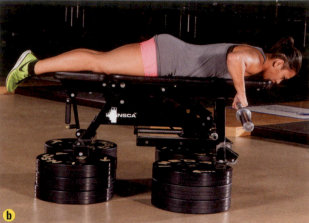

FIGURE 13.1 *(a)* Starting position and *(b)* top position of the bench pull.

13.3 1RM BACK SQUAT

Equipment

- A barbell, weight plates, and two safety locks; enough total weight to accommodate the maximum load of the strongest athlete; and a variety of plate sizes to allow for 5-pound (2.5 kg) gradations in weight
- A sturdy squat rack with adjustable spotting bars to support the weight of the bar if the athlete is unable to rise (as an alternative, one spotter can be used at each end of the bar)
- A flat and solid surface to stand on

Personnel

- Two spotters, one recorder

Procedure

1. Instruct the athlete in proper technique for the back squat as described in chapter 15.
2. Warm-up sets are performed as for the 1RM bench press test. However, the loads lifted are typically heavier than in the 1RM bench press test, so the load increments will be greater than those of the 1RM bench press.
3. Refer to figure 17.1 for a 1RM testing protocol.

Note: Normative and descriptive data for the 1RM back squat are presented in tables 13.1 through 13.4 near the end of the chapter.

13.4 1RM POWER CLEAN

Note: Because the power clean exercise has high technical demands, two athletes with the same muscular power capacity can differ greatly in their tested 1RM, lessening the value of the test for predicting athletic performance.

Equipment

- An Olympic-style barbell with a revolving sleeve, weight plates, and two safety locks; enough total weight to accommodate the maximum load of the strongest athlete; and a variety of plate sizes to allow for 5-pound (2.5 kg) gradations in weight
- A lifting platform or designated area set apart from the rest of the facility for safety

Personnel

- One tester/recorder

Procedure

1. Instruct the athlete in proper technique for the power clean as described in chapter 15.
2. Warm-up sets are performed and load increments are selected as for the 1RM bench press test.
3. Refer to figure 17.1 for a 1RM testing protocol.

Note: Normative and descriptive data for the 1RM power clean are presented in tables 13.1 through 13.4 near the end of the chapter.

13.5 STANDING LONG JUMP

Equipment

- A flat jumping area at least 20 feet (6 m) in length, which can be a gym floor, artificial turf, grass field, or a track
- A tape measure at least 10 feet (3 m) long
- Duct tape or masking tape
- Permissible alternative: a commercial jumping mat premarked in half-inch (1 cm) increments

Personnel

- One distance judge, one recorder

Procedure

1. Place a 2- to 3-foot (0.6-0.9 m) length of tape on the floor to serve as a starting line.
2. The athlete stands with the toes just behind the starting line.
3. The athlete performs a countermovement and jumps forward as far as possible.
4. The athlete must land on the feet for the jump to be scored. Otherwise the trial is repeated.
5. A marker is placed at the back edge of the athlete's rearmost heel, and the tape measure determines the distance between the starting line and the mark.
6. The best of three trials is recorded to the nearest 0.5 inches or 1 cm.

Note: Normative and descriptive data for the standing long jump are presented in tables 13.5 to 13.7 near the end of the chapter.

13.6   VERTICAL JUMP

Equipment

- A smooth wall with a ceiling higher than the highest jumper's jump height
- A flat floor with good traction
- Chalk of a different color than the wall
- Measuring tape or stick
- Permissible alternative: a commercial device for vertical jump testing (e.g., Vertec)

Personnel

- One tester/recorder

Procedure (Using a Wall and Chalk)

1. The tester rubs chalk on the fingertips of the athlete's dominant hand.

2. The athlete stands with the dominant shoulder about 6 inches (15 cm) from the wall and, with both feet flat on the floor, reaches as high as possible with the dominant hand and makes a chalk mark on the wall.

3. The athlete then lowers the dominant hand and, without a preparatory or stutter step, performs a countermovement by quickly flexing the knees and hips, moving the trunk forward and downward, and swinging the arms backward (figure 13.2a). During the jump, the dominant arm reaches upward while the nondominant arm moves downward relative to the body.

4. At the highest point in the jump, the athlete places a second chalk mark on the wall with the fingers of the dominant hand, using a swiping motion of the fingers. The score is the vertical distance between the two chalk marks.

5. The best of three trials is recorded to the nearest 0.5 inches or 1.0 cm.

Procedure (Using a Commercial Vertec Device)

1. The tester adjusts the height of the stack of movable color-coded horizontal plastic vanes to be within the athlete's standing reach height. The highest vane that can be reached and pushed forward with the dominant hand while the athlete stands flat-footed determines the standing touch height.

2. The vane stack is then raised by a measured distance (marked on the shaft holding the vanes) so that the athlete will not jump higher or lower than the set of vanes. This requires a rough estimate of how high the particular athlete will jump, but a correction can be made on the second attempt if necessary.

3. Without a preparatory or stutter step, the athlete performs a countermovement by quickly flexing the knees and hips, moving the trunk forward and downward, and swinging the arms backward (figure 13.2a). During the jump, the dominant arm reaches upward while the nondominant arm moves downward relative to the body.

4. At the highest point in the jump, the athlete taps the highest possible vane with the fingers of the dominant hand (figure 13.2b). The score is the vertical distance between the height of the highest vane tapped during the standing vertical reach and the vane tapped at the highest point of the jump.

5. The best of three trials is recorded to the nearest 0.5 inches or 1 cm (the distance between adjacent vanes).

Note: Descriptive data for the vertical jump are presented in table 13.7 near the end of the chapter.

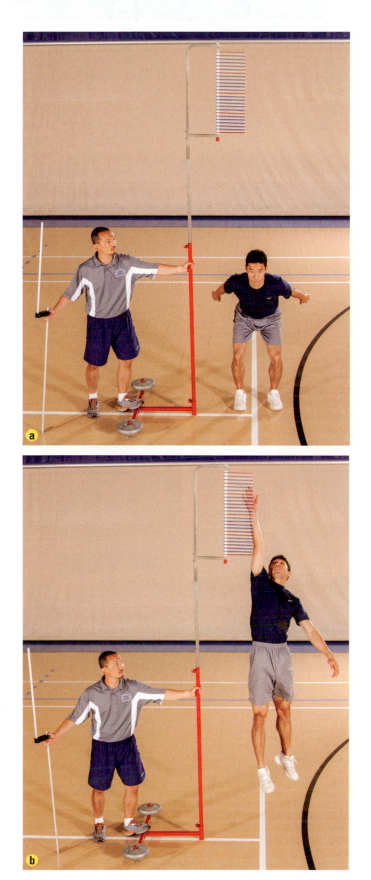

FIGURE 13.2 (a) Starting position and (b) maximum height of the vertical jump.

13.7 STATIC VERTICAL JUMP

Procedure (Using a Contact Mat System)

1. The test procedures are essentially the same as for the vertical jump, except that the countermovement is removed. Begin with the athlete standing on the mat (or force plate). *(Note: The vertical jump with countermovement can also be tested using a contact mat system.)*

2. The athlete descends into a squat position (knee angle approximately 110°) and holds this position for 2 to 3 seconds before jumping vertically (figure 13.3).

3. From the measuring device, obtain the jump height.

4. The takeoff and landing positions, as well as jumping strategy, should be the same for each trial.

5. The best of three trials is recorded. The ratio of the vertical jump height with countermovement to squat jump height can be calculated as the eccentric utilization ratio (69).

Note: Descriptive data for the static vertical jump are presented in table 13.7 near the end of the chapter.

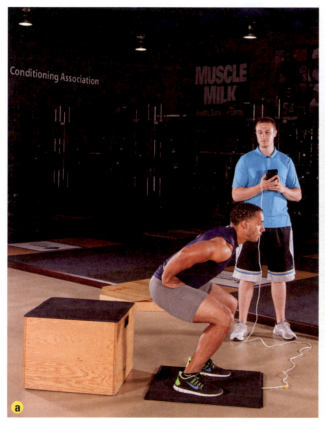 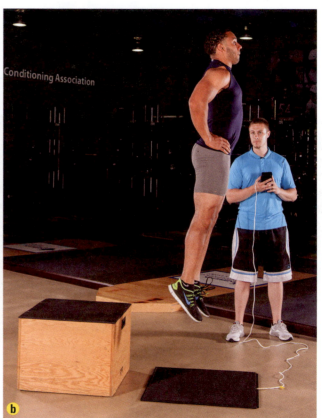

FIGURE 13.3 *(a)* Starting position and *(b)* maximum height of the static vertical jump.

13.8   REACTIVE STRENGTH INDEX

Equipment

- Boxes of varying heights—for example, 20 cm (7.9 inches), 30 cm (11.8 inches), and 40 cm (15.7 inches)
- A commercial device able to measure contact time—for example, a jump or contact mat (contact mat systems calculate jump height using flight time (37, 62, 122)

Personnel

- One tester/recorder

Procedure

1. Begin with the athlete standing on top of the drop box with the contact mat placed at least 0.2 m in front of the box.
2. Instruct the athlete to place hands on hips, to step forward off the box without stepping down or jumping up, and, upon contact with the ground, to jump as high as possible while minimizing contact time as much as possible (figure 13.4).
3. The takeoff and landing positions, as well as jumping strategy, should be the same for each trial.
4. From the measuring device, obtain the jump height and contact times.
5. The best of three trials is recorded.
6. Calculate the reactive strength index as jump height divided by contact time.
7. The procedure can be repeated from boxes of varying heights to obtain a stretch tolerance profile for the athlete.

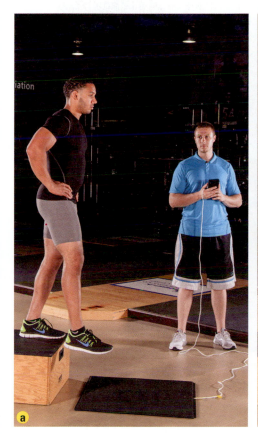 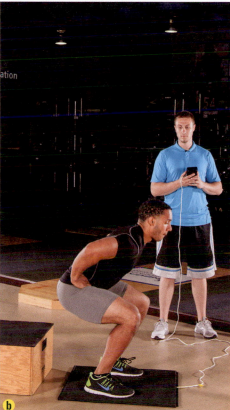 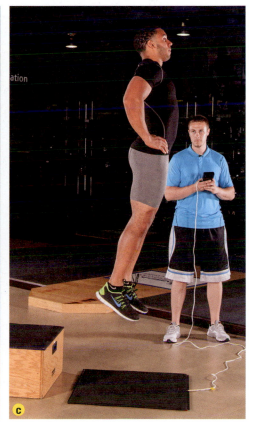

FIGURE 13.4   *(a)* Starting position, *(b)* contact on mat, and *(c)* maximum height of the drop jump test to measure reactive strength index.

13.9   MARGARIA-KALAMEN TEST

Equipment

- Staircase with nine or more steps, each approximately 7 inches (18 cm) high, and a straight and flat lead-up area 20 feet (6 m) or more in length (figure 13.5)
- Measuring tape or stick
- An electronic timing system with both a start and a stop switch mechanism
- Scale

Personnel

- One tester/recorder

Procedure

1. The height of each step is measured with a ruler or tape measure, and the elevation from the third step to the ninth step is calculated (6 × step height).
2. The timer start switch mechanism is placed on the third step, and the stop switch mechanism is placed on the ninth step.

3. The athlete to be tested is weighed on a scale, warms up, and practices running up the stairs three steps at a time.
4. When ready, the athlete sprints toward the stairs from a standing start 20 feet (6 m) from the base of the stairs and then up the staircase three steps at a time (third step to sixth step to ninth step) as fast as possible.
5. The time from third- to ninth-step contact is determined to the nearest 0.01 seconds using the timing system.
6. Power in watts is calculated as the athlete's weight *(w)* in newtons (pounds × 4.45 or kg × 9.807) times height *(h)* in meters (inches × 0.0254) from the third step to the ninth step divided by the measured time interval *(t)* in seconds; *P* (watts) = *(w × h) / t*.
7. Repeat the test two more times with a 2- to 3-minute recovery period between each trial.

Note: Normative data for the Margaria-Kalamen test are presented in table 13.8 near the end of the chapter.

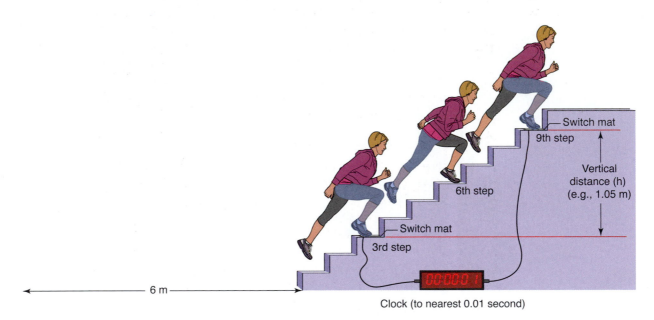

FIGURE 13.5   Margaria-Kalamen stair sprint test.

From E. Fox, R. Bowers, and M. Foss, 1993, *The physiological basis for exercise and sport*, 5th ed. (Dubuque, IA: Wm. C. Brown), 675. Reprinted with permission of McGraw-Hill companies.

13.10 300-YARD (274 m) SHUTTLE

Equipment

- A stopwatch with at least 0.1-second resolution
- Two parallel lines 25 yards (22.86 m) apart on a flat surface (figure 13.6)

Personnel

- One timer, two line judges

Procedure

1. Pair off athletes of similar ability.
2. Position two athletes immediately behind one line, facing the other line.
3. On an auditory signal, the athletes sprint to the line 25 yards (22.86 m) away, making foot contact with it, then immediately sprint back to the first line. Six such round trips are made as fast as possible without stopping (6 × 50 yards = 300 yards, or 274 m).
4. On completion of the first trial, record both athletes' times to the nearest 0.1 seconds and start a clock to time a 5-minute rest interval. As each pair of athletes completes the first trial, they may walk and stretch but must stay alert for the starting time on the second trial.
5. After the rest period, the pair of athletes does another trial.
6. The average of two trials is recorded to the nearest 0.1 second.

Note: Descriptive data for the 300-yard (274 m) shuttle are presented in table 13.9 near the end of the chapter.

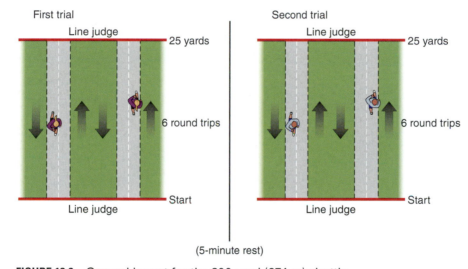

FIGURE 13.6 Ground layout for the 300-yard (274 m) shuttle.

Adapted, by permission, from Gilliam, 1983 (38).

13.11 PARTIAL CURL-UP

The partial curl-up test measures the muscular endurance of the abdominal muscles. It is favored over the sit-up test because it eliminates the use of the hip flexor muscles.

Equipment
- Metronome
- Ruler
- Masking tape
- Mat

Personnel
- One recorder/technique judge

Procedure
1. The athlete assumes a supine position on a mat with a 90° knee angle (figure 13.7a). The arms are at the sides, resting on the floor, with the fingers touching a 4-inch-long (10 cm) piece of masking tape positioned perpendicular to the fingers. A second piece of masking tape is situated parallel to the first tape at a distance determined by the age of the athlete (4.7 inches [12 cm] for those younger than 45 and 3.1 inches [8 cm] for those 45 or older).

2. Set a metronome to 40 beats per minute and have the individual do slow, controlled curl-ups to lift the shoulder blades off the mat (trunk makes a 30° angle with the mat; figure 13.7b) in time with the metronome (20 curl-ups per minute). The upper back must touch the floor before each curl-up. The athlete should avoid flexing the neck to bring the chin close to the chest.

3. The athlete performs as many curl-ups as possible without pausing, to a maximum of 75.

Note: Normative data for the partial curl-up are presented in table 13.10 near the end of the chapter.

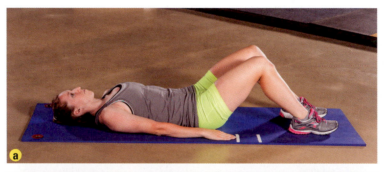

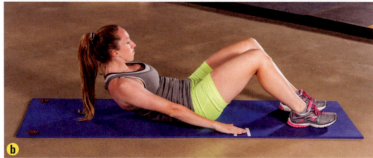

FIGURE 13.7 Curl-up: *(a)* beginning position and *(b)* end position.

13.12   PUSH-UP

Equipment

- A 4-inch (10 cm)-diameter foam roller (for female athletes)

Personnel

- One recorder/technique judge

Procedure

1. For both the Army and American College of Sports Medicine (ACSM) standards, men assume the standard push-up starting position with hands shoulder-width apart and elbows and body straight (figure 13.8a). For the Army standards, women assume the same position as the men. For the ACSM standards, women start similarly except that the knees rather than the feet contact the ground, with the knees flexed at 90° and the ankles crossed (figure 13.9a).

2. For the Army standards, the push-up low position is when the upper arms are parallel to the ground (figure 13.8b). For the ACSM standards, the low position for males is when the chest makes contact with the recorder's fist held vertically against the ground. There is no standard criterion for the female low position (30), but it has been suggested that females make torso contact with a foam roller on the ground rather than a fist (figure 13.9b). For either standard, repetitions that do not achieve the required low position are not counted.

3. For the Army standard, as many repetitions as possible are done within a timed 2-minute period. The athlete may pause only in the up position. For the ACSM standard, as many repetitions as possible are done continuously until failure.

Note: ACSM normative data for the push-up are presented in table 13.11 near the end of the chapter. Army push-up point scores are shown in table 13.12.

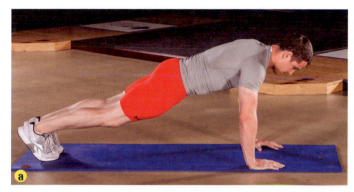
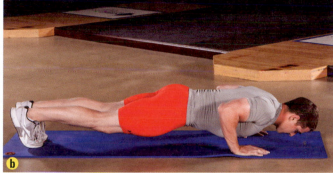

FIGURE 13.8   Push-up according to Army standard: *(a)* beginning position and *(b)* end position.

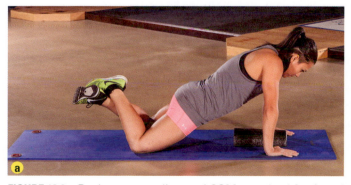
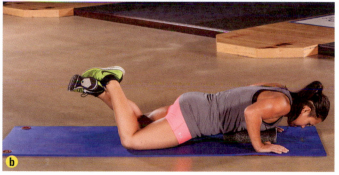

FIGURE 13.9   Push-up according to ACSM standard for females: *(a)* beginning position and *(b)* end position.

13.13 YMCA BENCH PRESS TEST

Equipment

- A barbell, weight plates, two safety locks, and enough total weight to assemble an 80-pound (36 kg) or a 35-pound (16 kg) load (including safety locks)
- Flat bench press bench (preferably with an upright rack to hold the barbell)
- Metronome

Personnel

- One spotter/recorder

Procedure

1. Instruct the athlete in proper technique for the flat barbell bench press as described in chapter 15.
2. The spotter/recorder stands at the head end of the bench throughout the test to help in raising the bar on a failed attempt and to help the athlete place the bar back on the rack.
3. Set the resistance at 80 pounds (36 kg) for males and 35 pounds (16 kg) for females.
4. Set the metronome cadence at 60 beats per minute to establish a rate of 30 repetitions per minute (one beat up, one beat down).
5. The athlete grips the bar at shoulder-width, lifts the bar off the rack, and extends the elbows. Then, in time with the metronome, the bar is repeatedly lowered to the chest and raised up again, so that the elbows are extended, until the athlete can no longer keep up with the metronome. The movement should be smooth and controlled, with the bar reaching its highest and lowest position with each beat of the metronome.

Note: Normative data for the YMCA bench press test are presented in table 13.13 near the end of the chapter.

13.14 1.5-MILE (2.4 km) RUN

Equipment

- Stopwatch
- Quarter-mile running track or measured and marked 1.5-mile (2.4 km) flat course with a good running surface. A 1.86-mile (3 km) course can also be used as an alternative.

Personnel

- One tester to call off each athlete's time, one recorder

Procedure

1. Have each athlete warm up and stretch before the test.
2. Each athlete should be recognizable to the scorer at the finish line. If that is not possible, numbers should be pinned to the athletes' shirts.
3. At the start, all runners should line up behind the starting line.
4. Instruct the athletes to complete the run as quickly as possible at a steady pace that they can barely maintain over the distance. (*Note:* Some athletes may have limited experience at pacing long efforts such as this, so some familiarization and prior pacing efforts in training are suggested.)
5. On an auditory signal, the athletes start running and cover the course as quickly as possible.
6. As the runners cross the finish line, each runner's time is recorded on a form as a timer calls off the time in minutes and seconds (00:00).

Note: Normative data for the 1.5-mile (2.4 km) run are presented in tables 13.14 through 13.17 near the end of the chapter. For each 1.5-mile (2.4 km) run time, the tables show an estimated maximal rate of oxygen consumption; the norms for athletes in various sports are shown in table 13.18 near the end of the chapter.

13.15 12-MINUTE RUN

Equipment

- A 400 m (437-yard) track or flat looped course with a marker at each 100 m
- Stopwatch

Personnel

- One tester to call out each athlete's position, one recorder

Procedure

1. Athletes line up at the starting line.
2. On an auditory signal, the athletes travel by foot as far as possible in 12 minutes, preferably by running, but if necessary by walking part or all of the time.
3. At 12 minutes, on an auditory signal, all the athletes stop in place.
4. The distance run by each athlete (laps $\times$ 400 m— e.g., 5.25 laps $\times$ 400 m = 2,100 m) is calculated and recorded.

Note: Normative data for the 12-minute run are presented in table 13.19 near the end of the chapter.

13.16 YO-YO INTERMITTENT RECOVERY TEST

The use of the Yo-Yo intermittent recovery tests (IRT1 and IRT2) is now commonplace in field testing protocols for team sports (9, 13, 58). It is suggested that these tests are more specific to team sports as they mimic the demands of short intensive bursts of exercise followed by short recovery periods. Both of the tests consist of 2 × 20 m shuttle runs at increasing speeds interspersed with a 10-second period of recovery, with the IRT1 starting at 10 km/h and the IRT2 starting at 13 km/h. It is recommended that strength and conditioning professionals use the IRT1.

Equipment

- Cones
- A tape measure at least 30 m long
- Audio software specifically for the Yo-Yo intermittent recovery test, IRT1 (available from a variety of commercial sources)
- Method of broadcasting the audio files (e.g., wireless speakers)
- Recording sheet
- Flat floor with good traction

Personnel

- One tester/recorder, one spotter

Procedure

1. Measure out a 20 m test course and arrange cones as seen in figure 13.10. Place markers 2 m apart at both ends of the test course at the start and turning lines. Also measure out a 5 m distance behind the start line.

2. Have the athletes warm up and stretch before the test. The athletes should run the course with a submaximal effort for practice.

3. The test begins with the athletes standing at the start line.

4. On an auditory signal, the athletes run forward to the turning line. At the sound of the second signal, athletes arrive at the turning line and then run back to the starting line, arriving in time with the next sound.

5. When the start marker is passed, the athletes jog toward the 5 m mark, then turn back to the start line. At this point the athletes stop and wait for the next sound.

6. The athletes are required to place one foot on or over the starting or turning line at the sound of each beep.

7. The athletes continue running for as long as they can maintain the increasing speed as indicated by the auditory signals.

8. The termination of the test is indicated by the inability of an athlete to maintain the required pace for two trials. A warning is given the first time the start or turning line is not reached.

9. At the end of the test, record the last level and number of 2 × 20 m intervals performed at that level on a recording sheet.

10. The final Yo-Yo intermittent recovery speed and interval score can be used to calculate the total distance covered by the athlete during the test.

Note: Descriptive data for the Yo-Yo intermittent recovery test are presented in table 13.20 near the end of the chapter.

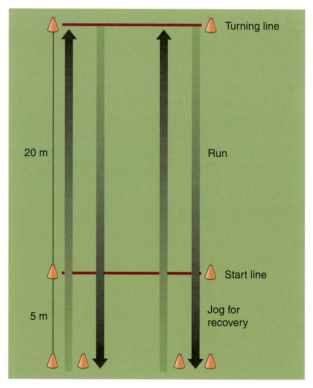

FIGURE 13.10 Setup for the Yo-Yo intermittent recovery test.

Aerobic Capacity

13.17 MAXIMAL AEROBIC SPEED TEST

Equipment

- Cones
- A tape measure at least 30 m long
- Audio software specifically for the MAS test
- Method of broadcasting the audio files (e.g., wireless speakers)
- Recording sheet
- Indoor or outdoor running track (at least 200 m)

Personnel

- One tester/recorder

Procedure

1. Marker cones are placed at 25 m intervals around the running track.
2. The initial speed of the test is set between 8 and 12 km/h depending on the fitness level of the athlete. It is generally recommended that athletes start at 10km/h.
3. The speed is then increased by 1 km/h every 2 minutes until the athlete cannot maintain the speed.
4. The last speed maintained for at least 2 minutes is considered the speed associated with $\dot{V}O_2$max or MAS.
5. The test is terminated if the athlete fails to reach the next cone on two consecutive occasions in the required time.
6. The speed at the last completed stage is increased by 0.5 km/h if the athlete is able to run a half stage.
7. The $\dot{V}O_2$max of the athlete can be calculated by multiplying 3.5 × MAS (speed in kilometers per hour) (60).
8. If the coach does not have access to the audio version, it is possible to conduct the test using a whistle. Calculate the timing of whistles using a set speed for reaching the next cone. For example, when the distance between cones is 25 m, the timing of whistles for 10 km/h would be every 9 seconds.

Note: Norms for the $\dot{V}O_2$max of athletes in various sports are shown in table 13.18 near the end of the chapter.

13.18 T-TEST

Equipment
- Four cones
- A tape measure at least 5 yards (4.6 m) long
- Stopwatch
- Flat floor with good traction

Personnel
- One tester/recorder, one spotter

Procedure
1. Arrange four cones as shown in figure 13.11 (points A, B, C, and D).
2. Have the athlete warm up and stretch before the test. The athlete may run the course with a submaximal effort for practice.
3. The test begins with the athlete standing at point A.
4. On an auditory signal, the athlete sprints forward to point B and touches the *base* of the cone with the right hand.
5. Then, while facing forward and not crossing the feet, the athlete shuffles to the left 5 yards (4.6 m) and touches the *base* of the cone at point C with the left hand.
6. The athlete then shuffles to the right 10 yards (9.1 m) and touches the *base* of the cone at point D with the right hand.
7. The athlete then shuffles to the left 5 yards and touches the *base* of the cone at point B with the left hand, and next runs backward past point A, at which time the watch is stopped.
8. For safety, a spotter and gym mat should be positioned several feet behind point A to catch an athlete who falls while running backward.
9. The best time of two trials is recorded to the nearest 0.1 seconds.
10. Reasons for disqualification of a trial: The athlete fails to touch the base of any cone, crosses one foot in front of the other instead of shuffling the feet, or fails to face forward for the entire test.

Note: Descriptive data for the T-test are presented in table 13.21 near the end of the chapter.

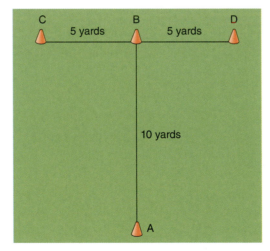

FIGURE 13.11   Floor layout for the T-test.

Adapted, by permission, from Semenick, 1990 (100).

13.19 HEXAGON TEST

Equipment

- Adhesive tape of a color that contrasts with the floor
- Measuring tape or stick
- Stopwatch
- Flat floor with good traction

Personnel

- One timer/recorder, one line judge

Procedure

1. Using the adhesive tape, create a hexagon on the floor with 24-inch (61 cm) sides meeting to form 120° angles (figure 13.12).
2. The athlete warms up and practices performance of the test at submaximal speed.
3. The test begins with the athlete standing in the middle of the hexagon.
4. On an auditory signal, the athlete begins double-leg hopping from the center of the hexagon over each side and back to the center, starting with the side directly in front of the athlete, in a continuous clockwise sequence until all six sides are covered three times (three revolutions around the hexagon for a total of 18 jumps) and the athlete is again standing at the center. The athlete remains facing the same direction throughout the test.
5. If the athlete lands on a side of the hexagon rather than over it, or loses balance and takes an extra step or changes the direction in which he or she is facing, the trial is stopped and restarted after the athlete is allowed time for full recovery.
6. The best time of three trials is recorded to the nearest 0.1 seconds.

Note: Descriptive data for the hexagon test are presented in table 13.21 near the end of the chapter.

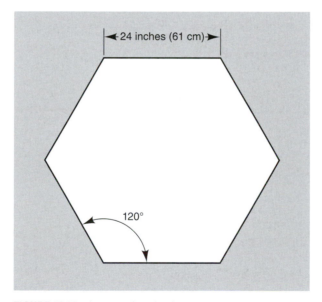

FIGURE 13.12 Layout for the hexagon test.

Adapted, by permission, from Pauole, et al., 2000 (86).

13.20 PRO AGILITY TEST

This test is also called the 20-yard (18.3 m) shuttle.

Equipment
- An American football field or other field marked with three parallel lines 5 yards (4.6 m) apart (figure 13.13)
- A stopwatch

Personnel
- One timer/recorder, one line judge

Procedure
1. The athlete straddles the centermost of the three parallel lines using a three-point stance.
2. On an auditory signal, the athlete sprints 5 yards (4.6 m) to the line on the left, then changes direction and sprints 10 yards (9.1 m) to the line on the right, then again changes direction and sprints 5 yards (4.6 m) to the center line. Hand (or foot) contact must be made with all indicated lines. (*Note:* It is important that this is kept consistent for both trials.)
3. The best time of two trials is recorded to the nearest 0.01 seconds.

Note: Normative data for the pro agility test are presented in table 13.22 near the end of the chapter.

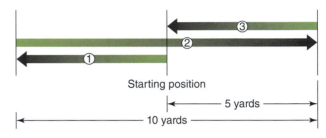

FIGURE 13.13 Layout for the pro agility test.

13.21 505 AGILITY TEST

Equipment
- 7 cones
- A stopwatch or timing lights

Personnel
- One timer/recorder, one line judge

Procedure
1. Arrange the cones as seen in figure 13.14. If timing lights are available, these can also be set up as shown.
2. Have the athlete warm up and stretch before the test. The athlete may run the course with a submaximal effort for practice.
3. The test begins with the athlete standing at the start line.
4. On an auditory signal, the athlete sprints forward 10 m to the first set of timing lights, then sprints a further 5 m to the turning line (one foot must be on or over the line), where he or she is required to turn and accelerate off the line.
5. The athlete may slow down only after passing through the timing lights for the second time.
6. The best time of two trials is recorded to the nearest 0.1 second.
7. The athlete completes the trials turning off the preferred leg. Alternatively, trials (at least two) can be given turning off either leg.

Note: Descriptive data for the 505 agility test are presented in table 13.21 near the end of the chapter.

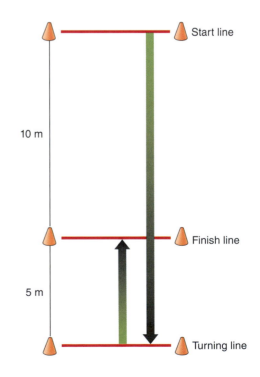

FIGURE 13.14 Layout for the 505 agility test.

13.22 STRAIGHT-LINE SPRINT TESTS

Equipment

- Stopwatch or timing lights
- Flat running surface with start and finish lines a specified distance apart (e.g., 40 yards or 37 m; 10 m, 20 m, 40 m), with at least 20 yards (18 m) after the finish line for deceleration

Personnel

- One timer/recorder

Procedure

1. Have the athlete warm up and dynamically stretch for several minutes.
2. Allow at least two practice runs at submaximal speed.
3. The athlete assumes a starting position using a three- or four-point stance.
4. On an auditory signal, the athlete sprints the specified distance at maximal speed.
5. The best split times of two trials are recorded to the nearest 0.1 second.
6. Allow at least 2 minutes of active recovery or rest between trials.

Note: Normative data for the 10 m, 20 m, 40 m, and 40-yard (37 m) sprint are presented in table 13.23 near the end of the chapter.

13.23 BALANCE ERROR SCORING SYSTEM (BESS)

Equipment
- Foam balance pad
- Stopwatch

Personnel
- One timer/recorder

Procedure
1. The six positions of the BESS are shown in figure 13.15.
2. The three stance positions are double-leg stance with feet together, single-leg stance on the nondominant foot with contralateral leg in approximately 90° of flexion, and tandem stance with the dominant foot in front of the nondominant foot (95). The test is conducted on a firm surface and on a soft surface.
3. The stances are held for 20 seconds with eyes closed for each condition and hands on hips.
4. Athletes are told to keep as steady as possible, and if they lose balance, they attempt to regain their initial position as quickly as possible.
5. Errors include opening eyes; lifting hands from hips; touchdown of nonstance foot; step, hop, or other movement of the stance foot or feet; lifting forefeet or heel; moving hip into more than 30° of hip flexion or abduction; or remaining out of position for more than 5 seconds.
6. The error scores from the BESS test are summed into a single score.

Note: Normative data for the BESS are presented in table 13.24 near the end of the chapter.

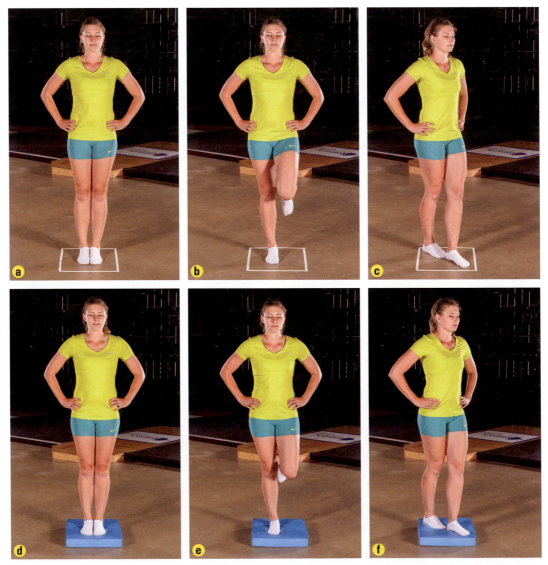

FIGURE 13.15 Balance error scoring system (BESS): *(a-c)* firm surface condition and *(d-f)* soft surface condition.

13.24 STAR EXCURSION BALANCE TEST (SEBT)

Equipment
- Adhesive tape

Personnel
- One recorder

Procedure
1. The athlete stands in the center of a grid with eight lines (120 cm) extending out at 45° increments as shown in figure 13.16 (83, 93).
2. The athlete maintains a single-leg stance facing in one direction while reaching with the contralateral leg as far as possible for each taped line, touching the farthest point possible and then returning to the bilateral position. Within a single trial, the athlete remains facing in the beginning direction and the stance leg remains the same, with the other leg doing all of the reaching.
3. The distance from the center of the star to the touch position is measured.
4. The starting direction and support leg are chosen randomly. Three trials are performed for each condition and averaged.
5. A 15-second rest is allowed between each of the reaches.
6. Trials are discarded if the athlete does not touch the line, lifts stance foot from the center grid, loses balance, or does not maintain start and return positions for 1 full second.
7. Athletes should be given a minimum of four practice trials before being tested (73).
8. It has been suggested that testing the anteromedial, medial, and posteromedial positions is sufficient for most situations (43).

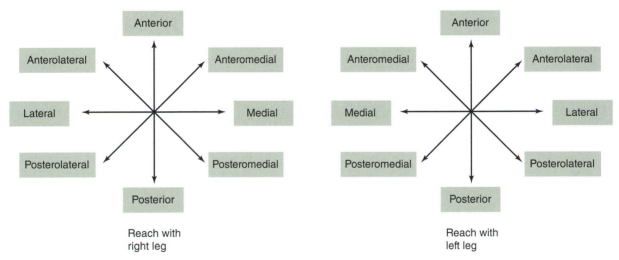

Reach with right leg

Reach with left leg

FIGURE 13.16 Directions for the star excursion balance test (SEBT).

Reprinted, by permission, from Reiman and Mankse, 2009 (93).

13.25 SIT-AND-REACH TEST

Note: A consistent method for the sit-and-reach test should be maintained if the test is done periodically. For example, if the test is performed with a measuring tape or stick during initial testing of the athlete, all subsequent testing of the athlete should be performed with a measuring tape or stick (i.e., a sit-and-reach box should not be used instead).

Equipment
- Measuring tape or stick
- Adhesive tape
- Permissible alternative: a standard sit-and-reach box

Personnel
- One tester/recorder

Procedure
1. Tape the measuring stick or tape measure to the floor. Place one piece of tape about 24 inches (61 cm) long across the measuring stick and at a right angle to it at the 15-inch (38 cm) mark.
2. Have the athlete warm up with nonballistic exercises involving the hamstrings and lower back (for example, by walking rapidly for 3 to 5 minutes); performing several repetitions of flexing forward from a standing, knees-straight position, reaching toward the toes, then reaching upward toward the ceiling (all without jerking); jogging in place while trying to kick the heels into the upper thighs from behind; and finishing with standing toe-touching or similar stretching on the floor.
3. Have the athlete sit shoeless with the measuring stick between the legs with its zero end toward the body, the feet 12 inches (30 cm) apart, the toes pointed upward, and the heels nearly touching the edge of the taped line at the 15-inch (38 cm) mark (figure 13.17*a*).
4. Have the athlete slowly reach forward with both hands as far as possible on the measuring stick, holding this position momentarily. To get the best stretch, the athlete should exhale and drop the head between the arms when reaching. Be sure the athlete keeps the hands adjacent to each other and does not lead with one hand. The fingertips should remain in contact with the measuring stick (figure 13.17*b*). The tester may hold the athlete's knees down, if necessary, to keep them straight. A score of less than 15 inches (38 cm) indicates that the athlete could not reach the bottom of the feet.
5. The best of three trials is recorded to the nearest 0.25 inches or 1 cm.

Note: Normative data for the sit-and-reach test are presented in tables 13.14 through 13.17 near the end of the chapter.

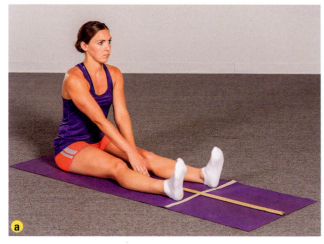
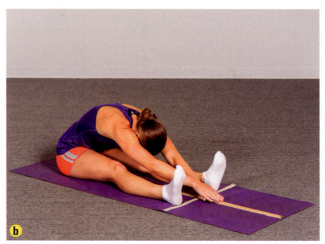

FIGURE 13.17 Sit-and-reach test: *(a)* starting position and *(b)* final position.

13.26 OVERHEAD SQUAT

Equipment

- Wooden dowel or barbell

Personnel

- One tester/recorder

Procedure

1. The athlete holds the wooden dowel overhead with the shoulders fully flexed and with elbows locked. The grip should be twice shoulder-width and the feet approximately shoulder-width apart and toes pointing forward or slightly out (figure 13.18).

2. The athlete then squats down; the initial action is flexion of the hips and knees. The heels remain in contact with the floor at all times.

3. The lowering continues until the crease of the hips is below the top of the knee.

4. The athlete should be able to hold this position with the torso remaining upright (parallel to the tibia) and the wooden dowel (or barbell) comfortably overhead.

5. The athlete performs a minimum of five repetitions, and the assessor views the movement from the side.

6. The assessment is qualitative and the goal is to assess the physical competency, with the movement scored as pass/fail.

7. It is important that the athlete be warmed up and familiarized with the movement patterns to increase the test validity.

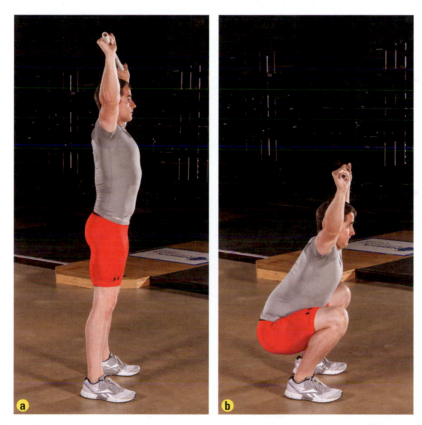

FIGURE 13.18 Body position for overhead squat: *(a)* starting position and *(b)* squat position.

13.27 SKINFOLD MEASUREMENTS

Equipment
- Skinfold calipers
- Flexible tape measure
- Marking pen

Personnel
- One tester, one recorder

Procedure (Obtaining a Skinfold Measurement)

1. Skinfold measurements should be made on dry skin, before exercise, to ensure maximum validity and reliability (10). The number of sites and equations should be selected based on the population tested (see table 13.25 near the end of the chapter).

2. Grasp the skin firmly with the thumb and index finger to form a fold of skin and subcutaneous fat.

3. Place the caliper prongs perpendicular to the fold 0.5 inch to 1 inch (approximately 1 to 2 cm) from the thumb and index finger.

4. Release the caliper grip so that its spring tension is exerted on the skinfold.

5. Between 1 and 2 seconds after the grip on the caliper has been released, read the dial on the caliper to the nearest 0.5 mm.

6. Obtain one measurement from each test site, and then repeat all test sites for a second trial. If the measurements do not differ by more than 10%, average the two measurements to the nearest 0.5 mm. Otherwise, take one or more additional measurements until two of the measurements are within 10%, and average those two measurements to the nearest 0.5 mm.

Procedure (Measuring the Selected Site and Calculating the Body Fat Percentage)

1. There are specific equations for estimating body density (Db) (then, in turn, percent body fat [%BF]) for different populations. First, select the equation appropriate for the athlete from table 13.25 near the end of the chapter.

2. Refer to the chosen equation and related instructions and mark the skin at the appropriate anatomical sites (45, 88):
   - Chest—a diagonal fold one-half the distance between the anterior axillary line and the nipple for men (figure 13.19a)
   - Thigh—a vertical fold on the anterior aspect of the thigh, midway between the hip and knee joints (figure 13.19b)
   - Abdomen—a vertical fold 1 inch (2.5 cm) to the right (relative to the athlete) of the umbilicus (figure 13.19c)
   - Triceps—a vertical fold on the posterior midline of the upper arm (over the triceps muscle), halfway between the acromion and the olecranon processes (the arm should be in anatomical position with the elbow extended and relaxed [figure 13.19d])
   - Suprailium—a diagonal fold above the crest of the ilium at the spot where an imaginary line would come down from the anterior axillary line (figure 13.19e) (some prefer the measure to be taken more laterally, at the midaxillary line)
   - Midaxilla—a vertical fold on the midaxillary line at the level of the xiphoid process of the sternum (figure 13.19f)
   - Subscapula—a fold taken on a diagonal line that extends from the vertebral border to a point 0.5 inch to 1 inch (1 to 2 cm) from the inferior angle of the scapula (figure 13.19g)
   - Calf—a vertical fold along the medial side of the calf, at the level of maximum calf circumference (figure 13.19h)

3. Using the appropriate population-specific equation from table 13.25, calculate the estimated body density from the skinfolds (45).

4. Enter the body density into the appropriate population-specific equation from table 13.26 near the end of the chapter to calculate the percent body fat from the body density (45).

5. Note that there are no universally accepted norms for body composition. When strength and conditioning professionals assess an athlete's body composition, they must account for a standard error of the estimate (SEE) and report a range of percentages that the athlete falls into. Note that the minimum SEE for population-specific skinfold equations is ±3% to ±5%. Therefore, if a 25-year-old male athlete's body fat is measured at 24%, there is a minimum of a 6% range (21-27%).

Note: Descriptive data for percent body fat are presented in tables 13.14 through 13.17 and table 13.27 near the end of the chapter.

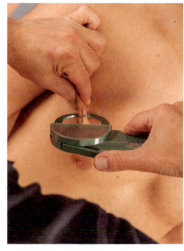

FIGURE 13.19a Chest skinfold.

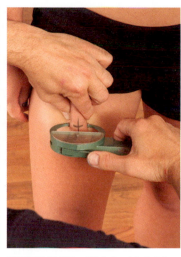

FIGURE 13.19b Thigh skinfold.

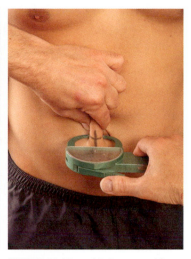

FIGURE 13.19c Abdomen skinfold.

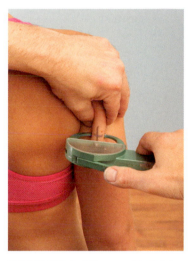

FIGURE 13.1d Triceps skinfold.

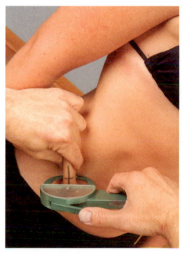

FIGURE 13.19e Suprailium skinfold.

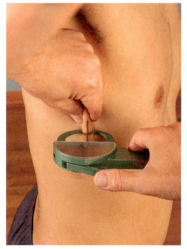

FIGURE 13.19f Midaxilla skinfold.

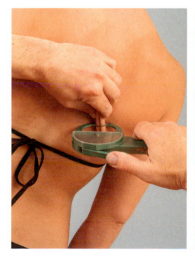

FIGURE 13.19g Subscapula skinfold.

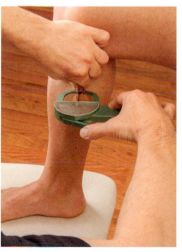

FIGURE 13.19h Calf skinfold.

13.28 GIRTH MEASUREMENTS

Equipment

- Flexible, spring-loaded tape measure (e.g., a Gulick tape)

Personnel

- One tester, one recorder

Procedure

1. Position the athlete in a relaxed anatomical position for each measurement (unless otherwise indicated for a particular measurement).
2. Measure the following sites (56); see figure 13.20:
   - Chest—at nipple level in males and at maximum circumference (above the breasts) in females
   - Right upper arm—at the point of maximal circumference with the elbow fully extended, palm up, and arm abducted to parallel with the floor
   - Right forearm—at the point of maximal circumference with the elbow fully extended, palm up, and arm abducted to parallel with the floor
   - Waist (abdomen)—at the level of the umbilicus
   - Hips (buttocks)—at the maximal protrusion of the buttocks with the heels together
   - Right thigh—at the point of maximal circumference, usually just below the buttocks
   - Right calf—at the point of maximal circumference between the knee and ankle

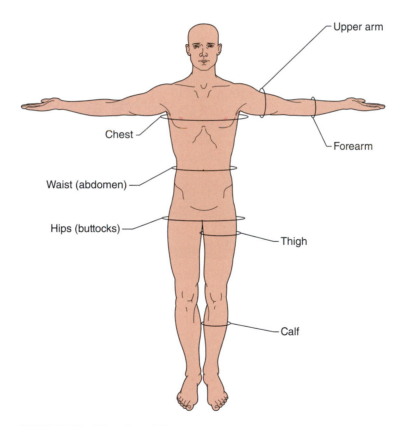

FIGURE 13.20 Sites for girth measurements.

Statistical Evaluation of Test Data

Once the proper test or tests have been chosen and administered and the scores collected, the next step may include any or all of the following: (1) analysis of the data to determine the change in performance of the individuals or group over the training period (weeks, months, or years); (2) analysis of the individual or group's performance relative to that of similar individuals or groups tested in the past; (3) analysis of the relationship of each athlete's scores to those of the group; and (4) comparison of individual scores to local, state, national, or international norms.

An important outcome of repeated performance testing is evaluation of both the improvement of individual athletes and the overall effectiveness of the physical conditioning program as determined by changes in test scores (73). A **difference score** is the difference between an athlete's score at the beginning and end of a training period or between any two separate testing times. The **percent change** is another measure that can be used. However, evaluating the effectiveness of a training program merely by degree of improvement has two major limitations. First, athletes who begin the training period at a higher training status will not improve as much as untrained athletes who perform poorly at the beginning of training. The window of adaptation for the various physical capacities is typically greater for less well-trained athletes (77). Secondly, athletes may deliberately fail to give maximal effort on pretraining tests to inflate their pre- to posttraining improvement scores. It is important to encourage athletes to give maximal effort on both the pre- and posttraining tests.

Types of Statistics

Statistics is the science of collecting, classifying, analyzing, and interpreting numerical data (18, 110). A working knowledge of statistics is helpful in making sound evaluations of test results. There are different branches of statistics such as descriptive and inferential. Recently, scientists and practitioners in strength and conditioning have made increasing use of magnitude-based approaches, which can be more meaningful as they provide information regarding the magnitude of change that matters to the athlete in the given sport.

Descriptive Statistics

Descriptive statistics summarizes or describes a large group of data. It is used when all the information about a population is known. For example, if all the members of a team are tested, statements can be made about the team with the use of descriptive statistics. There are three categories of numerical measurement in descriptive statistics: central tendency, variability, and percentile rank. In the sections that follow, these terms are defined and examples of how to calculate the values and scores are presented.

Central Tendency   Measures of **central tendency** are values about which the data tend to cluster. The three most common measures of central tendency (18, 110) are as follows:

Mean—the average of the scores (i.e., the sum of the scores divided by the number of scores). This is the most commonly used measure of central tendency.

Median—the middlemost score when a set of scores is arranged in order of magnitude. With an even number of scores, the median is the average of the two middlemost scores. Half a group of scores falls above the median and half falls below the median. Depending on the distribution of scores, the median can be a better measure of central tendency than the mean. This is particularly true when very high or very low scores of one or a few members of the group tested raise or lower the group mean to the extent that it does not adequately describe the ability of most group members.

Mode—the score that occurs with the greatest frequency. If each numerical score appears only once, there is no mode. If two or more scores are "tied" for greatest frequency, then all of the similar scores are modes. The mode is generally regarded as the least useful measure of central tendency.

Variability   The degree of dispersion of scores within a group is called **variability**. Two common measures of variability are the range and the **standard deviation**. The **range** is the interval from the lowest to the highest score. The advantage of the range is that it is easy to understand; the disadvantage is that it uses only the two extreme scores and so may not be an accurate measure of variability (110). For example, the range could be the same for a group of widely dispersed scores as for a group of scores that are narrowly dispersed except for one deviant score. The standard deviation is a measure of the variability of a set of scores about the mean. The formula for the standard deviation of a sample is as follows:

$$\text{SD} = \sqrt{\frac{\sum (x - \bar{x})^2}{n - 1}} \qquad \textbf{(13.1)}$$

where Σ refers to a summation, x is a score, $\bar{x}$ is the mean of the scores, and n is the sample size (number of scores). A relatively small standard deviation indicates that a set of scores is closely clustered about the mean; a large standard deviation indicates wider dispersion of the scores about the mean. The standard deviation is most useful when the group of scores is "normally distributed," forming the bell-shaped curve shown in figure 13.21 (18, 51).

The z score can be used to express the distance of any individual score in standard deviation (SD) units from the mean:

$$z = (x - \bar{x}) / SD \qquad (13.2)$$

For example, if an athlete runs the 40-yard (37 m) sprint in 4.6 seconds and the mean and standard deviation for the group tested are 5.00 and 0.33 seconds, respectively, equation 13.2 can be applied to determine that the z score for that athlete is −1.2. In other words, the athlete's score is 1.2 standard deviation units below (i.e., faster than) the group mean. Graphs can be a useful way of representing z scores visually. This can provide the strength and conditioning practitioner with a comparison

of different physical capacities and provide assistance with making decisions on which weaknesses to target with a training program (figure 13.22). In the example shown, the strength and conditioning practitioner may decide to focus on improving endurance and flexibility, while also improving body composition (figure 13.22).

Percentile Rank   An individual's **percentile rank** is the percentage of test takers scoring below that individual. As in calculation of the median, percentile ranking requires arranging scores ordinally (lowest to highest). For example, if an athlete is ranked in the 75th percentile, 75% of the group produced scores below that athlete's score. Norms based on large samples are sometimes expressed in evenly spaced percentiles. Several examples of percentile rank tables are shown in tables 13.1 to 13.3, table 13.5, table 13.10, tables 13.13 to 13.17, and table 13.22 near the end of the chapter.

Inferential Versus Magnitude Statistics

The use of **inferential statistics** allows one to draw general conclusions about a population from information collected in a population sample. For example, if a boys' 9th-grade gym class is put through a battery of tests and it is assumed that the class (sample) is representative of all the 9th-grade boys in the school (the population), then the results of these tests can be used to make inferences about the population as a whole. A basic assumption of inferential statistics is that the sample is truly representative of the population (18).

Magnitude statistics can provide a more useful approach for practitioners because it allows for inter-

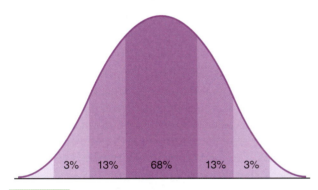

FIGURE 13.21   Normal bell curve.

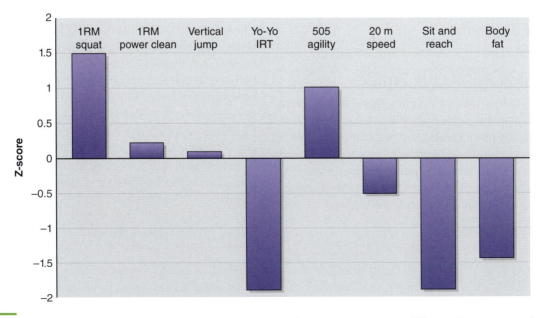

FIGURE 13.22 Z score column chart representing standardized test scores across different fitness tests for an individual athlete. The zero represents the team average.

pretation of the clinical significance of fitness testing (51). To describe and evaluate the magnitude of change in a fitness test, measures such as smallest worthwhile change and effect size are important.

Smallest worthwhile change refers to the ability of a test to detect the smallest practically important change in performance. The ability to track changes with a fitness test depends on the validity and reliability of that test. The smallest worthwhile change can be determined in a number of ways, but it is typically calculated as 0.2 of the between-subjects standard deviation (51). For example, if the standard deviation for a vertical jump test is 10 cm in a group of female athletes, this would mean that the smallest worthwhile change for this group of athletes is 2 cm (0.2 × 10 cm).

Effect size is a statistic that can be useful for calculating group performance following a training program or comparing between groups of athletes (29). The effect of the training program can be calculated as the difference or change in the mean score as a proportion of the pretest standard deviation (equation 13.3).

$$ES = (x \text{ posttest} - x \text{ pretest}) / SD \text{ pretest} \qquad \textbf{(13.3)}$$

For example, a group of athletes had a pretraining mean bench press 1RM of 104.5 kg (standard deviation of 5.7 kg), and after a 12-week training intervention the mean bench press is 111.7 kg. The calculated effect size would be equal to $(111.7 - 104.5)/5.7 = 1.26$.

Several scales have been provided to compare the magnitude of the effect (19, 73, 94), but reference values for small (0.2), moderate (0.6), large (1.2), and very large (2.0) can be a useful starting point for practitioners (29, 51). For the example just given, this would mean that the strength and conditioning professional would interpret the effect size of 1.26 as meaning that the training program had a large effect.

Developing an Athletic Profile

To determine the sport-specific training status of an athlete, the strength and conditioning professional can combine the results of selected tests to generate an **athletic profile**, which is a group of test results related to sport-specific abilities that are important for quality performance in a sport or sport position. When evaluating athletes, the strength and conditioning professional should follow these six steps:

1. Select tests that will measure the specific parameters most closely related to the physical characteristics of the sport or sports in question. For example, a testing battery for wrestlers should include

tests for pulling strength, pushing strength, and local muscular endurance.

2. Choose valid and reliable tests to measure these parameters, and arrange the testing battery in an appropriate order with sufficient rest between tests to promote test reliability. For example, appropriate tests for wrestling might include push-ups and sit-ups for maximum repetitions in a given time interval. These two tests should be separated by at least 10 minutes of rest to allow recovery from fatigue and thus promote accurate scores.

3. Administer the test battery with as many athletes as possible.

4. Determine the smallest worthwhile change for the tests and compare to normative data where appropriate. It is recommended that coaches store testing results and develop their own norms when standardized procedures are used.

5. Conduct repeat testing (e.g., pre- and posttraining program) and use the results to present a visual profile with figures.

6. Use the results of the testing in some meaningful way. Ideally the results will enable the strength and conditioning professional to identify the strengths and weaknesses of the athletes and to design the training program with these in mind.

Conclusion

Motor abilities and body composition variables that can be improved through strength and conditioning programs include maximum muscular strength, maximum muscular power, anaerobic capacity, local muscular endurance, aerobic capacity, agility, speed, flexibility, girths, percent body fat, and lean body mass. Performance testing can be used to evaluate basic motor abilities, as well as the improvement of individual athletes over time and the overall effectiveness of a physical conditioning program. Numerous tests are available to measure sport-specific physical capabilities and training status. Strength and conditioning professionals can either use existing normative data to evaluate athletic performance or develop their own normative data. Statistical measures of central tendency, variability, percentile rank, smallest worthwhile change, effect size, and standard scores are useful for evaluating physical abilities and the improvement of a group as well as the individuals within the group.

aerobic capacity
aerobic power
agility
anaerobic capacity
anaerobic power
anthropometry
athletic performance
athletic profile
balance
body composition
central tendency

descriptive statistics
difference score
effect size
flexibility
high-speed muscular strength
inferential statistics
local muscular endurance
low-speed muscular strength
magnitude statistics
maximal anaerobic muscular power
mean

median
mode
percent change
percentile rank
range
smallest worthwhile change
speed
stability
standard deviation
statistics
variability

STUDY QUESTIONS

1. Anaerobic capacity is quantified as the maximal power output achieved during activity lasting
   a. less than 10 seconds
   b. 30 to 90 seconds
   c. 2 to 3 minutes
   d. longer than 5 minutes

2. Which of the following tests is NOT used to measure maximum muscular power?
   a. Margaria-Kalamen test
   b. vertical jump
   c. 40-yard (37 m) sprint
   d. 1RM power clean

3. Flexibility of which of these muscle groups or body areas is assessed during the sit-and-reach test?
   I. hamstrings
   II. erector spinae
   III. lumbar spine
   IV. hip flexors
   a. I and III only
   b. II and IV only
   c. I, II, and III only
   d. II, III, and IV only

4. Which of the following is a reason for a trial of the T-test to be disqualified (see figure 13.11)?
   a. touching the base of cone D
   b. shuffling from cone C to cone D
   c. crossing the feet from cone B to cone C
   d. running forward from cone A to cone B

5. When compiling results from the volleyball team's vertical jump testing, the strength and conditioning professional notices that most scores are similar, but there are three scores that are much higher than the rest. Which of the following measures of central tendency is most appropriate for this group?
   a. mean
   b. median
   c. mode
   d. variance

TABLE 13.1 Percentile Values of the 1RM Bench Press, Squat, and Power Clean in NCAA Division I Female Collegiate Athletes

% rank	1RM bench press		1RM squat		1RM power clean		1RM bench press		1RM squat	
	lb	kg	lb	kg	lb	kg	lb	kg	lb	kg
	BASKETBALL						SWIMMING			
90	124	56	178	81	130	59	116	53	145	66
80	119	54	160	73	124	56	109	50	135	61
70	115	52	147	67	117	53	106	48	129	59
60	112	51	135	61	112	51	101	46	120	55
50	106	48	129	59	110	50	97	44	116	53
40	102	46	115	52	103	47	94	43	112	51
30	96	44	112	51	96	44	93	42	104	47
20	88	40	101	46	88	40	88	40	101	46
10	82	37	81	37	77	35	78	35	97	44
Mean	105	48	130	59	106	48	98	45	118	54
SD	18	8	42	19	20	9	15	7	19	9
n	120		86		85		42		35	
	SOFTBALL						VOLLEYBALL			
90	117	53	184	84	122	55	113	51	185	84
80	108	49	170	77	115	52	108	49	171	78
70	104	47	148	67	106	48	104	47	165	75
60	99	45	139	63	100	45	100	45	153	70
50	95	43	126	57	94	43	98	45	143	65
40	90	41	120	55	93	42	96	44	136	62
30	85	39	112	51	88	40	90	41	126	57
20	80	36	94	43	80	36	85	39	112	51
10	69	31	76	35	71	32	79	36	98	45
Mean	94	43	130	59	97	44	97	44	144	65
SD	18	8	42	19	20	9	14	6	33	15
n	105		97		80		67		62	

lb = pounds, SD = standard deviation, *n* = sample size

Adapted, by permission, from Hoffman, 2006 (47).

TABLE 13.2 Percentile Values of the 1RM Bench Press, Squat, and Power Clean in High School and College American Football Players

% rank	1RM bench press		1RM squat		1RM power clean		1RM bench press		1RM squat		1RM power clean	
	lb	kg	lb	kg	lb	kg	lb	kg	lb	kg	lb	kg
	HIGH SCHOOL 14-15 YEARS						HIGH SCHOOL 16-18 YEARS					
90	243	110	385	175	213	97	275	125	465	211	250	114
80	210	95	344	156	195	89	250	114	425	193	235	107
70	195	89	325	148	190	86	235	107	405	184	225	102
60	185	84	305	139	183	83	225	102	365	166	223	101
50	170	77	295	134	173	79	215	98	335	152	208	95
40	165	75	275	125	165	75	205	93	315	143	200	91
30	155	70	255	116	161	73	195	89	295	134	183	83
20	145	66	236	107	153	70	175	80	275	125	165	75
10	125	57	205	93	141	64	160	73	250	114	145	66
Mean	179	81	294	134	176	80	214	97	348	158	204	93
SD	45	20	73	33	32	15	44	20	88	40	43	20
n	214		170		180		339		249		284	
	NCAA DI						NCAA DIII					
90	370	168	500	227	300	136	365	166	470	214		
80	345	157	455	207	280	127	325	148	425	193		
70	325	148	430	195	270	123	307	140	405	184		
60	315	143	405	184	261	119	295	134	385	175		
50	300	136	395	180	252	115	280	127	365	166		
40	285	130	375	170	242	110	273	124	350*	159*		
30	270	123	355	161	232	105	255	116	335	152		
20	255	116	330	150	220	100	245	111	315	143		
10	240	109	300	136	205	93	225	102	283	129		
Mean	301	137	395	180	252	115	287	130	375	170		
SD	53	24	77	35	38	17	57	26	75	34		
n	1,189		1,074		1,017		591		588			

*Hoffman 2006 reported 365 lb, 166 kg, for the 40 percent rank of the NCAA DIII 1RM squat.

lb = pounds, SD = standard deviation, n = sample size.

Reprinted, by permission, from Hoffman, 2006 (47).

TABLE 13.3 Percentile Values of the 1RM Bench Press, Squat, and Power Clean in NCAA Division I Male Baseball and Basketball Athletes

% rank	1RM bench press		1RM squat		1RM power clean		1RM bench press		1RM squat		1RM power clean	
	lb	kg	lb	kg	lb	kg	lb	kg	lb	kg	lb	kg
	BASEBALL						BASKETBALL					
90	273	124	365	166	265	120	269	122	315	143	250	114
80	260	118	324	147	239	109	250	114	305	139	235	107
70	247	112	310	141	225	102	240	109	295	134	230	105
60	239	109	293	133	216	98	230	105	280	127	220	100
50	225	102	270	123	206	94	225	102	265	120	215	98
40	218	99	265	120	200	91	216	98	245	111	205	93
30	203	92	247	112	190	86	210	95	225	102	195	89
20	194	88	237	107	182	83	195	89	195	89	180	82
10	175	80	218	99	162	74	185	84	166	75	162	74
Mean	227	103	281	128	210	95	225	102	251	114	209	95
SD	41	19	57	26	36	16	33	15	57	26	34	15
n	170		176		149		142		131		122	

lb = pounds, SD = standard deviation, n = sample size.

Reprinted, by permission, from Hoffman, 2006 (47).

TABLE 13.4   1RM Squat, Bench Press, Power Clean, and Bench Pull Descriptive Data* for Various Groups

Group, sport, or position	Number of athletes	Body weight		Squat		Bench press		Power clean		Bench pull	
		lb	kg	lb	kg	lb	kg	lb	kg	lb	kg
National rugby league (7)	20	216.5 ± 21.8	98.2 ± 9.9	385.8 ± 59.5	175.0 ± 27.3						
State-level rugby league (7)	20	201.2 ± 18.5	91.3 ± 8.4	329.8 ± 30.9	149.6 ± 14.3						
National rugby league (8)	21	219.4 ± 19.2	99.5 ± 8.7			315.0 ± 33.5	142.7 ± 15.2				
State-level rugby league (8)	21	200.0 ± 19.6	90.7 ± 8.9			258.8 ± 35.9	117.4 ± 16.3				
National rugby league (5)	6	211.2 ± 32.2	95.8 ± 14.6			332.5 ± 2.6	150.8 ± 10.7				
National sailing (men) (87)	11	215.6 ± 27.6	97.8 ± 12.5			310.6 ± 58.6	140.9 ± 26.6			265.9 ± 37.3	120.6 ± 16.9
National canoe/rowing/wrestling/judo (men) (96)	75	167.6 ± 19.4	76.0 ± 8.8			199.0 ± 35.9	90.3 ± 16.3			176.8 ± 26.0	80.2 ± 11.8
National basketball (women) (105)	12	166.7 ± 32.2	75.6 ± 14.6			173.2 ± 6.6	78.6 ± 3.0				
NCAA Division IA college football (men) (12)	963					310.4	140.8				
NCAA Division IA college football (men) (12)	560			420.6	190.8						
National softball (women) (81)	10	158.1 ± 24.5	71.7 ± 11.1	183.6 ± 22.0	83.3 ± 10.0						
National ice hockey (women) (89)	22	155.2 ± 15.7	70.4 ± 7.1			144.0 ± 27.0	65.3 ± 12.2				
National soccer (men) (123)	17	168.7 ± 16.8	76.5 ± 7.6	378.5 ± 46.7	171.7 ± 21.2						
National soccer (men) (124)	14	169.5 ± 13.9	76.9 ± 6.3	362.9 ± 43.9	164.6 ± 21.8	182.3 ± 28.2	82.7 ± 12.8				
National soccer (men) (124)	15	169.6 ± 16.3	76.8 ± 7.4	297.6 ± 35.7	135.0 ± 16.2	170.036.4	77.1 ± 16.5				
NCAA Division IA college football (men) (82)	207	229.2 ± 48.7	104.0 ± 22.1			312.8 ± 58.6	141.6 ± 26.6				

Group, sport, or position	Number of athletes	Body weight		Squat		Bench press		Power clean		Bench pull	
		lb	kg	lb	kg	lb	kg	lb	kg	lb	kg
NCAA Division IA college football (men) (82)	88	226.0 ± 14.3	102.5 ± 6.5					267.4 ± 33.1	121.3 ± 15.0		
NCAA Division IA college football (men) (82)	86	226.0 ± 14.3	102.5 ± 6.5	397.9 ± 74.1	180.5 ± 33.6						
National handball (women) (40)	16	152.7 ± 18.1	69.3 ± 8.2			113.8 ± 14.8	51.6 ± 6.7				
National handball (men) (39)	15	207.0 ± 37.3	93.9 ± 16.9			235.7 ± 25.6	106.9 ± 11.6				
Under 16 rugby league (men) (114)	30	165.8 ± 24.5	75.2 ± 11.1	221.3 ± 48.3	100.4 ± 21.9	162.9 ± 29.1	73.9 ± 13.2			156.3 ± 22.3	70.9 ± 10.1
Under 17 rugby league (men) (114)	48	178.8 ± 20.7	81.1 ± 9.4	269.4 ± 41.2	122.2 ± 18.7	205.7 ± 29.5	93.3 ± 13.4			184.1 ± 22.5	83.5 ± 10.2
Under 18 rugby league (men) (114)	55	188.1 ± 22.0	85.3 ± 10.0	295.4 ± 34.2	134.0 ± 15.5	228.6 ± 33.7	103.7 ± 15.3			200.8 ± 22.3	91.1 ± 10.1
Under 19 rugby league (men) (114)	45	195.8 ± 21.8	88.8 ± 9.9	305.1 ± 43.2	138.4 ± 19.6	249.8 ± 36.2	113.3 ± 16.4			215.2 ± 27.3	97.6 ± 12.4
Under 20 rugby league (men) (114)	26	196.0 ± 18.7	88.9 ± 8.5	318.8 ± 48.7	144.6 ± 22.1	252.0 ± 33.7	114.3 ± 15.3			220.5 ± 24.7	100.0 ± 11.2
NCAA Division III lacrosse (women) (49)	11	132.3 ± 11.0	60.0 ± 5.0	158.5 ± 13.4	71.9 ± 6.1	96.8 ± 13.4	43.9 ± 6.1				
National rugby league forwards (men) (72)	63					271.2 ± 26.0	123.0 ± 11.8				
National rugby league backs (men) (72)	55					251.3 ± 37.5	114.0 ± 17.0				
National rugby union (men) (21)	30	236.1 ± 22.3	107.1 ± 10.1	351.6 ± 58.0	159.5 ± 26.3	308.6 ± 35.9	140.0 ± 16.3				
National rugby union (women) (10)	15	157.9 ± 21.8	71.6 ± 9.9	152.1 ± 19.4	69.0 ± 8.8						

*The values listed are means ± standard deviation. The data should be regarded as only descriptive, not normative.

TABLE 13.5 Norms for Standing Long Jump in Elite Male and Female Athletes

% rank	Males in.	Males cm	Females in.	Females cm
90	133	339	115	293
80	122	309	110	279
70	116	294	104	264
60	110	279	98	249
50	104	264	92	234
40	98	249	86	219
30	92	234	80	204
20	86	219	74	189
10	80	204	69	174

Reprinted, by permission, from J. Hoffman, 2006, *Norms for fitness, performance, and health* (Champaign, IL: Human Kinetics), 58. Adapted from D.A. Chu, 1996, *Explosive power and strength* (Champaign, IL: Human Kinetics).

TABLE 13.6 Rankings for Standing Long Jump in 15- and 16-Year-Old Male and Female Athletes

Category	Males in.	Males cm	Females in.	Females cm
Excellent	79	201	65	166
Above average	73	186	61	156
Average	69	176	57	146
Below average	65	165	53	135
Poor	<65	<165	<53	<135

Reprinted, by permission, from J. Hoffman, 2006, *Norms for fitness, performance, and health* (Champaign, IL: Human Kinetics), 58. Adapted from D.A. Chu, 1996, *Explosive power and strength* (Champaign, IL: Human Kinetics).

TABLE 13.7 Vertical Jump, Static Jump, and Broad Jump Descriptive Data* for Various Groups

Group, sport, or position	Number of athletes	Vertical jump in.	Vertical jump cm	Static jump in.	Static jump cm	Broad jump in.	Broad jump cm
College soccer (women) (118)	51	16.1 ± 2.2	40.9 ± 5.5				
High school soccer (women) (118)	83	15.6 ± 1.9	39.6 ± 4.7				
College lacrosse (women) (118)	79	15.8 ± 2.2	40.1 ± 5.6				
Under 18 Gaelic football (men) (22)	265	17.0 ± 2.0	43.3 ± 5.1			78.0 ± 8.1	198.2 ± 20.7
National soccer (women) (17)	21	12.4 ± 1.6	31.6 ± 4.0	11.9 ± 1.5	30.1 ± 3.7		
Under 19 soccer (women) (17)	20	13.5 ± 1.5	34.3 ± 3.9	12.9 ± 1.1	32.8 ± 2.9		
Under 17 soccer (women) (17)	21	11.4 ± 0.8	29.0 ± 2.1	11.1 ± 1.0	28.2 ± 2.5		
Under 21 soccer (men) (17)	18	15.9 ± 1.7	40.3 ± 4.3	14.6 ± 1.5	37.0 ± 3.9		
Under 20 soccer (men) (17)	17	15.8 ± 1.9	40.2 ± 4.7	15.0 ± 1.9	38.0 ± 4.9		
Under 17 soccer (men) (17)	21	16.1 ± 2.0	40.9 ± 5.1	14.7 ± 1.9	37.3 ± 4.7		
Division I Spain soccer (women) (99)	100	10.3 ± 1.9	26.1 ± 4.8				
National ice hockey (women) (89)	23	19.8 ± 2.2	50.3 ± 5.7#			84.6 ± 4.3	214.8 ± 10.9
National soccer (women) (42)	85	12.1 ± 1.6	30.7 ± 4.1				
Division I Norway soccer (women) (42)	47	11.1 ± 1.6	28.1 ± 4.1				
Ice hockey National Hockey League draftees (men) (15)	853	24.4 ± 3.0	62.0 ± 7.6#			100.0 ± 7.0	254.0 ± 17.8
College wrestling (men) (109)	20	20.5 ± 3.1	52.0 ± 8.0#				
National weightlifting (men) (32)	6	23.9 ± 1.5	60.8 ± 3.9				
National soccer (men) (123)	17	22.2 ± 1.6	56.4 ± 4.0				
National soccer (men) (124)	14	22.3 ± 2.6	56.7 ± 6.6				
National soccer (men) (124)	15	20.9 ± 1.6	53.1 ± 4.0				

Group, sport, or position	Number of athletes	Vertical jump		Static jump		Broad jump	
		in.	cm	in.	cm	in.	cm
National soccer (men) (106)	270	17.8 ± 0.7	45.1 ± 1.7	17.4 ± 0.5	44.1 ± 1.3		
National handball (women) (40)	16	15.1 ± 1.7	38.4 ± 4.4				
National handball (men) (39)	15	19.0 ± 2.8	48.2 ± 7.2				
Under 16 rugby league (men) (114)	67	18.0 ± 2.0	45.7 ± 5.2				
Under 17 rugby league (men) (114)	50	19.3 ± 2.3	49.1 ± 5.8				
NCAA Division I football (men) (31)	193	28.7 ± 3.7	72.8 ± 9.3#				
NCAA Division II football (men) (31)	181	27.3 ± 3.3	69.3 ± 8.5#				
NCAA Division III football (men) (31)	131	26.5 ± 3.5	67.4 ± 8.8#				
High school volleyball (women) (98)	27	18.5 ± 3.3	47.1 ± 8.5#				
NCAA Division I volleyball (women) (98)	26	20.8 ± 2.5	52.8 ± 6.3#				
National rugby league forwards (men) (20)	12	14.7 ± 1.7	37.3 ± 4.4				
National rugby league backs (men) (20)	6	15.9 ± 2.5	40.3 ± 6.4				
National rugby league (men) (35)	26	20.0 ± 2.9	50.7 ± 9.8#				
National rugby league (men) (34)	58	24.7 ± 2.2	62.8 ± 5.7#				
National rugby union (men) (21)	30					101.6 ± 7.9	258.0 ± 20.0
National rugby union (women) (10)	15	15.0 ± 1.6	38.0 ± 4.0	13.8 ± 1.2	35.0 ± 3.0		
High school track and field (women) (75)	8					83.4 ± 6.3	212.0 ± 16.0
NCAA Division I soccer (women) (67)	15	12.2 ± 2.0	31.0 ± 5.0			57.9 ± 4.3	147.0 ± 11.0
High school rugby league (men) (112)	302	16.3 ± 2.1	41.3 ± 5.3				
Junior national volleyball (men) (33)	14	21.5 ± 0.9	54.6 ± 2.2#				
Junior national volleyball (women) (33)	15	18.0 ± 0.6	45.7 ± 1.6#				
Under 18 Australian rules football (men) (127)	177	23.9 ± 2.2	60.6 ± 5.5#				
NCAA Division I lacrosse (women) (117)	84	15.8 ± 2.2	40.2 ± 5.6				
NCAA Division I soccer (men) (102)	27	24.3 ± 2.8	61.6 ± 7.1#				
National soccer (women) (1)	17	12.0 ± 0.5	30.5 ± 1.2				
National soccer (women) (76)	17	12.8 ± 1.5	32.6 ± 3.7				
National soccer (men) (76)	17	17.2 ± 0.9	43.7 ± 2.2				
National junior soccer (women) (76)	17	11.2 ± 0.8	28.4 ± 2.0				
National junior soccer (men) (76)	17	17.3 ± 1.9	43.9 ± 4.8				
National soccer (men) (2)	214	15.4 ± 2.0	39.2 ± 5.0	14.8 ± 1.9	37.6 ± 4.8		

*The values listed are means ± standard deviation. The data should be regarded as only descriptive, not normative.

#Jumps performed with arm swing.

TABLE 13.8   Margaria-Kalamen Stair Sprint Test Guidelines (Watts)

Classification	Age groups (years)				
	15-20	20-30	30-40	40-50	Over 50
MEN					
Excellent	Over 2,197	Over 2,059	Over 1,648	Over 1,226	Over 961
Good	1,844-2,197	1,726-2,059	1,383-1,648	1,040-1,226	814-961
Average	1,471-1,824	1,373-1,716	1,098-1,373	834-1,030	647-804
Fair	1,108-1,461	1,040-1,363	834-1,088	637-824	490-637
Poor	Under 1,108	Under 1,040	Under 834	Under 637	Under 490
WOMEN					
Excellent	Over 1,785	Over 1,648	Over 1,226	Over 961	Over 736
Good	1,491-1,785	1,383-1,648	1,040-1,226	814-961	608-736
Average	1,187-1,481	1,098-1,373	834-1,030	647-804	481-598
Fair	902-1,177	834-1,089	637-824	490-637	373-471
Poor	Under 902	Under 834	Under 637	Under 490	Under 373

Adapted from E. Fox, R. Bowers, and M. Foss, 1993, *The physiological basis for exercise and sport,* 5th ed. (Dubuque, IA: Wm. C. Brown), 676. Reprinted with permission of McGraw-Hill Companies.

TABLE 13.9   Descriptive Data for 300-Yard Shuttle Test*

Group, sport, or position	Number of athletes	Time (s)
High school volleyball (women) (98)	27	68.0 ± 6.3
NCAA Division 1 volleyball (women) (98)	26	67.7 ± 3.8
National soccer (men) (107)	18	56.7 ± 1.7
Recreational men and women (121)	81	72.8 ± 9.1
National badminton (men) (120)	12	73.3 ± 3.4

*The values listed are means ± standard deviation. The data should be regarded as only descriptive, not normative.

TABLE 13.10 Percentiles by Age Groups and Sex for Partial Curl-Up

Percentile*	20-29		30-39		40-49		50-59		60-69	
	M	F	M	F	M	F	M	F	M	F
90	75	70	75	55	75	55	74	48	53	50
80	56	45	69	43	75	42	60	30	33	30
70	41	37	46	34	67	33	45	23	26	24
60	31	32	36	28	51	28	35	16	19	19
50	27	27	31	21	39	25	27	9	16	13
40	24	21	26	15	31	20	23	2	9	9
30	20	17	19	12	26	14	19	0	6	3
20	13	12	13	0	21	5	13	0	0	0
10	4	5	0	0	13	0	0	0	0	0

*Descriptors for percentile rankings: 90 = well above average; 70 = above average; 50 = average; 30 = below average; 10 = well below average.

Reprinted, by permission, from American College of Sports Medicine, 2014, *ACSM's guidelines for exercise testing and prescription,* 9th ed. (Baltimore, MD: Lippincott, Williams, and Wilkins), 101.

TABLE 13.11 Fitness Categories by Age Groups and Sex for Push-Ups

Category	20-29		30-39		40-49		50-59		60-69	
	M	F	M	F	M	F	M	F	M	F
Excellent	36	30	30	27	25	24	21	21	18	17
Very good	35	29	29	26	24	23	20	20	17	16
	29	21	22	20	17	15	13	11	11	12
Good	28	20	21	19	16	14	12	10	10	11
	22	15	17	13	13	11	10	7	8	5
Fair	21	14	16	12	12	10	9	6	7	4
	17	10	12	8	10	5	7	2	5	2
Needs improvement	16	9	11	7	9	4	6	1	4	1

Source: Canadian Physical Activity, *Fitness & Lifestyle Approach: CSEP-Health & Fitness Program's Appraisal & Counselling Strategy,* Third Edition, © 2003. Reprinted with permission from the Canadian Society for Exercise Physiology.

TABLE 13.12 Push-Up Standards for U.S. Army Personnel

Age range	Push-up repetitions in 2 minutes									
MALES										
17-21	6	13	20	28	35	42	49	57	64	71
22-26	—	5	14	23	31	40	49	58	66	75
27-31	—	1	11	20	30	39	49	58	68	77
32-36	—	—	7	17	26	36	46	56	65	75
37-41	—	—	5	15	24	34	44	54	63	73
42-46	—	—	—	12	21	30	39	48	57	66
47-51	—	—	—	8	17	25	34	42	51	59
52-56	—	—	—	—	11	20	29	38	47	56
57-61	—	—	—	—	9	18	27	36	44	53
62+	—	—	—	—	8	16	25	33	42	50
Points awarded	10	20	30	40	50	60	70	80	90	100
FEMALES										
17-21	—	—	2	8	13	19	25	31	36	42
22-26	—	—	—	2	11	17	24	32	39	46
27-31	—	—	—	—	10	17	25	34	42	50
32-36	—	—	—	—	9	15	23	30	38	45
37-41	—	—	—	—	7	13	20	27	33	40
42-46	—	—	—	—	6	12	18	25	31	37
47-51	—	—	—	—	—	10	16	22	28	34
52-56	—	—	—	—	—	9	15	20	26	31
57-61	—	—	—	—	—	8	13	18	23	28
62+	—	—	—	—	—	7	12	16	21	25
Points awarded	10	20	30	40	50	60	70	80	90	100

60 points is passing; 90 points is excellent.

Data from U.S. Department of the Army, 1998 (24).

TABLE 13.13   YMCA Bench Press Norms

| Percentile | Age and sex | | | | | | | | | | | |
| | 18-25 | | 26-35 | | 36-45 | | 46-55 | | 56-65 | | >65 | |
	M	F	M	F	M	F	M	F	M	F	M	F
90	44	42	41	40	36	33	28	29	24	24	20	18
80	37	34	33	32	29	28	22	22	20	20	14	14
70	33	28	29	28	25	24	20	18	14	14	10	10
60	29	25	26	24	22	21	16	14	12	12	10	8
50	26	21	22	21	20	17	13	12	10	9	8	6
40	22	18	20	17	17	14	11	9	8	6	6	4
30	20	16	17	14	14	12	9	7	5	5	4	3
20	16	12	13	12	10	8	6	5	3	3	2	1
10	10	6	9	6	6	4	2	1	1	1	1	0

Score is number of repetitions completed in 1 minute using an 80-pound (36 kg) barbell for men and a 35-pound (16 kg) barbell for women.
Adapted from YMCA, 2000 (125).

TABLE 13.14   Maximal Rate of Oxygen Consumption, 1.5-Mile (2.4 km) Run Time, Sit-and-Reach Test, and Body Composition: Percentile Rankings for 20- to 29-Year-Old Males

| Percentile rank | $\dot{V}O_2$max ($ml \cdot kg^{-1} \cdot min^{-1}$) | 1.5-mile (2.4 km) run time, min:s | Sit-and-reach test* | | Body fat (%) |
			in.	cm	
99	60.5	8:29			4.2
90	54.0	9:34	22	55.9	7.9
80	51.1	10:09	20	50.8	10.5
70	47.5	10:59	19	48.3	12.6
60	45.6	11:29	18	45.7	14.8
50	43.9	11:58	17	43.2	16.6
40	41.7	12:38	15	38.1	18.6
30	39.9	13:15	14	35.6	20.7
20	38.0	14:00	13	33.0	23.3
10	34.7	15:30	11	27.9	26.6
01	26.5	20:58			33.4

*Sit and reach for 18- to 25-year-old men.

Adapted from American College of Sports Medicine, 2014, *ACSM's guidelines for exercise testing and prescription*, 9th ed. (Baltimore, MD; Lippincott, Williams, and Wilkins).

TABLE 13.15   Maximal Rate of Oxygen Consumption, 1.5-Mile (2.4 km) Run Time, Sit-and-Reach Test, and Body Composition: Percentile Rankings for 20- to 29-Year-Old Females

Percentile rank	$\dot{V}O_2$max (ml·kg⁻¹·min⁻¹)	1.5-mile (2.4 km) run time, min:s	Sit-and-reach test* in.	Sit-and-reach test* cm	Body fat (%)
99	54.5	9:30			11.4
90	46.8	11:10	24	61.0	15.1
80	43.9	11:58	22	55.9	16.8
70	41.1	12:51	21	53.3	18.4
60	39.5	13:24	20	50.8	19.8
50	37.8	14:04	19	48.3	21.5
40	36.1	14:50	18	45.7	23.4
30	34.1	15:46	17	43.2	25.5
20	32.3	16:46	16	40.6	28.2
10	29.5	18:33	14	35.6	33.5
01	23.7	23:58			38.6

*Sit and reach for 18- to 25-year-old women.

Adapted from American College of Sports Medicine, 2014, *ACSM's guidelines for exercise testing and prescription,* 9th ed. (Baltimore, MD; Williams & Wilkins).

TABLE 13.16   Maximal Rate of Oxygen Consumption, 1.5-Mile (2.4 km) Run Time, Sit-and-Reach Test, and Body Composition: Percentile Rankings for 30- to 39-Year-Old Males

Percentile rank	$\dot{V}O_2$max (ml·kg⁻¹·min⁻¹)	1.5-mile (2.4 km) run time, min:s	Sit-and-reach test* in.	Sit-and-reach test* cm	Body fat (%)
99	58.3	8:49			7.3
90	51.7	10:01	21	53.3	12.4
80	48.3	10:46	19	48.3	14.9
70	46.0	11:22	18	45.7	16.8
60	44.1	11:54	17	43.2	18.4
50	42.4	12:24	15	38.1	20.0
40	40.7	12:58	14	35.6	21.6
30	38.7	13:44	13	33.0	23.2
20	36.7	14:34	11	27.9	25.1
10	33.8	15:57	9	22.9	27.8
01	26.5	20:58			34.4

*Sit and reach for 26- to 35-year-old men.

Adapted from American College of Sports Medicine, 2014, *ACSM's guidelines for exercise testing and prescription,* 9th ed. (Baltimore, MD; Williams & Wilkins).

TABLE 13.17 Maximal Rate of Oxygen Consumption, 1.5-Mile (2.4 km) Run Time, Sit-and-Reach Test, and Body Composition: Percentile Rankings for 30- to 39-Year-Old Females

| Percentile rank | $\dot{V}O_2$max (ml·kg^{-1}·min^{-1}) | 1.5-mile (2.4 km) run time, min:s | Sit-and-reach test* | | Body fat (%) |
			in.	cm	
99	52.0	9:58			11.2
90	45.3	11:33	23	58.4	15.5
80	42.4	12:24	22	55.9	17.5
70	39.6	13:24	21	53.3	19.2
60	37.7	14:08	20	50.8	21.0
50	36.7	14:34	19	48.3	22.8
40	34.2	15:43	17	43.2	24.8
30	32.4	16:42	16	40.6	26.9
20	30.9	17:38	15	38.1	29.6
10	28.0	19:43	13	33.0	33.6
01	22.9	24:56			39.0

*Sit and reach for 26- to 35-year-old women.

Adapted from American College of Sports Medicine, 2014, *ACSM's guidelines for exercise testing and prescription*, 9th ed. (Baltimore, MD; Williams & Wilkins).

TABLE 13.18 $\dot{V}O_2$max Descriptive Data for Athletes in Various Sports

Classification	Typical $\dot{V}O_2$max of athletes playing the sport (ml·kg⁻¹·min⁻¹)		Sport
	Males	Females	
Extremely high	70+	60+	Cross-country skiing Middle-distance running Long-distance running
Very high	63-69	54-59	Bicycling Rowing Racewalking
High	57-62	49-53	Soccer Middle-distance swimming Canoe racing Handball Racquetball Speed skating Figure skating Downhill skiing Wrestling
Above average	52-56	44-48	Basketball Ballet dancing American football (offensive, defensive backs) Gymnastics Hockey Horse racing (jockey) Sprint swimming Tennis Sprint running Jumping
Average	44-51	35-43	Baseball, softball American football (linemen, quarterbacks) Shot put Discus throw Olympic-style weightlifting Bodybuilding

Data from Nieman, 1995 (78).

TABLE 13.19 Percentile Ranks for the 12-Minute Run

Percentile	Age (years) and distance					
	20-29		30-39		40-49	
	km	miles	km	miles	km	miles
MEN						
90	2.90	1.81	2.82	1.75	2.72	1.69
80	2.78	1.73	2.67	1.66	2.57	1.60
70	2.62	1.63	2.56	1.59	2.46	1.53
60	2.54	1.58	2.48	1.54	2.40	1.49
50	2.46	1.53	2.40	1.49	2.30	1.43
40	2.37	1.47	2.32	1.44	2.22	1.38
30	2.29	1.42	2.24	1.39	2.14	1.33
20	2.20	1.37	2.14	1.33	2.06	1.28
10	2.06	1.28	2.01	1.25	1.95	1.21
WOMEN						
90	2.59	1.61	2.53	1.57	2.43	1.51
80	2.46	1.53	2.40	1.49	2.27	1.41
70	2.35	1.46	2.27	1.41	2.20	1.37
60	2.27	1.41	2.19	1.36	2.11	1.31
50	2.20	1.37	2.14	1.33	2.04	1.27
40	2.12	1.32	2.04	1.27	1.96	1.22
30	2.03	1.26	1.95	1.21	1.90	1.18
20	1.95	1.21	1.88	1.17	1.82	1.13
10	1.82	1.13	1.75	1.09	1.70	1.05

Adapted, by permission, from ACSM, 2014, *ACSM's guidelines for exercise testing and prescription*, 9th ed. (Philadelphia: Wolters Kluwer Health/Lippincott Williams & Wilkins), 88.

TABLE 13.20 Descriptive Data for Yo-Yo for Various Populations*

Group, sport, or position	Number of athletes	Yo-Yo IR1	
		Distance (m)	Distance (yd)
National soccer (men) (74)	18	2260 ± 80	2472 ± 87
National soccer (men) (74)	24	2040 ± 60	2231 ± 66
National rugby league (men) (4)	23	1656 ± 403	1811 ± 441
Semiprofessional rugby league (men) (4)	27	1564 ± 415	1710 ± 454
National soccer (women) (76)	17	1224 ± 255	1339 ± 279
National soccer (men) (76)	17	2414 ± 456	2640 ± 499
National junior soccer (women) (76)	17	826 ± 160	903 ± 175
National junior soccer (men) (76)	17	2092 ± 260	2287 ± 284
Under 17 soccer (men) (25)	60	1556 ± 478	1702 ± 523
Under 16 rugby union (men) (85)	150	1150 ± 403	1258 ± 441
Under 14 elite basketball (men) (116)	15	1100 ± 385	1203 ± 421
Under 15 elite basketball (men) (116)	15	1283 ± 461	1403 ± 504
Under 17 elite basketball (men) (116)	17	1412 ± 245	1544 ± 268
Under 18 Gaelic football (men) (22)	265	1465 ± 370	1602 ± 405

*The values listed are means ± standard deviation. The data should be regarded as only descriptive, not normative.

TABLE 13.21 Descriptive Data for Agility Tests for Various Populations*

Group, sport, or position	Number of athletes	Time (s)			
		Pro Agility	T-test	505	Hexagon
College soccer (women) (118)	51	4.88 ± 0.20			
High school soccer (women) (118)	83	4.91 ± 0.22			
College lacrosse (women) (118)	79	4.99 ± 0.24			
National softball (women) (80)	10			2.66 ± 0.14	
National basketball (women) (105)	12			2.69 ± 0.28	
College students (women) (97)	34		11.92 ± 0.52		
College students (men) (97)	52		10.08 ± 0.46		
NCAA Division II college soccer (men) (63)	12	4.80 ± 0.33			
Recreational athletes (women) (108)	20	5.23 ± 0.25	11.70 ± 0.67		
Recreational athletes (men) (108)	24	4.67 ± 0.21	10.31 ± 0.46		
High school rugby league (men) (113)	70			2.42 ± 0.12	
High school rugby league (men) (36)	28			2.30 ± 0.13	
High school rugby league (men) (112)	302			2.49 ± 0.14	
High school rugby league (men) (112)	870			2.51 ± 0.15	
Junior national volleyball (men) (33)	14		9.90 ± 0.17		
Junior national volleyball (women) (33)	15		10.33 ± 0.13		
NCAA Division I college lacrosse (women) (117)	84	4.99 ± 0.23			
NCAA Division III college lacrosse (women) (49)	11	4.92 ± 0.22	10.50 ± 0.60		
MLB baseball (men) (50)	62	4.42 ± 0.90			
AAA baseball (men) (50)	52	4.53 ± 0.20			
AA baseball (men) (50)	50	4.42 ± 0.68			
A baseball (men) (50)	84	4.48 ± 0.54			
Rookie baseball (men) (50)	90	4.54 ± 0.19			
High school volleyball (women) (98)	27		10.96 ± 0.58		
NCAA Division I volleyball (women) (98)	26		10.65 ± 0.52		
Recreational athletes (women) (86)	52		12.52 ± 0.90		13.21 ± 1.68
Recreational athletes (men) (86)	58		10.49 ± 0.89		12.33 ± 1.47
College athletes (women) (86)	56		10.94 ± 0.60		12.87 ± 1.48
College athletes (women) (86)	47		9.94 ± 0.50		12.29 ± 1.39

*The values listed are means ± standard deviation. The data should be regarded as only descriptive, not normative.

TABLE 13.22 Percentile Ranks for the Pro Agility Test (Seconds) in NCAA Division I College Athletes

% rank	Women's volleyball	Women's basketball	Women's softball	Men's basketball	Men's baseball	Men's American football
90	4.75	4.65	4.88	4.22	4.25	4.21
80	4.84	4.82	4.96	4.29	4.36	4.31
70	4.91	4.86	5.03	4.35	4.41	4.38
60	4.98	4.94	5.10	4.39	4.46	4.44
50	5.01	5.06	5.17	4.41	4.50	4.52
40	5.08	5.10	5.24	4.44	4.55	4.59
30	5.17	5.14	5.33	4.48	4.61	4.66
20	5.23	5.23	5.40	4.51	4.69	4.76
10	5.32	5.36	5.55	4.61	4.76	4.89
Mean	5.03	5.02	5.19	4.41	4.53	4.54
SD	0.20	0.26	0.26	0.18	0.23	0.27
n	81	128	118	97	165	869

Data collected using electronic timing devices. SD = standard deviation, *n* = number of athletes.

Reprinted, by permission, from Hoffman, 2006 (47).

TABLE 13.23 Descriptive Data for Speed Testing for Various Populations*

Group, sport, or position	Number of athletes	Time (s) 10 m	Time (s) 20 m	Time (s) 40 m
College soccer (women) (118)	51		3.38 ± 0.17	5.99 ± 0.29
High school soccer (women) (118)	83		3.33 ± 0.15	5.94 ± 0.28
College lacrosse (women) (118)	79		3.37 ± 0.14	5.97 ± 0.27
NCAA Division I college soccer (women) (67)	15	2.31 ± 0.25		
Under 16 rugby league (men) (114)	67	1.82 ± 0.07	3.13 ± 0.00	
Under 17 rugby league (men) (114)	50	1.81 ± 0.06	3.12 ± 0.10	
Under 18 rugby league (men) (114)	56	1.80 ± 0.06	3.09 ± 0.10	
Under 19 rugby league (men) (114)	89	1.82 ± 0.07	3.11 ± 0.12	
Under 20 rugby league (men) (114)	22	1.79 ± 0.06	3.07 ± 0.12	
National soccer (men) (123)	17	1.82 ± 0.30	3.00 ± 0.30	
National rugby league (men) (7)	20	1.61 ± 0.06		5.15 ± 0.02
State rugby league (men) (7)	20	1.66 ± 0.06		5.13 ± 0.02
National rugby league forwards (men) (20)	12	1.66 ± 0.20	3.00 ± 0.08	
National rugby league backs (men) (20)	6	1.65 ± 0.15	2.91 ± 0.10	
State rugby league (men) (36)	26	2.06 ± 0.18	3.36 ± 0.23	5.83 ± 0.31
National rugby union (men) (21)	30	1.69 ± 0.10	2.93 ± 0.20	
National rugby league forwards (men) (72)	63			5.27 ± 0.19
National rugby league backs (men)	55			5.08 ± 0.20

Group, sport, or position	Number of athletes	Time (s)		
		10 m	20 m	40 m
National badminton (men) (120)	12	1.94 ± 0.18	3.35 ± 0.30	
National rugby league (men) (34)	58	1.73 ± 0.07		5.25 ± 0.17
Under 18 elite rugby league (men) (36)	28	1.81 ± 0.08	3.11 ± 0.12	5.56 ± 0.22
Under 18 subelite rugby league (men) (36)	36	1.94 ± 0.11	3.28 ± 0.18	5.83 ± 0.35
High school rugby league (men) (112)	302	1.88 ± 0.12	3.23 ± 0.16	
High school rugby league (men) (112)	870	1.90 ± 0.12	3.27 ± 0.19	
Junior national volleyball (women) (33)	20	1.90 ± 0.01		
Junior national volleyball (men) (33)	14	1.80 ± 0.02		
Under 18 Australian rules football (men) (127)	177		3.13 ± 0.09	
NCAA Division III college soccer (men) (63)	12	1.96 ± 0.11		5.79 ± 0.31
NCAA Division I college soccer (men) (102)	27	1.70 ± 0.10		4.90 ± 0.20
National Australian rules football (men) (126)	35	1.89 ± 0.07	3.13 ± 0.10	5.40 ± 0.17
National Australian rules football (men) (126)	30	1.70 ± 0.06	2.94 ± 0.08	
National soccer (women) (42)	85	1.67 ± 0.07		
National soccer (women) (42)	47	1.70 ± 0.07		
National soccer (women) (1)	17		3.17 ± 0.03	
National soccer (men) (106)	270	2.27 ± 0.40	3.38 ± 0.70	
Under 18 Gaelic football (men) (22)	265		3.22 ± 0.15	
		10 yd	20 yd	40 yd
NCAA Division I college lacrosse (women) (117)		1.99 ± 0.10	3.37 ± 0.14	5.97 ± 0.26
MLB baseball (men) (50)	62	1.52 ± 0.10		
AAA baseball (men) (50)	52	1.55 ± 0.09		
NCAA Divsion I football (men) (31)	281			4.88 ± 0.27
NCAA Division II football (men) (31)	282			4.92 ± 0.26
NCAA Division III football (men) (31)	205			4.96 ± 0.27

*The values listed are means ± standard deviation. The data should be regarded as only descriptive, not normative.

TABLE 13.24 Normative Data for the Balance Error Scoring System Test

Age	Women	Men
20-29	11.9 ± 5.1	10.4 ± 4.4
30-39	11.4 ± 5.6	11.5 ± 5.5
40-49	12.7 ± 6.9	12.4 ± 5.7
50-54	15.1 ± 8.2	13.6 ± 6.9
55-59	16.7 ± 8.2	16.4 ± 7.2
60-64	19.3 ± 8.8	17.2 ± 7.1
65-69	19.9 ± 6.6	20.0 ± 7.3

Data from Iverson and Koehle, 2013 (54).

TABLE 13.25   Equations for Calculating Estimated Body Density From Skinfold Measurements Among Various Populations

SKF sites[a]	Population subgroups	Sex	Age	Equation	Reference
S7SKF (chest + abdomen + triceps + subscapular + suprailiac + midaxilla + thigh)	Black or Hispanic	Women	18-55 years	Db (g/cc)[b] = 1.0970 − 0.00046971 (S7SKF) + 0.00000056 (S7SKF)^2 − 0.00012828 (age)	Jackson et al. (57)
S7SKF (chest + abdomen + triceps + subscapular + suprailiac + midaxilla + thigh)	Black or athletes	Men	18-61 years	Db (g/cc)[b] = 1.1120 − 0.00043499 (S7SKF) + 0.00000055 (S7SKF)^2 − 0.00028826 (age)	Jackson and Pollock (55)
S4SKF (triceps + anterior suprailiac + abdomen + thigh)	Athletes	Women	18-29 years	Db (g/cc)[b] = 1.096095 − 0.0006952 (S4SKF) − 0.0000011 (S4SKF)^2 − 0.0000714 (age)	Jackson et al. (57)
S3SKF (triceps + suprailiac + thigh)	White or anorexic	Women	18-55 years	Db (g/cc)[b] = 1.0994921 − 0.0009929 (S3SKF) + 0.0000023 (S3SKF)^2 − 0.0001392 (age)	Jackson et al. (57)
S3SKF (chest + abdomen + thigh)	White	Men	18-61 years	Db (g/cc)[b] = 1.109380 − 0.0008267 (S3SKF) + 0.0000016 (S3SKF)^2 − 0.0002574 (age)	Jackson and Pollock (55)
S2SKF (triceps + calf)	Black or white	Boys	6-17 years	% BF = 0.735 (S2SKF) + 1.0	Slaughter et al. (103)
S2SKF (triceps + calf)	Black or white	Girls	6-17 years	% BF = 0.610 (S2SKF) + 5.1	Slaughter et al. (103)
Suprailiac, triceps	Athletes	Women	High school and college age	Db (g/cc)[b] = 1.0764 − (0.00081 3 suprailiac) − (0.00088 3 triceps)	Sloan and Weir (104)
Thigh, subscapular	Athletes	Men	High school and college age	Db (g/cc)[b] = 1.1043 − (0.00133 3 thigh) − (0.00131 3 subscapular)	Sloan and Weir (104)
S3SKF (triceps + abdomen + thigh)	Athletes	Men or Women	18-34 years	%BF = 8.997 + 0.24658 (S3SKF) − 6.343 (gender[c]) − 1.998 (race[d])	Evans et al. (28)

[a]SSKF = sum of skinfolds (mm); Db = body density.

[b]Use population-specific conversion formulas (see table 13.26) to calculate %BF from Db.

[c]Male athletes = 1; female athletes = 0.

[d]Black athletes = 1; white athletes = 0.

Adapted, by permission, from V. H. Heyward, 1998, *Advanced fitness assessment and exercise prescription,* 3rd ed. (Champaign, IL: Human Kinetics), 155.

TABLE 13.26 Population-Specific Equations for Calculating Estimated Percent Body Fat From Body Density

Population	Age	Sex	%BF[a]
RACE			
American Indian	18-60	Female	$(4.81/Db) - 4.34$
Black	18-32	Male	$(4.37/Db) - 3.93$
	24-79	Female	$(4.85/Db) - 4.39$
Hispanic	20-40	Female	$(4.87/Db) - 4.41$
Japanese	18-48	Male	$(4.97/Db) - 4.52$
		Female	$(4.76/Db) - 4.28$
	61-78	Male	$(4.87/Db) - 4.41$
		Female	$(4.95/Db) - 4.50$
White	7-12	Male	$(5.30/Db) - 4.89$
		Female	$(5.35/Db) - 4.95$
	13-16	Male	$(5.07/Db) - 4.64$
		Female	$(5.10/Db) - 4.66$
	17-19	Male	$(4.99/Db) - 4.55$
		Female	$(5.05/Db) - 4.62$
	20-80	Male	$(4.95/Db) - 4.50$
		Female	$(5.01/Db) - 4.57$
LEVEL OF BODY FATNESS			
Anorexic	15-30	Female	$(5.26/Db) - 4.83$
Obese	17-62	Female	$(5.00/Db) - 4.56$
Athletes[b]	High school and college age	Male and female	$(4.57/Db) - 4.142$

BF = body fat; Db = body density.

[a]Multiply the value from this column's calculations by 100 to yield the percentage value.

[b]Use this formula with the Sloan and Weir formula (104) from table 13.25.

Adapted, by permission, from Heyward and Stolarczyk, 1996 (46).

TABLE 13.27   Percent Body Fat Descriptive Data for Athletes in Various Sports

| Classification | Typical percent body fat of athletes playing the sport | | Sport |
	Males	Females	
Extremely lean	<7	<15	Gymnastics Bodybuilding (at contest) Wrestling (at contest) Cross-country
Very lean	8-10	16-18	Men's basketball Racquetball Rowing Soccer Track and field decathlon (men) Track and field heptathlon (women)
Leaner than average	11-13	19-20	Men's baseball Canoeing Downhill skiing Speed skating Olympic-style weightlifting
Average	14-17	21-25	Women's basketball American football quarterbacks, kickers, linebackers Hockey Horse racing (jockey) Tennis Discus throw Volleyball Women's softball Powerlifting
Fatter than average	18-22	26-30	American football (linemen) Shot put

Data from Nieman, 1995 (78).

CHAPTER 14

Warm-Up and Flexibility Training

Ian Jeffreys, PhD

After completing this chapter, you will be able to

- identify the components and benefits of a preexercise warm-up,
- structure effective warm-ups,
- identify the factors that affect flexibility,
- use flexibility exercises that take advantage of proprioceptive neuromuscular facilitation, and
- select and apply appropriate static and dynamic stretching methods.

This chapter is devoted to two key areas, warm-up and training for flexibility. While these two areas have often been linked, it is important to differentiate between the two, as they have distinctly different key functions. A warm-up is designed to prepare an athlete for upcoming training or competition and can improve performance while potentially lessening the risk of injury. The chapter looks at the aims of a warm-up and suggests appropriate structures and protocols for designing effective warm-ups. Flexibility training, on the other hand, aims to increase the range of motion around a joint, normally through the use of different forms of stretching. The chapter looks at factors that affect flexibility and the use of different stretching protocols to facilitate enhancing flexibility.

Warm-Up

A warm-up period is now almost universally accepted as an integral part of any training session or competition (10). Essentially, its goal is to prepare the athlete mentally and physically for exercise or competition (51). A well-designed warm-up can confer a number of physiological responses that can potentially increase subsequent performance. These can be divided into temperature-related effects and non–temperature-related effects (10). Temperature-related effects include an increase in muscle temperature, core temperature (68), enhanced neural function, and the disruption of transient connective tissue bonds (33), while non–temperature-related effects can include increased blood flow to muscles, an elevation of baseline oxygen consumption, and postactivation potentiation (10). Warm-up effects are best elicited via an active type of warm-up rather than via passive warming techniques (33). The positive effects on performance may include the following:

- Faster muscle contraction and relaxation of both agonist and antagonist muscles (51)
- Improvements in the rate of force development and reaction time (3)
- Improvements in muscle strength and power (9, 33)
- Lowered viscous resistance in muscles and joints (33)
- Improved oxygen delivery due to the Bohr effect, whereby higher temperatures facilitate oxygen release from hemoglobin and myoglobin (68)
- Increased blood flow to active muscles (68)
- Enhanced metabolic reactions (33)
- An increased psychological preparedness for performance (10)

While the number of quality studies investigating the impact of warm-up on performance is surprisingly low, studies generally show a positive impact on subsequent performance (42). These include improvements in endurance performance (both aerobic and anaerobic) and improvements in performance on physical tasks such as jumping, as well as in actual sporting performance (42). What is also clear is that the major factors influencing the potential improvements are the structure of the warm-up and the specificity of the warm-up to the task(s) to be performed (42). It is likely that a range of warm-ups can be used, provided that they are structured in a way that addresses the specific physiological, biomechanical, and psychological requirements of the sport and of the athlete.

> **The structure of the warm-up influences potential improvements; as such, the warm-up needs to be specific to the activity to be performed.**

An effective warm-up has also traditionally been thought to decrease the risk of injury. While the influence of a warm-up on injury prevention is unclear, the evidence suggests that positive effects may exist (41, 85, 86). For example, increased muscle temperature can increase resistance to muscle tear (81).

Components of a Warm-Up

It is generally advised that a warm-up consist of a period of aerobic exercise, followed by stretching, and ending with a period of activity similar to the upcoming activity (42). A traditional warm-up program structure is built around these requirements and typically involves two key phases.

The first is a **general warm-up** period (21, 77), which may consist of 5 minutes of slow aerobic activity such as jogging, skipping, or cycling. The aim of this phase is to increase heart rate, blood flow, deep muscle temperature, respiration rate, and perspiration and decrease viscosity of joint fluids (30). This phase is typically followed by a period of general stretching that aims to replicate the ranges of motion required for the upcoming activity.

Following the general warm-up is the **specific warm-up** period, which incorporates movements similar to the movements of the athlete's sport. This phase should also include rehearsal of the skill(s) to be performed (100).

The whole warm-up should progress gradually and provide sufficient intensity to increase muscle and core temperatures without causing fatigue or reducing energy stores (68). Typically, it should last between 10 and 20 minutes; the shorter time periods are far more common in the majority of training sessions. Longer time periods are more common in cases in which aspects of the warm-up are an integral part of the main session, or when specific competition warm-ups are being carried out. The warm-up should end no more than 15 minutes before the start of the subsequent activity (after this time the positive effects of the warm-up start to dissipate) (33).

Targeted and Structured Warm-Ups

While the structure of general and specific warm-up is generally accepted, activities undertaken within warm-ups vary considerably. Consequently, although athletes may be undertaking a warm-up, it is difficult to ensure that the warm-up adequately addresses the key variables required to optimize subsequent performance (42). Effective planning needs to carefully consider how the warm-up will contribute to subsequent performance. Similarly, planning needs to delineate between warm-ups used before competition and the more ubiquitous warm-ups used within a training session. Whereas the warm-up for competition aims at maximizing performance in the subsequent competition, the training warm-up, as well as optimizing acute performance, can contribute to performance in other productive ways and should be planned appropriately. For optimal impact, this planning should also consider how the warm-up contributes to the overall development of the athlete; this planning should entail short-, medium-, and long-term considerations.

Medium- and long-term planning is a recent trend with regard to planning effective warm-ups. Athletes spend a great deal of training time warming up, and so structures that allow optimal use of this time provide a potentially powerful tool for the coach (54). Effective warm-ups should be thought of as an integral part of a training session, not as a separate entity (54). With most training warm-ups lasting from 10 to 20 minutes, over a training cycle this contributes to a significant amount of training time; with effective planning, this can contribute greatly to an athlete's overall development, as well as optimally preparing the athlete for the subsequent session.

> ▶ The warm-up is an integral part of the training session. Strength and conditioning professionals should plan warm-ups incorporating short-, medium-, and long-term considerations that will contribute to the overall development of the athlete.

It is likely that optimal levels of warm-up exist (89); these are related to the type of warm-up (training or competition), the task to be performed, the individual, and the environment. There is likely a range of potentially effective warm-ups; the key is that the coach has a structure around which to plan the warm-up. The structure of general and specific warm-up, though valid, may need to be supplemented by an approach that allows for greater targeting of both short- and long-term performance. One structure that has been adopted by many coaches and that addresses all of the key aspects of an effective warm-up is the **Raise, Activate and Mobilize, and Potentiate (RAMP)** protocol (54). This builds on the general and specific structure and provides a suitable approach via which performance can be maximized in the short, medium, and long term (54). As the name indicates, raise, activate and mobilize, and potentiate are its three key phases.

The first phase of RAMP involves activities that raise the level of key physiological parameters but also the levels of skill of the athletes. This phase is analogous to the general warm-up and has the aim of elevating body temperature, heart rate, respiration rate, blood flow, and joint fluid viscosity via low-intensity activities. However, a critical aspect is that unlike traditional general warm-up activities, these are not simply general aerobic exercises; instead, they attempt to simulate the movement patterns of the upcoming activity or develop the movement patterns or skill patterns the athlete will need to deploy within the sport. In this way, the session, from the outset, is targeted at key movement and skill capacities, as well as providing the required physiological effects of the activity. This also assists in the psychological preparation of the athlete for practice or competition as the session constantly addresses components that relate to performance.

The second phase, activating and mobilizing, is analogous to the stretching component of a typical warm-up. Key movement patterns required for athletic performance in both the subsequent session and in the athlete's overall development, such as squat patterns and lunge patterns, are performed. The focus on mobility, or actively moving through a range of motion, requires a combination of motor control, stability, and flexibility and more closely relates to the movements requirements an athlete will face (54). Great debate is still prevalent as to whether static stretching should be used within warm-up, and at present the evidence is equivocal. Some reviews of the literature on the effect of static stretching on performance question the practice (83, 84, 100), suggesting that it can compromise muscle performance (59). Studies have demonstrated negative effects of static stretching on performance in a range of parameters such as force production (8, 25-27, 35, 76), power performance (23, 92, 99, 100), running speed (38), reaction/movement time (7), and strength endurance (73). Other studies show no decrement in performance, and a more recent review by Kay and Blazevich (56) concludes that there is clear evidence that short-duration static stretching has no detrimental effect on subsequent performance unless stretches are held for greater than 60 seconds. However, a recent meta-analysis performed by Simic and colleagues (87) calls into question the work of Kay and Blazevich (56), suggesting that the authors did not use appropriate statistical measures to support their contentions. Simic and coworkers (87) report that shorter-duration (<45 seconds) static stretching bouts result in less performance decrement but that the performance decrement still exists and may affect competitive performance. Therefore, in deciding whether to use static stretching within this phase of the warm-up, it is important that the strength and conditioning professional perform a benefit–risk analysis (65). An important factor to consider in designing this phase of the warm-up is the range of motion required for the activity; athletes in sports that require greater ranges of motion may need to spend more time in this phase of warm-up than those with a low range of motion requirement (46, 97).

In relation to these decisions, the use of a mobilization and activation phase for warm-up rather than a stretching phase helps coaches select the activities. As no consistent link has been shown between stretching and injury prevention (47, 50, 75, 86, 89) or subsequent muscle soreness (55), the focus in warm-ups should shift to performance. Exercises should be designed to contribute to the preparation for the upcoming session but also enhance the athlete's overall movement capacities. Exercises that encourage the athlete to use key movement patterns, thus helping with the development of the required motor control as well as developing mobility, are ideal activities within this phase of the warm-up (54). Similarly, this phase provides a great opportunity via which to address any specific movement issues an athlete may demonstrate (54).

The use of a range of dynamic stretching and mobility exercises provides all of these key advantages. Additionally, dynamic stretching helps maintain the temperature-related benefits of the raising phase of the warm-up (54). Furthermore, a number of joints can be integrated into a single stretch, often including multiplanar movements similar to those that occur in sport. Thus, dynamic stretches are extremely time efficient, which can be important when training time is limited (49, 54). These advantages, together with the fact that dynamic stretching and mobility exercises have been shown to improve subsequent running performance (38, 66, 98), make these types of exercises the preferred activities during warming up for the majority of sports (54).

The third phase, **potentiation**, is analogous to the specific warm-up but importantly also focuses on the intensity of activities. This phase deploys sport-specific activities that progress in intensity until the athlete is performing at the intensity required for the subsequent competition or training session. This phase is important to subsequent performance, especially in activities that require high levels of speed, strength, and power, yet it is often omitted from traditional warm-ups. Indeed, the more power necessary for the sport or activity, the more important the potentiation phase of warm-up (17), and including high-intensity dynamic exercises can facilitate subsequent performance (11, 14, 36, 99). Competition warm-up should include a progression of sport-specific activities that enable the athlete to maximize performance physiologically and psychologically (11). For the training warm-up, this should be targeted to the upcoming session yet also address the longer-term requirements of the athlete. With effective planning, this phase of the warm-up can be a key part of the session, presenting an ideal opportunity to work on aspects of performance such as speed and agility (54). Effective planning of this phase can allow considerable training time to be spent on key components of fitness without an overall increase in training duration (54). Indeed, it is this phase that ultimately determines the optimal length of the warm-up, as the potentiation phase can become a key part of the session, allowing the delivery of elements such as speed training and agility training; in these instances the entire warm-up will be longer but will progress essentially seamlessly to the main session.

Flexibility

The degree of movement that occurs at a joint is called the **range of motion (ROM)**. **Flexibility** is a measure of ROM and has static and dynamic components. **Static flexibility** is the range of possible movement about a joint (22, 30) and its surrounding muscles during a passive movement (40, 44). Static flexibility requires no voluntary muscular activity; an external force such as gravity, a partner, or a machine provides the force for a stretch. **Dynamic flexibility** refers to the available ROM during active movements and therefore requires voluntary muscular actions. Dynamic ROM is generally greater than static ROM. The relationship between static and dynamic ROM has historically been questioned (52) and still remains largely unresolved, especially in relation to the fact that normal motion cannot guarantee normal movement (19). Therefore, the direct transfer between measures of static flexibility and sport performance cannot be determined.

In determining which type of flexibility is most crucial, it is important to look at the nature of sport itself. A key role of flexibility is its contribution to an athlete's movement. Thus, flexibility viewed in isolation can be misleading, as normal ROM does not guarantee normal movement (19). In this context the concept of mobility can be more enlightening, because it entails movement and therefore the integration of additional aspects such as balance coordination, postural control coordination, and perception (19). In this way, mobility frames flexibility as a dynamic quality, with the athlete required to demonstrate control, coordination, and force through any demonstrated ROM. This is advantageous when looking at the role of flexibility on performance. Indeed, enhanced ROM without appropriate motor control can never maximize performance (82).

Flexibility and Performance

The effects of flexibility on performance depend on the types of activity undertaken, and the most flexible athlete is not always the most successful (82). Therefore, optimizing flexibility in relation to the specific activity rather than simply maximizing flexibility is the main aim of training (71). Sports and activities have specific requirements for ROM, and it is likely that optimal levels of flexibility exist for each activity, with these related to the movements within the particular sport (45, 89). It is also important that the strength and conditioning professional keep in mind the kinetic and kinematic patterns required within the ROM, as this will dictate the types of development methods used. The development of greater ROM will be associated with the aim of enhancing performance, and this often involves the need to apply force over the required ROM and the ability to assume the key technical positions required for the sport. In some instances, greater ROM can be seen as the missing link in the athlete's power program, as the ability to apply force over a greater ROM can increase impulse, via extending the time over which the athlete can apply force, which in turn contributes to enhanced performance in a range of sports (67). Thus, the strength and conditioning professional should look at the optimal ROM required of the athlete, but also at the force patterns required through this ROM, and should develop these in tandem with enhanced ROM to ensure that the athlete is optimally prepared for performance.

There are optimal ranges of flexibility for different sports and activities, and injury risk may be increased when an athlete is unable to attain this range. It is also important to note that both inflexibility and hyperflexibility can result in higher risks of injury (78, 89). In addition, an imbalance in flexibility could predispose the individual to an increased risk of injury (57, 58).

Factors Affecting Flexibility

A number of anatomical and training-related factors affect flexibility. Training cannot alter some factors, such as joint structure, age, and sex. However, others can be manipulated and thus are important considerations in the design of flexibility development programs. A long-term program of stretching can have cumulative positive effects ranging from enhanced flexibility to enhanced

strength (82). Strength and conditioning professionals should consider each athlete's unique combination of factors and sport requirements when recommending flexibility development exercises and programs.

Joint Structure

The structure of a joint determines its ROM (66). **Ball-and-socket joints**, such as the hip and shoulder, move in all anatomical planes and have the greatest ROM of all joints (2). The wrist is an **ellipsoidal joint** (an oval-shaped condyle that fits into an elliptical cavity) primarily allowing movement in the sagittal and frontal planes; its ROM is significantly less than that of the shoulder or hip (2). In contrast, the knee is a modified **hinge joint**, with movement primarily in the sagittal plane; its ROM is less than that of either a ball-and-socket joint or the ellipsoidal wrist joint. The type of joint, the shapes of the joint's articulating surfaces, and the soft tissues surrounding the joint all affect its ROM.

Age and Sex

Young people tend to be more flexible than older people (95), and females tend to be more flexible than males (44). Differences in flexibility between young men and women may be due in part to structural and anatomical differences and the type and extent of activities performed. Older people undergo a process called **fibrosis**, in which fibrous connective tissue replaces degenerating muscle fibers (2). This is likely due to inactivity and a tendency to use less of the available ROM during movement. Just as older people can improve strength, they can improve flexibility with appropriate exercise.

Muscle and Connective Tissue

A range of body tissues can influence flexibility. For example, factors such as muscle tissue, the musculotendinous unit, tendons, ligaments, fascial sheaths, joint capsules, and skin may limit ROM (30). The relative contributions of these to increased flexibility, both acutely and chronically, remain unclear and reflect the impact of **elasticity** and **plasticity**. Elasticity (the ability to return to original resting length after a passive stretch) and plasticity (the tendency to assume a new and greater length after a passive stretch) of connective tissue are other factors that determine ROM (39, 96). Stretching exercises can positively affect connective tissues by taking advantage of their plastic potential, although the relative importance of each tissue type and the differences between individual responses remain unclear (12).

Stretch Tolerance

An important factor in determining an athlete's flexibility is stretch tolerance, or the ability to tolerate the discomfort of stretching (82). Individuals with a greater ROM tend to demonstrate a greater level of stretch tolerance and are thus able to tolerate a greater stretch load (12). One important feature of a regular stretching program is that it can increase an athlete's stretch tolerance, thus potentially permitting further increases in flexibility.

Neural Control

The control of an athlete's ROM is ultimately held at the level of the central and peripheral nervous system and less by structural elements (62). This system includes both afferent and efferent mechanisms resulting in both reflexive and conscious activities that ultimately control the ROM an athlete is able to attain. A key aspect of an effective flexibility program is the capacity to positively affect this system, allowing for elicitation of a greater ROM.

Resistance Training

A comprehensive and proper resistance training program may increase flexibility (60, 88) and also assist in the development of force capacity through the enhanced ROM. Effective strength training protocols should be seen as an important adjunct to a stretching program (82). However, this comes with a proviso: Heavy resistance training with limited ROM during the exercises may decrease ROM (30). To prevent loss of ROM, an athlete should perform exercises that develop both agonist and antagonist muscles (16) and should exercise through the full available ROM of the involved joints.

Muscle Bulk

A significant increase in muscle bulk may adversely affect ROM by impeding joint movement. An athlete with large biceps and deltoids, for example, may experience difficulty in stretching the triceps (30), racking a power clean, or holding a bar while performing the front squat. Although altering the training program can decrease the amount of muscle bulk, this may not be advisable for large power athletes such as shot putters or American football offensive linemen. Strength and conditioning professionals should always keep the requirements of the athlete's sport in mind: The need for large muscles may supersede the need for extreme joint mobility, but similarly, where ROM is crucial, the potential negative effects of muscle bulk should be considered and training programs planned accordingly.

Activity Level

An active person tends to be more flexible than an inactive one (44). This is particularly true if the activity includes flexibility exercises but is also true if the person performs other activities such as resistance training. Both men and women have successfully increased their flexibility as an outcome of a properly designed resistance training program (94). It is also important to understand that activity level alone does not improve flexibility; stretching exercises or exercises requiring the body to move through a full ROM are essential if joint flexibility is to be maintained or increased.

Frequency, Duration, and Intensity of Stretching

As with all forms of training, frequency, duration, and intensity are important issues in program design (28). Both static (13) and proprioceptive neuromuscular facilitation (34) stretching have been shown to increase joint flexibility around the knee, hip, trunk, shoulder, and ankle joints (89). Despite this, the exact mechanisms responsible for increased flexibility are still unclear. The acute effects of stretching on ROM are transient and are greatest immediately after the stretching session; then they decline, with the duration of significant improvements in flexibility ranging from 3 minutes (29) to 24 hours (31).

For longer-lasting effects, a dedicated flexibility program is required (89). Stretching twice per week, for a minimum of five weeks, has been shown to significantly improve flexibility (40). However, the literature provides limited guidelines regarding specific stretching parameters, especially for proprioceptive neuromuscular facilitation methods (30).

As to the appropriate duration for a static stretch, 15 to 30 seconds is generally recommended (78) and has been shown to be more effective than shorter durations (79, 93). Evidence supports the use of 30 seconds (4-6) and suggests that there are diminishing returns beyond this duration. Another consideration is the total stretch time throughout a day, which may be as important as the duration of a single stretch (17, 79). When performing static stretches, athletes should hold the stretch at a position of mild discomfort (not pain). Joint integrity should never be compromised in order to increase ROM. All stretching sessions should be preceded by a period of general activity to raise muscle temperature. Because neural and vascular structures are stretched during flexibility exercises, athletes should be monitored for a loss of sensation or radiating pain.

When Should an Athlete Stretch?

Stretching should be performed at the following times for optimal benefits:

- *Following practice and competition.* Postpractice stretching facilitates ROM improvements (43) because of increased muscle temperature (39).

It should be performed within 5 to 10 minutes after practice. The increased body temperature increases the elastic properties of collagen within muscles and tendons, which allows for a greater stretch magnitude. Postpractice stretching may also decrease muscle soreness (77), although the evidence on this is ambiguous (1, 61).

- *As a separate session.* If increased levels of flexibility are required, additional stretching sessions may be needed. In this case, stretching should be preceded by a thorough general warm-up to allow for the increase in muscle temperature necessary for effective stretching. This type of session can be especially useful as a recovery session on the day after a competition.

Proprioceptors and Stretching

Two important proprioceptors should be considered during stretching: **muscle spindles** and **Golgi tendon organs (GTOs)**. Muscle spindles, located within intrafusal muscle fibers that run parallel to extrafusal muscle fibers, monitor changes in muscle length (40). During a rapid stretching movement, a sensory neuron from the muscle spindle innervates a motor neuron in the spine. The motor neuron then causes a muscle action of the previously stretched extrafusal muscle fibers; this is the **stretch reflex**. Stimulation of the muscle spindle and the subsequent activation of the stretch reflex should be avoided during stretching, as motion will be limited by the reflexive muscle action. If the muscle spindles are not stimulated, the muscle relaxes and allows greater stretch. Because of the very slow movement during static stretching (see the next section, "Types of Stretching"), the stretch reflex is not invoked. Rapid (ballistic and dynamic) stretching movements may stimulate the muscle spindles, causing a stretch reflex.

The GTO, a **mechanoreceptor** located near the musculotendinous junction, is sensitive to increases in muscular tension. When stimulated, the GTO causes a muscle to reflexively relax. Relaxation that occurs in the same muscle that is experiencing increased tension is called **autogenic inhibition** (18, 22, 72). Autogenic inhibition is accomplished via active contraction of a muscle immediately before a passive stretch of that same muscle. Tension built up during the active contraction stimulates the GTO, causing a reflexive relaxation of the muscle during the subsequent passive stretch. Relaxation that occurs in the muscle opposing the muscle experiencing the increased tension is called **reciprocal inhibition** (18, 72). This occurs when one simultaneously contracts the muscle opposing the muscle that is being passively stretched. Here the tension in the contracting muscle stimulates the GTO and causes a simultaneous reflexive relaxation of the stretched muscle.

Types of Stretching

Stretching requires movement of a body segment to a point of resistance in the ROM. At the point of resistance, a force is applied. This stretching movement can be performed either actively or passively. An **active stretch** occurs when the person stretching supplies the force of the stretch. During the sitting toe touch, for example, the athlete contracts the abdominal muscles and hip flexors to flex the torso forward to stretch the hamstrings and low back. A **passive stretch** occurs when a partner or a stretching machine provides external force to cause or enhance a stretch.

Static Stretch

A **static stretch** is slow and constant, with the end position held for 15 to 30 seconds (4, 6). A static stretch includes the relaxation and concurrent elongation of the stretched muscle (37). Because it is performed slowly, static stretching does not elicit the stretch reflex of the stretched muscle (20); therefore, the likelihood of injury is less than during ballistic stretching (2, 39, 90). In addition, static stretching is easy to learn and has been shown to effectively improve ROM (13). Although injury to muscles or connective tissue may result if the static stretch is too intense, there are no real disadvantages to static stretching as long as proper technique is used. Static stretching is appropriate for all athletes in a variety of sports for increasing flexibility.

The sitting toe touch is a good example of a static stretch. To perform this stretch statically, the athlete sits on the ground with the lower extremities together and knees extended, leans forward from the waist, and slowly reaches toward the ankles. The athlete gradually increases the intensity of the stretch by leaning forward until he or she feels mild discomfort in the hamstrings or lower back. The athlete holds this position for 15 to 30 seconds and then slowly returns to an upright sitting position. The stretch is static because it is performed slowly and the end position is held without movement.

Ballistic Stretch

A **ballistic stretch** typically involves active muscular effort and uses a bouncing-type movement in which the end position is not held (70). Ballistic stretching is often used in the preexercise warm-up; however, if not appropriately controlled or sequenced, it may injure muscles or connective tissues, especially when there has been a previous injury (20). Ballistic stretching usually triggers the stretch reflex that does not allow the involved muscles to relax, which may limit ROM, so the strength and conditioning professional should monitor this during the session.

As an example, consider the sitting toe touch performed as a ballistic stretch rather than a static stretch. The athlete sits on the ground with knees extended, lower extremities together, and upper body perpendicular to the legs. The athlete reaches quickly toward the ankles, bounces at the end position, and immediately returns to a near-vertical upper body position. With each repetition, the end position extends farther than in the preceding repetition. Ballistic stretching has been shown to be just as effective as static stretching in enhancing ROM (63) and could play a role in a flexibility development program (24). However, care must be taken to ensure that the athlete is appropriately prepared for this type of exercise acutely and chronically, and special care should be taken when a previous injury has been reported.

Dynamic Stretch

A **dynamic stretch** is a type of functionally based stretching exercise that uses sport-generic and sport-specific movements to prepare the body for activity (64). Dynamic stretching—sometimes referred to as **mobility drills** (3)—places an emphasis on the movement requirements of the sport or activity rather than on individual muscles. This type of exercise can closely duplicate the movement requirements of a sport or activity (48); for example, a walking knee lift stretch mimics the knee lift of a sprinter. Essentially, one can think of dynamic stretching as actively moving a joint through the ROM encountered in a sport.

Dynamic and ballistic stretches may appear similar; however, a number of key differences significantly alter the effects of these activities such that dynamic stretching avoids the potential negative effects associated with ballistic stretching. Dynamic stretching avoids bouncing and is performed in a more controlled manner than ballistic stretching. The result is a controlled ROM that is often smaller than that produced by ballistic stretching but demonstrates the control required to be able to actively move through the full ROM and assume and hold the end position.

The ability to actively move a joint through a ROM is generally far more sport specific than the ability to statically hold a stretch. Advantages of dynamic stretching include its ability to promote dynamic flexibility and to replicate the movement patterns and ROM required for sport activities. As a consequence, dynamic stretches, as outlined in the discussion of warm-up, are increasingly the preferred method of stretching during warm-up.

In dynamic stretching, unlike static stretching, the muscle does not relax during the stretch but instead is active through the ROM; this is also more specific to the movement patterns that occur in sport. Even though it is an ideal warm-up activity, dynamic stretching may be less effective than static or proprioceptive neuromuscular facilitation stretching at increasing static ROM (5); in situations in which an increased static ROM is needed, static or proprioceptive neuromuscular facilitation methods may be preferred.

When one is designing a dynamic stretching program, the starting point should be a careful analysis of the major movement patterns within the given sport and the ROM required within these movements. One can then select exercises that replicate those movements via a series of dynamic stretches. In this way, it is possible to achieve a highly specific flexibility program.

Dynamic stretching provides the opportunity to combine movements (32, 49). This gives the strength and conditioning professional a large number of combinations that can be used to provide variety in the warm-up. Athletes can perform dynamic stretching exercises either for a series of repetitions in the same place (e.g., 10 lunges) or for a series of repetitions to cover a given distance (e.g., lunge for 15 m). Regardless of the method chosen, each drill should start slowly and gradually increase the ROM, the speed, or both during subsequent repetitions or sets. For example, athletes can perform the knee lift exercise over a distance of 15 m, starting at a walk, and build to a skip in subsequent repetitions. This progression provides for an increase in both speed and ROM. An effective warm-up using dynamic stretching can be achieved in 10 to 15 minutes (64).

In a dynamic stretch that mirrors a sport skill—such as a sprinter's knee lift drill—it is important that the stretch also emphasize the key skill factors required for the movement so that the most important mechanics of the drill are reinforced. For example, if the knee lift drill is used in the warm-up, effective body mechanics should be emphasized along with key joint positions such as dorsiflexion of the ankle of the lifted foot. The use of dynamic stretches must always be coordinated with appropriate sport techniques and never compromise proper technique.

Proprioceptive Neuromuscular Facilitation Stretch

Proprioceptive neuromuscular facilitation (PNF) stretching was originally developed as part of a neuromuscular rehabilitation program designed to relax muscles with increased tone or activity (90). It has since been expanded to athletics as a method of increasing flexibility. Proprioceptive neuromuscular facilitation techniques are usually performed with a partner and involve both passive movement and active (concentric and isometric) muscle actions. Proprioceptive neuromuscular facilitation stretching may be superior to other stretching methods because it facilitates muscular inhibition (21, 34, 53, 74, 80, 88, 91), although evidence for this has not been consistently shown (28). However,

PNF stretching is often impractical because most of the stretches require a partner and some expertise. This section serves as an introduction to PNF stretching.

During a PNF stretch, three specific muscle actions are used to facilitate the passive stretch. Both isometric and concentric muscle actions of the antagonist (the muscle being stretched) are used before a passive stretch of the antagonist to achieve autogenic inhibition. The isometric muscle action is referred to as *hold* and the concentric muscle action as *contract*. A concentric muscle action of the agonist, called **agonist contraction**, is used during a passive stretch of the antagonist to achieve reciprocal inhibition. Each technique also involves passive, static stretches that are referred to as *relax*.

There are three basic types of PNF stretching techniques:

- Hold-relax (15, 18, 21, 80, 88)
- Contract-relax (15, 21)
- Hold-relax with agonist contraction (18, 72)

The PNF techniques are completed in three phases. With each of the three techniques, the first phase incorporates a passive prestretch of 10 seconds. The muscle actions used in the second and third phases differ for the three techniques; the second and third phases give each technique its name. A stretch to improve hamstring flexibility provides an illustration (see figures 14.1 through 14.11).

Hold-Relax

The **hold-relax** technique begins with a passive prestretch that is held at the point of mild discomfort for 10 seconds (figure 14.3). The partner then applies a hip flexion force and instructs the athlete, "Hold and don't let me move the leg"; the athlete "holds" and resists the movement so that an isometric muscle action occurs and is held for 6 seconds (figure 14.4). The athlete then relaxes, and a passive stretch is performed and held for 30 seconds (figure 14.5). The final stretch should be of greater magnitude due to autogenic inhibition (i.e., activation of the hamstrings).

Contract-Relax

The **contract-relax** technique also begins with a passive prestretch of the hamstrings that is held at the point of mild discomfort for 10 seconds (figure 14.6). The athlete then extends the hip against resistance from the partner so that a concentric muscle action through the full ROM occurs (figure 14.7). The athlete then relaxes, and a passive hip flexion stretch is applied and held for 30 seconds (figure 14.8). The increased ROM is facilitated due to autogenic inhibition (i.e., activation of the hamstrings). In an alternative to this technique, the

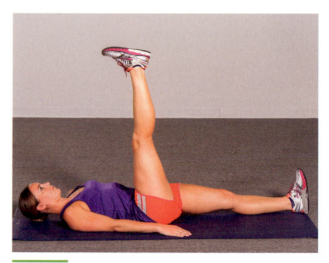

FIGURE 14.1   Starting position of PNF hamstring stretch.

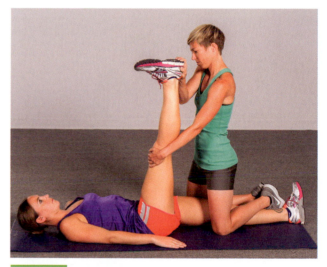

FIGURE 14.2   Partner and subject leg and hand positions for PNF hamstring stretch.

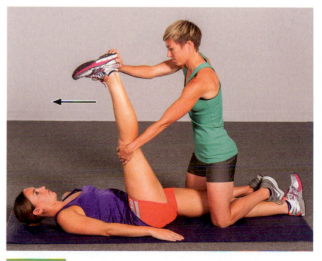

FIGURE 14.3   Passive prestretch of hamstrings during hold-relax PNF hamstring stretch.

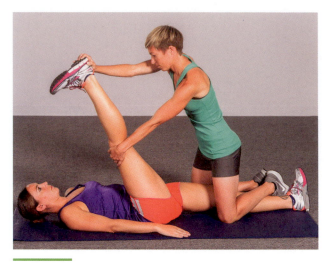

FIGURE 14.4 Isometric action during hold-relax PNF hamstring stretch.

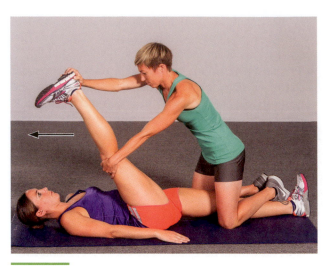

FIGURE 14.5 Increased ROM during passive stretch of hold-relax PNF hamstring stretch.

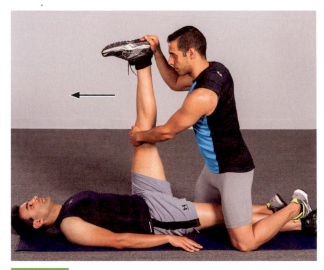

FIGURE 14.6 Passive prestretch of hamstrings during contract-relax PNF stretch.

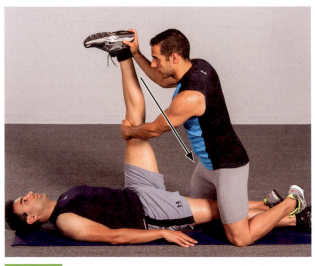

FIGURE 14.7 Concentric action of hip extensors during contract-relax PNF stretch.

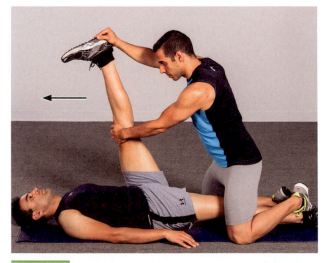

FIGURE 14.8 Increased ROM during passive stretch of contract-relax PNF stretch.

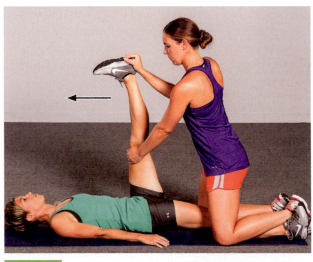

FIGURE 14.9 Passive prestretch during hold-relax with agonist contraction PNF hamstring stretch.

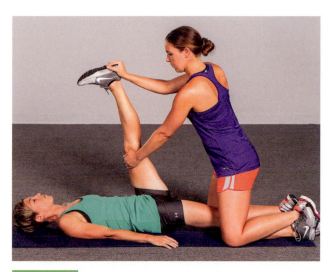

FIGURE 14.10 Isometric action of hamstrings during hold-relax with agonist contraction PNF hamstring stretch.

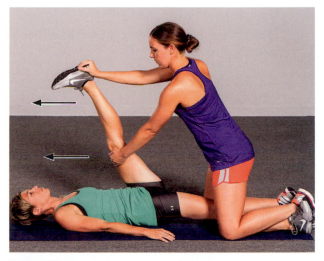

FIGURE 14.11 Concentric contraction of quadriceps during hold-relax with agonist contraction PNF hamstring stretch, creating increased ROM during passive stretch.

athlete attempts to extend the hip and the partner does not allow the movement (69). Because this is essentially the same as the hold-relax technique, the contract-relax method described here is preferred.

Hold-Relax With Agonist Contraction

The **hold-relax with agonist contraction** technique is identical to hold-relax in the first two phases (figures 14.9 and 14.10). During the third phase, a concentric action of the agonist is used in addition to the passive stretch to add to the stretch force (figure 14.11). That is, following the isometric hold, the athlete flexes the hip, thereby moving further into the new ROM. With this technique, the final stretch should be greater, primarily because of reciprocal inhibition (i.e., activation of the hip flexors) (69, 72) and secondarily because of autogenic inhibition (i.e., activation of the hamstrings) (72).

> The hold-relax with agonist contraction is the most effective PNF stretching technique due to facilitation via both reciprocal and autogenic inhibition.

Common PNF Stretches With a Partner

The following are common PNF stretches performed with a partner. Each is illustrated with a photo.

- Calves and ankles (figure 14.12)
- Chest (figure 14.13)

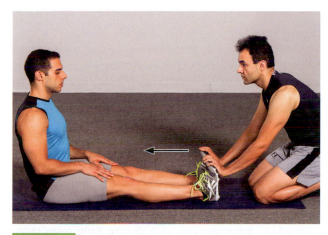

FIGURE 14.12 Partner PNF stretching for the calves.

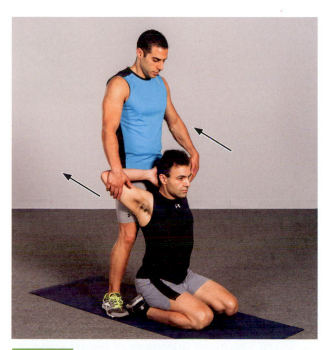

FIGURE 14.13 Partner PNF stretching for the chest.

- Groin (figure 14.14)
- Hamstrings and hip extensors (previously described)

- Quadriceps and hip flexors (figure 14.15)
- Shoulders (figure 14.16)

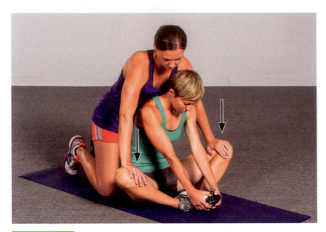

FIGURE 14.14   Partner PNF stretching for the groin.

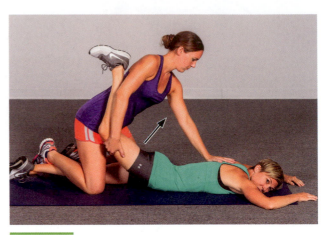

FIGURE 14.15   Partner PNF stretching for the quadriceps and hip flexors.

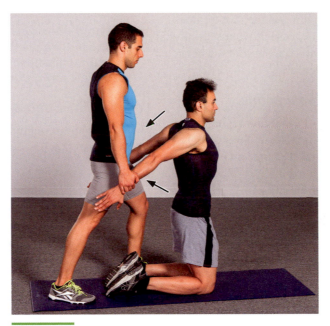

FIGURE 14.16   Partner PNF stretching for the shoulders.

Conclusion

A warm-up can provide benefits that enhance subsequent performance. Warm-up should be geared toward the particular sport or activity and should use an appropriate structure, ensuring that an athlete is optimally prepared for subsequent activity. Effective warm-up planning can ensure that the activities prepare the athlete for the upcoming session but do not induce undue fatigue. Additionally, the warm-up should be planned so that the activities contribute both to the goal of the upcoming session and to the development of the athlete in the medium and long term.

Optimal flexibility for performance varies from sport to sport and is closely related to the types of movements and actions an athlete will be required to perform. The concept of mobility may be more appropriate than flexibility with its focus on active movement through the required ROM. For athletes who need to increase flexibility, static and PNF stretching techniques will allow for an effective increase in ROM, and these techniques should be a key component of an extended training program. Strength and conditioning professionals should consider each athlete's unique combination of joint structure, age, sex, and sport requirements when recommending stretching protocols.

STATIC STRETCHING TECHNIQUES

Guidelines for Static Stretching

- Get into a position that facilitates relaxation.
- Move to the point in the ROM where you experience a sensation of mild discomfort. If performing partner-assisted PNF stretching, communicate clearly with your partner.
- Hold stretches for 15 to 30 seconds.
- Repeat unilateral stretches on both sides.

Precautions for Static Stretching

- Decrease stretch intensity if you experience pain, radiating symptoms, or loss of sensation.
- Use caution when stretching a hypermobile joint.
- Avoid combination movements that involve the spine (e.g., extension and lateral flexion).
- Stabilizing muscles should be active to protect other joints and prevent unwanted movements.

14.1   LOOK RIGHT AND LEFT

1. Stand or sit with the head and neck upright.
2. Turn the head to the right using a submaximal concentric muscle action.
3. Turn the head to the left using a submaximal concentric muscle action.

MUSCLE AFFECTED

sternocleidomastoid

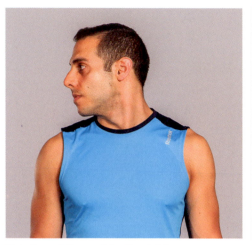 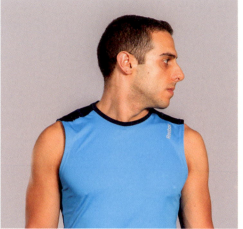

Rotation of the neck to the right   **Rotation of the neck to the left**

14.2   FLEXION AND EXTENSION

1. Standing or sitting with head and neck upright, flex the neck by tucking the chin toward the chest.
2. If the chin touches the chest, try to touch the chin lower on the chest.
3. Extend the neck by trying to come as close as possible to touching the head to the back.

MUSCLES AFFECTED

sternocleidomastoid, suboccipitals, splenae

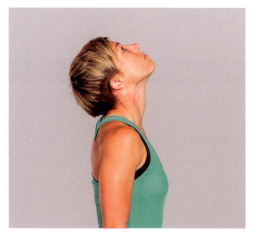 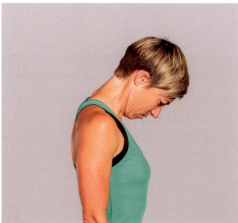

Neck extension   **Neck flexion**

14.3 | STRAIGHT ARMS BEHIND BACK

1. Standing, place both arms behind the back.
2. Interlock fingers with palms facing each other.
3. Straighten the elbows fully.
4. Slowly raise the arms, keeping the elbows straight.
5. Keep head upright and neck relaxed.

MUSCLES AFFECTED

anterior deltoid, pectoralis major

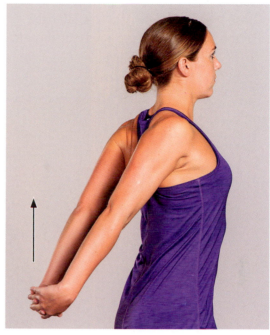

Stretching the shoulder joints—standing

14.4 | SEATED LEAN-BACK

1. Sitting with the legs straight and arms extended, place palms on the floor about 12 inches (30 cm) behind the hips.
2. Point the fingers away from the body (backward).
3. Slide the hands backward and lean backward.

MUSCLES AFFECTED

deltoids, pectoralis major

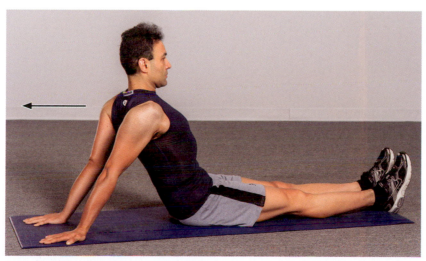

Stretching the shoulder joints—seated

14.5 BEHIND-NECK STRETCH (Chicken Wing)

1. Standing or sitting, abduct the right shoulder and flex the elbow.
2. Reach the right hand down toward the left scapula.
3. Grasp the right elbow with the left hand.
4. Pull the elbow behind the head with the left hand to increase shoulder abduction.

MUSCLES AFFECTED

triceps brachii, latissimus dorsi

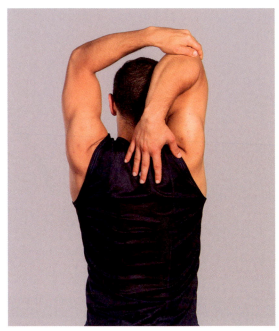

Stretching the triceps

14.6 CROSS ARM IN FRONT OF CHEST

1. Stand or sit with the left elbow slightly flexed (15°-30°) and the arm across the body (i.e., shoulder in horizontal adduction).
2. Grasp the upper arm just above the elbow, placing the right hand on the posterior side of the upper arm.
3. Pull the left arm across the chest (toward the right) with the right hand.

MUSCLES AFFECTED

posterior deltoid, rhomboids, middle trapezius

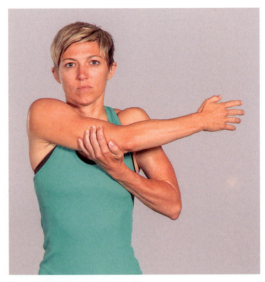

Stretching the upper back

14.7 ARMS STRAIGHT UP ABOVE HEAD (Pillar)

1. Stand with the arms in front of the torso, fingers interlocked with palms facing out.
2. Slowly straighten the arms above the head with the palms up.
3. Continue to reach upward with the hands and arms.
4. While continuing to reach upward, slowly reach slightly backward.

MUSCLE AFFECTED

latissimus dorsi

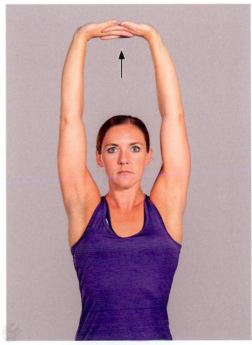

Stretching the upper back and forearms

333

14.8 SPINAL TWIST (Pretzel)

1. Sitting with the legs straight and the upper body nearly vertical, place the right foot to the left side of the left knee.
2. Place the back of the left elbow on the right side of the right knee, which is now bent.
3. Place the right palm on the floor 12 to 16 inches (30-40 cm) behind the hips.
4. Push the right knee to the left with the left elbow while turning the shoulders and head to the right as far as possible. Try to look behind the back.

MUSCLES AFFECTED

internal oblique, external oblique, piriformis, erector spinae

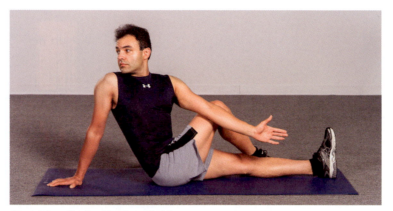

Stretching the low back and sides

14.9 SEMI-LEG STRADDLE

1. Sit with knees flexed 30° to 50°; let the legs totally relax.
2. Point the knees outward; the sides of the knees may or may not touch the floor.
3. Lean forward from the waist and reach forward with extended arms.

Note: Bending the knees and relaxing the legs decreases hamstring involvement and increases lower back stretch.

MUSCLE AFFECTED

erector spinae

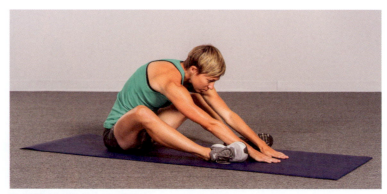

Stretching the low back from a seated position

14.10 FORWARD LUNGE (Fencer)

1. Standing, take a long step forward with the left leg and flex the left knee until it is directly over the left foot.
2. Keep the left foot flat on the floor.
3. Keep the right knee moderately flexed.
4. Keep the back foot pointed in the same direction as the front foot; it is not necessary to have the heel on the floor.
5. Keep the torso upright and rest the hands on the hips or the front leg (or allow them to hang at the sides).
6. Slowly lower the hips forward and downward.

MUSCLES AFFECTED

iliopsoas, rectus femoris

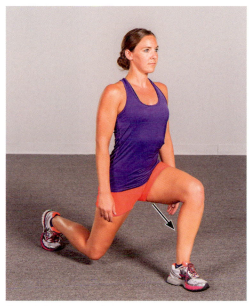

Stretching the hip flexors

14.11 SUPINE KNEE FLEX

1. Lie on the back with legs straight.
2. Flex the right knee and hip, bringing the thigh toward the chest.
3. Place both hands behind the thigh and continue to pull the thigh toward the chest.

MUSCLES AFFECTED

hip extensors (gluteus maximus and hamstrings)

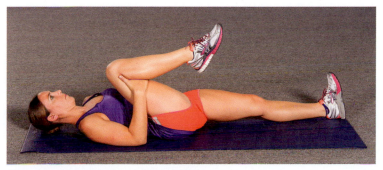

Stretching the gluteals and hamstrings

14.12 SIDE BEND WITH STRAIGHT ARMS

1. Stand with feet shoulder-width apart.
2. Interlace the fingers with the palms away from the torso and facing outward.
3. Reach upward with straight arms.
4. Keeping the arms straight, lean from the waist to the left side. Do not bend the knees.

MUSCLES AFFECTED

external oblique, latissimus dorsi, serratus anterior

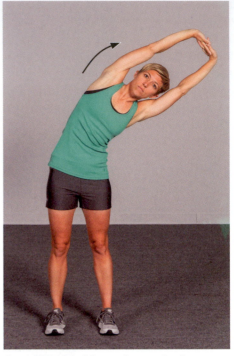

Stretching the sides and upper back

14.13 SIDE BEND WITH BENT ARM

1. Stand with feet shoulder-width apart.
2. Flex the right elbow and raise the elbow above the head.
3. Reach the right hand down toward the left shoulder.
4. Grasp the right elbow with the left hand.
5. Pull the elbow behind the head.
6. Keeping the arm bent, lean from the waist to the left side.
7. Do not bend the knees.

MUSCLES AFFECTED

external oblique, latissimus dorsi, serratus anterior, triceps brachii

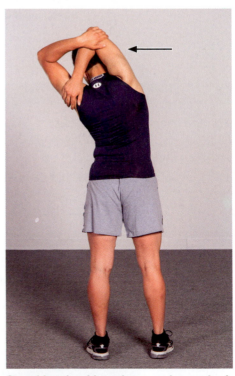

Stretching the sides, triceps, and upper back

14.14 SIDE QUADRICEPS STRETCH

1. Lie on the left side with both legs straight.
2. Place the left forearm flat on the floor and the upper arm perpendicular to the floor.
3. Place the left forearm at a 45° angle to the torso.
4. Flex the right leg (knee), with the heel of the right foot moving toward the buttocks.
5. Grasp the front of the ankle with the right hand and pull toward the buttocks.

Note: The stretch occurs as a result of knee flexion and hip extension.

MUSCLES AFFECTED

quadriceps, iliopsoas

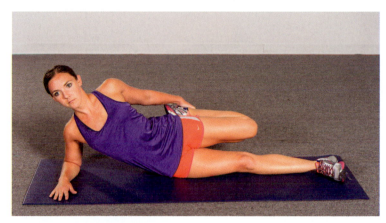

Stretching the quadriceps

14.15 SITTING TOE TOUCH

1. Sit with the upper body nearly vertical and legs straight.
2. Lean forward using hip flexion and grasp the toes with each hand. Slightly pull the toes toward the upper body and pull the chest toward the legs. If you have limited flexibility, try to grasp the ankles.

MUSCLES AFFECTED

hamstrings, erector spinae, gastrocnemius

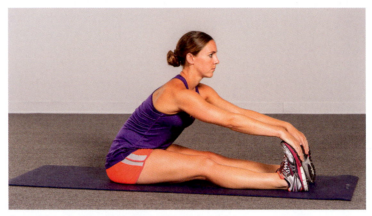

Stretching the hamstrings and lower back

14.16 SEMISTRADDLE (Figure Four)

1. Sit with the upper body nearly vertical and legs straight.
2. Place the sole of the right foot on the inner side of the left knee. The outer side of the right leg should be resting on the floor.
3. Lean forward using hip flexion and grasp the toes of the left foot with the left hand. Slightly pull the toes toward the upper body as the chest is also pulled toward the left leg.

MUSCLES AFFECTED

gastrocnemius, hamstrings, erector spinae

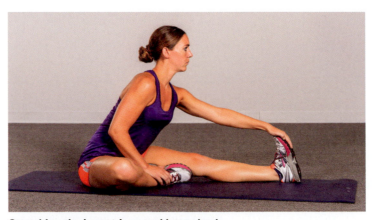

Stretching the hamstrings and lower back

14.17 STRADDLE (Spread Eagle)

1. Sit with the upper body nearly vertical and legs straight. Abduct the hips, spreading the legs as far as possible.
2. With both hands, grasp the toes of the left foot and pull on the toes slightly while pulling the chest toward the left leg.
3. Repeat toward the center by grasping the right toes with the right hand and the left toes with the left hand. Pull the torso forward and toward the ground.

MUSCLES AFFECTED

gastrocnemius, hamstrings, erector spinae, hip adductors, sartorius

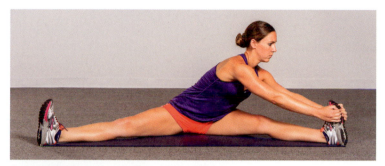

Stretching the hamstrings and hip adductors

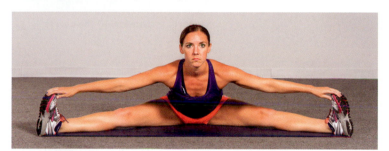

Stretching the hamstrings, hip adductors, and lower back

14.18 BUTTERFLY

1. Sitting with the upper body nearly vertical and legs straight, flex both knees, bringing the soles of the feet together.
2. Pull the feet toward the body.
3. Place the hands on the feet and the elbows on the legs.
4. Pull the torso slightly forward as the elbows push down, causing hip abduction.

MUSCLES AFFECTED

hip adductors, sartorius

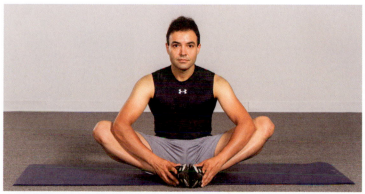

Stretching the hip adductors

14.19 WALL STRETCH

1. Stand facing the wall with feet shoulder-width apart and toes approximately 2 feet (0.6 m) from the wall.
2. Lean forward, placing the hands on the wall.
3. Step back approximately 2 feet (0.6 m) with the stretch leg while flexing the opposite knee.
4. Extend the knee of the stretch leg and lower the heel to the floor to apply the stretch.

MUSCLES AFFECTED

gastrocnemius, soleus; Achilles tendon

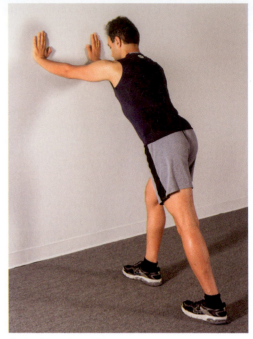

Stretching the calves

14.20 STEP STRETCH

1. Place the ball of one foot on the edge of a step or board 3 to 4 inches (8-10 cm) high, with the other foot flat on the step.
2. With straight legs, lower the heel of the foot on the edge of the step as far as possible.
3. Repeat with the other leg.

Note: To stretch the Achilles tendon, complete the same stretch with 10° of knee flexion.

MUSCLES AFFECTED

gastrocnemius, soleus, Achilles tendon

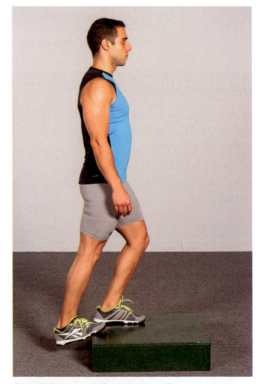

Stretching the calf while standing on a step

DYNAMIC STRETCHING TECHNIQUES

Guidelines for Dynamic Stretching

- Carry out 5 to 10 repetitions for each movement, either in place or over a given distance.
- Where possible, progressively increase the ROM on each repetition.
- Where appropriate, increase the speed of motion in subsequent sets, but always maintain control of the motion.
- Actively control muscular actions as you move through the ROM.
- Where appropriate, try to replicate the movements required for sport performance.

Precautions for Dynamic Stretching

- Move progressively through the ROM.
- Move deliberately through the motion but without bouncing (movement should be controlled at all times).
- Do not forsake good technique for additional ROM.

14.21 ARM SWINGS

1. Stand erect and raise the arms in front of the body until they are parallel to the floor.
2. While walking over a prescribed distance, swing the arms in unison to the right so the left arm is in front of the chest, the fingers of the left hand are pointing directly lateral to the left shoulder, and the right arm is behind the body.
3. Immediately reverse the direction of movement to swing the arms in unison to the left.
4. Movement should occur only at the shoulder joints (i.e., keep torso and head facing forward).
5. Alternate swinging the arms in unison to the right and left.

MUSCLES AFFECTED

latissimus dorsi, teres major, anterior and posterior deltoids, pectoralis major

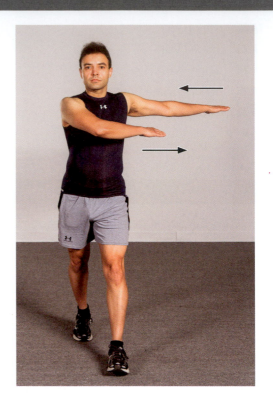

14.22 INCHWORM

1. Stand erect with the feet placed shoulder-width apart.
2. While slightly flexing the knees, bend forward at the waist and place hands shoulder-width apart flat on the floor.
3. The weight of the body should be shifted back (i.e., not directly over the hands), with the buttocks high in the air—imagine making an inverted V with the body.
4. Move the hands alternately forward, as if taking short steps with the hands, until the body is in the push-up position.
5. Walk the legs to the hands using small steps while keeping the knees slightly flexed.
6. Repeat the motion over a prescribed distance.

MUSCLES AFFECTED

erector spinae, gastrocnemius, gluteus maximus, hamstrings, soleus, anterior tibialis

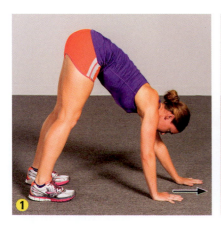
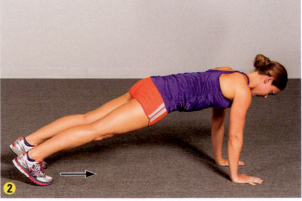
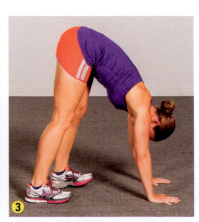

14.23   LUNGE WALK

1. Stand erect with the feet parallel to each other and shoulder-width apart.
2. Take an exaggerated step directly forward with the left leg, planting the left foot flat on the floor pointing straight ahead.
3. Allow the left hip and knee to slowly flex, keeping the left knee directly over the left foot.
4. Slightly flex the right knee and lower it until it is 1 to 2 inches (3-5 cm) above the floor; the right foot should be pointed straight ahead.
5. Balance the weight evenly between the ball of the right foot and the entire left foot.
6. Keep the torso perpendicular to the floor by "sitting back" on the right leg.
7. Forcefully push off of the floor by extending the left hip and knee.
8. Pick up the right foot and place it next to the left foot; do not stutter-step forward.
9. Stand erect, pause, and then step forward with the right leg, progressing forward with each step.

MUSCLES AFFECTED

gluteus maximus, hamstrings, iliopsoas, quadriceps

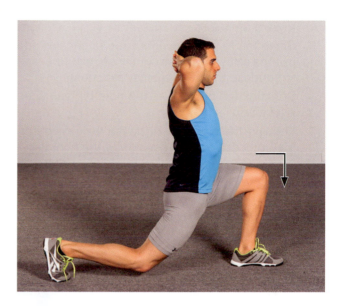

14.24   LUNGE WITH OVERHEAD SIDE REACH

1. Stand erect with the feet parallel to each other and shoulder-width apart.
2. Take an exaggerated step directly forward with the left leg, planting the left foot flat on the floor pointing straight ahead.
3. Allow the left hip and knee to slowly flex, keeping the left knee directly over the left foot.
4. Slightly flex the right knee and lower it until it is 1 to 2 inches (3-5 cm) above the floor; the right foot should be pointed straight ahead.
5. Reach up high with the right arm and bend the torso laterally toward the left leg.
6. Return to an erect torso position, and then forcefully push off the floor by extending the left hip and knee.
7. Pick up the right foot and place it next to the left foot; do not stutter-step forward.
8. Stand erect, pause, and then step forward with the right leg, progressing forward with each step.

MUSCLES AFFECTED

gluteus maximus, hamstrings, iliopsoas, latissimus dorsi, internal and external oblique, rectus femoris

14.25 WALKING KNEE LIFT

1. Stand erect with the feet parallel to each other and shoulder-width apart.
2. Step forward with the left leg and flex the right hip and knee to move the right thigh upward toward the chest.
3. Grasp the front of the right knee/upper shin and use the arms to pull the right knee up further and to squeeze the thigh against the chest.
4. Dorsiflex the left foot as the right hip and knee are flexed.
5. Keeping the torso erect, pause for a moment, then proceed to step down with the right leg.
6. Shift the body weight to the right leg and repeat the motion with the left leg.
7. Progress forward with each step, increasing the ROM and speed on subsequent steps.

MUSCLES AFFECTED

gluteus maximus, hamstrings

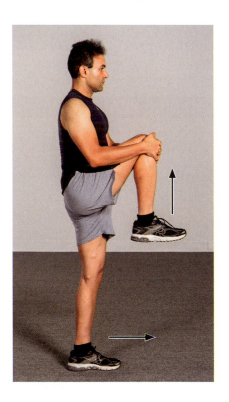

14.26 FORWARD LUNGE WITH ELBOW TO INSTEP

1. Stand erect with the feet parallel to each other and shoulder-width apart.

2. Take an exaggerated step directly forward with the left leg, planting the left foot flat on the floor pointing straight ahead.

3. Allow the left hip and knee to slowly flex, keeping the left knee directly over the left foot.

4. Slightly flex the right knee and lower it until it is 1 to 2 inches (3-5 cm) above the floor; the right foot should be pointed straight ahead.

5. Lean forward, bringing the left arm forward and touching the left elbow to the instep of the left foot; the right hand may be placed on the floor to maintain balance.

6. Lean back to return to an erect torso position, and then forcefully push off the floor by extending the left hip and knee.

7. Pick up the right foot and place it next to the left foot; do not stutter-step forward.

8. Stand erect, pause, and then step forward with the right leg, progressing forward with each step.

MUSCLES AFFECTED

biceps femoris, erector spinae, gastrocnemius, gluteus maximus, hamstrings, iliopsoas, latissimus dorsi, internal and external oblique, quadriceps, rectus femoris, soleus

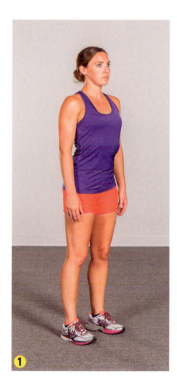
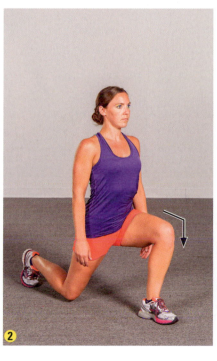
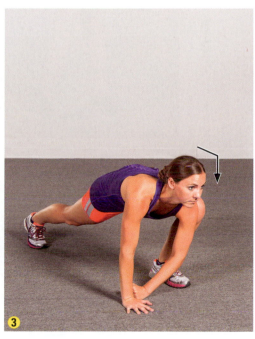

14.27 HEEL-TO-TOE WALK

1. Stand erect with the feet parallel to each other and shoulder-width apart.
2. Take a small step forward with the right leg; place the heel of the right foot on the ground first and then continue to dorsiflex the foot.
3. Immediately roll forward and rise up as high as possible onto the ball of the right foot.
4. Swing the left leg forward in order to take another small step.
5. Repeat with the left leg, progressing forward with each step.

MUSCLES AFFECTED

gastrocnemius, soleus, anterior tibialis

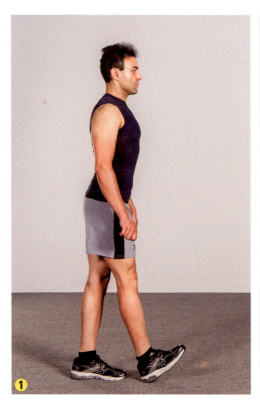

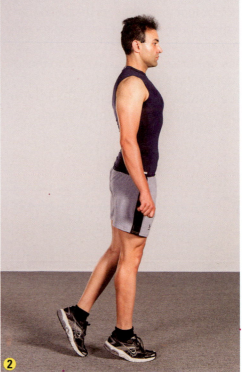

14.28 WALKING OVER AND UNDER

1. Stand erect with the feet parallel to each other and shoulder-width apart.
2. Flex the left hip and knee and then abduct the left thigh until it is parallel to the floor.
3. Step laterally to the left, stepping laterally over the first hurdle.
4. Place the left foot firmly on the ground, shift the body weight to the left leg, and then proceed to lift the right leg over the first hurdle.
5. After lifting the right leg over the hurdle and placing the right foot firmly on the ground, stand erect, pause, and then flex the hips and knees and dorsiflex the ankles to assume a full squat position.
6. Extend the left leg laterally, as if performing a lateral lunge.
7. Keeping the body weight low, move the body laterally, ducking under the second hurdle.
8. Stand erect, pause, and repeat the motion in the opposite direction, ducking under the second hurdle and stepping over the first.

Note: If hurdles are not available, athletes can perform the exercise can be performed by mirroring the motion of trying to step laterally and then under a hurdle.

MUSCLES AFFECTED

hip abductors, hip adductors, gastrocnemius, gluteus maximus, hamstrings, iliopsoas, rectus femoris, soleus

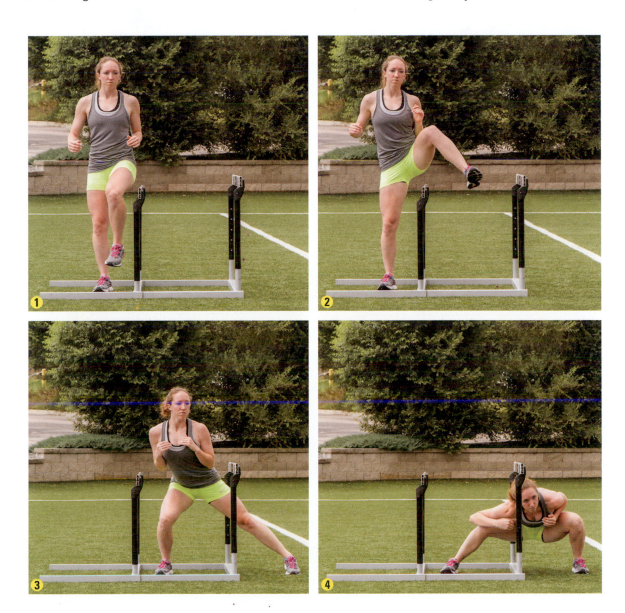

14.29 INVERTED HAMSTRING STRETCH

1. Stand tall and step a small step forward with the left leg.
2. Bend at the waist.
3. Reach forward with the left arm and simultaneously reach back with the right leg.
4. Try to keep the hips square.
5. Reach a position in which you feel a stretch in the hamstrings but eventually aim to attain a position in which the body is parallel to the floor.
6. Reach the right hand down toward the floor.
7. Return to the start by actively using the hamstrings and gluteals of the planted leg.
8. Take a step forward and repeat on the other leg.

MUSCLES AFFECTED

gluteus maximus, hamstrings, hip abductors, hip adductors, erector spinae

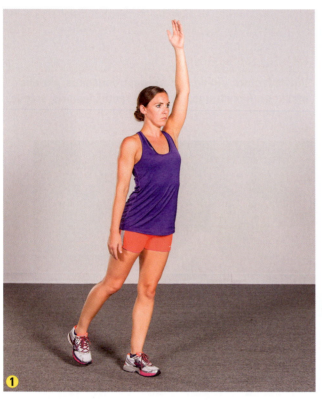

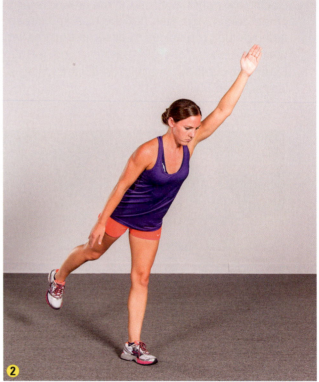

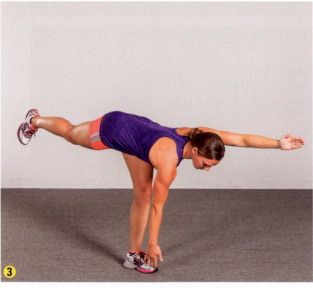

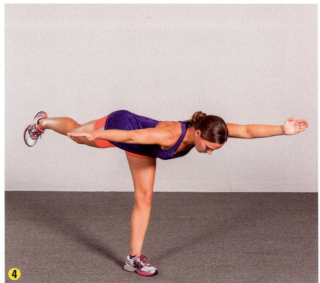

14.30 STRAIGHT-LEG MARCH

1. Assume a tall standing position with both arms outstretched in front of the chest.
2. Rise up onto the toes of the left leg and simultaneously, using a straight-leg action, raise the right leg forward and up, aiming to actively move it through as large a ROM as possible.
3. Once the highest point is reached, actively pull the leg back to the start position.
4. Maintain the tall standing posture throughout.
5. Repeat on alternate legs as you move forward.

MUSCLES AFFECTED

gluteus maximus, hamstrings, iliopsoas, rectus femoris

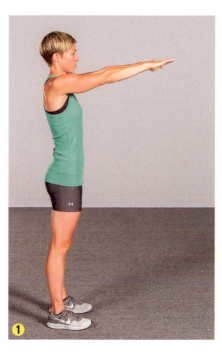
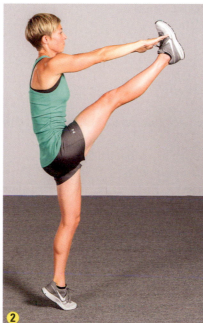
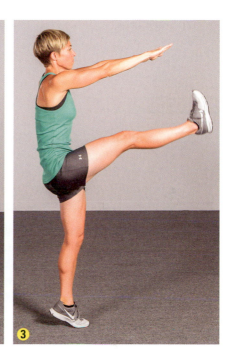

14.31 SPIDERMAN CRAWL

1. Assume a push-up position but with elbows bent so that the position is lower than normal.
2. Lift and externally rotate the left leg, bringing the knee forward at an angle outside the left elbow.
3. Walk the hands forward and across the body.
4. As this progresses, bring the right leg forward outside the right hand and repeat for the given distance.
5. Repeat, alternating sides, for the required distance.

MUSCLES AFFECTED

biceps femoris, erector spinae, gastrocnemius, gluteus maximus, hamstrings, iliopsoas, latissimus dorsi, internal and external oblique, quadriceps, rectus femoris, soleus

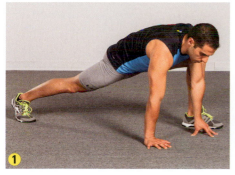
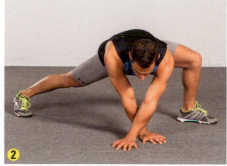
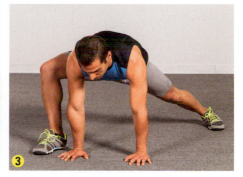

active stretch
agonist contraction
autogenic inhibition
ball-and-socket joint
ballistic stretch
contract-relax
dynamic flexibility
dynamic stretch
elasticity
ellipsoidal joint
fibrosis
flexibility

general warm-up
Golgi tendon organ (GTO)
hinge joint
hold-relax
hold-relax with agonist
  contraction
mechanoreceptor
mobility drills
muscle spindles
passive stretch
plasticity

potentiation
proprioceptive neuromuscular
  facilitation (PNF)
Raise, Activate and Mobilize, and
  Potentiate (RAMP)
range of motion (ROM)
reciprocal inhibition
specific warm-up
static flexibility
static stretch
stretch reflex

STUDY QUESTIONS

1. Which of the following is a nontemperature-related effect of a warm-up?
   a. enhanced neural function
   b. disruption of transient connective tissue bonds
   c. elevation of baseline oxygen consumption
   d. increase in muscle temperature

2. When stimulated during PNF stretching, Golgi tendon organs allow the relaxation of the
   a. stretched muscle by contracting the reciprocal muscle
   b. reciprocal muscle by contracting the stretched muscle
   c. reciprocal muscle by its own contraction
   d. stretched muscle by its own contraction

3. Which of the following stretching techniques decreases muscle spindle stimulation?
   a. dynamic
   b. ballistic
   c. static
   d. passive

4. Stimulation of muscle spindles induces a
   a. relaxation of GTOs
   b. relaxation of the stretched muscle
   c. contraction of the stretched muscle
   d. contraction of the reciprocal muscle

5. After performing the hold-relax with agonist contraction PNF stretch for the hamstrings, which of the following explains the resulting increase in flexibility?
   I. autogenic inhibition
   II. stretch inhibition
   III. reciprocal inhibition
   IV. crossed-extensor inhibition
   a. I and III only
   b. II and IV only
   c. I, II, and III only
   d. II, III, and IV only

CHAPTER 15

Exercise Technique for Free Weight and Machine Training

Scott Caulfield, BS, and Douglas Berninger, MEd

> **After completing this chapter, you will be able to**
>
> - understand the general techniques involved in properly performing resistance training exercises,
> - provide breathing guidelines,
> - determine the appropriateness of wearing a weight belt,
> - provide recommendations for spotting free weight exercises, and
> - teach proper resistance training exercise and spotting techniques.

The author would like to acknowledge the significant contributions of Roger W. Earle and Thomas R. Baechle to this chapter.

This chapter provides guidelines and strategies for performing and teaching safe and effective lifting and spotting techniques. At the core of safe and effective resistance training is proper exercise execution. Exercises that are performed and spotted correctly promote injury-free results and do so in a time-efficient manner.

The first half of this chapter summarizes the fundamental techniques involved in properly performing and spotting exercises and using a weight belt during lifting. The last section provides checklists and photographs depicting proper resistance training exercise and spotting techniques. It is assumed that the reader is familiar with these exercises. Therefore, the techniques presented are simply guidelines that represent the most commonly accepted method of performing the exercises. No attempt has been made to describe all variations for properly executing and spotting the exercises included in this chapter.

Fundamentals of Exercise Technique

There are several commonalities among resistance training exercise techniques. Most free weight and machine exercises involve some sort of handgrip on a bar, dumbbell, or handle; and absolutely all exercises require an optimal body or limb position, movement range and speed, and method of breathing. Additionally, some exercises may also warrant the use of a weight belt and certain procedures for lifting a bar off the floor.

Handgrips

Two common grips are used in resistance training exercises: (a) the **pronated grip**, with palms down and knuckles up, also called the **overhand grip**; and (b) the **supinated grip**, with palms up and knuckles down, also known as the **underhand grip** (figure 15.1). (A variation of either grip is the **neutral grip**, in which the knuckles point laterally—as in a handshake.) Two less common grips are the **alternated grip**, in which one hand is in a pronated grip and the other is in a supinated grip, and the **hook grip**, which is similar to the pronated grip except that the thumb is positioned under the index and middle fingers. The hook grip is typically used for performing exercises that require a stronger grip (power exercises, e.g., snatch). Note that the thumb is wrapped around the bar in all of the grips shown; this positioning is called a **closed grip**. When the thumb does not wrap around the bar, the grip is called an open or **false grip**.

Establishing the proper grip in an exercise involves placing the hands at the correct distance from each other (referred to as the **grip width**), from the center of the bar (i.e., to maintain balance). The three grip widths

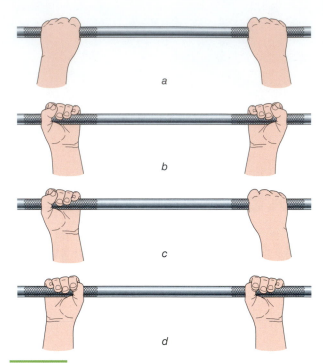

FIGURE 15.1   Bar grips: *(a)* pronated, *(b)* supinated, *(c)* alternated, and *(d)* hook (posterior view).

(shown in figure 15.2) are common, wide, and narrow. For most exercises, the hands are placed approximately shoulder-width apart. The hand positioning for all exercises should result in a balanced, even bar. Weightlifting exercises and their variations use two types of grips: (a) the **clean grip** or (b) the **snatch grip**. Both of these grips are pronated closed hand positions. The clean grip is slightly wider than shoulder-width apart, outside of the knees. The snatch grip is a wide grip and can be determined using two types of measurements: the fist-to-opposite-shoulder method and the elbow-to-elbow method (also known as the scarecrow method). Both the clean grip and the snatch grip are often used with a hook grip (mentioned previously) to assist in giving the athlete a stronger grip.

Stable Body and Limb Positioning

Whether an exercise requires lifting a barbell or dumbbell from the floor or pushing and pulling while one is positioned in or on a machine, establishing a stable position is critical for safety and optimal performance. A stable position enables the athlete to maintain proper

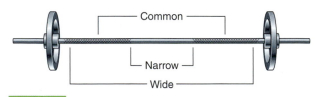

FIGURE 15.2   Grip widths.

body alignment during an exercise, which in turn places an appropriate stress on muscles and joints.

Exercises performed during standing typically require that the feet be positioned slightly wider than hip-width with the heels and balls of the feet in contact with the floor. Establishing a stable position in or on machines sometimes requires adjusting the seat or resistance arm and fastening belts snugly.

Seated or **supine** (lying face up) exercises performed on a bench require a specific posture. The athlete should position the body to achieve a **five-point body contact position**:

1. Head is placed firmly on the bench or back pad.
2. Shoulders and upper back are placed firmly and evenly on the bench or back pad.
3. Buttocks are placed evenly on the bench or seat.
4. Right foot is flat on the floor.
5. Left foot is flat on the floor.

Establishing and maintaining this five-point body contact position at the beginning and throughout the movement phases promotes maximal stability and spinal support (2, 9, 10).

> Exercises performed during standing typically require that the feet be positioned slightly wider than hip-width with the heels and balls of the feet in contact with the floor. Seated or supine exercises performed on a bench usually require a five-point body contact position.

Cam-, pulley-, or lever-based exercise machines that have an axis of rotation require specific positioning of the athlete's body, arms, or legs for reasons of safety and optimal execution. To align the primary joint of the body involved in the exercise with the axis of the machine, it may be necessary to move the seat; the ankle or arm roller pad; or the thigh, chest, or back pad. For example, adjust the ankle roller pad (up or down) and the back pad (forward or backward) to line up the knee joint with the machine axis before performing the leg (knee) extension exercise.

Range of Motion and Speed

When the entire **range of motion (ROM)** is covered during an exercise, the value of the exercise is maximized and flexibility is maintained or improved. Ideally, an exercise's full ROM should mimic the full ROM of the involved joint or joints in order for the greatest improvements to occur, but sometimes this is not possible (trailing leg knee joint during a lunge) or recommended (using intervertebral joints during a squat).

Repetitions performed in a slow, controlled manner increase the likelihood that full ROM can be reached. However, when power or quick-lift exercises (e.g., power clean, push jerk, and snatch) are performed, an effort should be made to accelerate the bar to a maximal speed while still maintaining control and proper form throughout the exercise.

Breathing Considerations

The most strenuous movement of a repetition—typically soon after the transition from the eccentric phase to the concentric phase—is referred to as the **sticking point**. Strength and conditioning professionals should typically instruct athletes to exhale *through* the sticking point and to inhale during the less stressful phase of the repetition (3, 6, 7). For example, since the sticking point of the biceps curl exercise occurs about midway through the upward movement phase (concentric elbow flexion), the athlete should exhale during this portion. Inhalation, then, should occur as the bar is lowered back to the starting position. This breathing strategy applies to most resistance training exercises.

There are some situations in which breath holding may be suggested, however. For experienced resistance-trained athletes performing **structural exercises** (those that load the vertebral column and therefore place stress on it) with high loads, the **Valsalva maneuver** can be helpful for maintaining proper vertebral alignment and support. As explained in chapter 2, the Valsalva maneuver involves expiring against a closed glottis, which, when combined with contracting the abdomen and rib cage muscles, creates rigid compartments of fluid in the lower torso and air in the upper torso (i.e., the "fluid ball"). The advantage of the Valsalva maneuver is that it increases the rigidity of the entire torso to aid in supporting the vertebral column, which in turn reduces the associated compressive forces on the disks during lifting (1, 4, 5, 8). It also helps to establish and maintain a normal lordotic lumbar spine position (also called a **neutral spine**) and erect upper torso position, described in the technique checklists for certain exercises. Be aware, however, that the resulting increase in intra-abdominal pressure has potentially detrimental side effects, such as dizziness, disorientation, excessively high blood pressure, and blackouts. This is why the breath-holding phase is—and should be—quite transient, only about 1 to 2 seconds (at most). Even a very well-trained individual should not extend the length of the breath-holding phase, as blood pressure can quickly rise to triple resting levels (7).

Strength and conditioning professionals involved in conducting 1-repetition maximum (1RM) tests in, for example, the squat, deadlift, hip sled, leg press, shoulder press, or power clean, need to be aware of the advantages and disadvantages of coaching athletes in the Valsalva maneuver. While it is obviously important that the vertebral column be internally supported during these movements for safety and technique reasons, it is recommended that an athlete not extend the breath-holding period.

> ▶ For most exercises, exhale through the sticking point of the concentric phase and inhale during the eccentric phase. Experienced and well-trained athletes may want to use the Valsalva maneuver when performing structural exercises to assist in maintaining proper vertebral alignment and support (6).

Weight Belts

The use of a weight belt may help maintain intra-abdominal pressure during lifting (5, 7). Its appropriateness depends on the type of exercise performed and the relative load lifted. It is recommended that a weight belt be worn for exercises that place stress on the lower back and during sets that use near-maximal or maximal loads. Adopting this strategy may reduce the risk of lower back injury when combined with proper lifting and spotting techniques. A drawback to weight belt use is that wearing a belt too often reduces opportunities for the abdominal muscles to be trained. Furthermore, no weight belt is needed for exercises that do not stress the lower back (e.g., biceps curl, lat pulldown), or for exercises that do stress the lower back (e.g., back squat or deadlift) but involve the use of light loads.

> ▶ Typically an athlete should wear a weight belt when performing exercises that place stress on the lower back and during sets that involve near-maximal or maximal loads. A weight belt is not needed for exercises that do not stress the lower back or for those that do stress the lower back but involve light loads.

Spotting Free Weight Exercises

A spotter is someone who assists in the execution of an exercise to help protect the athlete from injury. A spotter may also serve to motivate the athlete and help in the completion of forced repetitions (also referred to as partner-assisted reps), but the spotter's primary responsibility is the safety of the athlete being spotted. The spotter must realize that poor execution of this responsibility may result in serious injury, not only to the athlete being spotted, but also to the spotter and other individuals in close proximity. Although partner-assisted actions are valuable in helping an athlete benefit from

training, the importance of promoting safety cannot be overemphasized.

The remainder of this section offers additional insight on when and how to spot free weight exercises. This information provides a foundation for strength and conditioning professionals to apply to their specific training environment.

Types of Exercises Performed and Equipment Involved

Free weight exercises performed over the head (e.g., barbell shoulder press) or with the bar on the back (e.g., back squat), racked anteriorly on the shoulders or on the clavicles (e.g., front squat) or over the face (e.g., bench press, lying triceps extension), are more challenging for the athlete to correctly execute than those in which the bar or dumbbells are held or raised at the sides or in front (e.g., lateral shoulder raise or barbell biceps curl, respectively) and therefore should involve one or more spotters. The overhead, bar-on-the-back or bar-on-the-front-shoulders and over-the-face exercises (especially using dumbbells) also require more skill on the part of the spotter and are potentially the most dangerous to the athlete. Spotting dumbbell exercises typically requires more skill than spotting barbell exercises because there is an additional piece of equipment to observe and spot. Power exercises should not be spotted.

> ▶ With the exception of power exercises, free weight exercises performed with a bar moving over the head, positioned on the back, racked on the front of the shoulders, or passing over the face typically require one or more spotters.

Spotting Overhead Exercises and Those With the Bar on the Back or Front Shoulders

Ideally, to promote the safety of the athlete, the spotters, and others nearby, overhead exercises and those involving the bar on the back or front shoulders should be performed inside a power rack with the crossbars in place at an appropriate height. All plates, bars, locks, and weight-plate trees must be cleared from the lifting area so they cannot be tripped over or run into and cannot affect the movement of the bar. Athletes who are not lifting should be instructed to stay clear of the lifting area. Since the loads lifted in these exercises can be considerable, to exert sufficient leverage the spotter or spotters should be at least as strong and at least as tall as the athlete who is lifting. Out-of-the-rack exercises (e.g., forward step lunge or step-up) with heavy weights can result in serious injury. These exercises should be executed only by well-trained and skilled athletes and spotted by experienced professionals.

Spotting Over-the-Face Exercises

When spotting **over-the-face barbell exercises**, it is important for the spotter to grasp the bar with an alternated grip, usually narrower than the athlete's grip. Because of the bar's curved trajectory in some exercises (e.g., lying triceps extension, barbell pullover), the spotter will use an alternated grip to pick up the bar and return it to the floor but a supinated grip to spot the bar. This helps ensure that the bar does not roll out of the spotter's hands and onto the athlete's face or neck. Since the spotter may be called upon to catch the bar or assist in lifting moderate to heavy loads (usually from a higher vantage point), establishing a solid, wide base of support with the feet and a neutral spine position is critically important.

For dumbbell exercises, it is important to spot as close to the dumbbells as possible or, in a few exercises, to spot the dumbbell itself. Although some individuals advocate spotting dumbbell movements by placing the hands on the athlete's upper arms or elbows (figure 15.3a), this technique may lead to injury. If the athlete's elbows "collapse" (i.e., flex), the spotter will not be in a position to stop the dumbbells from striking the athlete's face or chest. Spotting at the forearms near the wrists (figure 15.3b) is a safer technique. Note that for some exercises (e.g., dumbbell pullover and overhead dumbbell triceps extension), it is necessary to spot with hands on the dumbbell itself.

Do Not Spot Power Exercises

Whereas spotting is recommended in the types of exercises previously described, it is not advised in power exercises. Instead of spotting these exercises, the strength and conditioning professional needs to teach athletes how to get away from a bar that is unmanageable. Spotting these types of exercises is too dangerous to both the spotter and athlete. Athletes should be instructed that when they miss the bar in front, they should push the bar away or simply drop it. They should be taught that if they lose the bar behind the head, they should release it and jump forward. For these reasons, the surrounding area or platform should be cleared of other athletes and equipment before such exercises are performed.

Number of Spotters

The number of spotters needed is largely determined by the load being lifted, the experience and ability of the athlete and spotters, and the physical strength of the spotters. With heavier loads, the likelihood and severity of an injury increase. Once the load exceeds the spotter's ability to effectively protect the athlete (and him- or herself), another spotter must become involved. On the other hand, one spotter is preferred if he or she can easily handle the load, because two or more spotters must coordinate their actions with those of the athlete. As the number of spotters increases, so does the chance that an error in timing or technique may occur.

Communication Between Athlete and Spotter

Communication is the responsibility of both the spotter and the athlete. Before beginning a set, the athlete should tell the spotter how the bar will initially be handled, how many repetitions will be performed, and when he or

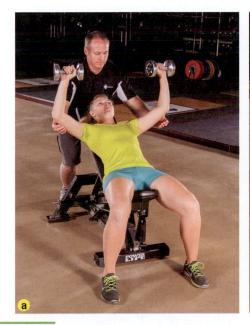 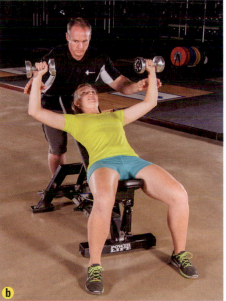

FIGURE 15.3 *(a)* Incorrect dumbbell spotting location. *(b)* Correct spotting location.

she is ready to move the bar into position. If spotters do not have this information they may take control of the bar improperly, too soon, or too late and consequently disrupt the exercise or injure the athlete.

Use of a Liftoff

The term **liftoff** refers to moving the bar from the upright supports to a position in which the athlete can begin the exercise. Usually the spotter helps place the barbell or dumbbells into the athlete's hands while the elbows are extended and helps to move the barbell or dumbbells to the proper starting position. Some athletes may want the spotter to provide a liftoff; others do not. If a liftoff is needed or requested, the athlete and spotter need to agree in advance on a verbal signal (e.g., the command "up" or "I will give it to you on the count of three"). Typically, the athlete signals that he or she is ready; the spotter says, "One, two, three," and on "three" the bar is moved into position. Liftoffs are normally used in the bench press (off the supports), shoulder press (off the supports or the shoulders), and squatting exercises if the supports are too low and nonadjustable. When two spotters are involved and the athlete wants a liftoff, as with a bench press, one spotter should assist with the

liftoff and then quickly move to the end of the bar to spot (the other spotter is already at the other end). The spotter providing the liftoff must be sure that the athlete has complete control of the bar at the conclusion of the liftoff. If two spotters are used, both should help the athlete place the bar back onto the supports on completion of the exercise.

Amount and Timing of Spotting Assistance

Knowing how much and when to help an athlete is an important aspect of spotting, and it requires the spotter to be experienced in proper spotting techniques. Most athletes typically need just enough help to successfully complete a repetition through a sticking point (i.e., a partner-assisted action); other times they might need the spotter to handle the entire load. At the first indication that a repetition will be missed, the athlete should quickly ask or signal the spotter (sometimes with just a grunt or sound) for help, and the spotter needs to immediately attempt to provide the amount of assistance needed. If the athlete cannot contribute anything to the completion of the repetition, the athlete should immediately tell the spotter to "take it" or use some other phrase agreed upon before the lift. Regardless of when or why the spotter

---

Guidelines for Spotting

Certain exercises that require spotting (over the face-neck and on the back) have a higher level of difficulty and thus warrant additional safety considerations. In any exercise where the potential for injury might occur, spotting should be used.

- Spotting is necessary on skillful multijoint exercises that involve a barbell or dumbbells being lifted over the head, on the back, on the front of the shoulders, or over the face.

- Exercises done overhead and with a bar racked on the back or in front of the shoulders may require more than one spotter, and multiple spotters must be taught how and where to spot the exercise.

- Spotting over-the-face exercises requires the spotter to grasp the implement being lifted or the athlete's wrists. Spotters must be trained to grasp the implement properly and even assist athletes in reracking the bar or returning dumbbells to the start position in case an exercise becomes too difficult to complete safely on their own.

- Power exercises are not spotted due to the safety factors for the athlete and the spotter(s), and athletes should be taught "how to miss" properly when learning these exercises.

- Determining the number of spotters for certain exercises depends on a number of factors, especially the amount of load being used, because the likelihood of injury can increase greatly with heavier loads.

- Both spotters and athletes must communicate properly before beginning an exercise requiring increased safety. They both must take part in this communication and be clear as to what exercise is being performed and how many repetitions. Therefore, communicating on exercises that require a liftoff is critical to safety in these exercises.

- The liftoff requires a spotter to assist the athlete in getting the implement(s) to the proper position before beginning the exercise and can require multiple spotters, depending on the exercise.

The spotting guidelines provided in this chapter should be a fundamental part of any strength and conditioning professional's training. Safety of athletes in the weight room is the most important part of supervising and conducting proper training programs and providing the best and safest atmosphere for athletes to be successful in training.

is needed to assist, he or she should take the bar—if possible—from the athlete quickly and smoothly, trying to avoid abrupt changes in the amount of load being handled by the athlete. The athlete should try to stay with the bar until it is racked or placed safely on the floor. This helps to protect both the spotter and athlete from injury.

The spotting guidelines provided in the exercise technique checklists are appropriate for a typical training environment. Spotting procedures may vary when excessively heavy loads are being used—such as 1RM attempts—because more spotters are typically needed.

Conclusion

It is critically important that the strength and conditioning professional provide athletes with proper instruction in resistance training exercise technique, including the fundamentals of breathing and weight belt use. In addition, the strength and conditioning professional needs to teach athletes how and when exercises should be spotted. Combined with quality supervision and ongoing feedback, this attention to proper instruction results in a safe training environment and an effective and appropriate training stimulus.

RESISTANCE TRAINING EXERCISES

Videos for exercises identified by this icon ▶ can be found online in HK*Propel*.

15.1   CURL-UP

Starting Position

- Lie in a supine position on a floor mat.
- Flex the knees to bring the heels near the buttocks.
- Fold the arms across the chest or abdomen.
- All repetitions begin from this position.

Upward Movement Phase

- Flex the neck to move the chin toward the chest.
- Keeping the feet, buttocks, and lower back neutral and stationary on the mat, curl the torso toward the thighs until the upper back is off the mat.

Downward Movement Phase

- Uncurl the torso back to the starting position.
- Keep the feet, buttocks, lower back, and arms in the same position.

MAJOR MUSCLE INVOLVED

rectus abdominis

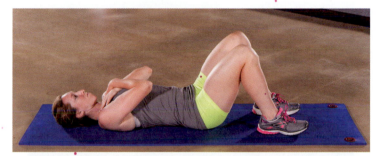

Starting position

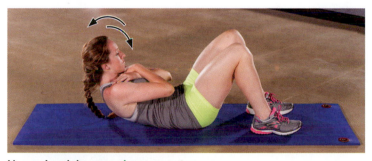

Upward and downward movements

15.2 ABDOMINAL CRUNCH

Starting Position

- Lie in a supine position on a floor mat.
- Place the heels on a bench with the hips and knees flexed to about 90°.
- Fold the arms across the chest or abdomen.
- All repetitions begin from this position.

Upward Movement Phase

- Flex the neck to move the chin toward the chest.
- Keeping the buttocks and lower back neutral and stationary on the mat, curl the torso toward the thighs until the upper back is off the mat.

Downward Movement Phase

- Uncurl the torso back to the starting position.
- Keep the feet, buttocks, lower back, and arms in the same position.

MAJOR MUSCLE INVOLVED

rectus abdominis

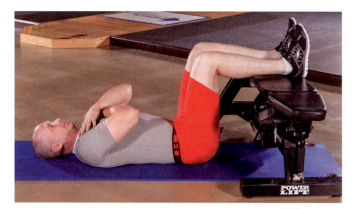

Starting position

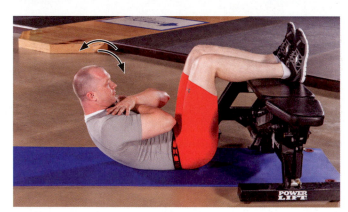

Upward and downward movements

15.3 ABDOMINAL CRUNCH (Machine)

Starting Position

- Sit down on the machine and press the back firmly against the back pad.
- Place the feet on the floor and the legs behind the roller pads.
- Position the legs parallel to each other.
- Reach back and grasp the handles with a closed, neutral grip with the back of the upper arms pressed against the arms pads.
- All repetitions begin from this position.

Forward Movement Phase

- Keeping the buttocks on the seat and the legs stationary, curl the torso forward toward the thighs.

Backward Movement Phase

- Uncurl the torso back to the starting position.
- Keep the feet, buttocks, lower back, and arms in the same position.

MAJOR MUSCLE INVOLVED

rectus abdominis

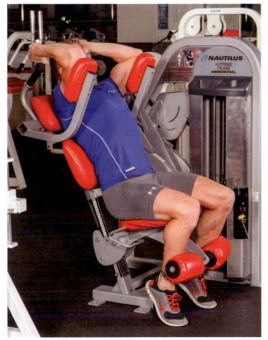

Starting position

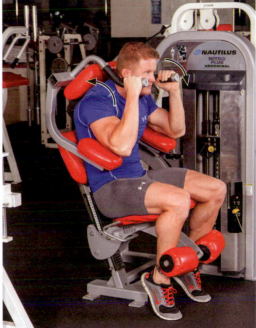

Forward and backward movements

15.4 BENT-OVER ROW

Before Beginning
- Grasp the bar with a closed, pronated grip.
- Grip should be wider than shoulder-width.
- Lift the bar from the floor as described for the deadlift exercise. Use a pronated grip, not an alternated grip.

Starting Position
- Position the feet in a shoulder-width stance with the knees slightly flexed.
- Flex forward at the hips so the torso is slightly above parallel to the floor.
- Create a neutral spine position.
- Focus the eyes a short distance ahead of the feet.
- Allow the bar to hang with the elbows fully extended.
- All repetitions begin from this position.

Upward Movement Phase
- Pull the bar toward the torso.
- Keep the torso rigid, back neutral, and knees slightly flexed.
- Do not jerk the torso upward.
- Touch the bar to the lower chest or upper abdomen.

Downward Movement Phase
- Lower the bar back to the starting position.
- Maintain the neutral spine and stationary torso and knee positions.
- At the end of the set, flex the hips and knees to place the bar on the floor and stand up.

MAJOR MUSCLES INVOLVED
latissimus dorsi, teres major, middle trapezius, rhomboids, posterior deltoids

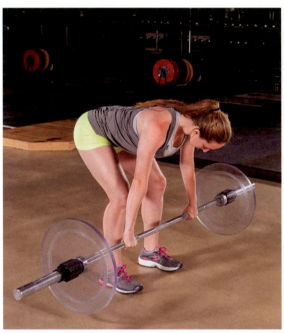

Starting position

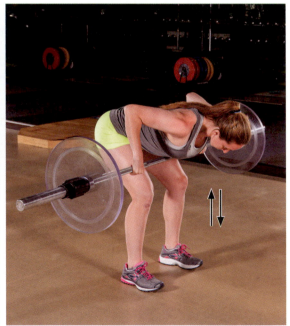

Upward and downward movements

15.5 ONE-ARM DUMBBELL ROW

Starting Position

- Position the feet in a shoulder-width stance with the knees slightly flexed.
- Flex forward at the hips so the torso is slightly above parallel to the floor.
- Create a neutral spine position.
- Grasp the dumbbell with a closed, neutral grip.
- Place the opposite hand on the bench for support.
- Allow the dumbbell to hang with the elbow fully extended.
- All repetitions begin from this position.

Upward Movement Phase

- Pull the dumbbell toward the torso, keeping the elbow close to the body.
- Keep the torso rigid, back neutral, and knees slightly flexed.
- Touch the dumbbell to the side of the torso.

Downward Movement Phase

- Lower the dumbbell back to the starting position.
- Maintain the neutral spine and stationary torso and flexed knee positions.

MAJOR MUSCLES INVOLVED

latissimus dorsi, teres major, middle trapezius, rhomboids, posterior deltoids

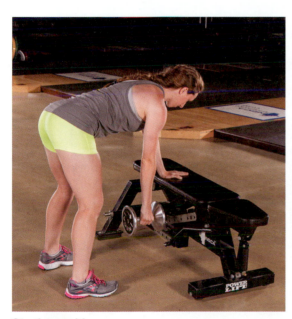

Starting position

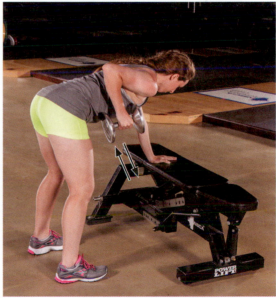

Upward and downward movements

15.6 LAT PULLDOWN (Machine)

Starting Position

- Grasp the bar with a closed, pronated grip.
- Grip should be wider than shoulder-width.
- Sit down on the seat facing the machine.
- Position the thighs under the pads with the feet flat on the floor. If necessary, adjust the seat and thigh pad.
- Lean the torso slightly backward.
- Extend the elbows fully.
- All repetitions begin from this position.

Downward Movement Phase

- Pull the bar down and toward the upper chest.
- Maintain the slight torso backward lean; do not jerk the torso backward.
- Touch the bar to the clavicle and upper chest area.

Upward Movement Phase

- Allow the elbows to slowly extend back to the starting position.
- Keep the torso in the same position.
- At the end of the set, stand up and return the bar to its resting position.

MAJOR MUSCLES INVOLVED

latissimus dorsi, teres major, middle trapezius, rhomboids, posterior deltoids

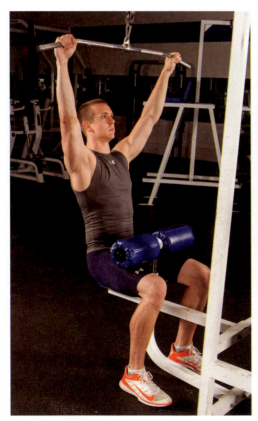

Starting position

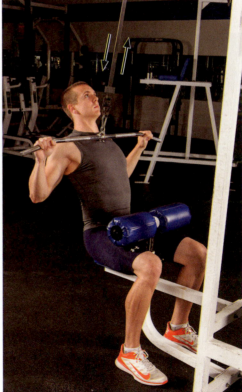

Downward and upward movements

15.7 SEATED ROW (Machine)

Starting Position

- Sit erect with the feet flat on the platform and press the torso against the chest pad.
- Grasp the handles with a closed grip, either pronated or neutral. If necessary, adjust the seat height to position the arms approximately parallel to the floor.
- Allow the elbows to extend fully.
- All repetitions begin from this position.

Backward Movement Phase

- Pull the handles toward the chest or upper abdomen.
- Maintain an erect torso position and keep the elbows next to the torso.
- Pull the handles as far back as possible.
- Do not jerk the torso backward.

Forward Movement Phase

- Allow the handles to move forward, back to the starting position.
- Keep the torso in the same position.

MAJOR MUSCLES INVOLVED

latissimus dorsi, teres major, middle trapezius, rhomboids, posterior deltoids

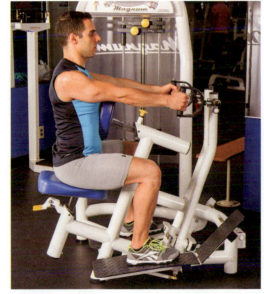

Starting position

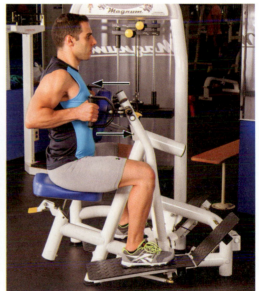

Backward and forward movements

15.8   LOW-PULLEY SEATED ROW (Machine)

Starting Position

- Sit on the long seat pad (or on the floor if the seat pad is not available) and place the feet on the foot supports or the machine frame.
- Grasp the handles with a closed grip, either neutral or pronated.
- Sit in an erect position with the torso perpendicular to the floor, knees slightly flexed, and the feet and legs parallel to each other.
- Allow the elbows to fully extend with the arms approximately parallel to the floor.
- All repetitions begin from this position.

Backward Movement Phase

- Pull the handles toward the abdomen.
- Maintain an erect torso position with the knees in the same slightly flexed position. Do not jerk the upper body or lean back.
- Continue pulling until the handles touch the abdomen.

Forward Movement Phase

- Allow the elbows to slowly extend back to the starting position.
- Maintain an erect torso position with the knees in the same slightly flexed position.
- At the end of the set, flex the knees and hips to return the weight to its resting position.

MAJOR MUSCLES INVOLVED

latissimus dorsi, teres major, middle trapezius, rhomboids, posterior deltoids

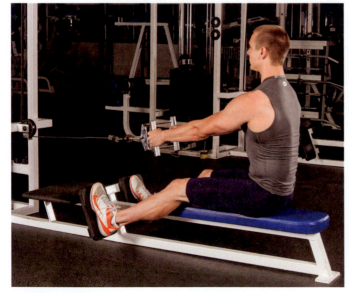

Starting position

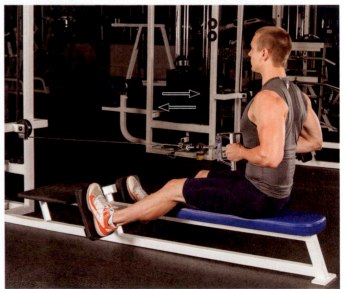

Backward and forward movements

15.9 BARBELL BICEPS CURL

Starting Position

- Grasp the bar with a closed, supinated grip.
- Grip should be shoulder-width so the arms touch the sides of the torso.
- Stand erect with the feet shoulder-width apart and the knees slightly flexed.
- Rest the bar on the front of the thighs with the elbows fully extended.
- All repetitions begin from this position.

Upward Movement Phase

- Flex the elbows until the bar is near the anterior deltoids.
- Keep the torso erect and the upper arms stationary.
- Do not jerk the body or swing the bar upward.

Downward Movement Phase

- Lower the bar until the elbows are fully extended.
- Keep the torso and knees in the same position.
- Do not bounce the bar on the thighs between repetitions.

MAJOR MUSCLES INVOLVED

biceps brachii, brachialis, brachioradialis

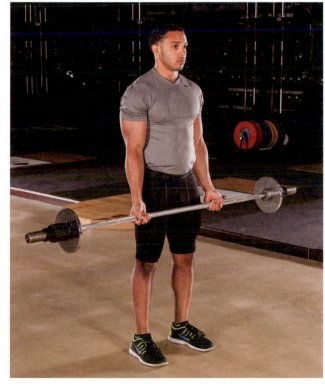

Starting position

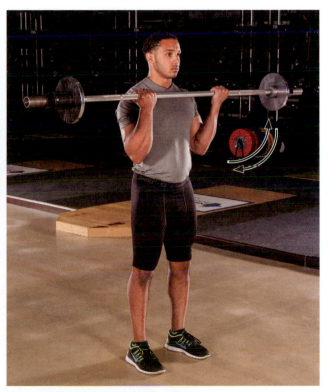

Upward and downward movements

15.10 HAMMER CURL

Starting Position

- Grasp two dumbbells using a closed, neutral grip.
- Stand erect with the feet shoulder-width apart and the knees slightly flexed.
- Position the dumbbells alongside the thighs with the elbows fully extended.
- All repetitions begin from this position.

Upward Movement Phase

- Keeping the dumbbell in a neutral grip, flex the elbow of one arm until the dumbbell is near the anterior deltoid. The other arm should be kept stationary at the side of the thigh.
- Keep the torso erect and the upper arm stationary.
- Do not jerk the body or swing the dumbbell upward.

Downward Movement Phase

- Lower the dumbbell until the elbow is fully extended.
- Keep the dumbbell in a neutral grip position.
- Keep the torso and knees in the same position.
- Repeat the upward and downward movement phases with the other arm (alternate arms).

MAJOR MUSCLES INVOLVED

brachialis, biceps brachii, brachioradialis

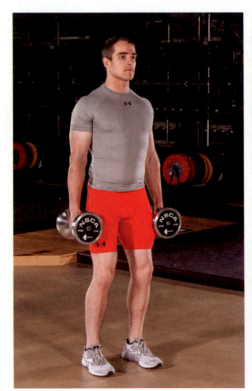

Starting position

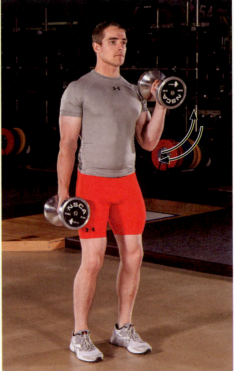

Upward and downward movements

15.11 STANDING CALF (HEEL) RAISE (Machine)

Starting Position

- Position the body evenly under the shoulder pads.
- Grasp the handles and place the balls of the feet on the nearest edge of the step with the legs and feet hip-width apart and parallel to each other.
- Stand erect with the knees fully extended but not forcefully locked out.
- Allow the heels to lower to a comfortable, stretched position.
- All repetitions begin from this position.

Upward Movement Phase

- Keeping the torso erect and the legs and feet parallel, push up as high as possible on the toes.
- Push up off the step; do not invert or evert the feet.
- Keep the knees extended but not locked out.

Downward Movement Phase

- Allow the heels to lower slowly back to the starting position.
- Maintain the same body position.

MAJOR MUSCLES INVOLVED

gastrocnemius, soleus

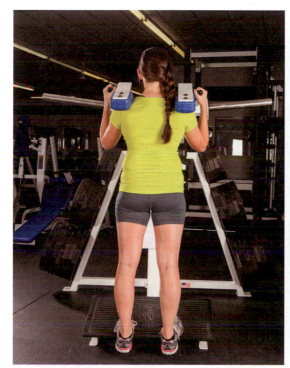

Starting position

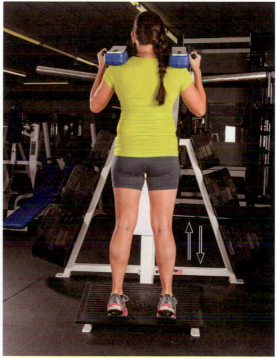

Upward and downward movements

15.12 SEATED CALF (HEEL) RAISE (Machine)

Starting Position

- Sit erect on the seat and place the balls of the feet on the nearest edge of the step with the legs and feet hip-width apart and parallel to each other.
- Lower the thigh–knee pad so it firmly presses against the knees and front of the lower thigh area.
- Plantar flex the ankles to remove the supports.
- Allow the heels to lower to a comfortable, stretched position.
- All repetitions begin from this position.

Upward Movement Phase

- Keeping the torso erect and the legs and feet parallel, push up on the toes as high as possible.
- Push up off the step; do not invert or evert the feet.

Downward Movement Phase

- Allow the heels to lower slowly back to the starting position.
- Maintain the same body position.
- At the end of the set, return the supports to the starting position and remove the feet.

MAJOR MUSCLES INVOLVED

soleus, gastrocnemius

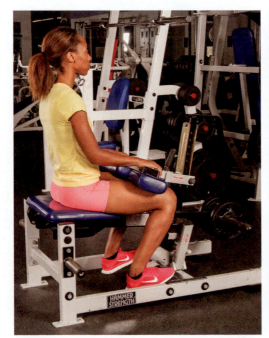

Starting position

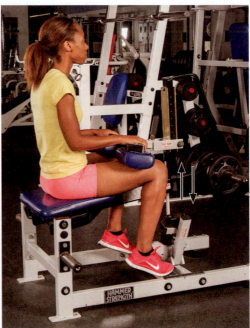

Upward and downward movements

15.13 FLAT BARBELL BENCH PRESS (and Dumbbell Variation)

This exercise can also be performed with two dumbbells, using a closed, pronated grip. When using dumbbells, the spotter assists by spotting the athlete's forearms near the wrists instead of the bar.

Starting Position: Athlete

- Lie in a supine position on a bench in the five-point body contact position.
- Place the body on the bench so that the eyes are below the racked bar.
- Grasp the bar with a closed, pronated grip slightly wider than shoulder-width apart.
- Signal the spotter for assistance in moving the bar off the supports.
- Position the bar over the chest with the elbows fully extended.
- All repetitions begin from this position.

Starting Position: Spotter

- Stand erect and very close to the head of the bench (but do not distract the athlete).
- Place the feet shoulder-width apart with the knees slightly flexed.
- Grasp the bar with a closed, alternated grip inside the athlete's hands.
- At the athlete's signal, assist with moving the bar off the supports.
- Guide the bar to a position over the athlete's chest.
- Release the bar smoothly.

Downward Movement Phase: Athlete

- Lower the bar to touch the chest at approximately nipple level.
- Keep the wrists stiff and the forearms perpendicular to the floor and parallel to each other.
- Maintain the five-point body contact position.

Downward Movement Phase: Spotter

- Keep the hands in the alternated grip position close to—but not touching—the bar as it descends.
- Slightly flex the knees, hips, and torso and keep the back neutral when following the bar.

Upward Movement Phase: Athlete

- Push the bar upward and very slightly backward until the elbows are fully extended.
- Keep the wrists stiff and the forearms perpendicular to the floor and parallel to each other.
- Maintain the five-point body contact position.
- Do not arch the back or raise the chest to meet the bar.
- At the end of the set, signal the spotter for assistance in racking the bar.
- Keep a grip on the bar until it is racked.

Upward Movement Phase: Spotter

- Keep the hands in the alternated grip position close to—but not touching—the bar as it ascends.
- Slightly extend the knees, hips, and torso and keep the back neutral when following the bar.
- At the athlete's signal, grasp the bar with an alternated grip inside the athlete's hands.
- Guide the bar back onto the supports.
- Keep a grip on the bar until it is racked.

MAJOR MUSCLES INVOLVED

pectoralis major, anterior deltoids, triceps brachii

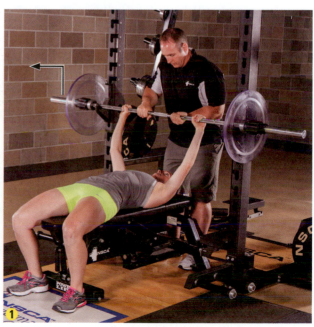

Liftoff

(continued)

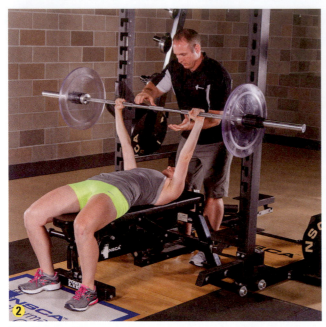

2 Starting positions

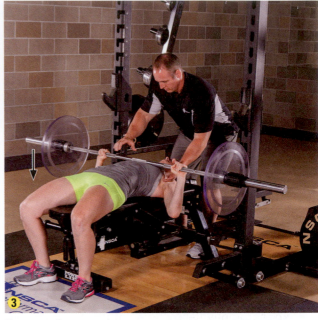

3 Downward movements

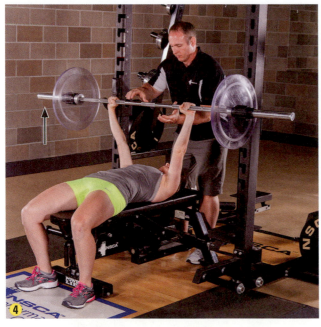

4 Upward movements

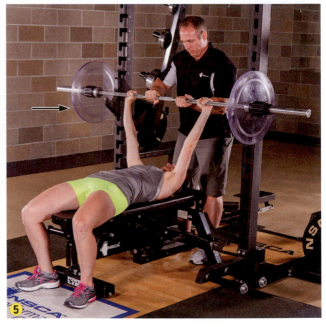

5 Racking the bar

15.14 INCLINE DUMBBELL BENCH PRESS (and Barbell Variation)

This exercise can also be performed with a barbell, using a closed, pronated grip slightly wider than shoulder-width. When using a barbell, the spotter assists by spotting the bar instead of the forearms near the athlete's wrists.

Starting Position: Athlete

- Grasp two dumbbells using a closed, pronated grip.
- Lie in a supine position on an incline bench in the five-point body contact position.
- Signal the spotter for assistance in moving the dumbbells into the starting position.
- Press the dumbbells in unison to an extended-elbow, parallel-arm position above the head and face.
- All repetitions begin from this position.

Starting Position: Spotter

- Stand erect and very close to the head of the bench (but do not distract the athlete).
- Place the feet shoulder-width apart with the knees slightly flexed.
- Grasp the athlete's forearms near the wrists.
- At the athlete's signal, assist with moving the dumbbells to a position over the athlete's head and face.
- Release the athlete's forearms smoothly.

Downward Movement Phase: Athlete

- Lower the dumbbells down and slightly out to be near the armpits and in line with the upper one-third area of the chest (between the clavicles and the nipples).

- Keep the wrists stiff and directly above the elbows, with the dumbbell handles aligned with each other.
- Maintain the five-point body contact position.
- Do not arch the back or raise the chest to meet the dumbbells.

Downward Movement Phase: Spotter

- Keep the hands near—but not touching—the athlete's forearms near the wrists as the dumbbells descend.
- Slightly flex the knees, hips, and torso and keep the back neutral when following the dumbbells.

Upward Movement Phase: Athlete

- Push the dumbbells upward at the same rate and very slightly toward each other until the elbows are fully extended.
- Keep the wrists stiff and directly above the elbows, with the dumbbell handles aligned with each other.
- Maintain the five-point body contact position.

Upward Movement Phase: Spotter

- Keep the hands near—but not touching—the athlete's forearms near the wrists as the dumbbells ascend.
- Slightly extend the knees, hips, and torso and keep the back neutral when following the dumbbells.

MAJOR MUSCLES INVOLVED

pectoralis major, anterior deltoids, triceps brachii

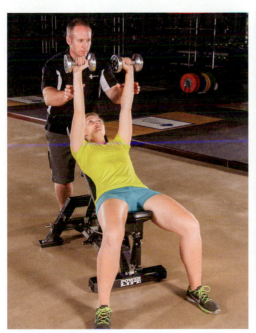

Starting positions

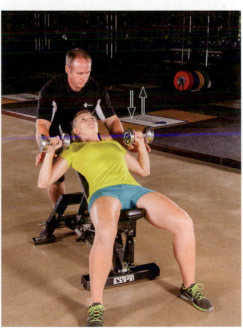

Downward and upward movements

15.15 FLAT DUMBBELL FLY (and Incline Variation)

This exercise can also be performed on an incline bench. If using the incline variation, begin by positioning the dumbbells over the head and face instead of over the chest.

Starting Position: Athlete
- Grasp two dumbbells using a closed, neutral grip.
- Lie in a supine position on a bench in the five-point body contact position.
- Signal the spotter for assistance in moving the dumbbells into the starting position.
- Press the dumbbells in unison to an extended-elbow position above the chest.
- Slightly flex the elbows and point them out to the sides.
- All repetitions begin from this position.

Starting Position: Spotter
- Position one knee on the floor with the foot of the other leg forward and flat on the floor (or kneel on both knees).
- Grasp the athlete's forearms near the wrists.
- At the athlete's signal, assist with moving the dumbbells to a position over the athlete's chest.
- Release the athlete's forearms smoothly.

Downward Movement Phase: Athlete
- Lower the dumbbells in a wide arc until they are level with the shoulders or chest.

- Keep the dumbbell handles parallel to each other as the elbows move downward.
- Keep the wrists stiff and the elbows held in a slightly flexed position.
- Keep the hands, wrists, forearms, elbows, upper arms, and shoulders in the same vertical plane.
- Maintain the five-point body contact position.

Downward Movement Phase: Spotter
- Keep the hands near—but not touching—the athlete's forearms near the wrists as the dumbbells descend.

Upward Movement Phase: Athlete
- Raise the dumbbells up toward each other in a wide arc back to the starting position.
- Keep the wrists stiff and the elbows held in a slightly flexed position.
- Keep the hands, wrists, forearms, elbows, upper arms, and shoulders in the same vertical plane.
- Maintain the five-point body contact position.

Upward Movement Phase: Spotter
- Keep the hands near—but not touching—the athlete's forearms near the wrists as the dumbbells ascend.

MAJOR MUSCLES INVOLVED
pectoralis major, anterior deltoids

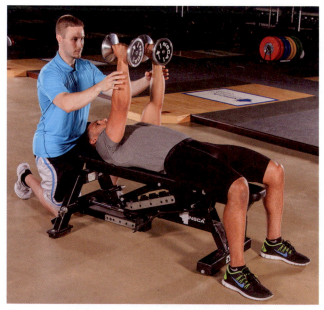

Starting positions

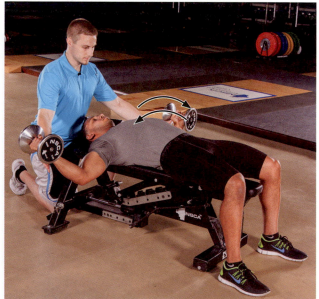

Downward and upward movements

15.16 VERTICAL CHEST PRESS (Machine)

Starting Position

- Sit down and lean back on the seat in the five-point body contact position.
- Grasp the handles with a closed, pronated grip.
- Align handles with the nipples. If necessary, adjust the seat height to correctly position the handles.
- All repetitions begin from this position.

Forward Movement Phase

- Push the handles away from the chest to a fully extended elbow position.
- Do not arch the lower back or forcefully lock out the elbows.
- Maintain the five-point body contact position.

Backward Movement Phase

- Allow the handles to slowly move backward to the starting position.
- Maintain the five-point body contact position.

MAJOR MUSCLES INVOLVED

pectoralis major, anterior deltoids, triceps brachii

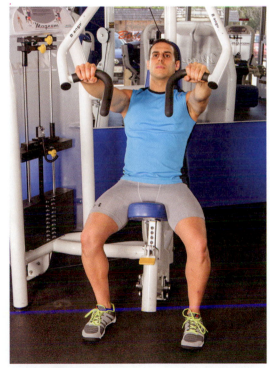

Starting position

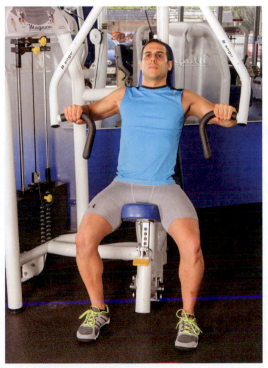

Forward and backward movements

15.17   PEC DECK (Machine)

Starting Position

- Sit down and lean back on the seat in the five-point body contact position. (*Note:* Some back pads are not long enough to allow the back of the head to be in contact with the bench.)
- Grasp the handles with a closed, neutral grip.
- Align the handles with the midchest so that the arms are parallel to the floor. If necessary, adjust the seat height to correctly position the handles.
- All repetitions begin from this position.

Forward Movement Phase

- Pull the handles toward each other while maintaining a slight bend in the elbow, until the fingers touch in front of the body.
- Do not arch the back or lock out the elbows.
- Maintain the five-point body contact position.

Backward Movement Phase

- Allow the handles to slowly move outward back to the starting position.
- Maintain the five-point body contact position.

MAJOR MUSCLES INVOLVED

pectoralis major, anterior deltoids, triceps brachii

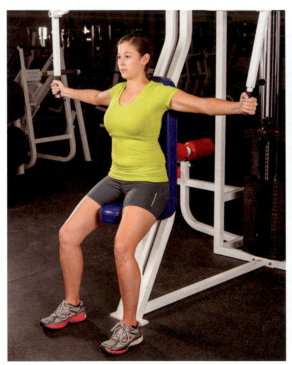

Starting position

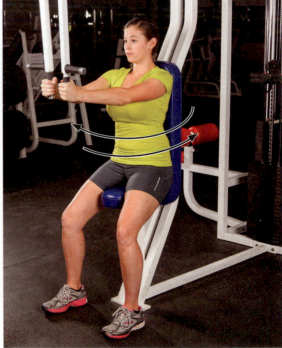

Forward and backward movements

15.18 WRIST CURL

Starting Position

- Sit on the end of a bench.
- Grasp the bar with a closed, supinated grip about hip- to shoulder-width apart.
- Position the feet and legs parallel to each other with the toes pointing straight ahead.
- Lean the torso forward and place the elbows and forearms on the top of the thighs.
- Move the wrists forward until they extend slightly beyond the patellae.
- Allow the wrists to extend and the hands to open so that the fingertips hold the bar.

Upward Movement Phase

- Raise the bar by flexing the fingers and then the wrists.
- Flex the wrists as far as possible without moving the elbows or forearms.
- Do not jerk the shoulders backward or swing the bar upward.

Downward Movement Phase

- Allow the wrists and fingers to slowly extend back to the starting position.
- Keep the torso and arms in the same position.

MAJOR MUSCLES INVOLVED

flexor carpi ulnaris, flexor carpi radialis, palmaris longus

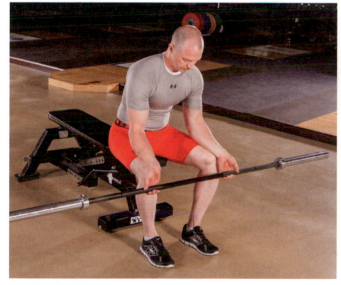

Starting position

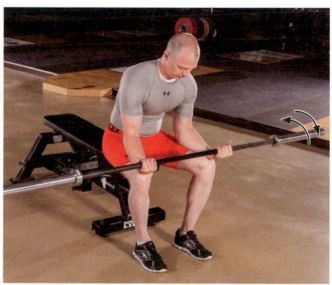

Upward and downward movements

15.19 WRIST EXTENSION

Starting Position

- Sit on the end of a bench.
- Grasp the bar with a closed, pronated grip about hip- to shoulder-width apart.
- Position the feet and legs parallel to each other with the toes pointing straight ahead.
- Lean the torso forward and place the elbows and forearms on the top of the thighs.
- Move the wrists forward until they are slightly beyond the patellae.
- Keep a closed grip on the bar but allow the wrists to flex toward the floor.

Upward Movement Phase

- Raise the bar by extending the wrists.
- Extend the wrists as far as possible without moving the elbows or forearms.
- Do not jerk the body backward or swing the bar upward.

Downward Movement Phase

- Allow the wrists to slowly flex back to the starting position.
- Keep the torso and arms in the same position.
- Maintain a closed grip.

MAJOR MUSCLES INVOLVED

extensor carpi ulnaris, extensor carpi radialis brevis (and longus)

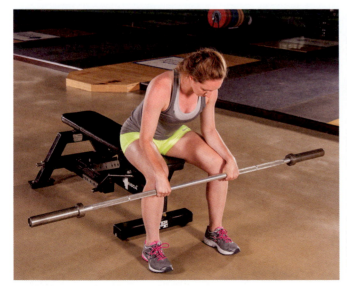

Starting position

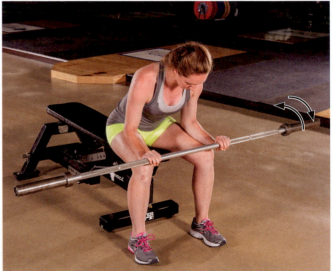

Upward and downward movements

15.20 HIP SLED (Machine)

Starting Position

- Sit in the machine with the lower back, hips, and buttocks pressed against their pads.
- Place the feet flat on the platform hip-width apart with the toes slightly angled out.
- Position the legs parallel to each other.
- Grasp the handles or the sides of the seat and move the hips and knees to a fully extended position, but do not forcefully lock the knees.
- Keep the hips on the seat and the back pressed firmly and evenly against the back pad.
- Remove the support mechanism from the foot platform and grasp the handles or the seat again.
- All repetitions begin from this position.

Downward Movement Phase

- Allow the hips and knees to slowly flex to lower the platform.
- Do not allow the platform to lower rapidly.
- Keep the hips and buttocks on the seat and the back pressed firmly and evenly against the back pad.
- Keep the knees aligned over the feet as they flex.

- Allow the hips and knees to flex until the thighs are parallel to the foot platform.
- Do not allow the buttocks to lose contact with the seat, the hips to roll off the back pad, or the heels to rise off the foot platform.

Upward Movement Phase

- Push the platform up by extending the hips and knees.
- Push to a fully extended position, but do not forcefully lock out the knees.
- Maintain the same hip and back position; do not allow the buttocks to rise.
- Keep the knees aligned over the feet as they extend.
- At the end of the set, return the supports to the starting position, remove the feet, and exit the machine.

MAJOR MUSCLES INVOLVED

gluteus maximus, semimembranosus, semitendinosus, biceps femoris, vastus lateralis, vastus intermedius, vastus medialis, rectus femoris

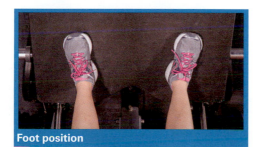

Foot position

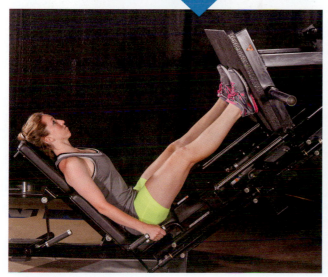

Starting position

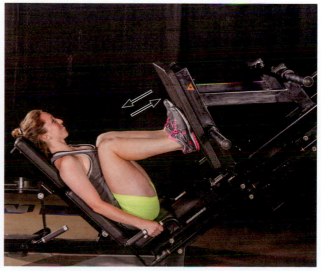

Downward and upward movements

▶ 15.21 BACK SQUAT

Starting Position: Athlete

- Grasp the bar with a closed, pronated grip (actual width depends on the bar position).
- Step under the bar and position the feet parallel to each other.
- Place the bar in a balanced position on the upper back and shoulders in one of two locations:
    1. *Low bar position*—across the posterior deltoids at the middle of the trapezius (using a handgrip wider than shoulder-width)
    2. *High bar position*—above the posterior deltoids at the base of the neck (using a handgrip only slightly wider than shoulder-width)
- Lift the elbows up to create a "shelf" for the bar using the upper back and shoulder muscles.
- Hold the chest up and out.
- Tilt the head slightly up.
- Once in position, signal the spotters for assistance in moving the bar off the supports.
- Extend the hips and knees to lift the bar.
- Take one or two steps backward.
- Position the feet shoulder-width apart (or wider), even with each other, with the toes pointed slightly outward.
- All repetitions begin from this position.

Starting Position: Two Spotters

- Stand erect at opposite ends of the bar with the feet shoulder-width apart and the knees slightly flexed.

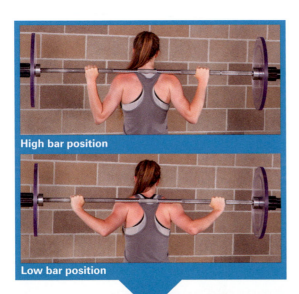

High bar position

Low bar position

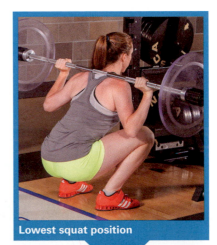

Lowest squat position

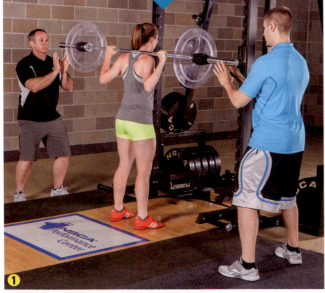

Starting positions with high bar position

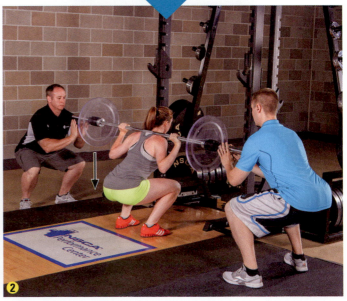

Downward movement positions

- Grasp the end of the bar by wrapping the hands around the bar with the thumbs crossed and palms facing the barbell.
- At the athlete's signal, assist with lifting and balancing the bar as it is moved off the supports.
- Release the bar smoothly.
- Hold the hands 2 to 3 inches (5-8 cm) below the ends of the bar.
- Move sideways in unison with the athlete as the athlete moves backward.
- Once the athlete is in position, get into a shoulder-width stance with the knees slightly flexed and the torso erect.

Downward Movement Phase: Athlete

- Maintain a position with the back neutral, elbows high, and the chest up and out.
- Allow the hips and knees to slowly flex while keeping the torso-to-floor angle relatively constant.
- Keep the heels on the floor and the knees aligned over the feet.
- Continue flexing the hips and knees until the tops of the thighs are parallel to the floor, the trunk begins to round or flex forward, or the heels rise off the floor.

Downward Movement Phase: Two Spotters

- Keep the thumbs crossed and hands close to—but not touching—the bar as it descends.
- Slightly flex the knees, hips, and torso to keep a neutral spine position when following the bar.

Upward Movement Phase: Athlete

- Maintain a position with neutral spine, high elbows, and the chest up and out.
- Extend the hips and knees at the same rate (to keep the torso-to-floor angle constant).
- Keep the heels on the floor and the knees aligned over the feet.
- Do not flex the torso forward or round the back.
- Continue extending the hips and knees to reach the starting position.
- At the end of the set, step forward toward the rack.
- Squat down until the bar rests on the supports.

Upward Movement Phase: Two Spotters

- Keep the thumbs crossed and hands close to—but not touching—the bar as it ascends.
- Slightly extend the knees, hips, and torso and keep the back neutral when following the bar.
- At the end of the set, move sideways in unison with the athlete back to the rack.
- Simultaneously grasp the bar and assist with balancing the bar as it is racked.
- Release the bar smoothly.

MAJOR MUSCLES INVOLVED

gluteus maximus, semimembranosus, semitendinosus, biceps femoris, vastus lateralis, vastus intermedius, vastus medialis, rectus femoris

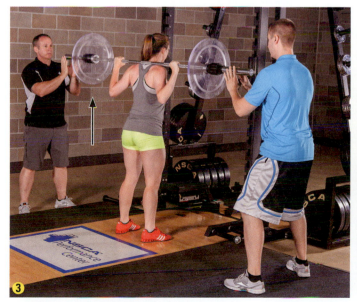

Upward movement positions

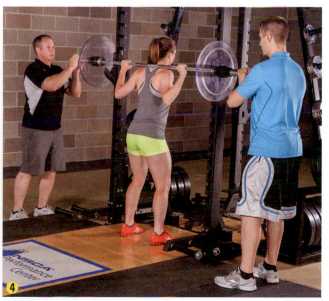

Racking the bar

15.22 FRONT SQUAT

Starting Position: Athlete

- Step under the bar and position the feet parallel to each other.
- Place the hands on the bar in one of two arm positions:
  1. Parallel-arm position
     - Grasp the bar with a closed, pronated grip.
     - Grip should be slightly wider than shoulder-width.
     - Move up to the bar to place it on top of the anterior deltoids and clavicles.
     - Fully flex the elbows to position the upper arms parallel to the floor.
  2. Crossed-arm position
     - Flex the elbows and cross the arms in front of the chest.
       - Move up to the bar to place it on top of the anterior deltoids.
       - Use an open grip with the hands on top of the bar and the fingers holding it in place.
       - Lift the elbows to position the arms parallel to the floor.
- Hold the chest up and out.
- Tilt the head slightly up.
- Once in position, signal the spotter for assistance in moving the bar off the supports.
- Extend the hips and knees to lift the bar.
- Take one or two steps backward.
- Position the feet shoulder-width apart (or wider), even with each other, with the toes pointed slightly outward.
- All repetitions begin from this position.

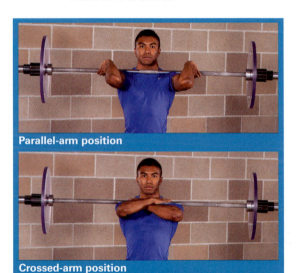

Parallel-arm position

Crossed-arm position

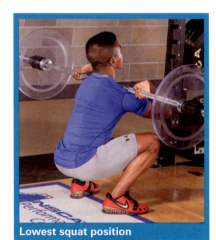

Lowest squat position

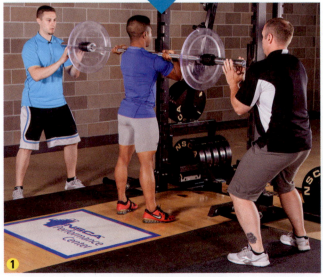

Starting positions with parallel-arm position

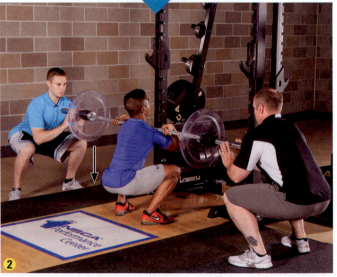

Downward movement positions

Starting Position: Two Spotters

- Stand erect at opposite ends of the bar with the feet shoulder-width apart and the knees slightly flexed.
- Grasp the end of the bar by wrapping the hands around the bar with the thumbs crossed and palms facing the barbell.
- At the athlete's signal, assist with lifting and balancing the bar as it is moved off the supports.
- Release the bar smoothly.
- Hold the hands 2 to 3 inches (5-8 cm) below the ends of the bar.
- Move sideways in unison with the athlete as the athlete moves backward.
- Once the athlete is in position, get into a shoulder-width stance with the knees slightly flexed and the torso erect.

Downward Movement Phase: Athlete

- Maintain a position with the back neutral, elbows high, and the chest up and out.
- Allow the hips and knees to slowly flex while keeping the torso-to-floor angle relatively constant.
- Keep the heels on the floor and the knees aligned over the feet.
- Do not flex the torso forward or round the back.
- Continue flexing the hips and knees until the tops of the thighs are parallel to the floor, the trunk begins to round or flex forward, or the heels rise off the floor.

Downward Movement Phase: Two Spotters

- Keep the thumbs crossed and hands close to—but not touching—the bar as it descends.

- Slightly flex the knees, hips, and torso and keep the back neutral when following the bar.

Upward Movement Phase: Athlete

- Maintain a position with the back neutral, elbows high, and the chest up and out.
- Extend the hips and knees at the same rate (to keep the torso-to-floor angle constant).
- Keep the heels on the floor and the knees aligned over the feet.
- Do not flex the torso forward or round the back.
- Continue extending the hips and knees to reach the starting position.
- At the end of the set, step forward toward the rack.
- Squat down until the bar rests on the supports.

Upward Movement Phase: Two Spotters

- Keep the thumbs crossed and hands close to—but not touching—the bar as it ascends.
- Slightly extend the knees, hips, and torso and keep the back neutral when following the bar.
- At the end of the set, move sideways in unison with the athlete back to the rack.
- Simultaneously grasp the bar and assist with balancing the bar as it is placed back on the supports.
- Release the bar smoothly.

MAJOR MUSCLES INVOLVED

gluteus maximus, semimembranosus, semitendinosus, biceps femoris, vastus lateralis, vastus intermedius, vastus medialis, rectus femoris

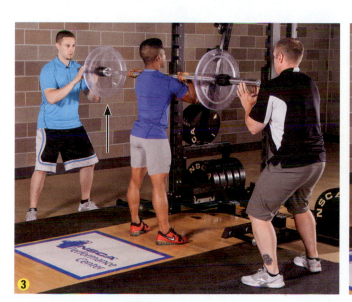

Upward movement positions

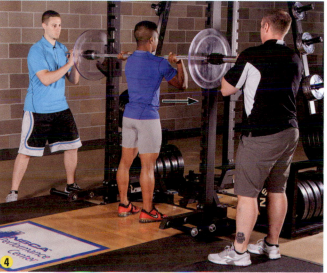

Racking the bar

15.23 FORWARD STEP LUNGE

This exercise can also be performed with two dumbbells, using a closed, neutral grip. The athlete allows the dumbbells to hang at arm's length alongside the body throughout the exercise. When using dumbbells, the spotter assists the athlete in the same manner as in the barbell version, although the task of helping the athlete rack the bar is not applicable. (*Note:* This exercise cannot be performed inside a typical power rack. The use of a tiered squat rack or a power rack that has supports on the outside is recommended. To allow an optimal view of the exercise technique, a rack is not shown in the photos.)

Starting Position: Athlete

- Step under the bar and position the feet parallel to each other.
- Grasp the bar with a closed, pronated grip.
- Place the bar in a balanced position on the upper back and shoulders above the posterior deltoids at the base of the neck (using a handgrip only slightly wider than shoulder-width).
- Lift the elbows up to create a "shelf" for the bar using the upper back and shoulder muscles.
- Hold the chest up and out.
- Tilt the head slightly up.
- Once in position, signal the spotter for assistance in moving the bar off the supports.
- Extend the hips and knees to lift the bar.

- Take two or three steps backward.
- All repetitions begin from this position.

Starting Position: Spotter

- Stand erect and very close to the athlete (but do not distract the athlete).
- Place the feet shoulder-width apart with the knees slightly flexed.
- At the athlete's signal, assist with lifting and balancing the bar as it is moved out of the rack.
- Move in unison with the athlete as the athlete moves backward to the starting position.
- Once the athlete is in position, get into a hip-width stance with the knees slightly flexed and the torso erect.
- Position the hands near the athlete's hips, waist, or torso.

Forward Movement Phase: Athlete

- Take one exaggerated step directly forward with one leg (the lead leg).
- Keep the torso erect as the lead foot moves forward and contacts the floor.
- Keep the trailing foot in the starting position, but allow the trailing knee to slightly flex.
- Plant the lead foot flat on the floor pointing straight ahead or slightly inward.

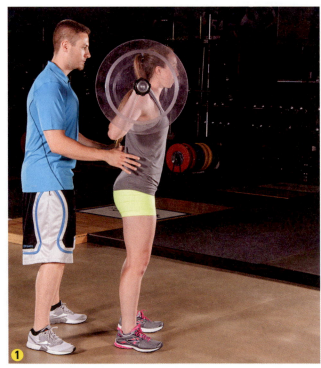

Starting positions

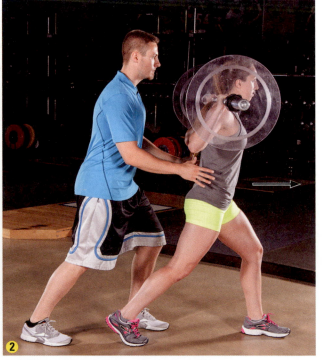

Beginning of forward movement positions

- Allow the lead hip and knee to flex slowly.
- Keep the lead knee directly over the lead foot.
- Continue to flex the trailing knee until it is 1 to 2 inches (3-5 cm) above the floor.
- Balance the weight evenly between the ball of the trailing foot and the whole lead foot.
- Keep the torso perpendicular to the floor by "sitting back" on the trailing leg.

Forward Movement Phase: Spotter

- Step forward with the same lead leg as the athlete.
- Keep the lead knee and foot aligned with the athlete's lead foot.
- Plant the lead foot 12 to 18 inches (30-46 cm) behind the athlete's lead foot.
- Flex the lead knee as the athlete's lead knee flexes.
- Keep the torso erect.
- Keep the hands near the athlete's hips, waist, or torso.
- Assist only when necessary to keep the athlete balanced.

Backward Movement Phase: Athlete

- Forcefully push off the floor by extending the lead hip and knee.

- Maintain the same erect torso position; do not jerk the upper body backward.
- Bring the lead foot back to a position next to the trailing foot; do not stutter-step backward.
- Stand erect in the starting position, pause, and then alternate lead legs for the next repetition.
- At the end of the set, step toward the rack and place the bar in the supports.

Backward Movement Phase: Spotter

- Push backward with the lead leg in unison with the athlete.
- Bring the lead foot back to a position next to the trailing foot; do not stutter-step backward.
- Keep hands near the athlete's hips, waist, or torso.
- Stand erect in the starting position, pause to wait for the athlete, and alternate lead legs for the next repetition.
- Assist only when necessary to keep the athlete balanced.
- At the end of the set, help the athlete rack the bar.

MAJOR MUSCLES INVOLVED

gluteus maximus, semimembranosus, semitendinosus, biceps femoris, vastus lateralis, vastus intermedius, vastus medialis, rectus femoris, iliopsoas

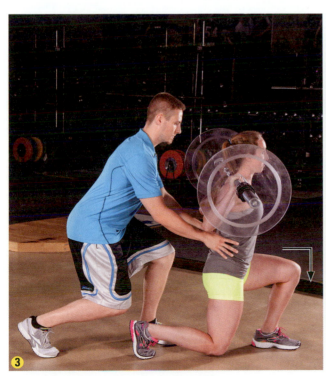

Completion of forward movement positions

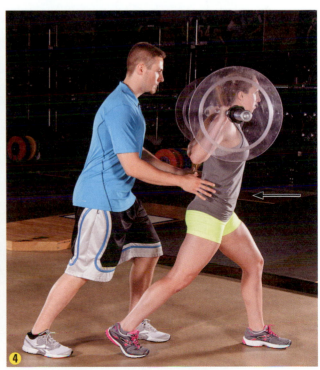

Middle of backward movement positions

15.24 STEP-UP

Note: The box used should be 12 to 18 inches (30-46 cm) high, or high enough to create a 90° angle at the knee joint when the foot is on the box. To allow an optimal view of the exercise technique, a rack is not shown in the photos.

Starting Position: Athlete

- Grasp the bar with a closed, pronated grip.
- Step under the bar and position the feet parallel to each other.
- Place the bar in a balanced position on the upper back and shoulders above the posterior deltoids at the base of the neck (using a handgrip only slightly wider than shoulder-width).
- Lift the elbows up to create a "shelf" for the bar using the upper back and shoulder muscles.
- Hold the chest up and out.
- Tilt the head slightly up.
- Once in position, signal the spotter for assistance in moving the bar off the supports.
- Extend the hips and knees to lift the bar.
- Move to a spot near the front of the box.
- All repetitions begin from this position.

Starting Position: Spotter

- Stand erect and very close to the athlete (but do not distract the athlete).
- Place the feet shoulder-width apart with the knees slightly flexed.
- At the athlete's signal, assist with lifting and balancing the bar as it is moved out of the rack.
- Move in unison with the athlete as the athlete moves to the starting position.
- Once the athlete is in position, get into a hip-width stance with the knees slightly flexed and the torso erect.
- Position the hands near the athlete's hips, waist, or torso.

Upward Movement Phase: Athlete

- Step up with one leg (the lead leg) to place the entire foot on the top of the box.
- Keep the torso erect; do not lean forward.
- Keep the trailing foot in the starting position, but shift the body weight to the lead leg.
- Forcefully extend the lead hip and knee to move the body to a standing position on top of the box.

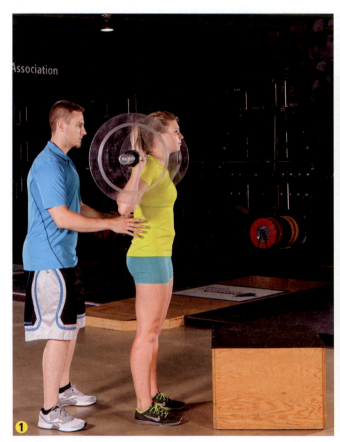

Starting positions

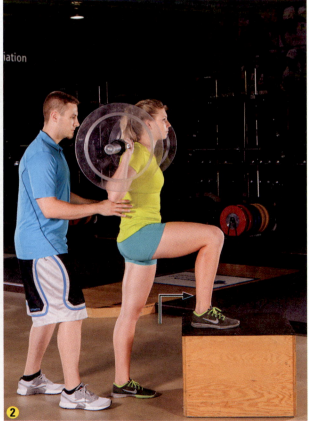

Initial contact of lead foot with top of box

- Do not push off or hop up with the trailing leg or foot.
- At the highest position, stand erect and pause before beginning the downward movement phase.

Upward Movement Phase: Spotter

- Take a small step forward with the lead leg as the athlete steps up on the box.
- As the athlete reaches the highest position, bring the trailing leg forward to be next to the lead leg.
- Keep the hands as near as possible to the athlete's hips, waist, or torso.
- Assist only when necessary to keep the athlete balanced.

Downward Movement Phase: Athlete

- Shift the body weight to the same lead leg.
- Step off the box with the same trailing leg.
- Maintain an erect torso position.
- Place the trailing foot on the floor the same distance from the box as the starting position.
- When the trailing foot is in full contact with the floor, shift the body weight to the trailing leg.
- Step off the box with the lead leg.

- Bring the lead foot back to a position next to the trailing foot.
- Stand erect in the starting position, pause, and then alternate lead legs for the next repetition.
- At the end of the set, step toward the rack and place the bar in the supports.

Downward Movement Phase: Spotter

- Take a small step backward with the same trailing leg, as the athlete steps back down to the floor.
- As the athlete steps off the box with the lead leg, take a step backward with the same lead leg.
- Keep the hands near the athlete's hips, waist, or torso.
- Stand erect in the starting position and pause to wait for the athlete.
- Assist only when necessary to keep the athlete balanced.
- At the end of the set, help the athlete rack the bar.

MAJOR MUSCLES INVOLVED

gluteus maximus, semimembranosus, semitendinosus, biceps femoris, vastus lateralis, vastus intermedius, vastus medialis, rectus femoris

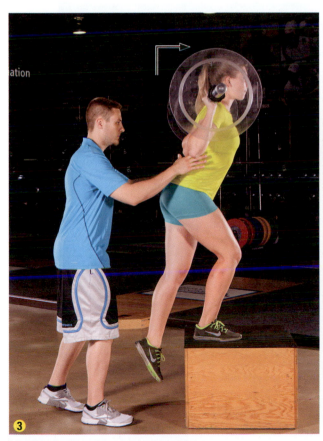

Middle of upward movement positions

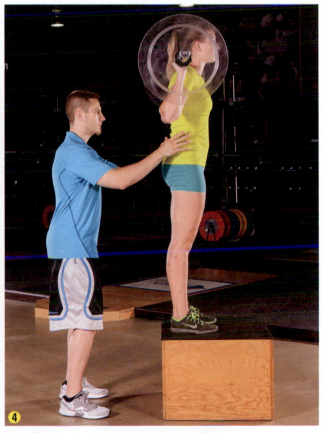

Completion of upward movement positions

15.25 GOOD MORNING

Note: To allow an optimal view of the exercise technique, a rack is not shown in the photos.

Starting Position

- Grasp the bar with a closed, pronated grip.
- Step under the bar and position the feet parallel to each other.
- Place the bar in a balanced position on the upper back and shoulders above the posterior deltoids at the base of the neck (using a handgrip only slightly wider than shoulder-width).
- Lift the elbows up to create a "shelf" for the bar using the upper back and shoulder muscles.
- Hold the chest up and out.
- Tilt the head slightly up.
- Position the feet shoulder-width apart (or wider), even with each other, with the toes pointed slightly outward.
- Extend the hips and knees to lift the bar off the supports.
- Take two or three steps backward.
- All repetitions begin from this position.

Downward Movement Phase

- Begin the exercise by slowly permitting the hips to flex. The buttocks should move straight back during the descent.
- Maintain a neutral spine and high elbow position; do not round the upper back during the descent.
- Keep the knees slightly flexed and the feet flat on the floor during the descent.
- Continue the downward movement until the torso is approximately parallel to the floor.

Upward Movement Phase

- Raise the bar by extending the hips.
- Keep the back neutral and the knees slightly flexed during the ascent.
- Continue extending the hips to reach the starting position.
- At the end of the set, step toward the rack and place the bar in the supports.

MAJOR MUSCLES INVOLVED

gluteus maximus, semimembranosus, semitendinosus, biceps femoris, erector spinae

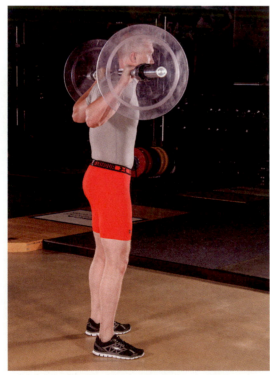

Starting position

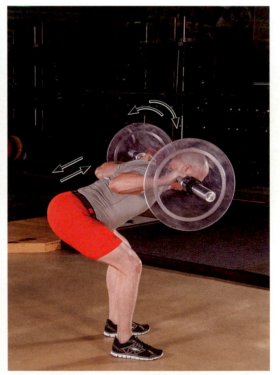

Downward and upward movements

15.26 DEADLIFT

Starting Position

- Stand with the feet flat and placed between hip- and shoulder-width apart with the toes pointed slightly outward.
- Squat down with the hips lower than the shoulders (farther than shown in the first photo), and grasp the bar with a closed, pronated grip. If the load is too heavy to hold the bar with a pronated grip, change to a closed, alternated grip.
- Place the hands on the bar slightly wider than shoulder-width apart, outside of the knees, with the elbows fully extended.
- Place the feet flat on the floor and position the bar approximately 1 inch (3 cm) in front of the shins and over the balls of the feet.
- Position the body with the
  - back neutral or slightly arched,
  - scapulae depressed and retracted,
  - chest held up and out,
  - head in line with the vertebral column or slightly hyperextended,
  - heels in contact with the floor,
  - shoulders over or slightly in front of the bar, and
  - eyes focused straight ahead or slightly upward.
- All repetitions begin from this position.

Upward Movement Phase

- Lift the bar off the floor by extending the hips and knees.
- Keep the torso-to-floor angle constant; do not let the hips rise before the shoulders.
- Maintain a neutral spine position.
- Keep the elbows fully extended and the shoulders over or slightly ahead of the bar.
- As the bar is raised, keep it as close to the shins as possible.
- As the bar rises just above the knees, keep the shoulders over the bar and extend the hips to keep the bar close to the body.
- Continue to extend the hips and knees until the body reaches a fully erect torso position.

Downward Movement Phase

- Allow the hips and knees to flex to slowly lower the bar to the floor.
- Maintain the neutral spine position; do not flex the torso forward.

MAJOR MUSCLES INVOLVED

gluteus maximus, semimembranosus, semitendinosus, biceps femoris, vastus lateralis, vastus intermedius, vastus medialis, rectus femoris

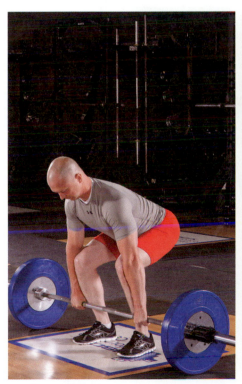

Starting position

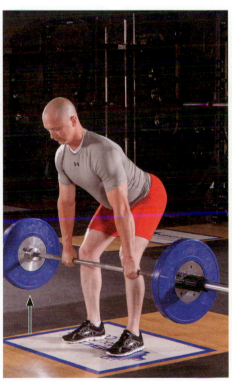

Middle position

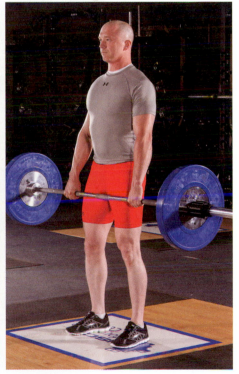

End position

15.27 STIFF-LEG DEADLIFT

Starting Position

- After performing the deadlift exercise to lift the bar off the floor, slightly to moderately flex the knees and keep them in this position throughout this exercise.
- All repetitions begin from this position.

Downward Movement Phase

- Begin the exercise by forming a neutral spine; then flex at the hips to lower the bar slowly, and under full control, toward the floor.
- Keep the knees in the same slightly or moderately flexed position with the back neutral or slightly arched and the elbows fully extended during the descent.
- Lower the bar until the plates touch the floor, the back cannot be held in the neutral position, the knees fully extend, or the heels rise off of the floor.

Upward Movement Phase

- Extend at the hips to return to the standing starting position.
- Keep the knees slightly flexed and the torso in a neutral spine position.
- Do not jerk the torso backward or flex the elbows.

MAJOR MUSCLES INVOLVED

gluteus maximus, semimembranosus, semitendinosus, biceps femoris, erector spinae

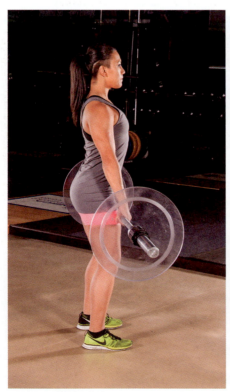

Starting position

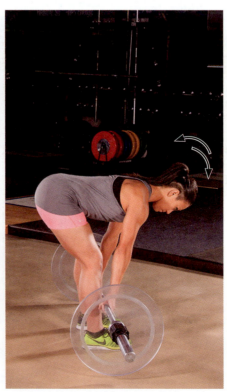

Downward and upward movements

15.28 ROMANIAN DEADLIFT (RDL)

Starting Position

- Place the hands on the bar in a closed, pronated position using either a clean or snatch grip.
- After performing the deadlift exercise to lift the bar off the floor, slightly to moderately flex the knees and keep them in this position throughout this exercise.
- All repetitions begin from this position.

Downward Movement Phase

- Begin the exercise by flexing the hips and pushing them backward, allowing the torso to move forward, keeping the bar in contact with the thighs.
- Keep the knees slightly flexed as the hips flex.
- Maintain a rigid torso, neutral spine, and keep the shoulders retracted until the barbell is aligned with the patella tendon and the torso is parallel to floor. (*Note:* If using a snatch grip with this exercise, the torso will be slightly below parallel, depending on the athlete's anthropometrics.)
- Keep a normal lordotic position throughout the movement.

Upward Movement Phase

- Extend the hips, raising the torso back to the starting standing position.
- Keep the knees slightly flexed and the torso in a neutral spine position.
- Make sure the barbell maintains contact with the thighs throughout the movement.
- Do not hyperextend the back or flex the elbows.

MAJOR MUSCLES INVOLVED

gluteus maximus, semimembranosus, semitendinosus, biceps femoris, erector spinae

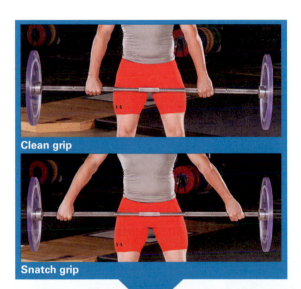

Clean grip

Snatch grip

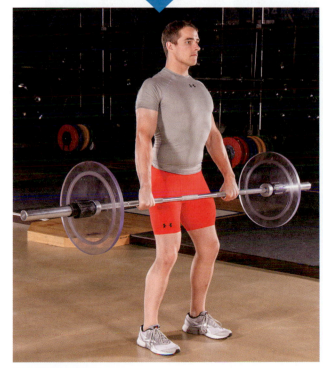

Starting position

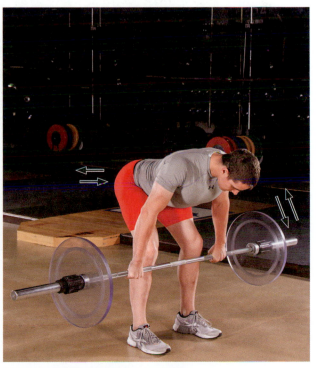

Downward and upward movements

15.29 LEG (KNEE) EXTENSION (Machine)

Starting Position

- Sit down in the machine and press the back firmly against the back pad.
- Place the feet behind and in contact with the roller pad.
- Position the legs parallel to each other.
- Align the knees with the axis of the machine. If necessary, adjust the back pad or the roller pad to position the legs correctly.
- Grasp the handles or the sides of the seat.
- All repetitions begin from this position.

Upward Movement Phase

- Raise the roller pad by fully extending the knees.
- Keep the torso erect and the back firmly pressed against the back pad.
- Keep the thighs, lower legs, and feet parallel to each other.
- Maintain a tight grip on the handles or the sides of the seat.
- Do not forcefully lock out the knees.

Downward Movement Phase

- Allow the knees to slowly flex back to the starting position.
- Keep the torso erect and the back firmly pressed against the back pad.
- Keep the thighs, lower legs, and feet parallel to each other.
- Do not allow the buttocks to lift off the seat.
- Maintain a tight grip on the handles or the sides of the seat.

MAJOR MUSCLES INVOLVED

vastus lateralis, vastus intermedius, vastus medialis, rectus femoris

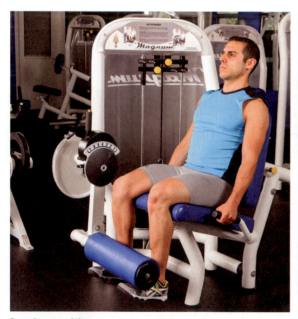

Starting position

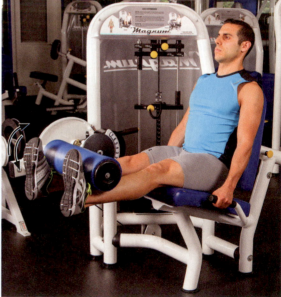

Upward and downward movements

15.30 **SEATED LEG (KNEE) CURL** (Machine)

Starting Position

- Sit down in the machine and press the back firmly against the back pad.
- Place the ankles on top of and in contact with the roller pad.
- Position the legs parallel to each other.
- Align the knees with the axis of the machine. If necessary, adjust the back pad to position the legs correctly.
- Grasp the handles or the sides of the seat.
- All repetitions begin from this position.

Downward Movement Phase

- Curl the roller pad below the seat by fully flexing the knees.
- Keep the torso stationary and the hips and torso firmly pressed against the pads.
- Do not allow the hips or low back to lift off the pads.
- Maintain a tight grip on the handles or the sides of the seat.

Upward Movement Phase

- Allow the knees to slowly extend back to the starting position.
- Keep the torso stationary and the hips and low back firmly pressed against the pads.
- Maintain a tight grip on the handles or the sides of the seat.
- Do not forcefully lock out the knees.

MAJOR MUSCLES INVOLVED

semimembranosus, semitendinosus, biceps femoris

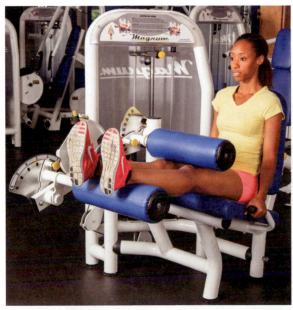

Starting position

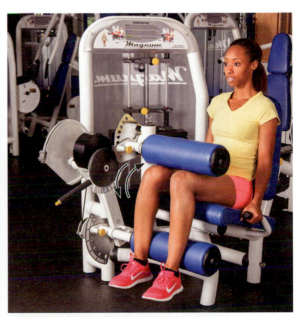

Downward and upward movements

15.31 SHOULDER PRESS (Machine)

Starting Position

- Sit down and lean back to place the body in the five-point body contact position.
- Grasp the handles with a closed, pronated grip.
- Align the handles with the top of the shoulders. If necessary, adjust the seat height to position the handles correctly.

Upward Movement Phase

- Push the handles upward until the elbows are fully extended.
- Maintain the five-point body contact position.
- Do not arch the lower back or forcefully lock out the elbows.

Downward Movement Phase

- Allow the elbows to slowly flex to lower the handles to the starting position.
- Maintain the five-point body contact position.

MAJOR MUSCLES INVOLVED

anterior and medial deltoids, triceps brachii

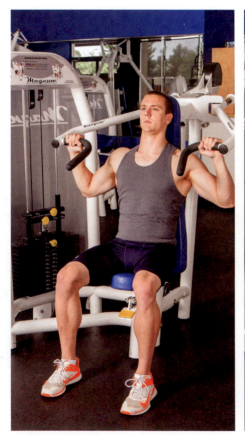

Starting position

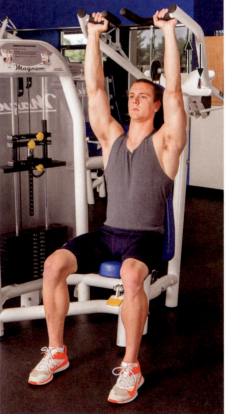

Upward and downward movements

15.32 **SEATED BARBELL SHOULDER PRESS** (and Dumbbell Variation)

This exercise can also be performed with two dumbbells, using a closed, pronated grip. When using dumbbells, the spotter assists by spotting the athlete's forearms near the wrists instead of the bar.

Starting Position: Athlete

- Sit down on a vertical shoulder press bench and lean back to place the body in the five-point body contact position.
- Grasp the bar with a closed, pronated grip.
- Grip should be slightly wider than shoulder-width.
- Signal the spotter for assistance in moving the bar off the supports.
- Press the bar over the head until the elbows are fully extended.
- All repetitions begin from this position.

Starting Position: Spotter

- Stand erect behind the bench with the feet shoulder-width apart and the knees slightly flexed.
- Grasp the bar with a closed, alternated grip inside the athlete's hands.
- At the athlete's signal, assist with moving the bar off the supports.
- Guide the bar to a position over the athlete's head.
- Release the bar smoothly.

Downward Movement Phase: Athlete

- Allow the elbows to slowly flex to lower the bar.
- Keep the wrists stiff and the forearms parallel to each other.
- Extend the neck slightly to allow the bar to pass by the face as it is lowered to touch the clavicles and anterior deltoids.
- Maintain the five-point body contact position.

Downward Movement Phase: Spotter

- Keep the hands in the alternated grip position close to—but not touching—the bar as it descends.
- Keep the knees slightly flexed and the back neutral when following the bar.

Upward Movement Phase: Athlete

- Push the bar upward until the elbows are fully extended.
- Extend the neck slightly to allow the bar to pass by the face as it is raised.
- Keep the wrists stiff and the forearms parallel to each other.
- Maintain the five-point body contact position.
- Do not arch the back or rise off the seat.
- At the end of the set, signal the spotter for assistance in racking the bar.
- Keep a grip on the bar until it is racked.

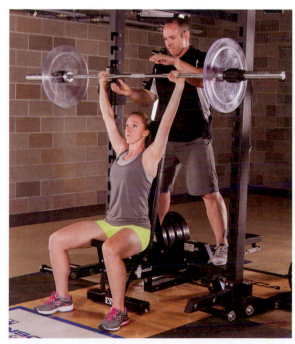

Starting positions

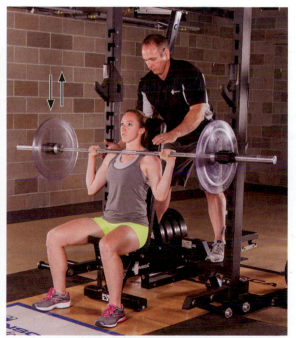

Downward and upward movements

(continued)

15.32 *(continued)*

Upward Movement Phase: Spotter

- Keep the hands in the alternated grip position close to—but not touching—the bar as it ascends.
- Slightly extend the knees, hips, and torso and keep the back neutral when following the bar.
- At the athlete's signal after the set is completed, grasp the bar with an alternated grip inside the athlete's hands.

- Guide the bar back onto the supports.
- Keep a grip on the bar until it is racked.

MAJOR MUSCLES INVOLVED

anterior and medial deltoids, triceps brachii

15.33   UPRIGHT ROW

Starting Position

- Grasp the bar with a closed, pronated grip approximately shoulder-width apart or slightly wider.
- Stand erect with feet shoulder-width apart, knees slightly flexed.
- Rest the bar on the front of the thighs with the elbows fully extended and pointing out to the sides.

Upward Movement Phase

- Pull the bar up along the abdomen and chest toward the chin.
- Keep the elbows pointed out to the sides as the bar brushes against the body.

- Keep the torso and knees in the same position.
- Do not rise up on the toes or swing the bar upward.
- At the highest bar position, the elbows should be level with or slightly higher than the shoulders and wrists.

Downward Movement Phase

- Allow the bar to slowly descend back to the starting position.
- Keep the torso and knees in the same position.

MAJOR MUSCLES INVOLVED

deltoids, upper trapezius

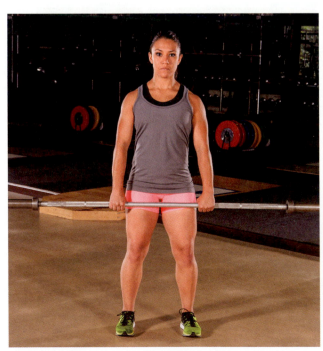

Starting position

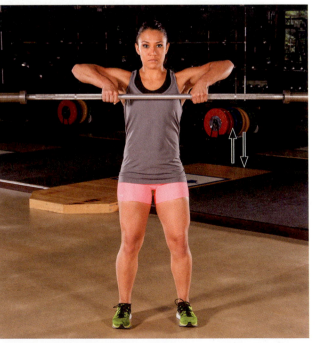

Upward and downward movements

15.34 LATERAL SHOULDER RAISE

Starting Position

- Grasp two dumbbells with a closed, neutral grip.
- Position the feet shoulder- or hip-width apart, with the knees slightly flexed, torso erect, shoulders back, and eyes focused ahead.
- Move the dumbbells to the front of the thighs, positioning them with the palms facing each other.
- Slightly flex the elbows and hold this flexed position throughout the exercise. (*Note:* The elbows should be slightly more flexed than shown in the photos.)

Upward Movement Phase

- Raise the dumbbells up and out to the sides; the elbows and upper arms should rise together ahead of the forearms, hands, and dumbbells.
- Maintain an erect upper body position with the knees slightly flexed and feet flat.
- Do not jerk the body or swing the dumbbells upward.
- Continue raising the dumbbells until the arms are approximately parallel to the floor or nearly level with the shoulders.

Downward Movement Phase

- Allow the dumbbells to descend slowly back to the starting position.
- Keep the torso and knees in the same position.

MAJOR MUSCLES INVOLVED

deltoids

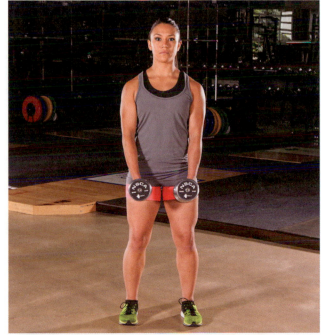

Starting position

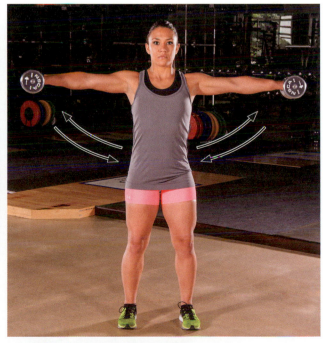

Upward and downward movements

15.35 **LYING BARBELL TRICEPS EXTENSION**

Starting Position: Athlete

- Lie in a supine position on a bench in the five-point body contact position.
- Grasp the bar from the spotter with a closed, pronated grip about 12 inches (30 cm) wide.
- Position the bar over the chest with the elbows fully extended and the arms parallel.
- Point the elbows toward the knees (not out to the sides).
- All repetitions begin from this position.

Starting Position: Spotter

- Stand erect and very close to the head of the bench (but do not distract the athlete).
- Place the feet shoulder-width apart in a staggered stance with the knees slightly flexed.
- Grasp the bar with a closed, alternated grip.
- Hand the bar to the athlete.
- Guide the bar to a position over the athlete's chest.
- Release the bar smoothly.

Downward Movement Phase: Athlete

- Keeping the upper arms stationary, allow the elbows to slowly flex to lower the bar toward the face.
- Keep the wrists stiff and the upper arms perpendicular to the floor and parallel to each other.
- Lower the bar until it almost touches the head or face.
- Maintain the five-point body contact position.

Downward Movement Phase: Spotter

- Place the hands in a supinated grip position close to—but not touching—the bar as it descends.
- Slightly flex the knees, hips, and torso and keep the back neutral when following the bar.

Upward Movement Phase: Athlete

- Push the bar upward by extending the elbows back to the starting position.
- Keep the wrists stiff and the elbows pointed toward the knees.
- Keep the upper arms parallel to each other and perpendicular to the floor.
- Maintain the five-point body contact position.
- At the end of the set, signal the spotter to take the bar.
- Keep a grip on the bar until the spotter removes it.

Upward Movement Phase: Spotter

- Keep the hands in a supinated grip position close to—but not touching—the bar as it ascends.
- Slightly extend the knees, hips, and torso and keep the back neutral when following the bar.
- At the athlete's signal after the set is completed, grasp the bar with an alternated grip, take it from the athlete, and set it on the floor.

MAJOR MUSCLE INVOLVED

triceps brachii

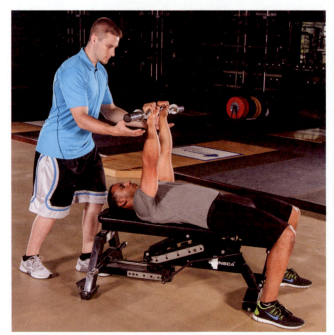

Starting positions

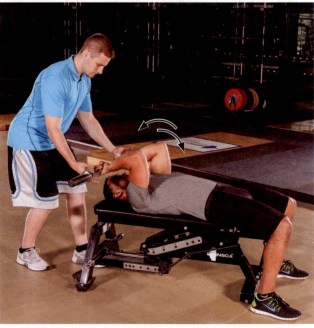

Downward and upward movements

15.36 TRICEPS PUSHDOWN (Machine)

Starting Position

- Grasp the bar with a closed, pronated grip 6 to 12 inches (15-30 cm) wide.
- Stand erect with feet shoulder-width apart, knees slightly flexed. Place the body close enough to the machine to allow the cable to hang straight down when it is held in the starting position.
- Pull the bar down to position the upper arms against the sides of the torso.
- Flex the elbows to position the forearms parallel to the floor or slightly above.
- All repetitions begin from this position.

Downward Movement Phase

- Push the bar down until the elbows are fully extended.
- Keep the torso erect and the upper arms stationary.
- Do not forcefully lock out the elbows.

Upward Movement Phase

- Allow the elbows to slowly flex back to the starting position.
- Keep the torso, arms, and knees in the same position.
- At the end of the set, return the bar to its resting position.

MAJOR MUSCLES INVOLVED

triceps brachii

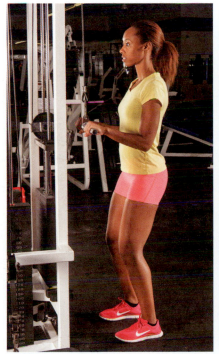

Starting position

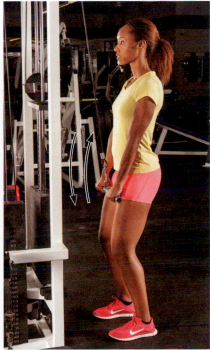

Downward and upward movements

15.37 PUSH PRESS

This exercise consists of quickly and forcefully pushing the bar from the shoulders to over the head. Although the ascent consists of two phases, the upward movement of the bar occurs in one continuous motion without interruption. Both the push press and the push jerk exercises involve a rapid hip and knee extension that accelerates the bar off the shoulders, followed immediately by movements that position the bar overhead. The technique used to attain this final bar position varies, however. In the push press, the hip and knee extension thrust is only forceful enough to drive the bar one-half to two-thirds the distance overhead. From this height, the bar is "pressed out" to the overhead position, with the hips and knees remaining fully extended after the thrust.

For either exercise, the athlete can begin with a bar taken from shoulder-height supports outside a power rack or by lifting a bar from the floor to the shoulders (via a repetition of the power clean exercise). Both exercises may be performed behind the neck using either a clean grip or a snatch grip. The following checklists describe the exercises using a power rack (although the rack is not shown).

Starting Position

- Grasp the bar with a closed, pronated grip.
- Grip should be slightly wider than shoulder-width (clean grip).
- Step under the bar and position the feet hip-width apart and parallel to each other.
- Move up to the bar to place it on top of the anterior deltoids and clavicles.
- Extend the hips and knees to lift the bar off the supports.
- Step back away from the supports and stand in the middle of the lifting platform.
- Position the feet hip- to shoulder-width apart and even with each other with the toes pointed slightly outward.
- All repetitions begin from this position.

Preparation Phase: Dip

- Flex the hips and knees at a controlled speed to move the bar in a straight path downward.
- Continue the dip to a depth not to exceed a quarter squat, the catch position of the power clean, or 10% of the athlete's height.
- Keep the feet flat on the floor, the torso erect, and the elbows underneath or slightly ahead of the bar.

Upward Movement Phase: Drive

- Immediately upon reaching the lowest position of the dip, reverse the movement by forcefully and quickly extending the hips, knees, and ankles and then the elbows to move the bar overhead.

Catch (for the Push Press)

- After the hips and knees are fully extended and the bar is overhead from the drive phase, press it up the rest of the way until the elbows are fully extended.
- In this position the torso is erect, the head is in a neutral position, the feet are flat on the floor, and the bar is slightly over or behind the ears.

Downward Movement Phase

- Lower the bar by gradually reducing the muscular tension of the arms to allow a controlled descent of the bar to the shoulders.
- Simultaneously flex the hips and knees to cushion the impact of the bar on the shoulders.
- At the end of the set, step toward the rack and place the bar in the supports.

MAJOR MUSCLES INVOLVED

gluteus maximus, semimembranosus, semitendinosus, biceps femoris, vastus lateralis, vastus intermedius, vastus medialis, rectus femoris, soleus, gastrocnemius, deltoids, trapezius

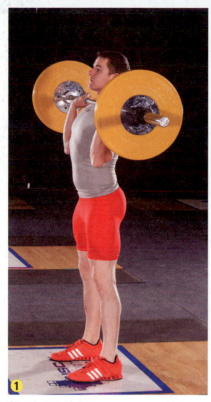

1 Starting position

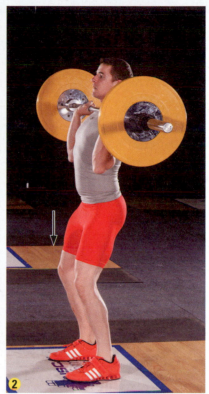

2 Dip

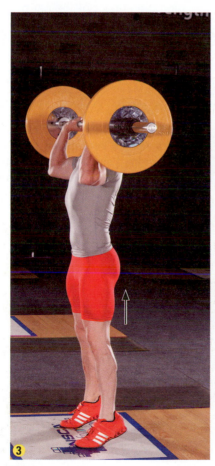

3 Drive

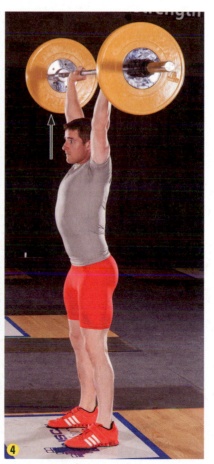

4 Catch (for the push press)

15.38 PUSH JERK

The push jerk involves a more forceful hip and knee thrust so that the bar is actually "driven" upward and caught with extended elbows in the overhead position with the hips and knees slightly flexed.

Starting Position

- Grasp the bar with a closed, pronated grip.
- Grip should be slightly wider than shoulder-width (clean grip).
- Step under the bar and position the feet hip- to shoulder-width apart and parallel to each other.
- Move close to the bar so that it is resting on the anterior deltoids and clavicles.
- Extend the hips and knees to lift the bar out of the supports.
- Step back away from the supports and stand in the middle of the lifting platform.
- Position the feet hip-width apart or slightly wider with toes pointed straight ahead or slightly outward.
- All repetitions begin from this position.

Preparation Phase: Dip

- Flex the hips and knees at a controlled speed to move the bar in a straight path downward.
- Continue the dip to a depth not to exceed a quarter squat.
- Keep the feet flat on the floor, the torso erect, and the elbows underneath or slightly ahead of the bar.

Upward Movement Phase: Drive

- Immediately upon reaching the lowest position of the dip, reverse the movement by forcefully and quickly extending the hips, knees, and ankles, and then the elbows to move the bar overhead.

Catch (for the Push Jerk)

- After the hips and knees are fully extended and the bar is being driven overhead, quickly flex the hips and knees to a dipped position while simultaneously fully extending the elbows so that the bar is received overhead at the same moment that the bar reaches its highest position.
- Catch the bar with the torso erect, the head in neutral position, feet flat on the floor, and the bar slightly behind the head, forming a straight line through the body.

Recovery Phase

- After gaining control and balance, stand up by extending the hips and knees to a fully erect position with the feet flat on the floor.
- Keep the elbows locked while the bar is stabilized overhead.

Downward Movement Phase

- Lower the bar by gradually reducing the muscular tension of the arms to allow a controlled descent of the bar to the shoulders.
- Simultaneously flex the hips and knees to cushion the impact of the bar on the shoulders.
- At the end of the set, step toward the rack and place the bar in the supports.

MAJOR MUSCLES INVOLVED

gluteus maximus, semimembranosus, semitendinosus, biceps femoris, vastus lateralis, vastus intermedius, vastus medialis, rectus femoris, soleus, gastrocnemius, deltoids, trapezius

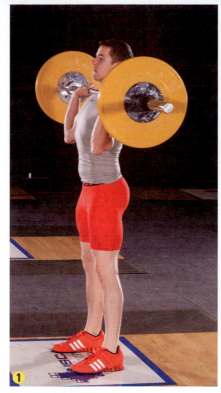

Starting position

Dip

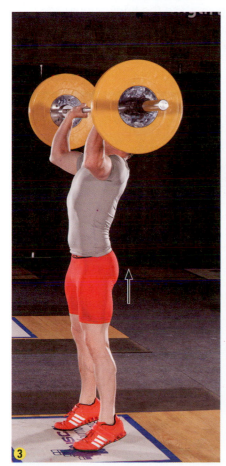

Drive

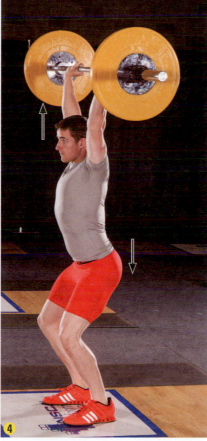

Catch (for the push jerk)

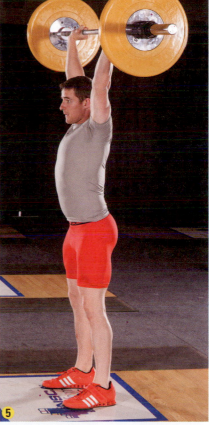

Recovery position

15.39 POWER CLEAN (and Hang Power Clean Variation)

This exercise consists of quickly and forcefully pulling the bar from the floor to the front of the shoulders—all in one movement. Although the ascent consists of four phases, the upward movement of the bar occurs in one continuous motion without interruption. The hang power clean is similar to the power clean exercise, except that the bar *begins* positioned at midthigh or slightly below or above the knees. In this variant of the power clean, the bar does not start on the floor or return to the floor between repetitions.

Starting Position

- Stand with the feet placed between hip- and shoulder-width apart with the toes pointed slightly outward.
- Squat down with the hips lower than the shoulders and grasp the bar evenly with a pronated grip. If a stronger grip is needed, use a hook grip.
- Place the hands on the bar slightly wider than shoulder-width apart, outside of the knees, with the elbows fully extended and pointing out to the side.
- Place the feet flat on the floor and position the bar approximately 1 inch (3 cm) in front of the shins and over the balls of the feet.
- Position the body with the
  - back neutral or slightly arched,
  - scapulae depressed and retracted,
  - chest held up and out,
  - head in line with the vertebral column or slightly hyperextended,
  - shoulders over or slightly in front of the bar, and
  - eyes focused straight ahead or slightly upward.
- All repetitions begin from this position.

Upward Movement Phase: First Pull

- Lift the bar off the floor by forcefully extending the hips and knees.
- Keep the torso-to-floor angle constant; do not let the hips rise before the shoulders.
- Maintain a neutral spine position.
- Keep the elbows fully extended, pointing out to the side, and the shoulders over or slightly ahead of the bar.
- As the bar is raised, keep it as close to the shins as possible.

Upward Movement Phase: Transition

- As the bar rises just above the knees, thrust the hips forward and slightly flex the knees to move the thighs against and the knees under the bar.
- Keep the back neutral or slightly arched and the elbows fully extended and pointing out to the sides.

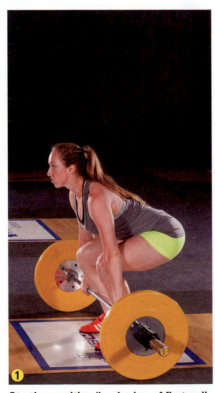

Starting position/beginning of first pull

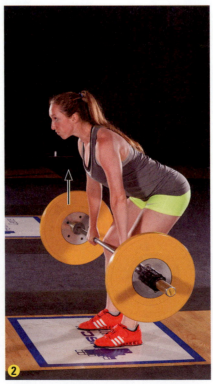

End of first pull/beginning of transition

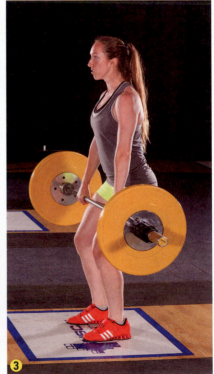

End of transition/beginning of second pull

Note: The transition phase is similar to the Romanian deadlift; in fact, weightlifters use the RDL to strengthen this movement pattern.

Upward Movement Phase: Second Pull

- Rapidly extend the hips, knees, and ankles. (*Note:* It is important that the heels stay in contact with the floor for as long as possible in order to maximize force transference to the barbell.)
- Keep the bar as close to the body as possible.
- Keep the back neutral and the elbows pointing out to the sides.
- Keep the shoulders over the bar and the elbows extended as long as possible.
- When the lower body joints reach full extension, rapidly shrug the shoulders upward with the elbows still fully extended and pointing to the sides.
- As the shoulders reach their highest elevation, flex the elbows to begin pulling the body under the bar.
- Due to the explosive nature of this phase, the torso is erect or slightly hyperextended, the head is tilted slightly back, and the feet may lose contact with the floor.

Upward Movement Phase: Catch

- After the lower body has fully extended, pull the body under the bar and rotate the arms around and under the bar.

- Simultaneously, flex the hips and knees to a quarter-squat position.
- Once the arms are under the bar, lift the elbows to position the upper arms parallel to the floor.
- Rack the bar across the front of the clavicles and anterior deltoids.
- Catch the bar with
  — a nearly erect torso,
  — the shoulders slightly ahead of the hips,
  — a neutral head position, and
  — flat feet.
- After gaining control and balance, stand up by extending the hips and knees to a fully erect position.

Downward Movement Phase

- Lower the elbows to unrack the bar from the anterior deltoids and clavicles; then slowly lower the bar down to the thighs.
- Simultaneously flex the hips and knees to cushion the impact of the bar on the thighs.
- Squat down with the elbows fully extended until the bar touches the floor or drop the bar to the platform if rubber bumper plates are being used.

MAJOR MUSCLES INVOLVED

gluteus maximus, semimembranosus, semitendinosus, biceps femoris, vastus lateralis, vastus intermedius, vastus medialis, rectus femoris, soleus, gastrocnemius, deltoids, trapezius

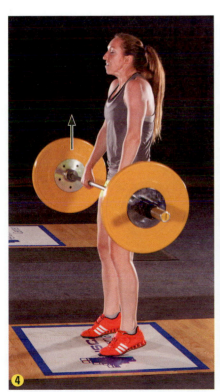

④ End of second pull

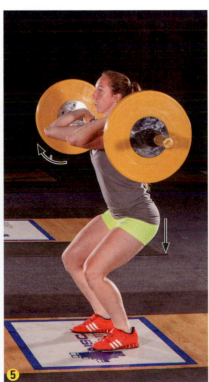

⑤ Catch

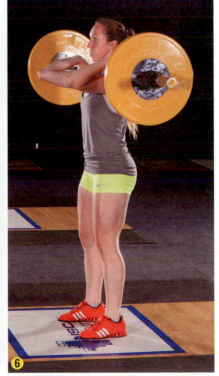

⑥ End position

15.40 POWER SNATCH (and Hang Power Snatch Variation)

This exercise consists of quickly and forcefully pulling the bar from the floor to over the head with the elbows fully extended—all in one movement. Although the ascent consists of multiple phases, the upward movement of the bar occurs in one continuous motion without interruption. The hang power snatch is similar to the power snatch exercise, except that the initial position of the bar is not on the floor, and it does *not* return to the floor between repetitions.

Starting Position

- Stand with the feet placed between hip- and shoulder-width apart with the toes pointed slightly outward.
- Squat down with the hips lower than the shoulders and grasp the bar evenly with a pronated grip. If a stronger grip is needed, use a hook grip.
- The grip width is wider than for other exercises; a way to estimate it is to measure and use one of these distances for spacing the hands: (1) the distance from the edge of the clenched fist of one hand to the opposite shoulder when the arm is straight out at the side, or (2) the elbow-to-elbow distance when the arms are straight out at the sides.
- Extend the elbows fully and point them out to the side.
- Place the feet flat on the floor and position the bar approximately 1 inch (3 cm) in front of the shins and over the balls of the feet.
- Position the body with the
  — back neutral or slightly arched,
  — scapulae depressed and retracted,
  — chest held up and out,
  — head in line with the vertebral column or slightly hyperextended,
  — feet flat on the floor,
  — shoulders over or slightly in front of the bar, and
  — eyes focused straight ahead or slightly upward.
- All repetitions begin from this position.

Upward Movement Phase: First Pull

- Lift the bar off the floor by forcefully extending the hips and knees.
- Keep the torso-to-floor angle constant; do not let the hips rise before the shoulders.
- Maintain the neutral spine position.
- Keep the elbows fully extended, pointing out to the side, and the shoulders over or slightly ahead of the bar.

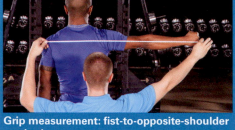

Grip measurement: fist-to-opposite-shoulder method

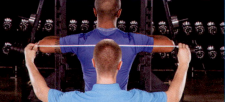

Grip measurement: elbow-to-elbow method

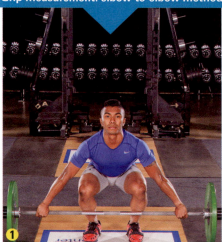

Starting position/beginning of first pull

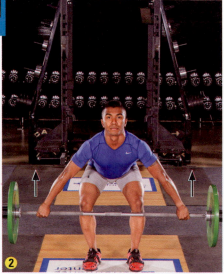

End of first pull/beginning of transition

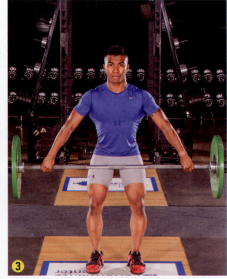

End of transition/beginning of second pull

- As the bar is raised, keep it as close to the shins as possible.

Upward Movement Phase: Transition

- As the bar rises just above the knees, thrust the hips forward and slightly flex the knees to move the thighs against, and the knees under, the bar.
- Keep the back neutral or slightly arched and the elbows fully extended and pointing out to the sides.

Note: The transition phase is similar to the Romanian deadlift; in fact, weightlifters use the RDL to strengthen this movement pattern.

Upward Movement Phase: Second Pull

- Rapidly extend the hips, knees, and ankles. (*Note:* It is important that the heels stay in contact with the floor for as long as possible in order to maximize force transference to the barbell.)
- Keep the bar as close to the body as possible.
- Keep the back neutral and the elbows pointing out to the sides.
- Keep the shoulders over the bar and the elbows extended as long as possible.
- When the lower body joints reach full extension, rapidly shrug the shoulders upward with the elbows still fully extended and out to the sides.
- As the shoulders reach their highest elevation, flex the elbows to begin pulling the body under the bar.
- Due to the explosive nature of this phase, the torso is erect or slightly hyperextended, the head is tilted slightly back, and the feet may lose contact with the floor.

Upward Movement Phase: Catch

- After the lower body has fully extended, pull the body under the bar and rotate the hands around and under the bar.
- Simultaneously, flex the hips and knees to a quarter-squat position.
- Once the body is under the bar, catch the bar over and slightly behind the ears with
  - fully extended elbows,
  - an erect and stable torso,
  - a neutral head position,
  - flat feet, and
  - the body's weight over the middle of the feet.
- After gaining control and balance, stand up by extending the hips and knees to a fully erect position.
- Stabilize the bar overhead.

Downward Movement Phase

- Lower the bar from the overhead position by gradually reducing the muscular tension of the shoulders to allow a controlled descent of the bar to the thighs.
- Simultaneously flex the hips and knees to cushion the impact of the bar on the thighs.
- Squat down with the elbows fully extended until the bar touches the floor or drop the bar to the platform if rubber bumper plates are being used.

MAJOR MUSCLES INVOLVED

gluteus maximus, semimembranosus, semitendinosus, biceps femoris, vastus lateralis, vastus intermedius, vastus medialis, rectus femoris, soleus, gastrocnemius, deltoids, trapezius

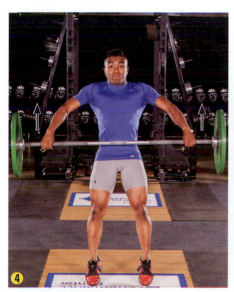

End of second pull

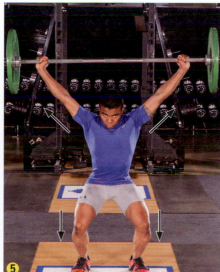

Catch

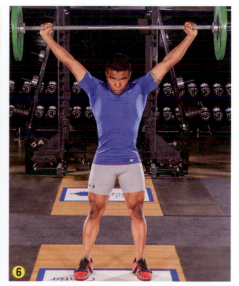

End position

KEY TERMS

alternated grip
clean grip
closed grip
false grip
five-point body contact position
forced repetitions
free weight exercises
grip width
hook grip

liftoff
neutral grip
neutral spine
out-of-the-rack exercises
overhand grip
over-the-face barbell exercises
partner-assisted reps
power exercises
pronated grip

range of motion (ROM)
snatch grip
spotter
sticking point
structural exercises
supinated grip
supine
underhand grip
Valsalva maneuver

STUDY QUESTIONS

1. Which of the following exercises requires a spotter?
   a. lat pulldown
   b. wrist curl
   c. power clean
   d. step-up

2. During which of the following exercises should a spotter's hands be placed on the athlete's forearms near the wrists?
   a. bench press
   b. incline dumbbell bench press
   c. upright row
   d. lying barbell triceps extension

3. Which of the following grips should be used during the deadlift exercise?
   I. overhand
   II. closed
   III. open
   IV. alternated
   a. I and III only
   b. II and IV only
   c. I, II, and IV only
   d. II, III, and IV only

4. Which of the following is the correct foot pattern in the step-up exercise?
   a. step up *left* foot, step up *right* foot, step down *left* foot, step down *right* foot
   b. step up *right* foot, step up *left* foot, step down *left* foot, step down *right* foot
   c. step up *left* foot, step down *left* foot, step up *right* foot, step down *right* foot
   d. step up *right* foot, step up *left* foot, step down *right* foot, step down *left* foot

5. The primary movement during the second pull phase of the power clean exercise is
   a. hip flexion
   b. hip extension
   c. knee flexion
   d. dorsiflexion

CHAPTER 16

Exercise Technique for Alternative Modes and Nontraditional Implement Training

G. Gregory Haff, PhD, Douglas Berninger, MEd, and Scott Caulfield, BS

> **After completing this chapter, you will be able to**
>
> - understand the basic guidelines for performing resistance exercise with alternative modes and nontraditional implements,
> - describe the benefits and limitations of bodyweight training activities,
> - identify the benefits and limitations associated with core training,
> - identify the appropriate technique and key technical flaws associated with the alternative mode exercises,
> - appropriately determine how to apply resistance bands and chains to traditional ground-based free weight exercise, and
> - determine the appropriate use of alternative methods and nontraditional implement exercises.

The use of alternative modes and nontraditional implement exercises has become increasingly popular in the strength and conditioning profession. Whenever implementing these types of training methods into training programs, one should consider some basic and specific guidelines to ensure that these methods are used safely.

General Guidelines

With the use of **alternative modes** and **nontraditional implement** exercises, the general guidelines are not very different from those used with traditional resistance training methods. A stable body position that allows the athlete to achieve and maintain safe and proper body alignment during the performance of the exercise is needed in order to appropriately stress the skeletal muscle system. Freestanding ground-based exercises typically use a position in which the feet are placed slightly wider than shoulder-width. With the use of instability devices, the body position may need to be modified in order to ensure that stability is achieved. The grip used with alternative modes and nontraditional implement exercises is typically one of the traditional grips presented in chapter 15. The choice of grip is based on the demands of the particular exercise. Additionally, with many nontraditional implements, the grip can be a limiting factor in the performance of the exercise.

As with more traditional exercises, the breathing pattern often recommended with these alternative methods is for the athlete to exhale through the **sticking point** (concentric portion) and to inhale during the less stressful portion (eccentric portion) of the movement. For example, athletes doing the dumbbell chest press on a stability ball would inhale as they lower the dumbbells to the chest and exhale as they push them away from the chest. With structural exercises (those that load the **axial skeleton**), breath holding may be warranted. However, when one is lifting loads greater than 80% of maximal voluntary contraction or lifting lighter loads to failure, the **Valsalva maneuver** (forced expiration against a closed glottis) may be unavoidable (32). The Valsalva maneuver allows for an increase in the intra-abdominal pressure that augments the stability of the spine, which may be beneficial for performing nontraditional exercises. For example, with the log clean, the athlete may perform the Valsalva maneuver during the pull and catch portion of the exercise. The athlete would then exhale after assuming an erect position. Chapter 15 presents more information on the Valsalva maneuver.

Bodyweight Training Methods

Bodyweight training methods are among the most basic methods for performing resistance training. Specifically, with these types of exercises, the body weight of the individual is used to provide resistance (37). Activities such as push-ups, pull-ups, chin-ups, sit-ups, and squat thrusts are typically mentioned in the context of bodyweight training. However, activities such as calisthenics, gymnastics, and yoga could all be classified as bodyweight training methodologies (37). As noted by Behm and colleagues (10), gymnastics was classically a part of the physical education system; and this type of training strongly promotes the development of the core musculature, which, when strengthened, appears to reduce injury potential. Bodyweight training appears to offer a low-cost training method that allows for the development of relative strength levels.

One of the issues related to bodyweight resistance training is the fact that the resistance load is limited to the individual's body weight. As such, bodyweight training tends not to significantly affect absolute strength levels (37). To increase the intensity of bodyweight exercises, one can do several things, including increasing the number of repetitions or changing the movement pattern. While increasing the number of repetitions will change the workload, it will shift the targeted outcome from strength toward strength-endurance, which shifts the targeted output away from the development of strength. Simple modifications to bodyweight exercises may obviate some of these limitations. Changing the movement pattern, for example, by elevating the legs while doing a push-up, will increase the resistance encountered. Suspension devices with bodyweight exercises could also be

---

General Guidelines for Alternative Modes and Nontraditional Implement Exercises

- Ensure proper body alignment via selection of a stable body position.
- If the exercise is a freestanding ground-based exercise, place the feet slightly wider than shoulder-width and keep them flat on the ground.
- Use the appropriate grip for the exercise based on the type of exercise (see chapter 15 for more detail).
- Exhale during the concentric portion of the exercise and inhale during the eccentric phase.
- With heavy loads (80% of maximal voluntary contraction or greater) or with lighter loads performed to failure, the Valsalva maneuver may be a useful technique for maintaining spinal stability.

Benefits of Bodyweight Training

The following are some of the benefits of bodyweight training (37):
- Is specific to each individual's anthropometrics
- Often includes closed chain–based exercises
- Strengthens several muscle groups at once
- Develops relative strength
- Improves body control
- Is a low-cost training alternative

---

used to increase training intensity (71, 72) as indicated by increases in muscle activation patterns (51). Snarr and Esco (72) report that **muscle activation** is significantly greater in push-ups performed in a suspension device when compared to traditional push-ups performed on stable ground.

Core Stability and Balance Training Methods

There is increasing interest in training the **core** in an attempt to improve overall health, rehabilitate from injuries, and enhance athletic performance (10). To target core stability and balance, interventions ranging from traditional **ground-based free weight exercises** to training on unstable devices have been advocated in the applied literature.

Anatomical Focus

The term *core* is commonly used in the popular media and in some training journals (10) to refer to the trunk, or more specifically the lumbopelvic region of the body (81). However, interpretation of the scientific literature appears to make an accurate or consistent definition of the core tenuous at best (10, 82). Typically, the **anatomical core** is defined as the axial skeleton and all the soft tissues with proximal attachments that originate on the axial skeleton (9, 10). It is important to note that the appendicular skeleton includes the pelvic and shoulder girdles, while the soft tissues include the articular cartilage and fibrocartilage, ligaments, tendons, muscles, and fascia (10). Ultimately the soft tissues act to generate forces (concentric muscle actions) and resist motion (eccentric and isometric muscle actions).

The muscles that are typically associated with the core allow for the transference of torques and angular momentum during the performance of integrated kinetic chain activities, such as kicking or throwing (81). In fact, Willardson (81) suggests that increasing an athlete's core stability will result in a better foundation for force production in the upper and lower extremities.

Isolation Exercises

Isolation exercises typically consist of dynamic or isometric muscle actions designed to isolate specific core musculature without the contribution of the lower and upper extremities (10). For example, common exercises performed to isolate the core are the prone plank (68) and side plank (78). There is evidence that these types of isolated exercises can increase muscle activation, which has been suggested to result in improvements in spinal stability and a reduction of injuries (56). While evidence suggests that these types of activities result in improvements in performance in untrained individuals and those recovering from an injury, there is limited support for the idea that these types of training activities translate to improvements in sport performance (65, 81). In fact, in a recent systematic review, Reed and colleagues (65) report that isolated core training is not very effective at improving sport performance. Additionally, according to Behm and coworkers (10) and Willardson (81), there is strong evidence that ground-based free weight exercises (e.g., squat, deadlift, push press, snatch, and exercises that involve trunk rotation) offer a greater benefit to actual sport performance compared to isolated core training. Ground-based free weight activities appear to offer activation of the core musculature that is similar to, or in most cases greater than, that with traditional isolation exercises designed to engage the core (35, 60). Isolation exercises may have the greatest benefit for injured athletes who are going through the rehabilitation process and are not able to adequately load traditional ground-based free weight exercises (81).

> ▶ **Ground-based free weight activities appear to offer similar or, in most cases, greater activation of the core musculature when compared to traditional isolation exercises designed to engage the core.**

Machines Versus Free Weight Exercises

When free weight training methods are compared to machine-based training methods, each has advantages and disadvantages (10, 34, 75). With regard to **machine-based training**, the stability provided by the machine may result in a better ability to target specific muscle groups; but in the context of sport performance, muscle rarely if ever functions in such an isolated fashion (10). With regard to the stabilizer muscles, it is generally accepted that activation of these muscles is greater during free weight training when compared with machine-based training (33). In partial support of this belief, Anderson and Behm (2) state that the activity of the back stabilizers was 30% lower during a Smith machine squat when compared to a free weight squat. Additionally, there is scientific support for the contention that machine-based strength gains exert a negligible or a possible detrimental effect on the muscle activation pattern in athletic movements (2, 15, 57). However, if instability is increased via performance of ground-based free weight training on unstable surfaces or devices, greater decrements in force production, the rate of force development, and power outputs have been noted (23, 49). Therefore, based on these data, it appears that free weight ground-based exercises offer the ideal combination of specificity and instability, especially when one is focusing on strength and power development. Ultimately, sufficient instability for the development of sport-specific adaptations can be stimulated via the use of traditional ground-based free weight strength training, and there appears to be no need to add increased instability to these types of exercises (10).

> ▶ **Free weight ground-based exercises offer the ideal combination of specificity and instability, especially when one is focusing on strength and power development.**

Instability Devices

Instability-based exercises are typically considered those that are performed on unstable surfaces or devices commonly found in strength and conditioning facilities. The increased popularity of training on instability devices seems to have stemmed from their use by physiotherapists in the rehabilitation process. These devices are used to promote postural disequilibrium or imbalance requiring a greater stabilizing function of the core musculature (10, 81). If perturbations are applied during use of these devices, a balance challenge can occur that requires activation of the core musculature in order to induce postural adjustments to remain upright (19).

Numerous instability devices are available to the strength and conditioning professional; the most common are the Swiss, physio, and pezzi gymnastics balls (10). Other instability options include hemispherical physioballs with one inflated dome side and a flat rubber side, inflatable disks, wobble boards, balance boards, foam tubes, and various foam platforms. Natural surfaces such as sand can also create scenarios that introduce instability into an athlete's movement pattern, creating an increased balance challenge that results in increased core muscle activation. Many strength and conditioning professionals believe that performing instability exercises trains the target agonist muscle group while simultaneously increasing core muscle activation (10). While there is some evidence to suggest that core muscle activation may be increased, it appears that this increase occurs in conjunction with reduced force generation by the agonist muscle (9, 23). During training with instability exercises, the overall agonist force-generating capacity (8) and overall power output (23) may be less than 70% of what can be achieved when the exercise is performed under stable conditions. Additionally, there can be a significant reduction in the rate of force development that is achieved during the exercise (60). Training with a reduced force production, power output, and rate of force development may not be the most advantageous method for preparing athletes, as these factors have a large impact on many aspects central to successful sport performance.

Overall, there is limited research that suggests the performance of resistance exercises on unstable devices by athletes results in significant performance improvements (21, 73). The lack of performance benefit noted in the literature might be expected based on the principle of diminishing returns, as it is very likely that trained athletes require a much greater adaptive stimulus in terms of force production, movement velocity, and rate of force development to realize performance gains than can be provided by instability exercise devices (10, 47). Therefore, the performance of static balance activities on instability devices may be considered an introductory training step to improve balance and core stability before the implementation of dynamic or explosive ground-based free weight exercises, such as the Olympic lifts, that are performed on stable surfaces (10).

> ▶ **Ground-based free weight exercises (e.g., squats, deadlifts, Olympic lifts) involve a degree of instability that allows for simultaneous development of all links of the kinetic chain, offering a much better training stimulus for the development of core stability and the enhancement of athletic performance than do instability device–based exercises (10).**

When used in the rehabilitation setting, unstable devices have been shown to reduce low back pain and improve the efficiency of the soft tissues that stabilize the knee and ankle joints (9, 10). Since several muscles related to the knee joint originate in the lumbopelvic region, the core of the body could be considered an important contributor to the prevention of **anterior cruciate ligament (ACL)** injuries (58). In fact, several studies provide evidence that using instability devices may reduce the likelihood of ACL injuries (58), especially after rehabilitation from an ACL injury (59). For example, Fitzgerald and colleagues (28) reported that activities that challenge the rehabilitating athlete using perturbations stimulated by tilt boards, roller boards, and other balance devices make a successful return to competitive sport activities five times more likely. Additionally, Caraffa and colleagues (18) suggest that the addition of balance training to traditional training methods results in a reduction of ACL injuries in amateur soccer players. However, in a systematic review, Grimm and coworkers (31) contest this contention and suggest that these types of interventions do not reduce ACL injury risk. In contrast, ground-based free weight activities seem to have a more balanced effect leading to improvements in performance while increasing core strength and balance abilities. Ultimately, the use of instability-based exercises to train the core seems to be an effective method for returning the injured athlete to competitive-based training.

Variable-Resistance Training Methods

Resistance training practices include three methods for applying overload to the body: **constant external**, **accommodating**, and **variable resistance** (30, 54). The most common method for applying resistance during training is to use a constant external load, which is best represented by traditional resistance training methods (e.g., free weights). In this scenario, the external load remains constant throughout the range of motion, better represents real-life activities, and allows for a more realistic skeletal muscle coordination and movement pattern (36, 54, 63). On the other hand, accommodating resistance (sometimes referred to as *semi-isokinetic resistance applications*) generally allows for the speed of movement or isokinetic resistance to be controlled throughout a range of motion (54, 75). Stone and coworkers (75) suggest that these types of devices have poor external validity. Additionally, these devices are unlikely to provide an adequate training stimulus when compared to more traditional methods such as those involving constant-loaded free weight movements, particularly when those movements are performed with multijoint movement patterns.

With traditional resistance training exercise, the external load remains constant, but the forces exerted by the muscle vary in accordance with the mechanical advantages associated with the joints involved in the movement (3, 13, 30). In order to combat the changing mechanical advantages and inertial properties associated with constant-loaded resistance, there has been a concerted effort to develop innovative training devices that allow the applied resistance to be varied in conjunction with changes in joint angle (30). These variable-resistance methods attempt to alter the resistance so the muscle maximizes force application throughout the full range of motion (29). For example, in the back squat the greatest muscle force production occurs at the midpoint of the movement, while the smallest forces are produced at the bottom. Thus variable-resistance methods would be used to reduce resistance at the bottom of the squatting motion and increase resistance as the athlete ascends from the bottom position. Another consideration is that during the concentric effort of a movement, a large portion of time is spent decelerating (30). Overall it has been suggested that variable-resistance methods may be able to match the changes in joint leverage (85), overcome the mechanical disadvantages associated with specific joint angles (24, 69, 70, 79), and provide for compensatory acceleration (69, 70).

With the use of a variable-loaded resistance model, the methodology most commonly seen in modern strength and conditioning facilities is the application of chains or rubber bands (30, 54). The combination of chains or bands with traditional free weight resistance training methods has been shown to alter the loading profile typically seen during these constant-loaded activities (30, 41). Specifically, the chains or bands allow for the resistance to be varied across the range of motion achieved during the activity.

> ► **With use of a variable-loaded resistance model, the most common methodology used in modern strength and conditioning facilities is application of chains or rubber bands (30, 54).**

Chain-Supplemented Exercises

One increasingly popular method of applying variable resistance is the addition of **chains** to traditional resistance training activities such as the bench press or back squat (4, 13, 39, 54). This method of force application is most popular among powerlifters (69, 70), but has become increasingly popular among strength and conditioning professionals working with a variety of sports (22). Despite the increasing popularity and the belief that these methods provide a training advantage, these beliefs are largely unsubstantiated in the scientific literature (13, 14, 39, 54). Some studies, however, demonstrate that the application of chains to traditional resistance training

Determining the Load to Use With Chains

To determine the load used with chains, the absolute chain resistance at the top and that at the bottom portion of the movement are summed and then averaged. For example, if athletes wanted to train at a 5-repetition maximum (5RM) load in the bench press, they would first determine the 5RM load without the chains. Then, if their 5RM is 120 kg (264 pounds), they would subtract the average chain resistance from this load. If at the bottom position the load is 0 kg and at the top the chain load is 11.1 kg (24.4 pounds), the average is 5.55 kg (12.2 pounds). Thus, the athlete would add 114 to 115 kg (251.8-253.0 pounds) to the barbell to achieve the appropriate loading.

methods such as the bench press can be advantageous (6). Careful inspection of these studies reveals that the means by which the chains are applied to the free weight exercise may influence their effectiveness. Specifically, these studies used a method in which the chain was suspended from the bar without touching the floor until the athlete had reached the lowest position in the squat or until the bar had reached chest height in the bench press (6). While some research seems to support this methodology, much more research is needed to explore the various methods of applying chains to traditional resistance training methods.

Determining Resistance With Chains

The resistance provided by chains is largely dictated by the structure, density, length, and diameter of the chain and must be quantified before the chain is used in a resistance training setting. Additionally, the number of links in a chain will affect the amount of resistance provided by the chain (13, 55). To quantify the loading provided by chains, Berning and colleagues (13) developed a practical chart that related chain link diameter and length to the resistance load provided by the chain. This chart was later modified by McMaster and colleagues (54) to show the relationship between the chain mass, length, and diameter (table 16.1).

As a means of deciding on the barbell resistance to use in conjunction with chains, the absolute load is determined for the top and the bottom portion of the

movement (4). The average of these two loads is then calculated and used to modify the barbell load in order to allow the athlete to train in the prescribed range.

As a general rule, Baker (4) recommends that the use of chains be reserved for experienced intermediate- and elite-level athletes who have stable exercise technique, as the addition of chains provides a loading challenge that can affect the athlete's technique.

Applying Chains to Free Weight Exercises

Generally, the application of chains to traditional resistance training methods allows for a linear increase in the applied resistance (54). Ways to apply chains include letting them touch the floor from the fully extended position during the movement (13) or hanging them from lighter chains (figure 16.1), which allows them to touch the floor only upon reaching the lowest portion (figure 16.2) of the movement pattern (i.e., bottom of the squat or at chest level during the bench press) (4, 6). Baker (4) suggests that the second method may affect the velocity of movement in three distinct ways. Firstly, the total barbell–chain complex comes into play only at the top of the movement (i.e., extend portion) when the chain links have been lifted off the floor. At the bottom of the movement, the links are in full contact with the floor, providing a reduction in load and allowing the athlete to accelerate the barbell at a faster rate. Secondly, it is possible that a within-repetition postactivation potentiation effect may occur in response to a greater

TABLE 16.1   Mass, Length, and Diameter of Chains

Chain diameters	Chain lengths				
	10 cm (4 in.)	50 cm (20 in.)	100 cm (40 in.)	150 cm (59 in.)	200 cm (79 in.)
6.4 mm (1/4 in.)	0.3 kg (0.6 lb)	1.3 kg (2.8 lb)	2.5 kg (5.5 lb)	3.8 kg (8.3 lb)	5.0 kg (11.0 lb)
9.5 mm (3/8 in.)	0.4 kg (0.8 lb)	1.9 kg (4.1 lb)	3.7 kg (8.1 lb)	5.6 kg (12.2 lb)	7.4 kg (16.3 lb)
12.7 mm (1/2 in.)	0.7 kg (1.6 lb)	3.7 kg (8.1 lb)	7.4 kg (16.3 lb)	11.1 kg (24.4 lb)	14.8 kg (32.6 lb)
19.1 mm (3/4 in.)	1.4 kg (3.1 lb)	7.0 kg (15.4 lb)	14.0 kg (30.8 lb)	21.0 kg (46.2 lb)	28.0 kg (61.6 lb)
22.2 mm (7/8 in.)	2.2 kg (4.8 lb)	10.8 kg (23.8 lb)	21.6 kg (47.5 lb)	32.4 kg (71.3 lb)	43.2 kg (95.0 lb)
25.4 mm (1 in.)	2.8 kg (6.2 lb)	14.0 kg (30.8 lb)	28.0 kg (61.6 lb)	42.0 kg (92.4 lb)	56.0 kg (123.0 lb)

Adapted, by permission, from McMaster, Cronin, and McGuigan, 2009 (54).

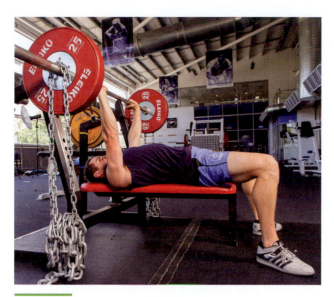

FIGURE 16.1 Bench press with added chain resistance. The links of the chains are draped over the lighter supporting chains, such that the chain does not contact the floor until the barbell reaches chest height. As the athlete lowers the barbell to the chest, the resistance progressively decreases as the chains furl onto the floor. Conversely, as the athlete moves the barbell concentrically away from the chest, the resistance progressively increases as the chains unfurl from the floor.

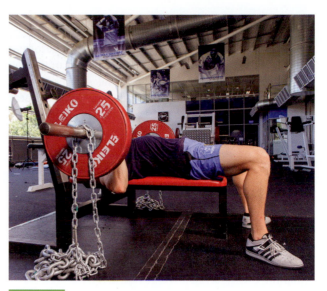

FIGURE 16.2 When the barbell is at chest height during the bench press, the chains are furled on the floor, with the result that their weight does not act on the barbell.

neural activation. Specifically, when the chains pile on the floor and the mass of the barbell decreases, a greater neuromuscular activation may occur, allowing for an enhancement in movement velocity. Finally, it is possible that the decreasing resistance at the bottom portion of the movement may cause a more rapid stretch–shortening cycle. Baker (4) suggests that this happens in response to the eccentric unloading that occurs when the chain links pile on the floor at the bottom of the movement and a quicker amortization phase occurs when the athlete shifts from eccentric to concentric muscle action.

Resistance Band Exercises

The use of **resistance bands** to augment traditional barbell resistances has become increasingly popular among strength and conditioning professionals (4, 27, 46, 77). There is some research support for the use of resistance bands combined with traditional resistance training exercises (1, 74, 79). For example, Wallace and coworkers (79) suggest that using bands to substitute 35% of the total load during a back squat can acutely increase peak power by approximately 13%. Additionally, Baker and Newton (5) suggest that the use of bands may result in a postactivation potentiation effect within each repetition. Support for this contention comes from the work of Stevenson and colleagues (74), who demonstrated that the use of bands to account for 20% of the training load

resulted in an acute increase in the concentric rate of force development when compared to a constant-loaded condition. While these data seem to suggest that the addition of bands to traditional resistance training methods may offer some benefit, especially to power or rate of force development, there is research contesting these findings (24, 41). For example, Ebben and Jensen (24) report no differences in integrated electromyography and mean ground reaction forces when resistance bands are used to apply 10% of the total loading during squats.

Currently, minimal research on the use of resistance bands, especially longitudinal studies, has been conducted to determine whether the acute effects noted by some authors translate into superior strength and power gains over time. More research is also needed to determine the optimal methodologies for using bands in the development of athletes.

Determining Resistance With Resistance Bands

In working with resistance bands, it is important to understand that their composition varies depending on the type of thermoplastic or elastomer used to produce them (54). The composition of resistance bands is important because it can exert an impact on their overall stiffness, density, yield, and tensile strength (54, 55, 77). Ultimately the tension (resistance) generated by a resistance band is determined by the overall stiffness of the band and the extent to which the band is stretched (deformation) (55). Specifically, based on Hooke's law, the tension generated by a band is equal to its stiffness (k) multiplied by the deformation (d):

$$\text{Tension} = \text{Stiffness } (k) \times \text{Deformation } (d)$$

As the band is stretched (i.e., increased deformation), there is a linear increase in the amount of tension placed on the band. However, several studies suggest that resistance bands exhibit both curvilinear and linear deformation regions (1, 55, 62).

When using bands in conjunction with traditional free weight training exercises such as the bench press or back squat, the strength and conditioning professional must be aware that there can be a 3.2% to 5.2% difference between two supposedly equal bands that could result in an 8% to 19% difference in mean tension between the bands (55). A basic length–tension relationship can be seen in table 16.2, and tension can be predicted based on the length of the band with the use of a prediction equation.

Similar to how resistance is applied with the use of chains, the use of bands requires the coach to determine how much load is provided by the free weight and how much is provided from the bands throughout the range of movement (4). Specifically, the coach must determine the load of the band at the bottom and top portions of the movement and create an average of these two loads. Based on the recommendations of Baker (4), an athlete who wants to train at a 5RM load of 150 kg (330 pounds) with bands would subtract the average of the two band positions (i.e., top and bottom) and reduce the load on the bar by that amount. So if the band exerts a zero resistance load at the bottom of the movement and a load of 26.6 kg (58.5 pounds) at the top position (i.e., lockout in the bench press), based on the length of the band achieved as it is stretched, the athlete would subtract 13.3 kg (29.2 pounds) from the total weight on the bar without the bands to get 136 to 137 kg (299.2-301.4 pounds).

Applying Resistance Bands to Free Weight Exercises

To apply bands to free weight resistance exercises, one can use a multitude of methods. The band may be attached to the barbell and either a customized attachment point on a squat rack or heavily weighted dumbbells (4). When the bands are applied, the highest tension and the total resistance load are provided to the athlete at the top position. Conversely, at the bottom position the applied load is reduced, as the bands will no longer be stretched and thus no longer apply resistance to the barbell. For example, in the squat at the lowest point (i.e., bottom position, figure 16.3), the bands are slack and do not actively create tension on the barbell, thus adding no additional resistance to the exercise. As the athlete ascends from the bottom position and approaches the lockout position, the bands will impart a larger stretch resistance and the athlete will experience the full load of both the bar and the bands (figure 16.4). It is important to note that as the athlete ascends from the bottom position the stretch load gradually increases. Conversely, as the athlete descends, the stretch load gradually decreases.

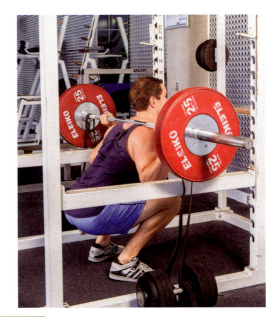

FIGURE 16.3   Bottom position of a squat performed with bands.

TABLE 16.2   Examples of Resistance Band Tension–Length Relationships

Width (mm)	Color	Length–tension relationships					Tension prediction equation
		110 cm (43.3 in.)	120 cm (47.2 in.)	130 cm (51.2 in.)	140 cm (55.1 in.)	150 cm (59.1 in.)	
14	Yellow	2.6 kg	5.7 kg	8.1 kg	9.8 kg	11.5 kg	$Y = -0.003x^2 + 0.98x - 69.82$
22	Red	4.6 kg	9.6 kg	13.3 kg	16.6 kg	19.2 kg	$Y = -0.004x^2 + 1.38x - 99.49$
32	Blue	8.5 kg	14.8 kg	19.5 kg	23.9 kg	27.3 kg	$Y = -0.004x^2 + 1.60x - 114.86$
48	Green	6.8 kg	16.5 kg	24.0 kg	30.0 kg	49.3 kg	$Y = -0.007x^2 + 2.43x - 179.56$
67	Black	15.4 kg	29.1 kg	40.0 kg	49.3 kg	57.2 kg	$Y = -0.010x^2 + 3.73x - 269.21$

Adapted, by permission, from: McMaster, Cronin, and McGuigan, 2010 (55).

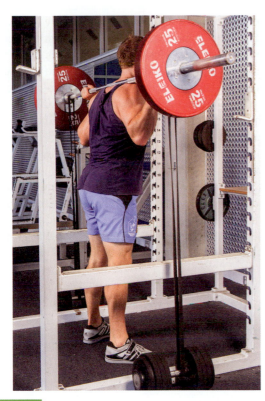

FIGURE 16.4   Top position of a squat performed with bands.

Nontraditional Implement Training Methods

Traditionally, resistance training interventions used in most modern strength and conditioning facilities have relied heavily on barbells, dumbbells, and various resistance training machines. More recently, strength and conditioning professionals have begun to incorporate nontraditional implements in order to add greater variation to the preparation of athletes. Nontraditional implements can include items that are typically associated with **strongman training** such as tires, logs, kettlebells, stones, weighted sleds, and other weighted implements (39). While nontraditional implement training is increasing in popularity, there is currently relatively little research directly exploring the efficacy of these types of training methods.

> While nontraditional implement training is increasing in popularity, there is currently relatively little research directly exploring the efficacy of these types of training methods.

Strongman Training

Strongman implement training has recently seen an increase in popularity as a proposed tool for enhancing sport performance (11, 53, 66, 80, 84, 86). Some of the most common strongman exercises are tire flipping, log (or keg) lifting, and farmer's walks. While research on these types of exercises is limited, some evidence suggests that they can be used to introduce a high-intensity stimulus resulting in an elevated blood lactate response (12, 44, 86). Additionally, it has been suggested that these types of exercises create a greater degree of instability that effectively challenges the athlete in different ways compared to traditional resistance training activities (53).

Tire Flipping

Tire flipping typically employs truck or heavy-equipment tires that can be modified via placement of an extra load in the center to address individual strength needs (39, 80). The selection of the appropriate tire size is dependent on numerous factors that the strength and conditioning professional must consider when designing a specific program for an athlete. Thought must be given to the tire's dimensions, including the height, width, and weight (16). As a general rule, the tire should not be taller than the athlete's upright standing height: The taller the tire, the harder it is for the athlete to flip because of the mechanical disadvantage and the greater overall lifting distance required. Additionally, the width of the tire can affect the athlete's ability to perform the flip. For example, narrow tires are generally considered harder to flip for taller athletes because of the limb length and depth requirements. Conversely, wider tires are more difficult for shorter athletes because of their shorter arm lengths (16). Another consideration is the tread on the tire; worn treads are more difficult to grip, and pronounced treads potentially contain cuts, debris, or exposed metal that could put the athlete at risk for injury (16, 80). Once the correct tire is selected based on the individual athlete's strength levels, appropriate exercise technique should be used to minimize risk of injury.

Three basic techniques can be used to flip tires; these include the sumo, the backlift style, and shoulders-against-the-tire technique (16, 80). The sumo-style flipping technique uses a traditional wider sumo deadlift stance coupled with the arms positioned in a narrower grip. This type of technique is typically used by powerlifters when deadlifting. With this technique, once the tire has been raised to hip or chest height, the hands are rotated so that a forward pressing action can be performed with the arms to flip the tire (16, 80). The backlift style is performed with a narrower, more conventional deadlift stance, ending with a forward pressing motion. This technique is initiated with feet placed in a hip-width stance, plus bending at the knees and hips, allowing the athlete to grab the base of the tire and pull in a fashion similar to that with a deadlift (80). As the tire is raised, the hands are repositioned so that a forward press can be used to flip the tire (16).

Currently no research has directly explored the overall safety of either tire-flipping techniques. However, some authors suggest that the sumo style is the safest, while more recently shoulders-against-the-tire has become the preferred technique in the practical literature (16). The tire lies on its side, and the athlete addresses the tire by kneeling behind it. The feet are placed in a hip-width position with the ankles dorsiflexed. In this position the athlete places the chin and shoulders onto the tire. This placement of the tire on the shoulders is similar to that seen in a traditional barbell front squat (see chapter 15). The tire is gripped with a supinated grip with a width that is largely dependent upon the size of the tire (i.e., wider tire = narrower grip). In this position, the athlete continues to dorsiflex the ankles so that he or she is on the balls of the feet while raising the knees from the ground. At this point the athlete's center of gravity should transition toward the tire, placing the majority of the athlete's body weight onto the tire. The athlete then raises the chest and contracts the musculature of the lower back (16) (see the photo of the starting position in the exercise technique section near the end of the chapter).

Next, the athlete initiates the flipping movement by extending the knees and hips followed by plantar flexing

Tire Flipping

Technique

Points to remember:

- Select a surface that is acceptable for tire flipping.
- While kneeling behind the tire, place the chin and anterior deltoid on the tire.
- Use a supinated grip with the arms extended but not locked out to grip the tire.
- Dorsiflex the ankles and raise the knees off the ground in order to get onto the balls of the feet.
- Raise the chest and contract the lower back musculature.

The movement technique:

- Extend the knees and hips and plantar flex the ankles while pushing the tire forward and up.
- Move forward explosively toward the tire by taking two or three steps.
- Flex one hip and forcefully strike the tire with the quadriceps of that leg.
- Immediately after striking the tire, reorient the hands into a pronated grip.
- Move the feet forward while extending the arms in order to flip the tire.

Common Technical Flaws and Their Corrections

- *Flaw: Placing the feet too close to the tire when initiating the movement.* When this occurs, athletes often have to round their back and position their knees close to their chest in order to initiate the movement. *Correction:* Have athletes move their feet away from the tire and instruct them to raise their chest while contracting the musculature of the lower back.
- *Flaw: Hips rise faster than the shoulders during the initial pushing motion.* This flaw is very similar to what can be seen during traditional deadlifting with incorrect technique. *Correction:* Instruct athletes to keep their hips low and drive the tire forward rather than lifting it. Additionally, encourage athletes to keep the hips slightly below the shoulders during this movement.
- *Flaw: A lifting motion is used instead of a pushing motion.* With heavier tires, this motion reduces the lifting speed; the tire will lose momentum as it is elevated to hip height, forcing the athlete to "muscle" the tire over. This is an extremely dangerous position, as the tire can easily fall onto the athlete, and should be corrected immediately. *Correction:* The athlete should be encouraged to drive the tire forward and move forward with the tire as it is elevated. One cue is to strike the tire with the quadriceps at hip height and continue a forward movement pattern.

Spotting the Tire Flip

In general, spotting the tire flip requires two spotters who are positioned on either side of the athlete. Spotters should do the following:

- Assist the athlete by pushing on the tire when needed.
- Pay close attention to ensure they can assist if the athlete loses grip on the tire.
- Be aware of the area around the athlete; in particular, the landing area needs to be monitored to ensure that the flipping path is clear of people and apparatus.

Adapted, by permission, from J.B. Bullock and D.M.M. Aipa, 2010, "Coaching considerations for the tire flip," *Strength & Conditioning Journal* 32: 75-78.

the ankles in order to push the tire forward and up. As this occurs, the shoulders and hips should rise at the same rate, ending in a triple extension, from which the athlete moves forward by taking two or three small steps. Once the tire reaches hip height, the athlete forcefully flexes the hip of one leg and strikes the tire with the quadriceps. The striking of the tire with the leg allows achievement of a forceful upward momentum (16). As this occurs, the athlete switches the hands into a pronated position. After reorienting the hands, the athlete runs the feet toward the tire while forcefully extending the arms to push the tire over. Photos of all of these positions can be found in the exercise technique section near the end of the chapter.

Log Lifting

One of the classic exercises that is a part of strongman training is the log lift, which is essentially a version of the clean. Other traditional lifting movements can also be performed with logs, such as cleans, presses, jerks, rows, squats, deadlifts, and lunges (39, 64, 83). **Logs** are typically designed to have weight added to them while offering a midrange grip support to accommodate a pronated grip position (64). Weight is typically added with the use of traditional plates, which eliminates the need for having a variety of logs (39). Information on how to effectively load log-based exercises is limited, but training loads may be based on traditional exercises. For example, Winwood and colleagues (83) used 70% of a 1RM for a traditional clean and jerk with log training. While the connection seems logical, it is likely that athletes will not be able to lift the same load as they could in the comparable traditional exercise because of the mechanical difficulties associated with lifting the log apparatus (39).

In another type of log, water can be used to provide the resistance (39, 64). Ratamess (64) suggests that with this type of log, the fluid inside will move, resulting in an increased activation of the stabilizer muscles. While this may seem logical, no scientific papers appear to have explored this contention.

While log-based training seems to be increasing in popularity, little research has explored the effectiveness of this training method or how best to apply this type of training in the preparation of athletes in various sports. Therefore, significantly more scientific inquiry is required to provide true understanding of the efficacy of log-based training.

Farmer's Walk

Another commonly used strongman exercise is the **farmer's walk**, in which the athlete holds a load at the sides in each hand while walking forward (53, 80). Winwood and colleagues (83) suggest that exercises such as the farmer's walk are useful training tools because they involve unstable and awkward resistances that have both unilateral and bilateral motions. Additionally, it has been suggested that the farmer's walk develops total body anaerobic endurance, back endurance, and grip strength (80). McGill and colleagues (53) suggest that the farmer's walk may enhance traditional resistance training programs because this exercise challenges body linkages and stabilizing systems in a different way than traditional resistance training. The farmer's walk can be performed with static loads (e.g., a heavy dumbbell) or variable loads (e.g., water-filled objects) (80). Regardless of the type load used, it appears that the farmer's walk offers a unique activation pattern of the core, although there is very limited research in the scientific literature supporting the use of this exercise as a strength and conditioning tool. Additionally, no available research has examined the safety of the farmer's walk, which makes it difficult to recommend safety precautions. Thus athletes should follow generally accepted safety principles and precautions: Only advanced athletes who possess high levels of strength should attempt this exercise. While this training modality may be popular in strength and conditioning environments, more research is required in order to determine its efficacy.

Kettlebell Training

Recently, strength and conditioning professionals have become interested in the use of **kettlebell** exercises (7, 17, 48). While seemingly a new phenomenon, the use of kettlebells dates back hundreds of years to when they were a popular training method in various Eastern Bloc countries (38). The word *kettlebell* comes from the Russian word *girya,* which refers to a cast iron cannonball with a handle on it (20). In Western literature the term *kettlebell* is used to refer to a weighted implement consisting of a ball with a handle, which is probably better termed a *kettleball* (20).

Along with the increasing interest in the use of kettlebell training has been an increase in the amount of scientific inquiry into the efficacy of using these implements with athletes and general populations. The majority of the scientific evidence supporting the use of kettlebells highlights their potential usefulness as a tool for general physical or fitness development (26, 40, 76). In these studies the most common exercise employed is the kettlebell swing, which can be performed with either one or two hands (40, 52, 76). While kettlebell swings appear to have a positive impact on cardiovascular fitness, it is important to note that this activity does not offer the same level of cardiovascular benefit as treadmill running or more traditional aerobic exercise (40).

Currently, limited research explores the efficacy of kettlebell training as a strength development tool. When used with clinical and recreationally trained populations,

Competition Kettlebell Dimensions

Following are the dimensions of competition kettlebells (20):

- Height: 228 mm (8.5 inches)
- Diameter: 210 mm (8.25 inches)
- Handle diameter: 35 mm (1.4 inches)

kettlebell training has been reported to increase muscular strength levels compared to no training (43, 61). Additionally, when a battery of kettlebell exercises (i.e., swings, goblet squats, accelerated swings) is performed across a six-week training intervention, there appears to be an increase in muscular strength and vertical jump performance in recreationally trained men (61). However, these strength gains are significantly lower than those typically seen with traditional weightlifting-based training methods. Specifically, Otto and colleagues (61) reported that six weeks of weightlifting training resulted in a 4% increase in vertical jump performance, while kettlebell swings increased jumping performance by only 0.8%. Additionally, back squat strength was increased by 13.6% after six weeks of traditional weightlifting training, while the kettlebell training resulted in only a 4.5% increase (61).

Based on the contemporary body of scientific knowledge, it appears that kettlebells are probably best used as general preparation exercise and that more traditional training methods such as weightlifting are more effective for developing maximal strength and jumping performance capacity. However, further scientific research is needed to develop a better understanding of the role that kettlebells may be able to play in the development of athletes.

Types of Kettlebells

When working with kettlebells, one must consider the type of kettlebell, as there are two major types: the cast iron (figure 16.5) and the sport kettlebell (figure 16.6) (20). The cast iron, or fitness, kettlebells are cast from iron and range in size depending on their weight. The

sport or competition kettlebells are made from steel and have universal design and measurements. Specifically, the size of the kettlebell does not change regardless of the weight, and the various weights are indicated by different colors (20). Besides the structural differences in the size and dimensions of the cast iron and sport kettlebell, the other difference is that the cast iron kettlebell is less expensive and probably more prevalent in strength and conditioning facilities.

Considerations for Selecting Kettlebells

The first major consideration in the selection of a kettlebell is the type of load provided. The two basic types of kettlebells are the fixed and the adjustable (20). With fixed-loaded kettlebells, such as cast iron or competition kettlebells, the load stays constant; thus a set of kettlebells, which range across several loads, is required in order to provide training variety. Adjustable kettlebells are either plate loaded or shot loaded. In actuality, a plate-loaded kettlebell is simply a handle that is attached to weight plates and is not really a kettlebell even though it is classified as one (20). In contrast, a shot-loaded kettlebell is a hollow version of the more traditional kettlebell. Historically, these kettlebells were filled with sand, water, lead, and even mercury (20). If this type of kettlebell is only partially filled, the shot moves around in the ball, causing an increased training stressor. While popular in the early 20th century, especially with circus strongmen such as the famous Arthur Saxon and Eugen Sandow, this type of kettlebell is not popular in contemporary strength and conditioning.

The second consideration relates to the handle, as it is the major interface between the athlete and the kettlebell.

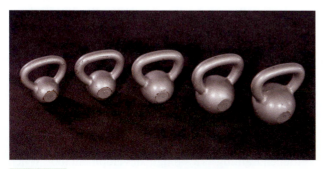

FIGURE 16.5 Cast iron class kettlebells.

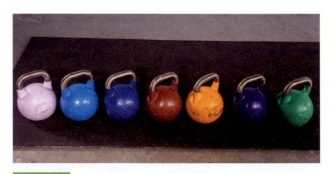

FIGURE 16.6 Competition kettlebells.

With cast iron kettlebells, the handle diameter changes slightly as the weight increases. For example a 20 kg (45 pounds) or heavier kettlebell has a handle between 33 (1.3 inches) and 35 (1.4 inches) mm; a smaller kettlebell may have a smaller handle diameter. Additionally, to facilitate the types of exercises that use kettlebells, the spacing between the handle and the top of the ball is standardized in good kettlebells. Typically, the space between the bottom of the handle and the top of the ball is 55 mm (2.2 inches), and the length of the handle is 186 mm (7.3 inches) (20). With regard to handle surface, some kettlebells come with smooth painted handles; others have polished steel handles, which have no paint and are basically bare medal. The polished steel handle tends to allow for a better grip because it holds chalk better and does not get as slippery as painted or polished handles do when athletes sweat on them (20).

Unilateral Training

When employing training methods, one can use unilateral or bilateral training interventions. These types of training methods can be performed with the upper body or lower body, depending on the targeted outcomes. Common lower body unilateral training exercises include lunges, step-ups, and the single-leg squat, which is sometimes referred to as the Bulgarian split squat. This exercise isolates one leg and is typically used in the preparation of athletes from numerous sports. Typically these types of exercises are integrated into training programs with varying degrees of emphasis (50) in an attempt to reduce **bilateral asymmetries** (45) or as a rehabilitation tool (25). They are often used to reduce a **bilateral deficit**, where there are asymmetries in force production between unilateral and bilateral movements (42). It has also been demonstrated that bilateral movements exhibit a **bilateral facilitation** in which there is an increase in voluntary activation of the agonist muscle group (8,

67). Trained or stronger individuals tend to exhibit a bilateral facilitation, while untrained, injured, or weaker athletes exhibit a bilateral deficit (10). Therefore, based on the bilateral facilitation response, trained individuals should not use unilateral methods for the development of strength. In contrast, unilateral training methods may be useful for strength development with untrained, weaker, and injured individuals (10).

> ▶ **Trained or stronger individuals exhibit a bilateral facilitation during bilateral exercises, while untrained, injured, or weaker individuals exhibit a bilateral deficit (10).**

Conclusion

In designing strength and conditioning interventions, one can use a variety of methods to apply overload. The use of alternative methods and nontraditional implements is increasing in popularity. When choosing to implement these methods, strength and conditioning professionals should consider the benefits and weaknesses of these types of training interventions. Additionally, the level of the athlete dictates whether use of these methods is warranted. For example, a novice athlete or untrained individual may derive a large benefit from doing bodyweight or core stability exercises. Conversely, the trained or elite athlete may experience greater gains with traditional ground-based free weight exercises. With the advanced athlete, the use of variable resistance may also allow for a greater training stimulus to be applied to traditional training methods. If choosing to employ alternative methods or nontraditional element–based training methods, strength and conditioning professionals must always ensure that they teach proper exercise techniques as well as constantly monitor their athletes in order to ensure that a safe training environment is maintained.

MODES AND NONTRADITIONAL EXERCISES

16.1   FRONT PLANK

Starting Position

- Kneel in a prone, quadruped position on the floor. The feet should be hip-width apart or slightly closer with the palms of the hands flat on the floor shoulder-width apart and the elbows pointing backward.
- Drop the elbows to the floor and position them directly under the shoulders.
- Move the feet back one at a time to allow the hips and knees to extend so the abdomen and the front of the hips and legs rest on the floor.

Ending Position

- Elevate the hips so the ankles, knees, hips, shoulders, and head are in a straight line.
- Isometrically hold the torso in a rigid position with the elbows under the shoulders and the head in a neutral position.

MAJOR MUSCLES INVOLVED

rectus abdominis, internal obliques, external obliques, erector spinae

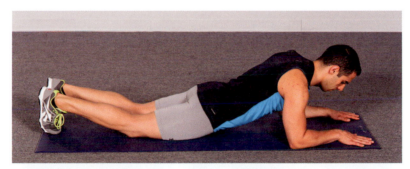

Starting position

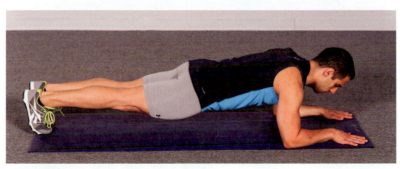

Ending position

16.2   SIDE PLANK

Starting Position

- Lie on the floor on the left side.
- Position the left elbow underneath the left shoulder with the left forearm perpendicular to the body.
- Stack the right foot on top of the left foot with the right leg evenly on top of the left leg or place the right foot on the floor immediately in front of the left foot. Also, stack the right arm evenly on top of the right side of the torso.
- Position the head in a neutral position with the eyes focused forward.

Ending Position

- Elevate the hips off the floor so the left ankle, knee, hip, and shoulder are in a straight line.
- Isometrically hold the torso in a rigid position with the left elbow under the left shoulder and the head in a neutral position.
- Switch and repeat the procedure for the right side.

MAJOR MUSCLES INVOLVED

internal obliques, external obliques

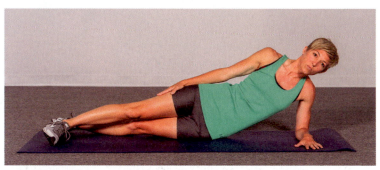

Starting position

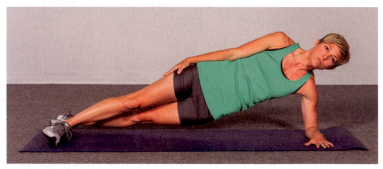

Ending position

16.3   STABILITY BALL ROLLOUT

Starting Position

- Kneel facing the stability ball with the upper body in an upright position, arms extended, and the hands touching the ball.
- While keeping the hands on the ball, create a 90-degree angle at the knees and ankles with the knees, hips, and shoulders in a near-vertical plane.

Ending Position

- Keep the knees and toes on the floor, elbows fully extended, arms parallel to each other, and knees, hips, and shoulders in a straight line. Extend the knees and flex the shoulders to roll the ball forward and the arms across the top of the ball until it comes very close to the face.
- Isometrically hold the torso in a rigid position; do not let the hips sag toward the floor.

MAJOR MUSCLES INVOLVED

rectus abdominis, iliopsoas

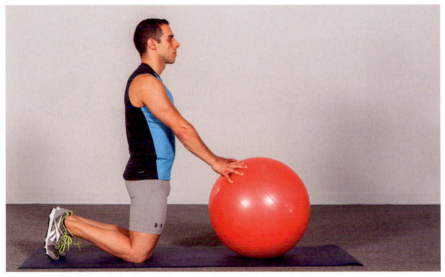

Starting position

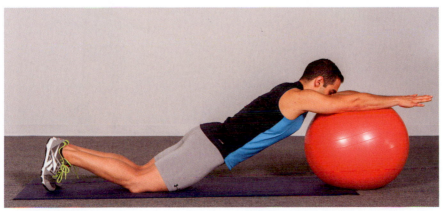

Ending position

16.4 STABILITY BALL PIKE

Starting Position

- Kneel down in front of a stability ball.
- Position the body facing away from the ball.
- In a quadruped position with the hands underneath the shoulders and the knees underneath the hips, place both feet on the stability ball.
- Isometrically hold the torso in a rigid position with the elbows fully extended and the head in a neutral position.
- All repetitions begin from this position.

Upward Movement Phase

- Keeping the knees and elbows fully extended and the torso in a rigid position, begin the exercise by flexing the hips to roll the ball toward the chest.
- Continue lifting the hips until the toes are on top of the ball and the hips are directly over the shoulders.
- Keep the head in a neutral position.

Downward Movement Phase

- Return to the starting position by allowing the hips to extend under control.
- Keep the knees and elbows fully extended and the torso held rigid.

MAJOR MUSCLES INVOLVED

rectus abdominis, iliopsoas

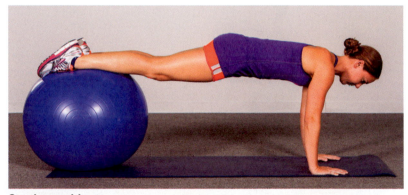

Starting position

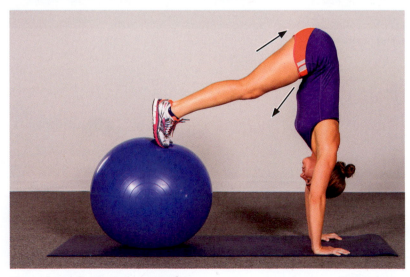

Upward and downward movements

16.5 STABILITY BALL JACKKNIFE

Starting Position

- Kneel down in front of a stability ball.
- Position the body facing away from the ball.
- In a quadruped position with the hands underneath the shoulders and the knees underneath the hips, place both feet on the stability ball.
- Isometrically hold the torso in a rigid position with the elbows fully extended and the head in a neutral position.
- All repetitions begin from this position.

Forward Movement Phase

- Keeping the knees and elbows fully extended and the torso in a rigid position, begin the exercise by raising the hips slightly and flexing the hips and knees to roll the ball toward the chest.
- Continue rolling the ball forward until the hips and knees are fully flexed.
- Keep the shoulders over the hands and the head in a neutral position.

Backward Movement Phase

- Return to the starting position by allowing the hips and knees to extend under control.
- Keep the elbows fully extended and the torso held rigid.

MAJOR MUSCLES INVOLVED

rectus abdominis, iliopsoas

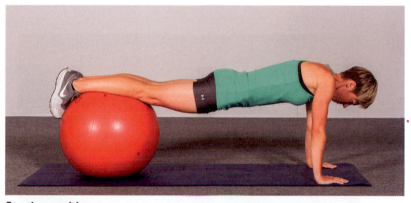

Starting position

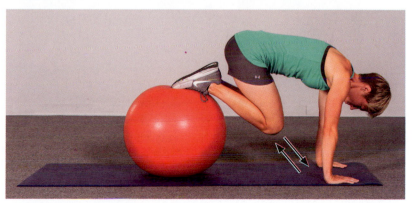

Forward and backward movements

16.6 TIRE FLIP

Starting Position

- Begin facing the tire with the feet hip- to shoulder-width apart.
- Squat down and lean into the tire so that the chin and the anterior deltoids are resting on the tire and the feet are positioned back far enough to maintain a neutral spine position.
- Keeping the arms outside the knees and the elbows fully extended, grasp the tire with a supinated grip.
- All repetitions begin from this position.

Upward Movement Phase

- Begin by extending the knees and hips and plantar flexing the ankles while pushing the tire forward.
- Move forward explosively toward the tire by taking two or three steps.
- Continue this movement until the body is aligned in a 45° angle to the tire.
- Flex the hip and knee of one leg fully to drive the knee upward and toward the tire.
- Immediately after striking the tire, reorient the hands into a pronated grip.
- While moving the feet forward, forcefully extend the arms in order to push the tire over in front of the body.

MAJOR MUSCLES INVOLVED

gluteus maximus, semimembranosus, semitendinosus, biceps femoris, vastus lateralis, vastus intermedius, vastus medialis, rectus femoris, soleus, gastrocnemius, deltoids, trapezius

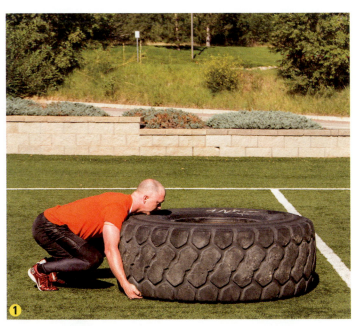

Starting position

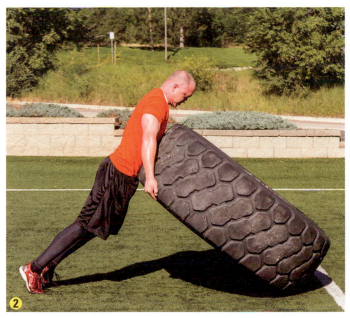

Triple extension

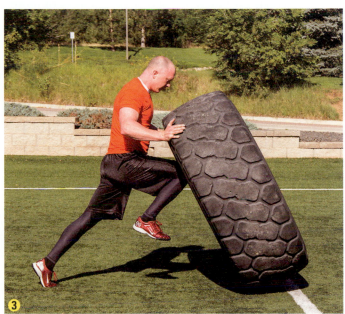

Strike position

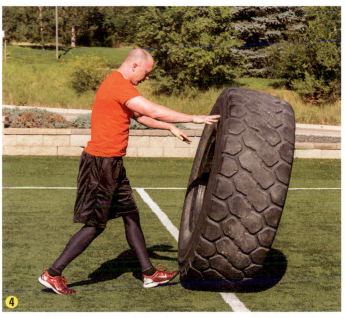

Push position

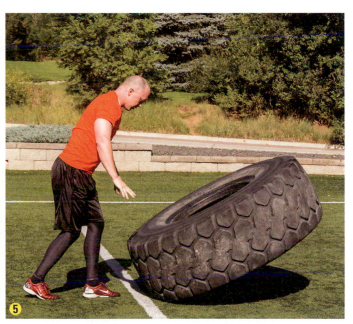

Walk forward

16.7   LOG CLEAN AND PRESS

This exercise comes from strongman training and consists of quickly and forcefully picking the log up from the ground to the front of the shoulders and then pressing it overhead. The log clean consists of three phases but occurs in two motions, with a pause of the log at the shoulders. The log can either be cleaned and pressed each rep or cleaned once and pressed for multiple repetitions.

Starting Position

- Stand with the feet placed between hip- and shoulder-width apart with the toes pointed forward or slightly outward.
- Squat down with the hips lower than the shoulders and grasp the log with a closed, neutral grip.
- Place the hands on the log handles with the arms slightly outside of the knees, with the elbows fully extended.
- Place the feet flat on the floor and position the log in front of the shins and over the balls of the feet.
- Position the body with the
  — back in a neutral spine position,
  — scapulae depressed and retracted,
  — head in line with the vertebral column, and
  — shoulders over or slightly in front of the log.
- All repetitions begin from this position.

Upward Movement Phase: First Pull

- Lift the log off the ground by extending the hips and knees.
- Keep the torso-to-floor angle constant; do not let the hips rise before the shoulders.
- Keep the elbows extended and the shoulders over or slightly ahead of the log.

Upward Movement Phase: Transition

- As the log passes the knees, pull the log into the body by flexing the knees and flexing at the elbows.
- Briefly pause in this position with the legs in a quarter-squat position and the log at or on the thighs.

Upward Movement Phase: Second Pull

- Forcefully jump upward by extending the hips and knees and plantar flexing the ankles.
- Keep the log close to the body and the elbows tucked into the body.
- When the lower body joints reach full extension, rapidly drive the elbows forward to keep rolling the log up the body.
- Because of the explosiveness of this movement, the torso is erect or slightly hyperextended, the

head is tilted slightly back, and the feet may lose contact with the floor.

Upward Movement Phase: Catch

- After the lower body has fully extended, pull the body under the log and rotate the arms around under the log.
- Simultaneously flex the hips and knees to a quarter- or half-squat position.
- Rack the log across the front of the clavicles and anterior deltoids.

Preparation Phase: Dip

- Flex the hips and knees at a slow to moderate speed to move the log in a straight path downward.
- Continue the dip to a depth not to exceed a quarter squat.
- Keep the feet flat on the floor, torso erect, and the upper arms directly under the log.

Upward Movement Phase: Drive

- Immediately upon reaching the lowest position of the dip, reverse the movement by forcefully and quickly extending the hips and knees and then the elbows to move the log overhead.

Downward Movement Phase

- Lower the log by gradually reducing the muscular tension of the arms to allow a controlled descent of the log to the shoulders.
- Simultaneously flex the hips and knees to cushion the impact of the log on the shoulders, and then return the log to the floor.

MAJOR MUSCLES INVOLVED

gluteus maximus, semimembranosus, semitendinosus, biceps femoris, vastus lateralis, vastus intermedius, vastus medialis, rectus femoris, deltoids, trapezius

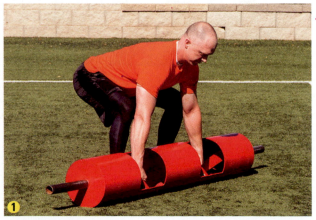

Starting position

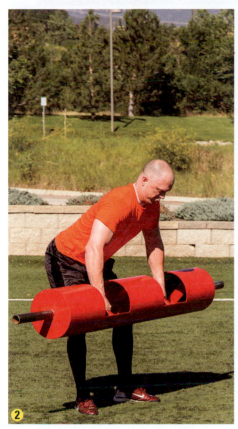

2

End of first pull/beginning of transition

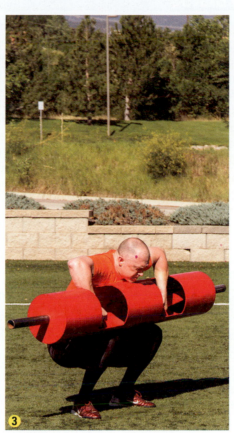

3

End of transition/beginning of second pull

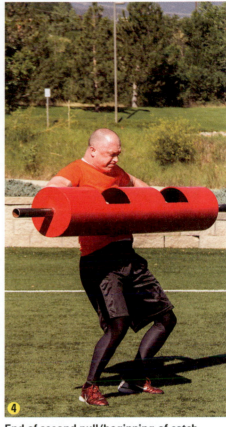

4

End of second pull/beginning of catch

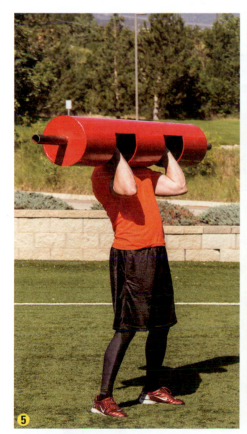

5

Catch/beginning of dip

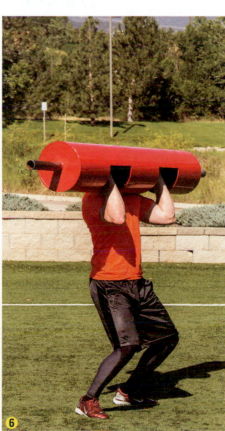

6

End of dip/beginning of drive

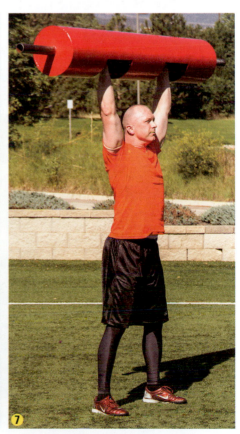

7

End of drive (final overhead position)

16.8 BACK SQUAT WITH BANDS

Band Placement

- Loop the ends of long elastic bands around the band pegs of each side of a power rack. If the rack does not have band pegs, loop the bands around the handles of heavy dumbbells that will not move during the exercise.
- Take the other ends of the bands and place them over the ends of the bar so they rest against the outside of the weight plates on either side.
- The bands should be loose enough that there is no tension at the bottom of the squat. Tension should be applied to the bar when the exercise is performed, but at the bottom of the range of motion, the bands should be slack to apply no load to the bar. (*Note:* Despite its appearance, the bands in the second photo are not creating any tension on the bar.)

Starting Position

- Grasp the bar with a closed, pronated grip.
- Step under the bar and position the feet parallel to each other.
- Place the bar in a balanced position on the upper back and shoulders; follow the guidelines for the back squat in chapter 15 regarding the high or low placement of the bar.
- Extend the hips and knees to lift the bar off the supporting pins or ledge, and take one or two steps backward.
- Position the feet shoulder-width apart or wider, even with each other, and the toes pointed slightly outward.

- Stand with an erect torso by positioning the shoulders back, tilting the head slightly back, and protruding the chest up and out to create a neutral or slightly arched back.
- All repetitions begin from this position.

Downward Movement Phase

- Begin the exercise by flexing the hips and knees slowly and under control while keeping the torso-to-floor angle relatively constant.
- Maintain a flat-foot position with the knees aligned over the feet as they flex.
- Continue flexing the hips and knees until the thighs are parallel to the floor, the torso begins to round or flex forward, or the heels begin to rise off the floor.

Upward Movement Phase

- Raise the bar by extending the hips and knees while keeping the torso-to-floor angle relatively constant.
- Keep the torso erect, shoulders back, and chest up and out.
- Keep the heels on the floor and the knees aligned over the feet.
- Continue extending the hips and knees until the body is fully erect.

MAJOR MUSCLES INVOLVED

gluteus maximus, semimembranosus, semitendinosus, biceps femoris, vastus lateralis, vastus intermedius, vastus medialis, rectus femoris

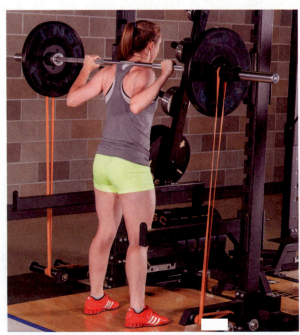

Starting position

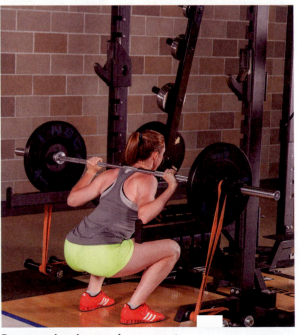

Downward and upward movements

Other Alternative Exercises

16.9 TWO-ARM KETTLEBELL SWING

Starting Position

- Stand with feet flat and placed between hip- and shoulder-width apart with the toes pointed straight ahead, straddling a kettlebell.
- Squat down with the hips lower than the shoulders and grasp the kettlebell with a closed, pronated grip.
- Place the hands on the kettlebell with index fingers touching or close together, inside of the legs, keeping the elbows fully extended.
- Position the body with the
  — back in a neutral spine position,
  — shoulders retracted and depressed,
  — feet flat on the floor, and
  — eyes focused straight ahead or slightly upward.
- Maintain a neutral spine or normal lordotic position while flexing the hips and knees to approximately a quarter-squat position, with the kettlebell hanging at arm's length between the thighs.
- All repetitions begin from this position.

Backward Movement Phase

- Begin the exercise by flexing at the hips to swing the kettlebell between the legs.
- Keep the knees in a moderately flexed position with the back neutral and the elbows extended.

- Keep swinging the kettlebell backward until the torso is nearly parallel to the floor and the kettlebell is past the vertical line of the body.

Forward/Upward Movement Phase

- When the backward swing reaches its end point, reverse the movement by extending the hips and knees to move the kettlebell in an upward arc.
- Allow momentum to raise the kettlebell to eye level, keeping the elbows extended and the back in a neutral spine position.

Downward/Backward Movement Phase

- Allow the kettlebell to drop into the downswing; flex the hips and knees to absorb the weight. Keep the elbows fully extended and the back neutral.
- Continue the downward-then-backward movement until the kettlebell passes under then behind the body, then begin the upward movement phase for the next repetition.

MAJOR MUSCLES INVOLVED

gluteus maximus, semimembranosus, semitendinosus, biceps femoris, vastus lateralis, vastus intermedius, vastus medialis, rectus femoris

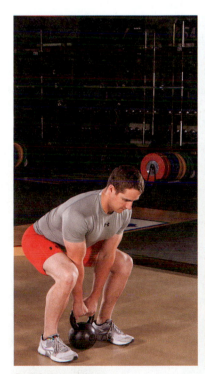

Starting position

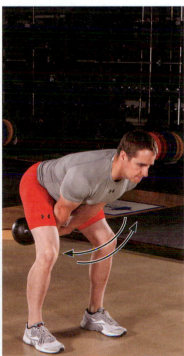

Initial backward movement and beginning of forward/upward movement

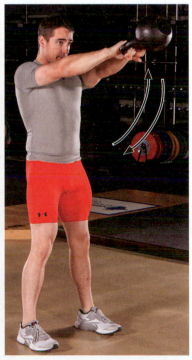

End of forward/upward movement and beginning of downward/backward movement

433

16.10 SINGLE-LEG SQUAT

Note: The single-leg squat is not typically done with a spotter. If spotting is needed, two spotters are used with one on each side of the bar. The positions of the spotters are not pictured in order to show the athlete's position at the various stages of the one-leg squat more clearly.

Starting Position: Athlete

- Grasp a barbell with a closed, pronated grip (for dumbbell variation, hold dumbbells with a closed, neutral grip with a dumbbell in each hand).
- Stand in front of a bench or box that is approximately knee-height with the feet approximately shoulder- to hip-width apart.
- Facing away from the bench or box, take a moderate step forward with one leg and place the instep of the back foot on top of the bench or box.
- Allow both knees to be slightly flexed, with the torso in a nearly erect position and the shoulders held back and chest up and out.
- All repetitions begin from this position.

Starting Position: Two Spotters

- The spotters should stand erect at opposite ends of the bar with the feet hip-width apart and the knees slightly flexed.
- Hold the hands 2 to 3 inches (5-8 cm) below the end of the bar.

Note: If dumbbells are used, no spotter is needed.

Downward Movement Phase: Athlete

- Flex the hip and knee of the forward leg simultaneously to lower the body in a vertical plane while keeping the torso-to-floor angle constant.

- Keep the heel of the forward foot flat on the floor and the instep of the back foot on top of the bench or box.
- Continue flexing the hip and knee until the front thigh is approximately parallel to the floor.

Downward Movement Phase: Two Spotters

- Keep the cupped hands close to but not touching the bar as it descends.
- Slightly flex the knees, hips, and torso to keep a neutral spine position when following the bar.

Upward Movement Phase: Athlete

- Raise the bar under control by actively extending the forward hip and knee; extend the other hip and knee also to keep the torso-to-floor angle constant.
- Maintain a neutral spine position and keep the torso upright.
- Keep the forward knee aligned over the forward foot.
- Do not flex the torso forward or round the spine.
- Continue extending the hip and knee of the forward leg to reach the starting position.
- Repeat for the desired number of repetitions and then switch the forward leg.

Upward Movement Phase: Two Spotters

- Keep cupped hands close to but not touching the bar as it ascends.
- Slightly extend the knees, hips, and torso and keep the back neutral when following the bar.

MAJOR MUSCLES INVOLVED

gluteus maximus, semimembranosus, semitendinosus, biceps femoris, vastus lateralis, vastus intermedius, vastus medialis, rectus femoris

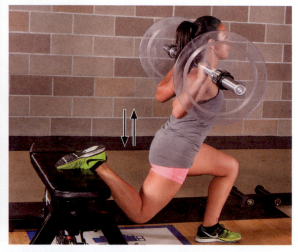

Starting position

Downward and upward movements

16.11 SINGLE-LEG ROMANIAN DEADLIFT (RDL)

Note: This exercise can be performed with the weight held in the hand of the same side of the body as the support leg (ipsilateral) or in the hand of the opposite side of the body as the support leg (contralateral). The description and the photos describe the contralateral single-leg RDL.

Starting Position

- With the right hand, grasp a dumbbell or kettlebell with a closed, pronated grip.
- Stand on the left leg (as the support leg) with the hips and shoulders over the left foot.
- Hold the dumbbell or kettlebell in front of the right thigh with the right elbow fully extended and the right foot slightly staggered back.
- All repetitions begin from this position.

Downward Movement Phase

- Allow the left support knee to flex until it reaches a moderately flexed position, and then rigidly hold that position throughout the movement.
- Begin the exercise by allowing the torso to flex forward at the hip of the left support leg.
- Keep the right shoulder, hip, knee, and ankle in one line as the torso flexes forward.
- Keep the back neutral and the right elbow still fully extended.
- Lower the dumbbell or kettlebell until the torso and right leg are approximately parallel to the floor.

Upward Movement Phase

- Extend the hip of the left support leg to return to the starting position.
- Do not hyperextend the torso or flex the elbow holding the dumbbell or kettlebell.
- Repeat for the desired number of repetitions and then switch the support leg.

MAJOR MUSCLES INVOLVED

gluteus maximus, semimembranosus, semitendinosus, biceps femoris

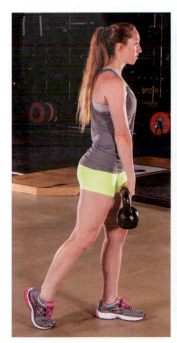

Starting position

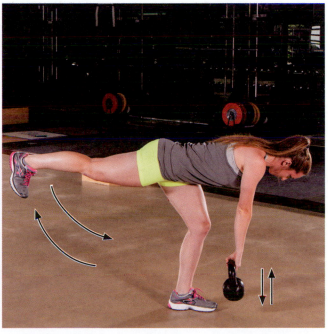

Downward and upward movements

16.12 ONE-ARM DUMBBELL SNATCH

Starting Position

- Straddle a dumbbell and place the feet between hip- and shoulder-width apart with the toes pointed slightly outward.
- Squat down with the hips lower than the shoulders; grasp the dumbbell with a closed, pronated grip with the elbow fully extended.
- Position the body with the
  — back neutral or slightly arched,
  — scapulae depressed and retracted,
  — chest held up and out,
  — head in line with the vertebral column or slightly hyperextended,
  — body's weight balanced between the middle and balls of the feet,
  — feet flat on the floor,
  — shoulders of the hand that is holding the dumbbell over or slightly in front of the dumbbell, and
  — eyes focused straight ahead or slightly upward.
- All repetitions begin from this position.

Upward Movement Phase

- Begin the exercise by extending the knees, hips, and ankles forcefully to accelerate the dumbbell.
- The dumbbell should slide up the thigh or remain very close to the thigh as it accelerates upward.
- Keep the elbow of the arm holding the dumbbell fully extended as the knees, hips, and ankles are extending.
- Once the knees, hips, and ankles reach full extension, rapidly shrug the shoulder of the arm holding the dumbbell.

- As the shoulder reaches its highest elevation, flex the elbow holding the dumbbell and keep it close to the torso.
- Keep the arm that is not holding the dumbbell on the opposite hip or held to the side.
- Continue pulling the dumbbell as high as possible.

Catch Phase

- Pull the body under the dumbbell by rotating the arm and hand holding the dumbbell around then under the dumbbell, and by flexing the hips and knees to approximately a quarter-squat position.
- Once the arm holding the dumbbell is under the dumbbell, extend the elbow quickly to push the dumbbell up and the body downward under the dumbbell.
- Catch the dumbbell in full extension at the same time the body reaches the quarter-squat position.
- Keep the arm that is not holding the dumbbell on the opposite hip or held to the side.
- After gaining control and balance, stand up to a fully erect position.

Downward Movement Phase

- Slowly allow the dumbbell to lower to the shoulder, then the thigh, and finally to the floor between the feet using a squatting movement.

MAJOR MUSCLES INVOLVED

rectus femoris, vastus medialis, vastus lateralis, vastus intermedius, gluteus maximus, semimembranosus, semitendinosus, biceps femoris, deltoids, trapezius

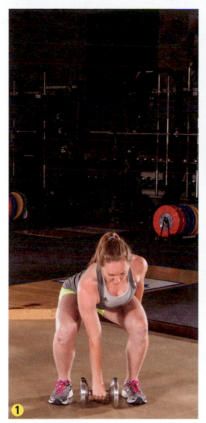

Starting position

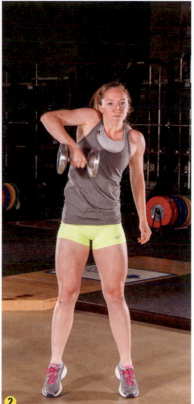

Upward movement

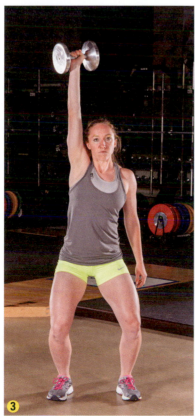

Catch

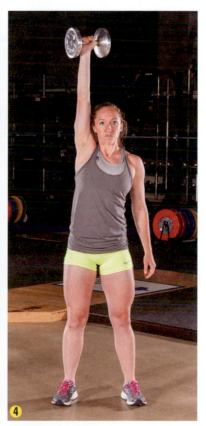

Standing position

KEY TERMS

accommodating resistance
alternative modes
anatomical core
anterior cruciate ligament (ACL)
axial skeleton
bilateral asymmetries
bilateral deficit
bilateral facilitation
bodyweight training

chains
constant external resistance
core
farmer's walk
ground-based free weight exercises
isolation exercises
kettlebells
logs

machine-based training
muscle activation
nontraditional implement
resistance band
sticking point
strongman training
Valsalva maneuver
variable resistance

STUDY QUESTIONS

1. If during the tire flip the athlete's hips rise faster than the shoulders during the initial pushing motion, what is an effective correction to give the athlete?
   a. Start with a higher hip position.
   b. Keep the hips slightly below the shoulders in this position.
   c. Lift the tire upward instead of driving it forward.
   d. Push with the arms first.

2. If a strong athlete incorporates only unilateral training into his or her program, what might the strength and conditioning professional expect to happen?
   a. A bilateral facilitation will occur.
   b. A bilateral deficit will be developed.
   c. A reduction in bilateral asymmetries will occur.
   d. Only unilateral strength will increase.

3. With regard to core training, when is instability exercise best applied?
   a. with untrained athletes who are relatively weak
   b. in trained athletes who are rehabilitating from an injury
   c. with trained athletes who are trying to optimize strength and power
   d. with untrained athletes who are new to the exercise

4. Which of the following is a rationale for using variable-resistance training methods?
   a. to accommodate the changing mechanical advantages associated with constant-loaded exercises
   b. to minimize force application throughout the full range of motion
   c. to increase the time spent decelerating during a lifting motion
   d. to keep the applied resistance constant during changes in joint angle

5. Training on instability devices can reduce the overall agonist force production capacity and power output of the athlete to less than _____ of what can be achieved in a stable condition.
   a. 20%
   b. 50%
   c. 70%
   d. 90%

CHAPTER 17

Program Design
for Resistance Training

Jeremy M. Sheppard, PhD, and N. Travis Triplett, PhD

 After completing this chapter, you will be able to

- evaluate the requirements and characteristics of a sport and assess an athlete for the purpose of designing a resistance training program;

- select exercises based on type, sport specificity, technique experience, equipment availability, and time availability;

- determine training frequency based on training status, sport season, load, exercise type, and other concurrent exercise;

- arrange exercises in a training session according to their type;

- determine 1-repetition maximum (1RM), predicted 1RM from a multiple RM, and RM loads;

- assign load and repetitions based on the training goal;

- know when and by how much an exercise load should be increased;

- assign training volumes according to the athlete's training status and the training goal; and

- determine rest period lengths based on the training goal.

The authors would like to acknowledge the significant contributions of Thomas R. Baechle, Roger W. Earle, and Dan Wathen to this chapter.

Effective training programs involve the coordination of many variables in a systematic fashion that enables the body to adapt and performance level to improve. Having a basic understanding of the physiological responses to various training stimuli is essential in order for the practitioner to be able to coordinate the various training aspects successfully. When focusing on the resistance training component of a comprehensive training program, it is helpful to approach the task one program element at a time, keeping in mind the primary principles of anaerobic exercise prescription.

Principles of Anaerobic Exercise Prescription

Resistance training programs for athletic populations require attention to the principles of specificity, overload, and progression. One of the most basic concepts to incorporate in all training programs is **specificity**. The term, first suggested by DeLorme in 1945 (14), refers to the method whereby an athlete is trained in a specific manner to produce a specific adaptation or training outcome. In the case of resistance training, *specificity* refers to aspects such as the muscles involved, the movement pattern, and the nature of the muscle action (e.g., speed of movement, force application), but does not always reflect the combination of all of these aspects. Importantly, it does not mean that all aspects of the training must mimic that of the sporting skill. For example, a squat movement is relevant to vertical jump because it involves overcoming resistance in the same movement and muscles that are involved in the vertical jump, yet the speed of movement and force application are disparate between the squat and vertical jump. Sometimes used interchangeably with *specificity* is the acronym **SAID**, which stands for *specific adaptation to imposed demands*. The underlying principle is that the type of demand placed on the body dictates the type of adaptation that will occur. For instance, athletes training for power in high-speed movements (e.g., baseball pitch, tennis serve) should attempt to activate or recruit the

same motor units required by their sport at the highest velocity possible (8, 86). Specificity also relates to the athlete's sport season. As an athlete progresses through the preseason, in-season, and postseason, all forms of training should gradually progress in an organized manner from generalized to sport specific (1). Although participation in the sport itself provides the greatest opportunity to improve performance in the sport, proper application of the specificity principle certainly increases the likelihood that other training will also positively contribute to performance.

Overload refers to assigning a workout or training regimen of greater intensity than the athlete is accustomed to. Without the stimulus of overload, even an otherwise well-designed program greatly limits an athlete's ability to make improvements. The obvious application of this principle in the design of resistance training programs involves increasing the loads assigned in the exercises. Other more subtle changes include increasing the number of sessions per week (or per day in some instances), adding exercises or sets, emphasizing complex over simple exercises, decreasing the length of the rest periods between sets and exercises, or any combination of these or other changes. The intent is to stress the body at a higher level than it is used to. When the overload principle is properly applied, overtraining is avoided and the desired training adaptation will occur.

If a training program is to continue producing higher levels of performance, the intensity of the training must become progressively greater. **Progression**, when applied properly, promotes long-term training benefits. Although it is customary to focus only on the resistance used, one can progressively increase training intensity by raising the number of weekly training sessions, adding more drills or exercises to each session, changing the type or technical requirements of the drills or exercises, or otherwise increasing the training stimulus. For example, an athlete may progress from the front squat to learning the hang power clean and eventually the power clean as a technical progression. The issue of importance is that progression is based on the athlete's training status and is introduced systematically and gradually.

Resistance Training Program Design Variables

1. Needs analysis
2. Exercise selection
3. Training frequency
4. Exercise order
5. Training load and repetitions
6. Volume
7. Rest periods

Designing a resistance training program is a complex process that requires the recognition and manipulation of seven **program design** variables (referred to in this chapter as steps 1 through 7). This chapter discusses each variable, shown in the sidebar, in the context of three scenarios that enable the strength and conditioning professional to see how training principles and program design guidelines can be integrated into an overall program.

The three scenarios include a basketball center (scenario A) in her preseason, an American football offensive lineman (scenario B) during his off-season, and a cross-country runner (scenario C) during his in-season. It is understood that in each scenario, the athlete is well conditioned for his or her sport, has no musculoskeletal dysfunction, and has been cleared for training and competition by the sports medicine staff. The athletes in scenarios A (basketball center) and B (American football lineman) have been resistance training since high school, are accustomed to lifting heavy loads, and are skilled in machine and free weight exercises. The high school cross-country runner in scenario C, in contrast, began a resistance training program in the preseason only four weeks ago, so his training is limited and his exercise technique skills are not well developed.

Step 1: Needs Analysis

The strength and conditioning professional's initial task is to perform a **needs analysis**, a two-stage process that includes an evaluation of the requirements and characteristics of the sport and an assessment of the athlete.

Evaluation of the Sport

The first task in a needs analysis is to determine the unique characteristics of the sport, which includes the general physiological and biomechanical profile, common injury sites, and position-specific attributes. This information enables the strength and conditioning professional to design a program specific to those requirements and characteristics. Although this task can be approached in several ways (30), it should at least include consideration of the following attributes of the sport (20, 43):

- Body and limb movement patterns and muscular involvement (**movement analysis**)
- Strength, power, hypertrophy, and muscular endurance priorities (**physiological analysis**)
- Common sites for joint and muscle injury and causative factors (**injury analysis**)

Other characteristics of a sport—such as cardiovascular endurance, speed, agility, and flexibility requirements—should also be evaluated. This chapter, however, focuses only on the physiological outcomes that specifically relate to resistance training program design: strength, power, hypertrophy, and muscular endurance.

For example, a movement analysis of the shot-put field event reveals that it is an all-body movement that begins with the athlete in a semicrouched stance, with many joints flexed and adducted, and culminates in an upright stance with many joints extended and abducted. The most heavily recruited muscles (not in order) are the elbow extensors (triceps brachii), shoulder abductors (deltoids), hip extensors (gluteals, hamstrings), knee extensors (quadriceps), and ankle plantar flexors (soleus, gastrocnemius). Physiologically, shot putting requires high levels of strength and power for a successful performance. Also, enhanced muscular hypertrophy is advantageous since the muscle's ability to produce force increases as its cross-sectional area becomes greater (40). The muscular endurance requirement is minimal, however. Due to the repetitive nature of training and competition, the muscles and tendons surrounding the shoulder and elbow joints tend to be injured due to overuse (98).

Assessment of the Athlete

The second task is to **profile** the athlete's needs and goals by evaluating training (and injury) status, conducting a

Athlete Scenarios

Scenario A		Scenario B		Scenario C	
Sex:	Female	Sex:	Male	Sex:	Male
Age:	20 years old	Age:	28 years old	Age:	17 years old
Sport:	Collegiate basketball	Sport:	Professional American football	Sport:	High school cross-country running
Position:	Center	Position:	Offensive lineman	Position:	(Not applicable)
Season:	Beginning of the preseason	Season:	Beginning of the off-season	Season:	Beginning of the in-season

variety of tests (e.g., maximum strength testing), evaluating the results, and determining the primary goal of training. The more individualized the assessment process, the more specific the resistance training program for each athlete can be.

Training Status

An athlete's current condition or level of preparedness to begin a new or revised program (**training status**) is an important consideration in the design of training programs. This includes an evaluation by a sports medicine professional of any current or previous injuries that may affect training. Also important is the athlete's **training background** or **exercise history** (training that occurred *before* he or she began a new or revised program), because this information will help the strength and conditioning professional better understand the athlete's training capabilities. An assessment of the athlete's training background should examine the

- type of training program (sprint, plyometric, resistance, and so on),
- length of recent regular participation in previous training program(s),
- level of intensity involved in previous training program(s), and
- degree of **exercise technique experience** (i.e., the knowledge and skill to perform resistance training exercises properly).

Table 17.1 provides an example of how such information might be used to classify athletes' training status as beginner, intermediate, or advanced. The strength and conditioning professional should realize that the three classifications exist on a continuum and cannot be definitively demarcated.

Physical Testing and Evaluation

Physical evaluation involves conducting assessments of the athlete's strength, flexibility, power, speed, muscular endurance, body composition, cardiovascular endurance, and so on. In this chapter, the needs analysis focuses on assessing maximal muscular strength, but a comprehensive assessment goes beyond that.

To yield pertinent and reliable data that can be used effectively to develop a resistance training program, the tests selected should be related to the athlete's sport, consistent with the athlete's level of skill, and realistically based on the equipment available. The result of the movement analysis discussed previously provides direction in selecting tests. Typically, major upper body exercises (e.g., bench press and shoulder press) and exercises that mimic jumping movements to varying degrees (e.g., power clean, squat, leg press) are used in testing batteries.

After testing is completed, the results should be compared with normative or descriptive data to determine the athlete's strengths and weaknesses. Based on this evaluation and the needs analysis of the sport, a training program can be developed to improve deficiencies, maintain strengths, or further develop physiological qualities that will enable the athlete to better meet the demands of the sport.

Primary Resistance Training Goal

The athlete's test results, the movement and physiological analysis of the sport, and the priorities of the athlete's sport season determine the primary goal or outcome for the resistance training program. Typically, this goal is to improve strength, power, hypertrophy, or muscular endurance. Despite a potential desire or need to make improvements in two different areas (e.g., strength *and* muscular endurance), an effort should be

TABLE 17.1   Example of Classifying Resistance Training Status

Resistance training status	Resistance training background				
	Current program	Training age	Frequency (per week)	Training stress*	Technique experience and skill
Beginner (untrained)	Not training or just began training	<2 months	≤1-2	None or low	None or minimal
Intermediate (moderately resistance trained)	Currently training	2-6 months	≤2-3	Medium	Basic
Advanced (well resistance trained)	Currently training	≥1 year	≥3-4	High	High

*In this example, "training stress" refers to the degree of physical demand or stimulus of the resistance training program.

made to concentrate on only one training outcome per season. An example of how the strength and conditioning professional may prioritize the resistance training emphases during the four main sport seasons is shown in table 17.2.

Step 2: Exercise Selection

Exercise selection involves choosing exercises for a resistance training program. To make informed exercise selections, the strength and conditioning professional

Application of the Needs Analysis
(Refer to the first scenario table in the chapter for a description of the scenario athletes.)

Scenario A Female collegiate basketball player **Preseason**	Scenario B Male professional American football lineman **Off-season**	Scenario C Male high school cross-country runner **In-season**
SPORT EVALUATION **Movement analysis** *Sport:* Running and jumping, ball handling, shooting, blocking, and rebounding *Muscular involvement:* All major muscle areas, especially the hips, thighs, and shoulders **Physiological analysis (primary requirement)** Strength/power	**SPORT EVALUATION** **Movement analysis** *Sport:* Grabbing, pushing, repelling, and deflecting opponents *Muscular involvement:* All major muscle areas, especially the hips, thighs, chest, arms, and low back **Physiological analysis (primary requirement)** Hypertrophy	**SPORT EVALUATION** **Movement analysis** *Sport:* Running, repetitive leg and arm movements *Muscular involvement:* All lower body muscle areas, postural muscles, shoulders and arms **Physiological analysis (primary requirement)** Muscular endurance
ATHLETE'S PROFILE **Training background** • Has resistance trained regularly since high school • Possesses excellent skill in performing free weight and machine exercises • Just completed a 4×/week resistance training program in the off-season consisting of *Upper body exercises* (2×/week): 6 exercises (2 core, 4 assistance), 3 sets of 10RM-12RM loads *Lower body exercises* (2×/week): 6 exercises (2 core, 4 assistance), 3 sets of 10RM-12RM loads	**ATHLETE'S PROFILE** **Training background** • Has resistance trained regularly throughout high school, college, and his professional career • Possesses excellent skill in performing free weight and machine exercises • Just completed a 2×/week resistance training program in the postseason[b] consisting of *All exercises performed in each session:* 8 exercises (3 core, 5 assistance; 2 lower body, 6 upper body), 2-3 sets of 12RM-15RM loads	**ATHLETE'S PROFILE** **Training background** • Just began resistance training in preseason • Has only limited skill in performing free weight and machine exercises • Just completed a 2×/week resistance training program in the preseason[c] consisting of *All exercises performed in each session:* 7 exercises (3 core, 4 assistance; 3 lower body, 4 upper body), 1-2 sets of 15RM loads
CLASSIFICATION OF RESISTANCE TRAINING STATUS Advanced	**CLASSIFICATION OF RESISTANCE TRAINING STATUS** Advanced	**CLASSIFICATION OF RESISTANCE TRAINING STATUS** Beginner
PRIMARY PRESEASON RESISTANCE TRAINING GOAL Strength/power[a]	**PRIMARY OFF-SEASON RESISTANCE TRAINING GOAL** Hypertrophy	**PRIMARY IN-SEASON RESISTANCE TRAINING GOAL** Muscular endurance
COMMENTS [a]The preseason will address both of these goals through a combination of appropriate exercise selection and volume-load assignments.	**COMMENTS** [b]Due to the extreme physical demands of American football, this athlete's postseason training volume was greater than is often assigned for the active rest phase of a typical program.	**COMMENTS** [c]Because this athlete just began his resistance training program, his frequency was limited to only 2×/week in the preseason rather than the 3 or 4 sessions/week typically completed by better-trained individuals.

The information in this table reflects one approach to evaluating the requirements of a sport and profiling an athlete.

TABLE 17.2   Example of General Training Priorities by Sport Season

Sport season	Priority given to		Resistance training goal*
	Sport practice	Resistance training	
Off-season	Low	High	Hypertrophy and muscular endurance (initially); strength and power (later)
Preseason	Medium	Medium	Sport and movement specific (i.e., strength, power, or muscular endurance, depending on the sport)
In-season	High	Low	Maintenance of preseason training goal
Postseason (active rest)	Variable	Variable	Not specific (may include activities other than sport skill or resistance training)

*The actual training goals and priorities are based on the specific sport or activity and may differ from the goals listed here.

must understand the nature of various types of resistance training exercises, the movement and muscular requirements of the sport, the athlete's exercise technique experience, the equipment available, and the amount of training time available.

Exercise Type

Although there are literally hundreds of resistance training exercises to select from when one is designing a program, most involve primary muscle groups or body areas and fall into categories based on their relative importance to the athlete's sport.

Core and Assistance Exercises

Exercises can be classified as either core or assistance based on the size of the muscle areas involved and their level of contribution to a particular sport movement. **Core exercises** recruit one or more large muscle areas (i.e., chest, shoulder, back, hip, or thigh), involve two or more primary joints (**multijoint exercises**), and receive priority when one is selecting exercises because of their direct application to the sport. **Assistance exercises** usually recruit smaller muscle areas (i.e., upper arm, abdominal muscles, calf, neck, forearm, lower back, or anterior lower leg), involve only one primary joint (**single-joint exercises**), and are considered less important to improving sport performance. Generally, all the joints at the shoulder—the glenohumeral and shoulder girdle articulations—are considered one *primary* joint when resistance training exercises are categorized as core or assistance. The spine is similarly considered a single primary joint (as in the abdominal crunch and back extension exercises).

A common application of assistance exercises is for injury prevention and rehabilitation, as these exercises often isolate a specific muscle or muscle group. The muscles that are predisposed to injury from the unique demands of a sport skill (e.g., the shoulder external rotators for overhand pitching) or those that require

reconditioning after an injury (e.g., a quadriceps contusion) can be specifically conditioned by an assistance exercise.

Structural and Power Exercises

A core exercise that emphasizes loading the spine directly (e.g., back squat) or indirectly (e.g., power clean) can be further described as a **structural exercise**. More specifically, a structural exercise involves muscular stabilization of posture during performance of the lifting movement (e.g., maintaining a rigid torso and a neutral spine during the back squat). A structural exercise that is performed very quickly or explosively is considered a **power exercise**. Typically, power exercises are assigned to athletes when they are appropriate for the athlete's sport-specific training priorities (45).

Movement Analysis of the Sport

In the needs analysis (step 1), the strength and conditioning professional has identified the unique requirements and characteristics of the sport. The exercises selected for a resistance training program that focus on conditioning for a particular sport need to be relevant to the activities of that sport in their body and limb movement patterns, joint ranges of motion, and muscular involvement. The exercises should also create muscular balance to reduce risk of injury from disproportionate training.

Sport-Specific Exercises

The more similar the training activity is to the actual sport movement, the greater the likelihood that there will be a positive transfer to that sport (8, 19, 20, 42, 72, 86). This is the specificity concept, also called the specific adaptation to imposed demands (SAID) principle. Table 17.3 provides examples of resistance training exercises that relate in varying degrees to the movement patterns of various sports. The strength and conditioning professional should find this table helpful when trying to identify sport-specific exercises. For example, the

TABLE 17.3   Examples of Movement-Related Resistance Training Exercises

Movement pattern	Related exercises
Ball dribbling and passing	Close-grip bench press, dumbbell bench press, triceps pushdown, reverse curl, hammer curl
Ball kicking	Unilateral hip adduction and abduction, single-leg squat, forward step lunge, leg (knee) extension, leg raise
Freestyle swimming (including start and turns)	Pull-up, lateral shoulder raise, forward step lunge, upright row, barbell pullover, single-leg squat
Vertical jumping	Snatch, power clean, push jerk, back squat, front squat, standing calf (heel) raise
Racket stroke	Flat dumbbell fly, lunge, bent-over lateral raise, wrist curl, wrist extension
Rowing	Power clean, clean pull, snatch pull, bent-over row, seated row, angled leg press, horizontal leg press, deadlift, stiff-legged deadlift, good morning
Running, sprinting	Snatch, clean, front squat, forward step lunge, step-up, leg (knee) extension, leg (knee) curl, toe raise (dorsiflexion)
Throwing, pitching	Lunge, single-leg squat, barbell pullover, overhead triceps extension, shoulder internal and external rotation

primary muscles involved in jumping for basketball are the hip and knee extensors. An athlete can exercise these muscles by performing the leg press or back squat, but which exercise is preferable? Certainly both exercises strengthen the hip and knee extensors, but because jumping is performed from an erect body position with balance and weight-bearing forces as considerations, the back squat is more relevant to jumping and is therefore preferred over the leg press (97). The power clean and snatch are relevant to jumping because of their quick movement characteristics, thereby applying a fast rate of force development and high power.

Muscle Balance

Exercises selected for the specific demands of the sport should maintain a balance of muscular strength across joints and between opposing muscle groups (e.g., biceps brachii and triceps brachii). Avoid designing a resistance training program that increases the risk of injury due to a disparity between the strength of the **agonist**, the muscle or muscle group actively causing the movement (e.g., the quadriceps in the leg [knee] extension exercise), and the **antagonist**, the sometimes passive (i.e., not concentrically involved) muscle or muscle group located on the opposite side of the limb (e.g., the hamstrings in the leg [knee] extension exercise). If an imbalance is created or discovered, exercises to restore an appropriate strength balance need to be selected. For example, if isokinetic testing reveals that the hamstrings are extremely weak compared with the quadriceps, additional hamstring exercises could be included to compensate for the imbalance (20, 72, 86). Note that **muscle balance** does not always mean equal strength, just a proper

ratio of strength, power, or muscular endurance of one muscle or muscle group relative to another muscle or muscle group.

Exercises to Promote Recovery

Exercises that do not involve high muscular stress and high stress on the nervous system but promote movement and restoration can be classified as **recovery exercise**. These exercises are generally included at the conclusion of the main resistance training session, or as a separate session within the microcycle, aimed at promoting recovery and restoration. They can take the form of lightly loaded resistance exercises or low-intensity aerobic exercise to assist the body in returning to its preexercise state (8). These exercises assist in the removal of metabolic wastes and by-products and maintain some amount of blood flow to the exercised muscles so the repair processes can be optimized.

Exercise Technique Experience

An important part of the needs analysis described earlier is evaluating the athlete's training status and exercise technique experience. If there is any question whether an athlete can perform an exercise with proper technique, the strength and conditioning professional should ask the athlete to demonstrate the exercise. If the athlete uses incorrect technique, the strength and conditioning professional should provide complete instruction. Often, unskilled individuals are introduced to machines and free weight assistance exercises (20) because these are considered easier to perform than free weight core exercises due to their lower balance and coordination requirements (20, 86). Despite this, one should not assume that the athlete will perform exercises correctly, even those that are relatively easy to perform.

Availability of Resistance Training Equipment

The availability of training equipment must be considered in the selection of exercises. A lack of certain equipment may necessitate selecting exercises that are not as sport specific. For example, the absence of Olympic-type barbells with revolving sleeves would preclude exercises such as the power clean, and an insufficient supply of barbell plates may result in substituting exercises that do not require as much resistance; for example, the back squat could be replaced by the front squat.

Application of the Exercise Selection Guidelines

(Refer to the first scenario table in the chapter for a description of the scenario athletes. Exercises are not listed in order of execution.)

Scenario A Female collegiate basketball player Preseason	Scenario B Male professional American football lineman Off-season	Scenario C Male high school cross-country runner In-season
CORE Hang clean (all body, power)[a] Snatch and clean (all body, power)[a] Push press (all body, power)[a] Front squat (hip and thigh) Incline bench press (chest) Pull-up (back, shoulders, arms)	**CORE**[b] Clean (all body, power) Tire flipping (all body, power) Back squat (hip and thigh) Deadlift (hip and thigh) Bench press (chest) Shoulder press (shoulders)	**CORE** Lunge (hip and thigh)[c] Vertical chest press (chest)[d] Rear leg elevated deadlift (hip and thigh)
ASSISTANCE Abdominal crunch (abdomen) Seated row (upper back) Stiff-leg deadlift (posterior hip and thigh Standing calf raise (posterior lower leg)	**ASSISTANCE** Towel-grip pull-up (forearm grip) Abdominal crunch (abdomen) Step-up (hip and thigh) Leg (knee) curl (posterior thigh) Bent-over row (upper back) Shoulder shrug (upper back and neck) Barbell biceps curl (anterior upper arm) Lying triceps extension (posterior upper arm) Seated calf (heel) raise (posterior lower leg)	**ASSISTANCE** Abdominal crunch (abdomen) Leg (knee) curl (posterior thigh) Lateral shoulder raise (shoulders) One-arm dumbbell row (upper back)[e] Toe raise (dorsiflexion) (anterior lower leg) Machine back extension (lower back) Cable hip flexion (hip flexors)
COMMENTS [a]These exercises are included to maximize power and match the jumping movements of basketball.	**COMMENTS** This athlete has extra time available to perform more resistance training exercises because sport skill practice is not the first priority in the off-season. [b]Greater training frequency allows more core exercises to be included (see step 3).	**COMMENTS** [c]Although not always considered a core exercise, the lunge recruits muscles and joints that have direct application to running. [d]This exercise also involves the triceps brachii muscle, so an assistance exercise to isolate the triceps is not needed. This reduces the time devoted to the resistance training portion of the in-season program. [e]This exercise also involves the biceps brachii muscle, so an assistance exercise to isolate the biceps is not needed. This reduces the time devoted to the resistance training portion of the in-season program.

Available Training Time per Session

The strength and conditioning professional should weigh the value of certain exercises against the time it takes to perform them. Some exercises take longer to complete than others. If time for a training session is limited, exercises that are more time efficient may need to be given priority over others. For example, the machine leg press could be selected instead of the free weight lunge to train the hips and thighs of a 100 m sprinter. The time required to move the machine pin to the correct slot in a weight stack and perform 10 repetitions of a machine leg press is much less than the time required for the lunge exercise, for which the athlete has to load both ends of a bar, attach the locks, back out of the power rack, establish a stable starting position, perform 10 repetitions of *each* leg, and rerack the bar. Although the machine leg press is less sport specific, the time saved may permit including other exercises or performing more sets. The benefit of including the more sport-specific lunge exercise, on the other hand, may be worth the additional time needed, although this depends on the goals of the training season and time available.

Step 3: Training Frequency

Training frequency refers to the number of training sessions completed in a given time period. For a resistance training program, a common time period is one week. When determining training frequency, the strength and conditioning professional should consider the athlete's training status, sport season, projected exercise loads, types of exercises, and other concurrent training or activities.

Training Status

The athlete's level of preparedness for training, which was determined during the needs analysis (step 1), is an influential factor in determining training frequency because it affects the number of rest days needed between training sessions. Traditionally, three workouts per week are recommended for many athletes, because the intervening days allow sufficient recovery between sessions (20). As an athlete adapts to training and becomes better conditioned, it is appropriate to consider increasing the number of training days to four and, with additional training, maybe five, six, or seven (see table 17.4). The general guideline is to schedule training sessions so as to include at least one rest or recovery day—but not more than three—between sessions that stress the same muscle groups (38). For example, if a strength and conditioning professional wants a beginning athlete to perform a total body resistance training program two times per week, the sessions should be spaced out evenly (e.g., Monday and Thursday or Tuesday and Friday).

TABLE 17.4   Resistance Training Frequency Based on Training Status

Training status	Frequency guidelines (sessions per week)
Beginner	2-3
Intermediate	3-4
Advanced	4-7

Data from references 24, 26, 27, 28, 37, and 47.

If the athlete trains only on Monday and Wednesday, the absence of a training stimulus between Wednesday and the following Monday may result in a *decrease* in the athlete's training status (16, 24, 38), although, for a short time in well-trained athletes, one session a week can maintain strength (16, 24).

More highly resistance-trained (intermediate or advanced) athletes can augment their training by using a **split routine** in which different muscle groups are trained on different days. Training nearly every day may seem to violate the recommended guidelines for recovery, but grouping exercises that train a portion of the body (e.g., upper body or lower body) or certain muscle areas (e.g., chest, shoulder, and triceps) gives the trained athlete an opportunity to adequately recover between similar training sessions (see table 17.5). For instance, a common lower body–upper body regimen includes four training sessions per week: lower body on Monday and Thursday and upper body on Tuesday and Friday (or vice versa). This way, there are two or three days of rest between each upper or lower body training session, even though the athlete trains on two consecutive days twice a week (39). For split routines with three distinct training days, the rest days are not on the same day each week.

Sport Season

Another influence on resistance training frequency is the sport season. For example, the increased emphasis on practicing the sport skill during the in-season necessitates a decrease in the time spent in the weight room and, consequently, reduces the frequency of resistance training (see tables 17.2 and 17.6). The problem is that there simply is not enough time to fit all the desired modes of training into each day. So, even though a well-trained athlete may be capable of completing four or more resistance training sessions per week, the other time demands of the sport may not permit this.

Training Load and Exercise Type

Athletes who train with maximal or near-maximal loads require more recovery time before their next training session (20, 74, 86). The ability to train more frequently may

TABLE 17.5 Examples of Common Split Routines

Training day	Body parts or muscle groups trained	Sample training week							Resulting training frequency
		Sun	Mon	Tues	Wed	Thurs	Fri	Sat	
1	Lower body	*Rest*	Lower body	Upper body	*Rest*	Lower body	Upper body	*Rest*	4 times per week
2	Upper body								
1	Chest, shoulders, triceps	*Rest*	Chest, shoulders, triceps	Lower body	Back, trapezius, biceps	*Rest*	Chest, shoulders, triceps	Lower body	5 times per week*
2	Lower body								
3	Back, trapezius, biceps								
1	Chest and back	Chest and back	Lower body	Shoulders and arms	*Rest*	Chest and back	Lower body	Shoulders and arms	6 times per week*
2	Lower body								
3	Shoulders and arms								

*Frequency varies between five times per week and six times per week, depending on the day of the week that is the first training day.

TABLE 17.6 Resistance Training Frequency Based on the Sport Season (for a Trained Athlete)

Sport season	Frequency guidelines (sessions per week)
Off-season	4-6
Preseason	3-4
In-season	1-3
Postseason (active rest)	0-3

Data from references 20, 87, and 90.

be enhanced by alternating lighter and heavier training days (20, 86). There is also evidence that upper body muscles can recover more quickly from heavy loading sessions than lower body muscles (37). The same is true regarding an athlete's ability to recover faster from single-joint exercises compared to multijoint exercises (85). These research findings may explain why, for example, powerlifters may schedule only one very heavy deadlift or squat training session per week.

Other Training

Exercise frequency is also influenced by the overall amount of physical stress, so the strength and conditioning professional must consider the effects of all forms of exercise. If the athlete's program already includes aerobic or anaerobic (e.g., sprinting, agility, speed-endurance, plyometric) training, sport skill practice, or any combination of these components, the frequency of resistance training may need to be reduced (13). Additionally,

the effects of a physically demanding occupation may be relevant. Athletes who work in manual labor jobs, instruct or assist others in physical activities, or are on their feet all day may not be able to withstand the same training frequency as athletes who are less active outside of their sport-related pursuits.

Step 4: Exercise Order

Exercise order refers to a sequence of resistance exercises performed during one training session. Although there are many ways to arrange exercises, decisions are invariably based on how one exercise affects the quality of effort or the technique of another exercise. Usually exercises are arranged so that an athlete's maximal force capabilities are available (from a sufficient rest or recovery period) to complete a set with proper exercise technique. Four of the most common methods of ordering resistance exercises are described in the following paragraphs.

Power, Other Core, Then Assistance Exercises

Power exercises such as the snatch, hang clean, power clean, and push jerk should be performed first in a training session, followed by other nonpower core exercises and then assistance exercises (20, 83, 88). The literature also refers to this arrangement as *multijoint exercises and then single-joint exercises* or *large muscle areas and then small muscle areas* (18, 20, 72, 86, 90). Power exercises require the highest level of skill and concentration of all the exercises and are most affected by fatigue (20).

Application of the Training Frequency Guidelines

(Refer to the first scenario table in the chapter for a description of the scenario athletes.)

Scenario A Female collegiate basketball player **Preseason**	Scenario B Male professional American football lineman **Off-season**	Scenario C Male high school cross-country runner **In-season**
ADVANCED TRAINING STATUS ALLOWS 4-7×/week	**ADVANCED TRAINING STATUS ALLOWS** 4-7×/week	**BEGINNER TRAINING STATUS ALLOWS** 2-3×/week
FREQUENCY GUIDELINE BASED ON THE SPORT SEASON 3-4×/week	**FREQUENCY GUIDELINE BASED ON THE SPORT SEASON** 4-6×/week	**FREQUENCY GUIDELINE BASED ON THE SPORT SEASON** 1-3×/week
ASSIGNED RESISTANCE TRAINING FREQUENCY 3×/week[a] • Monday, Wednesday, and Friday • All exercises performed each session	**ASSIGNED RESISTANCE TRAINING FREQUENCY** 4×/week (split routine[b]) • Monday and Thursday (lower body exercises) • Tuesday and Friday (upper body exercises)	**ASSIGNED RESISTANCE TRAINING FREQUENCY** 2×/week[c] • Wednesday and Saturday • All exercises performed each session
COMMENTS [a]Training frequency is decreased from the previous season (off-season) to allow for more time and physical resources to apply to basketball-specific sport skill training.	**COMMENTS** [b]A split routine allows for more overall exercises to be performed without an excessive increase in training time (per session) because the exercises are divided over more training days.	**COMMENTS** [c]The assigned training days need to be planned so they do not affect the athlete's performance on the scheduled days for cross-country meets.

Athletes who become fatigued are prone to using poor technique and consequently are at higher risk of injury. The explosive movements and extensive muscular involvement of power exercises also result in significant energy expenditure (86). This is another reason to have athletes perform such exercises first, while they are still metabolically fresh. If power exercises are not selected in step 2 (exercise selection), then the recommended order of exercises is core exercises and then assistance exercises.

Upper and Lower Body Exercises (Alternated)

One method of providing the opportunity for athletes to recover more fully between exercises is to alternate upper body exercises with lower body exercises. This arrangement is especially helpful for untrained individuals who find that completing several upper or lower body exercises in succession is too strenuous (20, 72). Also, if training time is limited, this method of arranging exercises minimizes the length of the rest periods required between exercises and maximizes the rest between body areas. The result is a decrease in overall training time, because the athlete can perform an upper body exercise and then immediately go to a lower body exercise without having to wait for the upper body to rest. If the exercises are performed with minimal rest periods (20-30 seconds), this method is also referred to as **circuit training**—a method sometimes also used to improve cardiorespiratory endurance (23), although to a lesser extent than conventional aerobic exercise training.

"Push" and "Pull" Exercises (Alternated)

Another method of improving recovery and recruitment between exercises is to alternate pushing exercises (e.g., bench press, shoulder press, and triceps extension) with pulling exercises (e.g., lat pulldown, bent-over row, biceps curl) (2). This push–pull arrangement ensures that the same muscle group will not be used in two exercises (or sets, in some cases) in succession, thus reducing fatigue in the involved muscles. In contrast, arranging several pulling exercises (e.g., pull-up, seated row, hammer curl) one after the other, even with a rest period between each, will compromise the number of repetitions performed because the biceps brachii muscle (involved in all three exercises) will become less responsive due to fatigue. The same result would occur if several pushing exercises (e.g., incline bench press, shoulder press, triceps pushdown) were sequentially arranged (all three engage the triceps brachii) (83). There are also push–pull arrangements for the lower body—for example, leg press and back squat as "push" and stiff-leg deadlift and leg (knee) curl as "pull"—but the classification of some exercises as "push" or "pull" is not as clear (e.g., leg [knee] extension). The alternation of push and pull exercises is also used in circuit training programs and is an ideal arrangement for athletes beginning or returning to a resistance training program (3, 20).

Supersets and Compound Sets

Other methods of arranging exercises involve having athletes perform one set of a pair of exercises with little to no rest between them. Two common examples are supersets and compound sets. A **superset** involves two sequentially performed exercises that stress two opposing muscles or muscle areas (i.e., an agonist and its antagonist) (2). For example, an athlete performs

Application of the Exercise Order Guidelines

(Refer to the first scenario table in the chapter for a description of the scenario athletes.)

Scenario A Female collegiate basketball player **Preseason**	Scenario B Male professional American football lineman **Off-season**	Scenario C Male high school cross-country runner **In-season**
ASSIGNED EXERCISE ORDER STRATEGIES • Power, other core, then assistance exercises • "Push" and "pull" exercises (alternated)	**ASSIGNED EXERCISE ORDER STRATEGIES** • Core and then assistance exercises • "Push" and "pull" exercises (alternated)	**ASSIGNED EXERCISE ORDER STRATEGIES** • Core and then assistance exercises • Upper and lower body exercises (alternated), circuit training
MONDAY, WEDNESDAY, AND FRIDAY Hang clean[a] Push jerk[b] Front squat[a] Incline bench press[b] Seated row Dumbbell alternating curl Triceps pushdown Abdominal crunch	**LOWER BODY (MONDAY AND THURSDAY)** Deadlift[c] Back squat[c] Step-up[c] Leg (knee) curl Seated calf (heel) raise **UPPER BODY (TUESDAY AND FRIDAY)** Bench press Bent-over row Shoulder press Barbell biceps curl[d] Shoulder shrug Lying triceps extension Abdominal crunch	**WEDNESDAY AND SATURDAY** Lunge Vertical chest press Leg (knee) curl One-arm dumbbell row Toe raise (dorsiflexion) Lateral shoulder raise Machine back extension[e] Abdominal crunch Complete one set of each exercise, then repeat[f]
COMMENTS [a,b]These exercises are alternated to provide relative rest between their similar movement patterns while still following the "power, other core, then assistance" exercise order strategy.	**COMMENTS** [c]These exercises do not follow the "push" and "pull" (alternated) exercise arrangement and could be performed in a variety of sequences (e.g., back squat, deadlift, step-up). [d]Although the barbell biceps curl exercise is a "pulling" movement and occurs before another "pull" exercise (shoulder shrug), it does not affect the athlete's ability to perform the shoulder shrug exercise.	**COMMENTS** [e]Exercises that concentrically train the lower back muscles should be performed after exercises that require an erect torso or a neutral spine position (e.g., lunge and lateral shoulder raise). Fatigue of the lower back muscles can result in incorrect and potentially injurious exercise technique in structural or standing exercises. [f]The eight exercises are performed one set at a time, one immediately after the other (i.e., in a "circuit").

10 repetitions of the barbell biceps curl exercise, sets the bar down, then goes over to the triceps pushdown station and performs 10 repetitions. A **compound set** involves sequentially performing two different exercises for the same muscle group (2). For instance, an athlete completes a set of the barbell biceps curl exercise, then switches to dumbbells and immediately performs a set of the hammer curl exercise. In this case, the stress on the same muscle is compounded because both exercises recruit the same muscle area. Both methods of arranging and performing pairs of exercises are time efficient and purposely more demanding—and consequently may not be appropriate for unconditioned athletes. Note, however, that sometimes the meanings of *superset* and *compound set* are interchanged (20).

Step 5: Training Load and Repetitions

Load most simply refers to the amount of weight assigned to an exercise set and is often characterized as the most critical aspect of a resistance training program (20, 63, 73, 86).

Terminology Used to Quantify and Qualify Mechanical Work

Mechanical work can be defined as the product of *force* and *displacement* (sometimes referred to as *distance*). An athlete can perform (external) mechanical work via demands made on the body to generate (internal) metabolic energy. Thus, it is important to quantify the amount of mechanical work or degree of metabolic demand in order to plan variation in the training program and to avoid the exhaustion phase of Selye's General Adaptation Syndrome associated with overtraining (8).

A quantity measure for resistance training "work" is needed. Traditionally, at least in the sport of Olympic weightlifting, this "work" is called the "load," and one can calculate it by multiplying each weight lifted by the number of times it is lifted and summing all such values over a training session.

However, **volume-load** (48, 77) may be a better term than just *load*. This quantity is highly related to mechanical work (59, 60, 62) and the associated metabolic energy demands and physiological stress, and also is distinguished from **repetition-volume** (rep-volume) (i.e., the total number of repetitions; see "Step 6: Volume" for more explanation).

To explain volume-load further, if a barbell that has 100 "weight units" is lifted 2 vertical "distance units" for 15 repetitions, the total concentric mechanical work is 3,000 "work units" ($100 \times 2 \times 15$). However, volume-load (1,500 units) does not include the distance value but is still directly related to the amount of mechanical work performed and the extent of the metabolic demand the athlete experiences to lift the weight for the required repetitions. Volume-load should be considered as *system mass volume-load* in the calculation of resistance training in which the athlete or a mass is moved (e.g., loaded jump squats) (10, 59, 61). For example, an 80 kg athlete with a 40 kg jump squat load for four sets of three is doing 120 kg $\times$ 12, or 1,440 kg. Volume-load approaches are also very useful in quantifying the nature of the total resistance training load, by separating the volume-load from core and assistance exercises or delineating between hypertrophy, maximal strength, and power training. In this way, the strength and conditioning practitioner can plan or determine not just the total volume-load for the session, but also what stimulus is achieved primarily from the session.

Note that the volume-load is not affected by the rep and set scheme (i.e., 15 sets of 1 repetition, 5 sets of 3 repetitions, 3 sets of 5 repetitions, or 1 set of 15 repetitions). Various repetition and set schemes affect the true **intensity** value for resistance exercise and indicate the *quality* of work performed. Instead of using time to calculate mechanical or metabolic power or intensity, it is more practical to use a value that is proportional to time, namely, rep-volume. The more repetitions performed, the longer the training session (rest period lengths are an additional consideration and are not directly accounted for). Dividing volume-load by rep-volume results in the average weight lifted per repetition per workout session (86). This is a good approximation for mechanical and metabolic power output, which are true intensity or quality of work parameters.

Relationship Between Load and Repetitions

The number of times an exercise can be performed (**repetitions**) is inversely related to the load lifted; the heavier the load, the lower the number of repetitions that can be performed. Therefore, focusing on one training goal automatically implies the use of a certain load and repetition regimen (e.g., training for muscular strength involves lifting heavy loads for few repetitions).

Before assigning training loads, the strength and conditioning professional should understand this relationship between loads and repetitions. Load is commonly described as either a certain percentage of a **1-repetition maximum (1RM)**—the greatest amount of weight that can be lifted with proper technique for only one repetition—or the most weight lifted for a specified number of repetitions, a **repetition maximum (RM)** (19). For instance, if athletes can perform 10 repetitions with 60 kg in the back squat exercise, the 10RM is 60 kg. It is assumed that the athlete provided a *maximal effort*; if he or she had stopped at nine repetitions but could have performed one more, a 10RM would not have been achieved. Likewise, if he or she lifted 55 kg for 10 repetitions (but could have performed more), the true 10RM was not accurately assessed because the athlete possibly could have lifted 60 kg for 10 repetitions.

Table 17.7 shows the relationship between a submaximal load—calculated as a percentage of the 1RM—and the number of repetitions that can be performed at that load. By definition, 100% of the 1RM allows the athlete to perform one repetition. As the percentage of the 1RM (i.e., the load lifted) decreases, the athlete will be able to successfully complete more repetitions. Other %1RM–repetition tables with slightly different %1RM values can be found in the literature (9, 49, 54, 65), but they vary by only about 0.5 to 2 percentage points from those provided in table 17.7.

Although %1RM–repetition tables provide helpful guidelines for assigning an athlete's training loads, research to date does not support the widespread use of such tables for establishing training loads for every exercise assigned to athletes, for the following reasons:

- Table 17.7 assumes there is a linear association between the loads lifted and the repetitions performed; however, several studies have reported a curvilinear relationship (51, 54, 56).
- Resistance-trained athletes may be able to exceed the number of repetitions listed in the table at any

given percentage of their 1RM, especially in lower body core exercises (35, 36).

- The number of repetitions that can be performed at a certain percent of the 1RM is based on a single set. When an athlete performs multiple sets, the loads may need to be reduced so that the desired number of repetitions can be completed in all of the sets (20).
- Despite the prevalence of 1RM research, athletes may not always perform the predicted number of repetitions at a specified percentage of a 1RM (20, 90). For instance, studies conducted by Hoeger and colleagues (35, 36) showed that subjects were able to perform two or three *times* more repetitions than are listed in table 17.7.
- A certain percentage of the 1RM assigned to a machine exercise can result in more repetitions at the same percentage of the 1RM than with a similar free weight exercise (35, 36).
- Exercises involving smaller muscle areas may not produce as many repetitions as seen in table 17.7, and exercises recruiting large muscle areas are likely to result in more repetitions performed (90).
- The most accurate relationship between percentages of the 1RM and the maximum repetitions possible is for loads greater than 75% of the 1RM and fewer than 10 repetitions (9, 84, 94). Empirical evidence further suggests that as the percentage of the 1RM decreases, the variability in the number of repetitions that can be completed increases.

Therefore, loads calculated from the %1RM in table 17.7 should be used only as a guideline for estimating a particular RM load for a resistance training exercise. Even with the inherent weaknesses just explained, it appears that it is still more accurate to assign loads based on a percentage of a test-established 1RM than it is to estimate a 1RM from a submaximal load (34, 35).

1RM and Multiple-RM Testing Options

To gather information needed to assign a training load, the strength and conditioning professional has the option of determining the athlete's

- actual 1RM (directly tested),
- estimated 1RM from a multiple-RM test (e.g., a 10RM), or
- multiple RM based on the number of repetitions planned for that exercise (the "goal" repetitions; e.g., five repetitions per set).

TABLE 17.7   Percent of the 1RM and Repetitions Allowed (%1RM–Repetition Relationship)

%1RM	Number of repetitions allowed
100	1
95	2
93	3
90	4
87	5
85	6
83	7
80	8
77	9
75	10
70	11
67	12
65	15

Data from references 9, 49, 54, and 65.

Once the actual 1RM is measured or estimated, the athlete's training load is calculated as a percentage of the 1RM. Alternatively, a multiple-RM test may be performed based on goal repetitions, thereby eliminating computations or estimations. In many cases, the strength and conditioning professional will use a variety of testing options depending on the exercises selected and the athlete's training background. A common strategy for testing sufficiently conditioned athletes is to conduct a 1RM test in several core exercises and use multiple-RM testing for assistance exercises.

Testing the 1RM

To assign training loads based on a percentage of the 1RM, the strength and conditioning professional must first determine the athlete's 1RM. This method of assessment is typically reserved for resistance-trained athletes who are classified as intermediate or advanced and have exercise technique experience in the exercises being tested. Individuals who are untrained, inexperienced, injured, or medically supervised may not be appropriate participants for 1RM testing. One-repetition maximum testing requires an adequate training status and lifting experience, as the assessment of maximal strength places significant stress on the involved muscles, connective tissues, and joints. Thus, it has been suggested that a 3RM test could be used instead of a maximal 1RM test (90). Ignoring an athlete's training status and exercise technique experience diminishes the safety and accuracy of 1RM test results.

When selecting exercises for 1RM testing, the strength and conditioning professional should choose core exercises, because the large muscle groups and multiple joints are better able to handle the heavy loads. Despite this guideline, an exercise should not be selected for 1RM testing if it cannot provide valid and reliable data (i.e., does not accurately and consistently assess maximal muscular strength). For instance, the large upper back musculature and multiple joints involved in the bent-over row exercise can probably tolerate the loads from a 1RM test, but maintaining a correct body position throughout testing would be extremely difficult. The weaker stabilizing muscles of the lower back might become very fatigued after several testing sets, resulting in a loss of proper exercise technique and invalid and potentially unreliable test data.

A variety of procedures can be used to accurately determine a 1RM; one method is described in figure 17.1. Despite an orderly testing sequence, variations in training status and exercise type will affect the absolute

---

1RM Testing Protocol

1. Instruct the athlete to warm up with a light resistance that easily allows 5 to 10 repetitions.
2. Provide a 1-minute rest period.
3. Estimate a warm-up load that will allow the athlete to complete three to five repetitions by adding
   - 10 to 20 pounds (4-9 kg) or 5% to 10% for upper body exercise or
   - 30 to 40 pounds (14-18 kg) or 10% to 20% for lower body exercise.
4. Provide a 2-minute rest period.
5. Estimate a conservative, near-maximal load that will allow the athlete to complete two or three repetitions by adding
   - 10 to 20 pounds (4-9 kg) or 5% to 10% for upper body exercise or
   - 30 to 40 pounds (14-18 kg) or 10% to 20% for lower body exercise.
6. Provide a 2- to 4-minute rest period.
7. Make a load increase:
   - 10 to 20 pounds (4-9 kg) or 5% to 10% for upper body exercise or
   - 30 to 40 pounds (14-18 kg) or 10% to 20% for lower body exercise
8. Instruct the athlete to attempt a 1RM.
9. If the athlete was successful, provide a 2- to 4-minute rest period and go back to step 7. If the athlete failed, provide a 2- to 4-minute rest period; then decrease the load by subtracting
   - 5 to 10 pounds (2-4 kg) or 2.5% to 5% for upper body exercise or
   - 15 to 20 pounds (7-9 kg) or 5% to 10% for lower body exercise.

   AND then go back to step 8.

Continue increasing or decreasing the load until the athlete can complete one repetition with proper exercise technique. Ideally, the athlete's 1RM will be measured within three to five testing sets.

FIGURE 17.1   A 1RM testing protocol.
Reprinted, by permission, from Earle, 2006 (18).

load increases in sequential testing sets. For example, the gradual load increase for 1RM attempts for an athlete who can back squat 495 pounds (225 kg) may be 20 to 30 pounds (9-14 kg) per testing set. For a weaker athlete with a back squat 1RM of 100 pounds (45 kg), a 20- or 30-pound testing load increment is too aggressive and is not precise enough to yield an accurate 1RM value. To improve the appropriateness and accuracy of the sequential testing sets, figure 17.1 also includes relative percentages that can be used instead of the absolute load adjustments.

Estimating a 1RM

When maximal strength testing is not warranted, testing with a 10RM load (and then estimating or predicting the 1RM) can be a suitable secondary option. This approach is appropriate for nearly all athletes, provided they can demonstrate the proper technique in the exercise tested. Core and assistance exercises can be selected for 10RM testing, but excessive warm-up and testing sets may fatigue the athlete and compromise the accuracy of the test. Additionally, power exercises do not lend themselves well to multiple-RM testing above five repetitions for repeated testing sets because technique can deteriorate rapidly (8, 86). Lower (and more accurate) multiple-RM determinations using heavier loads can be made once the athlete has sufficient training and technique experience.

The protocol for 10RM testing is similar to that for 1RM testing, but each set requires 10 repetitions, not one. After the completion of warm-up sets, the athlete's sequential load changes for the 10RM test are smaller than those listed in figure 17.1 (approximately one-half). Continue the process of testing until a load allowing only 10 repetitions is determined. An experienced strength and conditioning professional will be able to adjust the loads so that the 10RM can be measured within three to five testing sets.

Using a 1RM Table   To estimate the athlete's 1RM, consult table 17.8. In the "Max reps (RM)" = 10 (%1RM = 75) column, first find the tested 10RM load; then read across the row to the "Max reps (RM)" = 1 (%1RM = 100) column to discover the athlete's projected 1RM. For example, if an athlete's 10RM is 300 pounds, the estimated 1RM is 400 pounds. As noted in connection with table 17.7, the %1RM–repetition associations vary in the literature. This table is intended for use as a guide until the athlete has developed the neuromuscular attributes that will make testing with heavier loads (e.g., 1RM-5RM) safe and effective (20, 86).

Using Prediction Equations   Equations are also available to predict the 1RM from multiple-RM loads (9, 54). Researchers who have reviewed such equations report

that as the loads used in multiple-RM testing become heavier (i.e., bringing the loads closer to the actual 1RM), the accuracy of the 1RM estimation increases. Likewise, predictions are more accurate when the equations are based on loads equal to or less than a 10RM (9, 55, 84, 86, 94). Furthermore, the results obtained from lower multiple-RM testing (and subsequent predictions of the 1RM) are generally more accurate when an athlete has been consistently training with low multiple-RM resistances (i.e., heavy loads) for a few months before testing (8).

Multiple-RM Testing Based on Goal Repetitions

A third option for determining training loads requires the strength and conditioning professional to first decide on the number of repetitions (i.e., the **goal repetitions**) the athlete will perform in the actual program for the exercise being tested. For example, if the strength and conditioning professional decides that the athlete should perform six repetitions for the bench press exercise in the training program, the multiple-RM testing protocol should have the athlete perform the exercise with a load that will result in six repetitions (6RM). Core and assistance exercises can be selected for multiple-RM testing, but, as previously mentioned, high-repetition testing sets can create significant fatigue and may compromise the accuracy of the tested multiple RM. This effect seems to be more problematic for exercises that involve multiple joints and large muscle areas due to their high metabolic demand (86). Further, multiple-RM testing (and subsequent load assignments) for assistance exercises should be at or above an 8RM to minimize the isolative stress on the involved joint and connective tissue (2, 18). In other words, even if an athlete is following a muscular strength training program that involves 2RM loads for the core exercises, the heaviest load the assistance exercises should be assigned is an 8RM.

Assigning Load and Repetitions Based on the Training Goal

During the needs analysis, the strength and conditioning professional is challenged to choose the primary goal of the resistance training program based on the athlete's testing results, the movement and physiological analysis of the sport, and the priorities of the athlete's sport season. Once decided on, the training goal can be applied to determine specific load and repetition assignments via the RM continuum, a percentage of the 1RM (either directly tested or estimated), or the results of multiple-RM testing. As explained previously, the testing methods determine how the loads and repetitions are assigned for each exercise (i.e., loads are calculated

TABLE 17.8 Estimating 1RM and Training Loads

MAX REPS (RM)	1	2	3	4	5	6	7	8	9	10	12	15
%1RM	**100**	**95**	**93**	**90**	**87**	**85**	**83**	**80**	**77**	**75**	**67**	**65**
Load (pounds or kilograms)	10	10	9	9	9	9	8	8	8	8	7	7
	20	19	19	18	17	17	17	16	15	15	13	13
	30	29	28	27	26	26	25	24	23	23	20	20
	40	38	37	36	35	34	33	32	31	30	27	26
	50	48	47	45	44	43	42	40	39	38	34	33
	60	57	56	54	52	51	50	48	46	45	40	39
	70	67	65	63	61	60	58	56	54	53	47	46
	80	76	74	72	70	68	66	64	62	60	54	52
	90	86	84	81	78	77	75	72	69	68	60	59
	100	95	93	90	87	85	83	80	77	75	67	65
	110	105	102	99	96	94	91	88	85	83	74	72
	120	114	112	108	104	102	100	96	92	90	80	78
	130	124	121	117	113	111	108	104	100	98	87	85
	140	133	130	126	122	119	116	112	108	105	94	91
	150	143	140	135	131	128	125	120	116	113	101	98
	160	152	149	144	139	136	133	128	123	120	107	104
	170	162	158	153	148	145	141	136	131	128	114	111
	180	171	167	162	157	153	149	144	139	135	121	117
	190	181	177	171	165	162	158	152	146	143	127	124
	200	190	186	180	174	170	166	160	154	150	134	130
	210	200	195	189	183	179	174	168	162	158	141	137
	220	209	205	198	191	187	183	176	169	165	147	143
	230	219	214	207	200	196	191	184	177	173	154	150
	240	228	223	216	209	204	199	192	185	180	161	156
	250	238	233	225	218	213	208	200	193	188	168	163
	260	247	242	234	226	221	206	208	200	195	174	169
	270	257	251	243	235	230	224	216	208	203	181	176
	280	266	260	252	244	238	232	224	216	210	188	182
	290	276	270	261	252	247	241	232	223	218	194	189
	300	285	279	270	261	255	249	240	231	225	201	195
	310	295	288	279	270	264	257	248	239	233	208	202
	320	304	298	288	278	272	266	256	246	240	214	208
	330	314	307	297	287	281	274	264	254	248	221	215
	340	323	316	306	296	289	282	272	262	255	228	221
	350	333	326	315	305	298	291	280	270	263	235	228
	360	342	335	324	313	306	299	288	277	270	241	234
	370	352	344	333	322	315	307	296	285	278	248	241

(continued)

TABLE 17.8 *(continued)*

MAX REPS (RM)	1	2	3	4	5	6	7	8	9	10	12	15
%1RM	100	95	93	90	87	85	83	80	77	75	67	65
	380	361	353	342	331	323	315	304	293	285	255	247
	390	371	363	351	339	332	324	312	300	293	261	254
	400	380	372	360	348	340	332	320	308	300	268	260
	410	390	381	369	357	349	340	328	316	308	274	267
	420	399	391	378	365	357	349	336	323	315	281	273
	430	409	400	387	374	366	357	344	331	323	288	280
	440	418	409	396	383	374	365	352	339	330	295	286
	450	428	419	405	392	383	374	360	347	338	302	293
	460	437	428	414	400	391	382	368	354	345	308	299
	470	447	437	423	409	400	390	376	362	353	315	306
	480	456	446	432	418	408	398	384	370	360	322	312
	490	466	456	441	426	417	407	392	377	368	328	319
	500	475	465	450	435	425	415	400	385	375	335	325
	510	485	474	459	444	434	423	408	393	383	342	332
	520	494	484	468	452	442	432	416	400	390	348	338
	530	504	493	477	461	451	440	424	408	398	355	345
	540	513	502	486	470	459	448	432	416	405	362	351
	550	523	512	495	479	468	457	440	424	413	369	358
	560	532	521	504	487	476	465	448	431	420	375	364
	570	542	530	513	496	485	473	456	439	428	382	371
	580	551	539	522	505	493	481	464	447	435	389	377
	590	561	549	531	513	502	490	472	454	443	395	384
	600	570	558	540	522	510	498	480	462	450	402	390

as a percentage of a tested or estimated 1RM, or training loads are specifically determined from multiple-RM testing). The options for testing and assigning training loads and repetitions are summarized in figure 17.2.

Repetition Maximum Continuum

Figure 17.3 shows how RM ranges are associated with training goals; relatively heavy loads should be used if the goal is strength or power, moderate loads for hypertrophy, and light loads for muscular endurance (as indicated by the larger font sizes). To state this another way, low-multiple RMs appear to have the greatest effect on strength and maximum power training, and high-multiple RMs seem to result in better muscular endurance improvements (1, 20, 63, 90). The continuum concept effectively illustrates that a certain RM *emphasizes* a specific outcome, but the training benefits are blended at any given RM.

Percentage of the 1RM

Despite the physiological blend of training effects, the specificity principle still dictates the dominant outcome that is attained and enhanced with a particular training load. The relationship between the percentage of the 1RM and the estimated number of repetitions that can be performed at that load (table 17.7) allows the strength and conditioning professional to assign a specific resistance to be used for an exercise in a training session. In other words, the training goal is attained when the athlete lifts a load of a certain percentage of the 1RM for a specific number of repetitions (table 17.9).

How to Calculate a Training Load   For example, suppose an athlete's training goal is muscular strength and the tested 1RM in the bench press exercise is 220 pounds (100 kg). To increase strength, the athlete needs to handle loads of at least 85% of the 1RM (after

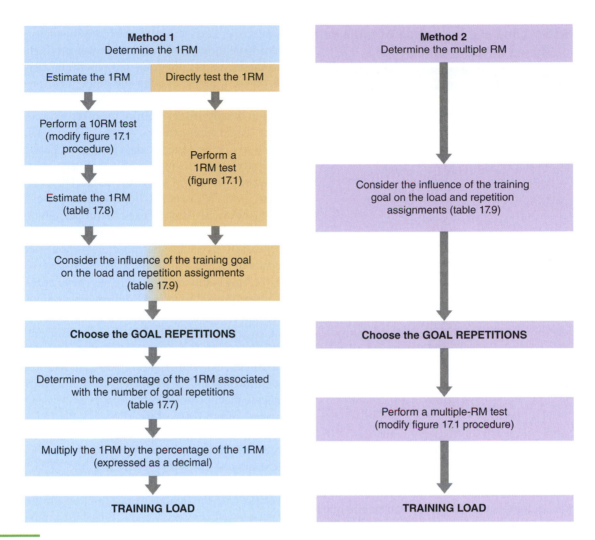

FIGURE 17.2 Summary of testing and assigning training loads and repetitions.

Reprinted, by permission, from Earle, 2006 (18).

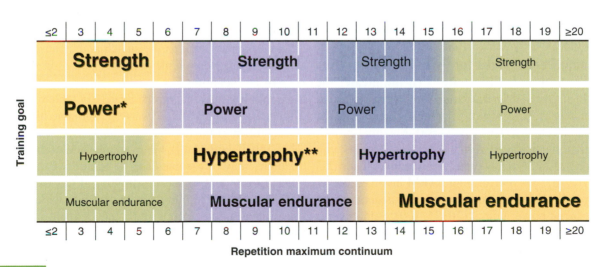

FIGURE 17.3 This continuum shows how RM ranges are associated with various training goals.

*The repetition ranges shown for power in this figure are not consistent with the %1RM–repetition relationship. Refer to the discussion of assigning percentages for power training for further explanation.

**While the existing repetition range for hypertrophy appears most efficacious, there is emerging evidence that some fiber types, depending on training status, may experience significant hypertrophy outside this range. It is too early to tell if these results would be experienced by the larger population.

Adapted from references 20 and 87.

TABLE 17.9   Load and Repetition Assignments Based on the Training Goal

Training goal	Load (%1RM)	Goal repetitions
Strength*	≥85	≤6
Power:**		
Single-effort event	80-90	1-2
Multiple-effort event	75-85	3-5
Hypertrophy	67-85	6-12
Muscular endurance	≤67	≥12

*These RM loading assignments for muscular strength training apply only to core exercises; assistance exercises should be limited to loads not heavier than an 8RM (2).

**Based on weightlifting-derived movements (clean, snatch, and so on). The load and repetition assignments shown for power in this table are *not consistent* with the %1RM–repetition relationship. In nonexplosive movements, loads equaling about 80% of the 1RM apply to the two- to five-repetition range. Refer to the discussion of assigning percentages of the 1RM for power training for further explanation.

Data from references 7, 20, 32, 33, 45, 86, 91, and 92.

warm-up) that typically allow performance of up to six repetitions per set (table 17.9). More specifically, if the strength and conditioning professional assigns four repetitions per set for this exercise, the corresponding load will be approximately 90% of the 1RM (table 17.7), or approximately 200 pounds (90 kg). Note that the strength and conditioning professional should make adjustments to assigned loads based on observation of the ease or difficulty an athlete experiences in lifting the load for the required repetitions.

Assigning Percentages for Power Training   The force–velocity curve illustrates that the greater the amount of concentric muscular force generated, the slower the muscle shortening and corresponding movement velocity (and vice versa). Maximal power, in contrast, is produced at intermediate velocities with the lifting of light to moderate, not maximal, loads (11, 12, 57, 61, 67, 68). Performing a 1RM involves slower movement velocities; maximum force is generated, but with reduced power output (20, 21, 100). Seldom is an athlete required to demonstrate a singular, maximal, slow-speed muscular strength effort in a sport (except in powerlifting, for example). Most sport movements are faster (66) and involve higher power outputs (41) than those produced during a 1RM test. This does not mean that an athlete's power capabilities are unaffected by maximal muscular strength training, however. Because speed- or power-related sport movements often begin

from zero or near-zero velocities, slow-velocity strength gains have direct application to power production (20). For these reasons, the load and repetition assignments for power training overlap the guidelines for strength training (table 17.9).

Non-weightlifting multijoint power exercise (jump squat, bench press throw, overhead press throw) and single-joint muscle action data reveal that peak power is generally reached with the lifting of very light loads— from body weight (0%) to 30% of the 1RM (11, 12, 21, 57, 61, 68). With such a light weight, however, these exercises are difficult to execute properly with typical resistance training equipment because the athlete cannot sufficiently overload the muscles without needing to decelerate at the end of the exercise range of motion. Performing some of these exercises (bench press throw, overhead press throw) in a Smith machine, for example, can help to address the safety issues. The jump squat is one exception and is best performed in a power rack (11, 12, 57, 59, 61, 68). On the other end of the load continuum, data from multiple national- and world-level weightlifting and powerlifting championships clearly indicate that power output increases as the weight lifted decreases from 100% of the 1RM (i.e., the 1RM) to 90% of the 1RM (21, 22, 81). In fact, for the back squat and deadlift exercises, power output for a load at 90% of the 1RM may be *twice* as high as with the 1RM load due to a large decrease in the time required to complete the exercise with the lighter load (22). Even for the already "fast" power exercises (weightlifting-based movements), there is still a 5% to 10% increase in power output as the load decreases from the 1RM to 90% of the 1RM (22). Considering these issues, the most effective and practical application is to assign loads that are about 75% to 90% of the 1RM for resistance training exercises that can be heavily loaded such as the snatch and clean and other weightlifting-derived movements (11, 21, 45, 57, 61).

To promote program specificity, particular load and repetition assignments are indicated for athletes training for *single-effort power events* (e.g., shot put, high jump, weightlifting) and for *multiple-effort power events* (e.g., basketball, volleyball). For example, single-effort event athletes may be assigned sets of one or two repetitions using loads that equal 80% to 90% of the 1RM, especially on heavy training days. For sports with multiple maximum-power efforts (e.g., the frequent maximum vertical jumping motions of a volleyball blocker), three to five repetitions per set with loads at 75% to 85% of the 1RM may be most appropriate (8, 11).

On the basis of the %1RM–repetition relationships shown in table 17.7, the strength and conditioning professional may question the load assignments for power training in table 17.9. The %1RM loads may appear to be too low compared to the goal number of repetitions.

For example, according to table 17.7, three to five repetitions are typically associated with loads 93% to 87% of the 1RM, not 75% to 85% of the 1RM or less as table 17.9 indicates. Power exercises cannot be maximally loaded at any repetition scheme, because the quality of the movement technique will decline before momentary muscle fatigue defines a true multiple-RM set (20). Therefore, lighter loads allow the athlete to complete repetitions with maximum speed to promote maximum power development. For example, power exercises are usually limited to five repetitions per set, but with loads up to and equal to a 10RM (i.e., approximately 75% of the 1RM) (45). This load adjustment to promote peak power output also applies to the RM continuum (figure 17.3). Power training can be emphasized across the range of five repetitions or fewer, but the strength and conditioning professional should realize that these loads are not true repetition *maximums*.

Variation of the Training Load

Training for muscular strength and power places a high physiological stress on an athlete's body. Intermediate and advanced resistance-trained athletes are accustomed to lifting heavy loads and possess the experience and motivation to exert to near failure on every set, but this should not always be the goal. Despite the high training status, this degree of training demand typically cannot be tolerated very long without contributing to an overtrained state. For example, an athlete may resistance train three days a week with muscular strength as the goal (e.g., Mondays, Wednesdays, and Fridays). It would be difficult for the athlete to perform the same high-load, low-volume regimen—especially in the power and other core exercises—with only one or two days of rest between sessions.

One strategy to counterbalance the overtraining associated with the heavy loads is to alter the loads (%1RMs) for the power and other core exercises so that only one training day each week (e.g., Monday) is a heavy day. These "heavy day" loads are designed to be full repetition maximums, the greatest resistance that can be successfully lifted for the goal number of repetitions. The loads for the other training days are reduced (intentionally) to provide recovery after the heavy day while still maintaining sufficient training frequency and volume. In the example of the three-days-a-week program, Wednesdays and Fridays are "light" and "medium" training days (respectively). For the light day, calculate 80% of the loads lifted in the power and other core exercises on the heavy day (Monday) and instruct the athlete to complete the same number of goal repetitions. Even if the athlete is able to perform more repetitions than the designated goal number, he or she should not do so. Similarly, calculate 90% of the loads lifted in the power

and other core exercises from Monday's training session for the "medium" day, and instruct the athlete to perform only the assigned number of goal repetitions (2, 8, 86). This approach can be used for any training frequency. For instance, a two-days-a-week program could have a heavy day and a light day, or an upper body–lower body split routine could consist of two heavy days (one upper body day and one lower body day) followed by two light days. Varying the training loads also works well with an athlete's other training, in that heavy lifting days can fall on light sport conditioning days, and light lifting days on heavy sport conditioning days (8). The strength and conditioning professional needs to monitor this schedule so that it does not lead to heavy training *every* day (86).

Progression of the Training Load

As the athlete adapts to the training stimulus, the strength and conditioning professional needs to have a strategy for advancing exercise loads so that improvements will continue over time (progression). Monitoring each athlete's training and charting his or her response to the prescribed workouts enable the strength and conditioning professional to know when and to what extent the loads should be increased.

Timing Load Increases

A conservative method that can be used to increase an athlete's training loads is called the **2-for-2 rule** (2). If the athlete can perform two or more repetitions over his or her assigned repetition goal for a given exercise in the last set in two consecutive workouts, weight should be added to that exercise for the next training session. For example, a strength and conditioning professional assigns three sets of 10 repetitions in the bench press exercise, and the athlete performs all 10 repetitions in all sets. After several workout sessions (the specific number depends on many factors), the athlete is able to complete 12 repetitions in the third (last) set for two consecutive workouts. In the following training session, the load for that exercise should be increased.

Quantity of Load Increases

The decision as to the size of the load increase can be difficult to make, but table 17.10 provides general recommendations based on the athlete's condition (stronger or weaker) and body area (upper or lower body). Despite these guidelines, the significant variation in training status, volume-loads, and exercises (type and muscular involvement) greatly influences the appropriate load increases. To contend with this variability, relative load increases of 2.5% to 10% can be used instead of the absolute values shown in table 17.10.

TABLE 17.10 Examples of Load Increases

Description of the athlete*	Body area exercise	Estimated load increase**
Smaller, weaker, less trained	Upper body	2.5-5 lb (1-2 kg)
	Lower body	5-10 lb (2-4 kg)
Larger, stronger, more trained	Upper body	5-10+ lb (2-4+ kg)
	Lower body	10-15+ lb (4-7+ kg)

*The strength and conditioning professional will need to determine which of these two subjective categories applies to a specific athlete.

**These load increases are appropriate for training programs using approximately three sets of 5 to 10 repetitions. Note that the goal repetitions per set remain constant as the loads are increased.

Application of the Training Load and Repetition Guidelines

(Refer to the first scenario table in the chapter for a description of the scenario athletes.)

Scenario A Female collegiate basketball player **Preseason**	Scenario B Male professional American football lineman **Off-season**	Scenario C Male high school cross-country runner **In-season**
PRIMARY PRESEASON RESISTANCE TRAINING GOAL Strength/power	**PRIMARY OFF-SEASON RESISTANCE TRAINING GOAL** Hypertrophy	**PRIMARY IN-SEASON RESISTANCE TRAINING GOAL** Muscular endurance
TESTING AND ASSIGNING LOADS AND REPETITIONS **Influence of the training goals** *Power exercises:* 75-85% of the 1RM; 3-5 repetitions[a] *Other core exercises:* >85% of the 1RM; <6 repetitions *Assistance exercises:* limited to loads not heavier than an 8RM	**TESTING AND ASSIGNING LOADS AND REPETITIONS** **Influence of the training goals** 67-85% of the 1RM; 6-12 repetitions	**TESTING AND ASSIGNING LOADS AND REPETITIONS** **Influence of the training goals** <67% of the 1RM; >12 repetitions
Number of goal repetitions *Power exercises:* 5 *Core exercises:* 6 *Assistance exercises:* 10	**Number of goal repetitions** *Core exercises:* 10 *Assistance exercises:* 10	**Number of goal repetitions** *Core exercises:* 12 *Assistance exercises:* 15

Testing methods
 	
3RM testing for power exercises[b]
  Hang clean
  Push jerk
 	
1RM testing for other core exercises[c]
  Front squat
  Incline bench press
 	
10RM testing for assistance exercises[d]
  Seated row
  Dumbbell alternating curl
  Triceps pushdown
	Testing methods
	
	1RM testing for core exercises
	  Deadlift
	  Back squat[i]
	  Bench press[i]
	  Shoulder press[i]
	
	10RM testing for new assistance exercises[j]
	  Step-up
	  Seated calf (heel) raise
	  Bent-over row
	  Shoulder shrug
		Testing methods
		
		12RM testing for core exercises[k]
		  Lunge
		  Vertical chest press
		
		15RM testing for new assistance exercises[k]
		  One-arm dumbbell row
		  Lateral shoulder raise

Scenario A	Scenario B	Scenario C
Female collegiate basketball player **Preseason**	**Male professional American football lineman** **Off-season**	**Male high school cross-country runner** **In-season**

Testing results

Scenario A

3RM hang clean	115 lb (53 kg)
Estimated 1RM[e]	*124 lb (56 kg)*
3RM push jerk	110 lb (50 kg)
Estimated 1RM[e]	*118 lb (54 kg)*
1RM front squat	185 lb (84 kg)
1RM incline bench press	100 lb (45 kg)
10RM seated row	90 lb (41 kg)
10RM dumbbell alternating curl	20 lb (9 kg)
10RM triceps pushdown	40 lb (18 kg)

Scenario B

1RM deadlift	650 lb (295 kg)
1RM back squat	675 lb (307 kg)
1RM bench press	425 lb (193 kg)
1RM shoulder press	255 lb (116 kg)
10RM step-up	205 lb (93 kg)
10RM seated calf (heel) raise	155 lb (70 kg)
10RM bent-over row	215 lb (98 kg)
10RM shoulder shrug	405 lb (184 kg)

Scenario C

12RM lunge	45 lb (20 kg)
12RM vertical chest press	70 lb (32 kg)
15RM one-arm dumbbell row	25 lb (11 kg)
15RM lateral shoulder raise	10 lb (5 kg)

Training loads

Scenario A

For power exercises:
- Assign 75% of the estimated 1RM

Hang clean	95 lb (43 kg)
Push jerk	90 lb (41 kg)

(All loads are rounded off to the nearest 5 lb.)

For other core exercises:
- Assign 85% of the tested 1RM

Front squat	155 lb (70 kg)
Incline bench press	85 lb (39 kg)

(All loads are rounded off to the nearest 5 lb.)

For assistance exercises:
- Assign loads equal to the loads from 10RM testing

Scenario B

For core exercises:
- Assign 75% of the tested 1RM

Deadlift	490 lb (223 kg)
Back squat	505 lb (230 kg)
Bench press	320 lb (145 kg)
Shoulder press	190 lb (86 kg)

(All loads are rounded off to the nearest 5 lb.)

For assistance exercises:
- Assign loads equal to the loads from the 10RM testing or
- Equal to the loads used in the postseason

Leg (knee) curl	190 lb (86 kg)
Barbell biceps curl	115 lb (52 kg)
Lying triceps extension	125 lb (57 kg)

Scenario C

For all exercises:
- Equal to the loads from 12RM (or 15RM) testing or
- Equal to the loads used in the preseason

Leg (knee) curl	65 lb (30 kg)
Toe raise (dorsiflexion)	20 lb (9 kg)
Machine back extension	50 lb (23 kg)

Weekly loading regimen (power/core exercises)[f]

Mondays ("heavy" day)
- Assign the full load assignments (calculated under "Training loads")

Wednesdays ("light" day)
- Assign only 80% of Monday's "heavy day" loads[g]

Fridays ("medium" day)
- Assign only 90% of Monday's "heavy day" loads[h]

(continued)

(continued)

Scenario A	Scenario B	Scenario C
Female collegiate basketball player **Preseason**	**Male professional American football lineman** **Off-season**	**Male high school cross-country runner** **In-season**

COMMENTS

[a]The load and repetition assignments shown for power exercises are based on basketball, a multiple-effort event, and are not consistent with the %1RM–repetition relationship.

[b]To test for power, a multiple-RM (3RM) protocol is used. From the result, the 1RM is estimated and load assignments are made by calculating a percent of the estimated 1RM.

[c]The athlete did perform these exercises in the off-season, but to raise the accuracy of the load assignments for the preseason, the athlete will be tested to determine the current 1RM.

[d]Even though some of these exercises were part of the off-season program, they all require multiple-RM testing because the preseason goal repetitions for these exercises is 10, rather than 12 from the previous season.

[e]Estimate the 1RM using table 17.8.

[f]The loads for the assistance exercises remain constant throughout the week; only the loads for the power and other core exercises change.

[g]Calculate 80% of the loads lifted in Monday's training session and perform the same number of goal repetitions. Even if the athlete is able to, do not allow more repetitions than the designated goal number (power, 5; other core, 6).

[h]Calculate 90% of the loads lifted in Monday's training session and perform the same number of goal repetitions. Even if the athlete is able to, do not allow more repetitions than the designated goal number (power, 5; other core, 6).

COMMENTS

[i]The athlete did perform these exercises in the postseason, but to raise the accuracy of the load assignments for the off-season, the athlete will be tested to determine the current 1RM.

[j]The exercises shown here were selected as new exercises for the off-season program and therefore require 10RM testing. The other assistance exercises were carried over from the postseason and do not require testing because the load and repetition assignments will be identical.

COMMENTS

[k]The exercises shown here were selected as new exercises for the in-season program and therefore require 12RM or 15RM testing. The other assistance exercises were carried over from the preseason and do not require testing because the load and repetition assignments will be identical.

Step 6: Volume

Volume relates to the total amount of weight lifted in a training session (20, 58, 69), and a **set** is a group of repetitions sequentially performed before the athlete stops to rest (20). Repetition-volume is the total number of repetitions performed during a workout session (4, 20, 75, 86), and volume-load is the total number of sets multiplied by the number of repetitions per set, then multiplied by the weight lifted per repetition. For example, the volume-load for two sets of 10 repetitions with 50 pounds (23 kg) would be expressed as $2 \times 10 \times 50$ pounds or 1,000 pounds (454 kg). (If different sets are performed with different amounts of weight, the volumes per set are calculated and then added to obtain the total training session volume.)

In the example just given (a volume-load of 1,000 pounds), multiplying each repetition by the additional factor of vertical displacement of the weight during that repetition would yield the concentric work performed. The displacement factor is fairly constant for a given athlete, so it is not used, but the resulting volume-load is still directly proportional to concentric work. As previously stated, volume-load divided by repetition-volume results in the average weight lifted per repetition, which is related to intensity or the quality of work. In running exercise, the common (rep) volume measure is distance. If an intensity value is known or measured (such as running pace, which relates to percent $\dot{V}O_2$max), then total metabolic energy cost (which is proportional to mechanical work done) can be calculated. This value is comparable to volume-load in resistance exercise. The same concepts are applicable to the number of foot or hand contacts (volume) in plyometric exercise, the number of strokes (volume) in swimming or rowing, or the number of throws or jumps (volume) for various sport activities.

Multiple Versus Single Sets

Some have advocated that one set of 8 to 12 repetitions (after warm-up) performed to volitional muscular failure is sufficient to maximize gains in muscular strength and hypertrophy. Additionally, others have reported increases in maximum strength after the performance of only one set per exercise per session (24, 52, 53).

Single-set training may be appropriate for untrained individuals (20) or during the first several months of training (24), but many studies indicate that higher volumes are necessary to promote further gains in strength, especially for intermediate and advanced resistance-trained athletes (44, 64, 89, 99). Further, the musculoskeletal system will eventually adapt to the stimulus of one set to failure and require the added stimulus of multiple sets for continued strength gains (20). Moreover, performing three sets of 10 repetitions *without going to failure* enhances strength better than one set to failure in 8 to 12 repetitions (46, 48), although the higher training volume with use of three sets is a contributing factor (4, 20, 86). Therefore, an athlete who performs multiple sets from the initiation of his or her resistance training program will increase muscular strength faster than with single-set training (48, 63). The strength and conditioning professional cannot expect, however, that an athlete will be able to successfully complete multiple sets with full RM loads at fixed repetition schemes for every exercise in each training session. Fatigue will affect the number of repetitions that can be performed in later sets.

Training Status

The training status of athletes affects the volume they will be able to safely tolerate. It is appropriate for an athlete to perform only one or two sets as a beginner and to add sets as he or she becomes better trained. As the athlete adapts to a consistent and well-designed program, more sets can gradually be added to match the guidelines associated with the given training goal.

Primary Resistance Training Goal

Training volume is directly based on the athlete's resistance training goal. Table 17.11 provides a summary of the guidelines for the number of repetitions and sets commonly associated with strength, power, hypertrophy, and muscular endurance training programs.

Strength and Power

In classic research, DeLorme (14) and DeLorme and Watkins (15) recommended sets of 10 repetitions as ideal to increase muscular strength, although the regimen was originally developed for injury rehabilitation. Later, Berger (6, 7) determined that three sets of six repetitions created maximal strength gains, at least in the bench press and back squat exercises. Although Berger's work seemed to be conclusive, his subsequent research (5) showed no significant difference among six sets of a 2RM load, three sets of a 6RM load, and three sets of a 10RM load, despite the differences in volume. Since then, many other studies have also been unable to

TABLE 17.11   Volume Assignments Based on the Training Goal

Training goal	Goal repetitions	Sets*
Strength	≤6	2-6
Power:		
Single-effort event	1-2	3-5
Multiple-effort event	3-5	3-5
Hypertrophy	6-12	3-6
Muscular endurance	≥12	2-3

*These assignments do not include warm-up sets and typically apply to core exercises only (2, 45).

**Based on weightlifting-derived movements (clean, snatch, and so on). The load and repetition assignments shown for power in this table are *not consistent* with the %1RM–repetition relationship. In nonexplosive movements, loads equaling about 80% of the 1RM apply to the two- to five-repetition range. Refer to the discussion of assigning percentages of the 1RM for power training for further explanation.

Data from references 20, 32, 86, 91, and 92.

support an exact set and repetition scheme to promote maximal increases in strength (17, 24, 25, 70, 80, 85). An important qualifier regarding these inconclusive reports is that most involved relatively untrained subjects, thus implying that nearly *any* type of program will cause improvements in strength for these individuals.

When training an athlete for strength, assigning volume begins with an examination of the optimal number of repetitions for maximal strength gains. As discussed earlier (and shown in figure 17.3 and table 17.9), this appears to be sets of six or fewer repetitions (at the corresponding RM load) for core exercises (20,

32, 33, 45, 86, 87, 91, 92). Comprehensive reviews of the literature by Fleck and Kraemer (20) and Tan (90) conclude that a range of two to five sets or three to six sets (respectively) promotes the greatest increases in strength. Specific set guidelines based on exercise type suggest that only one to three sets may be appropriate or necessary for assistance exercises (2, 45).

Volume assignments for power training are typically lower than those for strength training in order to maximize the quality of exercise. This reduction in volume results from fewer goal repetitions and lighter loads (figure 17.3 and table 17.9) rather than the recommended

Application of the Volume Guidelines

(Refer to the first scenario table in the chapter for a description of the scenario athletes.)

Scenario A Female collegiate basketball player **Preseason**		Scenario B Male professional American football lineman **Off-season**		Scenario C Male high school cross-country runner **In-season**	
Power exercises	4 sets of 5 repetitions	Core exercises	4 sets of 10 repetitions	Core exercises	3 sets of 12 repetitions
Other core exercises	3 sets of 6 repetitions	Assistance exercises	3 sets of 10 repetitions	Assistance exercises	2 sets of 15 repetitions
Assistance exercises	2 sets of 10 repetitions	(The number of sets does not include warm-ups.)		(The number of sets does not include warm-ups.)	
(The number of sets does not include warm-ups.)					

MONDAY, WEDNESDAY, AND FRIDAY		**LOWER BODY (MONDAY AND THURSDAY)**		**WEDNESDAY AND SATURDAY**	
Hang clean	4 × 5[a]	Deadlift	4 × 10	Lunge	3 × 12
Push jerk	4 × 5	Back squat	4 × 10	Vertical chest press	3 × 12
Front squat	3 × 6	Step-up	3 × 10	Leg (knee) curl	2 × 15
Incline bench press	3 × 6	Leg (knee) curl	3 × 10	One-arm dumbbell row	2 × 15
Seated row	2 × 10	Seated calf (heel) raise	3 × 10	Toe raise (dorsiflexion)	2 × 15
Dumbbell alternating curl	2 × 10	**UPPER BODY (TUESDAY AND FRIDAY)**		Machine back extension	2 × 15
Triceps pushdown	2 × 10	Bench press	4 × 10	Abdominal crunch	3 × 20
Abdominal crunch	3 × 20	Bent-over row	3 × 10	Complete one set of each exercise, then repeat.[b]	
		Shoulder press	4 × 10		
		Barbell biceps curl	3 × 10		
		Shoulder shrug	3 × 10		
		Lying triceps extension	3 × 10		
		Abdominal crunch	3 × 20		

COMMENTS	**COMMENTS**
[a]Represented as sets × repetitions here and in scenarios B and C.	[b]The eight exercises are performed one set at a time, one immediately after the other (i.e., in a "circuit"). Once two sets (circuits) are completed, the athlete performs the final sets of the lunge, vertical chest press, and abdominal crunch exercises in that order.

number of sets (11, 12, 45, 57, 61, 68). The common guideline is three to five sets (after warm-up) for power exercises included in a trained athlete's program (33, 86, 87).

Hypertrophy

It is generally accepted that higher training volumes are associated with increases in muscular size (31, 63). This is the result of both a moderate to higher number of repetitions per set (6 to 12; see figure 17.3 and table 17.9) and the commonly recommended three to six sets per exercise (20, 32, 33, 71, 91). Additionally, although research studies usually focus on only one or two exercises (total or per muscle group), empirical observations and interviews with elite bodybuilders, as well as more exhaustive prescriptive guidelines (20, 45), suggest that performing three or more exercises per muscle group is the most effective strategy for increasing muscle size (32). The effect on training volume from these assignments can be quite substantial.

Muscular Endurance

Resistance training programs that emphasize muscular endurance involve performing many repetitions—12 or more—per set (20, 45, 87, 91, 92). Despite this relatively high repetition assignment, the overall volume-load is not necessarily overly inflated since the loads lifted are lighter and fewer sets are performed, commonly two or three per exercise (45).

Step 7: Rest Periods

The time dedicated to recovery between sets and exercises is called the **rest period** or **interset rest**. The length of the rest period between sets and exercises is highly dependent on the goal of training, the relative load lifted, and the athlete's training status (if the athlete is not in good physical condition, rest periods initially may need to be longer than typically assigned).

The amount of rest between sets is strongly related to load; the heavier the loads lifted, the longer the rest periods the athlete will need between sets in order to safely and successfully complete the prescribed subsequent sets. For example, training for muscular strength with 4RM loads requires significantly longer rest periods between sets than training for muscular endurance in which lighter 15RM loads are lifted (20, 74, 86). Despite the relationship between training goals and the length of rest periods (e.g., long rest periods for muscular strength training programs), not all exercises in a resistance training program should be assigned the same rest periods. It is important that the strength and conditioning professional allocate rest periods based on

the relative load lifted and the amount of muscle mass involved in each exercise. An example of this specificity is for an assistance exercise as part of a muscular strength training program. Whereas a core exercise such as the bench press may involve a 4RM load and a 4-minute rest period, an assistance exercise such as the lateral shoulder raise may be performed with a 12RM load and therefore require only a 1-minute rest period (even though 1-minute rest periods generally apply to a hypertrophy training program). The recommended rest period lengths for strength, power, hypertrophy, and muscular endurance programs are shown in table 17.12.

Strength and Power

Training may enhance an athlete's ability to exercise with less rest (20, 86), but athletes who seek to perform maximal or near-maximal repetitions with a heavy load usually need long rest periods, especially for lower body or all-body structural exercises (95). For example, Robinson and colleagues (77) observed that, in the back squat exercise, 3 minutes of interset rest resulted in greater strength gains than a 30-second rest period. Common guidelines for rest period length are at least 2 minutes (45, 82, 93) or a range of 2 to 5 minutes (47, 50) or 3 to 5 minutes (20, 86, 96). These recovery intervals appear to apply equally to resistance training programs designed to improve maximal strength and those that focus on muscular power (45).

Hypertrophy

Athletes who are interested in gaining muscular size often use a short to moderate interset rest period (20, 45, 47, 74, 86). Some reviews of hypertrophy training

TABLE 17.12   Rest Period Length Assignments Based on the Training Goal

Training goal*	Rest period length
Strength	2-5 min
Power: Single-effort event Multiple-effort event	2-5 min
Hypertrophy	30 s to 1.5 min
Muscular endurance	≤30 s

*Because there are occasions when the prescribed percentage of the 1RM for assistance exercises falls outside the range associated with the training goal (e.g., ≥8RM loads are recommended for assistance exercises as part of a muscular strength training program [2]), the strength and conditioning professional should examine the loads used for each exercise when assigning rest periods rather than generally applying the guidelines for a training goal.

Data from references 20, 47, 50, 86, and 96.

programs support a limited rest period because they recommend that the athlete begin the next set before full recovery has been achieved (32, 91). Despite this, the high metabolic demand of exercises involving large muscle groups merits consideration (i.e., extra recovery time) when rest period lengths are being assigned (86). Typical strategies for the length of rest periods are less than 1.5 minutes (45) or a span of 30 seconds to 1 minute (47, 50, 92) or 30 seconds to 1.5 minutes (32, 91).

Muscular Endurance

A muscular endurance training program has very short rest periods, often less than 30 seconds. This restriction of the recovery time is purposeful; only a minimal

Application of the Rest Period Guidelines

(Refer to the first scenario table in the chapter for a description of the scenario athletes.)

Scenario A Female collegiate basketball player Preseason		Scenario B Male professional American football lineman Off-season		Scenario C Male high school cross-country runner In-season	
Power and core exercises	3 minutes	Core exercises	1.5 minutes	Core exercises	30 seconds[e]
Assistance exercises	60 seconds to 1.5 minutes	Assistance exercises	60 seconds	Assistance exercises	20 seconds[e]
MONDAY, WEDNESDAY, AND FRIDAY		**LOWER BODY (MONDAY AND THURSDAY)**		**WEDNESDAY AND SATURDAY**	
Hang clean	3 minutes	Deadlift	1.5 minutes	Lunge	30 seconds
Push jerk	3 minutes	Back squat	1.5 minutes	Vertical chest press	30 seconds
Front squat	3 minutes	Step-up	1.5 minutes[c]	Leg (knee) curl	20 seconds
Incline bench press	3 minutes	Leg (knee) curl	60 seconds	One-arm dumbbell row	20 seconds
Seated row	1.5 minutes[a]	Seated calf (heel) raise	60 seconds	Toe raise (dorsiflexion)	20 seconds
Dumbbell alternating curl	60 seconds[a]	**UPPER BODY (TUESDAY AND FRIDAY)**		Lateral shoulder raise	20 seconds
Triceps pushdown	60 seconds[a]	Bench press	1.5 minutes	Machine back extension	20 seconds
Abdominal crunch	20 seconds[b]	Bent-over row	60 seconds	Abdominal crunch	20 seconds
		Shoulder press	1.5 minutes	Complete one set of each exercise, then repeat.[f]	
		Barbell biceps curl	60 seconds		
		Shoulder shrug	60 seconds		
		Lying triceps extension	60 seconds		
		Abdominal crunch	20 seconds[d]		
COMMENTS		**COMMENTS**		**COMMENTS**	
[a]Despite following a muscular strength training program, the athlete is performing sets of 10 repetitions in this exercise, a volume assignment for hypertrophy training. Therefore, the length of the rest period should be 30 seconds to 1.5 minutes. The rest period for the single-joint exercises is slightly shorter because fewer muscles are involved. [b]Again, although this athlete is training for muscular strength, she is performing sets of 20 repetitions in this exercise, a volume assignment for muscular endurance. Therefore, the length of the rest period should be ≤30 seconds.		[c]This exercise is classified as an assistance exercise and, like the others, could be assigned a 60-second rest period. Despite this, the step-up is a unilateral exercise that requires more time for completion of each set. Therefore, a longer rest period is provided. [d]Although this athlete is training for hypertrophy, he is performing sets of 20 repetitions in this exercise, a volume assignment for muscular endurance. Therefore, the length of the rest period should be ≤30 seconds.		[e]Both of these rest period assignments fall within the guidelines for muscular endurance training. Due to the higher goal repetitions and lighter loads for assistance exercises, the rest period length was slightly shortened. [f]The eight exercises are performed one set at a time, one immediately after the other (i.e., in a "circuit"). Once two sets (circuits) are completed, the athlete performs the final sets of the lunge, vertical chest press, and abdominal crunch exercises in that order.	

amount of rest is allowed when light loads are being lifted for many repetitions. This type of program is designed to meet the guideline of the specificity principle for muscular endurance (2). Short rest periods are characteristic of circuit training programs (23, 29) in which it is common to alternate exercises and limit rest period lengths to 30 seconds or less (76, 78, 79).

Conclusion

Well-designed programs are based on the application of sound principles during each step of a process referred to as *program design*. The process begins with a needs analysis to determine the specific demands of the sport and the training status of the athlete. With this knowledge, appropriate exercises are selected and training frequency is established. The order of exercises in the workout is considered next, followed by load assignments and training volume choices based on desired training outcomes. Deciding on the length of the rest periods is the last step leading to the design of a sport-specific resistance training program. A composite view that includes all of the program design variables (steps 1-7) for the three scenarios is shown in the scenario table.

Application of All Program Design Variables (Steps 1-7)

(Refer to the first scenario table in the chapter for a description of the scenario athletes.)

Scenario A Female collegiate basketball player **Preseason**		Scenario B Male professional American football lineman **Off-season**		Scenario C Male high school cross-country runner **In-season**	
MONDAY ("HEAVY" DAY)		**LOWER BODY (MONDAY AND THURSDAY)[g]**		**WEDNESDAY AND SATURDAY**	
Hang clean[a]	4 × 5 @ 95 lb (43 kg)	Deadlift[b]	4 × 10 @ 490 lb (223 kg)	Lunge[e]	3 × 12 @ 45 lb (20 kg)
Push jerk[a]	4 × 5 @ 90 lb (41 kg)	Back squat[b]	4 × 10 @ 505 lb (230 kg)	Vertical chest press[e]	3 × 12 @ 70 lb (32 kg)
Front squat[a]	3 × 6 @ 155 lb (70 kg)	Step-up[b]	3 × 10 @ 205 lb (93 kg)	Leg (knee) curl[c]	2 × 15 @ 65 lb (30 kg)
Incline bench press[a]	3 × 6 @ 85 lb (39 kg)	Leg (knee) curl[d]	3 × 10 @ 190 lb (86 kg)	One-arm dumbbell row[c]	2 × 15 @ 25 lb (11 kg)
Seated row[b]	2 × 10 @ 90 lb (41 kg)	Seated calf raise[d]	3 × 10 @ 155 lb (70 kg)	Toe raise[c]	2 × 15 @ 20 lb (9 kg)
Dumbbell alternating curl[d]	2 × 10 @ 20 lb (9 kg)	**UPPER BODY (TUESDAY AND FRIDAY)[g]**		Lateral shoulder raise[c]	2 × 15 @ 10 lb (5 kg)
Triceps pushdown[d]	2 × 10 @ 40 lb (18 kg)	Bench press[b]	4 × 10 @ 320 lb (145 kg)	Machine back extension[c]	2 × 15 @ 50 lb (23 kg)
Abdominal crunch[c]	3 × 20	Bent-over row[d]	3 × 10 @ 215 lb (98 kg)	Abdominal crunch[c]	3 × 20
WEDNESDAY ("LIGHT" DAY)		Shoulder press[b]	4 × 10 @ 190 lb (86 kg)	Complete one set of each exercise, then repeat.[f]	
80% of Monday's load in power/core exercises		Barbell biceps curl[d]	3 × 10 @ 115 lb (52 kg)		
Hang clean[a]	4 × 5 @ 75 lb (34 kg)	Shoulder shrug[d]	3 × 10 @ 405 lb (184 kg)		
Push jerk[a]	4 × 5 @ 70 lb (32 kg)	Lying triceps extension[d]	3 × 10 @ 125 lb (57 kg)		
Front squat[a]	3 × 6 @ 125 lb (57 kg)	Abdominal crunch[c]	3 × 20		
Incline bench press[a]	3 × 6 @ 70 lb (32 kg)				
Seated row	2 × 10 @ 90 lb (41 kg)				
Dumbbell alternating curl[d]	2 × 10 @ 20 lb (9 kg)				
Triceps pushdown[d]	2 × 10 @ 40 lb (18 kg)				
Abdominal crunch	3 × 20				

(continued)

(continued)

Scenario A Female collegiate basketball player Preseason	Scenario B Male professional American football lineman Off-season	Scenario C Male high school cross-country runner In-season
FRIDAY ("MEDIUM" DAY) *90% of Monday's load in power/core exercises* Hang clean[a] 4 × 5 @ 85 lb (39 kg) Push jerk[a] 4 × 5 @ 80 lb (36 kg) Front squat[a] 3 × 6 @ 140 lb (64 kg) Incline bench press[a] 3 × 6 @ 75 lb (34 kg) Seated row[b] 2 × 10 @ 90 lb (41 kg) Dumbbell alternating curl[d] 2 × 10 @ 20 lb (9 kg) Triceps pushdown[d] 2 × 10 @ 40 lb (18 kg) Abdominal crunch 3 × 20		
COMMENTS Rest period lengths: [a]3 minutes [b]1.5 minutes [c]20 seconds [d]60 seconds [e]30 seconds	[g]Reduce the loads on Thursday and Friday by 5% to 10%.	[f]The eight exercises are performed one set at a time, one immediately after the other (i.e., in a "circuit"). Once two sets (circuits) are completed, the athlete performs the final sets of the lunge, vertical chest press, and abdominal crunch exercises in that order.

KEY TERMS

1-repetition maximum (1RM)
2-for-2 rule
agonist
antagonist
assistance exercise
circuit training
compound set
core exercise
exercise history
exercise order
exercise selection
exercise technique experience
goal repetitions
injury analysis
intensity

interset rest
load
mechanical work
movement analysis
multijoint exercise
muscle balance
needs analysis
overload
physiological analysis
power exercise
profile
program design
progression
recovery exercise
repetition

repetition maximum (RM)
repetition-volume
rest period
SAID
set
single-joint exercise
specificity
split routine
structural exercise
superset
training background
training frequency
training status
volume
volume-load

STUDY QUESTIONS

1. The basketball coach says his starting center needs to jump higher. In addition to beginning a plyometric program, which of the following resistance training exercises are MOST specific to this goal?
   I. power clean
   II. leg (knee) curl
   III. front squat
   IV. seated calf (heel) raise
   a. I and III only
   b. II and IV only
   c. I, II, and III only
   d. II, III, and IV only

2. The soccer team is transitioning from off-season to preseason training. How should the team's resistance training frequency be altered?
   a. Increase frequency to improve muscular endurance.
   b. Do not change frequency and add plyometrics.
   c. Decrease frequency to allow increased sport skill practice.
   d. Design a split routine with three days on and one day off.

3. An American football lineman has difficulty driving into defensive linemen and believes he has lost his explosive ability. Which of the following is the BEST exercise order to help this athlete improve his performance?
   a. back squat, hip sled, leg (knee) curl, power clean
   b. power clean, back squat, hip sled, leg (knee) curl
   c. leg (knee) curl, back squat, power clean, hip sled
   d. hip sled, power clean, leg (knee) curl, back squat

4. Which of the following volumes has the potential to increase muscular strength the MOST?
   a. 5 sets of 5 repetitions
   b. 1 set of 5 repetitions
   c. 5 sets of 15 repetitions
   d. 1 set of 15 repetitions

5. A female triathlete needs to improve the muscular endurance of her upper body. Using three sets of 15 repetitions per exercise, which of the following rest period lengths will MAXIMIZE her goal?
   a. 3 minutes
   b. 1.5 minutes
   c. 45 seconds
   d. 30 seconds

CHAPTER 18

Program Design and Technique for Plyometric Training

David H. Potach, PT, and Donald A. Chu, PhD, PT

After completing this chapter, you will be able to

- explain the physiology of plyometric exercise,
- identify the phases of the stretch–shortening cycle,
- identify the components of a plyometric training program,
- design a safe and effective plyometric training program,
- recommend proper equipment for use during plyometric exercise, and
- teach correct execution of lower and upper body plyometric exercises.

Plyometric exercise refers to those activities that enable a muscle to reach maximal force in the shortest possible time. *Plyometric* is a combination of Greek words that literally means to increase measurement (*plio* = more; *metric* = measure) (56). Practically defined, plyometric exercise is a quick, powerful movement using a pre-stretch, or countermovement, that involves the stretch–shortening cycle (SSC) (53). The purpose of plyometric exercise is to increase the power of subsequent movements by using both the natural elastic components of muscle and tendon and the stretch reflex. To effectively use plyometrics as part of a training program, it is important to understand (1) the mechanics and physiology of plyometric exercise, (2) principles of plyometric training program design, and (3) methods of safely and effectively performing specific plyometric exercises.

Plyometric Mechanics and Physiology

Functional movements and athletic success depend on both the proper function of all active muscles and the speed at which these muscular forces are used. The term used to define this force–speed relationship is **power**. When used correctly, plyometric training has consistently been shown to improve the production of muscle force and power (30, 50). This increased production of power is best explained by two proposed models: mechanical and neurophysiological (53).

Mechanical Model of Plyometric Exercise

In the *mechanical model*, elastic energy in the musculotendinous components is increased with a rapid stretch and then stored (3, 14, 31). When this movement is immediately followed by a concentric muscle action, the stored elastic energy is released, increasing the total force production (3, 14, 31). Hill (31) provides an excellent description (illustrated in figure 18.1) that helps with understanding the behavior of skeletal muscle. Of the mechanical model's many elements, it is the **series elastic component (SEC)** that is the workhorse of plyometric exercise. While the SEC includes some muscular components, it is the tendons that constitute the majority of the SEC. When the musculotendinous unit is stretched, as in an eccentric muscle action, the SEC acts as a spring and is lengthened; as it lengthens, elastic energy is stored. If the muscle begins a concentric action immediately after the eccentric action, the stored energy is released, allowing the SEC to contribute to the total force production by naturally returning the muscles and tendons to their unstretched configuration. If a concentric muscle action does not occur immediately following the

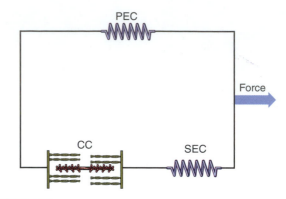

FIGURE 18.1 Mechanical model of skeletal muscle function. The series elastic component (SEC), when stretched, stores elastic energy that increases the force produced. The contractile component (CC) (i.e., actin, myosin, and crossbridges) is the primary source of muscle force during concentric muscle action. The parallel elastic component (PEC) (i.e., epimysium, perimysium, endomysium, and sarcolemma) exerts a passive force with unstimulated muscle stretch.

Based on Albert, 1995 (1).

eccentric action, or if the **eccentric phase** is too long or requires too great a motion about the given joint, the stored energy dissipates and is lost as heat.

Neurophysiological Model of Plyometric Exercise

The *neurophysiological model* involves the **potentiation** (change in the force–velocity characteristics of the muscle's contractile components caused by stretch [21]) of the concentric muscle action by use of the stretch reflex (figure 18.2) (8-11). The **stretch reflex** is the body's involuntary response to an external stimulus that stretches the muscles (27, 42). This reflexive component of plyometric exercise is primarily composed of muscle spindle activity. **Muscle spindles** are proprioceptive organs that are sensitive to the rate and magnitude of a stretch; when a quick stretch is detected, muscular activity reflexively increases (27, 42). During plyometric exercises, the muscle spindles are stimulated by a rapid stretch, causing a reflexive muscle action. This reflexive response potentiates, or increases, the activity in the agonist muscle, thereby increasing the force the muscle produces (8-11, 35). As in the mechanical model, if a concentric muscle action does not immediately follow a stretch (i.e., if there is too long a time between stretch and concentric action or movement over too large a range), the potentiating ability of the stretch reflex is negated.

While it is likely that both the mechanical and neurophysiological models contribute to the increased production of force seen during plyometric exercise (3, 8-11, 14, 31, 35), the degree to which each model con-

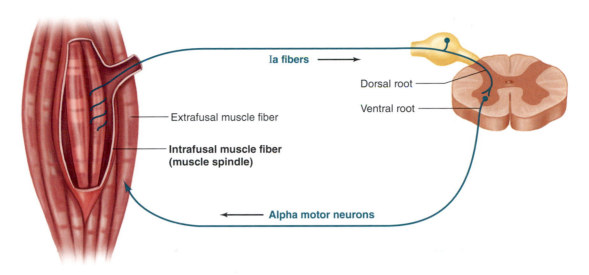

FIGURE 18.2   Illustration of the stretch reflex. When muscle spindles are stimulated, the stretch reflex is stimulated, sending input to the spinal cord via Type Ia nerve fibers. After synapsing with the alpha motor neurons in the spinal cord, impulses travel to the agonist extrafusal fibers, causing a reflexive muscle action.

Based on Wilk et al., 1993 (53).

tributes remains uncertain. Further research is needed to improve our understanding of both models and their respective roles in plyometric exercise.

Stretch–Shortening Cycle

The **stretch–shortening cycle (SSC)** employs the energy storage capabilities of the SEC and stimulation of the stretch reflex to facilitate a maximal increase in muscle recruitment over a minimal amount of time. The SSC involves three distinct phases as shown in table 18.1. While the table delineates the SSC's individual mechanical and neurophysiological events during each phase, it is important to remember that all of the events listed do not necessarily occur within the given phase. That is, some of the events may last longer or may require less time than allowed in the given phase. Phase I is the eccentric phase, which involves preloading the agonist muscle group(s). During this phase, the SEC stores elastic energy, and the muscle spindles are stimulated. As the muscle spindles are stretched, they send a signal to the ventral root of the spinal cord via the Type Ia

afferent nerve fibers (see figure 18.2). To visualize the eccentric phase, consider the long jump. The time from touchdown of the foot to the bottom of the movement is the eccentric phase (figure 18.3a).

Phase II is the time between the eccentric and **concentric phases** and is termed the **amortization** (or transition) **phase**. This is the time from the end of the eccentric phase to the initiation of the concentric muscle action. There is a delay between the eccentric and concentric muscle actions during which Type Ia afferent nerves synapse with the alpha motor neurons in the ventral root of the spinal cord (see figure 18.2). The alpha motor neurons then transmit signals to the agonist muscle group. This phase of the SSC is perhaps the most crucial in allowing greater power production; its duration must be kept short. If the amortization phase lasts too long, the energy stored during the eccentric phase dissipates as heat, and the stretch reflex will not increase muscle activity during the concentric phase (12). Consider the long jumper mentioned earlier. Once the jumper has touched down and movement has stopped, the amortization

TABLE 18.1   Stretch–Shortening Cycle

Phase	Action	Physiological event
I—Eccentric	Stretch of the agonist muscle	Elastic energy is stored in the series elastic component. Muscle spindles are stimulated.
II—Amortization	Pause between phases I and III	Type Ia afferent nerves synapse with alpha motor neurons. Alpha motor neurons transmit signals to agonist muscle group.
III—Concentric	Shortening of agonist muscle fibers	Elastic energy is released from the series elastic component. Alpha motor neurons stimulate the agonist muscle group.

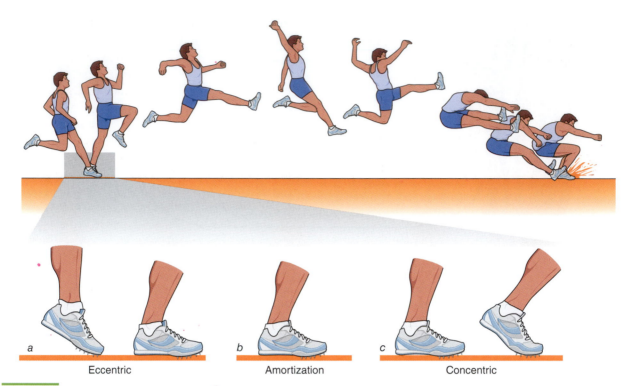

a   Eccentric   b   Amortization   c   Concentric

FIGURE 18.3   The long jump and stretch–shortening cycle. *(a)* The eccentric phase begins at touchdown and continues until the movement ends. *(b)* The amortization phase is the transition from eccentric to concentric phases; it is quick and without movement. *(c)* The concentric phase follows the amortization phase and comprises the entire push-off time, until the athlete's foot leaves the surface.

phase has begun. As soon as movement begins again, the amortization phase has ended (figure 18.3*b*).

The concentric phase, phase III, is the body's response to the eccentric and amortization phases. In this phase, the energy stored in the SEC during the eccentric phase either is used to increase the force of the subsequent movement or is dissipated as heat. This stored elastic energy increases the force produced during the concentric phase movement beyond that of an isolated concentric muscle action (13, 50). In addition, the alpha motor neurons stimulate the agonist muscle group, resulting in a reflexive concentric muscle action (i.e., the stretch reflex). The efficiency of these subsystems is essential to the proper performance of plyometric exercises. Again, visualize the long jumper. As soon as movement begins in an upward direction, the amortization phase has ended and the concentric phase of the SSC has begun (figure 18.3*c*). In this example, one of the agonist muscles is the gastrocnemius. Upon touchdown, the gastrocnemius undergoes a rapid stretch (eccentric phase); there is a delay in movement (amortization phase), and then the muscle concentrically plantar flexes the ankle, allowing the athlete to push off the ground (concentric phase).

The rate of musculotendinous stretch is vital to plyometric exercise (35). A high stretch rate results in greater muscle recruitment and activity during the SSC concentric phase. The importance of the stretch rate

may be illustrated by three different vertical jump tests: a static squat jump, a countermovement jump, and an approach jump with several steps. As the rate of stretch increases, an athlete's absolute performance in these tests improves; the static squat jump results in the lowest jump height, and the approach jump results in the highest. The static squat jump requires the athlete to get into a squatting position (i.e., 90° hip flexion and 90° knee flexion) followed by a jump up. This jump does not use stored elastic energy and is too slow to allow potentiation from the stretch reflex because there is essentially no eccentric phase. The countermovement jump uses a rapid eccentric element (i.e., partial squat) followed immediately by rapid concentric muscle activity (i.e., jump up). The rapid eccentric phase allows the athlete to store (and use) elastic energy in the stretched musculotendinous unit and stimulates the stretch reflex, thereby potentiating muscle activity (6, 29). The approach jump uses an even quicker, more forceful eccentric phase than

> The stretch–shortening cycle combines mechanical and neurophysiological mechanisms and is the basis of plyometric exercise. A rapid eccentric muscle action stimulates the stretch reflex and storage of elastic energy, which increase the force produced during the subsequent concentric action.

the countermovement jump; the increased rate of stretch during the eccentric phase allows a further increase in vertical jump height (4, 5, 7, 25).

Program Design

Plyometric exercise prescription is similar to resistance and aerobic exercise prescriptions—mode, intensity, frequency, duration, recovery, progression, and a warm-up period must all be included in the design of a sound plyometric training program. Unfortunately, there is little research demarcating optimal program variables for the design of plyometric exercise programs. Therefore, when prescribing plyometric exercise, practitioners must rely on the available research, practical experience, and the methodology used for designing resistance and aerobic training programs. The guidelines that follow are largely based on Chu's work (16, 18) and the National Strength and Conditioning Association's position statement (44).

Needs Analysis

To properly design a plyometric training program, the strength and conditioning professional must analyze the needs of the athlete by evaluating his or her sport, sport position, and training status. Each sport and position has its own unique requirements; some requirements are unique because of the movements involved while others have distinctive injury profiles and risks. Further, each athlete possesses a unique training status. Some may be new to training and have never performed plyometric exercises; others may have been injured. Each of these populations of athlete requires a different approach to plyometric training. By understanding each sport's individual requirements, the positions within the sport, and of the needs of each athlete, the strength and conditioning professional is better able to design a safe, effective plyometric training program.

Mode

The mode of plyometric training is determined by the body region performing the given exercise. For example, a single-leg hop is a lower body plyometric exercise, while a two-hand medicine ball **throw** is an upper body exercise. Modes of plyometric exercise are discussed in the paragraphs that follow.

Lower Body Plyometrics

Lower body plyometrics are appropriate for virtually any athlete and any sport, including track and field throwing and sprinting, soccer, volleyball, basketball, American football, baseball, and even endurance sports such as distance running and triathlons. Many of these sports require athletes to produce a maximal amount

of muscular force in a short amount of time. American football, baseball, and sprinting generally require horizontal or lateral movement during competition, while volleyball involves primarily horizontal and vertical movements. Soccer and basketball players must make quick, powerful movements and changes of direction in all planes to compete successfully. A basketball center is an example of an athlete who would benefit greatly from a plyometric training program, as the center is required to jump repeatedly for rebounds. To be successful, the center must be able to out-jump the opposing center in order to rebound more loose balls. Lower body plyometric training gives the player the ability to produce more force in a shorter amount of time, thereby allowing a higher jump. Further, participation in a plyometric training program improves running and cycling performance for endurance athletes by allowing muscles to produce more force with less energy.

The various lower body plyometric drills have differing intensity levels and directional movements. Types of lower body plyometric drills include **jumps in place**, **standing jumps**, **multiple hops and jumps**, **bounds**, **box drills**, and **depth jumps**. See table 18.2 for descriptions of these drills.

Upper Body Plyometrics

Rapid, powerful upper body movements are requisites for several sports and activities, including baseball, softball, tennis, golf, and throws in track and field (i.e., the shot put, discus, and javelin). As an example, an elite baseball pitcher routinely throws a baseball at 80 to 100 miles per hour (129-161 km/h). To reach velocities of this magnitude, the pitcher's shoulder joint must move at more than 6,000°/s (19, 22, 23, 46). Plyometric training of the shoulder joint would not only increase pitching velocity; it may also prevent injury to the shoulder and elbow joints, although further research is needed to substantiate the role of plyometrics in injury prevention.

Plyometric drills for the upper body are not used as often as those for the lower body and have been studied less extensively, but they are nonetheless essential to athletes who require upper body power (45). Plyometrics for the upper body include medicine ball throws, catches, and several types of **push-ups**.

Trunk Plyometrics

In general, it is difficult to perform true plyometric drills that directly target trunk musculature, because all the requisite plyometric elements may not be present. Plyometric exercise uses stored elastic energy (mechanical model) and potentiates muscle activity through stimulation of the stretch reflex (neurophysiological model). Following the eccentric phase of the SSC, there is likely some storage of elastic energy during "plyometric" trunk

TABLE 18.2   Lower Body Plyometric Drills

Type of drill	Rationale
Jumps in place	These drills involve jumping and landing in the same spot. Jumps in place emphasize the vertical component of jumping and are performed repeatedly, without rest between jumps; the time between jumps is the stretch–shortening cycle's amortization phase. Examples of jumps in place include the squat jump and tuck jump.
Standing jumps	These emphasize either horizontal or vertical components. Standing jumps are maximal efforts with recovery between repetitions. The vertical jump and jumps over barriers are examples of standing jumps.
Multiple hops and jumps	Multiple hops and jumps involve repeated movement and may be viewed as a combination of jumps in place and standing jumps. One example of a multiple jump is the zigzag hop.
Bounds	Bounding drills involve exaggerated movements with greater horizontal speed than other drills. Volume for bounding is typically measured by distance but may be measured by the number of repetitions performed. Bounding drills normally cover distances greater than 98 feet (30 m) and may include single- and double-leg bounds in addition to the alternate-leg bounds illustrated in this chapter.
Box drills	These drills increase the intensity of multiple hops and jumps by using a box. The box may be used to jump on or off. The height of the box depends on the size of the athlete, the landing surface, and the goals of the program. Box drills may involve one, both, or alternating legs.
Depth jumps	Depth jumps use gravity and the athlete's weight to increase exercise intensity. The athlete assumes a position on a box, steps off, lands, and immediately jumps vertically, horizontally, or to another box. The height of the box depends on the size of the athlete, the landing surface, and the goals of the program. Depth jumps may involve one or both legs.

drills. However, research supports the notion that the stretch reflex is not sufficiently involved during many trunk exercises to potentiate muscle activity. Stretch reflex latencies (time from reflex stimulation to the beginning of agonist muscle activity) largely depend on nerve conduction velocities and therefore increase with greater distances from the spinal cord (i.e., longer nerves) (34, 36, 38, 47). Quadriceps and gastrocnemius stretch reflexes typically range from 20 to 30 ms and from 30 to 45 ms, respectively (34, 47). Although no research has addressed abdominal stretch reflexes, it may be assumed that the latencies are shorter, as the muscles are closer to the spinal cord.

Exercises for the trunk may be performed "plyometrically," provided that movement modifications are made. Specifically, the exercise movements must be shorter and quicker to allow stimulation and use of the stretch reflex. The relatively large range of motion and the time needed to complete the movement do not permit reflexive potentiation of the abdominal muscles. The exercise can be modified to decrease both the range of motion and time, thereby allowing the agonist muscles to be potentiated and making the exercise more like a plyometric exercise.

Intensity

Plyometric intensity is the amount of stress placed on involved muscles, connective tissues, and joints and is controlled primarily by the type of drill performed. The intensity of plyometric drills covers a large range; skipping is relatively low in intensity, while depth jumps place high stress on the muscles and joints. In addition to the type of drill, several other factors also affect plyometric intensity (table 18.3). Generally, as intensity

TABLE 18.3   Factors Affecting the Intensity of Lower Body Plyometric Drills

Factor	Effect
Points of contact	The ground reaction force during single-leg lower body plyometric drills places more stress on an extremity's muscles, connective tissues, and joints than during double-leg plyometric drills.
Speed	Greater speed increases the intensity of the drill.
Height of the drill	The higher the body's center of gravity, the greater the force on landing.
Body weight	The greater the athlete's body weight, the more stress is placed on muscles, connective tissues, and joints. External weight (in the form of weight vests, ankle weights, and wrist weights) can be added to the body to increase a drill's intensity.

increases, volume should decrease (49). Because the intensity of plyometric exercise can vary significantly, careful consideration must be given to choosing proper drills during a specific training cycle.

Frequency

Frequency is the number of plyometric training sessions per week and typically ranges from one to three, depending on the sport, the athlete's experience with plyometric training, and the time of year. As with other program variables, research is limited on the optimal frequency for training plyometrically. Because the literature is sparse, strength and conditioning professionals often rely on practical experience when determining the frequency with which athletes train using plyometric exercise. Rather than concentrating on the frequency, many authors suggest relying more on the recovery time between plyometric training sessions (16). Forty-eight to 72 hours between plyometric sessions is a typical recovery time guideline for prescribing plyometrics (16); using these typical recovery times, athletes commonly perform two to three plyometric sessions per week. But the time of year, sport, and experience are more commonly used determinants of the frequency of plyometric training.

As previously mentioned, plyometric frequency may vary depending on the demands of the given sport, intensity and volume of daily workouts (e.g., practice, resistance training, running, and plyometrics), athlete experience with plyometric training, and time of the training cycle. For example, during the season, one session per week is appropriate for American football players, while two or three sessions per week are common for track and field athletes (2). During the off-season, plyometric training frequency may increase to two or three sessions per week for American football players and to three or four sessions per week for track and field athletes (2). Because research thus far is unfortunately insufficient to provide appropriate guidelines for plyometric training frequency, the use of proper recovery times between sessions and practical experience may be the best determinants of frequency.

Recovery

Because plyometric drills involve maximal efforts to improve anaerobic power, complete and adequate recovery (the time between repetitions, sets, and workouts) is required (44). Recovery for depth jumps may consist of 5 to 10 seconds of rest between repetitions and 2 to 3 minutes between sets. The time between sets is determined by a proper work-to-rest ratio (i.e., 1:5 to 1:10) and is specific to the volume and type of drill being performed. Drills should not be thought of as cardiorespiratory conditioning exercises but as power training. As with resistance training, recovery between workouts must be adequate to prevent overtraining (two to four days of recovery, depending on the sport and time of year). Furthermore, drills for a given body area should not be performed two days in succession (44). Although new research tangentially addresses recovery and training frequency (47), manipulation of recovery time between repetitions, exercises, and workouts has yet to be adequately explored in plyometric research; further work must be done in this area to provide more concrete times for recovery.

Volume

Plyometric volume is typically expressed as the number of repetitions and sets performed during a given training session. Lower body plyometric volume is normally given as the number of foot contacts (each time a foot, or the feet together, contact the surface) per workout (2, 16) but may also be expressed as distance, as with plyometric bounding. For example, an athlete beginning a plyometric training program may start with a double-leg bound for 98 feet (30 m) per repetition but may progress to 328 feet (100 m) per repetition for the same drill. Recommended lower body plyometric volumes vary for athletes of different levels of experience; suggested volumes are provided in table 18.4. Upper body plyometric volume is typically expressed as the number of throws or catches per workout.

Program Length

Research has yet to determine an optimal plyometric training program length. Currently, most programs range from 6 to 10 weeks (2, 30); however, vertical jump height improves as quickly as four weeks after the start of a plyometric training program (47). In general, plyometric training should be prescribed similarly to both resistance and aerobic training. For those sports requiring quick, powerful movements, it is beneficial to perform plyometric exercise throughout the training cycle (macrocycle). The intensity and volume of the chosen drills should vary with the sport and the season (i.e., off-season, preseason, or in-season).

TABLE 18.4   Appropriate Plyometric Volumes

Plyometric experience	Beginning volume*
Beginner (no experience)	80 to 100
Intermediate (some experience)	100 to 120
Advanced (considerable experience)	120 to 140

*Volume is given in contacts per session.

Steps for Implementing a Plyometric Training Program

1. Evaluate the athlete, including the athlete's sport and training history.
2. Establish sport-, position-, and athlete-specific goals.
3. Assign proper plyometric training program design variables, addressing intensity, frequency, recovery, volume, and program length.
4. Teach the athlete proper jumping, landing, and throwing technique.
5. Properly progress the plyometric training program.

Progression

Plyometrics is a form of resistance training and thus must follow the principles of progressive overload. *Progressive overload* is the systematic increase in training frequency, volume, and intensity in various combinations. Typically, as intensity increases, volume decreases. The sport, training phase, and design of the strength and conditioning program (resistance training, running, plyometrics, and time of year) determine the training schedule and method of progressive overload. An off-season plyometric program for American football, for example, may be performed twice a week. The program should progress from low to moderate volumes of low-intensity plyometrics, to low to moderate volumes of moderate intensity, to low to moderate volumes of moderate to high intensity.

Warm-Up

As in any training program, the plyometric exercise session must begin with a general warm-up, stretching, and a specific warm-up (refer to chapter 14 for a discussion of warming up). The specific warm-up for plyometric training should consist of low-intensity, dynamic movements. Refer to table 18.5 for a list and explanation of types of specific warm-up drills.

> ▶ **Effective plyometric programs include the same variables that are essential to any training program design: mode, intensity, frequency, recovery, volume, program length, progression, and warm-up.**

Age Considerations

It is becoming more common for younger and older individuals to want to augment the training programs for their sport with plyometric exercise. When these exercises are applied appropriately, these populations can experience the same positive outcomes as other age groups, with minimal risk of injury.

Adolescents

Although plyometrics have commonly been viewed as appropriate only for conditioning elite adult athletes, pre-

TABLE 18.5   Plyometric Warm-Up Drills

Drill	Explanation
Marching	Mimics running movements Emphasizes posture and movement technique Enhances proper lower body movements for running
Jogging	Prepares for impact and high-intensity plyometric drills • Toe jogging—not allowing heel to touch the ground (emphasizes quick reaction) • Straight-leg jogging—not allowing or minimizing leg flexion in preparation for impact of plyometric drills • "Butt-kickers"—flexing knee to allow heel to touch the buttocks
Skipping	Exaggerated form of reciprocal upper and lower extremity movements Emphasis on quick takeoff and landing, mimics plyometric activities
Footwork	Drills that target changes of direction Preparation for changes of direction during plyometric drills Examples: shuttle, shuffle, pattern, and stride drills
Lunging	Based on the forward step lunge exercise May be multidirectional (e.g., forward, side, backward)

pubescent and adolescent children may also benefit from training with plyometric and plyometric-like exercises. Besides providing the well-documented muscular power and bone strength adaptations, regular participation in an appropriately designed plyometric training program can better prepare young athletes for the demands of sport practice and competition (17) by enhancing neuromuscular control and performance. Research has yet to determine a universal age at which people are physically able to begin participating in a plyometric training program. An analysis of the body's development provides some insight into the issue. Because the epiphyseal plates of the bones of prepubescent children have yet to close (33, 40), depth jumps and other high-intensity lower body drills are contraindicated (2, 32, 39). While the growth plates are open, highly intense activity and injury may cause them to close prematurely, resulting in limb length discrepancies (32). Further, and as with all forms of exercise, boys and girls should have the emotional maturity to accept and follow directions and should be able to appreciate the benefits and concerns associated with this method of training. Empirically, 7- and 8-year-olds have been trained in progressive plyometric programs, and they continue to lead active lives as teenagers and adults (17).

Plyometric exercise programs for children should be used to develop the neuromuscular control and the anaerobic skills that will carry over to safer participation in sport and athletics, both during childhood and as they advance to higher levels of competition. As an example, several research studies cite the benefits of using proper landing technique as a method of reducing an athlete's risk of lower extremity injury (figure 18.4). Excessive inward (valgus) movement of the knees dramatically increases an athlete's risk of knee injury (see chapter 22 for a more detailed discussion on this topic).

It is extremely important that plyometric exercise programs for children gradually progress from relatively simple to more complex drills. It is important to focus on the quality of the movements (e.g., proper body alignment and speed of movement) to develop techniques that will be essential for more advanced exercises.

As with adults, recovery between workouts must be adequate to prevent overtraining. While the optimal amount of recovery needed between plyometric workouts is unknown, it should vary based on the intensity of the training program and the athlete's skills, abilities, and tolerances as well as on the time of year (i.e., off-season, preseason, or in-season). Therefore, a minimum of two or three days between plyometric workouts should be considered essential to optimize adaptations to the training program and minimize the athlete's risk of injury (17).

> **Under proper supervision and with an appropriate program, prepubescent and adolescent children may perform plyometric exercises. Special attention to valgus positioning must be given to reduce an athlete's risk of lower extremity injury. Depth jumps and high-intensity lower body plyometrics are contraindicated for this population.**

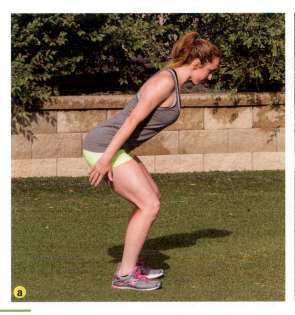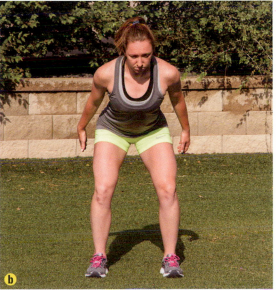

FIGURE 18.4   Proper plyometric landing position. *(a)* When viewed from the side, the shoulders are in line with the knees, which helps to place the center of gravity over the body's base of support. *(b)* When viewing from the front, note that the athlete's knees are over her toes; excessive inward (valgus) movement increases the athlete's risk of lower extremity injury.

Masters

Masters athletes find that they can maintain their physical capabilities late into life and are looking for additional training insights. When designing a plyometric training program for a masters athlete, the strength and conditioning professional needs to be specific in deciding on the goal or goals of the program. Some primary issues to consider are any preexisting orthopedic conditions (such as osteoarthritis or any sort of surgical joint intervention) or joint degeneration. These call for even greater caution and a more careful use of plyometric exercise. For example, a healthy masters athlete without surgical history who wants to improve his or her running performance should use depth jumps and single-leg exercises cautiously, so alternate-leg bounding and the double-leg hopping would be better choices. Similarly, a masters runner with a history of knee surgery such as partial meniscus removal, or with significant joint degeneration, should regard depth jumps and single-leg plyometric exercises as contraindicated and use other forms of plyometrics cautiously.

After consideration of the predispositions related to the masters athlete's physical condition, a plyometric program should be designed according to the same guidelines as outlined for adult athletes, with the following changes. The plyometric program should include no more than five low- to moderate-intensity exercises; the volume should be lower, that is, should include fewer total foot contacts than a standard plyometric training program; and the recovery time between plyometric workouts should be three or four days. With these guidelines in place—and as with all athletes—it is important to note how the masters athlete feels after training and recovery. Soreness may occur, but the program should be modified if chronic or excessive pain or discomfort is present.

Plyometrics and Other Forms of Exercise

Plyometric exercise is only one part of an athlete's overall training program. Many sports and activities use multiple energy systems or require other forms of exercise to properly prepare athletes for competition. Each energy system and sport-specific need must be included in a well-designed training program.

Plyometric Exercise and Resistance Training

A combination of plyometrics and resistance training during a training cycle should be structured to allow maximal efficiency and physical improvement. The following list and table 18.6 provide guidelines for developing a combined program.

- Combine lower body resistance training with upper body plyometrics, and upper body resistance training with lower body plyometrics.
- Performing heavy resistance training and plyometrics on the same day is not usually recommended (15, 20). However, some athletes may benefit from **complex training**, a combination of high-intensity resistance training followed by plyometrics. If athletes perform this type of training, adequate recovery is needed between plyometrics and other high-intensity training.
- Traditional resistance training exercises may be combined with plyometric movements to further enhance gains in muscular power (54, 55). For example, performing a squat jump with approximately 30% of one's squat 1-repetition maximum (1RM) as an external resistance further increases performance (54, 55). This is an advanced form of complex training that is appropriate only for athletes who have previously participated in high-intensity plyometric training programs.

Plyometric and Aerobic Exercise

Many sports—such as basketball and soccer—have both an anaerobic (i.e., power) and an aerobic component. Therefore, multiple types of training must be combined to best prepare athletes for these types of sports. Because aerobic exercise may have a negative effect on power production (15), it is advisable to perform plyometric exercise before aerobic endurance training. The design variables do not change and should complement each other to most effectively train these athletes for competition.

TABLE 18.6   Sample Schedule for Integrating Resistance Training and Plyometrics

Day	Resistance training	Plyometrics
Monday	High-intensity upper body	Low-intensity lower body
Tuesday	Low-intensity lower body	High-intensity upper body
Thursday	Low-intensity upper body	High-intensity lower body
Friday	High-intensity lower body	Low-intensity upper body

Safety Considerations

Plyometric exercise is not inherently dangerous; however, as with all modes of exercise, the risk of injury exists. Injuries can occur simply due to an accident, but they more typically occur when proper training procedures are violated and may be the result of an insufficient strength and conditioning base, inadequate warm-up, improper progression of lead-up drills, inappropriate volume or intensity for the phase of training, poor shoes or surface, or a simple lack of skill. The following sections identify and address these and other risk factors. Knowledge of risk factors can improve the safety of athletes performing plyometric exercise.

Pretraining Evaluation of the Athlete

To reduce the risk of injury and facilitate the performance of plyometric exercises, the athlete must understand proper plyometric technique and possess a sufficient base of strength, speed, and balance. In addition, the athlete must be sufficiently mature, both physically and psychologically, to participate in a plyometric training program. The following evaluative items can help determine whether an athlete meets these conditions.

Technique

Before adding any drill to an athlete's plyometric program, the strength and conditioning professional must demonstrate proper technique to the athlete in order to maximize the drill's effectiveness and minimize the risk of injury. For lower body plyometrics, proper landing technique is essential, particularly for depth jumps. If the center of gravity is offset from the base of support, performance is hindered and injury may occur. The shoulders should be over the knees and the knees over the toes during the landing, which the jumper accomplishes through flexion of the ankles, knees, and hips. In addition, when one views the frontal plane motion of the athlete performing lower body plyometrics, it is essential that the knees be positioned over the toes (figure 18.4). Inward movement of the knees—also termed *dynamic valgus*—is a significant risk factor for knee injuries of all types, including patellofemoral pain and tears or ruptures of the anterior cruciate ligament (ACL).

Strength

Consideration of the athlete's level of strength is necessary before he or she performs plyometrics. For lower body plyometrics, previous recommendations held that the athlete's 1RM squat should be at least 1.5 times his or her body weight (15, 20, 32, 44, 52). However, we would suggest that a more important consideration is technique. Many plyometric activities can be safely

taught to young athletes. It is our recommendation that plyometrics be included for all athletes whose sports require running, landing, jumping, or cutting. Teaching proper alignment and movement mechanics through the use of plyometric exercise has not been shown to cause injuries; instead, this type of training has been repeatedly shown to decrease the athlete's risk of injury during practices and games (43).

Balance

A less obvious lower body plyometric requirement is balance. **Balance** is the maintenance of a position without movement for a given period of time. Many lower body plyometric drills require the athlete to move in nontraditional patterns (e.g., double-leg zigzag hop and backward skip) or on a single leg (e.g., single-leg tuck jump and single-leg hop). These types of drills necessitate a solid, stable base of support upon which the athlete can safely and correctly perform the exercises. Three balance tests are provided in table 18.7, listed in order of difficulty; each test position must be held for 30 seconds (51). For example, an athlete beginning plyometric training for the first time would be required to stand on one leg for 30 seconds without falling. An experienced athlete beginning an advanced plyometric training program must maintain a single-leg half squat for 30 seconds without falling. The surface on which the balance testing is performed must be the same as that used in the plyometric drills.

Physical Characteristics

Athletes who weigh more than 220 pounds (100 kg) may be at an increased risk for injury when performing plyometric exercises (44, 52). Greater weight increases the compressive force on joints during the exercises, thereby predisposing these joints to injury. Therefore, athletes weighing over 220 pounds (100 kg) should avoid high-volume, high-intensity plyometric exercises and depth jumps from heights greater than 18 inches (46 cm) (44, 52). As with other forms of exercise, an athlete's joint structure and previous injuries must also be

TABLE 18.7   Balance Tests

Test	Variations
Standing	Double leg
	Single leg
Quarter squat	Double leg
	Single leg
Half squat	Double leg
	Single leg

examined before he or she begins a plyometric training program. Previous injuries or abnormalities of the spine, lower extremities, or upper extremities may increase an athlete's risk of injury during plyometric exercise. Specifically, athletes with a history of muscle strains, pathological joint laxity, or spinal dysfunction—including vertebral disk dysfunction or compression—should use caution when beginning a plyometric training program (24, 25, 32, 48).

Equipment and Facilities

In addition to participants' fitness and health, the area and equipment used for plyometric drills may significantly affect their safety.

Landing Surface

To prevent injuries, the landing surface used for lower body plyometrics must possess adequate shock-absorbing properties. A grass field, suspended floor, or rubber mat is a good surface choice (32). Surfaces such as concrete, tile, and hardwood are not recommended because they lack effective shock-absorbing properties (32). Excessively thick exercise mats (6 inches [15 cm] or thicker) may extend the amortization phase and thus not allow efficient use of the stretch reflex. Mini-trampolines are commonly used for beginning plyometric and balance training in rehabilitation (28). While these devices may provide a necessary introduction to plyometrics, especially for those recovering from musculoskeletal injury, mini-trampolines, like thick exercise mats, are not effective for plyometric training of uninjured athletes because the amortization phase is extended while the athlete is in contact with the elastic surface.

Training Area

The amount of space needed depends on the drill. Most bounding and running drills require at least 30 m (33 yards) of straightaway, though some drills may require a straightaway of 100 m (109 yards). For most standing, box, and depth jumps, only a minimal surface area is needed, but the ceiling height must be 3 to 4 m (9.8-13.1 feet) in order to be adequate.

Equipment

Boxes used for box jumps and depth jumps must be sturdy and should have a nonslip top. Boxes should range in height from 6 to 42 inches (15 to 107 cm) and should have landing surfaces of at least 18 by 24 inches (46 by 61 cm) (16). The box should be constructed of sturdy wood (e.g., 3/4-inch [1.9 cm] plywood) or heavy-gauge metal. To further reduce injury risk, there are several ways of making the landing surface nonslip: adding nonslip treads, mixing sand into the paint used

to cover the box, or affixing rubberized flooring to the top (16).

Proper Footwear

Participants must use footwear with good ankle and foot support, good lateral stability, and a wide, nonslip sole (44). Shoes with a narrow sole and poor upper support (e.g., running shoes) may invite ankle problems, especially with lateral movements. Shoes with insufficient foot support may lead to arch or lower leg injuries or both, while footwear without enough cushioning might lead to damage of more proximal joints (e.g., knee and hip joints).

Supervision

In addition to the safety considerations already outlined, close monitoring of athletes is necessary to ensure proper technique. Plyometric exercise is not intrinsically dangerous when performed correctly; but as with other forms of training, poor technique may unnecessarily predispose an athlete to injury.

Depth Jumping

There is a limit to the maximal height at which a depth jump can be effectively and safely performed. A height of 48 inches (1.2 m) would provide a significant overload on the muscles, but the resistance may be too great for many athletes to overcome while maintaining correct technique (40). Jumping from such a height increases the possibility of injury; furthermore, the amount of force to be overcome is so great that the amortization phase is extended and thus the purpose of the exercise defeated. The recommended height for depth jumps ranges from 16 to 42 inches (41 to 107 cm), with 30 to 32 inches (76 to 81 cm) being the norm (4, 18, 26, 37, 38, 41). Depth jump box height for athletes who weigh over 220 pounds (100 kg) should be 18 inches (46 cm) or less.

Conclusion

The major goal of plyometric training is to rapidly apply force to provide an overload to the agonist muscles. Although it has been repeatedly shown that plyometric exercise increases muscular power for participants in a formal training program (30, 47, 54, 55), research has yet to determine whether mechanical or neurophysiological adaptations account for the improvement. Plyometrics should be considered not an end in itself, but part of an overall program that includes strength, speed, aerobic, and flexibility training, and proper nutrition. After the athlete has begun a proper strength and conditioning program, plyometric training may be used to further develop power.

PLYOMETRIC DRILLS

18.1   TWO-FOOT ANKLE HOP

Intensity level: Low

Direction of jump: Vertical

Starting position: Get into a comfortable, upright stance with feet shoulder-width apart.

Arm action: None or double arm

Preparatory movement: Begin with a slight countermovement.

Upward movement: Hop up, with primary motion at the ankle joint.

Downward movement: Land in the starting position and immediately repeat hop.

Note: This drill should be performed with little horizontal (forward or backward) or lateral movement.

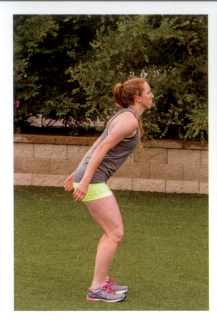
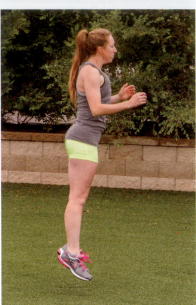

18.2   SINGLE-LEG ANKLE HOP

Intensity level: Medium

Direction of jump: Vertical

Starting position: Get into a comfortable, upright stance on one foot. The nonjumping leg is held in a stationary position with the knee flexed during the exercise.

Arm action: None or double arm

Preparatory movement: Begin with a slight countermovement.

Upward movement: Using the balancing foot, hop up, with primary motion at the ankle joint.

Downward movement: Land in the starting position and immediately repeat the hop using the same leg.

Repeat with the opposite leg after a brief rest.

Note: This drill should be performed with little horizontal (forward or backward) or lateral movement.

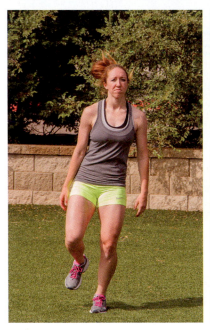
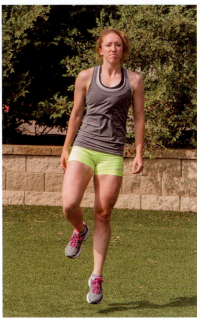

18.3   SQUAT JUMP

Intensity level: Low

Direction of jump: Vertical

Starting position: Get into a squat position (thighs slightly above parallel with the ground) with feet shoulder-width apart. Interlock fingers and place hands behind head.

Arm action: None

Preparatory movement: None

Upward movement: Explosively jump up to a maximum height.

Downward movement: Land in the squat position and immediately repeat the jump.

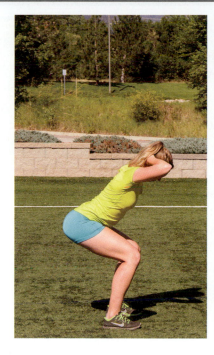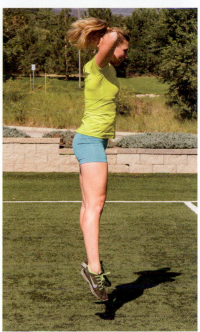

18.4   JUMP AND REACH

Intensity level: Low

Direction of jump: Vertical

Starting position: Get into a comfortable, upright stance with feet shoulder-width apart.

Arm action: Double arm with reach at top of jump

Preparatory movement: Begin with a countermovement.

Upward movement: Explosively jump up and reach for an object or target.

Downward movement: Land in starting position and immediately repeat jump.

Note: Emphasis is on vertical height with minimal delay between jumps.

Note: This drill should be performed with little horizontal (forward or backward) or lateral movement.

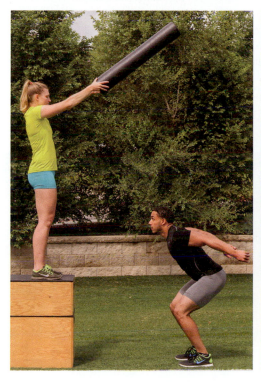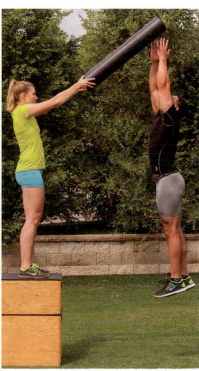

18.5   DOUBLE-LEG TUCK JUMP

Intensity level: Medium

Direction of jump: Vertical

Starting position: Get into a comfortable, upright stance with feet shoulder-width apart.

Arm action: Double arm

Preparatory movement: Begin with a countermovement.

Upward movement: Explosively jump up. Pull the knees to the chest, quickly grasp the knees with both hands, and release before landing.

Downward movement: Land in the starting position and immediately repeat the jump.

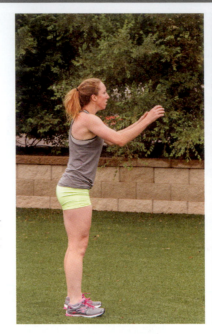
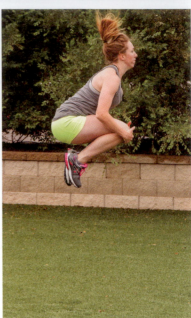

18.6   SPLIT SQUAT JUMP

Intensity level: Medium

Direction of jump: Vertical

Starting position: Get into a lunge position with one leg forward (hip and knee joints flexed approximately 90°) and the other behind the midline of the body.

Arm action: Double arm or none

Preparatory movement: Begin with a countermovement.

Upward movement: Explosively jump up, using the arms to assist as needed. Maximum height and power should be emphasized.

Downward movement: When landing, maintain the lunge position (same leg forward) and immediately repeat the jump.

Note: After completing a set, rest and switch front legs.

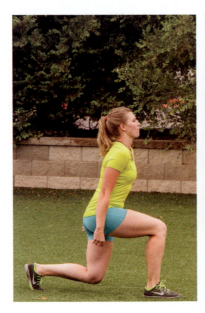
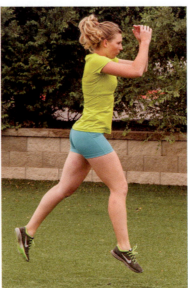
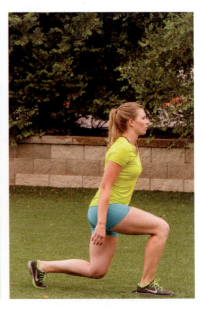

18.7   CYCLED SPLIT SQUAT JUMP

Intensity level: High

Direction of jump: Vertical

Starting position: Get into a lunge position with one leg forward (hip and knee joints flexed approximately 90°) and the other behind the midline of the body.

Arm action: Double arm or none

Preparatory movement: Begin with a countermovement.

Upward movement: Explosively jump up, using the arms to assist as needed. While off the ground, switch the position of the legs. Maximum height and power should be emphasized.

Downward movement: When landing, maintain the lunge position (opposite leg forward) and immediately repeat the jump.

Note: Be sure the lunge is not too deep (as in the third photo), as the SSC may not be able to effectively contribute to subsequent jumps.

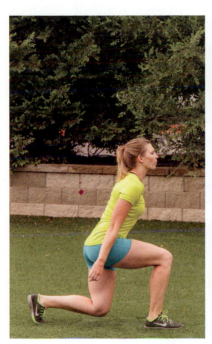
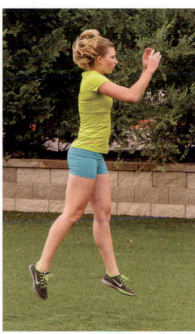
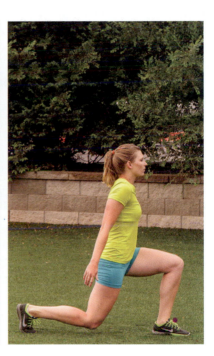

18.8 SINGLE-LEG TUCK JUMP

Intensity level: High

Direction of jump: Vertical

Starting position: Get into a comfortable, upright stance on one foot. The nonjumping leg is held in a stationary position with the knee flexed during the exercise.

Arm action: Double arm

Preparatory movement: Begin with a countermovement.

Upward movement: Explosively jump up. Pull the knee of the jumping leg to the chest, grasp the knee with both hands, and release before landing.

Downward movement: Land in the starting position and immediately repeat the jump using the same leg.

Repeat with the opposite leg after a brief rest.

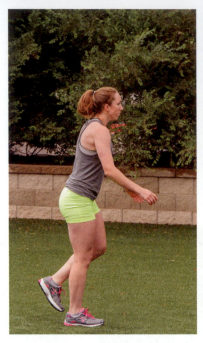
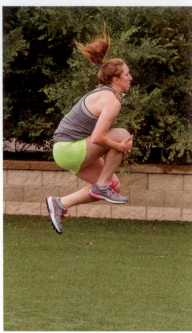

18.9 PIKE JUMP

Intensity level: High

Direction of jump: Vertical

Starting position: Get into a comfortable, upright stance with feet shoulder-width apart.

Arm action: Double arm

Preparatory movement: Begin with a countermovement.

Upward movement: Explosively jump up. Keeping the legs straight and together, try to lift them to the front and try to touch the toes with the hands.

Downward movement: Land in the starting position and immediately repeat the jump.

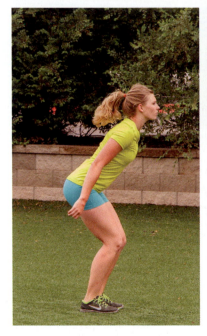
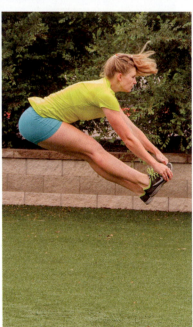

18.10 DOUBLE-LEG VERTICAL JUMP

Intensity level: Low

Direction of jump: Vertical

Starting position: Get into a comfortable, upright stance with feet shoulder-width apart.

Arm action: Double arm

Preparatory movement: Begin with a countermovement.

Upward movement: Explosively jump up, using both arms to assist, and reach for a target.

Downward movement: Land in the starting position and repeat the jump. Allow recovery time between jumps.

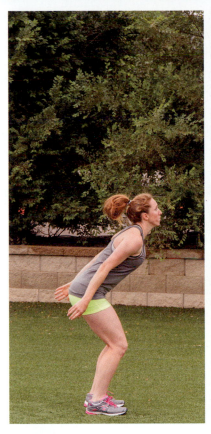
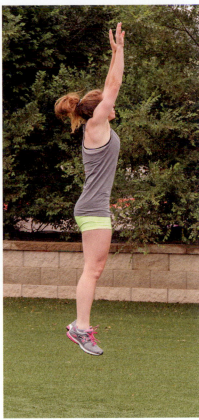

18.11 SINGLE-LEG VERTICAL JUMP

Intensity level: High

Direction of jump: Vertical

Starting position: Get into a comfortable, upright stance on one foot. The nonjumping leg is held in a stationary position with the knee flexed during the exercise.

Arm action: Double arm

Preparatory movement: Begin with a countermovement.

Upward movement: Explosively jump up, using both arms to assist, and reach for a target.

Downward movement: Land in the starting position and repeat the jump using the same leg. Allow recovery time between jumps.

Repeat with the opposite leg after a brief rest.

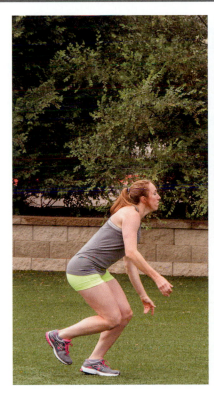
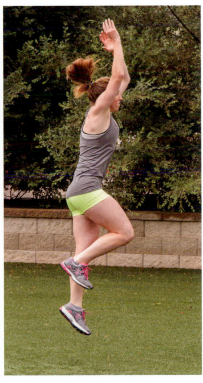

18.12 JUMP OVER BARRIER

Intensity level: Medium

Direction of jump: Horizontal and vertical

Equipment: A barrier such as a cone or hurdle

Starting position: Get into a comfortable, upright stance with feet shoulder-width apart.

Arm action: Double arm

Preparatory movement: Begin with a countermovement.

Upward movement: Jump over a barrier with both legs, using primarily hip and knee flexion to clear the barrier. Keep the knees and feet together without lateral deviation.

Downward movement: Land in the starting position and repeat the jump. Allow recovery time between jumps.

Note: The height of the barrier should be progressively increased (e.g., from a cone to a hurdle).

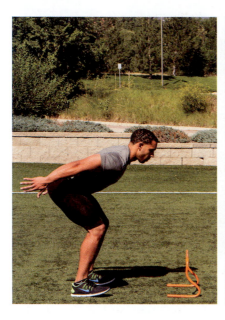 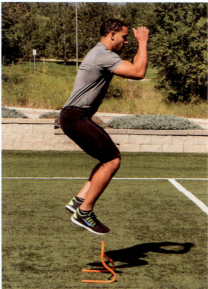 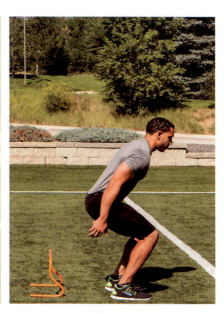

18.13 STANDING LONG JUMP

Intensity level: Low

Direction of jump: Horizontal

Starting position: Get into a comfortable, upright stance with feet shoulder-width apart.

Arm action: Double arm

Preparatory movement: Begin with a countermovement.

Upward movement: Explosively jump forward and up, using both arms to assist, with a goal of achieving maximal horizontal distance.

Downward movement: Land on both feet and repeat the jump. Allow recovery time between jumps.

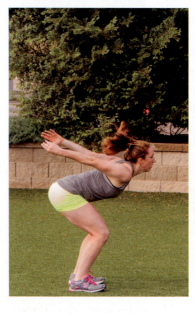 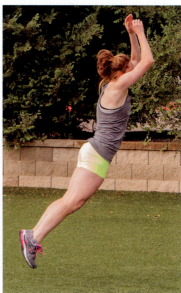

18.14 DOUBLE-LEG HOP

Intensity level: Medium

Direction of jump: Horizontal and vertical

Starting position: Get into a comfortable, upright stance with feet shoulder-width apart.

Arm action: Double arm

Preparatory movement: Begin with a countermovement.

Upward movement: Jump as far forward as possible.

Downward movement: Land in the starting position and immediately repeat the hop.

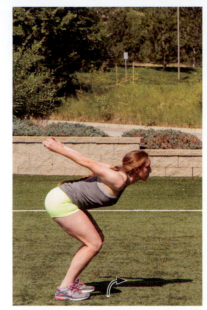
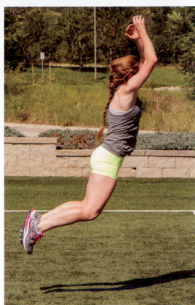

18.15 DOUBLE-LEG ZIGZAG HOP

Intensity level: High

Direction of jump: Diagonal

Equipment: Place about 10 hurdles 18 to 24 inches (45-60 cm) apart in a zigzag pattern.

Starting position: Get into a comfortable, upright stance with feet shoulder-width apart. Stand on the outside of the first hurdle. Elbows should be flexed at 90° and held at the sides of the body.

Arm action: Double arm

Preparatory movement: Begin with a countermovement.

Upward movement: Jump from the outside of the first hurdle to the outside of the second hurdle, keeping the shoulders perpendicular to an imaginary line through the center of all hurdles.

Downward movement: Immediately upon landing on the outside of the second hurdle, change direction and jump diagonally over the second hurdle to the outside of the third hurdle.

Continue hopping over all the hurdles.

Note: For a less intense version of this drill, set the hurdles in a straight line and hop over one hurdle at a time. Intensity of the zigzag hop can be increased by performing the hops with one leg only.

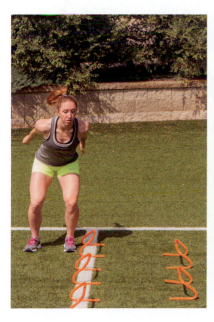
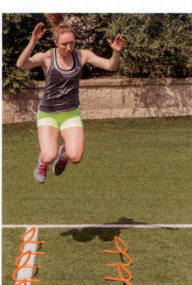
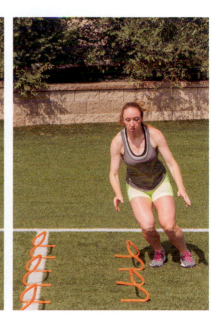

18.16   SINGLE-LEG HOP

Intensity level: High

Direction of jump: Horizontal and vertical

Starting position: Get into a comfortable, upright stance on one foot. The nonjumping leg is held in a stationary position with the knee flexed during the exercise.

Arm action: Double arm

Preparatory movement: Begin with a countermovement.

Upward movement: Explosively jump forward, using both arms to assist.

Downward movement: Land in the starting position and immediately repeat the hop using the same leg.

Repeat with the opposite leg after a brief rest.

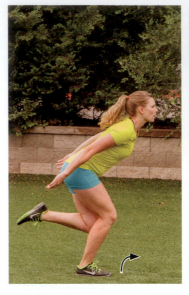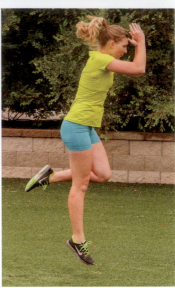

18.17   FRONT BARRIER HOP

Intensity level: Medium

Direction of jump: Horizontal and vertical

Equipment: Two barriers such as two cones or two hurdles

Starting position: Facing the first barrier, get into a comfortable, upright stance with feet shoulder-width apart.

Arm action: Double arm

Preparatory movement: Begin with a countermovement.

Upward movement: Jump over the first barrier with both legs, using primarily hip and knee flexion to clear the barrier. Keep the knees and feet together without lateral deviation.

Downward movement: Land in the starting position and immediately repeat the jump over the second barrier.

Note: Intensity level of the front barrier hop can be increased from medium to high by progressively increasing the height of the barrier (e.g., from a cone to a hurdle) or by performing the hops with one leg only.

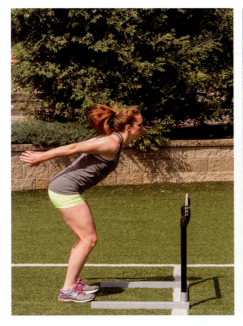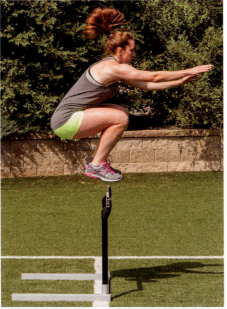

18.18   LATERAL BARRIER HOP

Intensity level: Medium

Direction of jump: Lateral and vertical

Equipment: A barrier such as a cone or hurdle

Starting position: With the barrier to one side, get into a comfortable, upright stance with feet shoulder-width apart.

Arm action: Double arm

Preparatory movement: Begin with a countermovement.

Upward movement: Jump over the barrier with both legs, using primarily hip and knee flexion to clear the barrier. Keep the knees and feet together.

Downward movement: Land on the opposite side of the barrier and immediately repeat the jump to the starting side.

Note: Intensity level of the lateral barrier hop can be increased from medium to high by progressively increasing the height of the barrier (e.g., from a cone to a hurdle) or by performing the hops with one leg only.

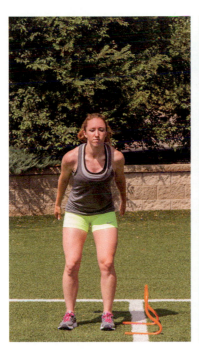
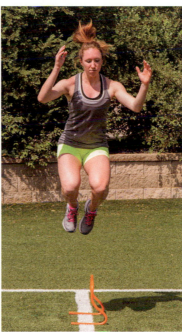
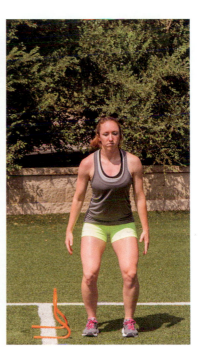

18.19 4-HURDLE DRILL

Intensity level: High

Direction of jump: Lateral and vertical

Equipment: Four hurdles: two pairs of hurdles. Each hurdle in the pair is separated by 12 inches (30 cm). Each pair is separated by 18 inches (46 cm).

Starting position: Get into a comfortable, upright stance on the right foot; the line of four hurdles will be to the athlete's left. The nonjumping leg is held in a stationary position with the knee flexed during the exercise.

Arm action: Double arm

Preparatory movement: Begin with a countermovement.

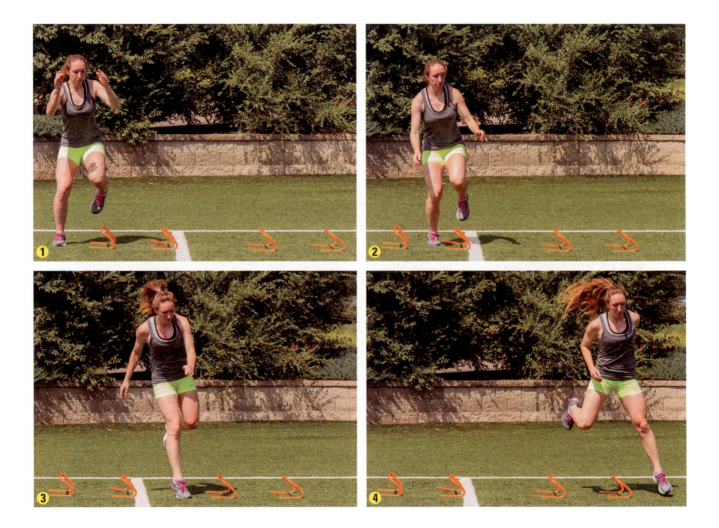

Movements:

1. Explosively jump left over the first hurdle with the right foot, using both arms to assist.
2. Land on the right foot and immediately repeat the hop over the next hurdle using the same leg.
3. Land on the right foot and immediately repeat the hop over the next **two** hurdles using the same leg.
4. Land on the left foot and immediately jump right over the first hurdle with the left foot, using both arms to assist.
5. Land on the left foot and immediately repeat the hop over the next hurdle using the same leg.
6. Land on the left foot and immediately repeat the hop over the next **two** hurdles using the same leg.
7. Land on the right foot.

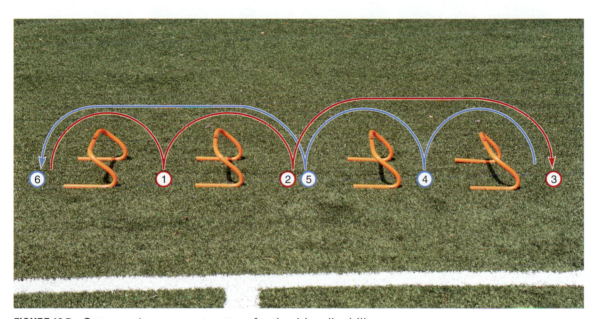

FIGURE 18.5 Setup and movement pattern for the 4-hurdle drill.

18.20   SKIP

Intensity level: Low

Direction of jump: Horizontal and vertical

Starting position: One leg is lifted to approximately 90° of hip and knee flexion.

Arm action: Reciprocal (as one leg is lifted, the opposite arm is lifted)

Preparatory movement: Begin with a countermovement on one leg.

Upward movement: Jump up and forward on one leg. The opposite leg should remain in the starting flexed position until landing.

Downward movement: Land in the starting position on the same leg. Immediately repeat the skip with the opposite leg.

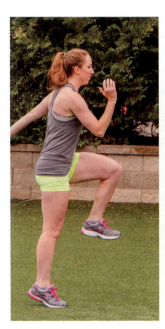
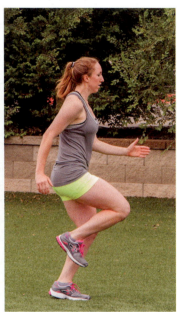
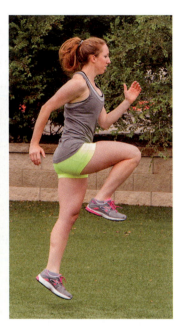

18.21 POWER SKIP

Intensity level: Low

Direction of jump: Vertical and horizontal

Starting position: One leg is lifted to approximately 90° of hip and knee flexion.

Arm action: Double arm

Preparatory movement: Begin with a countermovement on one leg.

Upward movement: Jump up and forward on one leg. Move the flexed, nonjumping leg up and into greater hip and knee flexion while jumping. Both arms should be used to assist with the upward movement.

Downward movement: Land in the starting position on the same leg. Immediately repeat the skip with the opposite leg.

Note: Emphasis is on the effectiveness of the skip.

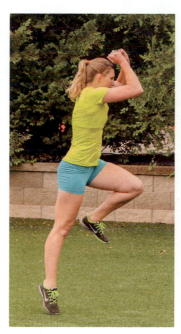
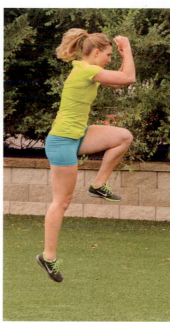
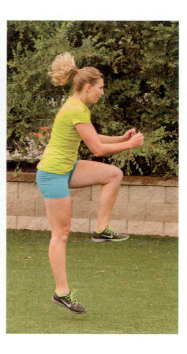

18.22 BACKWARD SKIP

Intensity level: Low

Direction of jump: Backward, horizontal, and vertical

Starting position: One leg is lifted to approximately 90° of hip and knee flexion.

Arm action: Double arm

Preparatory movement: Begin with a countermovement on one leg.

Upward movement: Jump backward with one leg and flex the hip and knee of the nonskipping leg to approximately 90°. Both arms should be used to assist with the movement.

Downward movement: Land in the starting position on the same leg. Immediately repeat the skip with the opposite leg.

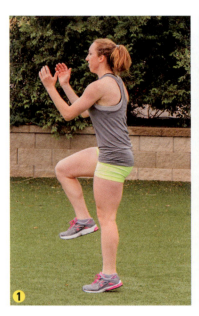
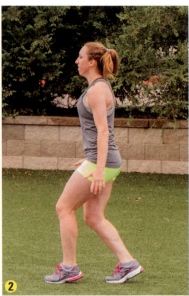
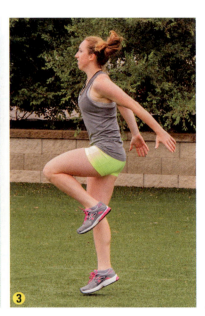

18.23 SIDE SKIP

Intensity level: Medium

Direction of jump: Vertical and lateral

Starting position: One leg is lifted to approximately 90° of hip and knee flexion.

Arm action: Reciprocal (as one leg is lifted, the opposite arm is lifted)

Preparatory movement: Begin with a countermovement on one leg.

Upward movement: Jump up and laterally on one leg. The opposite leg should remain in the starting flexed position until landing.

Downward movement: Land in the starting position on the same leg. Immediately repeat the skip with the opposite leg.

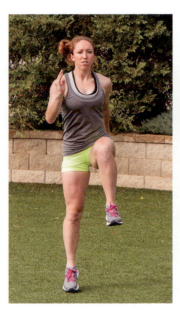 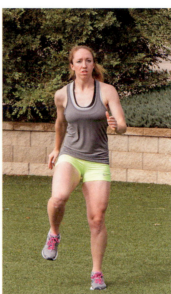 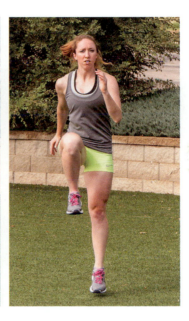

18.24 SINGLE-ARM ALTERNATE-LEG BOUND

Intensity level: Medium

Direction of jump: Horizontal and vertical

Starting position: Get into a comfortable, upright stance with feet shoulder-width apart.

Arm action: Single arm

Preparatory movement: Jog at a comfortable pace; begin the drill with the left foot forward.

Upward movement: Push off with the left foot as it contacts the ground. During push-off, bring the right leg forward by flexing the thigh to a position approx-imately parallel with the ground and the knee at 90°. During this flight phase of the drill, reach forward with the left arm.

Downward movement: Land on the right leg and immediately repeat the sequence on the opposite side upon landing.

Note: A bound is an exaggeration of the running gait; the goal is to cover as great a distance as possible during each stride.

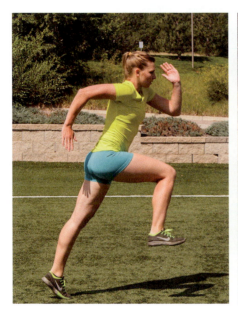
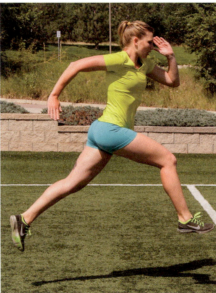
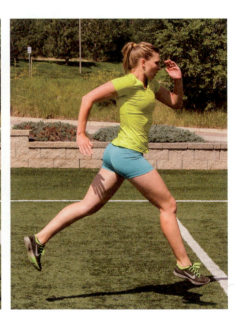

18.25 DOUBLE-ARM ALTERNATE-LEG BOUND

Intensity level: Medium

Direction of jump: Horizontal and vertical

Starting position: Get into a comfortable, upright stance with feet shoulder-width apart.

Arm action: Double arm

Preparatory movement: Jog at a comfortable pace; begin the drill with the left foot forward.

Upward movement: Push off with the left foot as it contacts the ground. During push-off, bring the right leg forward by flexing the thigh to a position approximately parallel with the ground and with the knee at 90°.

During this flight phase of the drill, reach forward with both arms.

Downward movement: Land on the right leg and immediately repeat the sequence on the opposite side upon landing.

Note: A bound is an exaggeration of the running gait; the goal is to cover as great a distance as possible during each stride.

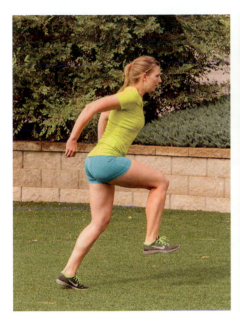 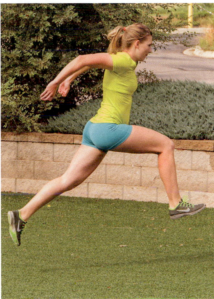 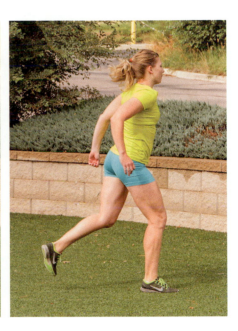

18.26 SINGLE-LEG PUSH-OFF

Intensity level: Low

Direction of jump: Vertical

Equipment: Plyometric box, 6 to 18 inches (15-46 cm) high

Starting position: Stand facing the plyometric box with one foot on the ground and one foot on the box. The heel of the foot on the box should be near the box's closest edge.

Arm action: Double arm

Preparatory movement: None

Upward movement: Jump up using the foot on the box to push off.

Downward movement: Land with the same foot on the box; this foot should land just before the ground foot. Immediately repeat the movement.

Note: Intensity may be increased by increasing the height of the box. Begin with a height of 6 inches (15 cm).

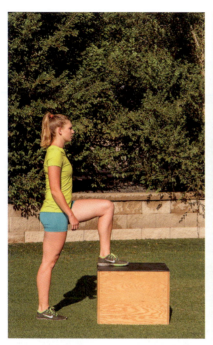
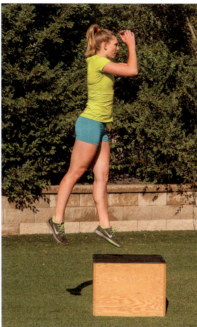
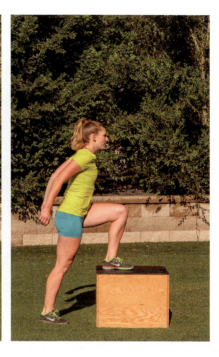

18.27 ALTERNATE-LEG PUSH-OFF

Intensity level: Low

Direction of jump: Vertical

Equipment: Plyometric box, 6 to 18 inches (15-46 cm) high

Starting position: Stand facing the plyometric box with one foot on the ground and one foot on the box. The heel of the foot on the box should be near the box's closest edge.

Arm action: Double arm

Preparatory movement: None

Upward movement: Jump up using the foot on the box to push off.

Downward movement: Land with the opposite foot on the box; this foot should land just before the ground foot. Immediately repeat the movement, reversing the feet each repetition.

Note: Intensity may be increased by increasing the height of the box. Begin with a height of 6 inches (15 cm).

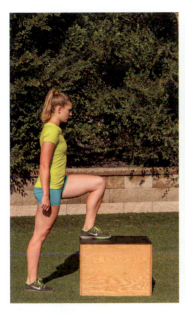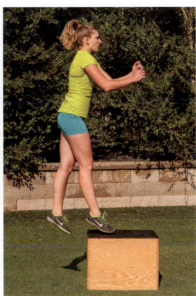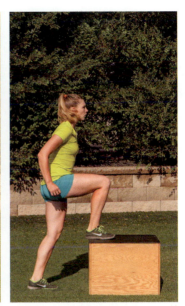

18.28 LATERAL PUSH-OFF

Intensity level: Low

Direction of jump: Vertical

Equipment: Plyometric box, 6 to 18 inches (15-46 cm) high

Starting position: Stand to one side of the plyometric box with one foot on the ground and one foot on the box. The inside of the foot on the box should be near the box's closest edge.

Arm action: Double arm

Preparatory movement: None

Upward movement: Jump up using the foot on the box to push off.

Downward movement: Land with the same foot on the box; this foot should land just before the ground foot. Immediately repeat the movement.

Note: Intensity may be increased by increasing the height of the box. Begin with a height of 6 inches (15 cm).

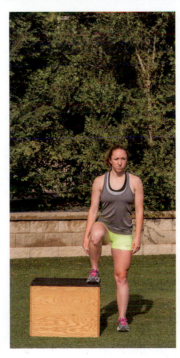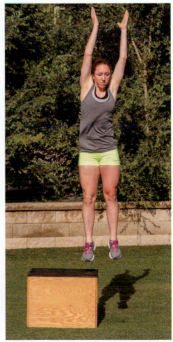

18.29   SIDE-TO-SIDE PUSH-OFF

Intensity level: Medium

Direction of jump: Vertical

Equipment: Plyometric box, 6 to 18 inches (15-46 cm) high

Starting position: Stand to one side of the plyometric box with one foot on the ground and one foot on the box. The inside of the foot on the box should be near the box's closest edge.

Arm action: Double arm

Preparatory movement: None

Upward movement: Jump up and over the box using the foot on the box to push off.

Downward movement: Land with the opposite foot on the opposite side of the top of the box; this foot should land just before the ground foot. Immediately repeat the movement to the opposite side.

Note: Intensity may be increased by increasing the height of the box. Begin with a height of 6 inches (15 cm).

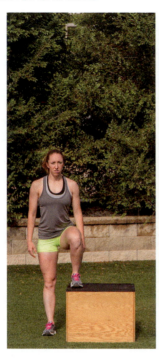
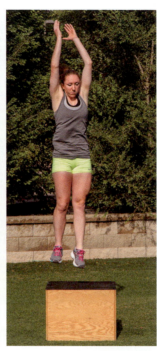
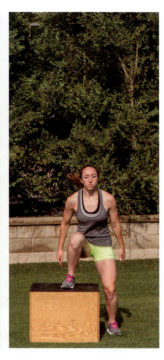

18.30   DOUBLE-LEG JUMP TO BOX

Intensity level: Low

Direction of jump: Vertical and slightly horizontal

Equipment: Plyometric box, 6 to 42 inches (15-107 cm) high

Starting position: Facing the plyometric box, get into a comfortable, upright stance with feet shoulder-width apart.

Arm action: Double arm

Preparatory movement: Begin with a countermovement.

Upward movement: Jump onto the top of the box using both legs.

Downward movement: Land on both feet in a half-squat position, step down from the box, and repeat.

Note: Intensity may be increased by increasing the height of the box. Begin with a height of 6 inches (15 cm).

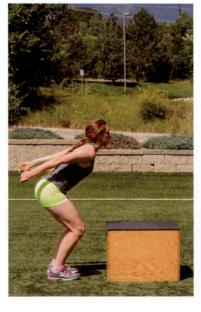
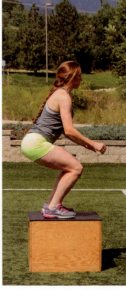

18.31 SINGLE-LEG JUMP TO BOX

Intensity level: High

Direction of jump: Vertical and slightly horizontal

Equipment: Plyometric box, 6 to 42 inches (15-107 cm) high

Starting position: Facing the plyometric box, get into a comfortable, upright stance on one foot. The non-jumping leg is held in a stationary position with the knee flexed during the exercise.

Arm action: Double arm

Preparatory movement: Begin with a countermovement.

Upward movement: Jump onto the top of the box using one leg.

Downward movement: Land on the same foot as used to jump in a half-squat position, step down from the box, and repeat.

Note: Intensity may be increased by increasing the height of the box. Begin with a height of 6 inches (15 cm).

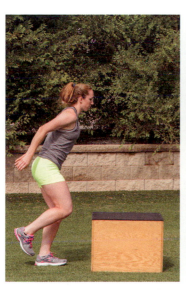
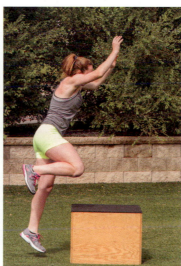
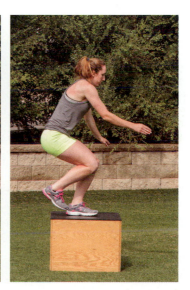

18.32 SQUAT BOX JUMP

Intensity level: Medium

Direction of jump: Vertical and slightly horizontal

Equipment: Plyometric box, 6 to 42 inches (15-107 cm) high

Starting position: Facing the plyometric box with hands clasped behind head, get into a comfortable, upright stance with feet shoulder-width apart.

Arm action: None

Preparatory movement: Begin with a countermovement.

Upward movement: Jump onto the top of the box using both legs.

Downward movement: Land on both feet in a half-squat position, step down from the box, and repeat.

Note: Intensity may be increased by increasing the height of the box. Begin with a height of 6 inches (15 cm).

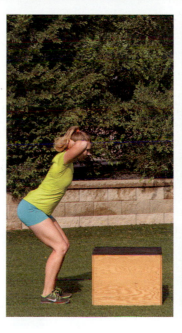
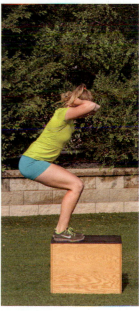

18.33 LATERAL BOX JUMP

Intensity level: Medium

Direction of jump: Vertical and slightly horizontal

Equipment: Plyometric box, 6 to 42 inches (15-107 cm) high

Starting position: Stand to one side of the plyometric box; get into a comfortable, upright stance with feet shoulder-width apart.

Arm action: Double arm

Preparatory movement: Begin with a countermovement.

Upward movement: Jump onto the top of the box using both legs.

Downward movement: Land on both feet in a half-squat position, step down from the box, and repeat in the opposite direction.

Note: Intensity may be increased by increasing the height of the box. Begin with a height of 6 inches (15 cm).

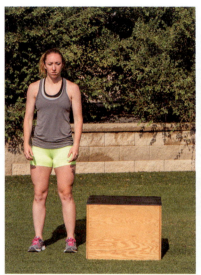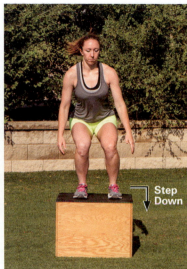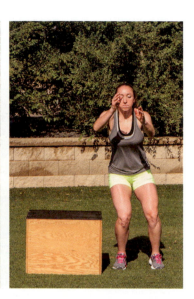

Step Down

18.34 DROP FREEZE

Intensity level: Medium

Direction of jump: Vertical

Equipment: Plyometric box, 12 to 42 inches (30-107 cm) high

Starting position: Get into a comfortable, upright stance with feet shoulder-width apart on the plyometric box; toes should be near the edge of the box.

Arm action: None

Preparatory movement: Step from the box.

Downward movement: Land on the floor with both feet, quickly absorbing the impact upon landing.

Step back onto the box and repeat.

Note: Intensity may be increased by increasing the height of the box. Begin with a height of 12 inches (30 cm).

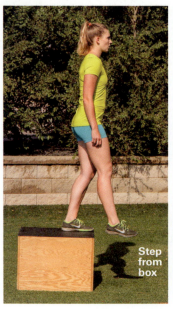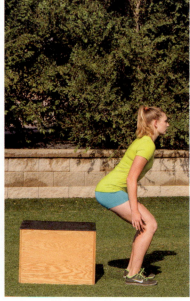

Step from box

18.35 DEPTH JUMP

Intensity level: High

Direction of jump: Vertical

Equipment: Plyometric box, 12 to 42 inches (30-107 cm) high

Starting position: Get into a comfortable, upright stance with feet shoulder-width apart on the plyometric box; toes should be near the edge of the box.

Arm action: Double arm

Preparatory movement: Step from the box.

Downward movement: Land on the floor with both feet.

Upward movement: Upon landing, immediately jump up as high as possible.

Note: When stepping from the box, step straight out. Do not first jump up or lower your center of gravity as you step down, as these adjustments will change the height from which the exercise is performed.

Note: Time on the ground should be kept to a minimum. Intensity may be increased by increasing the height of the box. Begin with a height of 12 inches (30 cm).

Note: Upon landing, emphasis should be on jumping up, with minimal horizontal movement. The third photo shows too much forward movement.

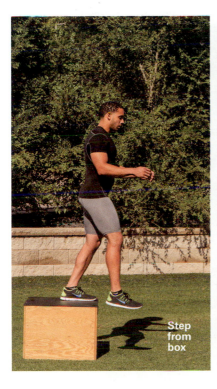 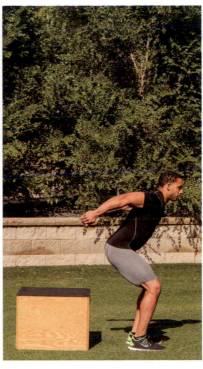 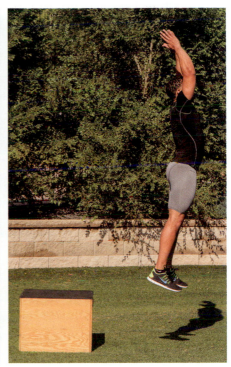

Step from box

Depth Jumps

18.36 DEPTH JUMP TO SECOND BOX

Intensity level: High

Direction of jump: Vertical and horizontal

Equipment: Two plyometric boxes, 12 to 42 inches (30-107 cm) high

Starting position: Get into a comfortable, upright stance with feet shoulder-width apart on the plyometric box, facing the second box; toes should be near the edge of the box.

Arm action: Double arm

Preparatory movement: Step from the box.

Downward movement: Land on the floor with both feet.

Upward movement: Upon landing, immediately jump onto the second box.

Note: When stepping from the box, step straight out. Do not first jump up or lower your center of gravity as you step down, as these adjustments will change the height from which the exercise is performed.

Note: Time on the ground should be kept to a minimum. Intensity may be increased by increasing the height of the box. Begin with a height of 12 inches (30 cm).

Note: The distance between boxes depends on experience and ability; the greater the distance between boxes, the higher the intensity of the jump. Begin with the boxes placed 24 inches (61 cm) apart.

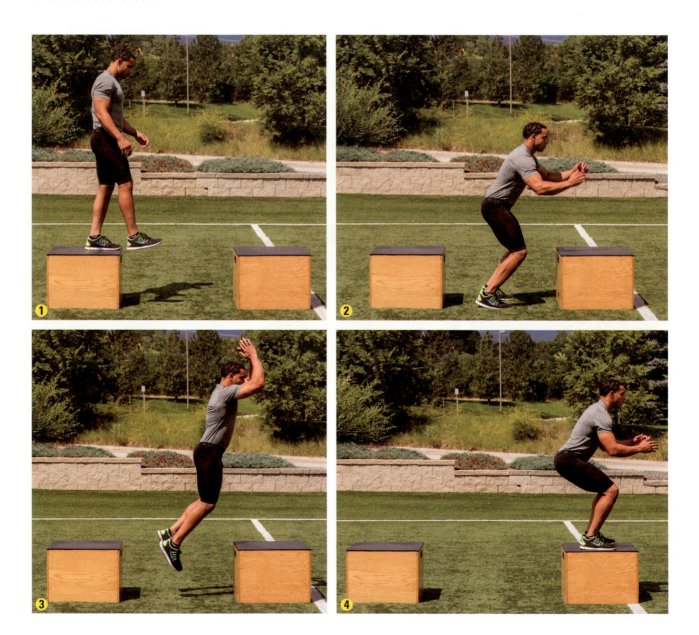

18.37 SQUAT DEPTH JUMP

Intensity level: High

Direction of jump: Vertical

Equipment: Plyometric box, 12 to 42 inches (30-107 cm) high

Starting position: Get into a comfortable, upright stance with feet shoulder-width apart on the plyometric box; toes should be near the edge of the box.

Arm action: Double arm or none

Preparatory movement: Step from the box.

Downward movement: Land on the floor in a squat position (90° of hip and knee flexion) with both feet. (The jumper in the second photo should have greater hip and knee flexion.)

Upward movement: Upon landing, immediately jump up as high as possible; land in the same squat position.

Note: When stepping from the box, step straight out. Do not first jump up or lower your center of gravity as you step down, as these adjustments will change the height from which the exercise is performed.

Note: Time on the ground should be kept to a minimum. Intensity may be increased by increasing the height of the box. Begin with a height of 12 inches (30 cm).

Note: Upon landing, emphasis should be on jumping up, with minimal horizontal movement.

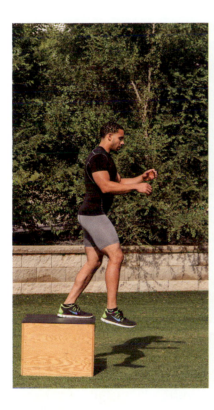 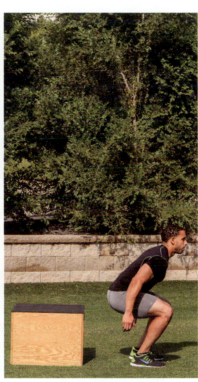 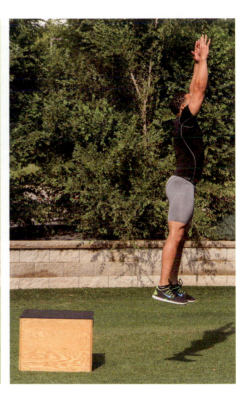

18.38 DEPTH JUMP WITH LATERAL MOVEMENT

Intensity level: High

Direction of jump: Vertical and lateral

Equipment: Plyometric box, 12 to 42 inches (30-107 cm) high; a partner

Starting position: Get into a comfortable, upright stance with feet shoulder-width apart on the plyometric box; toes should be near the edge of the box.

Arm action: Double arm

Preparatory movement: Step from the box.

Downward movement: Land on the floor with both feet. Have a partner point to the right or left just before you land.

Upward movement: Upon landing, immediately sprint in the direction determined by your partner.

Note: When stepping from the box, step straight out. Do not first jump up or lower your center of gravity as you step down, as these adjustments will change the height from which the exercise is performed.

Note: Time on the ground should be kept to a minimum. Intensity may be increased by increasing the height of the box. Begin with a height of 12 inches (30 cm).

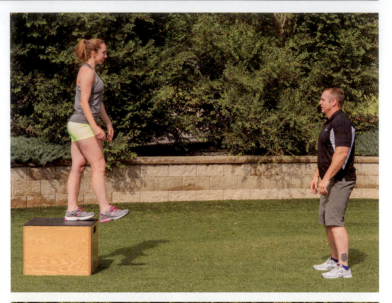

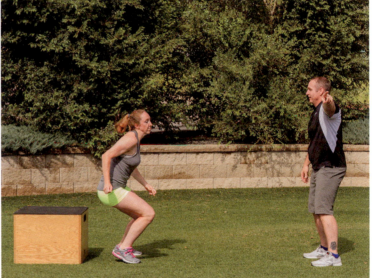

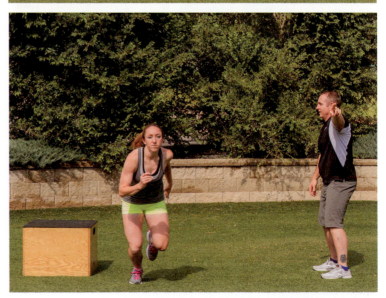

18.39 DEPTH JUMP WITH STANDING LONG JUMP

Intensity level: High

Direction of jump: Vertical and horizontal

Equipment: Plyometric box, 12 to 42 inches (30-107 cm) high

Starting position: Get into a comfortable, upright stance with feet shoulder-width apart on the plyometric box; toes should be near the edge of the box.

Arm action: Double arm

Preparatory movement: Step from the box.

Downward movement: Land on the floor with both feet.

Upward movement: Upon landing, immediately jump forward as far as possible with both feet.

Note: When stepping from the box, step straight out. Do not first jump up or lower your center of gravity as you step down, as these adjustments will change the height from which the exercise is performed.

Note: Time on the ground should be kept to a minimum. Intensity may be increased by increasing the height of the box. Begin with a height of 12 inches (30 cm).

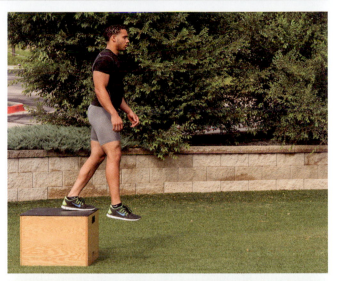

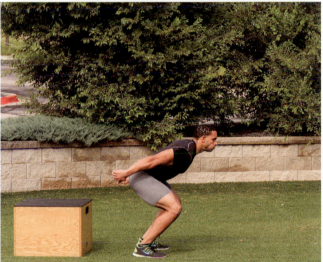

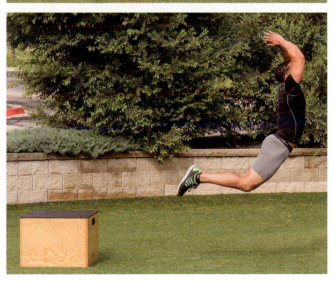

18.40 DEPTH JUMP TO 180° TURN

Intensity level: High

Direction of jump: Vertical and horizontal

Equipment: Plyometric box, 12 to 42 inches (30-107 cm) high

Starting position: Get into a comfortable, upright stance with feet shoulder-width apart on the plyometric box; toes should be near the edge of the box.

Arm action: Double arm

Preparatory movement: Step from the box.

Downward movement: Land on the floor with both feet.

Upward movement: Upon landing, immediately jump up as high as possible with both feet. While in the air, the athlete turns 180° to land facing the opposite direction.

Note: When stepping from the box, step straight out. Do not first jump up or lower your center of gravity as you step down, as these adjustments will change the height from which the exercise is performed.

Note: Time on the ground should be kept to a minimum. Intensity may be increased by increasing the height of the box. Begin with a height of 12 inches (30 cm).

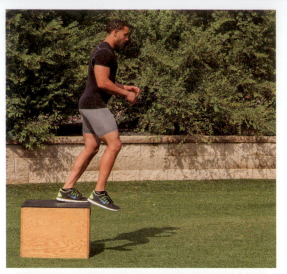

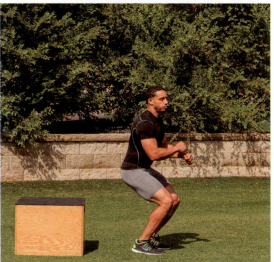

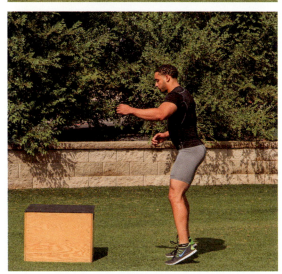

18.41 SINGLE-LEG DEPTH JUMP

Intensity level: High

Direction of jump: Vertical

Equipment: Plyometric box, 12 to 42 inches (30-107 cm) high

Starting position: Get into a comfortable, upright stance with feet shoulder-width apart on the plyometric box; toes should be near the edge of the box.

Arm action: Double arm

Preparatory movement: Step from the box.

Downward movement: Land on the floor with one foot.

Upward movement: Upon landing, immediately jump up as high as possible with the landing foot.

Note: When stepping from the box, step straight out. Do not first jump up or lower your center of gravity as you step down, as these adjustments will change the height from which the exercise is performed.

Note: Time on the ground should be kept to a minimum. Intensity may be increased by increasing the height of the box. Begin with a height of 12 inches (30 cm).

Note: This is a very advanced form of the depth jump and should be performed only by those with adequate experience and ability as demonstrated in other versions of the depth jump.

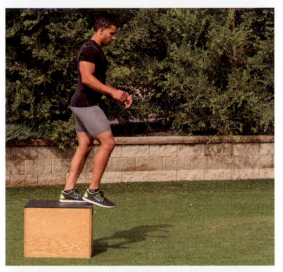

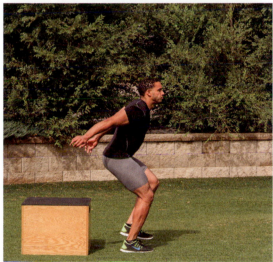

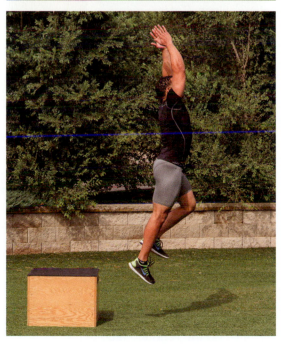

18.42 CHEST PASS

Intensity level: Low

Direction of throw: Forward

Equipment: Medicine or plyometric ball weighing 2 to 8 pounds (0.9-3.6 kg); rebounder or partner

Starting position: Get into a comfortable, upright stance with feet shoulder-width apart; face the rebounder or partner approximately 10 feet (3 m) away. Raise the ball to chest level with the elbows flexed.

Preparatory movement: Begin with a countermovement. (A countermovement for plyometric throws requires cocking the arms—that is, moving the arms slightly backward before the actual throw.)

Arm action: Using both arms, throw the ball to the rebounder or partner by extending the elbows. When the rebounder or partner returns the ball, catch it, return to the starting position, and immediately repeat the movement.

Note: Intensity may be increased by increasing the weight of the medicine ball. Begin with a 2-pound (0.9 kg) ball.

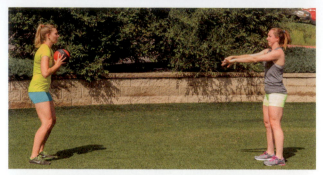

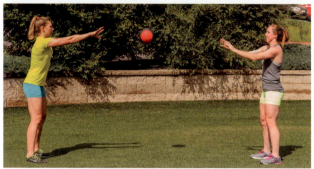

18.43 TWO-HAND OVERHEAD THROW

Intensity level: Low

Direction of throw: Forward and down

Equipment: Medicine or plyometric ball weighing 2 to 8 pounds (0.9-3.6 kg); rebounder or partner

Starting position: Get into a comfortable, upright stance with feet shoulder-width apart; face the rebounder or partner approximately 10 feet (3 m) away. Raise the ball overhead.

Preparatory movement: Begin with a countermovement. (A countermovement for plyometric throws requires cocking the arms—that is, moving the arms slightly backward before the actual throw.)

Arm action: Using both arms, throw the ball to the rebounder or partner, keeping the elbows extended. When the rebounder or partner returns the ball, catch the ball overhead and immediately repeat the throw. The partners can also bounce the ball on the ground between them, for a downward movement and a catch on the rebound (see photos).

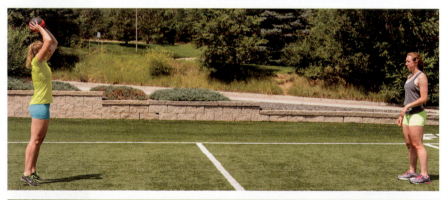

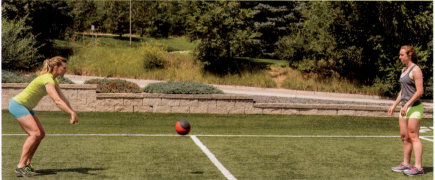

Note: Intensity may be increased by increasing the weight of the medicine ball. Begin with a 2-pound (0.9 kg) ball.

18.44 TWO-HAND SIDE-TO-SIDE THROW

Intensity level: Low

Direction of throw: Forward and diagonal

Equipment: Medicine or plyometric ball weighing 2 to 8 pounds (0.9-3.6 kg); rebounder or partner

Starting position: Get into a comfortable, upright stance with feet shoulder-width apart; face the rebounder or partner approximately 10 feet (3 m) away. Raise the ball in both hands to a position over one shoulder with the elbows flexed.

Preparatory movement: Begin with a countermovement. (A countermovement for plyometric throws requires cocking the arms—that is, moving the arms slightly backward before the actual throw.)

Arm action: Using both arms, throw the ball to the rebounder or partner by extending the elbows. When the rebounder or partner returns the ball, catch the ball over the opposite shoulder and immediately repeat the throw.

Note: Intensity may be increased by increasing the weight of the medicine ball. Begin with a 2-pound (0.9 kg) ball.

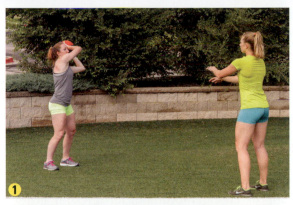

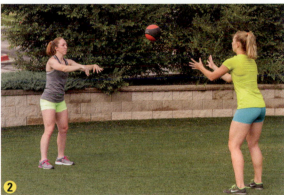

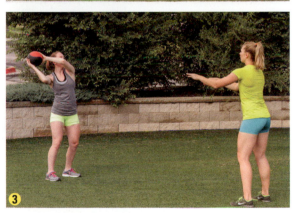

18.45 SINGLE-ARM THROW

Intensity level: Medium

Direction of throw: Forward

Equipment: Medicine or plyometric ball weighing 1 to 5 pounds (0.5-2.3 kg); rebounder or partner

Starting position: Get into a comfortable, upright stance with feet shoulder-width apart; face the rebounder or partner approximately 10 feet (3 m) away. Raise the ball in one hand to a position of 90° of shoulder abduction and 90° of elbow flexion, with arm rotated so the forearm is perpendicular to the floor.

Preparatory movement: Begin with a countermovement. (A countermovement for plyometric throws requires cocking the arm—that is, moving the arm slightly backward before the actual throw.)

Arm action: Using one arm, throw the ball to the rebounder or partner. When the rebounder or partner returns the ball, catch the ball in the starting position, allow the shoulder to externally rotate slightly, and immediately repeat the throw.

Note: Intensity may be increased by increasing the weight of the medicine ball. Begin with a 1-pound (0.5 kg) ball.

Note: This drill may also be performed using a natural throwing motion.

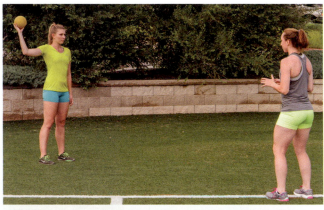

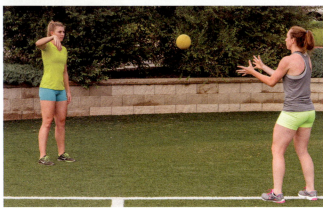

18.46 POWER DROP

Intensity level: High

Direction of throw: Upward

Equipment: Medicine or plyometric ball weighing 2 to 8 pounds (0.9-3.6 kg); partner; plyometric box 12 to 42 inches (30-107 cm) high

Starting position: Lie supine on the ground with elbows extended and both shoulders in approximately 90° of flexion; head should be near the base of the box. The partner should be on the box with the medicine ball held above the athlete's arms.

Preparatory movement: None

Arm action: When the partner drops the ball, catch it using both arms and immediately throw the ball back up to the partner.

Note: Intensity may be increased by increasing the weight of the medicine ball or by increasing the height of the box. Begin with a 2-pound (0.9 kg) ball and a height of 12 inches (30 cm).

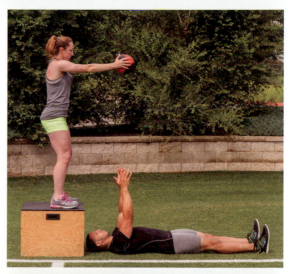

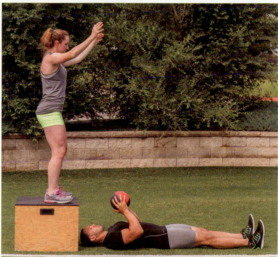

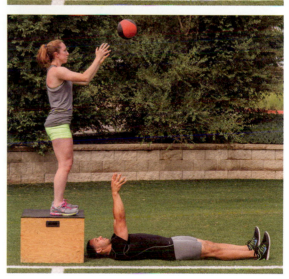

18.47 DEPTH PUSH-UP

Intensity level: Medium

Direction of movement: Vertical

Equipment: Medicine or plyometric ball weighing 5 to 8 pounds (2.3-3.6 kg)

Starting position: Lie in a push-up position, with the hands on the medicine ball and elbows extended.

Preparatory movement: None

Downward movement: Quickly remove the hands from the medicine ball and drop down. Contact the ground with hands slightly wider than shoulder-width apart and elbows slightly flexed. Allow the chest to almost touch the medicine ball by letting the elbows flex.

Upward movement: Immediately and explosively push up by fully extending the elbows. Quickly place the palms on the medicine ball and repeat the exercise.

Note: When the upper body is at maximal height during the upward movement, the hands should be higher than the medicine ball.

Note: Intensity may be increased by increasing the size of the medicine ball. Begin with a 5-pound (2.3 kg) ball.

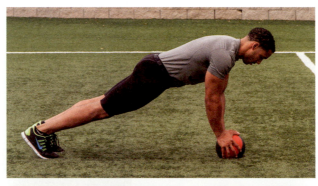

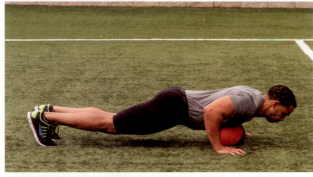

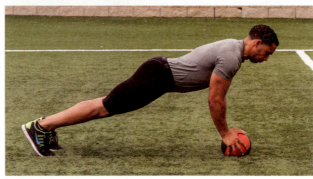

18.48 45° SIT-UP

Intensity level: Medium

Equipment: Medicine or plyometric ball weighing 2 to 8 pounds (0.9-3.6 kg); a partner

Starting position: Sit on the ground with the trunk at an approximately 45° angle. The partner should be in front with the medicine ball.

Preparatory movement: The partner throws the ball to your outstretched hands.

Downward action: Once the partner throws the ball, catch it using both arms, allow minimal trunk extension, and immediately return the ball to the partner.

Note: Intensity may be increased by increasing the weight of the medicine ball. Begin with a 2-pound (0.9 kg) ball.

Note: The force used to return the ball to the partner should come predominantly from the abdominal muscles.

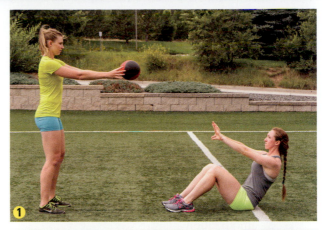

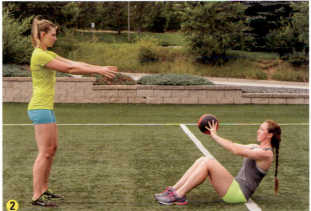

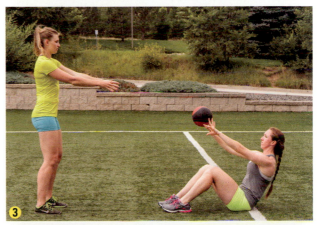

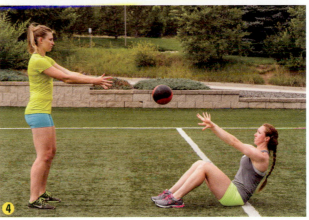

KEY TERMS

amortization phase
balance
bound
box drill
complex training
concentric phase
depth jump

eccentric phase
jumps in place
multiple hops and jumps
muscle spindle
potentiation
power

push-up
series elastic component (SEC)
standing jump
stretch reflex
stretch–shortening cycle (SSC)
throw

STUDY QUESTIONS

1. Which of the following is NOT a phase of the stretch–shortening cycle?
   a. amortization
   b. concentric
   c. eccentric
   d. isometric

2. Which of the following structures detects rapid movement and initiates the stretch reflex?
   a. Golgi tendon organ
   b. muscle spindle
   c. extrafusal muscle fiber
   d. Pacinian corpuscle

3. Which of the following should be assessed before beginning a lower body plyometric training program?
   I. balance
   II. strength
   III. training history
   IV. lean body mass
   a. I and III only
   b. II and IV only
   c. I, II, and III only
   d. I, II, III, and IV

4. Which of the following types of plyometric drills is generally considered to be the MOST intense?
   a. jumps in place
   b. bounds
   c. depth jumps
   d. box jumps

5. Which of the following work-to-rest ratios is the MOST appropriate to assign to a plyometric training workout?
   a. 1:5
   b. 1:4
   c. 1:3
   d. 1:2

Program Design and Technique for Speed and Agility Training

Brad H. DeWeese, EdD, and Sophia Nimphius, PhD

After completing this chapter, you will be able to

- describe the underlying biomechanical constructs of sprint, change-of-direction, and agility performance;

- apply sound movement principles to the coaching of locomotion modes and techniques;

- analyze the abilities and skills needed to perform specific movement tasks;

- effectively monitor the development of sprint, change-of-direction, and agility abilities;

- apply sound means and methods for developing speed, change of direction, and agility; and

- design and implement training programs to maximize athletic performance.

The authors would like to acknowledge the contributions of Steven S. Plisk to this chapter. Thanks also go to Matt L. Sams; Chris Bellon, MA, CSCS; Satoshi Mizuguchi, PhD; N. Travis Triplett, PhD, CSCS*D, FNSCA; Jared M. Porter, PhD, Adam Benz, MS, CSCS; and Tania Spiteri, MS.

This chapter addresses the development of speed, change-of-direction, and agility abilities. Although the term *speed* is often used when an athlete displays one or all of these aspects of physical performance, it is critical to understand that athlete development requires various underpinning physical capacities and skills as a result of differing biomechanical requirements. These three important aspects of physical performance can be defined as follows:

- Speed—the skills and abilities needed to achieve high movement velocities
- Change of direction—the skills and abilities needed to explosively change movement direction, velocities, or modes
- Agility—the skills and abilities needed to change direction, velocity, or mode in response to a stimulus

The ability to outrun the competition is a hallmark of most athletic endeavors. Further, the ability to change direction rapidly during an activity can mute the effect of an opponent's speed or provide both physical and tactical advantages on the field of play. Although it may seem that these scenarios all involve the "speed" of an athlete, this perceived "speed" may be a result of one quality or a combination of the three qualities just listed. Within sport, high-speed human locomotion can be categorized as linear or multidirectional. Generating high speeds linearly, more commonly referred to as sprinting, is the underlying requirement for success in many track and field events as well as open-field running in game-based contexts. While linear speed is important in team sports, play is primarily multidirectional. As a result, these athletes' success partially depends on responding to ever-changing game scenarios through fast, efficient changes of direction whereas **speed** requires the ability to accelerate and reach maximal velocity.

Because of the nature of most sports, there are scenarios in which athletes have a predetermined change of direction to make and they are limited only by their physical capacity to perform this activity (e.g., a route, play, or predetermined pattern). The physical capacity to change direction while decelerating and then reaccelerating, sometimes using a different mode of travel, is **change-of-direction** ability, whereas **agility** requires the use of perceptual–cognitive ability in combination with change-of-direction ability. This highlights the similar and contrasting qualities of speed, change of direction, and agility. For example, acceleration is a part of change-of-direction ability and agility, but additional aspects such as deceleration ability and mode of movement differentiate the training for speed from the training for change of direction and agility. The physical capacity to change direction may be a component of agility, but

the perceptual–cognitive component influences the physical demands of agility. Therefore, while reading this chapter, one should understand that although there is overlap between these qualities, differing physical, technical, or perceptual–cognitive development is required to improve each of these aspects of physical performance.

When athletes are sprinting or changing direction, their performance is a function of physical capacity and technical proficiency. While biomechanical and metabolic efficiency underpin performance in aerobic sport, effective application of force limits speed, change of direction, and agility. Simply put, an athlete's success in these explosive movements is the product of an athlete's strength capacity combined with the ability to use this strength within the constraints of the activity. **Strength** is often associated with an athlete's capacity to produce force, but it is important to understand that while high levels of maximal strength are desirable attributes in sport, sprint, change-of-direction, and agility events occur in periods that prevent athletes from producing and expressing their maximal strength.

Within sprinting, the application of force allows the athlete to accelerate, attain high velocities, and attempt to maintain the high velocities. In addition to the force application associated with acceleration and attainment of velocity in sprinting, change-of-direction ability requires effective application of force to decelerate and then reaccelerate in another direction. Further still, agility performance is considered a function of the athlete's ability not only to change direction, but also specifically to change direction in response to a stimulus (4) such as a defender or ball. For this reason, strength and conditioning professionals must be aware of their training choices regarding the development of physical characteristics that assist in promoting speed, change of direction, and agility on both the track and the field.

> Speed requires the ability to accelerate and reach maximal velocity, whereas agility performance requires the use of perceptual–cognitive ability in combination with the ability to decelerate and then reaccelerate in an intended direction.

Speed and Agility Mechanics

In order to execute movement techniques, athletes must apply force—the product of mass and acceleration. Due to the limited available time to produce force during most athletic activities, there are two variables that describe force relative to the time available to produce force:

- **Rate of force development (RFD)**—the development of maximal force in minimal time, typically used as an index of explosive strength (3)

- **Impulse**—the product of the generated force and the time required for its production, which is measured as the area under the force–time curve. According to the impulse–momentum relationship, impulse dictates the magnitude of change of momentum of an object.

Physics of Sprinting, Change of Direction, and Agility

Force represents the interaction of two physical objects. Force is a vector quantity, meaning that it has both magnitude (size) and direction. Traditionally, force is described as a push or a pull exerted on one object by another, which prevents both objects from occupying the same space. This movement of mass changes an object's velocity, causing **acceleration**.

Within the strength and conditioning profession, **velocity** and *speed* are often used interchangeably. For a proper discussion on sprint and agility performance, these terms need to be separated. Speed is a scalar quantity, which means that it describes only how fast an object is moving. Speed is the rate at which an object covers a distance. Like force, velocity is a vector quantity. Velocity describes both how fast an object is traveling and its direction. In short, velocity is speed with a direction.

Acceleration refers to the rate at which an object's velocity changes over time. Once a force acts upon a physical object, the mass will change direction and leave the space it was occupying. Acceleration of the object will continue as long as external forces continue to change velocity. In practical settings, *deceleration* replaces *negative acceleration* in describing a change from higher to lower velocity.

Rate of Force Development

Within the sporting context, the ability to produce force rapidly is arguably a more desirable trait than maximal force production (89). While the ability to generate high levels of maximal force has been shown to improve performance in jump height and other athletic measures, most competitive scenarios do not occur within a time frame that allows an athlete to generate maximal forces (19). Specifically, the generation of maximal contraction force takes at least 300 ms, while many sport activities consume 0 to 200 ms (see figure 19.1) (1). For this reason, in sport settings where success is restricted to timing of movement, RFD may be a more useful measure of an athlete's explosive ability (5). Rate of force development can be described as the change in force divided by the change in time (89).

The ability to accelerate a mass depends on a change in velocity resulting from the application of an external force. Therefore, from a practical standpoint, an athlete wishing to achieve higher acceleration capabilities should apply forces at a greater rate (73).

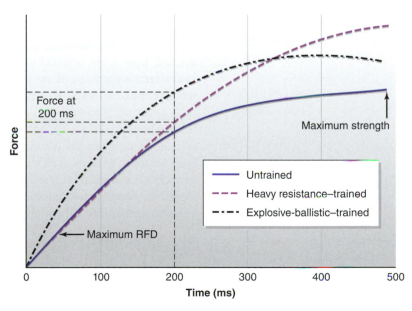

FIGURE 19.1 Force as a function of time, indicating maximum strength, rate of force development (RFD), and force at 0.2 seconds for untrained (solid blue line), heavy resistance–trained (dashed purple line), and explosive-ballistic–trained (dotted black line) subjects. Impulse is the change in momentum resulting from a force, measured as the product of force and time (represented by the area under each curve), and is increased by improving RFD. When functional movements are performed, force is typically applied very briefly—often for 0.1 to 0.2 seconds—whereas absolute maximum force development may require 0.6 to 0.8 seconds.

Reprinted, by permission, from Häkkinen and Komi, 1985 (46).

Impulse

In order for an object to change its location, forces must be applied to produce a change in velocity. Athletes attempting to increase speeds through the production of force never apply forces instantaneously. In fact, force is applied to the running surface over a period of time in the stance phase of sprinting (figure 19.2) or in the plant phase of changing direction. The length of time athletes are in this stance or plant phase is termed their *ground contact time*. The product of the time the force is applied to the ground and the amount of force applied is termed impulse and can be graphically represented as the area under a force–time curve. Changes in impulse result in changes of the athlete's momentum and therefore the ability to either accelerate or decelerate.

Figure 19.2 demonstrates how the vertical and horizontal forces differ in magnitude when the acceleration

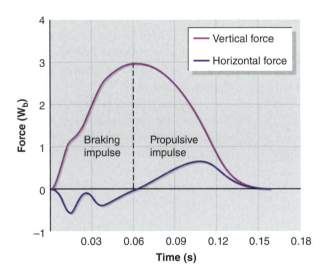

a

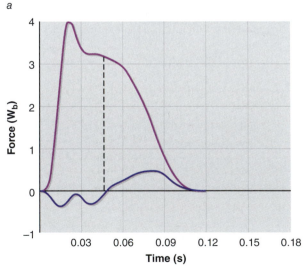

b

FIGURE 19.2   Sprint ground reaction force and impulse during the *(a)* acceleration phase and *(b)* maximal-velocity phase. W_b = body weight.

phase (figure 19.7, later in the chapter) is compared to the maximal-velocity phase (figure 19.8), which reflects the two different body positions used to produce force through maximal extension. Further, these two diagrams demonstrate the concept of impulse (represented as the area under the force–time curve) during the braking phase, indicated by a negative horizontal force, or during the propulsive phase that occurs where there is a positive horizontal force. These two phases of impulse are indicated by the vertical dotted line. It should be noted that during maximal-velocity phases, there is an asymmetrical production of force and the RFD is very high, resulting in much shorter ground contact times in comparison to the acceleration phase.

Momentum is defined as the relationship between the mass of an object and the velocity of movement. During a sprint, an athlete's body mass remains constant. Thus, given the same time frame, the only way to achieve a greater impulse is to generate greater force. This increase in impulse leads to an increase in momentum or a decrease in momentum, depending on whether the athlete is intending to accelerate or reaccelerate or decelerate before a change of direction. In other words, a change in impulse results in a change in momentum and is the cause of an object's movement.

Within human locomotion, the magnitude of the force coupled with the length of time the force is produced during an individual step is paramount to success. Changes in these forces can increase or decrease the athlete's momentum. For this reason, training should focus on impulse—the area under the force–time curve—in addition to RFD.

Power has not been discussed here because it is derived from force and velocity. Therefore, power is considered a mechanical construct that does not truly indicate maximal explosive performance (32). Practically speaking, a power value does not give insight into the performance in a way that is fully useful to professionals, because it is unclear whether a power value has been achieved as a result of the force or of the velocity. In understanding that force, RFD, and impulse are direct measures, one does not require a more complex derived value to gain additional insight.

Practical Implications for Speed

In order to displace their body mass down a track or field, athletes must produce forces sufficient to overcome the effects of gravity and create a positive change in velocity. Within a short sprint, force is the effort needed to accelerate an athlete up to his or her highest achievable speeds, which are largely determined by physiological factors. These forces or efforts are produced rapidly, with time constraints that are often shorter than the time needed for maximal voluntary force production. For this reason, rate of force production may be a more important factor for sprinting success. Moreover, since sprinting success is largely dependent on the production of forces within a short amount of time, impulse is an important underlying factor.

Practical Implications for Change of Direction and Agility

In addition to the requirement for acceleration, the production of braking forces over certain periods of time, termed *braking impulse*, should be considered during change-of-direction and agility maneuvers. The amount of impulse required to change momentum effectively and efficiently is a direct reflection of the physical requirements for change of direction. For example, as the angle of directional change required or the velocity of entry into the change of direction increases, so does the impulse required to change momentum; therefore it is physically more demanding to perform such activities. Further, the time restraints placed on a performer due to the perceptual–cognitive aspects of agility can influence the physical demands by limiting the time available to produce the required force (and impulse) to successfully change direction in response to a stimulus.

Neurophysiological Basis for Speed

Sprinting, agility, and change of direction are all dynamic displays of force production in the athletic setting. Because strength and conditioning professionals are often asked to assist in the development of these competitively advantageous qualities, an overview of how these force measures are produced during movement is warranted.

Nervous System

Neuromuscular function is vital to sprint performance, because the activity and the interaction of the central nervous system with the muscles ultimately influence the rate and strength of muscle contraction. Research has shown that the combination of strength, plyometric, and sprint training produces several adaptations within the neuromuscular system that may contribute to improved sprint performance. Strength training enhances *neural drive,* the rate and amplitude of impulses being sent from the nervous system to the target muscles (1). Increases in neural drive, which are indicative of an increase in the rate at which action potentials occur, are related to increases in both muscular force production and the rate of force production. Similarly, plyometric training demonstrates increases in excitability of high-

threshold motor neurons. Increased excitability ultimately enhances neural drive. Taken together, increases in neural drive may contribute to increases in the athlete's RFD and impulse generation.

Stretch–Shortening Cycle

Many functional tasks begin with preparatory countermovements involving spring-like actions referred to as the **stretch–shortening cycle (SSC)**—an eccentric–concentric coupling phenomenon in which muscle–tendon complexes are rapidly and forcibly lengthened, or stretch loaded, and immediately shortened in a reactive or elastic manner. Practically speaking, the SSC is demonstrated in movements in which a rapid transition from an eccentric action to a concentric action occurs. Therefore, SSC actions are particularly prevalent in sports involving running, jumping, and other explosive changes in velocity. Their performance is a distinct capability that is independent of maximal strength in elite athletes (35, 45, 46, 71, 72, 80, 87, 99).

Stretch–shortening cycle actions exploit two phenomena: (1) intrinsic muscle–tendon behavior and (2) force and length reflex feedback to the nervous system (3, 4, 9, 14, 25). Acutely, SSC actions tend to increase mechanical efficiency and impulse via elastic energy recovery, whereas chronically, they upregulate muscle stiffness and enhance neuromuscular activation (35, 45, 46, 71, 72).

Training activities aimed at improving SSC performance should fulfill two criteria (36, 71, 72, 80, 87):

- They should involve skillful, multijoint movements that transmit forces through the kinetic chain and exploit elastic–reflexive mechanisms.

- In order to manage fatigue and emphasize work quality and technique, they should be structured around brief work bouts or clusters separated by frequent rest pauses.

In practice, a combination of progressive plyometric and heavy resistance methods can accomplish these objectives. An intriguing example of this strategy is **complex training**, in which alternating SSC tasks with heavy resistance exercises within the same session enhances their working effect. The basis of this method is an acute aftereffect phenomenon referred to as **postactivation potentiation** (37, 66, 69). This training modality is becoming increasingly popular as a means of enhancing advanced athletes' performance but may be inappropriate for novices or youths.

Spring–Mass Model

Exposure to strength and speed training may be linked to a rise in the preactivation of the musculature used in sprinting (43, 46). The onset of pre-tension may be related to an increase in the sensitivity of associated muscle spindles. The improvement in the time needed for feedback from muscle spindles results in greater muscle stiffness and tendon compliance (44, 48, 68). This physiological condition provides support to the SSC, which underpins the **spring–mass model (SMM)**. The SMM (figure 19.3) is a mathematical model that depicts sprinting as a type of human locomotion in which the displacement of a body mass is the aftereffect from energy produced and is delivered through the collective coiling and extension of spring-like actions within muscle architecture (10, 21, 27, 29). During a complete

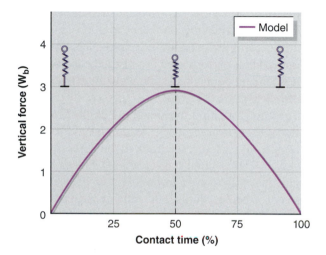

a

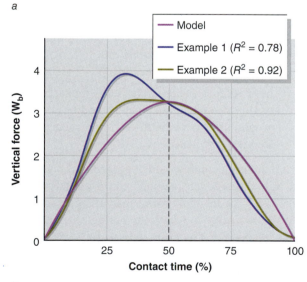

b

FIGURE 19.3 A simple spring–mass model relative to the ground reaction force during the stance phase of a sprint. During the stance phase, the model demonstrates how the leg (represented as a spring) is uncompressed at initial contact and then is compressed (represented by the change in length of the spring) during midstance or as vertical ground reaction force increases.

Reprinted, by permission, from Clark and Weyand, 2014 (17).

running cycle, one spring compresses and propels the sprinter's body forward. Simultaneously, the other spring swings forward in preparation for ground contact.

Within an upright sprint, compression of the spring begins at foot strike, resulting in horizontal braking forces. This sudden and brief deceleration assists in propelling the swing leg forward in preparation for the subsequent step. As the center of mass moves ahead of the foot, the sprinter is in midstance. Within the SMM, the spring is compressed to the lowest point, which coincides with a lowered center of mass at midstance. Finally, the model describes the push-off segment of the stance phase as the return of energy through the extension of the coiled spring. This resultant energy and return of force projects the sprinter forward.

While the SMM provides a conceptual framework for highlighting the actions involved in upright high-speed running, recent investigations suggest that there are limitations to the model's ability to describe the stance phase of elite sprinters. As illustrated in figure 19.2, during the maximal-velocity phase, elite sprinters tend to deviate from a classic SMM by producing much of their vertical force in the first half of a ground contact. In contrast, most nonelite sprinters, such as those involved in many team or field-based sports, display stance phases that are described by the SMM (17), where the vertical force curve is more symmetrical, as shown in figure 19.3. As such, the SMM should be used as a means to describe the relationship between the SSC, muscle stiffness, and sprinting. In fact, as stride frequency increases at a given running speed, one of the most important features of the leg spring is an increase in muscle stiffness (29).

> **Because sprinting requires an athlete to move at high speeds, strength and conditioning professionals should emphasize the prescription of exercises that have been shown to increase neural drive while overloading musculature of the hip and knee regions involved in the SSC.**

Additional Neurophysiological Considerations for Change-of-Direction and Agility Development

In addition to the neurophysiological aspects of speed performance previously discussed, there are other factors to consider with regard to change-of-direction and agility performance. During the plant phase, depicted in figure 19.4, the length of ground contact time of either an agility (0.23 to 0.25 seconds) (7) or a change-of-direction movement (0.44 to 0.722 seconds) (8, 39, 54) exceeds the typical ground contact time of both the acceleration phase of sprinting (0.17 to 0.2 seconds)

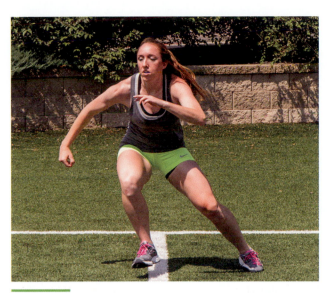

FIGURE 19.4 Plant phase, termed *stance phase* in the context of sprinting, of a change-of-direction movement. This is the point in a change-of-direction movement that represents the transition between the deceleration step and the acceleration step. Body positioning and the ability to maintain strong trunk positions during the deceleration of momentum and reorientation of the body to run in a new direction are critical for performance.

(4) and the maximal-velocity phase of sprinting (0.09 to 0.11 seconds) (92, 93). In view of this, most change of direction requires longer SSC activities.

Since effective braking is an important part of agility performance (83, 84), neuromuscular development with respect to high-velocity and high-force eccentric contractions should be considered, for two reasons. First, the adaptations or motor unit recruitment pathways called upon during an eccentric contraction are different than those called upon during concentric contractions (28). Secondly, the adaptations to eccentric training appear to be specific to the velocity of eccentric loading (62). In addition, training athletes for effective agility performance requires knowledge of perceptual–cognitive demands over and above the neurophysiological requirements for changing direction. Not only are the perceptual–cognitive demands on athletes related to their abilities in the areas of visual search scanning, anticipation, decision making, and reaction time (76), but also the tactical situation (offensive vs. defensive) changes the brain processing strategy required (82, 85).

The training required to improve agility becomes clearer as one begins to understand the various demands required for change of direction and agility with respect to neurophysiological factors, including the SSC, eccentric muscle action neuromuscular training, and implications of the length of time or the demand of the change-of-direction maneuver on the SMM. Further, neurophysiological requirements of agility performance extend beyond physical requirements to perceptual–cognitive requirements that are specific to the tactical situation.

Running Speed

Sprinting is a series of coupled flight and support phases, known as strides, orchestrated in an attempt to displace the athlete's body down the track at maximal acceleration or velocity (or both), usually over brief distances and durations. Sprinting has been described as rapid, unpaced, maximal-effort running of 15 seconds or less (67). However, the classic definition of sprint speed concerns the relationship between stride length and stride frequency (53).

Based on this understanding, sprint speed can be increased by an increase in stride length or an increase in stride frequency (figure 19.5). Although these changes in performance variables are logical, the underlying component to maximizing stride length and stride frequency is related to rapid force production.

- The differences between elite and novice sprinters can be traced to a single component. Much of the current literature on sprinting (13, 52, 93, 94) suggests that the amount of vertical force applied to the ground during the stance phase may be the most critical component to improving speed. In addition, these greater forces must be applied to the ground in the shortest period possible (RFD).

- Application of force is needed to displace a mass. In sprinting, stride length represents the displacement of mass. Elite male sprinters achieve a stride length of 2.70 m, whereas novice sprinters display a stride length of 2.56 m at maximum velocity (figure 19.6*a*) (52).

- Since contact with the ground is needed to continue force production and subsequent alterations in velocity, increasing the stride rate would theoretically maximize the time available to produce force. Elite male sprinters demonstrate stride rates near 4.63 steps per second compared to novice sprinters, who produce a lesser stride rate of 4.43 steps per second (figure 19.6*b*) (52). In other words, an elite sprinter needs less ground contact time to exert the effort needed to displace his or her mass. Thus these faster sprinters spend more time in the air due to their more frequent stride rate. Interestingly, elite sprinters display times to reposition the swing leg that are similar to those of their slower counterparts (52, 94).

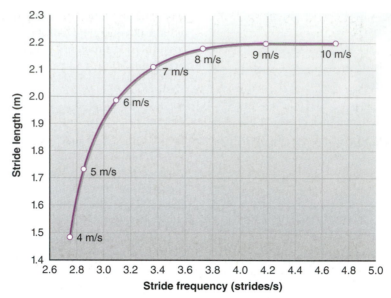

FIGURE 19.5   Stride length–frequency interaction as a function of running velocity.

Adapted from Dillman, 1975 (26).

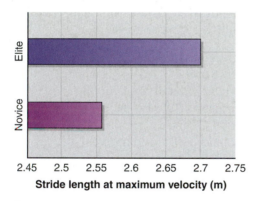

a

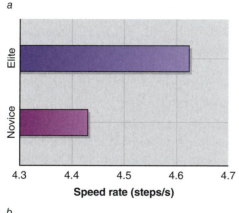

b

FIGURE 19.6   *(a)* Stride length and *(b)* stride rate in sprinters with varying qualifications.

Data from Mann (52).

Although the time required for staging the subsequent ground contact is similar between elite and novice sprinters, elite sprinters are able to propel themselves farther down the track due to properly directed vertical forces. Mann (52) suggests that these vertical forces are better directed toward the track due to an optimized knee height at maximal flexion of the recovering leg. This higher knee position provides a greater time period for force production and subsequent ground clearance. This technical advantage may be further evidence for why elite sprinters tend to produce most of their force within the first half of the stance phase.

In addition, faster sprinters are able to achieve higher velocities through the continuous application of high forces in a short stance phase, which results in longer strides occurring at a higher rate. Within the elite setting, this results in male sprinters achieving velocities near 12.55 m/s, whereas novices are limited to 11.25 m/s. While force production is arguably the limiting factor, technical efficiency and properly designed training also limit sprint speed.

> Sprint speed is determined by an athlete's stride length and stride rate; more successful sprinters tend to have longer stride lengths as a result of properly directed forces into the ground while also demonstrating a more frequent stride rate. These findings suggest that RFD and proper biomechanics are two of the primary limiting factors influencing sprint performance.

Sprinting Technique Guidelines

Linear sprinting is composed of a series of subtasks that can be divided into the start, acceleration (figure 19.7), and top speed (figure 19.8). While these phases of a sprint are technically distinct, they all require the athlete

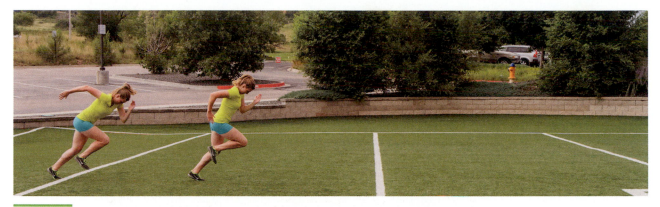

FIGURE 19.7   Sprinting technique during the initial acceleration (start) and acceleration.

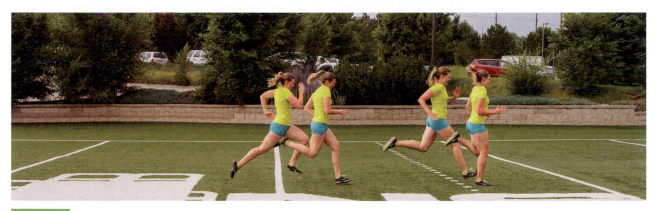

FIGURE 19.8   Sprinting technique at maximum velocity includes the late flight to early support, early support, late support, and toe-off phases.

to volitionally move the lower limbs at maximal speeds through a series of stance and flight phases. The stance phase can be broken down further into an eccentric braking period followed by a concentric propulsive period. In contrast, the flight phase consists of the **recovery** and **ground preparation** segments of the swing leg.

Figure 19.9 is a sprint technique checklist that accompanies figures 19.7 and 19.8. These recommendations are based on linear sprinting and may be useful for both instruction and evaluation of the movements. Figure 19.10 describes the fundamental movements occurring in maximum-velocity sprinting.

Technical Errors and Coaching

Table 19.1 highlights many common sprinting errors as well as possible causes and coaching corrections. Quite often, these errors are the result of the misapplication of forces due to improper coaching cues, insufficient mobility, or disruption to an athlete's normal gait caused by external interference. For instance, an athlete may demonstrate overstriding due to a coaching drill (such as reaching to successively longer marks along the track in order to gain speed) or the belief that acutely increasing stride length will allow one to "catch up" to a competitor

in a race. Regardless of the reason, the aim of coaches should be to promote an athlete's speed through the proper transmission of forces into the ground that will optimize the athlete's gait cycle.

Training Goals

The overarching goal of sprinting is to achieve optimal stride length and stride frequency through the correct application of force into the ground. The transmission of high forces must occur within a short stance phase, also known as ground contact time. During the acceleration phase, propulsive forces assist in elevating the hips above the ground to a point at which speed is no longer increasing at large rates. This portion of the sprint, known as maximum velocity, uses the SSC (through stiffness regulation) to propel the athlete's center of mass down the track horizontally.

The following fundamental training objectives regarding performance enhancement and injury prevention should be considered during the development of speed in practical settings:

- *Emphasize brief ground support times as a means of achieving rapid stride rate.* As previously

Sprinting Technique Checklist: Start, Acceleration, and Maximum Velocity

Start (Figure 19.7)

The athlete should attempt to distribute a balanced body weight through a set position (blocks, three- or four-point staggered start) that uses segment angles critical for the production of forces necessary to deliver explosive forces from the start.

- Front lower leg angle is ~90° in elite sprinters.
- Rear lower leg angle is ~133° in elite sprinters.

Aggressive extension with both legs

- Goal should be to generate high horizontal velocities through a maximal exertion (push) against blocks or ground.
- During start clearance (0.28 seconds), the legs combine to produce ~905 N of force.
- In order to overcome static start position, the sprinter must rely on the production of vertical forces to support the body weight in addition to moving the body's center of gravity into an upward running position.
- Vertical velocity is greatest during block clearance and the subsequent two steps due to the need for appropriate rise in the body's center of gravity.

Start clearance occurs once the leg set in the front block position nears extension at the knee joint.

- The exit angle of the front lower leg extension (measured at knee) during block clearance is ~160° in elite male sprinter populations.
- Optimal length of touchdown of first step is 0.5 m from start line.
- Initial starting velocity of elite sprinters can reach 5 m/s.

Acceleration (Figure 19.7)

Initial steps

- During both the start clearance and initial steps of the acceleration, the recovery of the swing legs should be low to the ground to a point where the toes are barely off the ground.
- Elite male sprinters display a stride rate of 5.26 steps/second during the second step compared to novice sprinters, who move at a rate of 3.45 steps/second.
- Elite male sprinters display a stride length of 1.13 to 1.15 m during the first two steps of block clearance compared to novices, who average 1.21 to 1.50 m.
- Stride length is shorter in elite sprinters due to the need for less flight time so that horizontal velocity is increased through more frequent ground contact times.
- Elite male sprinters average ground times of ~0.123 seconds during the second step of start clearance, while novice sprinters average 0.223 seconds.

By ~20 m, the body's center of gravity has been raised to a point at which sprinting is nearly upright. The head is in a relaxed, neutral position and will rise at the same rate as the torso.

Maximum Velocity (Figure 19.8)

The sprinter displays stacked joints with the shoulders appearing to sit directly above the hips, which sit above the foot during stance phase. The head continues to stay in a relaxed, neutral position with eyes focused directly ahead. The shoulders stay down and relaxed to allow the arms to move at the same rate as legs cycle through the phases of stance and swing.

- Elite male sprinters attain horizontal velocities ~12.55 m/s compared to novice sprinters, who reach velocities of 11.25 m/s.
- At maximum velocity, top sprinters display higher stride rates than their competitors. Specifically, elite males demonstrate a stride rate of 4.63 steps/second while novice sprinters take 4.43 steps/second.
- Elite male sprinters produce stride lengths of 2.70 m at maximum velocity compared to their novice counterparts, who achieve 2.56 m per stride.
- Elite male sprinters minimize ground contact time to 0.087 seconds, while novice sprinters maintain ground contact times of 0.101 during maximum velocity.

FIGURE 19.9 A checklist for sprinting at start, acceleration, and maximum velocity.

Adapted from Mann, 2011 (52).

Fundamental Movements Occurring in Maximum-Velocity Sprinting

Early Flight
- *Eccentric hip flexion:* decelerates backward rotation of thigh
- *Eccentric knee extension:* decelerates backward rotation of leg/foot

Midflight
- *Concentric hip flexion:* accelerates thigh forward
- *Eccentric knee extension → eccentric knee flexion*

Late Flight
- *Concentric hip extension:* rotates thigh backward in preparation for foot contact
- *Eccentric knee flexion:* accelerates leg backward, limiting knee extension; stops before foot strike (aided by concentric knee flexion to minimize braking at touchdown)

Early Support
- *Continued concentric hip extension:* minimizes braking effect of foot strike
- *Brief concentric knee flexion followed by eccentric hip extension:* resists tendency of hip/ankle extension to hyperextend knee; absorbs landing shock
- *Eccentric plantarflexion:* helps absorb shock and control forward rotation of tibia over ankle

Late Support
- *Eccentric hip flexion:* decelerates backward thigh rotation; rotates trunk in preparation for forward takeoff
- *Concentric knee extension:* propels center of gravity forward
- *Concentric plantarflexion:* aids in propulsion

FIGURE 19.10   List of the fundamental movements of the flight and support phases in maximum-velocity sprinting.
From Putnam and Kozey 1989 (65); Wood 1987 (95).

TABLE 19.1   Common Sprinting Technique Errors, Causes, and Corrections

Error	Cause	Coaching recommendations
START AND ACCELERATION		
Hips too high in start of crouch position.	Misunderstanding of setup	Instruct athlete to space feet by 1.5 to 2 foot lengths, then lower into starting position by dropping the shin of back leg to be more parallel with sprint surface.
Athlete is stepping out laterally during the initial drive phase.	Improper distribution of forces	Instruct athlete to push or drive through the ground to initiate the sprint.
Athlete's arm movement is abnormally short and tight.	Misunderstanding of natural arm swing	Instruct the athlete to either (a) drive the elbow down and back or (b) pull the hands down and back so as to simulate pulling on a rope. In addition, cue the athlete to allow the hands to fully break the waist while also allowing the arms to recover at midline of the body (invisible line from nose through navel).
Unnecessary tension in dorsal muscles; neck hyperextension.	Misunderstanding of movement	Instruct athlete to keep head in line with spine, as the torso and head should rise at the same rate during the acceleration and transition phases of the sprint.
Athlete "jumps" first stride or steps over the knee of stance leg.	Push-off angle too high; upward thrust too steep	Instruct the athlete to initiate movement by driving through the ground and allow the swing leg to horizontally "cut" the stance leg shin, rather than stepping over the stance leg. In addition, one may cue the athlete to keep the foot of swing leg close to the ground in order to set up a proper acceleration phase.

(continued)

TABLE 19.1   *(continued)*

Error	Cause	Coaching recommendations
Premature upright posture.	Inadequate push-off force; improper carriage of head	Instruct the athlete to continue pushing into the ground while maintaining a natural trunk lean. Also cue the athlete to keep the head in line with the spine, as lifting the head may result in a sudden lifting of the torso, ultimately minimizing acceleration patterns.
MAXIMUM VELOCITY		
Athlete is superficially attempting to maintain an acceleration phase when the shins are clearly vertical.	Improper understanding of movement patterns	Instruct the athlete that as the shins and hips come up to vertical, so should the torso and head. Encourage the athlete to feel for the rise in the hips so that the joints (shoulders to hips to ankles) stay stacked or in line. This position allows for the proper transmission of forces into the running surface.
Athlete is not displaying optimal front side mechanics with regard to the height of swing leg knee.	Inadequate force production	Recall that the swing leg's knee height (traditionally called front side mechanics) is purely a display of ground reaction forces. Improper cueing an athlete to lift the knees may result in further improper transmission of forces and ultimately change the musculature naturally used during the sprint event.
Athlete is overstriding.	Misunderstanding of force application	Success in sprint events results from the ability to produce high vertical forces in a short amount of time. An athlete overstriding is attempting to increase speed via larger ground contact times, which ultimately dampens the effects of the stretch–shortening cycle. Instruct athletes to "run in their lane" and maintain their natural gait cycle.
Athlete is displaying chronic hamstring injury or pain.	Insufficient mobility, improper positioning of pelvis	A high likelihood of hamstring injury occurs during the swing phase of the sprint event as a result of eccentric (lengthening) forces. An athlete is further compromised when displaying anterior pelvic tilt during the sprint event. Before training or competition, mobility and soft tissue therapy may be warranted in order to stabilize the pelvis in a neutral position.
Athlete is attempting to "cycle" the leg action, resulting in an increased time to complete the swing phase. This is made apparent by the open gap between the knees during the stance phase.	Improper force application	Instruct the athlete to drive the foot down and back into the track, not paw. Due to the seemingly horizontal movement of the foot during a sprint, coaches often miscue athletes to paw the foot into the track. Pawing the foot horizontally against the track prevents the athlete from using vertical forces, overloading the stretch–shortening cycle to move down the track.
Athlete is displaying erroneous arm movement in the transverse plane.	Improper understanding of movement pattern	While traditionally coaches would claim that erratic arm movement is a symptom of fatigue, much literature suggests that speed is limited by mechanical force application, not metabolic efficiency. Under this newer model, coaches should emphasize driving the arms down and back while maintaining an upright torso. In addition, the coach should recommend to the athlete that the arm swing recover near the midline of the body in order to take advantage of the glenohumeral joint's natural range of motion.

mentioned, this requires high levels of explosive strength. This quality is developed systematically through consistent exposure to speed training as well as properly designed strength training programs.

- *Emphasize the further development of the SSC as a means to increase the amplitude of impulse for each step of the sprint.* Specifically, high achievers at top-speed sprinting produce high forces in a shorter stance phase using the SSC. The complete weightlifting movements and their derivatives are key exercises for overloading the SSC with forces greater than those produced during an open sprint.

Agility Performance and Change-of-Direction Ability

In both field and court sports, there are a substantial number of preplanned change-of-direction movements as well as changes in direction in response to the ball, the game, or opponents. In sports such as baseball, softball, American football, and basketball, athletes decide before commencement of movement on the path they will run. Such patterns often including a quick or sudden change of direction—for example, exploding into a sprint out of a shuffle off a base or running a route before receipt of a ball. However, many sports also include rapid changes of direction in response to opponents or tactical situations. Such responses can occur in an offensive or a defensive scenario, and the physical movement and perceptual–cognitive aspects of such performances impose different demands on the athlete. Therefore, one should thoroughly understand the factors associated with agility performance from a physical standpoint

▶ **Athletes improve change-of-direction ability through development of a number of physical factors and technical skills during a variety of speeds and modes of movement. The development of agility also requires improving perceptual–cognitive abilities in relation to the demands of the sport.**

(change-of-direction ability) and in combination with the perceptual–cognitive aspects (agility).

Factors Affecting Change of Direction and Perceptual–Cognitive Ability

It is becoming increasingly clear that the ground contact time and ground reaction force during the plant phase (figure 19.4) of a movement provide valuable insight into the physical factors that affect change-of-direction performance, while perceptual–cognitive factors must also be considered with regard to agility. Change-of-direction and agility movements performed at shallow cutting angles (less than 75°) and associated with shorter ground contact times (less than 250 ms) (83) will benefit from training similar to speed training with regard to the physical demands but will still require additional perceptual–cognitive training. On the other hand, when a change of direction involves a more aggressive cutting angle (equal to or greater than 75°), the length of ground contact time can often exceed 250 ms (8, 38, 54) due to the greater braking requirements. Therefore, one should consider increasing emphasis on eccentric strength and maximal strength alongside the concentric explosiveness required during the reacceleration. Figure 19.11 provides an example of how various requirements (angle of change of direction or perceptual–cognitive requirement of agility) may affect the ground reaction force and ground contact times of athletes. Of particular interest is the effect of various methods of changing direction (for the same-degree cut) on ground reaction force and ground contact times. The effect of method of changing direction can be seen in figure 19.11: The

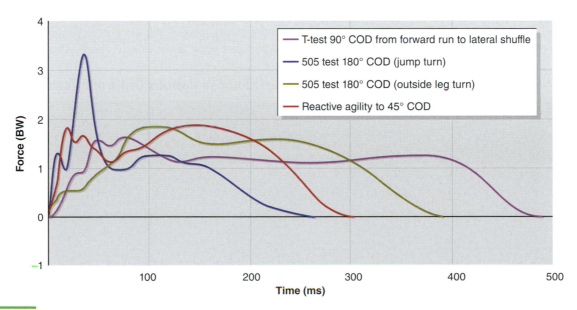

FIGURE 19.11 Comparison of ground reaction force and contact times during various change-of-direction (COD) and agility maneuvers.

505 was performed either with a single-leg change of direction (outside leg turn) or with a "jump turn" that can be performed in a testing environment but is not commonly performed on the field of play. Nevertheless, this demonstrates that the technique chosen will dictate the demands; therefore, if trying to elicit a specific adaptation from an athlete, one should provide specific instructions.

The test used for assessment of agility performance will have an impact on perceived agility ability of the athlete. A plethora of tests are used to assess "agility," but tests without a reactive aspect should be considered change-of-direction tests, and a test that includes a reactive stimulus is now by definition a test of agility for most sports. Further, the requirements of the test may result in assessment of factors other than change-of-direction ability or perceptual–cognitive requirements. Therefore, one must be informed about and critical regarding a test used to assess "agility" or "change-of-direction ability." For example, if the Illinois agility test, often performed with soccer athletes (91), was used after pre-season training, improvements in performance during the Illinois agility test may be due to improved metabolic capacity and not necessarily improved change-of-direction ability. This is attributed to the length of the Illinois test, which imposes a higher metabolic demand than shorter tests.

However, it should be noted that even similar-length tests such as the traditional 505 test, the modified 505 test (the 505 without the initial 10 m run-up), and the L-run used on the same athletes have only a moderate relationship (31), indicating they are not all assessing the same type of change-of-direction ability or the same underpinning physical requirements. This becomes more apparent when one realizes that some tests require a rapid change of direction while others require multiple changes of direction. Tests with multiple changes of direction often require more bending around an object or cone, while maintaining as much velocity as possible, in comparison to a sharp change of direction that demands a rapid deceleration. Therefore, tests such as the Illinois agility or L-run that require a bend to maintain velocity instead of an aggressive change of direction could be considered tests of maneuverability (58). With this said, table 19.2 gives examples of change-of-direction and agility tests and drills that address different physical requirements within the realm of "agility." One should consider the aspect most important to the given sport when determining change-of-direction and agility abilities and consider testing and monitoring various types of change-of-direction abilities and perceptual–cognitive abilities required during true agility tests.

Change-of-Direction Ability

As just stated, one must understand that an athlete's measured change-of-direction ability may vary depending on the demand imposed by the chosen change-of-direction test. Therefore, it may be beneficial to choose different tests that measure this ability under a high-velocity braking requirement; with multiple changes of direction; or, as will be discussed, in reaction to a scenario, opponent, or stimulus. Another consideration regarding change-of-direction ability is the orientation of the body leading into the deceleration, through the transition phase as the athlete comes to a stop, and then the positioning as he or she subsequently reaccelerates out of the change of direction. Therefore, the positioning of the trunk will influence the performance of the change of direction. Therefore, it is a combination of the ability to decelerate, reorient the body to face or partially face the direction of intended travel, and then explosively reaccelerate that truly determines change-of-direction ability.

Considering the requirements for rapidly changing momentum, increased muscle mass in combination with decreased body fat has been regarded as a predictor of

TABLE 19.2   Aspects of Agility Tested or Trained in Various Drills and Tests

	Change-of-direction speed	Maneuverability	Perceptual–cognitive ability	Metabolic requirement* (average length of test)
Reactive agility tests	✓		✓	< 3 s
505	✓			< 3 s
Pro agility	✓			< 5 s
T-test	✓	✓		< 12 s*
Illinois agility			✓	< 12 s*
L-run			✓	< 6 s

*The length of the test has a large influence on the metabolic requirements and whether changes in test performance can become a function of enhanced conditioning instead of directly related to improvements in change-of-direction or agility ability.

Data from references 31, 60, 63, 75, 79, 90, 91, and 97.

change-of-direction performance when assessed by the T-test in elite basketball players (16). Other anthropometrics and their relationship to change-of-direction ability are not discussed here, as aspects such as height and limb length are not modifiable by the strength and conditioning professional. Instead, body center of mass height is related to improved lateral change-of-direction performance (78), and this can be actively targeted during training.

Overall, change-of-direction ability among a variety of movement patterns (various degrees of cutting) has been shown to improve with increased hip extension velocity (rapid application of force by the hip extensors), low center of mass height, increased braking impulse and propulsive impulse, increased knee flexion entering the change of direction, minimized trunk angular displacement entering the change of direction (deceleration phase), and increased lateral trunk tilt (during 180° changes) (15, 70, 78, 83, 84, 86). As the ability to decelerate, hold body position, and then reaccelerate is important in change-of-direction tasks as described by the kinetic and kinematic requirements of faster change-of-direction and agility performances, it is clear that a well-rounded approach to strength development involving dynamic, isometric, and in particular eccentric strength capacities is needed for the development of better change-of-direction performances (41, 86). In contrast to sprint development, it is recommended that athletes undergo training that allows for the neuromuscular system to effectively adapt to the rate of loading required during the braking phase, with the understanding that the neuromuscular requirements for braking capacity must be specifically trained using high-velocity eccentric contractions (28) such as those during drop landings, landing from a loaded jump, or the catch phase of a power clean or power snatch. All of these place different eccentric loading demands on the hips, knees, and ankles (56).

Perceptual–Cognitive Ability

When the physical ability to change direction rapidly is present, one can focus on the components of perceptual–cognitive ability that must be developed to bring together the ability to perform both physically and mentally on the field of play. There are several components of perceptual–cognitive ability: visual scanning, anticipation, pattern recognition, knowledge of the situation, decision-making time and accuracy, and reaction time (75, 77, 83, 97, 98). Many of these aspects of development are sport specific, and a comprehensive discussion is beyond the scope of this text. However, general drills to help improve these skills are discussed in the section on methods of developing agility.

Technical Guidelines and Coaching

In comparison to sprinting, change of direction and agility have a large number of degrees of freedom due to the multitude of movements that occur during a change of direction. Further, agility performance as restricted or determined by opponents or other tactical restraints and scenarios cannot be trained through the use of a single technique. Nevertheless, the following are some technical guidelines and coaching suggestions.

Visual Focus

- When changing direction in response to an opponent (either offensive or defensive), the athlete should focus on the shoulders, trunk, and hip.
- Following the anticipation of the event, unless deception is intended, the athlete should quickly redirect attention to a new area to help lead the transition of the body.

Body Position During Braking and Reacceleration

- Control the trunk leading into the deceleration (decrease large amounts of trunk motion) (70).
- Through the stance phase, reorient the trunk and hips toward the direction of intended travel to allow for a more effective reacceleration (15).
- Just as with acceleration mechanics, body lean is paramount in allowing proper force application through the ground with strong alignment of the ankle, knee, and hip and through to the trunk and shoulders.
- Enter and exit changes in direction with a lower center of mass; when performing side-shuffling changes of direction, maintaining this low center of mass is critical (78).

Leg Action

- Ensure that the athlete can effectively dissipate or tolerate the eccentric braking loads through an effective range of motion at the knee and avoid a stiff-legged braking style (81, 83).
- Emphasize "pushing the ground away" in order to enhance performance, especially while learning in closed drills. External focus of attention—through instructions to concentrate on the ground instead of a body part—has been shown to improve change-of-direction performance (64).

Arm Action

- Powerful arm actions should be used to facilitate leg drive.
- Ensure that the action of the arms is not counterproductive (i.e., does not cause a decrease in speed

or efficiency), particularly during transitioning between difficult changes of direction (e.g., from a backpedal to a sprint).

Training Goals

The three goals of agility performance are enhanced perceptual–cognitive ability in various situations and tactical scenarios, effective and rapid braking of one's momentum, and rapid reacceleration toward the new direction of travel. To meet these goals, one should emphasize the following:

- Directing visual focus toward the opponent's shoulders, trunk, and hips to increase perceptual ability to anticipate the movement of a defensive or offensive opponent (75)

- Orienting the body into a position that allows for effective application of forces into the ground to maximize braking capacity, and increasing the speed from which one can rapidly stop as well as the direction of movement one must brake from (running forward, running backward, or shuffling laterally) (15, 70, 78, 83, 84, 86)

- The ability to maintain a good position after braking, reorient the body into a position that faces the new direction, and effectively use acceleration mechanics to reaccelerate (58)

Methods of Developing Speed

From a practical standpoint, the demonstration of proper speed is the result of well-organized programming that organically develops and matures the required skill sets within the athlete. This organic approach to sprint training results from a schema of development that is based on the emphasis and de-emphasis of certain qualities, such as acceleration and maximum velocity, within each training phase. Furthermore, the training plan should coordinate these singular qualities through phasic progression. A well-constructed training plan highlights specific components that will assist in fully maximizing an athlete's movement potential.

Sprinting

Although a variety of training stimuli are important for the optimization of athletic performance, it can be argued that no exercise improves running velocity more than maximum-velocity sprinting. An athlete's sprint prowess depends on the generation of high forces in short periods of time (52, 93). Neurological adaptations resulting from long-term training plans that emphasize maximal strength and movement velocity improve both RFD and impulse generation (1, 89). In the strength and conditioning setting, weightlifting movements and jump training are prescribed to develop RFD and impulse at varying loads, as these movements use the SSC. Similarly, upright sprinting uses the SSC, defining it as a plyometric movement. Chronic exposure to movements eliciting the SSC can increase muscle stiffness, which is a potential physiological advantage for sprint ability (29).

In addition, sprinting requires near-maximum to maximum muscle activation, which depends on high central nervous system activity. This activity is often referred to as *rate coding* (47, 68). When signal frequency reaches a threshold, skeletal muscle may not completely relax between stimulations (47). Incomplete relaxation results in more forceful contractions and a greater RFD in subsequent contractions (57). Therefore, chronic exposure to sprinting may lead to improvements in musculoskeletal control via the central nervous system. This would result in a cyclical dose–response relationship, as neurophysiological adaptations from previous practices would bolster subsequent training. In an effort to either enhance the force required or target potential neuromuscular adaptations for sprinting improvement, resisted and assisted sprint training techniques are often employed. The proposed benefits, potential drawbacks, and coaching considerations are outlined in table 19.3.

Strength

As noted throughout the chapter, sprint speed is underpinned by an athlete's ability to produce large forces within a brief period of time. These forces must be large enough to (a) support the body weight in the presence of gravity and (b) displace the body through an increase in velocity (52). Thus many strength and conditioning professionals are aware of the importance of weight training in the development of a sprint-based athlete. Central to the discussion of strength training is how best to transfer newly developed strength qualities from the weight room to the track (96). The transfer of strength improvements to sprinting may require an emphasis on the specificity of training. This transfer of training effect deals with the degree of performance adaptation and may result from the similarities between the movement patterns, peak force, RFD, acceleration, and velocity patterns of an exercise and the sporting environment (87).

While maximal strength training may be beneficial, training should emphasize agendas that merge maximal strength and speed–strength qualities (34). The selection of exercises and movements that provide opportunities to display forces and velocities similar to those found in sprinting may have the most benefit with regard to enhancing rate coding and firing frequency, alongside alterations to Type II muscle fibers such as cross-sectional area and fascicle length (30, 33). For instance, evidence suggests that weightlifting movements and

TABLE 19.3   Assistance and Resistance Training for Speed Development

Type of training	Example exercise modalities	Potential benefits	Potential disadvantages	Practical use suggestion
Assistance training (e.g., overspeed training)	Inclusive of modalities such as rope towing, bungee cord pulls, or downhill running with the intention of allowing the athlete to run at supramaximal speeds	Theoretically, these training tools are used in hopes of exposing the athlete to higher velocities than one can achieve in unassisted sprinting by inducing an increased stride rate. This increased stride rate is hypothesized to have potential for neuromuscular adaptations to increase maximal sprint velocity.	Assisted sprinting may prematurely rush an athlete's stance phase, thus removing time needed to exert proper forces, and has been shown to result in decreased muscle activation and propulsive force production in comparison to maximal running (55). Therefore what can be described as "chop" steps may often be observed. Exercises that rely on the towing of athletes may increase braking forces in comparison to maximal running (55) as athletes attempt to tolerate velocities they cannot naturally create or accommodate to as a result of biomechanical efficiency, training state, or both. Downhill sprinting may expose the athlete to unnecessary eccentric forces through a modified stance leg that results from having to "find the ground." This may also affect the SSC, which is optimized through the foot placement occurring just in front of the center of mass upon ground contact in flat-surface upright sprinting (55). To date, very little research supports the implementation of overspeed training, as sprint success results from an athlete's ability to produce large forces in a short ground contact time.	Top-speed sprinting should be developed through more natural and safer training tools that consider an athlete's training status and support optimal biomechanics. Coaches should carefully assess the implications of assistance modalities before implementation.
Resistance training	Inclusive of training modalities such as sled towing, wind resistance, incline sprinting, and sled pushing with the intention of improving an athlete's accelerative abilities	Accentuates the biomechanics of the acceleration phase by placing the athlete in a position that promotes lowered torso, hips, and shin angles. Resisted sprinting may optimize an athlete's ability to cover short distances quickly by overloading the acceleration phase, resulting in ground contact times that produce higher propulsive forces. Improving acceleration, which is a change in velocity, may lead to an increase in top speed through enhanced rate of force development.	Sprint efforts against a load that is too great may lead to longer ground contact times in addition to shorter stride lengths that are not task specific (49). Slopes of incline that are too great may modify proper sprinting biomechanics, resulting in rehearsal of improper technique and thus limiting transfer of training effect. Sled pushing may alter the natural sprinting gait cycle due to the removal of arm action that synchronizes and counterbalances the leg action occurring at the hip.	Coaches and athletes attempting to improve the acceleration phase of a sprint may adopt resistance training modalities that maintain normal biomechanics involved in unresisted sprints. Loads should be chosen based on the sporting context while also considering the athlete's physical status. For instance, track and field sprinters may use loads that do not decrease running velocity by more than 10% to 12% (2, 39, 51, 42). In contrast, field sport athletes who overcome external resistance while blocking, tackling, and scrimmaging can use loads 20% to 30% of body weight to improve the initial 5-10 m of movement (20, 42).

SSC = stretch-shortening cycle.
Data from references 2, 20, 40, 42, 49, 51, and 55.

their derivatives such as the clean, snatch, and midthigh pulls may enhance sprint performance through physiological adaptations such as muscular stiffness, enhanced RFD, and coactivation of the musculature surrounding the hips and knees (6, 18, 24).

Mobility

While not a kinetic variable, soft tissue manipulation has become an increasingly used practice in the development of speed athletes. Coaches and trainers rely on tools such as stretching, chiropractic care, massage, and myofascial release in an attempt to achieve optimal mobility within the dynamic state. Mobility is the freedom of an athlete's limb to move through a desired range of motion, whereas flexibility is a joint's total range of motion. With an understanding that positional characteristics are among several limiting factors in performance, coaches should ensure that proper postural integrity is in place before the onset of practice or competition.

Based on the previously described constructs of speed, the currently accepted model of sprint success is based on the athlete's ability to produce and overcome ground reaction forces in a short amount of time. Moreover, while these ground reaction forces assist in producing optimal stride length through forward propulsion, the sprinter's position in flight may be limited by insufficient mobility. Specifically, an athlete may possess the physical characteristics necessary to yield high rates of force in a short amount of time, but compromises in a joint's freedom of movement will result in misplaced forces. The improper placement of forces due to erroneous ground contact will result in dampened sprint speed and an increased likelihood for injury.

Methods of Developing Agility

As discussed throughout the chapter, a multifactorial approach is warranted to develop both the physical and the perceptual–cognitive aspects required for continual improvement in agility performance. Therefore, one should consider a plan that addresses underpinning physical capacities using various strength development strategies, technical competence in a closed skill environment with movement-specific actions (change-of-direction ability), and improvement of perceptual–cognitive capacity through agility drills and inherent aspects of skills practice (58).

Strength

Similar to aspects of strength development for speed, strength development for agility should emphasize relative strength and a variety of speed–strength qualities along the force–velocity spectrum. However, additional

development of the eccentric strength of the athlete due to the large braking forces during change-of-direction and agility movements should be considered. This means that training exercises can include a spectrum of load–velocity profiles in the weight room (32) as well as a variety of load–velocity profile activities in the field, such as squat jumps, countermovement jumps, and drop jumps of various heights in combination with the change-of-direction and agility drills themselves. The multifactorial nature of agility warrants a well-rounded approach to strength development. Table 19.4 provides an example of how training in the weight room and on the field can satisfy the strength requirements underlying agility performance. Understanding that athletes will develop the physical requirements before being able to transfer newly gained strength into technical competence helps both coaches and athletes realize that performance gains will lag behind fundamental physical requirements for a given technical skill (88).

Change-of-Direction Ability

Similar to the progressions of plyometric activities based on intensity and difficulty of each drill, closed skill change-of-direction drills can progress from beginner to intermediate to advanced levels based on the physical loading demands that have been discussed in this chapter. Table 19.5 presents an example of a progression of drills for change-of-direction ability (both rapid changes of direction and those associated with maneuverability), as well as a progression plan for agility drills. The physical loading during agility drills will be higher than beginner change-of-direction drills. Therefore, table 19.5 provides practitioners with a series of drills and a guideline for safely and effectively advancing athletes so they can build on their physical and technical attributes as they improve.

Perceptual–Cognitive Ability

During years of skills training (within the sport), athletes continually enhance visual scanning, pattern recognition, and knowledge of the situation, while in drills used to improve agility (outside of skills practice) they primarily focus on improving anticipation, decision-making time, and accuracy. In the same way one would regularly increase the demands of a physical task to continually improve performance, one can train perceptual–cognitive ability (table 19.5). Therefore, agility activities should begin by adding a perceptual–cognitive component to common closed skill change-of-direction drills. For example, decelerations or the Z-drill can evolve into agility drills by including a generic stimulus such as a whistle, a coach command, or a flashing arrow or light (76, 97). Following success with the aforementioned

TABLE 19.4   Comparison of Focus for Agility Development in Novice and Advanced Athletes

Strength requirement	Novice athletes (weight room associated)	Novice athletes (field and court drills)	Advanced athletes (weight room associated)	Advanced athletes (field and court drills)
Dynamic strength Required to provide base strength for all subsequent training as well as to ensure adequate mobility during body weight and loaded training	Body weight exercises	"Body awareness" work such as leaning drills	Squat (and variations) Pulls (and variations)	Various change-of-direction drills
Concentric explosive strength (may include isometric strength work) Required to effectively reaccelerate after the braking phase or maintain strong position through the transition phase of change of direction and agility	Box jumps	Acceleration drills	Box jumps Olympic lifts Squat jumps (loaded)	Advanced acceleration drills (e.g., sled push)
Eccentric strength Required to develop the ability to effectively absorb load required during the braking phase of change of direction and agility	Drop landing	Deceleration drills (forward emphasis)	Drop landings and receiving strength required during the catch phase of Olympic lifts Accentuated eccentric training	Decelerations drills (high velocity and various angles)
Reactive strength Required to increase the ability to transfer from high eccentric load to concentric explosiveness	—	Beginner plyometrics	Loaded jumps Drop jumps Complex training	Advanced plyometrics
Multidirectional strength Required to hold body position strongly during multitude of movement demands	Lunges	Low-velocity COD (e.g., Z-drill) Lateral, backward, and forward COD drills	Unilateral lifts Greater degree of freedom lifts (e.g., land mine exercises)	High-velocity COD drills Challenging cutting-angle COD drills
Perceptual–cognitive abilities Required to progress in visual scanning, effective anticipation, and decision making	—	Simple reaction drills: introduction to increasing either temporal or spatial uncertainty	—	Small-sided games Agility drills with severely restricted temporal and spatial aspects

COD = change of direction.
Adapted, by permission, from Nimphius, 2014 (58).

agility drills, progression requires activities that have sport-specific stimuli such as evasive drills and small-sided games, which have been said to have better transfer to performance (76, 97). Both generic and specific stimuli can be made more difficult within a given agility drill through progressive increases in either temporal (time) or spatial (space or area) stress on the athlete.

Program Design

Program design involves planning at several levels, each with its own set of considerations: microcycles (short-term), mesocycles (medium-term), and macrocycles (long-term). The process is referred to as periodization. **Periodization** is the strategic manipulation of an athlete's preparedness through the employment of sequenced training phases defined by cycles and stages of workload. These planned workloads are varied in order to facilitate the integration of planned programming tactics that will harmonize the relationship between training-induced fatigue and accommodation (22). Furthermore, the periodization process is guided by information collected during the athlete monitoring process. Specifically, as an athlete progresses through a training phase, consistent information acquired through various monitoring strategies helps to show how the athlete is responding to the training stimulus in the short term and how the athlete should be further developed in

TABLE 19.5 Change-of-Direction and Agility Drill Progressions

Agility component	Beginner	Intermediate	Advanced
Change of direction	Deceleration drills (forward) progressing to higher entry velocity or shorter distance to stop Basic movement patterns for forward, backward, and lateral shuffling Change-of-direction drills that involve low velocities (less than 5 yards of acceleration into change of direction)—Z-drill, for example	Deceleration drills (lateral) with same progressions as forward Expand to include a broad range of cutting angles less than 75° May increase entry velocity during drills (up to 10 yards of acceleration leading into change of direction)	Deceleration to reacceleration in both forward and lateral directions Expand further to a comprehensive range of cutting angles including those greater than 75°
"Maneuverability"	Basic drills or tests such as the Illinois agility that require nearly straight-line running with slight bends	Drills that increase the difficulty of the "bend" involved such as the L-run Drills that require transition between modes of movement (shuffling, sprinting, and backpedaling) such as the T-test	
Agility	Physical and technical competence should occur before agility drills are incorporated.	Change-of-direction drills in beginner and intermediate categories with the addition of simple stimuli (arrow, pointing in a certain direction) These drills present a limited number of options for the athlete to have to react to (e.g., right or left, forward or back) on the signal	Expand into large degrees of spatial and temporal uncertainty (and therefore greater perceptual–cognitive stress) Small-sided games Evasion games and drills

Adapted, by permission, from Nimphius, 2014 (58).

the long term—that is, how the original training program should be modified to reflect responses to the training.

At each level of training plan development, strength and conditioning professionals must manipulate certain variables. While these are useful in characterizing the training agenda as well as quantifying workloads, coaches should also keep in mind that each variable must be considered individually as well as with regard to how it affects the collective system. Moreover, individual athlete training responses, which athlete monitoring reveals, should be used in the manipulation of these variables.

- Exercise (or work) interval—the duration or distance over which a repetition is executed
- Exercise order—the sequence in which a set of repetitions is executed
- Frequency—the number of training sessions performed in a given time period (e.g., day or week)
- Intensity—the effort with which a repetition is executed (% of maximum)

- Recovery (rest) interval—the time period between repetitions and sets
- Repetition—the execution of a specific workload assignment or movement technique
- Series—a group of sets and recovery intervals
- Set—a group of repetitions and rest intervals
- Volume—the amount of work (e.g., three sets of five repetitions) performed in a given training session or time period
- Work-to-rest ratio—the relative density of exercise and relief intervals in a set, expressed as a ratio
- Volume load—the density of volume performed at prescribed intensities—for example, three sets of five repetitions at 100 kg results in a volume-load of 1,500 kg

Chapter 21 explains periodization of resistance training programs, and the same concepts can be applied to sprint, change-of-direction, and agility training.

Speed Development Strategies

The planning process for speed development is very similar to that used by strength and conditioning professionals in the weight room. Specifically, planning tactics should be periodized in a manner that addresses the physical and psychological components of sprinting through emphasis and de-emphasis on particular qualities in a phasic manner. An athlete's capability to sprint can be improved through the incorporation of training periods that are designed to fully maximize and saturate a fitness quality, which may bolster the effects of future training agendas.

In order to enhance speed, a practitioner should consider the relationship between human locomotion and force production. Throughout this chapter the authors have pointed to a link between sprint success and certain physiological phenomena. Elite sprinters produce large amounts of force within a short amount of time. This high level of force allows the sprinter to produce longer stride lengths at a faster rate. This display of movement on the track is a reflection of enhanced neuromuscular factors, namely maximal strength, RFD, and impulse. These variables are the product of well-designed training protocols that aim to enhance qualities such as the hypertrophy of task-specific motor units, firing frequency, rate coding, and muscle–tendon stiffness.

The example of speed development provided in the application table demonstrates how sequenced phases of training may seamlessly develop sprint potential through the maturation of accelerative abilities before the execution of maximal-velocity efforts. This model, which can be referred to as a *short to long method* of sprint training, is a conceptual progression that attempts to merge the relationship between larger rates of acceleration and greater sprint velocities (discussed earlier in this chapter) (23). Specifically, an athlete taking part in a short to long model will begin the training year with an emphasis on improving propulsive force output through short sprints that maintain the biomechanics associated with the acceleration phase of a sprint. Later, the athlete bridges into longer sprint work that aims to enhance top

Application of Speed Development Strategies: Phasic Development of a Short-Distance (100 m) Sprinter

Block and emphasis	Training tool and notes	Load prescription (rest periods between sets) for week 1 for each block
BLOCK 1: *Primary aim:* Acceleration development	1. Use incline sprinting in order to place athlete into proper acceleration mechanics, which provides an opportunity to maximize propulsion forces in the initial stages of a sprint. 2. Emphasize low heel recovery; driving the foot "down and through" the ground; aggressive and complete arm action; neutral head position "in line with the spine."	**MONDAY AND WEDNESDAY:** **Incline sprints** 1 × 3 × 15 m (1.5 min) 1 × 4 × 20 m (2 min) **FRIDAY:** **Incline sprints** 1 × 2 × 15 m (1.5 min) 1 × 3 × 20 m (2 min) 1 × 2 × 25 m (2.5 min)
BLOCK 2: *Primary aim:* Long acceleration development *Secondary aim:* Improve transition to upright sprinting *Tertiary aim:* Exposure to speed endurance	1. Steadily remove the athlete from the incline by gradually introducing flat-ground sprinting from a low starting position or towing mechanism. 2. Promote the correct biomechanics of transition sprinting from acceleration to maximal velocity through the inclusion of acceleration holds.*	**MONDAY:** **Incline sprints** 1 × 3 × 30 m (3 min) 1 × 3 × 40 m (4 min) **WEDNESDAY:** **Push-up starts** 1 × 4 × 15 m (2 min) **Sled tows** 2 × 3 × 20 m (2 min /4 min) **FRIDAY:** **Crouch starts** 1 × 4 × 15 m (2 min) **Acceleration holds** 1 × 3 × 40 m (4 min)

(continued)

(continued)

Block and emphasis	Training tool and notes	Load prescription (rest periods between sets) for week 1 for each block
BLOCK 3: *Primary aim:* Introduction to max speed training *Secondary aim:* Maintain accelerative ability *Tertiary aim:* Continued exposure to speed endurance; introduction to special endurance	1. Maintain acceleration abilities through inclusion of short sprints at beginning of almost every session. 2. Begin exposure to maximum speed training through exercises that use upright sprinting mechanics. 3. Prescribe speed endurance or special endurance sessions later in the week when effects of summated fatigue may dampen neural drive.	**MONDAY:** **Block starts** 1 × 2 × 20 m (2.5 min) 1 × 2 × 30 m (3.5 min) **Accelerations from crouch stance** 1 × 3 × 40 m (5 min) **WEDNESDAY:** **High-stance starts** 1 × 3 × 20 m (2.5 min) **Fly-ins** 1 × 4 × 15 m build/20 m fly (4 min) **FRIDAY:** **Block starts** 1 × 4 × 25 m (3 min) **Accelerations from crouch stance** 1 × 2 × 45 m (5 min) **Speed endurance from high stance** 1 × 2 × 60 m (5.5 min)
BLOCK 4: *Primary aim:* Enhance maximal speed ability *Secondary aim:* Maintain accelerative ability *Tertiary aim:* Continued exposure to speed endurance and special endurance	1. Continue exposure to maximum speed training through longer fly-in zones or race-modeling practices. 2. Maintain acceleration abilities through inclusion of short sprints at beginning of almost every session. 3. Prescribe speed endurance or special endurance sessions that are relevant to the athlete's primary events.	**MONDAY:** **Push-up starts** 1 × 3 × 15 m (2 min) **Block starts** 1 × 2 × 20 m (2.5 min) 1 × 2 × 30 m (3.5 min) **Acceleration holds** 1 × 2 × 40 m (5 min) **WEDNESDAY:** **High-stance starts** 1 × 3 × 20 m (2 min) **Fly-float-fly** 1 × 4 × 20/20/20 (7 min) **FRIDAY:** **Block starts** 1 × 3 × 25 m (3 min) **Accelerations from crouch stance** 1 × 1 × 40 m (5 min) **Speed endurance from high stance** 1 × 1 × 70 m (6.5 min) 1 × 2 × 90 m (8.5 min)

*An acceleration hold is a sprint drill for which the coach places a cone on the track near or slightly before the point at which an athlete's shin typically rises to a vertical position, which is indicative of upright sprinting. The athlete is then instructed to maintain the speed achieved up to the cone through the remainder of the sprint. For instance, an athlete may be prescribed acceleration holds for 40 m, but the coach's mark ending the acceleration zone is placed at the 20 m mark on the track. The athlete then maintains that speed from the 20 m to the 40 m. This drill is used to begin to focus on improving transitional mechanics as well as a method to introduce speed endurance.

speed through upright running mechanics. The concept behind this proposed model is that an athlete may see greater improvements in top speed if force production can occur at the ideal rate and moment through an investment in acceleration development and optimization (52).

Monitoring Sprint Ability

The longstanding method of assessing an athlete's speed ability has typically involved a test of maximal-effort linear sprinting. Much of the time, the maximal-effort sprint test is carried out over a distance, such as 40 yards (36.6 m), that is believed to be relevant to the athlete's sport. While time to completion is an effective tool to evaluate changes in sprint performance, these tests do not fully address the minute changes regarding an athlete's progression toward race or field readiness. In addition, testing error in the form of hand timing and various start tactics confound the interpretation of testing results. As a result, strength and conditioning professionals may consider the adoption of additional monitoring tools as part of their battery of assessments.

One such method of evaluation comes from the assistance of high-speed cameras or optical timing systems that use interruptions of infrared light to capture data from an athlete's collective foot strike (12). This technology provides coaches with additional insight into the sprint capabilities of the athlete. Table 19.6 provides a description of key variables that may be beneficial in the monitoring of speed development.

TABLE 19.6   Monitoring Speed Development

Measure	Description	Interpretation
Ground contact time	The total time allotted for a single stance phase.	In general, decreased ground contact times coupled with improved sprint completion times may suggest that an athlete has improved the ability to generate high rates of force in a shorter amount of time. However, an athlete may demonstrate slightly longer ground contact times at the initial stages of the sprint due to acceleration mechanics.
Step length	The distance between the toe and heel of two consecutive footsteps. Example: centimeters between the toe of right foot and the heel of left foot.	Improvements in step length (increases in distance covered) may occur through improved sprint mechanics or posture and ultimately enhanced force output.
Stride length	The distance between the heel in two consecutive steps of the same foot. Example: meters between the heel of the right foot and the heel of the next ground contact made by the right foot.	Improvements in stride length (increases in distance covered by two successive steps) may occur through improved sprint mechanics or posture, and ultimately enhanced force output.
Flight time	The duration of time that an athlete is not in contact with the ground. This occurs between the end of one step and the beginning of the subsequent step.	Increases in flight time can be interpreted two ways: (1) An athlete is producing higher vertical forces over a shorter amount of time, resulting in proper horizontal displacement of the athlete's mass down the track. (2) An athlete is producing higher forces over a longer amount of time, which may result in unnecessary vertical amplitude of the center of mass.
Stride angle	The angle at which the foot leaves the track.	The angle of stride may provide the coach with an ability to determine if the athlete is producing forces at the right moment, which is achieved through proper sprint mechanics. Furthermore, data on the stride angle elucidate what stage of sprint the athlete is attaining (acceleratory, transitory, maximum speed) and may relate to ground contact times.
Speed	The relationship between steps and the sum of the first step's ground contact time and the flight time leading to the subsequent ground contact.	Speed dictates how fast an athlete can move the body mass over a specific distance.
Acceleration	The change in speed as determined by the delta of two steps (e.g., right heel to left heel) and the sum of ground contact times and flight times of each step.	Acceleration provides insight into how well the athlete changes speed (increasing velocity in a direction) over a prescribed distance. For most athletes, furthering the length an athlete can accelerate will lead to higher top speed, provided that postural integrity and mechanics are sound.

Sample Program of Agility Development

The following is an example of steps for determining the appropriate tests, analyzing the results, and using them to program agility development of an athlete. As agility performance is underpinned by multiple factors, one should target the largest window of opportunity through direct assessment of the strengths and weakness of the athlete.

Step 1: Perform a needs analysis of the sport and match tests appropriately to assess these qualities (see the table).

Step 2: Determine strengths and weaknesses by comparing results as a standardized score to performance standards or team mean (see figure 19.12).

Step 3: Plan the development of a primary area of need and a secondary area of need for the athlete.

Step 4: Distribute the time available for this development based on need identification.

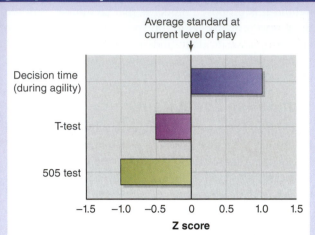

FIGURE 19.12 **Strengths and weaknesses of an athlete through representation of standardized scores for perceptual–cognitive ability, maneuverability, and change-of-direction ability. Negative values indicate performance lower than average whereas positive values indicate performance better than average.**

Needs Analysis for Agility Development

Sport	Basketball
Time frame	12 weeks (8 weeks off-season and 4 weeks preseason training)
Sport-specific agility needs analysis	High-velocity changes of direction • Backdoor cuts, cuts through the lane, fast break, and possession changes Maneuverability (multiple modes of change-of-direction movement) • Defensive shuffling, backpedaling, and bending changes of direction around screens to lose defender Agility (perceptual-cognitive) • Decision-making time (provides great advantages both offensively and defensively) • Ability to move in reaction to play or opponent
Recommended tests	505, T-test, agility test (decision time measured)

Step 5: Provide a preliminary plan for transition of percent distribution through the training blocks (see the table). Determine if this progression is appropriate by monitoring the development of change of direction and agility as described in table 19.7 (e.g., change-of-direction deficit).

Planned Distribution of Training Blocks for Agility Development

	Change of direction Primary aim	Maneuverability Secondary aim	Agility (perceptual-cognitive) Tertiary aim
Estimated % time allotted through blocks	Block 1 ~65% Block 2 ~60% Block 3 ~50%	Block 1 ~35% Block 2 ~30% Block 3 ~25%	Block 1 N/A Block 2 ~20% Block 3 ~25%
Additional comments	Check strength or specifically load absorption ability with drop landings.	Assess body positioning during lateral shuffling and changes of direction.	May be reliant on their perceptual–cognitive ability. This may have previously masked the identification they could improve their physical change-of-direction ability.

With the information provided by the testing as well as taking into account other physical fitness capacities, one can implement an appropriate periodized plan. The application table for agility shows an example of three blocks of training (four weeks each). The length of time for a training session is between 10 and 15 minutes inclusive of work and rest time and can be completed one to three times per week dependent on additional requirements of the athletes (such as skills training increasing in the preseason). A variety of drills can replace the examples given here; however, they should be chosen based on their classification (table 19.2) and ability to address the athlete needs.

Agility Development Strategies

The development of agility is best achieved using a periodized programming method. Random programming or the development of agility using only "sport-specific methods" such as small-sided games has not been found to be as effective (11). Although agility is a constant element on the field of play or during skills practices, it is recommended that agility development begin with the use of change-of-direction drills (preplanned) and progress in difficulty through increases in the physical demands; this is followed by the addition of drills involving perceptual–cognitive stress or what are typically termed "agility" drills (50, 97). In line with this

Application of Agility Development Strategies

Block and emphasis	Training tool and notes	Load prescription (rest periods between sets) for week 1 for each block
BLOCK 1: *Primary aim:* Change of direction (deceleration capacity—linear) *Secondary aim:* Maneuverability (body position)	1. Braking tasks are eccentric focused; therefore start with low volumes similar to those used to introduce eccentric tasks (plyometrics). 2. Focus on athlete staying low; sacrifice speed for positioning.	2-3 sessions per week **COD DRILL:** Decelerations** (forward) 2 × 4 (30 s; 2 min) (Alternate nonpreferred and preferred leg finish braking.) **MANEUVERABILITY DRILL:** Lateral shuffling @ height 1 × 4 × 10 m (30 s) (Use a rope or other object set at head height during athletic stance to provide feedback to athletes if they are "standing" instead of holding low center of mass.)
BLOCK 2: *Primary aim:* Change of direction (deceleration capacity—lateral) *Secondary aim:* Maneuverability (transition between modes of change of direction— shuffle to sprint to shuffle)	1. Ensure that athlete can use body position to effectively brake when oriented both forward and laterally; focus on athlete absorbing into stop. Expand to a single effort in reaction to generic stimulus. 2. Promote effective application of force into the ground ("pushing the ground away"); watch shank angle for visual feedback.	2-3 sessions per week **COD DRILL:** Decelerations** (forward) 1 × 4 (30 s; 2 min) **As with week 1** Decelerations (lateral) 1 × 4 (30 s; 2 min) **MANEUVERABILITY DRILL:** Z-drill (forward) 2 × 4 (30 s; 2 min) (Always alternate start direction, left to right vs. right to left direction.) **AGILITY** Deceleration 1 × 4 (decelerate on whistle) (30 s)
BLOCK 3: *Primary aim:* Change of direction (effective deceleration to reacceleration) *Secondary aim:* Maneuverability (combine effective transition and body positioning) *Tertiary aim:* Agility (focus on keeping change-of-direction performance and body position even in response to a generic stimulus)	1. Focus on "braking in" and "exploding out" of the change of direction. 2. Focus on footwork and keeping low, with steps that promote a "drop and drive" out of change of direction. 3. This is used to check the "transfer" of physical training to a more specific (yet still generic) stimulus. Focus on the "decide and go," checking for athletes to reorient effectively or "to move as effectively as they decide."	1-2 sessions per week (dependent on skills volume) **COD DRILL:** Modified 505 drill 2 × 4 (30 s; 2 min) (Alternate plant foot.) **MANEUVERABILITY DRILL:** T-test 1 × 4 (30 s; 2 min) **AGILITY** Reactive agility (Y agility drill) 1 × 4 (30 s) (Same direction in response to pointing in a direction) Skills training will also inherently contain sport-specific stimulus trainingd

COD = change of direction.

**Speed should progressively increase for deceleration drills through the weeks—for example, half speed to three-quarters speed entry velocity.

Note: There is not a separate emphasis on acceleration ability here, as it is expected this will be addressed in conjunction with speed sessions.

recommendation, the development of agility should start with a needs analysis based on assessment of the athlete's change-of-direction ability and agility. The agility test should specifically evaluate perceptual–cognitive ability, as previously described in table 19.2. Further, dependent on the additional movement requirements of the sport, one may also choose to use a test that is more dependent on maneuverability. The following is an example of using this type of testing information to create an informed agility program.

Monitoring Agility and Change-of-Direction Ability

In line with the concepts considered in monitoring sprint performance, simply assessing performance modification in either change of direction or agility according to time to completion of the chosen test does not isolate the physical quality or perceptual–cognitive quality that one is trying to examine—the actual ability to change direction (59, 61, 81, 85). Therefore, when monitoring change-of-direction or agility performance, the strength and conditioning professional may consider the measures in table 19.7. Although these aspects of performance have been measured using expensive devices such as three-dimensional motion analysis equipment, readily available high-speed cameras (collecting more than 100 frames per second) could easily be used in conjunction with the usual timing methods (hand or electronic) and in the absence of high-end biomechanical equipment.

TABLE 19.7 Monitoring Agility Development

Measure	Description	Interpretation
Change-of-direction deficit	The difference in time between a straight-line sprint and a change-of-direction test of equal length.	Assessing the COD deficit provides insight into the additional amount of time required by the athlete due to the demands of change of direction. An example is subtraction of 10 m sprint time from 505 change-of-direction time (a common COD test 10 m in length).
Ground contact time	The total time the foot is in contact with the ground during the change of direction (length of the plant phase).	Assessing the ground contact time in conjunction with other variables can determine if the athlete is effectively improving the actual change of direction independent of the total time required to complete a COD test, which usually requires a greater percentage of straight-line sprinting.
Exit velocity	The horizontal velocity of the athlete during the initial step out of the plant of the change in direction. Considered the first step of reacceleration from toe-off of the plant foot to foot strike of subsequent step.	Unlike the situation for total time, using a high-speed video camera to assess the velocity of the athlete (at the hip or center of mass) can give a direct measure of the ability to change direction. Improved exit velocity in conjunction with either the same or faster ground contact times implies greater rate of force development relevant to improving change-of-direction ability.
Entry velocity	Velocity of the athlete before the plant phase; can be measured over several steps or as the last step is entering the plant phase of the change of direction.	Similar methods can be used by practitioners to assess entry velocity as suggested for exit velocity. This allows the coach to understand the demand of the change of direction that should be considered when tracking the exit velocity.
Decision-making time	Measurement of the time between two events is considered decision-making time and can either be a positive or a negative value. Decision-making time can be broken down into two different orientations to comprehensively assess how athletes respond during game scenarios: (1) defensive (move in the same direction as the stimulus); (2) offensive (move in the opposite direction to the stimulus).	Similar to the measurement of entry and exit velocity, a high-speed camera can be positioned to the side of the directional change to capture both the stimulus and the athlete's first definitive foot plant to change direction in response. If the decision-making time is negative, this indicates that the athlete anticipated the directional change before the stimulus finalized the movement. Negative decision-making time is observed only during response to movements of another person (video or human stimulus), highlighting the importance of stimulus specificity during agility protocols. The measurement of decision-making time in both defensive and offensive situations allows coaches to identify whether athletes need to develop perceptual–cognitive ability in a specific game scenario.

COD = change of direction.

Conclusion

Speed, change of direction, and agility are well-established measures of athletic prowess in most sporting contexts. For this reason, strength and conditioning professionals should be aware of how these abilities are established and modified through training plan design and execution. These components of athletic movement and game play are underpinned by task-specific force application. This task-specific force production must be large enough to stabilize the athlete's body weight in the presence of gravity, displace the athlete from one point to another, and continue moving the athlete at high velocities.

Running speed is associated with the relationship between stride length and rate. Sprinting is a near-maximum to maximum run that is defined by large rates of force developed within a short stance time. Better sprinters spend more time in the air as a result of increased stride lengths that occur at faster rates than those of their slower counterparts. Agility encompasses the skills and abilities needed to explosively change movement velocities or modes in response to a stimulus. Both sprinting and agility use the SSC and greater neuromuscular efficiency compared to slower movements. However, agility includes perceptual–cognitive demands such as visual search scanning, decision making, anticipation, and reaction times that make it a separate training quality.

Strength and conditioning coaches aiming to improve these performance attributes should do so through the cyclic and sequential arrangement of training phases that harmonize strength training with speed, agility, or change-of-direction practice or some combination of these. This training effect may best result from the incorporation of exercises that are task specific and promote proper movement mechanics. The training prescribed should reflect the results of a needs analysis assessment at the beginning of a long phase or year. Furthermore, subsequent training plans should be optimized through an ongoing athlete monitoring program, which can assist the strength and conditioning professional in determining how the athlete is responding to the programmed agenda.

SPEED AND AGILITY DRILLS

19.1　A-SKIP

The A-skip is a commonly prescribed sprint drill that is used to simulate upright sprinting mechanics and vertical force production.

Starting Position

- Begin the exercise in a tall stance with torso directly above the hips, knees, and ankles (stacked joints).

Movement Phase

- Initiate movement by lifting one leg to a bent knee position in which the top of the thigh is near parallel. The foot of the lifted leg (swing leg) should be approximately at knee height of the stance leg, with the heel pulled up under the buttocks. This will result in the appearance of a "figure 4" at the legs. Swing leg will always accord with this description
- Begin the first skip by aggressively driving the swing leg down to the ground through an active foot, established through slight dorsiflexion. "Lift the big toe up" to establish appropriate dorsiflexion.

- Complete the aggressive drive down of the swing leg through the forefoot until near triple extension of the new stance leg occurs.
- The fore- to midfoot of the new stance leg should land under the hips, maintaining the stacked joints appearance.
- At the initiation of contact, the opposing leg should pop up rapidly to create a swing leg.
- The force generated from the active push down should coincide with a skipping motion that will result in a horizontal displacement of the body down the track.

Technique Tips

- Maintain a tall posture with relaxed shoulders through the entire duration.
- The arms should move at the same rate as the legs, with minimal to no pausing of arm action between cycles.

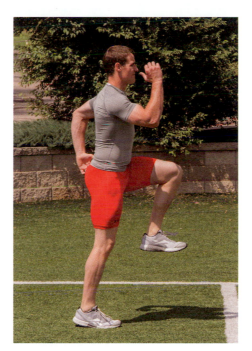

The "figure 4" at the legs

19.2   FAST FEET

This drill is designed to enhance the stride frequency of a sprinter.

Starting Position

- Athlete begins exercise in a tall stance with torso directly above the hips, knees, and ankles (stacked joints).

Movement Phase

- Athlete initiates movement by lifting one leg to a bent knee position, with the foot of the lifted leg approximately at the halfway point of the shank in order to replicate a swing leg. Swing leg will always accord with this description.
- Once this position has been achieved, the athlete alternates stance and swing legs as quickly as possible while maintaining stacked joints.
- The quick and aggressive drive down of the swing leg should be completed through the forefoot, ensuring that the feet do not rise above the halfway point of the shank. The aim of the shortened rise of the swing leg is to ensure quicker stepping frequency.
- The fore- to midfoot of the new stance leg should land under the athlete's hips, maintaining the stacked joints appearance.
- The athlete's arm should move at the same rate as the legs, with minimal to no pausing of arm action between cycles.

Technique Tips

- While this drill has traditionally been prescribed to increase a sprinter's stride frequency, remember that stride frequency is a by-product of high vertical forces occurring in a short ground contact time. In other words, an athlete cannot artificially improve stride frequency by moving the feet faster during a sprint event.

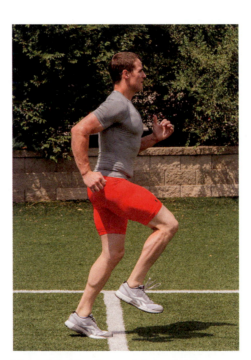

The quick drive down of the swing leg

19.3   SPRINT RESISTANCE: INCLINE FOR ACCELERATION

Incline sprinting is a type of resisted sprinting that is prescribed to promote improvements within the acceleration phase of a sprint.

Starting Position

- Begin the exercise by placing the athlete in the correct starting position (commonly called a crouched start). First, instruct the sprinter to split the stance position by placing the dominant leg forward and to drop the back/swing leg by one to two foot lengths.

- The length of split between the drive and swing leg is largely determined by the compromise between the athlete's (a) ability to generate sufficient forces needed to overcome a lower center of gravity and (b) comfort. In addition, the feet should be split in such a manner that the front and back legs are in line with the pelvis, so that no unnecessary twisting of the hips occurs.

- Once the split stance has been established, instruct the athlete to drop the back knee "straight down" so that the shank (shin) is nearer (more parallel) to the ground. This aids in promoting the proper driving position needed to begin acceleration.

- With a tall and rigid torso, the athlete should then raise the arm that is opposite to the front/drive leg to a position near or slightly above the forehead. The hand should be spaced approximately 6 to 8 inches (15 to 20 cm) away from the forehead. The rear arm (opposite to the rear/swing leg) should be pulled back to a point at which the hand is near the lateral aspect of the buttocks with an elbow angle that may range from 100°

to 120°. This position allows for the arm action to assist in producing sufficient propulsive forces to overcome static inertia.

- Upon completion of setup, instruct the athlete to lean the entire body forward so that 60% of the body weight is on the front leg. Ensure that the athlete does not "break at the waist" during this shift. The athlete should continue to feel balanced and stable.

Movement Phase

- After body weight has been transferred, the athlete can initiate the sprint through an aggressive push down and through the ground via the front/drive leg. The back leg should also assist in force production but will leave the ground earlier due to starting stance position. Arm action should be synchronous with leg action.

Technique Tips

- Cue the athlete to maximize accelerative mechanics through a low heel recovery of the rear/swing leg. This should be staged through the proper setup of the crouched starting position described earlier.

- Coach the athlete to continue aggressive pushing against the ground alongside an arm swing that may be cued to emphasize a hand that is pulled down and back. Recall that arm action often parallels movements of the legs.

- The torso should remain tall and tight with the head in a neutral position. The torso and head are in line and will rise at the same rate as the hips gradually rise.

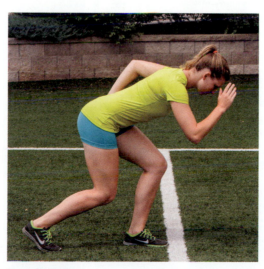

Crouched start

19.4   DECELERATION DRILL

Deceleration drills are intended to improve the braking ability of the athlete and assist in transfer of training from eccentric strength exercises in the weight room toward a more movement-specific pattern on the field. The exercise should be performed first with just forward running to deceleration and can then be expanded to forward running into a lateral deceleration. In forward deceleration drills, the athlete rapidly accelerates and then, in a fixed number of steps, controls the body into a stopped lunge position. In lateral deceleration drills, the athlete rapidly accelerates and then decelerates before a set position, braking while facing perpendicular to the original running direction and actively absorbing the force.

Movement Phase

- Depending on the physical and technical competence of the athlete, have him or her run forward at half speed and then decelerate and stop within three steps.
- If the athlete effectively absorbs the load by the third step, increase to running at three-quarters

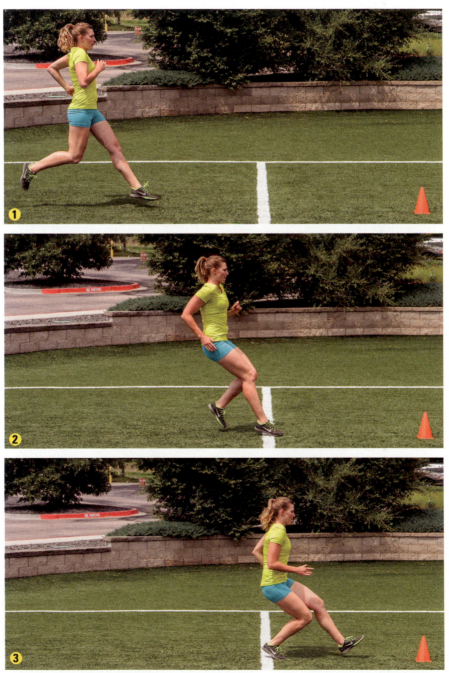

Forward deceleration drill

speed (more than 10 yards [9 m] of acceleration) and then decelerating within five steps.

- The most advanced version of this drill requires braking from top speed and decelerating within seven steps.

- The most demanding braking step or the step resulting in the greatest deceleration occurs one or more steps before stopping and does not typically occur only on the final deceleration or change-of-direction step.

Technique Tips

- Variations of this drill can be used during lateral movement and backward running. An intermediate version of this drill would require the athlete to accelerate for 5 to 15 yards (4.6 to 13.7 m) (similar to what the 505 and modified 505 tests call for) and come to a complete stop while facing perpendicular to the original direction of running. This allows for progression into reaccelerating out of the deceleration.

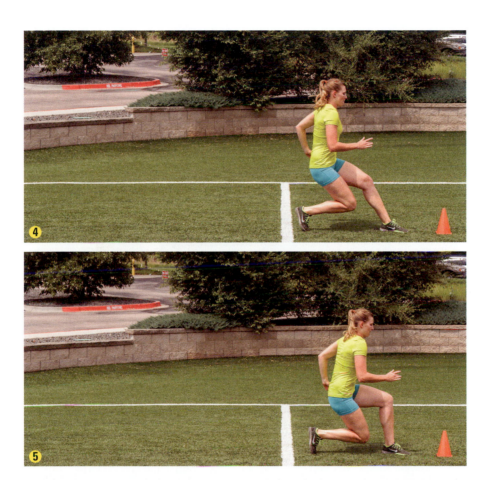

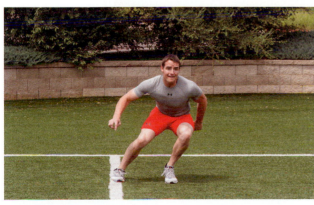
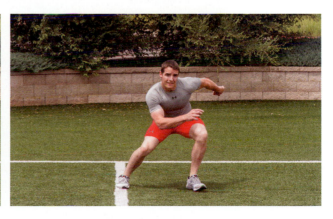

Lateral deceleration drill

19.5   Z-DRILL

The Z-drill is intended as a beginning-level change-of-direction drill to develop proficiency in the patterns of side shuffling, accelerating out of a change of direction, and decelerating into a change of direction. See the diagram for cone arrangement and running direction.

Starting Position

- Begin the exercise by starting at the first cone in the athletic ready position with a lowered center of mass and a stance wider than shoulder-width.

Movement Phase

- Side shuffle to the next cone while keeping the center of mass at a constant height (as low as the original center of mass height during the start position). Emphasize pushing the ground away. Coaches may look at the angle of the shank to ensure that it is directed toward the direction of intended travel.

- The athlete should plant at or near the cone and rapidly transition into a sprint toward the cone located on the diagonal.

- Approaching this cone, the athlete should effectively decelerate and transition into another shuffle (as with the second step).

Technique Tips

- This drill can be modified to run the Z formation in reverse, which would require the athlete to backpedal, adding another basic movement pattern that is important in the beginning stages of change-of-direction development. Throughout the movement, one should evaluate the ability to control the trunk effectively during changes and transitions as well as effective and efficient development of force during decelerations and accelerations.

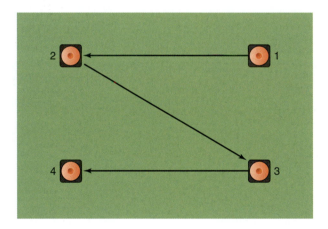

Z-DRILL SETUP

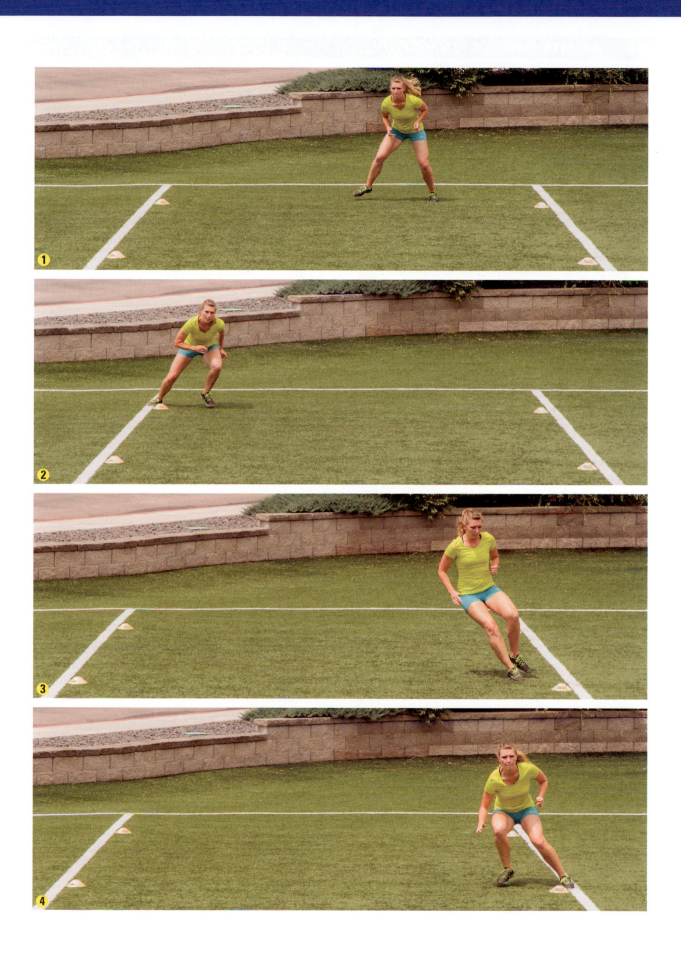

19.6   AGILITY DRILL (Y-SHAPED AGILITY)

This drill is intended to be the starting point for working on agility by using a generic stimulus followed by a specific stimulus to work on incorporating a perceptual–cognitive requirement in conjunction with a change of direction.

Starting Position

- Start at a cone 10 yards (9 m) away from a person who will act as the stimulus or director.

Movement Phase

- Run toward the stimulus and change direction based on the direction in which the stimulus points or the audible signal the stimulus provides (these two options are considered generic stimuli).
- The director should point left or right when the athlete reaches the 5-yard (4.6 m) (mark this with another cone for the director to refer to).
- The athlete should plant and change direction as soon as possible, accelerating to one of the two cones that are placed at an angle of 45 degrees and distance of 3 yards (2.7 m) to the left and right of the stimulus.

Technique Tips

Variations of this drill to adapt for more specific stimuli (advanced-level drill):

- Have the athlete move in the direction opposite to the generic stimulus (offensive).
- Have the stimulus take either a single step or two steps, with the athlete responding either offensively or defensively (instruct the athlete as to which before each repetition). A two-step addition option will increase the temporal difficulty of the drill, as one can cross over with an initial left then right step to confuse the athlete as to the final direction of the stimulus.
- Have the stimulus pass an implement relevant to the sport to either of two teammates standing on the right and left of the stimulus.

acceleration
agility
change of direction
complex training
force
ground preparation

impulse
momentum
periodization
postactivation potentiation
rate of force development (RFD)
recovery

speed
spring–mass model (SMM)
sprinting
strength
stretch–shortening cycle (SSC)
velocity

STUDY QUESTIONS

1. What does the term *impulse* refer to?
   a. the relationship between power and velocity
   b. the relationship between acceleration and velocity
   c. the relationship between force and velocity
   d. the relationship between force and time

2. Elite sprinters produce _____ forces in a _____ ground contact time as compared to their novice counterparts.
   a. larger, longer
   b. similar, shorter
   c. larger, shorter
   d. smaller, longer

3. In upright sprinting, an athlete's stride length is largely dependent on _____.
   a. the amount of vertical force produced during the stance phase
   b. the athlete's flexibility
   c. the athlete's stride rate
   d. the amount of horizontal force produced during the toe-off of the stance phase

4. Drills or tests that require the athlete to move rapidly in response to a stimulus such as a whistle, arrow, or opponent are best for measuring which of the following?
   a. change of direction
   b. maneuverability
   c. agility
   d. acceleration

5. Select the aspect of training that requires additional emphasis when the aim is to improve change-of-direction ability.
   a. strength
   b. eccentric strength
   c. reactive strength
   d. rate of force development

Program Design and Technique for Aerobic Endurance Training

Benjamin H. Reuter, PhD, and J. Jay Dawes, PhD

 After completing this chapter, you will be able to

- discuss the factors related to aerobic endurance performance;
- select the mode of aerobic endurance training;
- set aerobic endurance training frequency based on training status, sport season, and recovery requirements;
- assign aerobic endurance training duration and understand its interaction with training intensity;
- assign aerobic endurance exercise intensity and understand the various methods used to monitor intensity;
- describe the various types of aerobic endurance programs;
- apply the program design variables based on the sport season; and
- address the issues of cross-training, detraining, tapering, supplemental resistance training, and altitude when designing an aerobic endurance training program.

The authors would like to acknowledge the significant contribution of Patrick S. Hagerman to this chapter.

Designing an aerobic training program has many similarities to anaerobic exercise prescription. This chapter discusses the general principles of program design as they apply to aerobic endurance training and a stepwise approach to designing a safe and effective program.

Improvements in aerobic endurance performance can be derived only when sound principles are applied during training. Although the fundamental mechanisms responsible for inducing adaptations during training are undefined, it is clear that in order to adapt, the various systems of the body must be challenged by an exercise stimulus (e.g., specificity and overload). The physiological systems that are not involved during the training session or not stressed sufficiently by exercise will not adapt to the training program (47, 48).

Training specificity refers to the distinct adaptations to the physiological systems that arise from the training program. A training effect is limited to the physiological systems used and overloaded during training (48, 73). Unless training programs are strictly designed to involve and stress a physiological system, there will be very limited or possibly no adaptations in that system. To improve aerobic endurance performance, training programs must be designed to enhance the function of the respiratory, cardiovascular, and musculoskeletal systems.

For a training adaptation to occur, a physiological system must be exercised at a level beyond that to which it is presently accustomed (72). During continued overload, the physiological systems of the body adapt to the exercise stress. Adaptations within the physiological systems occur until the tissues are no longer overloaded. This necessitates use of a greater overload. Exercise frequency, duration, and intensity are the variables most often manipulated to provide overload to the systems of the body.

Successful performance in aerobic endurance competitions involving running, cycling, and swimming is dependent on the athlete's ability to cover a fixed distance in the shortest time possible. This requires athletes to be in peak physical condition for the competition. To reach this level of performance, athletes must train hard, yet intelligently, to maximize the physiological adaptations derived from training. In fact, the physical condition of the aerobic endurance athlete is of primary importance if that athlete is to perform at optimal levels during competition (15, 24, 54, 77, 82). A common trend with many aerobic endurance athletes is to adopt and embrace the training practices of other highly successful or well-known aerobic endurance athletes. Although this strategy may be effective for a few, most aerobic endurance athletes would likely be better served by constructing their own training regimen based on a good working knowledge of sound training principles and an understanding of their own physical limitations and needs.

Numerous types of training programs have been designed for aerobic endurance athletes. These training programs vary in the mode, frequency, duration, and intensity of the activity. What successful aerobic endurance athletes have in common is a training program designed to enhance their strengths and improve their weaknesses. This chapter is designed to provide the strength and conditioning professional with a good working knowledge of the scientific principles of aerobic endurance training and conditioning. Specifically, the chapter includes information about the factors related to performance, aerobic endurance training program design variables, and the various types of programs. Additional discussion focuses on sport season training and special issues related to aerobic endurance training. As it would be exhausting to review relevant information about training for all possible aerobic endurance sports, only basic aerobic endurance training topics are presented, with specific examples as they relate to running, cycling, and swimming.

Factors Related to Aerobic Endurance Performance

When designing aerobic endurance training programs, it is important to understand those factors that influence and play a significant role in successful aerobic endurance performance. This allows for the development of sound training programs while minimizing unnecessary training that may lead to counterproductive adaptations, fatigue, overwork, or overtraining.

Maximal Aerobic Capacity

As the duration of the aerobic endurance event increases, so does the proportion of the total energy demand that must be met by aerobic metabolism. Therefore, high **maximal aerobic capacity ($\dot{V}O_2max$)** is necessary for success in aerobic endurance events (59). A high correlation has been shown to exist between $\dot{V}O_2max$ and performance in aerobic endurance events (1, 19, 32, 59, 60). Consequently, aerobic endurance training programs should be designed to improve $\dot{V}O_2max$. However, although a high $\dot{V}O_2max$ is important for successful performance, other factors may be equally or even more important. These factors include a high lactate threshold, good exercise economy, high efficiency in using fat as a fuel source, and a high percentage of Type I muscle fibers.

For well-trained endurance athletes, improving $\dot{V}O_2max$ may benefit performance only up to a certain point, especially since these individuals typically already possess excellent aerobic capacity. Consequently, the ability to sustain higher velocities during competition and training may have a greater impact on performance than attempting to make marginal improvements in aerobic capacity. For this reason, many athletes use high-intensity interval training (HIIT). While the issue is not well understood, HIIT may contribute to performance in highly trained endurance athletes via improvements in peak power output, ventilatory threshold, hydrogen ion buffering, and utilization of fat as a fuel source (55).

Lactate Threshold

In aerobic endurance events, the best competitor among athletes with similar $\dot{V}O_2$max values is typically the person who can sustain aerobic energy production at the highest percentage of his or her $\dot{V}O_2$max without accumulating large amounts of lactic acid in the muscle and blood (54). Although numerous terms have been used to refer to this phenomenon, **lactate threshold** is the one most commonly employed in the literature. The lactate threshold is that speed of movement or percentage of $\dot{V}O_2$max at which a specific blood lactate concentration is observed or the point at which blood lactate concentration begins to increase above resting levels (82). Several studies have shown that an athlete's lactate threshold appears to be a better indicator of his or her aerobic endurance performance than $\dot{V}O_2$max (21, 22). The **maximal lactate steady state** is another term that often appears in the aerobic endurance training literature. The maximal lactate steady state is defined as the exercise intensity at which maximal lactate production is equal to maximal lactate clearance within the body (4). The maximal lactate steady state is considered by many to be a better indicator of aerobic endurance performance than either $\dot{V}O_2$max or the lactate threshold (4, 34). What is clear from this information is that aerobic endurance athletes must improve their lactate threshold or maximal lactate steady state. This requires athletes to conduct some training at elevated levels of blood and muscle lactate to maximize training improvements.

Exercise Economy

A measure of the energy cost of activity at a given exercise velocity is referred to as the **exercise economy**. Athletes with a high exercise economy expend less energy during exercise to maintain a given exercise velocity (e.g., running speed). Several investigators have suggested that exercise economy is an important factor in successful performance in running events (14, 31), with better performers having a slightly shorter stride length and greater stride frequency compared to less successful performers (12). During cycling, exercise economy can be affected by body mass size, cycling velocity, and aerodynamic positioning (22, 61, 78). For cyclists, an increase in body mass and cycling velocity and an inefficient body position generate greater wind resistance, resulting in a decrease in exercise economy. It has been demonstrated that elite swimmers are much more economical than nonelite swimmers (81) and use less oxygen at any given swimming velocity. The most profound impact on exercise economy during swimming can be observed when swimming technique becomes more efficient. As improvements in stroke mechanics occur, energy demand for a given swimming velocity is reduced (80). Training to improve exercise economy is critical for aerobic endurance athletes.

> ▶ **An improvement in exercise economy can enhance maximal aerobic capacity ($\dot{V}O_2$max) and lactate threshold.**

Designing an Aerobic Endurance Program

An effective aerobic endurance training program must include an exercise prescription specifically developed for the individual athlete. This requires manipulation of the primary program design variables. The sidebar lists the design variables as steps 1 through 5. Unfortunately, coaches and athletes often use the training practices or programs of current successful coaches or athletes in their sport. This does not carefully consider the strengths and weaknesses of the athlete and may lead to development of an ineffective or potentially harmful training program. The optimal way to develop a sound training program is to have the factors related to aerobic endurance performance evaluated and then use that information to generate a training program specific to the athlete. For example, an athlete with poor exercise economy should place emphasis on training to improve

---

Aerobic Training Program Design Variables

Step 1: Exercise mode

Step 2: Training frequency

Step 3: Training intensity

Step 4: Exercise duration

Step 5: Exercise progression

exercise economy. This might include interval training with a focus on technique, as well as using long rest periods. Conversely, athletes who need to increase lactate threshold might consider performing more high-intensity training.

Training programs for female athletes do not have to be different from those used to train male athletes; evidence indicates that males and females respond similarly to training programs (10, 60, 67). Refer to chapter 7 for a discussion on sex-related differences and their implications for exercise.

Step 1: Exercise Mode

Exercise **mode** refers to the specific activity performed by the athlete: cycling, running, swimming, and so on. When training to improve aerobic endurance performance, the athlete should select activities that mimic as closely as possible the movement pattern employed in competition. This will cause positive adaptations in specific physiological systems of the body. For example, the recruitment of specific muscle fibers and the adaptation of the energy systems within those fibers must be challenged during aerobic endurance training. Selecting the appropriate exercise mode during training ensures that the systems used in competition are challenged to improve. Remember that the more specific the training mode is to the sport, the greater the improvement in performance. For an athlete involved in multiple aerobic endurance sports, or one who is interested in a general aerobic endurance fitness program, cross-training or participation in multiple aerobic endurance activities may be warranted (35).

Step 2: Training Frequency

Training **frequency** refers to the number of training sessions conducted per day or per week. The frequency of training sessions depends on an interaction of exercise intensity and duration, the training status of the athlete, and the specific sport season. Higher exercise intensity and longer duration may necessitate less frequent training to allow sufficient recovery from exercise sessions. The training status of the athlete can influence training frequency, with lesser-trained athletes requiring more recovery days at the beginning of a training period than more highly trained athletes. The sport season that the athlete is currently in can also influence training frequency; an off-season program may include five training days per week, but training frequency may progress to daily workouts (or even multiple workouts per day for a triathlete) in the preseason. Additionally, fewer training sessions may be required to maintain an achieved level of physiological function or performance than to attain that level initially (77). Appropriate training frequency is important for the aerobic endurance athlete, because too much training may increase the risk of injury, illness, or overtraining. A number of studies have shown increased injury rates with training sessions more frequent than five times per week (49, 69); however, these studies used active individuals in a wide age range, not only young and healthy athletes, as subjects. Conversely, too little training will not result in positive adaptations to the various systems of the body. Research has shown that it is necessary to train more than twice per week in order to increase $\dot{V}O_2max$ (38, 83). Many coaches recognize that multiple training sessions per day may be needed to improve performance in some endurance athletes. Research conducted by Hansen and colleagues (43) showed that time to exhaustion, resting muscle glycogen concentrations, and citrate synthase activity increased among seven healthy untrained men after 10 weeks of training twice every other day versus once daily. It was speculated that training in a glycogen-depleted state may improve glycogen resynthesis via an increase in the transcription and transcription rate of certain genes responsible for training adaptations. However, the researchers cautioned that these results should not necessarily be used by coaches and practitioners to guide practice, as low glycogen concentrations may reduce the period of time an athlete is able to train and may increase risk of overtraining. This is one reason why it is important to monitor the effects of the training load on athletes.

Recovery from individual training sessions is essential if the athlete is to derive maximum benefits from the subsequent training session. Exercise performance has been shown to improve following relative rest from difficult training sessions (2). Obtaining sufficient rest, becoming rehydrated, and restoring fuel sources are critical issues for the athlete during recovery. Relaxation and avoidance of strenuous physical activity are particularly important following days of high-intensity or long-duration training. Postexercise ingestion of adequate fluids is important for replacing the fluid lost during training. If the training session was especially long or intense, then postexercise carbohydrate intake is important for replacing the muscle and liver glycogen stores that were likely depleted. More detailed information on this topic can be found in chapter 10, "Nutrition Strategies for Maximizing Performance."

Step 3: Training Intensity

Central to causing training adaptations in the body is the interaction of training intensity and duration. Generally, the higher the exercise intensity, the shorter the exercise duration. Adaptations in the body are specific to the **intensity**, or effort expended during a training session. High-intensity aerobic exercise increases cardiovascular and respiratory function and allows for improved oxygen delivery to the working muscles (72). Increasing exercise intensity may also benefit skeletal muscle adaptations by affecting muscle fiber recruitment (28). As exercise intensity is increased, greater recruitment of Type II muscle fibers occurs to meet the increased power needs. This training stimulus allows those fibers to become more aerobically trained, thereby possibly improving overall aerobic performance.

The regulation of exercise intensity is critical to the success of each training session and ultimately the entire program. An exercise intensity that is too low does not **overload** the body's systems and induce the desired physiological adaptations, whereas an intensity that is too high results in fatigue and a premature end to the training session (70). In either instance, the training session will be poor and ineffective.

The most accurate methods for regulating exercise intensity are to monitor oxygen consumption during exercise to determine its percentage of $\dot{V}O_2$max and to periodically measure the blood lactate concentration to determine the relationship to the lactate threshold. If $\dot{V}O_2$max testing is not available, exercise prescriptions can use heart rate, ratings of perceived exertion, metabolic equivalents, or exercise velocity to monitor exercise intensity. Cycling power–measuring devices are frequently used by professional and top-level amateur competitors.

Heart Rate

Heart rate is likely the most frequently used method for prescribing aerobic exercise intensity. The reason is the close relationship between heart rate and oxygen consumption, especially when the intensity is between 50% and 90% of **functional capacity** ($\dot{V}O_2$max), also called **heart rate reserve (HRR)**, which is the difference between an athlete's maximal heart rate and his or her resting heart rate (5).The most accurate means of regulating intensity using this method is to determine the specific heart rate associated with the desired percentage of $\dot{V}O_2$max or the heart rate associated with the lactate threshold. For the greatest precision, this necessitates laboratory testing to identify these exercise intensities. If laboratory testing is unavailable, then the individual's **age-predicted** (estimated) **maximal heart rate (APMHR)** can be used as the basis for determining exercise intensity. Refer to the sidebar "Target Heart Rate Calculations" for formulas and sample calculations for determining aerobic endurance exercise heart rate ranges using the **Karvonen method** and the **percentage of maximal heart rate (MHR) method**. The relationship between $\dot{V}O_2$max, HRR, and MHR is shown in table 20.1.

Although the Karvonen and percentage of maximal heart rate formulas provide practical intensity assign-

TABLE 20.1 Relationship Between $\dot{V}O_2$max, HRR, and MHR

% $\dot{V}O_2$max	% HRR	% MHR
50	50	66
55	55	70
60	60	74
65	65	77
70	70	81
75	75	85
80	80	88
85	85	92
90	90	96
95	95	98
100	100	100

HRR = heart rate reserve; MHR = percentage of maximal heart rate.

ments, basing them on age-predicted maximal heart rates may entail some inaccuracies (vs. laboratory-tested maximal heart rates) when exercise intensity is being monitored during cycling or running (65). It has been determined that age contributes 75% of the variability of heart rate; the effects of other factors such as mode of exercise and fitness level must also be considered with the use of heart rate to monitor intensity (65). Additionally, using estimations of exercise intensity via estimated maximal heart rate equations provides no information about the intensity associated with the lactate threshold. Without some knowledge of an athlete's lactate threshold, a highly effective aerobic endurance training program cannot be developed.

Ratings of Perceived Exertion Scales

Ratings of perceived exertion (RPE) scales can also be used to regulate intensity during aerobic endurance training (26, 39). It appears that RPE can be used to accurately regulate intensity when there are changes in fitness level (6); however, researchers have demonstrated that the RPE–intensity relationship can be influenced by various external environmental factors such as passive distracters and environmental temperature (13, 71). According to Haddad, Padula, and Chamari (41), various subject characteristics such as age, sex, training status, and fitness level may influence RPE. Furthermore, a few environmental factors that may influence RPE are listening to music, watching television or video, environmental temperature, altitude, nutritional considerations, and external feedback. However, these authors suggest that despite the potential influence of these factors, RPE is still a valid monitoring tool (see table 20.2).

Target Heart Rate Calculations

Karvonen Method

Formula:

- Age-predicted maximum heart rate (APMHR) = 220 − age
- Heart rate reserve (HRR) = APMHR − resting heart rate (RHR)
- Target heart rate (THR) = (HRR × exercise intensity) + RHR

Do this calculation twice to determine the target heart rate range (THRR).

Example:

A 30-year-old athlete with an RHR of 60 beats/min is assigned an exercise intensity of 60% to 70% of functional capacity:

- APMHR = 220 − 30 = 190 beats/min
- RHR = 60 beats/min
- HRR = 190 − 60 = 130 beats/min
- Lowest number of the athlete's THRR = (130 × 0.60) + 60 = 78 + 60 = 138 beats/min
- Highest number of the athlete's THRR = (130 × 0.70) + 60 = 91 + 60 = 151 beats/min

When monitoring heart rate during exercise, divide the THRR by 6 to yield the athlete's THRR in number of beats for a 10-second interval:

138 ÷ 6 = 23   151 ÷ 6 = 25

The athlete's THRR is 23 to 25 beats per 10 seconds.

Percentage of Maximal Heart Rate Method

Formula:

- Age-predicted maximum heart rate (APMHR) = 220 − age
- Target heart rate (THR) = (APMHR × exercise intensity)

Do this calculation twice to determine the target heart rate range (THRR).

Example:

A 20-year-old athlete is assigned an exercise intensity of 70% to 85% of maximal heart rate:

- APMHR = 220 − 20 = 200 beats/min
- Lowest number of the athlete's THRR = 200 × 0.70 = 140 beats/min
- Highest number of the athlete's THRR = 200 × 0.85 = 170 beats/min

When monitoring heart rate during exercise, divide the THRR by 6 to yield the athlete's THRR in number of beats for a 10-second interval:

140 ÷ 6 = 23   170 ÷ 6 = 28

The athlete's THRR is 23 to 28 beats per 10 seconds.

TABLE 20.2   Rating of Perceived Exertion (RPE) Scale

Rating	Description
1	Nothing at all (lying down)
2	Extremely little
3	Very easy
4	Easy (could do this all day)
5	Moderate
6	Somewhat hard (starting to feel it)
7	Hard
8	Very hard (making an effort to keep up)
9	Very very hard
10	Maximum effort (can't go any further)

Reprinted, by permission, from NSCA, 2012, Aerobic endurance training program design, by P. Hagerman. In *NSCA's essentials of personal training,* 2nd ed., edited by J.W. Coburn and M.H. Malek (Champaign, IL: Human Kinetics), figure 16.1, 395.

Metabolic Equivalents

Metabolic equivalents may also be used to prescribe exercise intensity. One **metabolic equivalent (MET)** is equal to 3.5 ml·kg^{-1}·min^{-1} of oxygen consumption and is considered the amount of oxygen required by the body at rest (1). Metabolic equivalent values have been determined for a variety of physical activities; a brief list is shown in table 20.3. For example, an activity with a MET value of 10.0 requires 10 times the oxygen uptake that is required by an individual at rest. Assigning MET values as part of an aerobic exercise prescription requires the strength and conditioning professional to know (or estimate) an athlete's maximal oxygen uptake in order to be able to calculate an exercise MET level (40).

Power Measurement

Cyclists may use power-measuring cranks and hubs to monitor exercise intensity (25). Due to cost, these devices are probably suitable only for professionals and top-level amateurs. Research studies have indicated

TABLE 20.3 Metabolic Equivalents (METs) for Physical Activities

METs	Activity
1.0	Lying or sitting quietly, doing nothing, lying in bed awake
2.0	Walking, <2 miles per hour (<3.2 km/h), level surface
2.5	Walking, 2 miles per hour (3.2 km/h), level surface
3.0	Resistance training (free weight, Nautilus or Universal type), light or moderate effort
3.5	Stationary cycling, 30-50 W, very light effort
3.0	Walking, 2.5 miles per hour (4 km/h)
3.5	Walking, 2.8-3.2 miles per hour (4.5-5.2 km/h), level surface
3.5	Calisthenics, home exercise, light or moderate effort
4.3	Walking, 3.5 miles per hour (5.6 km/h), level surface
4.8	Stair stepping (with a 4-inch [10 cm] step height), 30 steps per minute
5.0	Aerobic dance, low impact
5.0	Walking, 4 miles per hour (6.4 km/h), level surface
5.0	Elliptical trainer, moderate effort
5.5	Step aerobics (with a 4-inch [10 cm] step height)
5.5	Water aerobics, water calisthenics
5.8	Swimming laps, freestyle, slow, moderate or light effort
6.0	Outdoor cycling, 10 to 11.9 miles per hour (16.1-19.2 km/h)
6.0	Resistance training (free weight, Nautilus or Universal type), powerlifting or bodybuilding, vigorous effort
6.3	Stair stepping (with a 12-inch [31 cm] step height), 20 steps per minute
6.3	Walking, 4.5 miles per hour (7.2 km/h), level surface
6.8	Stationary cycling, 90-100 W, light effort
6.9	Stair stepping (with an 8-inch [20 cm] step height), 30 steps per minute
7.0	Rowing, stationary, 100 W, moderate effort
7.3	Aerobic dance, high impact
7.5	Step aerobics (with a 6- to 8-inch [15-20 cm] step)
8.0	Calisthenics (e.g., push-ups, sit-ups, pull-ups, jumping jacks), vigorous effort
8.0	Circuit training, including some aerobic stations, with minimal rest
8.0	Outdoor cycling, 12 to 13.9 miles per hour (19.3-22.4 km/h)
8.3	Walking, 5 miles per hour (8.0 km/h)
8.5	Rowing, stationary, 150 W, moderate effort
8.8	Stationary cycling, 101-160 W, moderate effort
9.0	Running, 5.2 miles per hour (8.4 km/h) (11.5 minutes per mile)
9.0	Stair aerobics (with a 10-12-inch [31 cm] step height)
9.8	Running, 6 miles per hour (9.7 km/h) (10 minutes per mile)
9.5	Step aerobics (with a 10- to 12-inch [25.4-31 cm] step)
9.8	Swimming laps, freestyle, fast, vigorous effort
10.0	Outdoor cycling, 14 to 15.9 miles per hour (22.5-25.6 km/h)
10.5	Running, 6.7 miles per hour (10.8 km/h) (9 minutes per mile)

(continued)

TABLE 20.3 *(continued)*

METs	Activity
11.0	Running, 7 miles per hour (11.3 km/h) (8.5 minutes per mile)
11.0	Stationary cycling, 161-200 W, vigorous effort
11.0	Rope skipping, general
11.8	Running, 7.5 miles per hour (12.1 km/h) (8 minutes per mile)
11.8	Running, 8 miles per hour (12.9 km/h) (7.5 minutes per mile)
12.0	Outdoor cycling, 16 to 19 miles per hour (25.7-30.6 km/h)
12.0	Rowing, stationary, 200 W, moderate effort
12.3	Running, 8.6 miles per hour (13.7 km/h) (7 minutes per mile)
12.8	Running, 9 miles per hour (14.5 km/h) (6 minutes 40 seconds per mile)
14.0	Stationary cycling, 201-270 W, very vigorous effort
14.5	Running, 10 miles per hour (16.1 km/h) (6 minutes per mile)
15.8	Outdoor cycling, >20 miles per hour (>32.2 km/h)

Based on Ainsworth et al., 2011, "Compendium of physical activities: A second update of codes and MET values," *Medicine and Science in Sports and Exercise* 43: 1575-1581.

that at least two of these devices provide valid and reliable power measures (36, 57). Using power to monitor intensity in cycling has an advantage over other measures because metabolic rate is closely related to mechanical power production (25). Using power as an intensity measure also allows reproducible intensity efforts regardless of environmental conditions, which may influence other measurements of intensity such as heart rate and training velocity (25).

Step 4: Exercise Duration

Exercise **duration** refers to the length of time of the training session. The duration of a training session is often influenced by the exercise intensity: the longer the exercise duration, the lower the exercise intensity (74). For example, exercise that is conducted at an intensity above the maximal lactate steady state (e.g., 85% of $\dot{V}O_2max$) will have a relatively short duration (20-30 minutes) because the accumulation of lactate within the muscle will contribute to fatigue. Conversely, exercise that is performed at a much lower intensity (e.g., 70% of $\dot{V}O_2max$) may be performed for several hours before the athlete experiences fatigue.

> ▶ The duration of a training session is often influenced by the exercise intensity; the longer the exercise duration, the lower the exercise intensity.

Step 5: Exercise Progression

Once athletes begin an aerobic endurance exercise program, they need to continue the program to either maintain or advance their aerobic fitness level. Research seems to indicate that aerobic fitness does not decrease for up to five weeks when intensity of training is maintained and frequency decreases to as few as two times per week (46).

Depending on the goals of the athlete, progression of an aerobic endurance exercise program initially involves increasing the frequency, intensity, and duration of exercise. General recommendations are that individuals always include at least one recovery or active rest day in each week of training. Most athletes have the goal of attempting to increase rather than just maintain aerobic fitness. This requires regular progression of the training program. Typically, exercise frequency, intensity, or duration should not increase more than 10% each week (42). At higher levels of fitness, athletes will reach a point where it is not feasible to increase either the frequency or the duration of exercise. When this occurs, progressions in training will occur only through exercise intensity manipulation (42).

As shown by the sidebar titled "Examples of Aerobic Exercise Progression," athletes and strength and conditioning professionals can manipulate combinations of frequency, intensity, and duration. Progression of training frequency may be limited by constraints such as

Examples of Aerobic Exercise Progression

Example A

- *Week 1:* Four times per week at an intensity of 70% to 85% THR for 40 minutes
- *Week 2:* Five times per week at an intensity of 70% to 85% THR for 45 minutes
- *Week 3:* Three times per week at an intensity of 70% to 85% THR for 40 minutes, one time per week for 50 minutes at 60% to 75% THR
- *Week 4:* Four times per week at an intensity of 70% to 85% THR for 45 minutes, one time per week for 50 minutes at 60% to 75% THR
- *Week 5:* Four times per week at an intensity of 70% to 85% THR for 45 minutes, one time per week for 55 minutes at 60% to 75% THR

Example B

- *Week 1:* Three times per week at an intensity of 60% to 70% THR for 30 minutes
- *Week 2:* Four times per week at an intensity of 60% to 70% THR for 35 minutes
- *Week 3:* Three times per week at an intensity of 65% to 75% THR for 30 minutes
- *Week 4:* Four times per week at an intensity of 65% to 70% THR for 35 minutes
- *Week 5:* Three times per week at an intensity of 70% to 75% THR for 30 minutes

school and work. It may not be possible for the athlete to incorporate more than one training session each day. Training intensity measurement should use the same methods as used in the original exercise intensity prescription. The best method is determined by the equipment available to monitor intensity (heart rate monitor, RPE charts, or machines that provide MET workloads). Progression of training intensity should be monitored very carefully to avoid overtraining. The duration of each training session is limited by the same constraints as training frequency. Athletes who train predominantly outdoors are also limited by the number of daylight hours, especially in the late fall, winter, and early spring.

Types of Aerobic Endurance Training Programs

There are several types of aerobic endurance training programs, each with varying frequency, intensity, duration, and progression parameters. Each type incorporates the five design variables and results in regimens created for specific outcomes. Table 20.4 summarizes the types of aerobic endurance training and their common prescriptive guidelines. Sample training programs for each type of aerobic endurance training are included after the sections that follow; the specific training mode being discussed is boldfaced in the sample training chart.

TABLE 20.4   Types of Aerobic Endurance Training

Training type	Frequency per week*	Duration (work bout portion)	Intensity
Long, slow distance (LSD)	1-2	Race distance or longer (~30-120 minutes)	~70% of $\dot{V}O_2max$
Pace/tempo	1-2	~20-30 minutes	At the lactate threshold; at or slightly above race pace
Interval	1-2	3-5 minutes (with a work:rest ratio of 1:1)	Close to $\dot{V}O_2max$
High-intensity interval training	1	30-90 seconds (with a work:rest ratio of 1:5)	Greater than $\dot{V}O_2max$
Fartlek	1	~20-60 minutes	Varies between LSD and pace/tempo training intensities

*The other days of the week are composed of other training types and rest–recovery days.
Data from references 15, 24, 54, 77, and 82

Long, Slow Distance Training

Traditionally, endurance coaches and athletes have used the term **long, slow distance (LSD)** to refer to training at intensities equivalent to approximately 70% of $\dot{V}O_2max$ (or about 80% of maximum heart rate). The fitness professional and athlete should remember that the term *slow* refers to a pace that is slower than typical race pace. The LSD terminology is probably due for a change to better reflect the intention of the activity. We have kept the term *LSD* to match terminology that is commonly used. In a LSD training session, the training distance should be greater than race distance, or the duration should be at least as long as 30 minutes to 2 hours (24). This intensity and duration is typically characterized as "conversation" exercise, with the athlete able to talk without undue respiratory distress. The physiological benefits derived from LSD training primarily include enhanced cardiovascular and thermoregulatory function, improved mitochondrial energy production and oxidative capacity of skeletal muscle, and increased utilization of fat as a fuel (7, 11, 16, 18, 28, 33, 40, 47, 48, 52, 73, 82). These changes are likely to improve the lactate threshold intensity by enhancing the body's ability to clear lactate. Chronic use of this type of training also causes a change in the metabolic characteristics of the involved muscles (40, 50) and an eventual shift of Type IIx fibers to Type I fibers (68, 76).

The increase in fat utilization may also cause a sparing of muscle glycogen (20, 23, 44, 48, 52, 58, 82). The intensity during LSD training is lower than the intensity used during competition, and this may be a disadvantage if too much of this type of training is performed. Additionally, LSD training does not stimulate the neurological patterns of muscle fiber recruitment that are required during a race (82), and this may result in adaptations in muscle fibers that are not used during competition.

Pace/Tempo Training

Pace/tempo training employs an intensity at or slightly higher than race competition intensity. The intensity corresponds to the lactate threshold; therefore, this type of training is also often called *threshold training* (24) or *aerobic–anaerobic interval training* (15). There are two ways to conduct pace/tempo training: steady and intermittent (24). Steady pace/tempo training is continuous training conducted at an intensity equal to the lactate threshold for durations of approximately 20 to 30 minutes. The purpose of pace/tempo training is to stress the athlete at a specific intensity and improve energy production from both aerobic and anaerobic metabolism. Intermittent pace/tempo training is also referred to as *tempo intervals*, *cruise intervals*, or *threshold training* (24). During intermittent pace/tempo training, the intensity is the same as for a steady-threshold workout, but the training session consists of a series of shorter intervals with brief recovery periods between work intervals. During pace/tempo training, it is important to avoid exercising at a higher intensity than the prescribed pace. If the workout seems relatively easy, it is better to increase the distance than to increase the intensity. The primary objective for this type of training is to develop a sense of race pace and enhance the body systems' ability to sustain exercise at that pace. Pace/tempo training involves the same pattern of muscle fiber recruitment as is required in competition. The benefits derived from this type of training include improved running economy and increased lactate threshold.

Interval Training

Interval training involves exercise at intensities close to $\dot{V}O_2max$. The work intervals should last between 3 and 5 minutes, although they can be as short as 30 seconds (1). The rest intervals for 3- to 5-minute work intervals should be equal to the work interval, thereby keeping the work:rest ratio (W:R) at 1:1. Interval training permits the athlete to train at intensities close to $\dot{V}O_2max$ for a greater amount of time than would be possible in a single exercise session at a continuous high intensity. This type of training should not be performed until a firm base of aerobic endurance training has been attained (54). Interval training is very stressful on the athlete and should be used sparingly. The benefits derived from interval training include an increased $\dot{V}O_2max$ and enhanced anaerobic metabolism.

High-Intensity Interval Training

High-intensity interval training, or HIIT, is a form of training that uses repeated high-intensity exercise bouts interspersed with brief recovery periods (9). According to Buchheit and Laursen (9), for an optimal stimulus it is necessary for athletes to spend several minutes within the HIIT session above 90% of the $\dot{V}O_2max$. Both short (<45 seconds) and long (2- to 4-minute) HIIT intervals can be used to elicit different training responses. As the work duration for a single exercise bout is increased, the energy contribution from anaerobic glycolysis will likely increase along with blood lactate levels. Additionally, HIIT training may be beneficial for improving running speed and economy. This may be particularly important toward the later stages of an aerobic endurance race when the "final kick" or "push" is needed to pass a competitor or set a record or personal best time.

In performing HIIT, the appropriate amount of rest between repetitions is critical. If the relief intervals are too short, the athlete will be unable to put forth a quality effort on subsequent exercise bouts and also will be at a greater risk for injury. If the rest periods are too long, many of the benefits experienced from challenging the anaerobic glycolytic energy system will likely diminish. An example of an appropriate work-to-rest ratio for long-interval HIIT training is ≥ 2 to 3 minutes at or above 90% $\dot{V}O_2$max, with relief bouts of ≤ 2 minutes (8, 9, 55).

Fartlek Training

Fartlek training (the word *Fartlek* originates from the Swedish term for speed play) is a combination of several of the previously mentioned types of training. Although Fartlek training is generally associated with running, it can also be used for cycling and swimming. A sample Fartlek run involves easy running (~70% $\dot{V}O_2$max) combined with either hill work or short, fast bursts of running (~85-90% $\dot{V}O_2$max) for short time periods. Athletes can apply this basic format to cycling and swimming by simply combining long, slow distance training, pace/tempo training, and interval training. A Fartlek training workout challenges all systems of the body and may help reduce the boredom and monotony associated with daily training. This type of training is likely to enhance $\dot{V}O_2$max, increase the lactate threshold, and improve running economy and fuel utilization.

Sample LSD Training Program for a Beginning Marathon Runner

Sunday	Monday	Tuesday	Wednesday	Thursday	Friday	Saturday
Rest day	45-min Fartlek run	**60-min LSD run**	45-min interval run	60-min run at race pace over hills and flats	45-min repetition run	**120-min LSD run**

Comments

- Frequency: To help combat overtraining or overuse, the two LSD training days should be spread out evenly during the week to allow recovery between sessions.
- Duration: Since the athlete's race distance is a marathon (26.2 miles, 42 km), the duration or running distance of the LSD training sessions should approach that of the marathon (for a trained athlete), at least for one of the two LSD sessions.
- Intensity: To complete the extended LSD sessions, the athlete should run at a lower intensity or training pace (minutes per mile or per kilometer); high respiratory stress is not required.

Sample Pace/Tempo Training Program for a Beginning 50 km Cyclist

Sunday	Monday	Tuesday	Wednesday	Thursday	Friday	Saturday
Rest day	60-min LSD ride	**30-min pace/ tempo ride**	45-min Fartlek ride	45-min easy ride	**30-min pace/ tempo ride**	90-min LSD ride

Comments

- Frequency: Because the pace/tempo rides are stressful, these two training days should be spread out during the week to allow recovery between sessions.
- Duration: For *steady* pace/tempo training, exercise duration is shorter than race distance or duration to allow for a higher training intensity.
- Intensity: The athlete should cycle at a high intensity or training pace (minutes per mile or per kilometer); high respiratory stress is required to simulate race pace.

Sample Interval Training Program for an Intermediate 10 km Runner

Sunday	Monday	Tuesday	Wednesday	Thursday	Friday	Saturday
Rest day	**10 reps of 0.5 km intervals at race pace with a 1:1 W:R ratio**	10 km easy run	45-min LSD run	HIIT 3 min @ 90% $\dot{V}O_2$max/2 min passive recovery × 6 reps	45-min LSD run	45-min Fartlek run on flat course

Comments

- Frequency: Because the interval runs are stressful, these two training days should be spread out during the week to allow recovery between sessions.
- Duration: The total distance or duration of the training portion of the session (i.e., the sum of the interval work bouts) should approach the competition distances as the athlete becomes more highly trained.
- Intensity: The athlete should run at an intensity (pace) close to $\dot{V}O_2$max when completing the work bout portions of the interval training sessions.

Sample High-Intensity Interval Training Swim Program for an Intermediate 140.6 Triathlete (Swim Training Portion; Race Distance Is 2.4 Miles)

Sunday	Monday	Tuesday	Wednesday	Thursday	Friday	Saturday
Rest day	60-min LSD swim	**HIIT 2 min @ 95% $\dot{V}O_2$max/2 min passive recovery × 8 reps**	45-min LSD swim	Rest day (no swim workout)	1-mile swim at race pace	60-min LSD swim

Comments

- Frequency: Because the HIIT workouts are stressful, only one HITT training day should occur during the week.
- Duration: Work bouts >2 to 3 minutes with ≤2-minute passive recovery between repetitions.
- Repetitions: Six to 10 reps × 2 minutes, 5 to 8 reps ≥ 3 minutes.
- Intensity: The athlete should swim at an intensity (pace) at or above 90% $\dot{V}O_2$max when completing the work bout portions of the HIIT sessions.

Sample Fartlek Training Program for a Female 5 km Collegiate Cross-Country Runner

Sunday	Monday	Tuesday	Wednesday	Thursday	Friday	Saturday
Rest or easy run	60-min LSD run	**45-min Fartlek run of hard/easy work on hills and flats**	25-min pace/tempo run	45-min LSD run	25-min LSD run	Competition

Comments

- Frequency: Because the Fartlek runs are stressful, only one Fartlek training day should occur during the week.
- Duration: The total distance or duration of the training portion of the session (i.e., the sum of the interval work bouts) should approach the competition distance as the athlete becomes more highly trained.
- Intensity: The athlete should run at an intensity (pace) close to $\dot{V}O_2$max when completing the work bout portions of the Fartlek training sessions.

> **The various types of training induce different physiological responses. Ideally a sound program would incorporate all types of training into the athlete's weekly, monthly, or yearly training schedule.**

Application of Program Design to Training Seasons

The program design variables and the various types of aerobic endurance training are often applied to athletes' sport seasons to create a yearly training program. Typically, the training year is divided into phases that include the off-season (sometimes called **base training**), preseason, in-season (sport competition), and postseason (active rest). Table 20.5 summarizes the main objectives and the typical program design assignments for each training season.

Off-Season (Base Training)

The priority in **off-season** training is to develop a base of cardiorespiratory fitness. Initially, the training program should be composed of long-duration and low-intensity workouts. As the off-season continues, intensity and, to a lesser extent, duration are increased; however, the increase in training duration should not be more than 5% to 10% per week (87). Increasing the training duration too much can actually lead to decreases in aerobic endurance performance (18). Periodic increases in exercise intensity occur when an athlete has adapted to the training stimulus and requires additional overload for continued improvements.

Preseason

During the **preseason**, the athlete should focus on increasing intensity, maintaining or reducing duration, and incorporating all types of training into the program. The strengths and weaknesses of the individual athlete should determine the amount and frequency of each type of training.

In-Season (Competition)

The **in-season** training program needs to be designed to include competition or race days in the training

TABLE 20.5   Sport Season Objectives and Program Design Assignments

Sport season	Objective	Frequency per week	Duration	Intensity
Off-season (base training)	Develop sound conditioning base	5-6	Long	Low to moderate
Preseason	Improve factors important to aerobic endurance performance	6-7	Moderate to long	Moderate to high
In-season (competition)	Maintain factors important to aerobic endurance performance	5-6 (training and racing)	Short (training)	Low (training)
			Race distance	High (racing)
Postseason (active rest)	Recovery from competitive season	3-5	Short	Low

Data from references 15, 24, 54, 77, and 82.

schedule. Low-intensity and short-duration training days should precede scheduled competitions so that the athlete is fully recovered and rested. The types of training employed during the in-season are based on the continued goal of improving weaknesses and maintaining strengths of the athlete.

Postseason (Active Rest)

During the **postseason**, the main focus should be on recovering from the previous competitive season. Low training duration and intensity are typical for this active rest phase, but enough overall exercise or activity should be performed to maintain a sufficient level of cardiorespiratory fitness, muscular strength, and lean body mass. During the postseason, the aerobic endurance athlete should focus on rehabilitating injuries incurred during the competitive season and improving the strength of weak or underconditioned muscle groups.

> A sound year-round aerobic endurance training program should be divided into sport seasons with specific goals and objectives designed to improve performance gradually and progressively.

Special Issues Related to Aerobic Endurance Training

In addition to the program design variables, it is important to consider other related issues when developing an aerobic endurance training program. These include cross-training, detraining, tapering, and supplemental resistance training. The strength and conditioning professional should contemplate these issues when adapting the types of aerobic endurance training programs to an individual athlete or developing an aerobic endurance program based on the sport season.

Cross-Training

Cross-training is a mode of training that can be used to maintain general conditioning in athletes during periods of reduced training due to injury or during recovery from a training cycle (33). Cross-training may reduce the likelihood of overuse injuries because it distributes the physical stress of training to muscle groups different from those used during training (87). Multiple-event athletes also use cross-training to maximize performance in swimming, cycling, and running. The benefits derived from cross-training include adaptations of the respiratory, cardiovascular, and musculoskeletal systems (53, 57, 87). It seems reasonable to expect that cross-training would maintain some level of conditioning in single-event athletes who perform another mode of training (e.g., runners who perform cycling or swimming). To be effective in maintaining $\dot{V}O_2$max, cross-training must be equal in intensity and duration to the athlete's primary mode of exercise (37, 56, 85); however, cross-training will not improve single-event performance to the same magnitude as mode-specific training only (33).

Detraining

Detraining occurs when the athlete reduces the training duration or intensity or stops training altogether due to a break in the training program, injury, or illness. In the absence of an appropriate training stimulus, the athlete experiences a loss of the physiological adaptations brought about by training. It has been demonstrated that most of the physiological adaptations attained with training regress rapidly toward pretraining levels when the training stimulus is removed (27, 29, 52). To avoid some of the effects of detraining, the use of other training modes may be beneficial; however, cross-training may only attenuate some of the loss of physiological adaptation normally seen during complete cessation of training. Aerobic endurance athletes can minimize the effects of detraining by continuing to use their primary mode of exercise at reduced frequency and intensity, if possible (82).

Tapering

Tapering is an important component of the training program as aerobic endurance athletes prepare for major competition. Tapering involves the systematic reduction of training duration and intensity, combined with an increased emphasis on technique work and nutritional intervention. The objective of tapering the training regimen is to attain peak performance at the time of competition. While the duration of the taper is dependent on numerous factors, a typical tapering period may last between 7 and 28 days (63). Although most of the available research on tapering has been conducted on swimmers (17, 46, 79), the use of tapering is not limited to these aerobic endurance athletes. Research among runners and cyclists has shown that these endurance athletes also benefit from a well-planned tapering regimen (63, 64, 75). Tapering before competition helps facilitate recovery and rehydration and promotes increases in muscle and liver glycogen stores (63).

There are several types of tapering models that may be employed by athletes in order to restore impaired physiological capacities resulting from the rigors of training. The most common tapering models are linear, step, and progressive tapers (79). The linear taper is characterized by a gradual decrease in the overall daily training volume throughout the duration of the taper. In contrast, a step taper is typified by an abrupt and considerable reduction (normally ≥50%) in training volume that is maintained throughout the duration of the taper without fluctuation. The progressive taper uses a combination of the linear and step tapering models. This model is associated with a rapid 10% to 15% immediate reduction in training volume, with smaller, more gradual reductions in volume at each tier. Training volume is systematically reduced while intensity and frequency are maintained.

Resistance Training

Resistance training is an important but often overlooked factor in improving performance in aerobic endurance athletes. Overall, research on the effects of resistance training on performance in trained aerobic endurance athletes is limited; however, some data suggest that benefits can be derived from performing resistance training during aerobic endurance training. Of particular importance, Hickson and colleagues (45) demonstrated that although the $\dot{V}O_2$max of highly trained aerobic athletes did not improve as a result of resistance training, there was an improvement in short-term exercise performance during both cycling and running. Benefits that

aerobic endurance athletes may obtain from performing resistance training include faster recovery from injuries, prevention of overuse injuries, and reduction of muscle imbalances. Increased strength is important for various aspects of aerobic endurance competition, including hill climbing, bridging gaps between competitors during breakaways from groups, and the final sprint (87). More recently Mikkola and colleagues (62) examined the influence of a variety of resistance training programs on the running performance of recreational runners. Muscle endurance training and explosive resistance and heavy resistance training programs all improved running performance on a treadmill.

Chapter 17 provides guidelines for designing resistance training programs that can apply to aerobic endurance athletes; refer to scenario C for a sample program that focuses on a high school cross-country runner.

Altitude

Altitude can be defined as the height above sea level. **Altitude** is classified into several categories, ranging from sea level (>500 m) to low (>500-2,000 m), moderate (>2,000-3,000 m), high (>3,000-5,500 m), and extreme (>5,500 m) (30). Contrary to popular belief, the percentage of oxygen is the same at different altitudes (66). However, as altitude increases, the atmospheric pressure drops, causing a reduction in partial pressure (PO_2), which acts as the driving force for gas exchange in the lungs (30, 66). This leads to a cascade of physiological responses to compensate for the reduction in PO_2. Subsequently, aerobic endurance performance decrements upon acute altitude exposure may begin to occur at altitudes as low as 700 m (86).

Acclimatization to altitude may occur between 12 and 14 days at moderate altitudes up to 2,300 m; however, it has been found that this process may take up to several months (86). According to Wyatt (86), recommendations for optimizing performance at altitude vary dramatically, from arriving immediately before competition (24-48 hours) to 12 weeks of altitude exposure.

Many elite and subelite athletes train at altitude to produce an ergogenic effect. In order to experience a benefit from this type of training, it has been reported that an athlete must receive a hypoxic dose of training ≥12 hours/day for a minimum of three weeks at moderate altitude (approximately 2,100-2,500 m) (51, 86). "Live high, train low" (LHTL) is a method commonly used by athletes seeking to benefit from altitude training. The LHTL requires individuals to live at moderate altitudes, between 2,000 and 3,000 m, and train at near sea level (51). This method of training allows athletes to simultaneously experience the benefits of altitude acclimatization and training at sea level (84). Thus,

LHTL may potentially provide an ergogenic benefit by allowing athletes to take advantage of the metabolic and hematological adaptations experienced when living at altitude to augment neuromuscular development at lower altitudes (30, 84).

Conclusion

Training to improve aerobic endurance performance requires a well-developed and scientifically based program. The training program should be developed in conjunction with periodic performance assessment and should be structured to enhance the strengths and improve the weaknesses of the athlete. A combination of a variety of the training types described in this chapter should be used so that all physiological systems involved in successful performance are overloaded and challenged to respond with positive adaptations.

Training programs should be developed far enough in advance and with enough structure to ensure enhancement of performance, but with enough flexibility to avoid overuse injuries and overtraining. Although other forms of training can be employed to avoid boredom and overtraining, activity-specific training results in the best adaptations to training and ultimately the most improvement in performance.

AEROBIC ENDURANCE TRAINING EXERCISES

The following section discusses some basic technique considerations for performance of aerobic endurance training. General guidelines for both common cardiorespiratory training machines and nonmachine activities are provided. These exercise instructions are largely adapted from Beck (3).

20.1   TREADMILL

Starting Position

- Begin by attaching the security clip to the clothing where it will not interfere with the action of the lower or upper limbs.
- Straddle the belt by placing the feet on the right and left platform.
- Read the instructions on the console of the treadmill to gain an understanding of how to adjust the speed and incline of the specific treadmill being used.
- Turn on the machine and adjust the speed of the belt so that it is at the desired warm-up speed.

Movement Phase

- While holding the handrails, allow one leg to swing freely, and using a pawing action, strike the treadmill with the midfoot.
- Once comfortable with the speed of the belt, begin walking/running on the treadmill.
- Run/walk, keeping toward the front portion of the machine while remaining in the center of the treadmill deck.
- Release the hands from the handrails and adjust the speed and incline until the desired training level is attained.
- Avoid holding on to the console or front handrails or leaning backward while walking or running.

Ending Position

- Reduce the speed of the treadmill and perform a 3- to 5-minute cool-down to prevent blood pooling and improve venous return.
- Step onto the platforms on either side of the belt and turn the machine off (3).

20.2 STATIONARY BIKE

Starting Position

- Begin by adjusting the seat height so the knee of the extended leg is slightly bent (25°-30°) at the bottom of the pedal stroke.
- The foot of the down leg should be flat and parallel to the floor with the balls of the feet in contact with the pedals.
- Adjust the seat so that the knee is over the center of the pedal on the extended leg and the hips do not rock back and forth during pedaling.
- While maintaining a neutral spine position, lean slightly forward at the hips.
- Adjust the handlebars so that when the arms are extended at a downward angle there is a slight bend in the elbows. Ideally the upper arm and torso will form an angle of approximately 90°.

Movement Phase

- Begin pedaling while keeping the balls of the feet in contact with the pedals throughout the duration of the exercise.

- Maintain a neutral posture and do not round the shoulders.
- With "bullhorn" handlebars, a variety of hand positions may be used. These include
  - pronated, palms-facing downward grip, allowing a more upright posture;
  - neutral palms-facing grip on the sides of the handlebars, encouraging a greater forward lean; and
  - racing position, with the forearms resting on the handlebars, creating maximum forward lean.

Ending Position

- Slow down until the pedals have come to a complete stop, and step off of the bike.

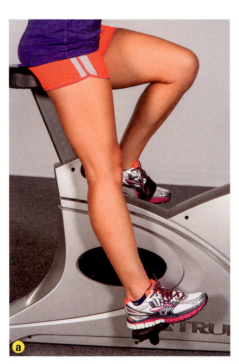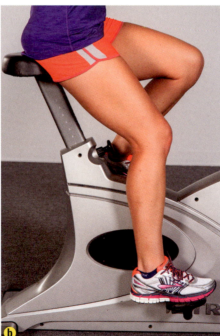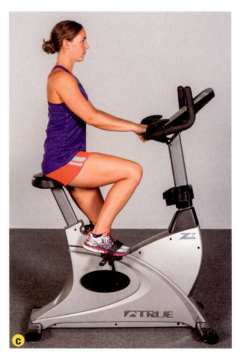

Proper seat height adjustment: *(a)* leg straight with knee locked and heel on pedal; *(b)* knee slightly bent with ball of foot on pedal; *(c)* with the pedal at 12 o'clock, the knee is about even with the hips and approximately parallel with the floor.

20.3 ROWING MACHINE

Starting Position (Start)

- Keep the back upright, not rounded, with a slight lean forward from the hips.
- Hold the head upright while looking straight ahead.
- Extend the arms in front of the body and grab the rower handle while flexing the hips and knees until the shins are approximately vertical.

Movement Phase (Drive)

- Extend the hips and knees while using the arms to pull the handle toward the abdomen just below the rib cage.
- Adjust the air vent to increase (more air admitted) or decrease (less air admitted) the resistance provided.

Ending Position (Finish)

- The legs should be fully extended with the torso leaning slightly backward.
- Arms are bent at the elbows and the handle is at the abdomen just below the rib cage.

Recovery is the movement from finish back to the start.

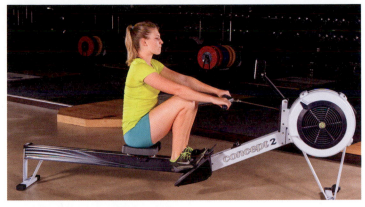

Starting position (and the catch)

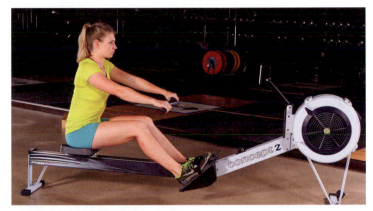

The drive

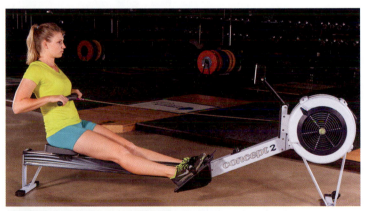

The finish

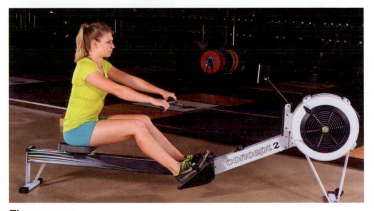

The recovery

20.4   STAIR STEPPER

Starting Position

- Hold the handrails while stepping forward onto the pedals.
- Place the whole foot in contact with each pedal.

Movement Phase

- Begin stepping, using the handrails for support.
- While maintaining an upright posture, take deep (4- to 8-inch [10 to 20 cm]) steps.
- Do not allow the steps to contact the floor or the upper-limit stop of the machine.
- Continue to hold the handrails lightly while looking straight ahead, keeping an upright posture with the shoulders squared and relaxed, the torso over the hips, the knees aligned with the feet, and toes pointed forward.

Ending Position

- Hold the handrails while stepping backward off the pedals.

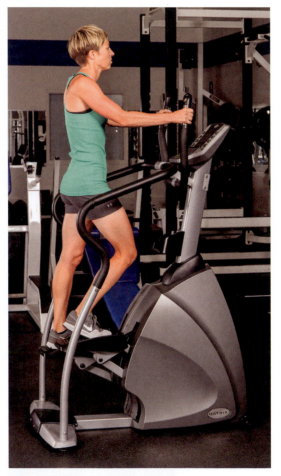

Proper position on a stair stepper

20.5 ELLIPTICAL TRAINER

Starting Position

- Facing the center console of the elliptical, place one foot on each pedal.
- While standing upright and looking forward, grasp the handrails with the torso upright and properly balanced directly over the hips, head held high, and shoulders relaxed (but not rounded).

Movement Phase

- Begin pedaling forward moving the arms and legs in a reciprocating fashion.
- The feet should remain in full contact with the pedals throughout the duration of the exercise unless the design of the machine causes the rear heel to lift.
- The knees should not be allowed to come forward past the toes when in the flexed position.
- Hold on to the handrails in order to maintain balance. If handrail holding is unnecessary, it is a good idea to release the hold on the handrails and pump the arms similarly to the way they move in walking or running.
- The incline of the elliptical may be increased to more closely simulate a running motion or reduced to replicate a walking motion.
- Performing this exercise with a forward motion may place greater emphasis on the quadriceps; performing it with a backward motion may increase the stress on the hamstrings and gluteals.

Ending Position

- Slow down until the machine has come to a complete stop then step off the pedals.

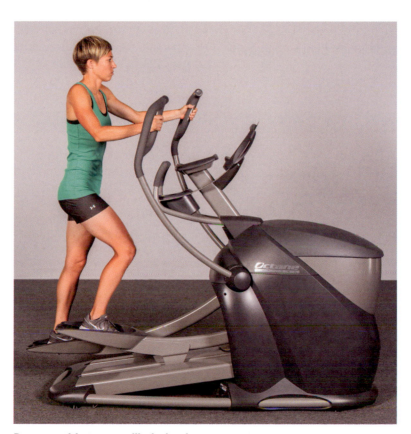

Proper position on an elliptical trainer

Aerobic Endurance Training Exercises

20.6 WALKING (GAIT)

Body Position

- Hold the head upright with the eyes looking straight ahead.
- Relax the shoulders, and do not allow them to round.
- Position the upper body directly over the hips while keeping the ear, shoulder, and hip aligned.

Foot Strike

- The heel should strike the ground first, followed by a gentle "rolling" heel-to-ball action, allowing the weight to be spread over the foot.
- The weight should transfer from the outer side of the heel and continue to shift forward and slightly inward toward the middle of the ball of the foot at push-off.

Stride

- Without rolling the pelvis (unless racewalking), allow the hips to move freely to increase stride length.
- Lift the knees and engage the hips and gluteals in the movement.

Arm Action

- The arms should swing forward and backward in a reciprocating fashion with the lower body (i.e., when the left arm is forward, the right leg is extended, and vice versa).
- The shoulders should be relaxed, allowing the arms to swing freely.
- At faster walking speeds, the actions should be as follows:
  - The arms should be bent at the elbows 90° with arm movement originating at the shoulders.
  - The arms and hands should swing backward and forward, not crossing the midline of the body, in order to create forward propulsion.
  - The hands should stay relaxed, with the hand coming up to the level of the chest at the nipple line on the forward swing, and the hip bone at the side of the body on the backward swing.

Note: Racewalkers must increase hip rotation with each stride to create a pelvic roll. This enables them to increase stride length while keeping one foot in contact with the ground at all times.

20.7 RUNNING (GAIT)

Body Position

- Hold the head upright with the eyes looking straight ahead.
- Relax the shoulders, but do not allow them to round.
- Position the upper body directly over the hips while keeping the ear, shoulder, and hip aligned.

Foot Strike

- The heel should strike the ground first, followed by a gentle "rolling" heel-to-ball action, allowing the weight to be spread over the foot.
- The weight should transfer from the outer side of the heel and continue to shift.

Stride

- Without rolling the pelvis (unless racewalking), allow the hips to move freely to increase stride length.
- Lift the knees and engage the hips and gluteals in the movement.

- With each running step, the foot should land approximately under the hips to avoid "braking" and spending too much time in the air.

Arm Action

- The arms should swing forward and backward in a reciprocating motion with the lower body (i.e., when the left arm is forward, the right leg is extended, and vice versa).
- The shoulders should be relaxed, allowing the arms to swing freely.
- In contrast to what occurs in walking, the majority of arm movement comes from the lower arm, as too much shoulder movement wastes energy.
- The forearms should be carried between the waist and the chest.
- The arms and hands should swing backward and forward, not crossing the midline of the body, in order to create forward propulsion.

age-predicted maximal heart
  rate (APMHR)
altitude
base training
cross-training
detraining
duration
exercise economy
Fartlek training
frequency
functional capacity
heart rate reserve (HRR)

high-intensity interval training
in-season
intensity
interval training
Karvonen method
lactate threshold
long, slow distance training (LSD)
maximal aerobic capacity ($\dot{V}O_2max$)
maximal lactate steady state
metabolic equivalent (MET)
mode
off-season

overload
pace/tempo training
percentage of maximal heart
  rate (MHR) method
postseason
preseason
ratings of perceived exertion
  (RPE)
recovery
resistance training
tapering

STUDY QUESTIONS

1. Which of the following adaptations occur as an outcome of an aerobic endurance training program?
   - I. increased oxygen delivery to working tissues
   - II. higher rate of aerobic energy production
   - III. greater utilization of fat as a fuel source
   - IV. increased disturbance of the acid–base balance
   - a. I and III only
   - b. II and IV only
   - c. I, II, and III only
   - d. II, III, and IV only

2. Which of the following types of training is conducted at an intensity equal to the lactate threshold?
   - a. pace/tempo
   - b. interval
   - c. high-intensity interval training (HIIT)
   - d. Fartlek

3. Which of the following is the method most commonly used to assign and regulate exercise intensity?
   - a. oxygen consumption
   - b. heart rate
   - c. ratings of perceived exertion
   - d. race pace

4. The loss of physiological adaptations upon the cessation of training is an example of
   - a. specificity of training
   - b. cross-training
   - c. detraining
   - d. tapering

5. The longest aerobic endurance training sessions should be performed during which of the following sport seasons?
   - a. postseason
   - b. preseason
   - c. in-season
   - d. off-season

Periodization

G. Gregory Haff, PhD

After completing this chapter, you will be able to

- understand the central concepts that underpin the periodization of training;
- appreciate the value, role, and application of periodization in strength and conditioning programs;
- describe the four periods of the traditional periodization model;
- describe the two phases of the preparatory period of the traditional periodization model;
- relate the four sport seasons to the four periods of the traditional periodization model; and
- apply the program design variables to create a periodized strength training program.

The author would like to acknowledge the significant contributions of Dan Wathen, Thomas R. Baechle, and Roger W. Earle to this chapter.

The ability of strength and conditioning programs to stimulate the physiological adaptations necessary to enhance performance is largely related to modulating training stressors to enhance adaptive responses while reducing the potential for performance plateaus or overtraining. When training loads are mismanaged, there is an increased risk of injury and the potential for overtraining (46). Ultimately, as athletes become more trained or have a greater training age, it becomes more difficult to stimulate performance gains. Thus increased variation is often required in the training program of more advanced athletes in order to facilitate long-term training and performance gains (3, 59). To meet this requirement, training programs need to be logically designed so that they are structured in a systematic and preplanned manner, allowing variation of training volume, intensity, frequency, density, foci, mode, and exercise selection in accordance with the athlete's needs and the sport's requirements. Central to the effective programming of training interventions is the concept of **periodization** (28). Periodization is often attributed to Leonid Matveyev (43), who proposed the basic theories that underpin periodization in the 1960s. But though Matveyev is often considered the father of periodization, several other individuals were exploring the concept at the same time, including László Nádori (48), Tudor Bompa (2), and Yuri Verkoshansky (64). Later on, American sport scientists Michael H. Stone, Harold O'Bryant, and John Garhammer adapted the concepts of the early periodization theorists with special application to strength and power athletes (57, 58). Ultimately, periodization is a theoretical and practical construct that allows for the systematic, sequential, and integrative programming of training interventions into mutually dependent periods of time in order to induce specific physiological adaptations that underpin performance outcomes.

This chapter discusses the concept of periodization and its application within a strength and conditioning program. In order to understand periodization theories and how they are applied to training program design, it is essential to develop an understanding of how the body responds to training (i.e., stressors) (24, 28); this topic is discussed first. Second, the basic hierarchal structure of a periodized training program is discussed in order to demonstrate how the training year is broken into smaller blocks of training, each with its own training goals and priorities. It is important to note that this overall schedule of training encompasses all aspects of the athletes' training program, including general conditioning, sport-specific activities, and resistance training. Finally, the second half of this chapter presents detailed examples of a yearlong periodized strength and conditioning

program. To understand the intricacies of the program, the reader is encouraged to read chapter 17 first.

Central Concepts Related to Periodization

A successful training program allows for management of the adaptive and **recovery** responses to specific interventions that are delivered in a structured way (28). The ultimate success of any training program centers on its ability to induce specific physiological adaptations and translate those adaptations into increases in performance. At the center of this process is the ability to manage the adaptive response, handle accumulated fatigue, and capitalize on the aftereffects established from the various training factors encountered. The strength of a periodized training plan lies in its ability to sequence and structure the training interventions in order to manage all of these factors and peak performance at appropriate time points (4-6, 51, 59, 63). Ultimately, peak performance can be optimized only for short periods of time (7-14 days), and the average time it can be maintained is inversely related to the average intensity of the training plan (17, 33, 59). In order to elucidate how periodized training models can manage these factors, three basic mechanistic theories have been established: the **General Adaptation Syndrome (GAS)**, **stimulus-fatigue-recovery-adaptation theory**, and the **fitness–fatigue paradigm** (22, 28, 59, 65).

> **Periodization is the logical and systematic process of sequencing and integrating training interventions in order to achieve peak performance at appropriate time points.**

The General Adaptation Syndrome

In 1956, Hans Selye, a pioneering researcher on the biological effects of exposure to stressful stimuli, presented the basic concepts of the GAS in which a three-stage response to stress (alarm, resistance, and exhaustion) was defined (54, 55). While not originally conceptualized in the context of physical training, over time the GAS has become one of the foundational concepts from which periodization theories have been developed (21, 59). Any time the body experiences a novel, new, or more intense stress than previously applied (e.g., lifting a heavier training load or a greater volume-load; see chapter 17), the initial response, or alarm phase, is an accumulation of fatigue, soreness, stiffness, or reduction in energetic stores that results in a reduction in performance capacity (59). Depending on the magnitude of the stress encountered by the athlete, this response may last several hours, days, or weeks. After this initial response, the body moves into the resistance phase, in which it adapts to the stimulus and returns to a normal functional capacity. If the training stress is appropriately structured and not excessive, these adaptive responses can result in specific biochemical, structural, and mechanical adjustments that further elevate the athlete's performance capacity, resulting in what is termed **supercompensation** (58).

If, however, the stress persists for an extended period of time, the athlete can move into the exhaustion phase. If this occurs, the athlete is demonstrating an inability to adapt to the imposed stressors and will present some of the same symptoms noted in the alarm phase. Ultimately, when athletes reach the exhaustion phase they are most likely experiencing overreaching or overtraining responses (20). From a training perspective, excessive loading, monotonous training, and overly varied training can all result in the occurrence of the exhaustion phase. Additionally, the responses to training can be affected by other nontraining-related stress (e.g., occupational issues, insufficient sleep, relationship, poor diet) that can contribute to the overall stress level experienced by the athlete. Ultimately, the strength and conditioning professional should strive to avoid the occurrence of this phase of the GAS through the proper planning and management (periodization) of training stressors.

Although the actual dimensions (i.e., slope, magnitude, and timing) of the curve shown in figure 21.1 are highly individualized, the figure represents the basic application of the GAS to training responses.

Stimulus-Fatigue-Recovery-Adaptation Theory

The stimulus-fatigue-recovery-adaptation theory is an extension of the GAS and suggests that training stimuli produce a general response (figure 21.2) that is influenced by the overall magnitude of the training stressor (59). Specifically, the greater the overall magnitude of the workload encountered, the more fatigue accumulates and the longer the delay before complete recovery and adaption can occur. As the athlete recovers from and adapts to the training stimuli, fatigue will dissipate, and preparedness and performance increase. If no new training stimulus is introduced, a state of involution or detraining (i.e., a reduced overall capacity, to below the current baseline) is observed. In contrast, if a new training stimulus is introduced, the process is repeated. This basic pattern is present whenever an athlete is exposed to a training exercise, session, day, or cycle within a periodized training plan. It should be noted that while recovery is an important part of the training process, it is not always necessary to reach a state of complete recovery

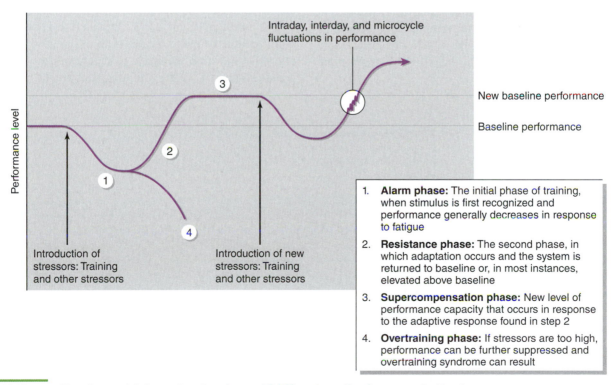

FIGURE 21.1   The General Adaptation Syndrome (GAS) and application to periodization.

Adapted, by permission, from Haff and Haff, 2012 (28).

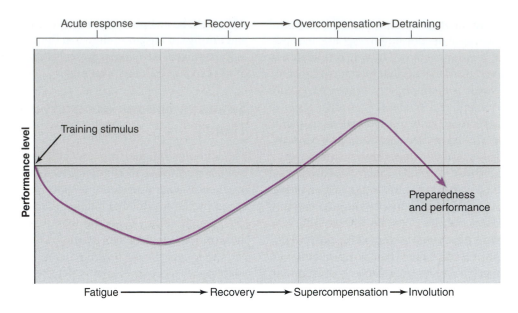

FIGURE 21.2 The stimulus-fatigue-recovery-adaptation theory, with interchangeable terminology.

Adapted, by permission, from Haff and Haff, 2012 (28).

before engaging in a new bout or session of training (49). The manipulation of workloads and training intensities through use of light and heavy sessions or days of training can be used to modulate fatigue and recovery responses (9, 19) while allowing for fitness to be either increased or maintained. Conceptually, this theory serves as the foundation for sequential periodization models in that these models allow for the manipulation of various training factors to modulate the athlete's overall fatigue levels, rate of recovery, and adaptive response to the training stimuli.

Fitness–Fatigue Paradigm

Generally, there is a summation of the two primary training aftereffects (i.e., fitness and fatigue) in response to training interventions that influence the athlete's level of preparedness (3, 14, 66). Zatsiorsky (65) presents the classic explanation of these relationships as the fitness–fatigue paradigm (figure 21.3). Ultimately, every training bout, session, or cycle creates both fatigue and fitness aftereffects, which summate to create a state of preparedness (14, 65). When training loads are the highest,

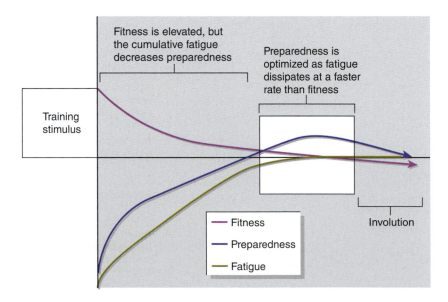

FIGURE 21.3 The fitness–fatigue paradigm.

Adapted, by permission, from Haff and Haff, 2012 (28).

fitness becomes elevated; but because of the high training loads, a concomitant increase in fatigue occurs. When fitness and fatigue are summed in this case, the level of fatigue results in a reduction in preparedness. On the other hand, when training workloads are low, little fatigue occurs and minimal fitness is developed, resulting in a low level of preparedness. Thus the sequencing of training loads becomes important in that it allows for training workloads to be varied in a systematic manner. An important thing to remember is that fatigue dissipates at a faster rate than fitness, thus allowing preparedness to become elevated if appropriate training strategies are used to retain fitness while reducing fatigue (25, 28). While the fitness–fatigue paradigm is classically represented as one fatigue, fitness, and preparedness curve, it is likely that each training factor stimulates its own individual fitness, fatigue, and preparedness aftereffect response (14, 59). These aftereffects are often considered to be residual training effects and serve as a fundamental concept underlying the use of sequential periodization models (25, 28). Ultimately, the residual training effects of one training period have the potential to affect the level of preparedness in subsequent training periods, depending on the overall structure of the periodized training plan (28).

Periodization Hierarchy

Ultimately periodization is simply a means of organizing the planning of a training intervention so that the program is partitioned into specific time periods (table 21.1) (22, 24). The multiyear training plan covers the most time but is the least detailed plan within a periodized training structure. For example, it may involve the basic progression of a collegiate football player from his freshman to senior year and contain key developmental goals that are targeted within each year of training. This multiyear training structure is then subdivided into more detailed individual **annual training plans** that are developed based on the athlete's progression through the various stages or benchmarks associated with the multiyear training plan. In sports that have only one competitive season such as American football, an annual training plan would be represented as a **macrocycle**. However, in a sport like college track and field, the annual plan would be divided into two macrocycles because of the indoor and outdoor seasons typical of this college sport. Typically the macrocycle lasts several months up to a year, depending on the sport. Within each macrocycle are

> ► Periodization of training begins with general global training targets set forth in the multiyear or annual training plan and becomes more specific as the program is developed for the macro-, meso-, and microcycles. For example, annual training plans set the general pathway for a training year, while the other cycles set the means, methods, and modes used to get to the primary competitive targets.

TABLE 21.1 Periodization Cycles

Period	Duration	Description
Multiyear plan	2-4 years	A 4-year training plan is termed a quadrennial plan.
Annual training plan	1 year	The overall training plan can contain single or multiple macrocycles. Is subdivided into various periods of training including preparatory, competitive, and transition periods.
Macrocycle	Several months to a year	Some authors refer to this as an annual plan. Is divided into preparatory, competitive, and transition periods of training.
Mesocycle	2-6 weeks	Medium-sized training cycle, sometimes referred to as a block of training. The most common duration is 4 weeks. Consists of microcycles that are linked together.
Microcycle	Several days to 2 weeks	Small-sized training cycle; can range from several days to 2 weeks in duration; the most common duration is 1 week (7 days). Composed of multiple workouts.
Training day	1 day	One training day that can include multiple training sessions is designed in the context of the particular microcycle it is in.
Training session	Several hours	Generally consists of several hours of training. If the workout includes >30 min of rest between bouts of training, it would comprise multiple sessions.

Adapted, by permission, from G.G. Haff and E.E. Haff, 2012, Training integration and periodization. In *NSCA guide to program design*, edited by J. Hoffman (Champaign, IL: Human Kinetics), 220.

mesocycles, each lasting several weeks to months; two to six weeks is the most typical duration. The number of mesocycles within each macrocycle is dependent on the training targets and the length of the macrocycle within the annual training plan. Each mesocycle is then broken down into individual microcycles that last from several days to weeks; the most common duration is one week (22, 28). Within each **microcycle** are training days that are further subdivided into training sessions.

Periodization Periods

The overall variation and structure of the program design variables within each individual meso- and microcycle are constructed based on the periods included in the macrocycle or annual training plan (22, 25). Across these periods of the training plan, the volume and intensity of the training and conditioning program generally receive the greatest attention; but the time spent acquiring and perfecting sport-specific technique must also be considered when one is constructing the overall periodized training plan (57). Ultimately, periodized training plans systematically shift training foci from general nonspecific activities of high volume and low intensity toward activities of lower volume and higher intensities over a period of many weeks or months to help reduce the potential for overtraining while optimizing performance capacities.

The basic sequencing of periodized training programs and how training progresses through the various phases for specified training targets are very similar to the sequencing and evolution of learning academic concepts. For example, in academics we start with simple concepts

and skills that progress to more complex concepts. Ultimately we are building on the simple skills in order to provide a sound foundation for the more complex items. Ultimately the periods within a periodized training plan serve as the pathway for developing simple skills into more complex sport-specific targets.

In the classic periodization literature, the major divisions of training are classified as the preparatory, competitive, and transition periods (24, 43). Stone, O'Bryant, and Garhammer (57) modified this classic model to include a "first transition" between the preparatory and competitive periods of training. Based on this structure, contemporary periodization models often contain four distinct but interrelated training periods: preparatory, first transition, competitive, and second transition. Figure 21.4 presents the basic periodization model described by Stone, O'Bryant, and Garhammer (57). This model is often applied for novice athletes with a lower training status. Generally, in this application, intensity begins lower and gradually increases, while volume starts higher and slowly decreases as the athlete becomes more conditioned. It is important to note that not all novice athletes are able to tolerate large changes in these variables and that smaller fluctuations may be required (58, 61, 62). It is also important to note that even though these fluctuations are often represented graphically as straight lines, the volume and intensity progressions are in fact nonlinear because of the fluctuations in the loadings that occur at the micro- and mesocycle levels (22, 24, 25, 51). This basic misunderstanding of the classic models of periodization has resulted in these types of models being falsely termed *linear periodization models* (25, 51).

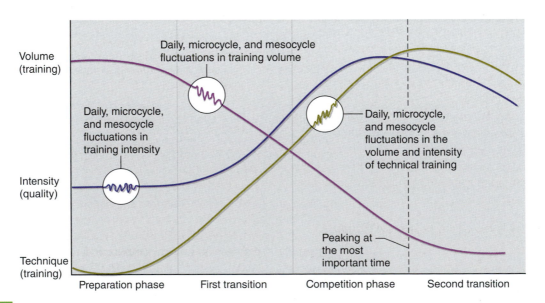

FIGURE 21.4   Matveyev's model of periodization (appropriate for novices).

Reprinted, by permission, from G.G. Haff and E.E. Haff, 2012, Training integration and periodization. In *NSCA's guide to program design*, edited by J. Hoffman (Champaign, IL: Human Kinetics), 223; adapted from figure 11.7, p. 2239. Reprinted from *Weight training: A scientific approach*, 2nd edition, by Michael H. Stone and Harold St. O'Bryant, copyright © 1987 by Burgess.

Advanced athletes tend to train closer to their abilities and have smaller adaptation windows. Therefore, these athletes require greater training variation as well as higher volumes and intensities in order to allow them to continue to experience appropriate training stimuli (51). For example, Zatsiorsky and Kraemer (66) demonstrate that a stimulating load for a novice athlete would be a maintenance load at best for advanced athletes. To address this issue, the shift from higher-volume to higher-intensity training can occur earlier in the preparatory phase, with higher overall training volumes as compared to those in the base model presented in figure 21.4.

Preparatory Period

In outlining a periodized training plan, the starting point is usually the **preparatory period**. This period occurs when there are no competitions, and technical, tactical, or sport-specific work is limited. This period often corresponds to what is termed the off-season. The central goal of this period of training is to develop a base level of conditioning in order to increase the athlete's ability to tolerate more intense training. Based on the model presented in figure 21.4, the conditioning activities would begin with relatively low intensities and high volumes: long, slow distance running or swimming; low-intensity plyometrics; and high-repetition resistance training with light to moderate resistances. Traditionally, the preparatory period is subdivided into general and specific phases. The **general preparatory phase** typically occurs during the early part of the period and often targets the development of a general physical base (3). This early part of the preparatory period includes high training volumes, low training intensities, and a larger variety of training means that are structured to develop general motor abilities and skills (36, 44). The **specific preparatory phase** occurs after the completion of the general preparatory phase and involves a shift in training focus. From the training base that has been established, this phase expands the athlete's training base through an increased emphasis on sport-specific training activities that prepare the athlete for the competitive period (15). During the preparatory period, resistance training phases can be created in order to depict more refined differences in training intensity and volume. In order, these are the hypertrophy/strength endurance and basic strength phases (57, 58).

Hypertrophy/Strength Endurance Phase

The **hypertrophy phase**, which is also referred to as the **strength endurance phase**, generally occurs during the early portion of the preparatory period (i.e., the general preparatory phase) (18, 27, 28). During this phase, the training intensity is low to moderate and the overall volume is high. The primary goals during this phase are (a) to increase lean body mass, (b) to develop an endurance (muscular and metabolic) base, or (c) to do both. This development will serve as the foundation for the higher-intensity training in subsequent phases and periods (29, 30). With strength/power athletes, the primary target might be to stimulate hypertrophic effects while increasing strength endurance. With endurance athletes, the primary goal would be to increase strength endurance without significantly increasing hypertrophy. Regardless of the sport or athlete being trained, it is generally accepted that during the general preparatory phase, sport conditioning activities may not be specific to the athlete's sport. However, as the athlete moves into the specific preparatory phase, over several weeks the training activities will become more sport specific. For example, sprinters may begin the general preparatory phase with longer-distance runs (longer than their competitive distance, not traditional distance running; for example, a 100 m sprinter may do 400 m runs to establish a foundation) at slower speeds in conjunction with lower-intensity plyometrics such as double-leg bounding and hopping, as well as more basic resistance exercises that are not necessarily biomechanically or structurally similar to running (back squat, leg curl, and so on.). Generally, the athlete performs resistance training with low to moderate intensities for high volumes (table 21.2).

However, it is important to note that throughout this phase, daily variations in training intensity and workload will facilitate recovery (27). Additionally, recovery weeks or microcycles may be placed throughout the phase and most often at the end of the phase before the next phase of training begins.

> The hypertrophy/strength endurance phase involves low to moderate intensity (50-75% of the 1-repetition maximum [1RM]) and high volumes (three to six sets of 8-20 repetitions).

Basic Strength Phase

In the later portion of the preparatory period, during the specific preparatory phase, the primary aim of the **basic strength phase** is to increase the strength of the muscles that are essential to the primary sport movements (11-13). For example, the sprinter's running program would progress to include interval sprints of a moderate distance and more complex and specialized plyometric drills. The resistance training program also becomes more specific to the sport (e.g., squats, power cleans, one-leg squats) and involves heavier loads performed at lower volumes than in the hypertrophy/strength

TABLE 21.2   A Periodization Model for Resistance Training

Period	Preparatory		First transition	Competition			Second transition
Subperiod	General preparatory	Specific preparatory	Precompetitive	Main competitive			Postcompetitive
Season	Off-season		Preseason	In-season			Postseason
Phase	Hypertrophy/ strength endurance	Basic strength	Strength/power	Peaking	Or	Maintenance	Active rest
Intensity	Low to moderate	High	Low to very high	Very high to very low		Moderate to high	Recreational activities (may not involve resistance training)
	50-75% of 1RM	80-95% of 1RM	87-95% of 1RM*	50% to ≥93% of 1RM		85-93% of 1RM	
			30-85% of 1RM**				
Volume	High	Moderate to high	Low	Very low		Low to moderate	
	3-6 sets***	2-6 sets***	2-5 sets***	1-3 sets***		~2-5 sets***	
	8-20 repetitions	2-6 repetitions	2-5 repetitions	1-3 repetitions		3-6 repetitions	

*These percentages of 1RM apply to nonpower core exercises.

**These percentages of 1RM apply to power exercises. The actual percentage used to elicit power development depends on the exercise that is used. For more information see Kawamori and Haff (39).

***These recommendations do not include warm-up sets and represent only target sets for core exercises (2); they also do not include lower-intensity recovery days that are often part of a periodized training plan (27).

Adapted from 27, 56, 57, 58, 59.

endurance phase (table 21.2). As with the hypertrophy/ strength endurance phase, daily variations in training load facilitate recovery (27, 28).

> The basic strength phase involves higher intensity (80-95% of 1RM) and moderate to high volumes (two to six sets of two to six repetitions).

First Transition Period

As originally described by Stone and colleagues (56-58), the **first transition period** is a link between the preparatory and competitive periods. Classically the resistance training in this period focuses on the development of strength and power as noted in Stone, O'Bryant, and Garhammer's (57) seminal paper on the periodization of strength training. The central aim of this period is to shift training focus toward the elevation of strength and its translation into power development (56, 57). In order to maximize this process and facilitate recovery, there are variations in training intensity and workload at the microcycle level (27, 28). Additionally, the last week of the period is marked by reduced volume, intensity, or

both in order to achieve recovery before the beginning of the competition period.

Strength/Power Phase

The main phase within the first transition period is the **strength/power phase**. In this phase, the sprinter's interval and speed training intensifies to near competitive pace; speed drills are performed (e.g., sled towing, sprints against resistance, and uphill sprints); plyometric drills mimic sprinting; and the resistance training program involves performing power/explosive exercises at low to very high loads with low volumes. As explained in chapter 17, the load assignments for power exercises do not follow the typical %RM–repetition relationship, but their relative intensities are elevated during this phase (table 21.2). Specifically, the exercises selected in this phase can dictate the loading that is used (39). For example, the development of power may be facilitated with a load of 80% of 1RM with hang power cleans (38), while a load of 50% to 70% of 1RM may be used with the bench press throw when the aim is to maximize power development (39). Ultimately, in order to address both strength and power development, a mixed training approach is warranted in which heavy- and low-load training is used to optimize both attributes (31).

> **The strength/power phase involves low to very high loads (30-95% of 1RM, depending on the exercise) and low volumes (two to five sets for two to five repetitions).**

Competitive Period

The central training target during the **competitive period** is preparing the athlete for competition by further increasing strength and power via additional increases in training intensity while decreasing volume. This process can be a delicate balancing act, as adequate volume and intensity of training are needed in order to maintain competitive preparedness, and reductions in volume, intensity, or both are needed to optimize performance. To understand this conundrum, consider the fitness–fatigue paradigm presented earlier. If training workloads (volume or intensity) are reduced too much, fatigue will be reduced, but there will be a concomitant decrease in overall fitness that results in a reduction in competitive preparedness. Also during this period, time spent practicing sport-specific skills and tactics increases dramatically, and a proportional decrease occurs in time spent performing physical conditioning activities such as resistance training. For example, a sprinter places even more emphasis on speed, reaction time, sprint-specific plyometric drills, and technique training. The competition period may last for one or two weeks for some sports in which a peaking program is employed (7, 23). **Peaking** programs attempt to place the athlete in peak condition for about one or two weeks. Trying to extend this to longer durations ultimately results in reduced performance capacity as a result of reduction in fitness or potential overtraining (3, 23). Depending on the load reduction strategy employed, peaking programs result in a progressive shift from higher-intensity training toward lower-intensity work designed to reduce fatigue as the athlete moves through the taper before competition (23). As shown in table 21.2, resistance training may range between 50% and ≥93% of 1RM, depending on where athletes are in the peaking program.

For team sports, this period spans an entire season and may last for many months, requiring the use of a **maintenance** program (3). Because of the prolonged duration of the competitive period in this situation, the intensity and volume of training must be manipulated on a microcycle basis in order to maintain strength and power while managing the fatigue associated with a frequent-competition schedule. Generally, a maintenance program is marked by moderate- to high-intensity training (e.g., 85-93% 1RM) at low to moderate volumes. At the microcycle level, the training loads are modulated based on the training, travel, and competitive schedule. Careful monitoring of the athlete's performance capacity and recovery is critical during the team sport athlete's competitive period.

> **The competitive period includes peaking and maintenance. For peaking, athletes use very high to low intensities (50% to ≥93% of the 1RM) and very low volume (one to three sets of one to three repetitions) for one to two weeks. For maintenance, athletes modulate training between moderate and high intensities (85-93% of 1RM) with moderate volumes (about two to five sets of three to six repetitions).**

Second Transition Period (Active Rest)

Between the competitive season and the next annual training plan or the preparatory period of a macrocycle, a **second transition period** is often used to create a linkage (57). This period is sometimes referred to as an **active rest** or **restoration** period and generally lasts for one to four weeks (3). It is important to note that if active rest is extended for a prolonged duration, athletes will require a much longer preparatory period in order to regain their performance capacities (26). Therefore, it is generally recommended that the second transition period last no longer than four weeks unless an athlete requires additional time to recover from an injury. During this period, aggressive training immediately after the peak performance or end of the maintenance phase should be avoided so athletes can rehabilitate injuries and rest physically and mentally (11-13). For example, a sprinter may engage in recreational activities such as volleyball, racket sports, and swimming in a leisurely manner and perform very low-volume, nonsport-specific resistance training with very low loads. A secondary use of the active rest concept is to structure one-week breaks between long phases (three weeks) or periods of training. The purpose is to create an unloading week in order to prepare the body for the subsequent phase or period of

> **The second transition (active rest) provides a period of time in which athletes can rehabilitate injuries and refresh both physically and mentally before beginning a new annual training plan or macrocycle. This period should not last longer than four weeks, because long periods with reduced training will require the athlete to engage in a longer preparatory period in order to regain sporting form.**

training. The practice of reducing the training load via the reduction of training intensity and volume is believed by many strength and conditioning professionals to reduce overtraining potential.

Applying Sport Seasons to the Periodization Periods

In practical terms, periodization involves a logical, systematic variation and integration of training in order to direct the training responses while managing fatigue and optimizing performance in accordance with the seasonal demands of the sport and athletes. Based on the competitive season, the overall annual plan or macrocycle is structured in order to sequentially develop specific attributes required by the athlete. In order to avoid monotony, staleness, and overtraining potential, the training program must involve structured variation of key training variables (e.g., volume, intensity, training frequency, training foci, exercise selection) (28). Classically, most intercollegiate and professional sports have an annual schedule that includes an off-season, preseason, in-season, and postseason. These seasons are easy to relate to the periods in a periodized training model (see figure 21.5).

Off-Season

The off-season should be considered the preparatory period; it typically lasts from the end of the postseason to the beginning of the preseason, which can be about six weeks before the first major competition (although this varies greatly). This preparatory period is subdivided into general and specific preparatory phases that are broken down into mesocycles; these interlink to prepare the athlete for the subsequent competitive season. For example, the athlete may complete several rotations of mesocycles that focus on hypertrophy/strength endurance and basic strength (see figure 21.5). Ultimately, these cyclical rotations are selected based on the sport and the athlete's needs. For example, if an American football player needs to gain muscle mass, more mesocycles that target the hypertrophy phase will be prescribed.

Preseason

After the completion of the off-season, the preseason is used to lead into the first major competition. The first transition period is often undertaken at this time with a focus on the strength/power phase of resistance training. This time is used to prepare the athlete for the subsequent competitive period. It is very important to note that the preseason is not the time to build the foundational physical capacities needed for the sport; this should occur primarily in the off-season. The preseason is designed to capitalize on the off-season and elevate the athlete's performance capacity during the competitive period.

In-Season

The competition, or in-season, period contains all the contests scheduled for the given year, including any tournament games. Most sports have a long season that requires multiple mesocycles arranged around key contests. Thus, a long competition season (12-16+ weeks)

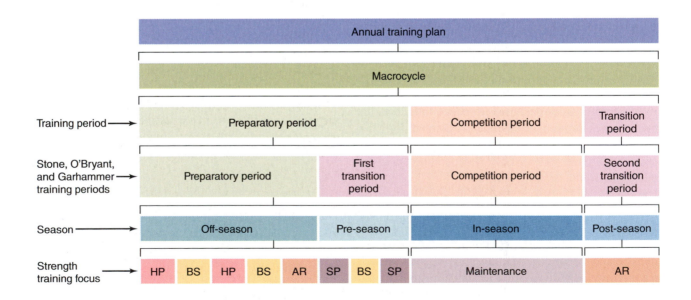

FIGURE 21.5 Relationship of periodization periods to seasons and strength training focus. HP = hypertrophy/strength endurance; BS = basic strength; AR = active rest; SP = strength/power.

presents unique programming challenges. One solution is to structure three- or four-week mesocycle blocks that unload the athlete in the last microcycle in order to allow for fatigue reduction and performance supercompensation before critical contests (28). This does not mean that the athlete is in poor condition for the other contests, as varying training intensities and volumes across the mesocycle can modulate preparedness. Specifically, training intensity and volume are increased or decreased in order to maintain physical capacities while reducing fatigue and peaking preparedness before the competitive engagements. The other approach is to design a maintenance program that modulates moderate intensities with low to moderate volumes.

Postseason

After the final contest, the postseason or second transition period provides the athlete with a relative or active rest before the beginning of the next year's off-season or preparatory period. It is important to remember that the longer the postseason, the greater the chance for detraining, which results in an increased need for a longer general preparatory phase during the next off-season (3).

Undulating Versus Linear Periodization Models

For better or worse, contemporary periodization literature has adopted the terms *linear* and *nonlinear* when referring to periodization models. However, it should be noted that a central tenet of periodization is the removal of linearity from training (25, 32, 37, 43, 49, 51). Often the traditional resistance training model is falsely referred to as linear due to the gradual and progressive mesocycle increases in intensity over time (8, 37, 51). However, a closer look at the traditional model as described by Stone, O'Bryant, and Garhammer (57, 58) and within the literature (37) shows that the traditional model contains nonlinear variation in training intensity and volume-load at the microcycle level and throughout the mesocycle. Regardless of this, an alternative model termed the **nonlinear periodization** model has been introduced in the strength and conditioning industry (42, 53). This model is probably better described as an undulating or **daily undulating periodization** model, because it involves large daily (i.e., within the microcycle) fluctuations in the load and volume (e.g., repetitions and volume-load) of assigned core resistance training exercises. For example, using this model you might perform four sets with a 6RM load (strength focus) on the first day of the week (e.g., Tuesday), three sets with a 10RM (hypertrophic focus) on the next training day (e.g., Thursday), and five sets with a 3RM load (power

focus) on the last training day (e.g., Saturday). In this case the load, volume (e.g., repetitions and volume-load), and training focus are all modified within the microcycle. These modifications are in contrast to what occurs with the **traditional periodization** model, falsely referred to as the **linear periodization** model, according to which the athlete performs the same number of sets and repetitions across the training days and varies the training load. For example, the athlete may perform four sets of six at 85% of 1RM on the first day of training, at 75% of 1RM on the second day, and at 65% of 1RM on the third day to basically train using a heavy-to-light training structure. While the traditional model appears to vary only intensity because the repetitions do not change, one must remember that the volume-load changes in this model result in undulations in workload and training volume, supporting the idea that the traditional model is in fact nonlinear and should not be classified as linear (37).

Some research studies suggest that the undulating model is more effective than the traditional model (16, 41, 45, 47, 53), although other evidence suggests that there is no difference between the models (1, 10, 52) or that the traditional model is superior (34, 35, 50). Proponents of the undulating model suggest that one of its strengths is the absence of accumulated neural fatigue caused by extended, ever-increasing training intensities common to the traditional model (40). Conversely, proponents of the traditional model suggest that the overall high volume-loads of training in the undulating model result in greater peripheral fatigue and increased risk of injury because of the high levels of metabolic fatigue this type of programming can stimulate (50). Additionally, examination of the fatigue–fitness paradigm (figure 21.3) and the stimulus-fatigue-recovery-adaptation theory (figure 21.2) indicates that the undulating model has the potential to decrease athlete preparedness because of accumulated fatigue that occurs with higher volume-load training sessions. Some authors suggest that, based upon the GAS, this response may actually increase the potential for overtraining with higher-level athletes (25, 60) and result in an increased injury risk for athletes using this model in conjunction with their sport-based training.

Example of an Annual Training Plan

An example of one approach to designing a full annual training plan (i.e., macrocycle for sports with one competitive season) spanning all four sport seasons is presented in the four application tables near the end of this chapter. The program is based on the preseason resistance training program for scenario A from chapter

17, "Program Design for Resistance Training," which concerns a female collegiate basketball center. Background information and initial testing information about this athlete are provided in chapter 17.

The annual plan example provided in this chapter begins where the preseason program from chapter 17 left off and shows a continuation of the training program through the in-season, the postseason, and the following year's off-season. The primary focus of the annual training plan example is the resistance training component of scenario A. Although other modes of training are described briefly (e.g., plyometrics, anaerobic conditioning, aerobic endurance), this example is not intended to illustrate every aspect of variation for a strength and conditioning program for basketball. Also, although this example is divided into four sport seasons that are made up of two- to four-week mesocycles, an alternative approach is to structure each season as an individual macrocycle.

Preseason

After undertaking one or two unloading weeks following the cessation of the off-season training period, the athlete begins the preseason period of training. For this example, the period covers about 3.5 months (mid-August until the first game, possibly mid-November). The goals of the preseason are to increase the intensity of sport-specific training and the attention given to basketball drills and skills. The resistance training portion is planned for three days per week and focuses primarily on strength and power outcomes. Other training modes (e.g., plyometrics and anaerobic conditioning) hold high priority, especially if they directly contribute to basketball training. Although chapter 17 does not show microcycle progressions, it describes the resistance training portion of this season in detail; therefore, please refer to the table titled "Application of All Program Design Variables" in that chapter for the preseason program example. The same method of applying the periodization concepts described in this chapter can be used to design the remainder of the preseason period.

In-Season

After an unloading week following the preseason, the athlete is ready to begin the competition period of training. The in-season period lasts approximately 20 weeks, spanning a time period from November until April (including a four-week tournament period, although it could last longer). The goals for the in-season are to maintain and possibly improve strength, power, flexibility, and anaerobic conditioning. The time constraints of games, skill and strategy practice, and travel result in a lower volume of off-court training activities.

Due to multiple games each week, resistance training may be limited to 30 minutes, one to three times per week, consisting of an undulating regimen of varying volume-loads and relative intensities. Power and basketball-specific nonpower core exercises predominate, with assistance exercises added for balance. See the sample in-season program near the end of this chapter. Plyometric sessions should be alternated with resistance training and conducted once or twice weekly, depending on the number of games.

On days when no resistance training is scheduled, 15 to 20 minutes of various short sprint intervals could be performed once or twice weekly during practice. Speed, agility, and other running conditioning can be incorporated into practice time, and flexibility training can be part of the practice and game warm-up and cool-down. Two or three days of rest should be afforded between resistance training, plyometrics, and sprint interval sessions, depending on the game schedule. This period is similar to the previous training period in that the majority of the athlete's time is spent on skill and strategy development, with the remainder devoted to conditioning.

The athlete is in good condition from the previous mesocycles, so she should be able not only to maintain that condition but also to peak again if the team continues in the conference tournament. In that case, she would revert back to mesocycle 2 and progress to mesocycle 3 if the team qualifies for a tournament to be held after the conference tournament. If the tournament game schedule does not allow for more than one resistance training session per week, the athlete should perform all the week's power and core exercises (if time allows) and omit the assistance exercises. Two examples of specific weekly tournament schedules are presented near the end of this chapter.

Postseason (Active Rest Period)

Following the completion of the competitive season is a (second) transition period of active rest with no formal or structured workouts. For this example, the transition period lasts a month (from April 4 until May 1). The goal of the period is for the athlete to recuperate physically and psychologically from the long in-season. Recreational games and fitness activities include swimming, jogging, circuit weight training, volleyball, racquetball, and informal basketball. *All activities are performed at low intensities with low volumes.*

Off-Season

Following the postseason active rest period, the athlete should be rested and ready to begin off-season (preparatory period) training. For this example, this preparatory period lasts about 14 weeks, from the beginning of May to the beginning of August. The goal of this period is to establish a base level of conditioning to increase the athlete's tolerance for more intense training in later phases and periods. During the first week, testing should be performed so the strength and conditioning professional can determine initial training loads for the exercises in the first mesocycle. In later mesocycles, when more or other exercises are added, the training loads can be estimated from loads used in similar exercises or can be determined from RM testing. For example, the strength and conditioning professional can reasonably predict training load for the hang clean from the tested power clean maximum, or the actual RM load could be measured. Other monitoring tests related to basketball are shoulder and hip flexibility tests, 12-minute run, 300-yard (274 m) shuttle, line drill, T-test, vertical jump, and skinfold measurements (see chapter 13 for testing protocols).

The resistance training component holds higher priority in the off-season, and an athlete may follow a split routine of four or more training days per week. In this example, the basketball player begins the off-season with an all-body, three times per week regimen but soon progresses to four training days per week with variations in training intensity across the microcycle to allow fatigue to be managed. These advancements also involve a gradual increase in loading, with associated decreases in training volume. Other training includes aerobic endurance exercises to maintain or improve body composition and cardiovascular fitness. These conditioning workouts are scheduled on nonresistance training days, and flexibility training can be emphasized in the warm-up and cool-down portions of each training session.

Reviewing the Annual Plan Example

For any periodization model to function optimally, the sport coach and the strength and conditioning professional must plan the program together in order to share goals and strategies. This is a critical issue in that working together allows all the training factors that the athlete will engage in to be integrated so as to better manage the training stress and modulate fatigue and recovery. Without the cooperation of all involved professionals, optimal performance cannot be fully achieved.

The example in this chapter is a representation of only one periodization model that could be used to structure training for a sample athlete. Other athletes or sports may require subtle to radical variations in the structure presented here. It is important to remember that a multitude of periodization models can be adapted to meet the needs of the various athletes and sports.

Conclusion

Periodization is a process through which the athlete's training is logically and systematically organized in order to promote peak condition (preparedness) for the most important competitions. The annual training plan (year of training) is divided into macrocycles that contain preparatory, competition, and transition periods. Each period is subdivided into mesocycles that target specific phases of development: hypertrophy/strength endurance, basic strength, or strength/power. Transitions are used to link mesocycles or macrocycles and provide the athlete with an unloading period that enhances recovery. The overall structure of the macrocycle, mesocycle, and individual microcycles is dictated by the individual sport's competitive season and demands.

In-Season (Competitive Period)
Female college basketball center
5 months (20 weeks): November 21-April 3 (including tournament play)
(Beginning after an unloading week; November 15-21)

Mesocycle 1
4 Weeks: November 22-December 19; Unload Week December 20-26

Session	Exercises	Sets	Reps	TRAINING LOADS				
				Week 1	Week 2	Week 3	Week 4	Week 5
1	High pull	1	4	75% 1RM	80% 1RM	85% 1RM	90% 1RM	60% 1RM
	Back squat	1	6	80% 6RM	85% 6RM	90% 6RM	95%6RM	65% 6RM
	Incline bench press	1	6	80% 6RM	85% 6RM	90% 6RM	95%6RM	65% 6RM
	Lateral shoulder raise	1	10	75% 10RM	80% 10RM	85% 10RM	90% 10RM	70% 10RM
	Abdominal crunch	Max in 60 s						
2	Push press	1	6	70% 6RM	75% 6RM	80% 6RM	85% 6RM	60% 6RM
	Hip sled	1	6	70% 6RM	75% 6RM	80% 6RM	85% 6RM	60% 6RM
	Closed-grip bench press	1	6	70% 6RM	75% 6RM	80% 6RM	85% 6RM	60% 6RM
	Seated low pulley row	1	6	70% 6RM	75% 6RM	80% 6RM	85% 6RM	60% 6RM
	Supine leg raise	Max in 60 s						

Mesocycle 2
4 Weeks: December 27-January 23; Unload Week January 24-30

Session	Exercises	Sets	Reps	TRAINING LOADS				
				Week 1	Week 2	Week 3	Week 4	Week 5
1	Hang clean	1	3	70% 1RM	75% 1RM	80% 1RM	85% 1RM	65% 1RM
	Front squat	1	5	75% 5RM	80% 5RM	85% 5RM	90% 5RM	60% 5RM
	Standing shoulder press	1	5	75% 5RM	80% 5RM	85% 5RM	90% 5RM	60% 5RM
	Lying triceps extension	1	10	75% 10RM	80% 10RM	85% 10RM	90% 10RM	70% 10RM
	Abdominal crunch	Max in 60 s						
2	Push jerk	1	3	65% 1RM	70% 1RM	75% 1RM	80% 1RM	60% 1RM
	Step-up	1	5	70% 5RM	75% 5RM	80% 5RM	85% 5RM	60% 5RM
	Closed-grip bench press	1	10	65% 10RM	70% 10RM	75% 10RM	80% 10RM	60% 10RM
	Lat pull-down	1	10	65% 10RM	70% 10RM	75% 10RM	80% 10RM	60% 10RM
	Supine leg raise	Max in 60 s						

Mesocycle 3

4 Weeks: January 31-February 27; Unload Week February 28-March 6

Session	Exercises	Sets	Reps	TRAINING LOADS				
				Week 1	Week 2	Week 3	Week 4	Week 5
1	Power clean	1	2	75% 1RM	80% 1RM	85% 1RM	90% 1RM	70% 1RM
	Back squat	1	4	75% 4RM	80% 4RM	85% 4RM	90% 4RM	65% 4RM
	Bench press	1	4	75% 4RM	80% 4RM	85% 4RM	90% 4RM	65% 4RM
	Barbell biceps curl	1	8	75% 8RM	80% 8RM	85% 8RM	90% 8RM	65% 8RM
	Abdominal crunch	Max in 60 s						
2	Hang snatch	1	3	65% 1RM	70% 1RM	75% 1RM	80% 1RM	60% 1RM
	Forward step lunge	1	4	65% 4RM	70% 4RM	75% 4RM	80% 4RM	60% 4RM
	Closed-grip decline bench press	1	8	65% 8RM	70% 8RM	75% 8RM	80% 8RM	60% 8RM
	Upright row	1	8	65% 8RM	70% 8RM	75% 8RM	80% 8RM	60% 8RM
	Supine leg raise	Max in 60 s						

Tournament Mesocycle

4 Weeks: March 7-April 3

Go back to mesocycle 2; progress again to mesocycle 3 if tournament play extends beyond four weeks.

Comments:

- Each mesocycle is considered a block of training and contains five individual microcycles, with the fifth microcycle constituting an unloading microcycle.
- This in-season program incorporates a nonlinear approach with variations in volume-load, training intensity (kg), and targeted training exercises.
- Repetition maximum loads are not used, as training to failure has been shown to reduce power output and increase the risk of overtraining. Therefore, percentages of RM loads are used to deal with the accumulated fatigue associated with in-season training and competitions.
- It is important to note that these are the target sets and that three to five warm-up sets should be performed in order to provide an appropriate specific warm-up for the targeted loadings.
- Refer to table 17.7 for the relationship between the %RM and the number of repetitions allowed and table 17.8 for the estimation of 1RM.
- Refer to table 17.12 for rest period length assignment based on repetition goal.

Tournament Week A (Two Games)

Sunday	Monday	Tuesday	Wednesday	Thursday	Friday	Saturday
Practice (or rest)	Practice	Practice	Practice	Game	Practice	Game
	Resistance training		Plyometric session		Interval sprints	

Tournament Week B (Three Games)

Sunday	Monday	Tuesday	Wednesday	Thursday	Friday	Saturday
Game	Practice (or rest)	Practice	Practice	Game	Practice	Game
		Resistance training			Interval sprints	

Off Season (Preparation Period)
Female College Basketball Center
3 1/2 months (14 weeks): May 2-August 7

Initial Pretesting

(For Mesocycle 1) Microcycle 1: May 2-8

5RM POWER EXERCISE
1. Power clean

10RM FOR ASSISTANCE EXERCISES
1. Leg (knee) curl
2. Lat pull-down
3. Biceps curl
4. Lying triceps extension
5. Upright row

OTHER TESTING
1. Sit and reach
2. Shoulder elevation
3. 1.5-mile (2.4 km) run
4. 200-yard (274 m) shuttle run
5. Line drill
6. T-test
7. Vertical jump
8. Body composition (skinfolds)

10RM FOR NONPOWER CORE EXERCISES
1. Back squat
2. Bench press

Mesocycle 1

2 Weeks: May 9-22: Hypertrophy/Strength Endurance Phase 1

Day	Exercise	WEEK 1			WEEK 2		
		Sets	Reps	Intensity	Sets	Reps	Intensity
Mon/Fri	Power clean	2	10/2*	65% 5RM	3	10/2*	70% 5RM
	Back squat	2	10	65% 10RM	3	10	70% 10RM
	Leg (knee) curl	2	10	65% 10RM	3	10	70% 10RM
	Bench press	2	10	65% 10RM	3	10	70% 10RM
	Lying triceps extension	2	10	65% 10RM	3	10	70% 10RM
	Upright row	2	10	65% 10RM	3	10	70% 10RM
	Abdominal crunch	2	20		3	20	
	Note: Friday workout should use a load 10% less than Monday's.						
Wed	Clean pull (floor)**	2	10	60% 5RM	3	10	65% 10RM
	Romanian deadlift**	2	10	60% 5RM	3	10	65% 10RM
	Lat pulldown	2	10	60% 10RM	3	10	65% 10RM
	Biceps curl	2	10	60% 10RM	3	10	65% 10RM
	Abdominal crunch	2	20		3	20	

*Performed as cluster sets with a 20-second rest between clusters of two repetitions.
**Training loads are based on the 5RM power clean test.

Mesocycle 2

2 Weeks: May 23-June 5; Basic Strength Phase 1

Day	Exercise	WEEK 1			WEEK 2		
		Sets	Reps	Intensity	Sets	Reps	Intensity
Mon/Fri	Power clean	3	5	80% 5RM	3	5	85% 5RM
	Back squat	3	5	80% 5RM	3	5	85% 5RM
	Leg (knee) curl	3	5	80% 5RM	3	5	85% 5RM
	Bench press	3	5	80% 5RM	3	5	85% 5RM
	Lying triceps extension	2	10	70% 10RM	3	10	75% 10RM
	Upright row	2	10	70% 10RM	2	10	75% 10RM
	Abdominal crunch	2	25		3	25	
	Note: Friday workout should use a load 10% less than Monday's.						
Wed	Clean pull (floor)**	3	5	85% 5RM	3	5	90% 5RM
	Romanian deadlift**	3	5	75% 5RM	3	5	80% 5RM
	Lat pulldown	2	10	70% 10RM	3	5	75% 10RM
	Barbell biceps curl	2	10	70% 10RM	3	5	75% 10RM
	Abdominal crunch	2	25		2	10	

**Training loads are based on the 5RM power clean test.

Unloading Week

1 Week: June 6-12

Day	Exercise	Sets	Reps	Intensity
Mon/Fri	Power clean	3	5	70% 5RM
	Back squat	3	5	70% 5RM
	Bench press	3	5	70% 5RM
	Abdominal crunch	3	20	
Wed	Clean pull (floor)**	3	5	70% 5RM
	Romanian deadlift	3	5	70% 5RM
	Lat pulldown	2	10	60% 10RM
	Abdominal crunch	3	20	

**Training loads are based on the 5RM power clean test.

Mesocycle 3

2 Weeks: June 13-26; Hypertrophy/Strength Endurance Phase 1

Day	Exercise	WEEK 1			WEEK 2		
		Sets	Reps	Intensity	Sets	Reps	Intensity
Mon/ Thurs	Hang snatch	3	10	55% 10RM	3	10	60% 10RM
	Back squat	3	10	70% 10RM	3	10	75% 10RM
	Incline bench press	3	10	70% 10RM	3	10	75% 10RM
	Lunge	3	10	70% 10RM	3	10	75% 10RM
	Leg (knee) curl	3	10	70% 10RM	3	10	75% 10RM
	Seated calf raise	3	10	70% 10RM	3	10	75% 10RM
	Note: Thursday workout should use a load 15% less than Monday's.						
Tues/Fri	Push jerk	3	10	60% 10RM	3	10	65% 10RM
	Clean pull (floor)**	3	10	65% 10RM	3	10	70% 10RM
	Bent-over row	3	10	65% 10RM	3	10	70% 10RM
	Shoulder press	3	10	65% 10RM	3	10	70% 10RM
	Barbell biceps curl	3	10	65% 10RM	3	10	70% 10RM
	Triceps pushdown	3	10	65% 10RM	3	10	70% 10RM
	Abdominal muscles	3	20		3	20	
	Note: Friday workout should use a load 10% less than Tuesday's.						

**Training loads are based on the power clean test.

Mesocycle 4

2 Weeks: June 27-July 10: Basic Strength Phase 2

Day	Exercise	WEEK 1			WEEK 2		
		Sets	Reps	Intensity	Sets	Reps	Intensity
Mon/ Thurs	Hang snatch	4	5	80% 5RM	4	5	85% 5RM
	Back squat	3	5	80% 5RM	3	5	85% 5RM
	Incline bench press	3	5	80% 5RM	3	5	85% 5RM
	Lunge	3	6	80% 6RM	3	6	85% 6RM
	Leg (knee) curl	3	6	80% 6RM	3	6	85% 6RM
	Seated calf raise	3	6	80% 6RM	3	6	85% 6RM
	Note: Thursday workout should use a load 15% less than Monday's.						

Day	Exercise	WEEK 1			WEEK 2		
		Sets	Reps	Intensity	Sets	Reps	Intensity
Tues/Fri	Push jerk	4	5	75% 5RM	4	5	80% 5RM
	Clean pull (floor)**	3	5	75% 5RM	3	5	80% 5RM
	Bent-over row	3	6	75% 6RM	3	6	80% 6RM
	Shoulder press	3	6	75% 6RM	3	6	80% 6RM
	Barbell biceps curl	3	6	75% 6RM	3	6	80% 6RM
	Triceps pushdown	3	6	75% 6RM	3	6	80% 6RM
	Abdominal muscles	3	20		3	20	
	Note: Friday workout should use a load 10% less than Tuesday's.						

**Training loads are based on the power clean test.

Unloading Week

1 Week: July 11-17

Day	Exercise	Sets	Reps	Intensity
Mon/ Tues	Hang snatch	4	5	70% 5RM
	Back squat	3	5	70% 5RM
	Abdominal muscles	3	20	
	Note: Thursday workout should use a load 15% less than Monday's.			
Thurs/ Fri	Push jerk	4	5	70% 5RM
	Clean pull (floor)**	3	5	70% 5RM
	Incline bench press	3	5	70% 5RM
	Shoulder press	3	5	70% 5RM
	Note: Friday workout should use a load 10% less than Tuesday's.			

**Training loads are based on the 5RM power clean test.

Mesocycle 5

2 Weeks: July 18-31: Strength/Power Phase 1

Day	Exercise	WEEK 1			WEEK 2		
		Sets	Reps	Intensity	Sets	Reps	Intensity
Mon/ Thurs	Power clean	4	3	90% 3RM	4	3	95% 3RM
	Front squat	5	3	85% 3RM	5	3	90% 3RM
	Push jerk	4	3	85% 3RM	4	3	90% 3RM
	Bench press	5	3	85% 3RM	5	3	90% 3RM
	Hammer curl	2	6	80% 6RM	2	6	85% 6RM
	Lying triceps extension	2	6	80% 6RM	2	6	85% 6RM
	Standing calf (heel) raise	2	6	80% 6RM	2	6	85% 6RM
	Note: Thursday workout should use a load 15% less than Monday's.						
Tues/Fri	Hang snatch	4	3	80% 3RM	4	3	85% 3RM
	Clean pull (floor)	5	3	80% 3RM	5	3	85% 3RM
	Bent-over row	3	6	75% 6RM	3	6	80% 6RM
	Lat pulldown	3	6	75% 6RM	3	6	80% 6RM
	Romanian deadlift	3	5	75% 6RM	3	5	80% 6RM
	Abdominal muscles	3	20		3	20	
	Note: Friday workout should use a load 10% less than Tuesday's.						

**Training loads are based on the power clean test.

Unloading Week

1 Week: August 1-7

Day	Exercise	Sets	Reps	Intensity
Mon/ Tues	Hang snatch	4	3	70% 3RM
	Back squat	5	3	70% 3RM
	Abdominal muscles	3	20	
	Note: Thursday workout should use a load 15% less than Monday's.			
Thurs/ Fri	Push jerk	4	3	70% 3RM
	Clean pull (floor)**	5	3	70% 3RM
	Incline bench press	5	3	70% 3RM
	Note: Friday workout should use a load 10% less than Tuesday's.			

**Training loads are based on the 5RM power clean test.

Posttesting

(Before In-Season) Microcycle: August 8-14

1RM POWER EXERCISE	1RM FOR NONPOWER CORE EXERCISES	OTHER TESTING
1. Power clean 2. Hang snatch 3. Push jerk 4. Push press	1. Back squat 2. Front squat 3. Bench press	1. Sit and reach 2. Shoulder elevation 3. 1.5-mile (2.4 km) run 4. 200-yard (274 m) shuttle run 5. Line drill 6. T-test 7. Vertical jump 8. Body composition (skinfolds)

Other exercises to test based on in-season program

Comments:

- It is important to note that these are the target sets and that three to five warm-up sets should be performed in order to provide an appropriate specific warm-up for the targeted loadings.
- Refer to table 17.7 for the relationship between the %RM and the number of repetitions allowed and table 17.8 for the estimation of 1RM.
- Refer to table 17.12 for rest period length assignment based on repetition goal.

active rest
annual training plan
basic strength phase
competitive period
daily undulating periodization
first transition period
fitness–fatigue paradigm
General Adaptation Syndrome (GAS)
general preparatory phase
hypertrophy/strength endurance phase

linear periodization
macrocycle
maintenance
mesocycle
microcycle
nonlinear periodization
peaking
periodization
preparatory period
recovery

restoration
second transition period
specific preparatory phase
stimulus-fatigue-recovery-
    adaptation theory
strength/power phase
supercompensation
traditional periodization

STUDY QUESTIONS

1. During which stage of the General Adaptation Syndrome does the body physiologically adapt to heavier training loads?

    a. alarm
    b. resistance
    c. exhaustion
    d. restoration

2. When relating the season terminology to periodization periods, which season corresponds to the preparatory period of training?

    a. in-season
    b. preseason
    c. off-season
    d. postseason

3. During which of the following periods are sport-specific activities performed in the greatest volume?

    a. preparatory
    b. first transition
    c. competition
    d. second transition

4. The medium-sized training cycle that lasts two to six weeks in duration is referred to as a

    I. block of training
    II. macrocycle
    III. microcycle
    IV. mesocycle
    a. II and III only
    b. I and IV only
    c. I, II, and IV only
    d. III and IV only

5. Which of the following phases is (are) commonly used to vary workouts during the preparatory period?

    I. hypertrophy
    II. cardiovascular
    III. basic strength
    IV. supercompensation
    a. I and III only
    b. II and IV only
    c. I, II, and III only
    d. II, III, and IV only

Rehabilitation and Reconditioning

David H. Potach, PT, and Terry L. Grindstaff, PhD, PT, ATC

> **After completing this chapter, you will be able to**
>
> - identify the members of the sports medicine team and their responsibilities during the rehabilitation and reconditioning of injured athletes,
> - recognize the types of injuries athletes sustain,
> - comprehend the timing and events of tissue healing,
> - understand the goals of each tissue healing phase, and
> - describe the role of the strength and conditioning professional during injury rehabilitation and reconditioning.

As the employment of strength and conditioning professionals continues to increase, their role will expand to allow more active participation in the rehabilitation and reconditioning of injured athletes. The strength and conditioning professional has unique knowledge and insight regarding optimal athletic function and can serve a vital role during the final stages of an advanced rehabilitation program by preparing the athlete for a return to competition. These abilities give the strength and conditioning professional distinct responsibilities during rehabilitation from athletic injury. To fully understand how the strength and conditioning professional can best augment the rehabilitation of injured athletes, one must first recognize the role of each member of the sports medicine team. Furthermore, an understanding of different types of injury and the physiological healing process is essential to hastening the recovery from injury.

This chapter is not intended to provide the reader with rehabilitation protocols for specific injuries. Rather, the aim is to explain the physiological events that follow a musculoskeletal injury, thereby allowing optimal goal setting by the strength and conditioning professional to improve injury outcomes. The information in this chapter should ultimately be used to maximize function of the injured athlete. The rehabilitation and reconditioning approach follows five basic principles, listed in the sidebar.

Sports Medicine Team

The sports medicine team provides health care services, with athlete needs and concerns as the primary focus (8). All members of the sports medicine team are responsible for educating coaches and athletes regarding injury risks, precautions, and treatments; they must also prevent injuries and rehabilitate those athletes who have sustained injury. Several different professionals play important roles in assisting the injured athlete's return to the playing field, necessitating effective communication.

Sports Medicine Team Members

The **team physician** provides medical care to an organization, school, or team. The team physician is most often a medical doctor (MD) or doctor of osteopathy (DO). The team physician may have specialized training (residency or fellowship) in a variety of fields, including family medicine, internal medicine, pediatrics, and orthopedics (43, 60), but should be proficient in the care of musculoskeletal injuries and sport-related medical conditions (20). Specific responsibilities of the team physician may include preparticipation examinations, on-field emergency care, injury and illness evaluation and diagnosis, and referral to other health care professionals as needed

(43). Although not responsible for daily rehabilitation, the team physician most often makes the final determination of an athlete's readiness for return to competition (20, 43). Another important role of the team physician is the prescription of medications as needed, including anti-inflammatory, pain, and cold and flu medications.

The person typically responsible for the day-to-day physical health of the athlete is the **athletic trainer** or athletic therapist. In the United States, an athletic trainer is certified by the National Athletic Trainers' Association Board of Certification as a *Certified Athletic Trainer* (ATC). The athletic trainer works under the supervision of the team physician and is employed primarily by secondary schools, colleges, or professional teams but may also work in an outpatient physical therapy clinic. Primary responsibilities of this individual include management and rehabilitation of injuries resulting from physical activity and prevention of injuries through the prescription of sport-specific exercise and the application of prophylactic equipment (e.g., tape and braces). Specifically, the athletic trainer evaluates injuries, provides the injured athlete with therapeutic exercise to hasten the rehabilitation process, treats injuries with therapeutic modalities, and serves as an administrator for the sports medicine team (8). Because the athletic trainer has a significant amount of contact with the athlete, he or she plays a key role in promoting communication between members of the sports medicine team, the coach, and the athlete (8).

A **physical therapist** (or **physiotherapist**) with specialization in orthopedics or sports medicine can play a valuable role in reducing pain and restoring function to the injured athlete. Although physical therapists are typically based in outpatient physical therapy clinics, many collegiate and professional teams now directly employ physical therapists as members of the sports medicine staff. A physical therapist may help develop specific treatment strategies or manage long-term rehabilitation. In the United States, physical therapists with expertise in sport injury management may become board certified through the American Board of Physical Therapy Specialties (ABPTS) and obtain the *Sports Certified Specialist* (SCS) credential. These board-certified specialists are more commonly becoming participants in the evaluation, treatment, and rehabilitation of acutely injured athletes and often serve in the dual capacity of team athletic trainer and sports physical therapist.

The **strength and conditioning professional** typically focuses on strength, power, and performance enhancement. The strength and conditioning professional also plays a valuable role within the sports medicine team and is an integral part of the rehabilitation and reconditioning process. Ideally, this person should be certified by the National Strength and Conditioning Association

Principles of Rehabilitation and Reconditioning

- Healing tissues must not be overstressed.
- The athlete must fulfill specific criteria to progress from one phase to another during the rehabilitative process.
- The rehabilitation program must be based on current clinical and scientific research.
- The program must be adaptable to each individual and his or her specific requirements and goals.
- Rehabilitation is a team-oriented process requiring all the members of the sports medicine team to work together toward a common goal of returning the athlete to unrestricted competition as quickly and safely as possible.

as a *Certified Strength and Conditioning Specialist* (CSCS) to ensure that he or she has the knowledge and background to contribute to the rehabilitation process. In consultation with the athletic trainer or sports physical therapist, this professional uses an understanding of the proper technique and application of several types of exercise (e.g., resistance, plyometric, and aerobic exercise) to develop a reconditioning program to ready the injured athlete for return to competition. Furthermore, strength and conditioning professionals possess an extensive understanding of the role that biomechanics play in a wide variety of sports and activities, which may allow them to suggest exercises for advanced rehabilitation and reconditioning of many injuries.

Additionally, the sports medicine team often includes specialized members who assist with the postacute rehabilitation and reconditioning of injured athletes. An **exercise physiologist** has a formal background in the exercise sciences and uses his or her expertise to assist with the design of a conditioning program that carefully considers the body's metabolic response to exercise and the ways in which that reaction aids the healing process. Because proper nutrition is crucial in recovery from injury, a **nutritionist** or a registered dietician with a background in sport nutrition may provide guidelines regarding proper food choices to optimize tissue recovery. Ideally, the nutritionist has been formally trained in food and nutrition sciences and may be a registered dietitian (RD) recognized by the Academy of Nutrition and Dietetics Commission on Dietetic Registration. Finally, recovering from an injury may be mentally traumatic for an athlete; a licensed **counselor**, **psychologist**, or **psychiatrist** with a background in sport may provide strategies that help the injured athlete better cope with the mental stress accompanying an injury.

Communication

Communication between members of the sports medicine team is essential (8, 65). Most often the injured athlete has the most contact with coaches, the athletic trainer, and the strength and conditioning professional.

In some instances, athletes disclose the initial onset of an injury to a sport coach or strength and conditioning professional before consulting with the athletic trainer. Thus consistent communication between these individuals is imperative. This does not negate communication with other members of the sports medicine team (physician, physical therapist, nutritionist, sport psychologist) who may not have as frequent interactions over the course of a week. A weekly meeting of the sports medicine team can provide a forum so all members are able to discuss the training requirements and necessary restrictions for each injured athlete. Relevant questions for discussion could include the following: What is the current status of the athlete (no participation, limited participation, full participation)? What exercises or activities is the athlete currently performing? Are any restrictions or modifications necessary? How is the athlete progressing? Do any program changes need to be made?

To most effectively develop training programs for an injured athlete, the strength and conditioning professional must understand the diagnosis of the given injury and exercise indications and contraindications. An **indication** is a form of treatment required by the rehabilitating athlete. For example, a softball outfielder with shoulder impingement must maintain lower extremity function, so the athletic trainer may request that the athlete continue to perform lower extremity strength, speed, agility, and power exercises during shoulder rehabilitation. Therefore, lower body exercise is indicated. A **contraindication** is an activity or practice that is inadvisable or prohibited due to the given injury. For example, during the later phases of rehabilitation from an anterior shoulder dislocation, an American football player may require upper body strengthening before being cleared to play. The athletic trainer requests that the athlete initiate upper body strengthening, but the bench press exercise may be contraindicated because it can place the injured shoulder in a vulnerable position in the presence of anterior instability. To clarify the role of the strength and conditioning professional during this process, it may be beneficial to have the sports medicine team use a form that specifies the indications and contraindications for exercises, providing for safe and efficient conditioning (figure 22.1). Additionally, the strength and conditioning professional can use a similar form (figure 22.2) to communicate the components of a given program and the athlete's subjective and objective responses to those components.

> The sports medicine team includes a large number of professionals working together to provide an optimal rehabilitation and reconditioning environment. Thus, the relationship of the sports medicine team members requires thoughtful communication to ensure a safe, harmonious climate for the injured athlete.

Types of Injury

Macrotrauma is a specific, sudden episode of overload injury to a given tissue, resulting in disrupted tissue integrity. Trauma to the bone can lead to either a con-

tusion or a fracture. Skeletal fractures can result from a direct blow to a bone and can be given a variety of classifications (e.g., closed, open, avulsed, incomplete). Joint trauma is manifested as either a **dislocation** (complete displacement of the joint surfaces) or a **subluxation** (partial displacement of the joint surfaces) and may result in joint laxity or instability. Ligamentous trauma is termed a **sprain** and is assigned a classification of *first degree* (partial tear of the ligament without increased joint instability), *second degree* (partial tear with minor joint instability), or *third degree* (complete tear with full joint instability).

Musculotendinous trauma is classified as either a **contusion** (if the trauma was direct) or a strain (if the trauma was indirect). A muscle contusion is an area of excess accumulation of blood and fluid in the tissues surrounding the injured muscle; it may severely limit the function of the injured muscle. Muscle **strains** are tears of muscle fibers and are further assigned grades, or degrees. A *first-degree* strain is a partial tear of individual fibers and is characterized by strong but painful muscle activity. A *second-degree* strain is a partial tear with

---

Rehabilitation Referral

Date: January 2, 2016

Name: Allison Pierson   Sport and position: Volleyball setter

Injury date: November 22, 2015

Surgery date: December 3, 2015

Diagnosis: Left ACL reconstruction

Indications

Stationary bicycle   Progress gradually up to 60 minutes. No running at this time.

Single-leg hip sled   Less than 90° left knee flexion, begin without resistance, progress only after

consultation with athletic training staff.

Upper extremity resistance exercises

Contraindications

Leg extension exercise

Full squats

Plyometrics

Running

Jonah Grey, ATC   January 2, 2016

FIGURE 22.1   A sample rehabilitation referral form, which communicates indications and contraindications to sports medicine team members.

Strength and Conditioning Summary

Date: October 22, 2015

Name: Molly Jackson

Sport: Soccer

Position: Midfield

Diagnosis: Grade II right MCL sprain

Injury date: October 8, 2015

Activity Summary

Number of sessions: 7

Date begun: October 15, 2015

Current Activities

Activity	Sets	Reps	Resistance
1/2 squats	3	10	115
Leg extension	3	10	60
Leg flexion	3	10	50
Heel raise	3	15	95

	Time		Speed
Stationary bicycle	20 minutes		80 rpm
Stair stepper	20 minutes		70 feet per minute
Jogging	10 minutes		5.0 mph

Assessment

No difficulty with 1/2 squats; may increase squat depth to 3/4.

Suggestions

Increase squat depth, increase jogging speed and time.

Jill Michaels, CSCS   October 22, 2015

FIGURE 22.2 A sample strength and conditioning summary form, which records the athlete's current activities and responses to those activities.

weak, painful muscle activity. A *third-degree* muscle strain is a complete tear of the fibers and is manifested by very weak, painless muscle activity. A tendon, like a muscle, can also rupture if the tensile load applied to it exceeds its limit. Typically, tendon collagen fibers are significantly stronger than the muscle fibers to which they attach, so failure is more likely to occur within the muscle belly, at the musculotendinous junction, or at the tendon attachment to the bone than within the substance of the tendon.

Microtrauma, or overuse injury, results from repeated, abnormal stress applied to a tissue by continuous training or training with too little recovery time. Overuse injuries may be due to training errors (e.g., poor program design, excessive volume), suboptimal training surfaces (e.g., too hard or uneven), faulty biomechanics or technique during performance, insufficient motor control, decreased flexibility, or skeletal malalignment and predisposition (54, 66). Two common overuse injuries involve bone and tendon. The most common overuse injury to bone is a stress fracture. Although body type and structure, nutrition, and metabolic factors play a large role, stress fractures are often the result of a rapid increase in training volume or excessive training volume on hard training surfaces (3, 66). **Tendinitis** is an inflammation of a tendon (52), and if the cause of the inflammation is left uncorrected, chronic tendinitis or tendinopathy may develop. (A term with the suffix -*itis* refers to an inflammatory condition [e.g., tendinitis, arthritis].) Tendinopathy is a degenerative condition characterized by minimal inflammation and neovascularization (52).

Tissue Healing

The process of returning to competition following injury involves the healing of the injured tissues and the preparation of these tissues for the return to function. To better understand the role of the strength and conditioning professional during rehabilitation and reconditioning, it is necessary to review the general phases of tissue healing following musculoskeletal injury (22, 24). The timing of the events occurring within each phase of tissue healing differs for each tissue type and is affected by a variety of systemic and local factors, including age, lifestyle, degree of injury, and the structure that has been damaged. However, all tissues follow the same basic pattern of healing (table 22.1).

> The process of returning to competition following injury involves healing of the injured tissues, preparation of these tissues for the return to function, and use of proper techniques to maximize rehabilitation and reconditioning.

TABLE 22.1 Tissue Healing

Inflammatory response phase	Pain, swelling, and redness
↓	Decreased collagen synthesis
	Increased number of inflammatory cells
Fibroblastic repair phase	Collagen fiber production
↓	Decreased collagen fiber organization
	Decreased number of inflammatory cells
Maturation–remodeling phase	Proper collagen fiber alignment
	Increased tissue strength

Inflammatory Response Phase

Inflammation is the initial reaction to injury (22, 24) and is necessary in order for normal tissue healing to occur. Both local and systemic inflammation occur during the **inflammatory response** phase, allowing the eventual healing and replacement of damaged tissue. During the inflammatory phase, several events transpire that contribute to both tissue healing and an initial decrease in function. The injured area becomes red and swollen due to changes in vascularity, blood flow, and capillary permeability. After tissues are damaged, a locally hypoxic environment leads to a certain amount of tissue death that allows the release of several chemical mediators, including histamine and bradykinin. These substances further increase blood flow and capillary permeability in this local area, thereby allowing edema, the escape of fluid into the surrounding tissues. **Edema** inhibits contractile tissues and can significantly limit function. Tissue debris and pathogens are removed from the injured area by increased blood flow and a process called *phagocytosis*; phagocytosis allows the release of macrophages, which search for and remove cellular debris that may slow healing.

The inflammatory substances present during this phase may result in stimulation of pain fibers, causing the injured athlete to sense pain, further contributing to decreased function. This phase typically lasts two to three days following an acute injury but may last longer with a compromised blood supply and more severe structural damage. Though the inflammatory phase is critical to tissue healing, if it does not end within a reasonable amount of time, the phases that follow may not occur, thereby delaying the rehabilitation process. Typically this phase lasts less than one week.

Fibroblastic Repair Phase

Once the inflammatory phase has ended, tissue **repair** begins (22, 24); the **fibroblastic repair** phase is characterized by catabolism (tissue breakdown) and replacement of tissues that are no longer viable following injury. In an attempt to improve tissue integrity, new capillaries and connective tissue (scar tissue) form in the area. Type III collagen is randomly deposited along the injured structure and serves as the framework for tissue regeneration. This newly formed tissue is weaker than the original tissue; thus optimal strength of the new tissue is not yet achieved. Collagen fibers are strongest when they lie longitudinally to the primary line of stress, yet many of the new fibers are positioned transversely, which limits their ability to efficiently transmit force. This phase of tissue healing begins as early as two days after injury and may last up to two months.

Maturation–Remodeling Phase

The weakened tissue produced during the repair phase is strengthened during the **maturation–remodeling** phase of healing (22, 24). Production of collagen fibers has shifted to a stronger Type I collagen, allowing the newly formed tissue the opportunity to improve its structure, strength, and function. With increased loading, the collagen fibers of the newly formed scar tissue begin to hypertrophy and align themselves along the lines of stress (18). The thicker and more optimally aligned collagen fibers become stronger, allowing a return to function. Although strength of the collagen fibers and healing tissue improves, this tissue is not as strong as the tissue it has replaced. Tissue **remodeling** in the maturation–remodeling phase can last months to years after injury (22, 24, 32).

> ► Following injury, all damaged tissues go through the same general phases of healing: inflammation, repair, and remodeling. The timing of the events occurring within each phase of tissue healing differs for each tissue type and is affected by a variety of systemic and local factors, including age, lifestyle, degree of injury, and the structure that has been damaged. Characteristic events define each phase and separate one phase from another.

Goals of Rehabilitation and Reconditioning

The strength and conditioning professional must consider both the athlete's subjective response to injury and the physiological mechanisms of tissue healing; both are essential in relation to an athlete's return to optimal performance. The process of re turning to competition following injury involves healing of the injured tissues, preparation of these tissues for the return to function, and use of proper techniques to maximize rehabilitation and reconditioning. While the goal is often a rapid resumption of activity, it is important to remember that each athlete responds differently to injury and thus progresses uniquely during rehabilitation.

As a preface to discussion of the goals of treatment during injury rehabilitation, two points must be made. First, healing tissue must not be overstressed (44). During tissue healing, controlled therapeutic stress is necessary to optimize collagen matrix formation (4, 18), but too much stress can damage new structures and significantly slow the athlete's return to competition. This means choosing a level of loading that provides neither too much stress nor too little stress to the ath-

lete's healing tissue. It should be obvious that when one is choosing the load, it is necessary to consider the phase of healing and athlete type. For example, an exercise that provides too little tissue loading during the maturation–remodeling phase may provide too much loading (increased tissue stress) during the inflammatory response phase. Further, an exercise that provides too little stress to a professional basketball center may be excessive for an amateur cross-country runner. The plane of movement is another necessary consideration. As an example, the medial collateral ligament of the knee is subject to the greatest stress when loaded in the frontal plane (i.e., valgus stress) during terminal knee extension. Therefore, if the athlete has a medial collateral ligament injury, frontal plane movements (valgus stress) should be avoided during early healing phases. However, those frontal plane movements should probably be included in some form during the later phases.

Second, the athlete must meet specific objectives to progress from one phase of healing to the next (67, 68). These objectives may depend on range of motion, strength, or activity. It is the responsibility of the team physician, athletic trainer, physical therapist, or a combination of these professionals to establish these guidelines.

> ► Healing tissue must not be overstressed, but controlled therapeutic stress is necessary to optimize collagen matrix formation. The athlete must meet specific objectives to progress from one phase of healing to the next.

Inflammatory Response Phase

The first response to an injury is inflammation, a reaction that is essential for subsequent healing but also important to manage properly so as to not retard the rehabilitation process.

Treatment Goal

The primary goal for treatment during the inflammatory response phase is to prevent disruption of new tissue. A healthy environment for new tissue regeneration and formation is essential for preventing prolonged inflammation and disruption of new blood vessel and collagen production, which can prolong the injury. Relative rest and **physical agents** (e.g., modalities) including ice, compression, elevation, and electrical stimulation are often primary treatment options to minimize tissue damage and decrease acute pain, but results on efficacy have been mixed (40, 62).

It is also important to realize that a quick return to function relies on the health of other body tissues.

Therefore, the power, strength, and endurance of the musculoskeletal tissues and the function of the cardiorespiratory system must be maintained. The strength and conditioning professional can provide significant knowledge and expertise in this area. To accomplish these tasks, the strength and conditioning professional should consult with the athletic trainer to determine which types of exercises are indicated and contraindicated for the specific injury. Maximal protection of the injured structures is the primary goal during this phase. Assuming that this requirement is fulfilled, exercises may include general aerobic and anaerobic training and resistance training of the uninjured extremities. If movement of the injured limb is not contraindicated, isolated exercises that target areas proximal and distal to the injured area may also be permissible provided that they do not stress the injured area. Examples include hip abduction and rotation exercises following knee injury (14, 26, 41) or scapula stabilizing exercises following glenohumeral joint injury (35, 64, 69).

Exercise Strategies

Although a rapid return to competition is often a goal, passive rest of the injured area is initially necessary to protect the damaged tissue from additional injury. Therefore, exercise directly involving or stressing the injured area is not recommended during this phase. Exercises that do not directly involve or stress the injured area can still be performed (e.g., upper extremity exercises for lower extremity injury, single-leg exercises with the uninvolved limb).

Fibroblastic Repair Phase

After the inflammatory response phase, the body begins to repair the damaged tissue with similar new tissue; however, the resiliency of this new tissue is low at this time. Repair of the weakened injury site can take up to eight weeks if the proper amount of restorative stress is applied, or longer if too much or too little stress is applied.

Treatment Goal

The treatment goal during the fibroblastic repair phase is to prevent excessive muscle atrophy and joint deterioration of the injured area. In addition, a precarious balance must be maintained in which disruption of the newly formed collagen fibers is avoided but low-load stresses are gradually introduced to allow increased collagen synthesis and prevent loss of joint motion. To protect the new, relatively weak collagen fibers, the athlete should avoid active resistive exercise involving the damaged tissue. Too little activity, though, can also have a deleterious effect, as newly formed fibers will

not optimally align and may form adhesions, thereby preventing full motion. Early protected motion hastens the optimal alignment of collagen fibers and promotes improved tissue mobility. As in the inflammatory phase, therapeutic modalities are permissible, but their goal during repair is to promote collagen synthesis and manage pain. Ultrasound, electrical stimulation, and ice are continued in order to support and hasten new tissue formation (5, 27, 51). Again, maintenance of muscular and cardiorespiratory function remains essential for the uninjured areas of the body. The strength and conditioning professional has considerable expertise to offer the other members of the sports medicine team regarding selection of the appropriate activities. Possible exercise forms during the repair phase include strengthening of the uninjured extremities and areas proximal and distal to the injury, aerobic and anaerobic exercise, and improving strength and neuromuscular control of the involved areas.

Exercise Strategies

The following exercises should be used during the repair phase only after consultation with the team physician, athletic trainer, or physical therapist. Isometric exercise may be performed, provided that it is pain free and otherwise indicated by the physician or athletic trainer. Submaximal isometric exercise allows the athlete to maintain neuromuscular function and improve strength with movements performed at an intensity low enough that the newly formed collagen fibers are not disrupted. Unfortunately, isometric strengthening is joint angle specific; that is, strength gains occur only at the angles used (28). Therefore, if indicated, it may be appropriate for the athlete to perform isometric exercises at multiple angles (28). Isokinetic exercise uses equipment that provides resistance to movement at a given speed (e.g., 60°/s or 120°/s). Because sport is not performed at a single consistent speed, isokinetic exercise is limited in real-world application. Furthermore, most isokinetic equipment allows single-joint exercise only, which permits concentration on a specific muscle or joint but is not always the most functional method of strengthening.

While isotonic exercise (i.e., concentric and eccentric) involves movements with constant external resistance, the amount of force required to move the resistance varies, depending primarily on joint angle and the length of each agonist muscle. Isotonic exercise uses several different forms of resistance, including gravity (i.e., exercises performed without equipment, with gravitational effects as the only source of resistance), dumbbells, barbells, and weight stack machines. Concentric and eccentric muscle actions can be used to increase strength and appropriately stress healing tissues. Eccentric exercise allows for greater force production and requires less energy expenditure compared to concentric exercise (38). Loads may be increased to provide greater challenge as tissue healing progresses. The speed at which the movement occurs is controlled by the athlete; movement speed can be a program design variable, with more acute injuries calling for slower movement and the later phases of healing amenable to faster, more sport-specific movement.

Neuromuscular control is the ability of muscles to respond to afferent sensory information to maintain joint stability (53). This afferent sensory information is referred to as **proprioception** and occurs in response to stimulation of sensory receptors in skin, muscles, tendons, ligaments, and the joint capsule. Proprioception contributes to the conscious and unconscious efferent control of posture, balance, stability, and sense of position (53). For example, when running on an uneven surface, cross-country runners rely on sensory input (proprioception) from their lower extremities to adjust to the ground to prevent falls and injuries; that ability to adjust is neuromuscular control. After an injury, neuromuscular control, like strength and flexibility, is usually impaired (13). Specific types of exercises exist to improve neuromuscular control following injury and can be manipulated through alterations in surface stability, vision, and speed. Mini-trampolines, balance boards, and stability balls can be used to create unstable surfaces for upper and lower extremity training. Athletes can perform common activities such as squats and push-ups on uneven surfaces to improve neuromuscular control. Exercises may also be performed with eyes closed, thus removing visual input, to further challenge balance. Finally, increasing the speed at which exercises are performed provides additional

challenges to the system. Specifically controlling these variables within a controlled environment will allow the athlete to progress to more challenging exercises in the next stage of healing.

Maturation–Remodeling Phase

The outcome of the repair phase is the replacement of damaged tissue with collagen fibers. After those fibers are laid down, the body can begin to remodel and strengthen the new tissue, allowing the athlete to gradually return to full activity.

Treatment Goal

The primary goal during the maturation–remodeling phase is optimizing tissue function while transitioning to return to play or activity. Athletes improve function by continuing and progressing the exercises performed during the repair phase and by adding more advanced, sport-specific exercises that allow progressive stresses to be applied to the injured tissue. The athlete can be tempted to do "too much too soon," which may further damage the injured tissues. It is important to remember that, while there may be less pain with activity at this point, the injured tissues have not fully healed and require further attention to achieve complete recovery (figure 22.3). Progressive tissue loading allows improved collagen fiber alignment and fiber hypertrophy (4, 18). Return-to-play or activity decisions should be based on an understanding of normal tissue healing time frames as well as a criteria-based progression with predetermined objectives. These objectives usually include measures of range of motion and strength, functional testing, and

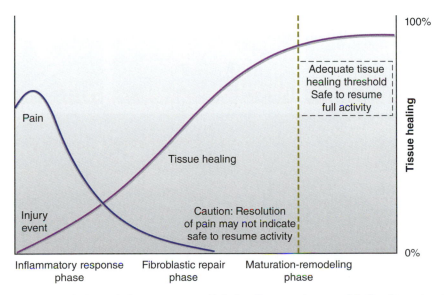

FIGURE 22.3 Profile of a typical soft tissue injury response. Pain is often used as a guide for tissue health. Pain levels (blue line) often decrease well before tissue healing (purple line) is complete, which may lead athletes to inappropriately believe adequate tissue healing has occurred (vertical yellow line) and it is safe to resume full activity.

patient-reported function using established patient-reported outcome forms (1, 35, 69). It is important for the sports medicine team members to communicate, have clearly defined roles, and use return-to-play metrics to ensure a safe return to play.

Exercise Strategies

Ultimately, as with other aspects of strength and conditioning, rehabilitation and reconditioning exercises must be functional and must mimic activity demands—that is, reflect specificity. Examples of functionally specific training include joint angle–specific strengthening, velocity-specific muscle activity, closed kinetic chain exercises, and exercises designed to further enhance neuromuscular control. Strengthening should transition from general exercises to sport-specific exercises designed to replicate movements common in given sports. For example, for a basketball guard who sprained an ankle,

rehabilitation exercises may progress from a general single-joint exercise to those more specific to the sport and position (figure 22.4). Specificity of movement speed is another important program design variable. Strengthening exercises performed during rehabilitation should also mimic sport speed requirements; that is, activities that require greater speeds (e.g., sprinting) should include exercises performed at higher velocities. Using the example in figure 22.4, the exercises progress from the relatively slow and controlled balance and strength exercises to the faster plyometric and sprinting exercises. Similarly, consider a sprinter with a hamstring muscle strain. Whereas initial reconditioning may concentrate on the recovery of flexibility and strength of the injured muscles, the nature of this athlete's sport necessitates exercises performed at rapid speeds during the later phases of rehabilitation and reconditioning. Exercise selection for a sprinter with an improving hamstring

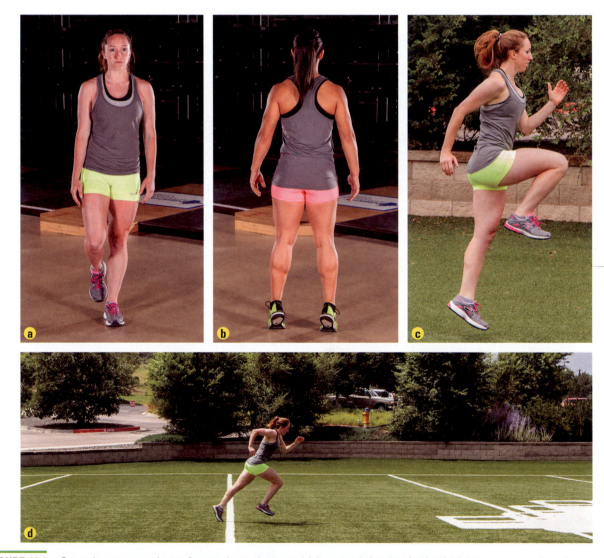

FIGURE 22.4 Sample progression of exercises that could be used for basketball players recovering from ankle sprains. Exercises progress from general to basketball specific.

muscle strain might progress from hamstring flexibility to eccentric strength to concentric strength to dynamic stretching and finally to rapid isotonic strengthening. Examples of velocity-specific exercise include manually resisted strengthening and plyometric and speed training. Refer to chapters 18 and 19 for a thorough discussion of plyometric and speed training, respectively.

The kinetic chain is the collective effort or involvement of two or more sequential joints to create movement (56). A **closed kinetic chain** exercise is one in which the terminal joint meets with considerable resistance that prohibits or restrains its free motion (56); that is, the distal joint segment is stationary. Lower extremity closed kinetic chain exercises have often been classified as a more functional form of exercise than open kinetic chain exercises (23, 63) because most sport-related activities are performed with the feet "fixed" to the surface. For example, during the closed kinetic chain squat exercise, the feet are "fixed" to the floor and essentially do not move, providing a base upon which movement occurs (figure 22.5a). Closed kinetic chain exercises have several advantages, including increased joint stability and functional movement patterns; during sport activity, joints are not typically used in isolation but rather work in concert with the adjacent joints and surrounding musculature. Although closed kinetic chain

exercises are commonly viewed as lower extremity exercises, closed chain upper extremity exercises exist as well (figure 22.5b) (35, 69).

An **open kinetic chain** exercise uses a combination of successively arranged joints in which the terminal joint is free to move; open kinetic chain exercises allow for greater concentration on an isolated joint or muscle (23). An example is the leg (knee) extension exercise, during which the feet and lower legs are allowed to move freely (figure 22.6). The leg extension allows greater concentration on the quadriceps at the knee joint; in comparison, the squat, which also uses the quadriceps muscles and knee joint, relies on muscle activity at both the hip and ankle joints as well (figure 22.5a). Although closed kinetic chain exercises are often viewed as more functional, most activities involve both closed and open kinetic chain movements. In sprinting, for example, while one lower extremity is on the ground (closed kinetic chain), the other is in the air (open kinetic chain), which means that both types of movement can occur simultaneously (figure 22.7). In some situations,

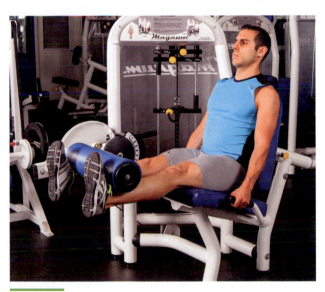

FIGURE 22.6 Example of an open kinetic chain exercise— leg (knee) extension exercise.

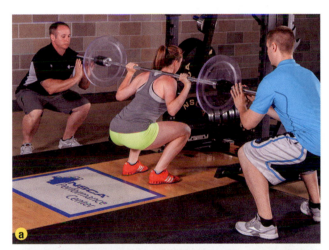

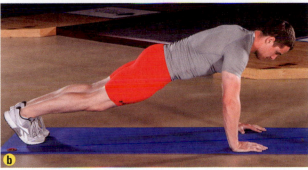

FIGURE 22.5 Closed kinetic chain exercises: *(a)* squat exercise (downward movement) and *(b)* push-up exercise.

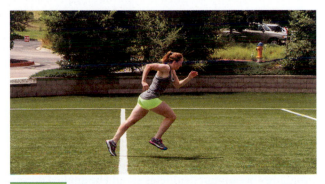

FIGURE 22.7 Sprinting offers an example of open and closed kinetic chain movement occurring together.

Rehabilitation and Reconditioning Goals and Strategies

Although rehabilitation and reconditioning programs must be individualized, the following are lists of general goals and approaches for each phase.

Inflammatory Response Phase

- Prevention of new tissue disruption and prolonged inflammation with the use of relative rest and passive modalities
- Maintenance of function of the cardiorespiratory and surrounding neuromusculoskeletal systems
- No active exercise for the injured area

Fibroblastic Repair Phase

- Prevention of excessive muscle atrophy and joint deterioration of the injured area
- Maintenance of function of the neuromusculoskeletal and cardiorespiratory systems
- Possible exercise options:
  - Submaximal isometric, isokinetic, and isotonic exercise
  - Balance and proprioceptive training activities

Maturation–Remodeling Phase

- Optimization of tissue function
- Progressive loading of the neuromusculoskeletal and cardiorespiratory systems as indicated
- Possible exercise options:
  - Joint angle–specific strengthening
  - Velocity-specific muscle activity
  - Closed and open kinetic chain exercises
  - Proprioceptive training activities

---

an open chain exercise may therefore be an equally appropriate choice.

Exercises designed to improve neuromuscular control, which were introduced during the repair phase, should be continued and progressed as appropriate during the maturation–remodeling phase. Rehabilitation and reconditioning goals and strategies are summarized in the sidebar.

Program Design

The area in which strength and conditioning professionals can best contribute to the rehabilitation and reconditioning process is the provision of resistance and aerobic training programs designed for the injured athlete. Their experience in prescribing exercise for uninjured athletes gives strength and conditioning professionals the ability to properly adapt training programs for those recovering from injury. Although protocols do exist for exercise prescription following injury, many do not incorporate sport-specific program design variables; the same principles used to design resistance and aerobic training programs for uninjured athletes should be applied during rehabilitation and reconditioning.

Resistance Training

Several programs have been developed to assist with the design of resistance training programs (9, 12, 29, 57, 73), and many of these programs have been advocated for use in the rehabilitation setting (9, 29, 36, 42, 73). Both the De Lorme (9) and Oxford (73) programs use three sets of 10 repetitions with a pyramid-type design. De Lorme's program progresses from light to heavy resistance. The initial set involves 10 repetitions of 50% of the athlete's 10-repetition maximum (10RM); the second set increases the resistance to 75% of the 10RM; and the final set requires 100% of the 10RM (9, 10). The Oxford system (73) is the reverse of De Lorme's system; that is, it progresses from heavy to light resistance. The first set performed is 100% of the athlete's 10RM; the second is 75% of the 10RM; and the third is 50% of the 10RM (73).

Knight's (30) **daily adjustable progressive resistive exercise (DAPRE)** system requires and allows more manipulation of intensity and volume than either the De Lorme or the Oxford system (9, 10, 73); DAPRE involves four sets, with repetitions ranging from 10 to possibly only one during the final set. The first set requires 10 repetitions of 50% of the estimated 1RM, and the second set requires six repetitions of 75% of the estimated 1RM. The third set in the DAPRE requires the maximum number of repetitions of 100% of the estimated 1RM; the number of repetitions performed during the third set determines the adjustment to be made in resistance for the fourth set (table 22.2) (30). The De Lorme, Oxford, and Knight systems are protocols that have been shown to increase muscle strength (10, 30, 36, 42, 73) and may be appropriate when one is designing rehabilitation resistance training programs. However, athletes require rehabilitation and reconditioning programs tailored to the demands of their respective sports. Although these protocols (10, 30, 73) are established strengthening programs, they may be too strict to allow individualization for athletes in different sports.

Programs for both the healthy and the damaged tissues of an injured athlete require the same basic design principles provided in chapter 17. According to the specific adaptation to imposed demands (SAID) principle, the system will adapt to the demands placed on it. Therefore, the goal of training (specific adaptation) should dictate the design of the resistance training program (imposed demands). For example, during the remodeling phase of an injured marathoner's patellofemoral rehabilitation, his or her quadriceps muscles should be trained with an emphasis on muscular endurance. Therefore, the athlete should perform many repetitions of the rehabilitation exercises to prepare the muscles for the demands of long-distance running. Conversely, an Olympic weightlifter rehabilitating from the same injury requires fewer repetitions of high-intensity rehabilitation and reconditioning exercises during the later portions of the remodeling phase to prepare the muscles for the power demands of this sport. Refer to the application table for a comparative example of the rehabilitation strategies for these two athletes.

Aerobic and Anaerobic Training

Although research has yet to determine an optimal aerobic training program for use in the rehabilitation setting, it is generally accepted that the program should mimic specific sport and metabolic demands as closely as possible. The strength and conditioning professional, having a background in designing and implementing conditioning exercises for healthy athletes, is the ideal member of the sports medicine team to prescribe and supervise the aerobic training portion of the injured athlete's reconditioning program. As with the resistance training program, the strength and conditioning professional must consider the demands that the given sport places on the injured athlete. Keeping these demands and the contraindications of the injury in mind, the strength and conditioning professional can use the prescription guidelines in chapters 17 and 20 to create an appropriate training program to allow an uncomplicated return to competition.

Again consider rehabilitation from a patellofemoral injury for a marathon runner, a wrestler, and an Olympic lifter; the metabolic energy demands of their rehabilitation and reconditioning are markedly different. For the marathon runner's goals, aerobic fitness is of much greater concern and must be addressed immediately. The metabolic demands for the wrestler involve a combination of aerobic and anaerobic systems; therefore, interval training is more appropriate (16). In contrast, the Olympic lifter's program would focus on maintaining anaerobic fitness. Selecting the appropriate training device depends on the region of the body that is injured. While specificity of training is important, gains in exercise capacity can be made through exercise of other body regions (i.e., upper extremity exercise to improve oxygen consumption) (61). A variety of options exist to modify aerobic and anaerobic training, including the upper body ergometer, deep-water running, lower extremity cycling, and elliptical machines. Strategies to maintain cardiorespiratory fitness can be implemented early, even during the inflammatory response phase. As already emphasized, it is important to remember that to allow optimal healing, attempts should be made to initially minimize stress to healing tissues, but relevant stresses can be applied to uninjured areas. An example would be for a soccer player with an acute right knee injury.

TABLE 22.2 Resistance Adjustments for Daily Adjustable Progressive Resistance Exercise (DAPRE) Protocol

Number of repetitions performed during set 3	Adjusted resistance for set 4	Resistance for next exercise session
0-2	− 5 to 10 lb (2.3 to 4.5 kg)	− 5 to 10 lb (2.3 to 4.5 kg)
3-4	− 0 to 5 lb (0 to 2.3 kg)	Same resistance
5-6	Same resistance	+ 5 to 10 lb (2.3 to 4.5 kg)
7-10	+ 5 to 10 lb (2.3 to 4.5 kg)	+ 5 to 15 lb (2.3 to 6.8 kg)
11	+ 10 to 15 lb (4.5 to 6.8 kg)	+ 10 to 20 lb (4.5 to 9 kg)

Application of Design Principles for Resistance Training Programs During Rehabilitation and Reconditioning From Patellofemoral Injury

Phase of healing	Design variable	ATHLETE	
		Marathon runner	Olympic lifter
Inflammatory response phase	Goals and exercises	• None that require quadriceps activity—relative rest of this area needed to reduce inflammation • Maintenance of muscular strength and endurance of adjacent areas (i.e., hip extensors, knee flexors, and plantar flexors) • Maintenance of cardiorespiratory fitness	• None that require quadriceps activity—relative rest of this area needed to reduce inflammation • Maintenance of muscular strength and power of adjacent areas (i.e., hip extensors, knee flexors, and plantar flexors) • Maintenance of upper body muscular strength and power
Fibroblastic repair phase	Goals and exercises	• Isometric quadriceps strengthening at full knee extension (progressing to multiple angles) • Progress to pain-free isotonic quadriceps strengthening (following consultation with sports medicine team) • Continue exercise of adjacent areas • Continue aerobic exercise; may begin stationary bicycle or stair stepper (per recommendation of sports medicine team)	• Isometric quadriceps strengthening at full knee extension (progressing to multiple angles) • Progress to pain-free isotonic quadriceps strengthening (following consultation with sports medicine team) • Continue exercise of adjacent areas • Continue upper body muscular strength and power exercises
	Sets × repetitions	2-3 × 15-20	3-4 × 8-10
	Intensity	Submaximal (≤50% 1RM)	Submaximal (≤50% 1RM)
Maturation–remodeling phase	Goals and exercises	• Begin more sport-specific activities, movements, and speeds • Return to running, gradually increasing distance and speed as tolerated • Add lunge and squat (increase knee range of motion as able)	• Begin more sport-specific activities, movements, and speeds • Increase movement speeds to those similar to competition • Add Romanian deadlift and squat (increase knee range of motion as able)
	Sets × repetitions	2-3 × 15-20	4-5 × 3-8
	Intensity	Progress to maximal intensity (50-75% 1RM)	Progress to maximal intensity (>75% 1RM)

Although options for right lower extremity strengthening may be initially limited, exercises may still be performed for the upper extremity as well as the uninvolved left lower extremity (e.g., single-leg squat with weights). The strength and conditioning professional may need to modify uninvolved left lower extremity exercises to ensure that the involved right lower extremity is protected. Exercises targeting the uninvolved limb can improve muscle strength in the involved limb (33, 34).

> **Designing strength and conditioning programs for injured athletes requires the strength and conditioning professional to examine the rehabilitation and reconditioning goals to determine what type of program will allow the quickest return to competition.**

Thus it is important for injured athletes to continue to perform strength and conditioning exercises for the uninvolved body regions.

Reducing Risk of Injury and Reinjury

In addition to using strength training and conditioning strategies when rehabilitating athletes from injuries, strength and conditioning professionals can implement research findings to reduce both risk for initial injury and risk of reinjury following injury (49, 58). Structured programs have been developed for the lower (15, 17, 21, 48) and upper extremities (35, 71). These programs are often sport specific and address common risk factors for injury.

Previous injury is one of the most substantial risk factors for future injury in active individuals (19, 47, 54, 59). Risk factors for upper extremity injury include decreased glenohumeral range of motion, scapular dyskinesis, and decreased shoulder strength (6, 7, 70). Range of motion exercise and the Throwers Ten are often used as a structured program to reduce upper extremity injury risk (71). Risk factors for lower extremity injury include decreased balance, decreased neuromuscular control during jump landing, and decreased lower extremity muscle strength (2, 31, 72). Structured lower extremity programs to reduce injury risk should be sport specific and should focus on neuromuscular control during activities such as landing from a jump and cutting. Two exercises that may be used to reduce this risk of injury to the lower extremities are proper jumping and landing technique during plyometric exercise (figure 22.8a) and a single-leg squat to emphasize unilateral strength (figure 22.8b).

> **Previous injury is one of the most substantial risk factors for future injury in active individuals. Lower extremity programs designed to reduce injury risk should be specific to a sport's demands and should focus on the neuromuscular control required during specific activities such as landing from a jump and cutting.**

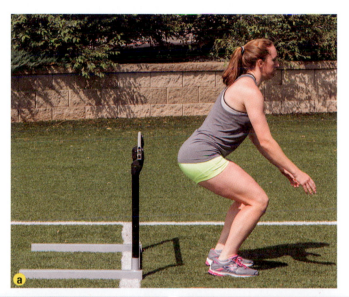

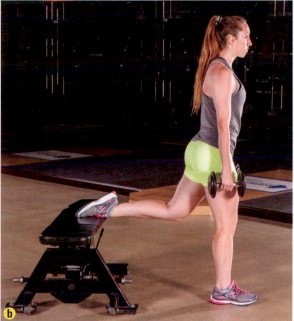
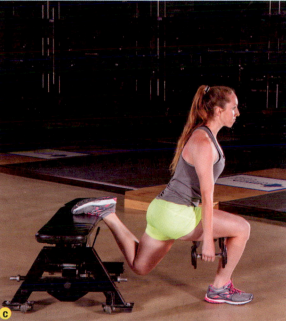

FIGURE 22.8   Two exercises that may be used to reduce risk of injury to the lower extremities are *(a)* proper jumping and landing technique during plyometric exercise and *(b, c)* a single-leg squat to emphasize unilateral strength.

While upper extremity injury risk reduction programs exist (71), much of the research has focused on the prevention of lower extremity injuries, specifically anterior cruciate ligament (ACL) injuries. Two examples of structured programs designed to reduce injury risk are Sportsmetrics (21) and PEP (Prevent Injury and Enhance Performance) (39). While using slightly different foci, each of these programs introduces exercises and movements shown to address risk factors for injury and reduce lower extremity injury rates, especially ACL injuries and ankle sprains (15, 17, 21, 48). In addition, using eccentric exercise has been shown to dramatically reduce risk of hamstring injury (46, 50).

After return to sport, individuals may continue to demonstrate deficits in strength, biomechanics, and functional performance (45, 55). Deficits may often be compared to the contralateral limb (37) or established normative values (11, 25). Side-to-side differences in strength and functional performance less than 10% may be considered acceptable (37). The transition between supervised rehabilitation for an injury and unrestricted activity participation is a critical time when members of the sports medicine team need to be in communication regarding how deficits in strength and performance will be managed.

Conclusion

Effective athletic injury rehabilitation and reconditioning require efficient communication between the members of the sports medicine team. Each member plays a distinct role in ensuring the injured athlete's return to function; although the job of each professional is different, the tasks of each complement those of the others on the team. Goals are established for each athlete, and therapeutic exercise programs must be designed, administered, and progressed according to the tissue healing sequence. The program must be individualized to effectively return the athlete to normal function and competitive athletics. Early rehabilitation for initial tissue protection and strengthening is more structured than later rehabilitation phases; the latter allow for progression to functional activities that are specific to the athlete's sport and position. Designing reconditioning programs for injured athletes necessitates a careful examination of the sport requirements and a thorough understanding of both the healing process and therapeutic exercise.

KEY TERMS

athletic trainer
closed kinetic chain
contraindication
contusion
counselor
daily adjustable progressive
  resistive exercise (DAPRE)
dislocation
edema
exercise physiologist
fibroblastic repair
indication

inflammation
inflammatory response
macrotrauma
maturation-remodeling
microtrauma
neuromuscular control
nutritionist
open kinetic chain
physical agent
physical therapist
physiotherapist
proprioception

psychiatrist
psychologist
remodeling
repair
sprain
strain
strength and conditioning
  professional
subluxation
team physician
tendinitis

STUDY QUESTIONS

1. All of the following individuals can provide medical supervision during a college soccer match EXCEPT the
   a. athletic trainer
   b. team physician
   c. Certified Strength and Conditioning Specialist
   d. Sports Certified Physical Therapist

2. Which of the following is NOT typically the result of overuse?
   a. stress fracture
   b. grade III joint sprain
   c. tendinitis
   d. microtraumatic injury

3. Which of the following is NOT one of the phases of healing following an injury?
   a. inflammatory response
   b. reconditioning hypertrophy
   c. maturation-remodeling
   d. fibroblastic repair

4. Which of the following types of activity is inappropriate during the inflammatory response phase of a medial collateral ligament sprain?
   a. lower extremity plyometrics
   b. submaximal isometric quadriceps strengthening
   c. hip joint stretching
   d. upper extremity ergometry

5. The rotator cuff muscles act as stabilizers to the shoulder joint. During the maturation–remodeling phase of rotator cuff (supraspinatus muscle) tendinitis rehabilitation of a basketball player, what exercise repetition range is MOST appropriate for improving the muscular endurance of the rotator cuff muscles?
   a. 3-5
   b. 5-8
   c. 8-12
   d. 12-20

Facility Design, Layout, and Organization

Andrea Hudy, MA

 After completing this chapter, you will be able to

- identify the aspects of new facility design, including the four phases (predesign, design, construction, and preoperation);

- identify the aspects of modification of an existing facility, along with the differences between design of a new facility and modification or renovation of an existing facility;

- explain how to assess an athletic program's needs in order to design a facility that is well suited to these needs;

- explain how to design specific facility features, including supervision location, access, ceiling height, flooring, environmental factors, electrical service, and mirrors;

- explain how to arrange equipment in organized groups, creating better traffic flow throughout the facility; and

- explain the maintenance and cleaning needs for the surfaces and equipment in a strength and conditioning facility.

The author would like to acknowledge the significant contributions of Michael Greenwood and Lori Greenwood to this chapter.

Organizing the construction and design of a strength and conditioning facility requires a well-thought-out plan created by a committee of experienced professionals. This chapter provides information on the different phases of planning a new facility, along with information about the facility's design and organization and about maintenance of the equipment. The chapter also outlines the phases of construction or remodeling of a facility. The design must account for the needs of the athletic programs or athletes and the staff in order for the layout to be most efficient.

General Aspects of New Facility Design

Building a facility from the ground up takes a long time and a lot of planning. One of the first things to do is assemble a committee of professionals. The committee should consist of a contractor, architect, designers, lawyers, and people involved in using the facility. At least one of the instructors, coaches, strength and conditioning professionals, or other experts who will be working in the facility should also be considered for the committee to include another perspective that will help maximize the space's utility and safety. This committee will assist with the facility design as well as considering the economic aspects of opening a new facility. One of the main challenges in designing a strength and conditioning facility is tailoring the facility to the intended audience. Figure 23.1 outlines the four phases of designing a new facility, along with the main objectives for each phase.

Predesign Phase

The **predesign phase** is the first step in building a new facility. This phase should consist of a needs analysis, a feasibility study, and master plan formation. At the end of the predesign phase, a reputable architect should be hired—likely through a bid process—and begin making a basic blueprint for the facility.

The **needs analysis** is the step in which the designers and experts collaborate and determine the needs of the athletic program (5). Examples of questions are "How much space do you need?" and "What needs to fit into the allotted space?" The needs analysis should be consistent with the philosophy of the strength and conditioning professional and the athletic program. For example, if a coach regularly programs plyometrics or prescribes conditioning, an area needs to be set aside for those activities.

The second part of the predesign phase is called a **feasibility study**. The feasibility study should analyze strengths, weaknesses, opportunities, and threats (known as a SWOT analysis) (5). The goal of the feasibility study is to ensure that the financial investment will yield a viable and sustainable return. The feasibility study should also look at the location, the strengths and weaknesses of any ideas, and the potential for growth for both the athletic and the strength and conditioning programs. The potential opportunities and competition threats also need to be considered. This includes market evaluation to identify the best opportunity to train more athletes most efficiently, as well as analyzing any competing facility's target market and growth potential. The aim of this step of the feasibility study is to help determine if the facility will have an opportunity for success against competing businesses.

The **master plan** is the general plan for all phases of the new facility. The master plan should include the building and construction plan, facility design, budget information, and an operational plan to act on once the facility is actually complete (5). The operational plan should consist of short-term and long-term goals that will enhance the facility's success both in the near term and down the road. The operational plan also needs to entail staff development and a plan for the hiring process.

The last step of the predesign phase is hiring an architect. Selecting an architect is crucial for meeting the administration's and coaches' goals. It is important to select from a list of architects who have a positive reputation based on previous work. If possible, it is best to choose an architect who has had previous experience in the strength and conditioning industry. The architect will likely be hired through a bid process, meaning that the architect who is hired is usually the one who submitted the lowest price. Bid plans require efficient use

Predesign phase		Design phase	Construction phase		Preoperation phase	
Needs analysis	Feasibility study	Finalize committee	Follow master plan	Arrange equipment	Hire staff	Create cleaning schedule
Master plan	Hire architect	Create blueprint	Check construction progress		Assign duties	Create plan for operation

FIGURE 23.1   Phases and objectives of designing a new facility.

of resources so that the money is spent on what is most useful for the users of the facility.

Design Phase

The **design phase** is the second phase in the process of building a new facility. In the design phase the committee's ideas come together with regard to the facility's structure and design elements. It is extremely important to plan around the flow of the facility while adhering to all relevant regulations and codes. City codes are often highly specific with regard to aspects of a design. The city planning department can provide the local guidelines and codes.

The first step in the design phase is finalizing the design committee. To reiterate, the committee should include strength and conditioning professionals with experience in facility production and design. This is also the phase in which the designers need to work closely with the architect to produce a blueprint of the facility.

The blueprint and design need to consider the equipment specifications. This will help with the flow of the facility and will influence how effectively people can move from one area of the facility to another once it is operational. Traffic flow is one of the more important aspects of designing the facility. Creating easy access for people will have the greatest effect on the facility's function and safety when multiple groups of athletes are present at the same time. The flow of traffic should also allow coaches or supervisors to have a clear view of the whole floor. For ease of access, and to create a space with a clear view in the middle of the room, low machines and dumbbell racks can be placed in the center.

Construction Phase

The **construction phase** is the period of time from the beginning of construction to the end. This is usually the longest phase of the process. During construction, the committee needs to continually refer to the master plan to ensure that the project is on track with regard to the established goals and design. Keeping the project on track in relation to the deadline must also become a priority. Costs of delays may have to be borne by the builder or architect if deadlines are not met and the owners lose potential revenue. This situation usually leads to a lawsuit so that money can be made back, or the owners are reimbursed and the price from the initial bid is reduced.

Preoperation Phase

The **preoperation phase** consists of the final steps before the facility can open. These steps include finishing the interior decor (note that aesthetics can greatly enhance the experience of users) and hiring a qualified staff. The staff should have at least the minimum required certifications and education. The National Collegiate Athletic Association is now enforcing legislation that requires strength and conditioning professionals to be Certified Strength and Conditioning Specialists. Finding hardworking, knowledgeable, loyal, and trustworthy employees is crucial to running a successful strength and conditioning program. During the preoperation phase it is important to include a plan for staff development as well. This could vary from semiannual workshops to a weekly staff meeting.

During the preoperation phase it is vital to create a plan that will make opening the facility easy. For example, duties such as cleaning and maintenance should be delegated to the staff on a weekly basis. This is easier to do when a cleaning and maintenance schedule has been created and is followed as soon as the facility is operating.

Also during preoperation, a plan for administrative and clerical duties should be created to organize work related to matters such as liability insurance, scheduling, and budgeting. Details such as choosing a scheduling software package and delegating clerical duties need to be taken care of before the facility opens.

Existing Strength and Conditioning Facilities

Modifying an existing strength and conditioning facility is similar to designing a new facility, minus the process of building from the ground up. In some cases, modifying an existing facility is a long process. A committee can also be formed for an existing facility, but members such as a contractor and architect may not be necessary. An existing facility may also use a different hiring process. Sometimes strength and conditioning professionals continue to work in the same facility regardless of a change of ownership or management. However, there should still be a focus on standards, education, professionalism, and staff development. Figure 23.2 outlines the main steps in modifying an existing facility.

> ▶ The strength and conditioning professional should assess existing equipment based on the needs of all athletes and teams who use the facility.

Assessing Athletic Program Needs

One of the more important considerations in building a strength and conditioning facility is the needs and

First steps	Form committee	Feasibility study	Needs analysis
Second steps	Create operational plan	Remodel and/or upgrade	Finalize design and decorations
Third steps	Arrange equipment	Create employee duties and schedule	Hire/keep staff

FIGURE 23.2   Steps in modifying an existing facility.

requirements of the athletes and athletic program. The number of athletes, the coaches' philosophies, the athletes' ages and training experience, the athletes' schedules, and the equipment available can affect the design of the facility (6). When it comes time to assess such needs, the facility designers should be able to answer these questions:

• *How many athletes will be using the facility?* This is an important consideration because the facility size will be greatly influenced by the number of athletes using the facility at the same time and the total number who use it per day, week, and season. The number of athletes will also affect the scheduling and flow of the facility if two or more groups are training simultaneously. Based on regulations such as fire codes or other occupational health and safety regulations, the city's planning department will specify how many athletes can be allowed to use the facility at one time.

• *What are the training goals for the athletes, coaches, and administration?* The training goals of the coaches or athletes will affect which equipment is chosen for the facility. For example, if a coach wants athletes to focus on plyometrics and agility, the facility will need an area (turf or field) designated for this purpose. The strength and conditioning professional should also use his or her philosophy as a guideline for ordering equipment. If resistance training is to be programmed, weightlifting racks and platforms are more space efficient compared to bench or incline bench press setups that serve only one purpose.

• *What are the demographics of the athletes?* The demographics of the users are important when one is determining the equipment needs of the facility. Are the users primarily older, younger, male, female, high school, college, or professional? A facility with primarily older populations may not need as much free weight equipment as it does machines. In a collegiate or team environment, use of the equipment may be more efficient if it is grouped into sections so that multiple groups can work out simultaneously without interference.

• *What will the training experience of the athletes be?* Answering this question will help the strength and conditioning professional devise training plans, which in turn will dictate the equipment needed. Training will vary according to the experience of the athlete. Athletes with no previous lifting experience may do more bodyweight exercises than advanced athletes, who may do more weightlifting. It is also important to assess whether needs will change over time and whether equipment requirements will vary depending on the season. For example, in a high school or collegiate setting, athletes with little lifting experience may enter the facility at the start of every academic year.

• *How will the athletes be scheduled?* The scheduling of athletes or groups of athletes can be one of the more difficult aspects of running a facility. The number of people on staff, the layout, and the design of the facility can all be affected by the athletes' schedules. If more than one group will likely be coming into the facility at one time, it would make sense to divide the facility into sections so the amount of overlap is limited. Athletes should be scheduled to arrive throughout the day so that they do not flood the facility all at once. This will help maintain suggested staff-to-athlete ratios and ensure that enough equipment is available. (See chapter 24 for additional detail.)

• *What equipment needs to be repaired or modified?* No equipment in a facility should have issues such as holes, cuts, or missing pieces. If a cable is frayed or damaged, discontinue using the cable column until the cable is replaced. All existing equipment should be repaired or replaced if broken. Existing equipment should be cleaned regularly and repaired promptly or should be sold to provide funds for new equipment. In some cases, a piece of equipment is in good repair but needs an accessory for an upgrade. For example, cable columns may require new attachments to be fully functional.

Once all of these questions are answered, the process of designing the facility will be much easier. Ideally the facility designers should have a solution for every problem; this would allow for an optimal training environment. In reality, however, budget and space limitations often stand in the way. It is important to focus on what will affect the facility the most and to design from there. For example, not having enough space will have a larger impact on the training environment and scheduling than not having enough of a specialized piece of equipment. The recommended minimum amount of space per athlete is 100 square feet (9.3 m²) per participant.

Designing the Strength and Conditioning Facility

Before arranging and positioning equipment, one must consider the design of the strength and conditioning facility, whether new or existing. The strength and conditioning professional should pay particular attention to facility location and access, structural and functional considerations, environmental factors, and safety and supervision.

Location

The strength and conditioning facility should ideally be located on the ground floor away from offices and classrooms. This will prevent interruptions elsewhere in the building that are caused by dropped weights, music, or other noises common to strength and conditioning facilities. If the facility is not located on the ground floor, the floor must be stable enough to support heavy equipment and equipment that is dropped. The load-bearing capacity should be at least 100 pounds per square foot (488 kg/m²).

Supervision Location

The facility supervisor's station or office should be in a central location with a clear line of sight and mirrors providing the opportunity to look out and see everyone. One option is to place the office at an elevation over the floor of the weight room for better viewing.

Access

The facility should be accessible to people with disabilities, with either a ramp or a wheelchair lift for any change in height exceeding 0.5 inches (13 mm). A ramp should run 12 inches for every 1-inch rise (30.5 cm run for every 2.5 cm rise), and steps should have a rough strip on the edge to help prevent anyone from falling. Another option for persons with disabilities is a mechanical lift or an elevator. A weight room should also have double doors so that large equipment and machines can be moved in and out. However, if the hallway is too narrow, the size of the doors will not make a difference (8), as an outside wall will have to temporarily be removed, or a garage door opened, when moving equipment.

Ceiling Height

The ceiling should be high enough to accommodate any jumping or explosive activities. This includes the athlete's height plus the space required for box jumps, vertical jumps, and Olympic lifting exercises. A recommended height is 12 to 14 feet (3.66 m to 4.27 m), which should give enough clearance to allow athletes to comfortably perform these activities (8).

Flooring

Several types of flooring options are available for a strength and conditioning facility. The most common option is some type of rubber flooring and an antifungal carpet. Another option is indoor turf, which can be useful if the strength and conditioning professional plans to have people do plyometric, agility, or conditioning exercises. Turf is also a good surface for ground-based movements and sled pushes. Although usually more expensive, rubber flooring can be easier to clean than carpet. Rubber flooring is typically available in the form of rolls, insert tiles, and a poured surface.

Ideally, weightlifting platforms should have a middle portion made of wood and outer sections made of rubber. Wood does not allow shoes to get caught or slide, so the wood portion creates a safe lifting surface for weightlifting movements.

Environmental Factors

The facility's lighting should include artificial and natural lighting. The lights should be between 50 and 100 lumens, depending on the height of the ceilings and the amount of natural light. Natural light is the light coming from the sun through windows. Windows help make a facility feel more open and modern, and mirrors can enhance the amount of light that comes in by reflecting it to spots in the room where natural light is not present (2).

A strength and conditioning facility needs to maintain a comfortable training temperature. The heating, ventilation, and air conditioning (HVAC) system should ideally have the capability to heat and cool individual sections of the facility. Most sources indicate that anywhere between 68 °F and 78 °F (20-25 °C) is a good temperature range, with many suggesting that operation is optimal in the 72 °F to 78 °F (22-25 °C) range (2, 4). If the facility is too hot or too cold, the athletes may be uncomfortable and the quality of training will be affected.

Relative humidity should also be monitored in the strength and conditioning facility. In any space where there is physical activity, relative humidity should not exceed 60%. This helps to prevent bacterial and microbial growth, avoiding the spread of infections and disease (2).

Circulation should also be a primary concern with regard to the facility's design and HVAC system. An HVAC system, a fresh air exchange system, and ceiling or box fans can provide the necessary circulation. The air should be exchanged anywhere from 8 to 12 times per hour to prevent odors caused by stagnant air (4). If fans are used, a general guideline is two to four fans for every 1,200 square feet (111.5 m²). Fans help keep the air from feeling stagnant and muggy, which makes for a better training environment.

Many facilities have sound systems that help create a training environment conducive to hard work. While not essential, music helps athletes get motivated and into a rhythm. Two considerations for installing a sound system are speaker volume and placement. The sound should be less than 90 decibels so that athletes can hear instructions and cues (2). Speakers should also be elevated and in a corner to prevent any damage and to project sound toward the middle of the room so that it is more evenly distributed.

Background noise and excess external noise are other issues to consider. Such sounds can emanate from sources ranging from the HVAC system to the people in the next building. In a facility that has yoga or dance classes, sound-absorbing material should be used in the floors and walls to prevent excess noise from reaching others in the facility. Absorbent rubber flooring can be used to mute noise caused by people jumping, running, or dropping things (4).

Electrical Service

A strength and conditioning facility typically requires more outlets than other buildings. Some outlets may require relatively higher voltage for more powerful equipment, such as stair climbers, elliptical machines, and treadmills. The electrical service also needs to be properly grounded to protect the system from a lightning strikes or power surges. Ground-fault circuits are also necessary to ensure athlete safety in the event of an electrical short (1).

Mirrors

Mirrors can be used for many purposes in a strength and conditioning facility. They can be used as a coaching tool if racks and platforms are placed in the right position, as they provide immediate visual feedback to the athlete (8). Mirrors can also be used to enhance a room aesthetically, making it feel larger than it really is by reflecting light from windows or from artificial lighting.

Mirrors should be placed at least 6 inches (15 cm) away from any equipment and a minimum of 20 inches (51 cm) above the floor. The purpose of the height guideline is to ensure that weights do not roll, bounce, or slide into the bottom of the mirror and cause it to break. The standard weight plate is 18 inches (46 cm) in diameter, giving mirrors a 2-inch (5 cm) clearance in the event that the plate is dropped near the mirror or leaned against the wall behind the mirror (8).

Other Considerations

Drinking fountains are a positive addition to a strength and conditioning facility. They should be located away from the training area and should not interrupt traffic flow. Drinking fountains are often placed next to the entrance of the facility or next to the bathrooms and lockers.

Locker rooms can also be a nice addition to a facility. At the very least, having a shower located somewhere in the building ensures that cleaning up after a workout will be convenient. Good hygiene is important for preventing the spread of infections and disease. Although not everyone will use the showers or lockers, having them available for on-the-go athletes may boost morale and hopefully give them a reason to push themselves during a workout.

Every facility should have at least one phone that is accessible to persons in wheelchairs. This complies with the Americans with Disabilities Act (ADA); it also provides safety in the event of an emergency if the only person who could help is in a wheelchair. Ideally the phone should be at the front of the facility in or outside of an office so that a supervisor can call emergency services as soon as possible following an accident (2).

Bumper rails or padding may be useful for places that require protection, such as a mirror or drywall. Rails help prevent damage from people or objects falling or bumping against such surfaces. Rails are also used in rooms such as dance or yoga studios. People can hold on to them for balance when necessary.

A strength and conditioning facility needs a space in which to store items such as extra equipment, cleaning supplies, tools, or broken equipment. A bigger facility with more equipment requires a larger storage room than a small facility. The largest amount of space in the storage room is more than likely occupied by unused equipment.

Arranging Equipment in the Strength and Conditioning Facility

It is essential to consider particular requirements when placing equipment in the available space. A floor plan can be drawn to help with visualizing how to arrange equipment, especially since there are safety and efficiency recommendations for each type of equipment and mode of exercise.

Equipment Placement

Equipment should be grouped into sections such as a stretching and warm-up area, agility and plyometrics, free weights, aerobic area, and resistance machines. Ideally, free weights and racks should be organized along the wall, and there should be walkways between the free weights and machines (1). This allows for improved flow through the weight room, preventing congestion and maximizing space for more utilization.

Machines can be lined up in the middle of the weight room to make a walkway on each side of the room. Planning ahead and organizing the equipment so it can be used as a circuit will also help with traffic flow. Tall machines should be bolted to the floor or a column or a wall so there is no chance that they will tip over.

Cardiorespiratory machines should be in their own section and should be lined up and organized such that the treadmills, elliptical machines, stair machines, and bikes are grouped together. Keep in mind that most machines requiring electricity will have to be along a wall unless there are electrical outlets in the floor or on a column. Equipment should also be placed away from the walkway to minimize the chances of someone tripping over it or on associated electrical cords.

Barbells and dumbbells should have a minimum of 36 inches (91 cm) of space between other barbells and dumbbells to allow for movement between racks without danger to the lifter or spotter(s). If a spotter is likely to be needed (e.g., on a rack), more space should be provided to allow more than one spotter access to the rack. Weight trees should be placed in close proximity to plate-loaded equipment, while the distance between lifting equipment and trees should be 36 inches (91 cm).

Racks are better placed along a wall unless there is a row of two racks with the backs of the racks facing each other. In any case, there should be at least 36 inches (91 cm) of space for walking around the entire rack.

Use visibility as a guideline. Shorter equipment is better placed in the middle of the room so that coaches or trainers can easily see across the facility. Tall equipment can be bolted on the walls, preferably along portions of the wall with no windows or mirrors.

Traffic Flow

Traffic flow is heavily influenced by equipment placement. Most facilities are one big room, and walkways can be created via arrangement of the equipment. As just mentioned, most racks or machines are best placed lined up in a row running the length of the facility. This usually creates two or three main walkways that should be at least 36 inches (91 cm) wide.

> ▶ Safety and function are top priorities when one is deciding on placement of equipment in a facility.

Stretching and Warm-Up Area

A stretching and warm-up area is an open area with soft tissue instruments, mats, or bands. This area should include foam rollers; bands; PVC pipes; tennis balls, golf balls, and softballs; and possibly even jump ropes. If possible, there should be at least 49 square feet (4.6 m²) of open space so that athletes can perform a dynamic warm-up (7), as well as enough room for multiple people to be using the area at the same time. Mats are sometimes used so that athletes do not have to lie on a hard floor, but this is not necessary.

Circuit Training Area

A circuit training area is typically a space with machines lined up or grouped together to make it easy for people to switch from one machine to the next. There are several ways to group the machines. Examples of different groupings include upper body and lower body, pushing actions and pulling actions, and various body part groupings. In many facilities, injured athletes use the circuit machines to exercise the body parts that are still healthy. Ease of access between machines should be kept in mind so that injured athletes can move freely.

The circuit training machines should be at least 24 inches (61 cm)—preferably 36 inches (91 cm)—away from each other in order to provide a wide enough walk space and some extra space for safety called a **safety cushion**. Any designated walkways in the circuit training area should be between 4 and 7 feet (1.2 and 2.1 m) wide to provide enough space to move freely (7).

Free Weights

Free weight equipment includes dumbbells, barbells, benches, kettlebells, farmer's walk handles, hexagonal bars, squat racks, and any other equipment necessary to use these items. As stated earlier, the racks and dumbbells should be lined up along a wall with enough room to walk between the wall and weights and with at least 36 inches (91 cm) between the ends of racked bars. This not only gives staff more space for cleaning but also prevents weights from crashing into the wall or mirrors. Kettlebells can either be lined up under a dumbbell rack or in their own section. Since most activities with a kettlebell are dynamic and take up lots of space, this section should be large.

Weightlifting Area

A weightlifting area generally contains racks with platforms or a platform standing alone. It could also be an open area where weightlifting is performed without a platform. This is typically done on a rubber floor with a concrete foundation. To keep things organized, weight trees or racks and bar holders can be used when the equipment is not in use.

Racks and platforms should have enough room between them that if someone were to fall, people nearby would not be injured. Racks and platforms should be spaced 3 to 4 feet (0.9 to 1.2 m) apart.

The weightlifting racks should be bolted to the floor to ensure that they do not move when in use. If a rack is portable, it should be moved to a designated storage area when not in use.

Aerobic Area

The aerobic area is where the cardiopulmonary training equipment is grouped together. This equipment consists of stationary bicycles, stair climbers, elliptical machines, treadmills, rowers, and so on. Floor space requirements for the aerobic equipment and the space between pieces of equipment are provided in table 23.1 (7). These requirements outline the amount of space needed for each piece of equipment, along with the required amount of space to allow for room to move and prevent accidents caused by falling into equipment.

Organizing a facility begins with arranging the equipment in a safe, functional space. The guidelines in this chapter provide the tools necessary to properly arrange the equipment. Taking a blank floor plan of the facility and sketching the equipment arrangement on the blank plan will help with equipment placement. Figures 23.3 and 23.4 near the end of the chapter show examples of weight room layouts for secondary school and university settings. Notice the walkway spacing and arrangement, as well as the organization and grouping of the equipment. Also note the placement of the supervisor's office and window placement. Table 23.2 provides calculations to determine the space needs for various types of equipment.

Maintaining and Cleaning Surfaces and Equipment

Surfaces in the strength and conditioning facility should be cleaned consistently to ensure that the equipment is safe and functional. Proper maintenance will save money in the long run, because cleaning materials are cheaper than replacing padding, flooring, and so on. Microbes will begin to grow if the surfaces are not wiped down with a germicidal cleaner. Equipment that is used more often and has a greater chance of developing bacterial growth (e.g., padding, vinyl) should be cleaned every day or every other day. It is important that any germicidal cleaner used in the strength facility have the ability to prevent the spread of HIV and hepatitis. Nonabsorbent floors should be regularly mopped for removal of dust

TABLE 23.1　Aerobic Equipment Space Requirements

Equipment	Space needed
Bikes	24 ft² (2.2 m²)
Stair steppers	24 ft² (2.2 m²)
Skiers	6 ft² (0.6 m²)
Rowers	40 ft² (3.7 m²)
Treadmills	45 ft² (4.2 m²)

Adapted, by permission, from Kroll, 1991 (7).

and grime buildup. Wood weightlifting platforms should also be checked for splintering and cracking and cleaned with an appropriate cleaner to remove dust and dirt that could cause foot slippage. During cleaning around racks and machinery, the bolts and screws that hold the equipment to the floor should also be tightened or checked regularly. Machines that have cables and pulleys should be regularly checked and should be repaired if the cables and pulleys are loose or fraying. If the facility has a tiled or rolled rubber floor, there should be minimal gaps between the pieces and no visible glue extruding between the cracks. Carpet should be vacuumed and cleaned regularly to prevent mold, mildew, or fungal growth.

Walls and ceilings should also be cleaned at least once every week or two. The walls and ceilings should have no dirt buildup, and there should not be any dust in the corners. Cobwebs tend to build up high in the corners where the walls meet the ceiling and should be removed. If the facility has windows and mirrors, they should be regularly checked for cracking and replaced as soon as a crack is noticed. Clean windows and mirrors also enhance the aesthetics of the facility. Use a window cleaner and microfiber towel to leave the surface streak free. Dirt and dust can build up on flat edges of items affixed to the wall or fixtures hanging from the ceiling. Any windowsills, shelves, or anything hanging from the ceiling should be regularly dusted. If exercise equipment is hanging from the ceiling, it should be regularly checked to ensure that it is tightly secured and will not fall down (3). Figure 23.5 near the end of the chapter presents a list for the floors, walls, and ceilings to refer to when one is creating a cleaning schedule.

> **Scheduling frequent maintenance and cleaning ensures safe training, protects investments, and maintains the strength and conditioning facility's appearance.**

Maintenance should include not only the surface materials but also the equipment. The equipment should

TABLE 23.2   Calculations for Space Needs

Area	Examples	Formula
Prone and supine exercises	Bench press Lying triceps extension	**Formula:** Actual weight bench length (6-8 ft [1.8-2.4 m]) + safety space cushion of 3 ft (0.9 m) *multiplied by* a suggested user space for a weight bench width of 7 ft (2.1 m) + a safety space cushion of 3 ft (0.9 m)
		Example 1: If using a 6-foot-long weight bench for the bench press exercise, (6 ft + 3 ft) × (7 ft + 3 ft) = 90 ft²
		Example 2 (metric approximations): If using a 2 m long weight bench for the bench press exercise, (2 m [bench] + 1 m [safety space]) × (2 m [user space] + 1 m [safety space]) = 9 m²
Standing exercises	Biceps curl Upright row	**Formula:** Actual bar length (4-7 ft [1.2-2.1 m]) + a double-wide safety space cushion of 6 ft (1.8 m) *multiplied by* a suggested user space for a standing exercise "width" of 4 ft (1.2 m)
		Example 1: If using a 4-foot curl bar for the biceps curl exercise, (4 ft + 6 ft) × (4 ft) = 40 ft²
		Example 2 (metric approximations): If using a 1 m curl bar for the biceps curl exercise, (1 m [bar] + 2 m [safety space]) × (1 m [user space]) = 3 m²
Standing exercises in a rack	Back squat Shoulder press	**Formula:** Actual bar length (5-7 ft [1.5-2.1 m]) + a double-wide safety space cushion of 6 ft (1.8 m) *multiplied by* a suggested user space for a standing exercise (from a rack) "width" of 8 to 10 ft (2.4-3 m)
		Example 1: If using a 7-foot Olympic bar for the back squat exercise, (7 ft + 6 ft) × (10 ft) = 130 ft²
		Example 2 (metric approximations): If using a 2 m Olympic bar for the back squat exercise, (2 m [bar] + 2 m [safety space]) × (3 m [safety space]) = 12 m²
Olympic lifting area	Power clean	**Formula:** Lifting platform height (typically 8 ft [2.4 m]) + a perimeter walkway safety space cushion of 4 ft (1.2 m) *multiplied by* a lifting platform width (typically 8 ft [2.4 m]) + perimeter walkway safety space cushion of 4 ft (1.2 m)
		Example 1: (8 ft + 4 ft) × (8 ft + 4 ft) = 144 ft²
		Example 2 (metric approximations): (2.5 m [platform] + 1 m [safety space]) × (2.5 m [platform] + 1 m [safety space]) = 12.25 m²

be regularly checked for broken or damaged parts, particularly those that affect the equipment's functionality. If the equipment is used often and not cleaned enough, residue can build up that may cause functional or health issues. Nonfunctional equipment should be labeled with an "Out of Order" sign (2). If fixing broken equipment will take a while, it should be removed from the floor and placed in storage. As with surfaces, equipment can end up costing a lot more if it is not maintained and cleaned properly.

The National Strength and Conditioning Association's safety checklist for exercise facility and equipment maintenance (figure 23.6) is helpful for determining the maintenance needs of the facility's equipment. A cleaning schedule should be made that specifies the equipment to be cleaned daily, weekly, biweekly, or monthly. The checklist also covers facility layout issues, especially those relating to safety.

Cleaning and maintenance materials should be kept in storage or in a closet. If possible, the cleaning materials should be locked, and they should be used only when needed. Any tools should be kept in a toolbox that is put away and out of sight of the weight room. Tools and cleaning materials should also be regularly inventoried and restocked. A list of maintenance equipment and cleaning supplies is provided in table 23.3.

Conclusion

Designing a strength and conditioning facility is a long process that involves extensive designing and planning. The process begins with the formation of a committee that will aid in the construction and design of the facility. The next step involves assessing the athletic program's needs. This is the phase in which the number of athletes, athletes' training experience, coaches' needs, scheduling, and equipment

TABLE 23.3 Equipment and Supplies for Maintenance and Cleaning

Maintenance equipment	Cleaning supplies
File	Disinfectant (germicide)
Hammer	Specialty cleaners (wood, walls, upholstery, and so on)
Pliers	Glass cleaner
Screwdrivers	Lubrication
Wrench set	Paper towels
Knife	Spray bottles
Stapler	Cloth towels and rags
Duct tape	Sponges
Extra nuts, bolts, and washers	Brooms and dustpans
Heavy-duty glue	Vacuum cleaner
Drill and drill bit set	Mop and bucket
Vise grips	Stain remover

needs should be determined. After these determinations have been made, the process of designing the facility and arranging the equipment should begin. Care should be taken and guidelines followed in arranging and spacing equipment.

After the design process is complete, the facility and the equipment must be properly maintained and cared for to ensure safe training and protect investments. Regular maintenance and cleaning of equipment and surfaces are vital for the longevity of the facility. Cleaning and maintenance should focus the most on the equipment that is used more often. This will help to prevent the spread of infections among the facility users as well as promote proper hygiene and maintain the aesthetics of the environment.

construction phase
design phase
feasibility study

master plan
needs analysis
predesign phase

preoperation phase
safety cushion

STUDY QUESTIONS

1. What is the order of the four phases involved in designing a new strength and conditioning facility?
   a. construction, predesign, design, preoperation
   b. preoperation, design, construction, predesign
   c. predesign, construction, design
   d. predesign, design, construction, preoperation

2. A master plan should be created in which of the following phases?
   a. predesign phase
   b. design phase
   c. construction phase
   d. preoperation phase

3. What is the recommended minimum distance between the floor and the bottom of mirrors on the walls?
   a. 16 inches (41 cm)
   b. 18 inches (46 cm)
   c. 20 inches (51 cm)
   d. 22 inches (56 cm)

4. Which of the following is NOT a key consideration when determining the space requirements of a college strength and conditioning facility?
   a. accessibility for the athletes
   b. amount and type of equipment
   c. number of athletes using the facility
   d. number of athletic teams desiring to use the facility

5. What is the minimum recommended space between the ends of racks to provide room for spotters?
   a. 1 foot (30 cm)
   b. 2 feet (61 cm)
   c. 3 feet (91 cm)
   d. 4 feet (123 cm)

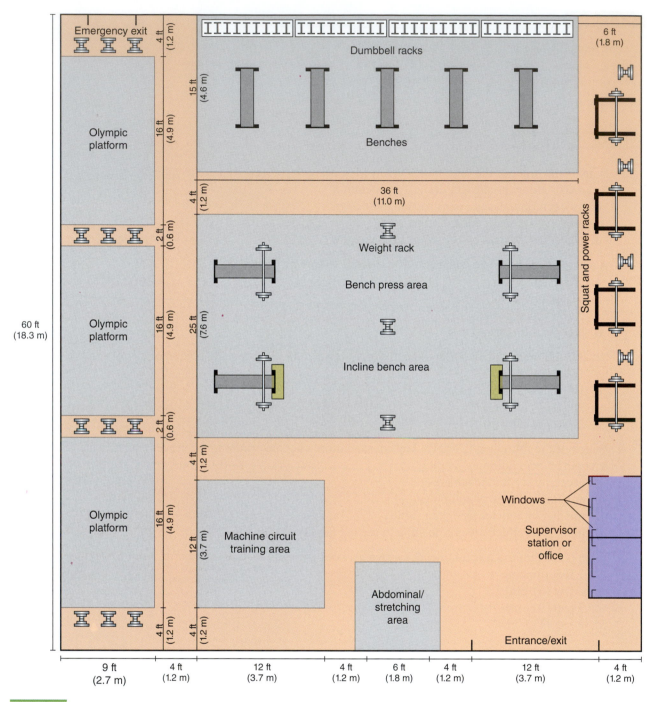

FIGURE 23.3 Example of a secondary school strength and conditioning facility floor plan (3 feet [ft] = 1 m).

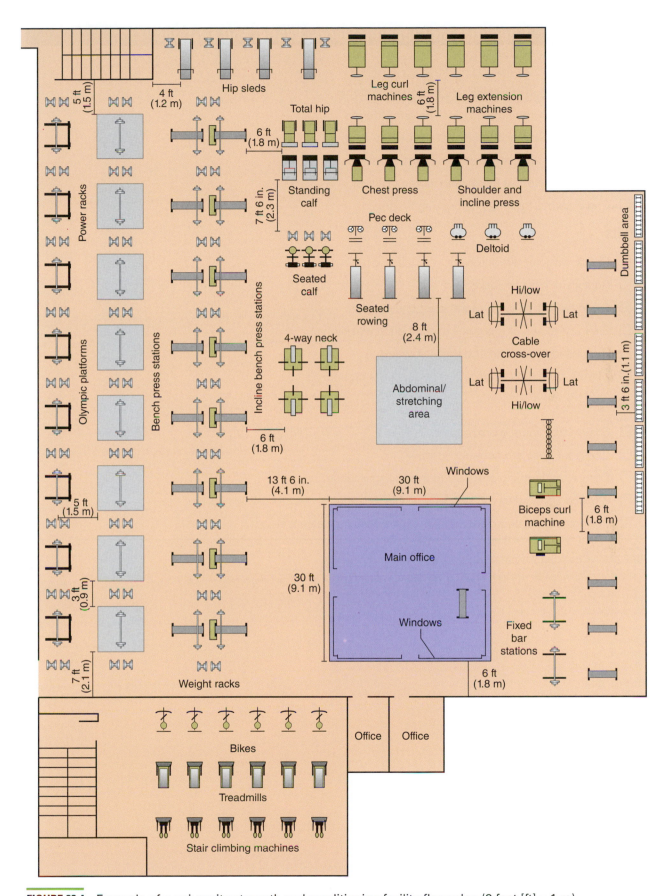

FIGURE 23.4 Example of a university strength and conditioning facility floor plan (3 feet [ft] = 1 m).

Checklist for Cleaning Floors, Walls, and Ceilings

Floors

☐ Check for large cracks and standing dirt or grime.

☐ Check for splintering and breaking on platforms.

☐ Check any bolts or screws that go into the floor.

☐ Ensure that no glue is extruding from the floor.

☐ Ensure that floor is sturdy and locked in place.

☐ Check carpet for mold, mildew, and tears.

Walls

☐ Check walls for dirt buildup.

☐ Replace mirrors if cracked.

☐ Clean mirrors of smudges at least once weekly.

☐ Clean windows of smudges at least once weekly.

☐ Dust windowsills and any shelving weekly.

☐ Mirrors should be at least 20 inches off the ground.

Ceilings

☐ Ensure that lights work properly.

☐ Check for dust and cobweb buildup.

☐ Ensure that nothing attached to the ceiling is loose.

☐ Replace ceiling tiles as soon as possible if needed.

☐ Ceilings should be at least 12 feet high to ensure clearance.

FIGURE 23.5 Checklist for cleaning floors, walls, and ceilings.

From NSCA, 2016, *Essentials of strength training and conditioning*, 4th ed., edited by G. Haff and T. Triplett (Champaign, IL: Human Kinetics).

NSCA's Safety Checklist for Exercise Facility and Equipment Maintenance

Exercise Facility

Floor

- ☐ Inspected and cleaned daily
- ☐ Wooden flooring free of splinters, holes, protruding nails, and loose screws
- ☐ Tile flooring resistant to slipping; no moisture or chalk accumulation
- ☐ Rubber flooring free of cuts, slits, and large gaps between pieces
- ☐ Interlocking mats secure and arranged with no protruding tabs
- ☐ Nonabsorbent carpet free of tears; wear areas protected by throw mats
- ☐ Area swept and vacuumed or mopped on a regular basis
- ☐ Flooring glued or fastened down properly

Walls

- ☐ Wall surfaces cleaned two or three times a week (or more often if needed)
- ☐ Walls in high-activity areas free of protruding appliances, equipment, or wall hangings
- ☐ Mirrors and shelves securely fixed to walls
- ☐ Mirrors and windows cleaned regularly (especially in high-activity areas, such as around drinking fountains and in doorways)
- ☐ Mirrors placed a minimum of 20 inches (51 cm) off the floor in all areas
- ☐ Mirrors not cracked or distorted (replace immediately if damaged)

Ceiling

- ☐ All ceiling fixtures and attachments dusted regularly
- ☐ Ceiling tile kept clean
- ☐ Damaged or missing ceiling tile replaced as needed
- ☐ Open ceilings with exposed pipes and ducts cleaned as needed

Exercise Equipment

Stretching and Body Weight Exercise Area

- ☐ Mat area free of weight benches and equipment
- ☐ Mats and bench upholstery free of cracks and tears
- ☐ No large gaps between stretching mats
- ☐ Area swept and disinfected daily
- ☐ Equipment properly stored after use
- ☐ Elastic cords secured to base with safety knot and checked for wear
- ☐ Surfaces that contact skin treated with antifungal and antibacterial agents daily
- ☐ Nonslip material on the top surface and bottom or base of plyometric boxes
- ☐ Ceiling height sufficient for overhead exercises (12 feet [3.7 m] minimum) and free of low-hanging apparatus (beams, pipes, lighting, signs, and so on)

(continued)

FIGURE 23.6 The National Strength and Conditioning Association's safety checklist for exercise facility and equipment maintenance.

From NSCA, 2016, *Essentials of strength training and conditioning*, 4th ed., edited by G. Haff and T. Triplett (Champaign, IL: Human Kinetics). Adapted, by permission, from National Strength and Conditioning Association, 2004, *NSCA's essentials of personal training*, edited by R.W. Earle and T.R. Baechle (Champaign, IL: Human Kinetics) 604-606.

Resistance Training Machine Area

☐ Easy access to each station (a minimum of 2 feet [61 cm] between machines; 3 feet [91 cm] is optimal)

☐ Area free of loose bolts, screws, cables, and chains

☐ Proper selectorized pins used

☐ Securing straps functional

☐ Parts and surfaces properly lubricated and cleaned

☐ Protective padding free of cracks and tears

☐ Surfaces that contact skin treated with antifungal and antibacterial agents daily

☐ No protruding screws or parts that need tightening or removal

☐ Belts, chains, and cables aligned with machine parts

☐ No worn parts (frayed cable, loose chains, worn bolts, cracked joints, and so on)

Resistance Training Free Weight Area

☐ Easy access to each bench or area (a minimum of 2 feet [61 cm] between machines; 3 feet [91 cm] is optimal)

☐ Olympic bars properly spaced (3 feet [91 cm]) between ends

☐ All equipment returned after use to avoid obstruction of pathway

☐ Safety equipment (belts, collars, safety bars) used and returned

☐ Protective padding free of cracks and tears

☐ Surfaces that contact skin treated with antifungal and antibacterial agents daily

☐ Securing bolts and apparatus parts (collars, curl bars) tightly fastened

☐ Nonslip mats on squat rack floor area

☐ Olympic bars turn properly and are properly lubricated and tightened

☐ Benches, weight racks, standards, and the like secured to the floor or wall

☐ Nonfunctional or broken equipment removed from area or locked out of service

☐ Ceiling height sufficient for overhead exercises (12 feet [3.7 m] minimum) and free of low-hanging apparatus (beams, pipes, lighting, signs, and so on)

Weightlifting Area

☐ Olympic bars properly spaced (3 feet [91 cm]) between ends

☐ All equipment returned after use to avoid obstruction of lifting area

☐ Olympic bars rotate properly and are properly lubricated and tightened

☐ Bent Olympic bars replaced; knurling clear of debris

☐ Collars functioning

☐ Sufficient chalk available

☐ Wrist straps, belts, and knee wraps available, functioning, and stored properly

☐ Benches, chairs, boxes kept at a distance from lifting area

☐ No gaps, cuts, slits, splinters in mats

☐ Area properly swept and mopped to remove splinters and chalk

☐ Ceiling height sufficient for overhead exercises (12 feet [3.7 m] minimum) and free of low-hanging apparatus (beams, pipes, lighting, signs, and so on)

Aerobic Exercise Area

☐ Easy access to each station (minimum of 2 feet [61 cm] between machines; 3 feet [91 cm] is optimal)

☐ Bolts and screws tight

(continued)

☐ Functioning parts easily adjustable

☐ Parts and surfaces properly lubricated and cleaned

☐ Foot and body straps secure and not ripped

☐ Measurement devices for tension, time, and revolutions per minute properly functioning

☐ Surfaces that contact skin treated with antifungal and antibacterial agents daily

Frequency of Maintenance and Cleaning Tasks

Daily

☐ Inspect all flooring for damage or wear.

☐ Clean (sweep, vacuum, or mop and disinfect) all flooring.

☐ Clean and disinfect upholstery.

☐ Clean and disinfect drinking fountain.

☐ Inspect fixed equipment's connection with floor.

☐ Clean and disinfect equipment surfaces that contact skin.

☐ Clean mirrors.

☐ Clean windows.

☐ Inspect mirrors for damage.

☐ Inspect all equipment for damage; wear; loose or protruding belts, screws, cables, or chains; insecure or nonfunctioning foot and body straps; improper functioning or improper use of attachments, pins, or other devices.

☐ Clean and lubricate moving parts of equipment.

☐ Inspect all protective padding for cracks and tears.

☐ Inspect nonslip material and mats for proper placement, damage, and wear.

☐ Remove trash and garbage.

☐ Clean light covers, fans, air vents, clocks, and speakers.

☐ Ensure that equipment is returned and stored properly after use.

Two or Three Times per Week

☐ Clean and lubricate aerobic machines and the guide rods on selectorized resistance training machines.

Once per Week

☐ Clean (dust) ceiling fixtures and attachments.

☐ Clean ceiling tile.

As Needed

☐ Replace light bulbs.

☐ Clean walls.

☐ Replace damaged or missing ceiling tiles.

☐ Clean open ceilings with exposed pipes or ducts.

☐ Remove (or place sign on) broken equipment.

☐ Fill chalk boxes.

☐ Clean bar knurling.

☐ Clean rust from floor, plates, bars, and equipment with a rust-removing solution.

CHAPTER 24

Facility Policies, Procedures, and Legal Issues

Traci Statler, PhD, and Victor Brown, MS

 After completing this chapter, you will be able to

- develop or clarify the goals and objectives of a strength and conditioning program,

- understand the daily operational practices of a strength and conditioning program and facility that help to achieve the goals and objectives,

- establish a standard of practice that leads to a safe and effective strength and conditioning program,

- identify common areas of potential liability exposure and implement appropriate risk management strategies,

- create a policies and procedures manual for a strength and conditioning program and facility, and

- properly schedule the strength and conditioning facility, along with formulating guidelines on seasonal planning and staff-to-athlete ratios.

The authors would like to acknowledge the significant contributions of Boyd Epley, John Taylor, Michael Greenwood, and Lori Greenwood to this chapter.

The strength and conditioning profession continues to evolve. Typically, a practitioner's knowledge and skill development involves competencies in exercise science, administration, management, teaching, and coaching (20). With student-athlete safety and welfare at the forefront, developing a policies and procedures manual provides a blueprint for implementing safe and effective programs and services.

Policies are essentially a facility's rules and regulations; they reflect the goals and objectives of the program. **Procedures** describe how policies are met or carried out. It is necessary to examine program goals and objectives, because they are the basis on which policies and procedures are created. Additionally, specific policies and procedures should include elements that protect the program and its employees from a risk of **litigation**; issues such as guidelines for supervision and instruction, facility administration, and emergency action planning and response should be included. The goal of this chapter is to identify areas of risk exposure and means of increasing safety, as well as to guide the strength and conditioning professional in providing and enhancing the quality of services and programs.

Mission Statement and Program Goals

A **mission statement** is an organization's statement of purpose (2). Creating a mission statement requires forward thinking with the end result in mind. A good mission statement provides the strength and conditioning program with focus and direction and is the foundation of effective administration. According to the Drucker Foundation (22), the following are suggested criteria for an effective mission statement:

- It should be short and sharply focused.
- It should be clear and easy to understand.
- It defines why the organization exists.
- It does not prescribe means.
- It is broad in scope.
- It provides direction for upholding code of ethics.
- It addresses and matches the organization's scope of practice.
- It inspires commitment.

The mission statement addresses three important components: target clientele (key market), what service is being provided (contribution), and what makes the service unique (distinction) (2).

The following is an example of a mission statement of a strength and conditioning program:

To provide to athletes the means by which they can train consistently, sensibly, and systematically over designated periods of time in a safe, clean, and professional environment to help prevent injury and improve athletic performance.

Program goals are the desired end products of a strength and conditioning program, stated in a broad, general manner. An effective strength and conditioning program should be based on scientific principles to enhance performance and increase injury resistance with intended outcomes specific to the sport and the athlete's position within the sport (7).

Developing a standard of care is a collaborative responsibility. Therefore, developing a mission statement and a list of program objectives should involve not only the strength and conditioning department, but also the institution, including but not limited to athletic administration and the sports medicine department. The more people participating the better, so that all involved groups and individuals take ownership and commit to achieving the strength and conditioning program's mission, goals, and objectives.

> A mission statement is an organization's statement of purpose, providing the strength and conditioning program with focus and direction.

Program Objectives

Program objectives are specific means of attaining program goals. If program goals are stated but the ways in which these goals might be attained are not specified, the result may be that athletes never achieve them. Program objectives should encompass all areas of the program to ensure that the goals are attained. Following is a sample list of objectives that can lead to reaching program goals and prepare a strength and conditioning professional to handle the job requirements.

- Design and administer strength, flexibility, aerobic, plyometric, and other training programs that reduce the likelihood of injuries and improve athletic performance. More precisely, design training programs that create the desired results in body composition, hypertrophy, strength, muscular endurance, cardiovascular endurance, speed, agility, coordination, balance, and power.

- Develop training programs to account for biomechanical and physiological differences between individual athletes, taking into consideration their ages, sex, training status, physical limitations, and injury status.

- Recognize acute and chronic physiological responses and adaptations to training and their implications for the design of sport-specific training programs.
- Educate athletes on the importance of good nutrition as well as sleep and its role in health and performance.
- Educate athletes about the effects of performance-enhancing substances and their abuse, relevant school policy, and legislation.

The performance team concept—that is, the use of individuals with specific areas of expertise as resources—can be applied in the creation of a strength and conditioning program that works toward meeting the preceding objectives. For example, when an athlete requires rehabilitation and reconditioning, the sports medicine staff should be consulted. The director of strength and conditioning needs to establish written policies and procedures for determining appropriate utilization of staff in the delivery of safe, effective, and efficient service. Additionally, an annual orientation meeting should be held at the beginning of the school year or sport season to familiarize staff, sport coaches, and participants with the established goals, objectives, policies, and procedures. Periodically reevaluate and review goals and objectives.

Strength and Conditioning Performance Team

The responsibilities of the strength and conditioning professional are continually changing as the field grows and becomes better recognized (14). The strength and conditioning staff can be aligned through the hiring of practitioners with formal education and specialization in specific scientific foundations (e.g., anatomy, exercise physiology, biomechanics). An assembled team allows for cooperative expertise by practitioners with complementary skills and provides an educational opportunity for staff members to gain knowledge outside of their specialization. Table 24.1 provides a practical example of a strength and conditioning performance team. The director of strength and conditioning is responsible for delineating the appropriate duties and responsibilities to the strength and conditioning staff for program design, exercise technique, organization and administration, and testing and evaluation.

Although job responsibilities vary according to institution, it would be prudent to consult *Strength and Conditioning Professionals Standards and Guidelines* (20) when one is developing the strength and conditioning performance team. Guideline 2.3 of this document states the following:

The productivity of a Strength and Conditioning staff, as well as learning and skill development of individual members, should be enhanced by aligning a performance team comprised of qualified practitioners with interdependent expertise and shared leadership roles. Once the team is assembled, respective activities and responsibilities from the "Practical/Applied" domain identified in the Certified Strength and Conditioning Specialist Examination Content Description, as well as the appropriate liaison assignments, should be delegated according to each member's particular "Scientific Foundations" expertise.

TABLE 24.1   Sample Strength and Conditioning Performance Team

Scientific foundations Education and expertise	Practical and applied activities and responsibilities	Liaison assignment(s)
Exercise and sport anatomy; biomechanics	Exercise techniques; testing and evaluation; rehabilitation and reconditioning	Exercise and sport science faculty; team coaches; sports medicine team
Exercise and sport physiology	Program design; testing and evaluation	Exercise and sport science faculty; team coaches
Exercise and sports nutrition	Nutritionist	Exercise and sport science faculty
Exercise and sport pedagogy	Program design; exercise technique; organization and administration	Exercise and sport science faculty; athletic administration
Exercise and sport psychology; motor learning	Exercise technique; rehabilitation and reconditioning	Exercise and sport science faculty; sports medicine team
Training methodology	Program design; organization and administration	Exercise and sport science faculty; athletic administration
Kinesiology; physiotherapy; sports medicine	Rehabilitation and reconditioning	Sports medicine team

Adapted, by permission, from NSCA, 2009 (20).

Director of Strength and Conditioning (Head Strength and Conditioning Coach)

The director of strength and conditioning (referred to hereafter as *director*)—also commonly referred to as the head strength and conditioning coach—is both a practitioner and an administrator. This person is responsible for the overall strength and conditioning program, facility, equipment, staff, and such administrative tasks as preparing a budget, purchasing equipment, preparing proposals, and working with administration and media. Figure 24.1 shows a sample job listing for such a position. Figure 24.2 provides a general job description for the director of strength and conditioning.

Director of Strength and Conditioning Job Listing

Responsibilities and duties as assigned by the director of athletics include developing and monitoring performance training programs for athletic teams, implementing safe and effective program design based on scientific principles, instructing proper resistance training exercise techniques, speed and agility development, and testing and evaluation. The head strength and conditioning professional will oversee policies and procedures, facility organization, and risk management for the strength and conditioning performance team in collaboration with the institution. The strength and conditioning professional should work cooperatively with the medical staff in the interest of student-athlete development, health, and well-being. A bachelor's degree is required, with a master's degree preferred (with emphasis in the exercise sciences). The strength and conditioning professional must possess certification from an independent accreditation agency (e.g., Certified Strength and Conditioning Specialist by the National Strength and Conditioning Association) and maintain continuing education requirements. First aid, cardiopulmonary resuscitation, and automated external defibrillator certifications required. Two years' experience is required in progressively responsible positions involving development and management of sport-specific individual and group performance training programs. Excellent management, supervisory, and management skills are required. Salary is commensurate with background and experience.

FIGURE 24.1   A job announcement similar to this can be used to attract quality applicants.

Based on Casa et al. 2012 (6).

Responsibilities of the Strength and Conditioning Director

- Direct all facets of staff, program, and facility operations.
- Design (or have final review of) all training programs.
- Oversee the athletic performance operation to ensure compliance with institutional, conference, and governing bodies' rules and regulations.
- Develop and submit the annual budget and ensure budgetary compliance through efficient financial management.
- Generate income and budget available funds for maintenance and improvement of the facility.
- Oversee the selection, installation, and maintenance of performance equipment, including cleaning and repair.
- Conduct orientation meetings for student-athletes on such issues as facility rules, the value of proper training and nutrition, and the dangers of banned substances.
- Develop staff work and supervision schedules, assign duties, and evaluate performance.
- Coordinate time schedules for use of the facility by each sport team and individual student-athletes.
- Assist with on-campus recruiting activities for prospective student-athletes.
- Serve on various departmental, institutional, conference, governing body, and professional committees and task forces.
- Work and communicate with coaches in the athletic department.
- Travel with sport teams (if applicable) and provide remote-site performance training programs, including pregame warm-up.
- Maintain a performance training library for professional development.
- Achieve and maintain professional certification(s) with continuing education requirements and a code of ethics, such as the CSCS credential offered through the NSCA. Depending on the professional's scope of activities, responsibilities, and knowledge requirements, relevant certifications offered by other governing bodies may also be appropriate (5).
- Perform other duties and special projects as requested by supervisor.
- Perform the duties of the assistant strength and conditioning professional and facility supervisor as needed.

FIGURE 24.2   A sample job description for a strength and conditioning director.

Adapted from Earle 1993 (7); Epley 1998 (8).

The director is also responsible for developing, presenting, and enforcing the written policies and procedures of the staff and participants in the program. It is the responsibility of the director to ensure that staff are properly trained and prepared. He or she achieves this by having staff and student-athlete orientation meetings and by periodically evaluating the staff's professional performance as well as determining and evaluating the attainment of professional goals. A sample form for the evaluation of student staff members is provided in figure 24.3. This form could be used to evaluate student interns and adapted to apply more specifically and effectively to members of the strength and conditioning performance team.

Student Staff Evaluation

Evaluation of staff member:_____

For period: _____   to   _____

The evaluation process is a method of assessing individual performance. It is an opportunity to bring to light any outstanding contributions or deficiencies among student staff members, improve individual job performance, determine appropriate personnel actions, and stimulate individual development.

Communication

Has the respect of the athletes while maintaining discipline	1	2	3	4	5	N/A
Teaches proper resistance training exercise technique	1	2	3	4	5	N/A
Has the ability to motivate athletes and elicit team unity	1	2	3	4	5	N/A
Enforces the weight room rules	1	2	3	4	5	N/A
Exhibits courtesy to athletes of both sexes	1	2	3	4	5	N/A
Does not subject athletes to verbal or physical abuse	1	2	3	4	5	N/A

Assumes Responsibility and Leadership

Follows instructions	1	2	3	4	5	N/A
Is adaptable to new ideas	1	2	3	4	5	N/A
Is always trying to learn	1	2	3	4	5	N/A
Does not delegate authority without permission	1	2	3	4	5	N/A
Demonstrates a high level of integrity	1	2	3	4	5	N/A
Adjusts training activity to fit skill or age level of the athlete	1	2	3	4	5	N/A
Demonstrates good judgment	1	2	3	4	5	N/A
Demonstrates consistent attendance and promptness	1	2	3	4	5	N/A
Submits paperwork on time as requested	1	2	3	4	5	N/A
Possesses the ability to get the project done, large or small	1	2	3	4	5	N/A
Submits high-quality work	1	2	3	4	5	N/A
Possesses an appropriate appearance	1	2	3	4	5	N/A

Attitude

Functions compatibly with all staff, athletes, and other departments	1	2	3	4	5	N/A
Is trustworthy with sensitive information	1	2	3	4	5	N/A
Does not gossip about coaches, athletic trainers, or athletes	1	2	3	4	5	N/A
Strives for objectives as stated in department's role and mission statement	1	2	3	4	5	N/A

Key

1 = Significantly below performance expectations
2 = Minimally acceptable performance
3 = Meets performance expectations
4 = Exceeds performance expectations
5 = Clearly exceptional performance

FIGURE 24.3   This sample student staff evaluation form can be used to assess staff competencies.

From NSCA, 2016, *Essentials of strength training and conditioning,* 4th ed., edited by G. Haff and T. Triplett (Champaign, IL: Human Kinetics). Reprinted, by permission, from R.W. Earle, 1993, *Staff and facility policies and procedures manual* (Omaha, NE: Creighton University).

Strength and Conditioning Staff (Personal Qualifications)

The possession of a certification from an independently accredited organization, such as the Certified Strength and Conditioning Specialist certification, establishes a standard of care. On August 1, 2015, National Collegiate Athletic Association (NCAA) Division I adopted legislation "To specify that a strength and conditioning coach shall be certified and maintain current certification through a nationally accredited strength and conditioning certification program" (p. 1) (16). Continuing education is a necessary part of maintaining a professional certification and reducing liability exposure, especially in the area of supervision and instruction (1). Litigation issues in this area often involve questions of "professional instructor qualifications," which include continuing education (19). Thus, assistant strength and conditioning professionals should also achieve and maintain a professional certification including standard first aid, cardiopulmonary resuscitation (CPR), and automated external defibrillation (AED). (See figure 24.4 for points of preparedness required of each staff member.)

Additionally, each staff member needs to understand the strength and conditioning program's goals and objectives, cooperatively work with others' responsibilities and schedules (such as the other members of the sports medicine team), and maintain a professional code of conduct.

Appendix A of *Strength and Conditioning Professional Standards and Guidelines* defines the strength and conditioning professional:

Certified Strength and Conditioning Specialists are professionals who practically apply foundational knowledge to assess, motivate, educate, and train athletes for the primary goal of improving sports performance. They conduct sport-specific testing sessions, design and implement safe and effective strength training and conditioning programs, and provide guidance for athletes in nutrition and injury prevention. Recognizing their area of expertise is separate and distinct from the medical, dietetic, athletic training, and sport coaching fields, Certified Strength and Conditioning Specialists consult with and refer athletes to these professionals when appropriate. (p. 13)

Staff Preparedness

1. Maintenance of professional certification
2. Maintenance of certification in standard first aid, CPR, and AED
3. Review of emergency response procedures
   a. Rudimentary first aid procedures annually
   b. Common training facility injuries and their prevention
   c. Building evacuation plan
4. Knowledge and understanding of program policies and procedures
   a. Review of room capacity and safe supervision ratios
   b. Review of preparticipation screening and clearance procedure
   c. Review of personal and professional liability, negligence, and insurance coverage issues
5. Knowledge and understanding of governing body rules and regulations
   a. Review of general knowledge of regulations
   b. Review of rules specific to administering the strength and conditioning program
6. Knowledge and understanding of cleaning and maintenance issues and needs
7. Knowledge and understanding of program philosophy and instruction methods
   a. Technique and drill instruction.
   b. Body composition guidelines and nutritional consultation
   c. Motivational issues
      - Pushing athletes beyond physical limits
      - Athletes who overtrain
      - Athletes who refuse to follow program recommendations

FIGURE 24.4 Points of preparedness required of each staff member.

Adapted from Taylor, 2006 (23).

Legal and Ethical Issues

Everyone involved in athletic activities, including the strength and conditioning professional, must be cognizant of legal liability. The risk of injury cannot be totally eliminated, but it can be effectively managed by the strength and conditioning professional. **Risk management** is the employment of strategies to decrease and control the risk of injury from athletic participation and therefore the risk of liability exposure. The first steps in risk management are to understand integral key terms and identify the areas of potential liability exposure that could cause injuries and lead to litigation. Although each facility is unique, recognizable areas of potential liability are present in all strength and conditioning facilities. The following sections discuss these risk areas and the need for an emergency care plan, reliable record keeping, and liability insurance.

Common Legal Terminology

To understand the potential legal ramifications of running a strength and conditioning facility, the strength and conditioning professional must first understand the following common legal terms.

Informed consent—The process by which a procedure or activity is described to a participant, with an explanation of the inherent risks and benefits involved, allowing the individual to determine if he or she desires to participate.

Liability—A legal responsibility, duty, or obligation. Strength and conditioning professionals have a duty to the athletes they serve by virtue of their employment not only to act when an injury occurs but also to prevent injury (5).

Standard of care—What a reasonable and prudent person would do under similar circumstances. A strength and conditioning professional is expected to act according to his or her education, level of training, and certification status (e.g., Certified Strength and Conditioning Specialist [CSCS], National Strength and Conditioning Association Certified Personal Trainer [NSCA-CPT], Emergency Medical Technician [EMT], CPR, AED, first aid).

Negligence—Failure to act as a reasonable and prudent person would under similar circumstances. Four elements must exist in order for a strength and conditioning professional to be found negligent: **duty**, **breach of duty**, **proximate cause**, and **damages** (20). The strength and conditioning professional must be found to have had a duty to act and to have failed to act (a breach) with the appropriate standard of care, resulting in damages (physical or economic injury) to another person because of the natural and continuous

sequence of reasonably foreseeable events (proximate cause). For example, a strength and conditioning professional sees that a cable is excessively worn on a resistance training machine and notes it, but does not post an "Out of Order" sign. An athlete uses the machine and incurs an injury. In this case, the strength and conditioning professional could be found negligent: His or her duty was to fix the cable or post a sign, but he or she failed to act, and an athlete sustained an injury because of the potentially injurious situation of a cable that was ready to break.

Assumption of risk—Knowing that an inherent risk exists with participation in an activity and voluntarily deciding to participate anyway (11). All athletic activities, including strength and conditioning, involve a certain level of risk; athletes must be thoroughly informed of the risk and should sign a statement to that effect.

Preparticipation Screening and Medical Clearance

Before an athlete is allowed access to the strength and conditioning facility, preparticipation screening and clearance in accordance with relevant governing bodies (e.g., NCAA, institution sports medicine staff, and high school athletic associations) are required. This requirement is established under Section 1 of *Strength and Conditioning Professional Standards and Guidelines* (20). Standard 1.1 "requires participants to undergo health care provider screening and clearance before participation." The strength and conditioning professional does not need an actual copy of the physical examination but should require a signed statement to show proof of medical clearance to participate. Athletes who are returning from an injury or illness or who have special needs (e.g., have diabetes, asthma, epilepsy, hypertension) should also be required to show proof of medical clearance before beginning or returning to a strength and conditioning program.

Procedures should therefore be in place to ensure that documentation confirming that each athlete was screened and cleared to participate by the sports medicine staff is on record in the main office of the strength and conditioning program before athletes are allowed to participate. Note, however, that it is the responsibility of the sports medicine staff (e.g., the team or program's certified athletic trainer, physician, or physical therapist) to allow an athlete to begin formal involvement in the strength and conditioning program. In the case of a school location, this applies to both athletes who are new to the school or program and athletes who are just recovering from an injury or illness. This stipulation is important because it is not in the strength and conditioning professional's

scope of practice (i.e., proper legal parameters and professional duties) to diagnose or evaluate an individual's medical or health condition. Therefore, only the sports medicine staff can provide medical clearance (and proof thereof) and answer any questions about participation.

Eligibility Criteria

To focus the attention and efforts of the strength and conditioning staff on a target training population, certain eligibility requirements should be established. The following is a list of typical individuals or groups who are allowed to use the strength and conditioning facility at an institution:

- Full- or part-time student-athletes participating in an athletic department-sponsored sport
- Newly incoming and just-transferred student-athletes who have registered for school and have confirmation of team status as designated by the head sport coach
- Students in physical education classes
- All athletic department coaching and administrative staff
- All sports medicine department staff
- Alumni athletes who participated in an athletic department–sponsored sport and completed their eligibility
- Individuals and groups approved by the athletic director or director of strength and conditioning

Other individuals or groups may request access to the strength and conditioning facility. These persons or groups must receive prior approval by the athletic director or director of strength and conditioning and should have a prearranged schedule that specifies when they will use the facility so proper supervision can be provided. To be consistent and objective, it is advantageous to have a policy in place to refer to rather than having to decide on this on a case-by-case basis. This policy is especially important as it relates to the facility fee, if any. The following are examples of common criteria by which to determine whether outside organizations can use a strength and conditioning facility:

- Use must be preapproved by the athletic director.
- Use must be preapproved by the strength and conditioning director.
- The program or session must be supervised by strength and conditioning department staff.
- The program or session must be scheduled during off-hours when athletes are not present.
- The individual or organization must supply written proof of additional liability insurance.

- All participants must sign a release agreement form. Figure 24.5 shows a sample release of liability form. Check any such form for compliance with current local and national laws before using it.
- All participants must follow the rules and regulations of the strength and conditioning facility.
- The athletic director and the strength and conditioning director have the right to limit an individual's or group's access, if warranted.

Record Keeping

Documentation is fundamental to the effective management of a strength and conditioning facility. Secure records should be kept on file of cleaning and maintenance, safety procedures, manufacturer's warranties and guidelines, assumption-of-risk or other informed consent forms, medical waivers and clearance forms, personnel credentials, professional guidelines and recommendations (e.g., use of weight belts, resistance training techniques), and injury report forms (20). Injury report forms should be maintained as long as possible in case an injury suit is filed. The time during which individuals can file a lawsuit (i.e., the **statute of limitations**) varies (from state to state in the United States as well as throughout the world), so it is a good practice to maintain files indefinitely or to check with a legal authority (12).

Liability Insurance

Because of the potential for injury in athletic participation, it is essential for strength and conditioning staff members to purchase professional liability insurance, especially if they are not covered under the facility policy. Liability insurance is a contractual promise by which the insurer promises to defend and indemnify the insured, up to the defined limits of liability, from certain defined liability risks at the insurer's cost in exchange for payment of a premium. Strength and conditioning professionals should consult their human resource manager, legal consultant, or professional organization (e.g., NSCA) for further information.

> **Insurance is a contractual promise by which the insurer promises to defend and indemnify the insured, up to the defined limits of liability, from certain defined liability risks at the insurer's cost in exchange for payment of a premium.**

Product Liability

Product liability refers to the legal responsibilities of those who manufacture or sell products if a person sustains injury or damage as a result of using the product (1).

Sample Release Agreement Form for Facility Use by an Outside Individual or Group

(School Name)

Release Agreement

I, the undersigned, do hereby acknowledge and understand that I will be using the ____(school name)____ strength and conditioning facility.

I further acknowledge that I have been advised of the risks involved in the use of the strength and conditioning facility and its equipment, and I further acknowledge that I have been warned that my use of the strength and conditioning facility and its equipment could result in injury or harm to myself.

I acknowledge and assume any such risk to my person should I use the strength and conditioning facility and its equipment.

In the event that I should sustain injury to myself as a result of my use of the strength and conditioning facility and its equipment, I hereby agree to hold harmless the _____(school name)_____ , the coaches, athletic trainers, supervisors, or any other employees.

I have read and fully understand the contents of this "hold harmless" agreement and execute same as my own voluntary act.

I agree to modify my workout to conform to the recommendations of the _____(school name)_____ strength and conditioning staff if asked to do so, and I agree to leave the strength and conditioning facility if asked to do so by a member of the _____(school name)_____ strength and conditioning staff.

Signature: _____

Date: _____

Name (printed): _____

FIGURE 24.5 All participants must sign a liability waiver, which should be modified as needed to comply with local and national laws. Reducing liability for on-premise injuries during use of the facility is critical in any risk management strategy.

Adapted from Earle 1993 (7); Epley 1998 (8).

Although strength and conditioning professionals may not manufacture or sell a product, they can be named as codefendants in product liability suits. Therefore, it is important for strength and conditioning professionals to understand the concept of product liability and actions that could place them at risk for litigation. Although product liability applies only to those who are in the business of manufacturing or selling products, there are behaviors that can void liability of the manufacturer or seller and place responsibility in the hands of the strength and conditioning professional. Two key considerations that determine whether the manufacturer or seller is liable are whether the product has been changed from the condition in which it was originally sold and whether the product is used as intended by the manufacturer (5). To avoid injury to athletes caused by strength and conditioning equipment, the following steps should be taken:

- Use equipment only for the purpose intended by the manufacturer. Refer to the manufacturer's instructional materials that accompany the equipment, including user age and size specifications.

- Be certain that equipment meets existing professional standards and guidelines. Do not purchase and use equipment that has been deemed unsafe or ineffective by professional organizations and experts. Be aware of equipment recalls, and return such equipment to the manufacturer immediately.

- Buy only from reputable manufacturers. Strength and conditioning professionals must do their homework to check on the safety record of a manufacturer or seller and any claims that may have been filed against that manufacturer or seller. Organizations such as the Better Business Bureau in the United States, other strength and conditioning colleagues, and professional organizations are good resources for this information.

- Do not modify equipment unless such adaptations are clearly designated and instructions for doing so are included in the product information. Some equipment is designed to be modified for specific needs, such as fitting, but directions for modifying the product must be followed exactly.

- Apply all warning labels that accompany a new equipment purchase. If such labels are not placed on the machine in plain view and an individual is injured (and the injury relates to what the warning label addresses), the strength and conditioning professional can be held liable.

- Continually inspect equipment for damage and wear that may place an athlete at risk for injury. To recognize potential problems, the strength and conditioning professional must understand the purpose, capabilities, and limitations of equipment and how equipment can cause injury. Always inspect newly purchased equipment before use. If new equipment arrives damaged, immediately notify the manufacturer or seller and have it replaced. If currently owned equipment becomes damaged, remove it for repair or replacement. If equipment is too large to remove or no storage space exists, affix a sign to the equipment stating that it should not be used.

- Do not allow unsupervised athletes to use equipment. Constant supervision of the athletes by the strength and conditioning professional ensures that equipment is used for its intended purpose and with proper technique (20).

Discipline

To ensure that athletes adhere to the facility rules, the strength and conditioning director may want to require them to sign and date a copy of the facility rules and guidelines to acknowledge that they understand and will adhere to all rules before facility use. This process will reduce the possibility of claims that they did not know the repercussions of aberrant behavior. The facility rules need to be enforced, with possible disciplinary actions posted, documented, and levied in proportion to the offense. The use of exercise and conditioning activities as punishment is discouraged. According to The Inter-Association Task Force for Preventing Sudden Death in Collegiate Conditioning Sessions best practice recommendations, "no additional physical burden that would increase the physical risk of injury or sudden death should be placed on the athlete under any circumstance" (p. 478). Following is an example of a tiered penalty system applied to a repeated violation (7). (Note that this type of policy must be established with full support and involvement of the athletic director and all sport coaches. Typically, the strength and conditioning staff does not have to pursue disciplinary actions past the first or second offense, because most sport coaches want to handle such a situation.)

- *First offense*: A verbal warning by a staff member, an explanation of the nature and importance of the

rule or guideline that was broken, and a reminder of the disciplinary action that will result from a second offense.

- *Second offense*: Dismissal from the facility for one day, documentation of the offense by the staff member, correspondence with the athlete's sport coach, and a reminder of the disciplinary action that will result from a third offense.

- *Third offense*: Dismissal from the facility for one week, documentation of the offense by the staff member, correspondence with the athlete's sport coach, and a reminder of the disciplinary action that will result from a fourth offense.

- *Fourth offense*: Dismissal from the facility for the remainder of the year, documentation of the offense by the staff member, correspondence with the athlete's sport coach and the athletic director, and a reminder of the disciplinary action that will result from a fifth offense.

- *Fifth offense*: Permanent dismissal from the facility, documentation of the offense by the staff member, and correspondence with the athlete's sport coach and the athletic director.

Supplements, Ergogenic Aids, and Banned Substances

Strength and conditioning professionals are commonly approached for nutrition and supplement advice. The strength and conditioning professional is expected to uphold the NSCA Code of Ethics. Standard 9.1 in *Strength and Conditioning Professional Standards and Guidelines* states:

> Strength and Conditioning professionals must not prescribe, recommend or provide drugs, controlled substances or supplements that are illegal, prohibited or harmful to participants for any purpose including enhancing athletic performance, conditioning or physique. Only those substances that are lawful and have been scientifically proven to be beneficial, or at least not harmful, may be recommended or provided to participants by Strength and Conditioning professionals, and only to individuals age 18 or above.

Rules and regulations may differ between various sport governing bodies (e.g., NCAA, United States Olympic Committee, Major League Baseball, National Basketball Association, National Football League, National Hockey League). It is the responsibility of the strength and conditioning professional to stay up to date and seek out the related rules and regulations, as well as the scientific evidence that supports or refutes the efficacy of nutritional supplements. It is recommended that strength and conditioning professionals consult with a sports nutritionist or dietitian on matters regarding nutritional supplements.

Staff Policies and Activities

Discussed here are various policies typically established and activities typically observed in a strength and conditioning facility. This information is provided for reference only; each strength and conditioning facility is unique and may have certain characteristics that dictate the specific application of these policies and activities.

Orientation Meeting

Typically, at the beginning of the school year or sport season, an orientation meeting is held for the athletes and sport coaches before their first use of the strength and conditioning facility. At this meeting the director provides the phone numbers of the facility and staff and explains the services of the staff (goals, objectives, and mission of the program), hours of operation including team training schedule, facility rules and regulations including disciplinary actions, and emergency procedures. Preparticipation and eligibility requirements should be explained. A strength training orientation should cover proper equipment use including spotting techniques when appropriate, correct exercise execution, and common risks associated with incorrect or inattentive exercise technique or spotting.

Reporting and Documentation

As discussed earlier, proper documentation and record keeping are essential to the management and monitoring of the strength and conditioning programs and facilities. In cases of emergency or incidents of injury, it is important to establish a chain of command for risk management. This may include coaches, the director of strength and conditioning, sports medicine personnel, and the athletics director. Significant efforts should be made to protect the privacy and confidentiality of participants. In compliance with federal regulatory laws such as the Health Insurance Portability and Accountability Act (HIPAA), a participant's health care information may not be released without written authorization; this includes injury reports provided by the sports medicine staff. An incident–injury report form should be completed and kept on file when an injury has occurred (19).

Additional records that should be developed and maintained and that are crucial to the operation of the strength and conditioning programs and facilities include the following (20):

- Personnel credentials
- Professional standards and guidelines
- Policies and procedures for operation and safety (written emergency plan)
- Equipment user manuals provided by the manufacturer (warranties, operating guidelines, installation, setup)
- Equipment and facility maintenance (inspection, maintenance, cleaning, and repair)
- Preparticipation medical clearance
- Return-to-participation clearance
- Protective legal documents such as informed consent, waiver of claim, personal contract
- Training logs, evaluation entries, instruction notes

Participants should complete and sign such legal documents at the annual orientation meeting.

Code of Ethics and Professionalism

A code of ethics comprises the standards and principles for which the professional will be held accountable. Most professional organizations have codes of ethics or codes of conduct that members must agree to adhere to and apply in their professional practices (17). These codes are intended to establish professionalism and high standards of ethical behavior while protecting the rights and dignity of individuals. Strength and conditioning professionals should become familiar with the NSCA Code of Ethics as well as their institution's code of ethics and student-athlete code of conduct if applicable. Athlete welfare is generally the primary focus. Bullying, hazing, and social media guidelines may also be addressed. Additionally, consider designating specific policies for appearance or dress code, telephone use, personal workouts, and personal use of company equipment, as well as standards for the coach–athlete, coach–intern, and coach–sport coach relationships and athlete conduct in the weight room (4, 18). These written principles are intended to enhance the strength and conditioning program's effectiveness while promoting high standards of integrity.

Instruction and Supervision

A qualified strength and conditioning professional must properly instruct athletes in safe and effective strength and conditioning techniques. Instruction involves teaching an athlete a skill in a safe manner and correcting the athlete if necessary. Emphasizing safety and proper technique for resistance training rather than the amount of weight lifted helps reduce the incidence of injury and therefore liability exposure. Instructional methods, procedures, and progressions that are consistent with professional guidelines and standards should be used (5).

Furthermore, direct supervision is required to achieve maximum performance, safety, and instruction. Staff members should have the ability to clearly communicate and view both the athlete and the zone being supervised (if not the entire facility). Spotting, in conjunction with the use of appropriate safety equipment, is critical (19). Staff should effectively communicate with the athlete to ensure safe, proper, and effective spotting when athletes are performing exercises in which free weights are sustained on the trunk or moved over the face and head. Principles of supervision include the following (5):

- Always be there.
- Be active and hands on.
- Be prudent, careful, and prepared.
- Be qualified.
- Be vigilant.
- Inform participants of safety and emergency procedures.
- Know participants' health status.
- Monitor and enforce rules and regulations.
- Monitor and scrutinize the environment.

Guideline 3.1 in *Strength and Conditioning Professional Standards and Guidelines* states the following:

Strength and Conditioning activities should be planned, and the requisite number of qualified staff should be available such that recommended guidelines for minimum average floor space allowed per participant (100 ft²), professional-to-participant ratios (1:10 junior high school, 1:15 high school, 1:20 college), and number of participants per barbell or training station are achieved during peak usage times. (p. 10)

Supervision was cited in an estimated 80% of court cases in which athletic injuries occurred (5). Inadequate instruction or supervision is often a main cause. All athletes should be constantly supervised, which requires the physical presence of a qualified strength and conditioning professional for overseeing all activities (12, 13, 15). To provide proper supervision, supervisor stations need to be located where a clear view of the facility and athletes is possible (19). Suggested staff-to-athlete ratios should be also be adhered to, but these can vary depending on the type of training. For instance, if a group of athletes is performing a machine circuit training workout, they do not need as much supervision as athletes who are lifting with free weights. Also, athletes with a low training age need more supervision than athletes who are experienced in the weight room.

Regarding the influence of supervision on performance, strength gains are greater in subjects training under lower supervision ratios (10). Employers and practitioners must understand the importance of staffing for safety and performance gains and, in instances in which optimal ratios are not possible for various reasons, continually work toward a goal of meeting appropriate ratios as soon as is practical.

Strength and conditioning professionals are commonly approached to attend team practices and competitions as well as to travel with the sport teams. They should be encouraged to attend as long as this does not adversely affect the facility's coach-to-athlete ratio.

> ► **The risk of injury cannot be totally eliminated but can be effectively managed by the strength and conditioning professional.**

Program Design

An effective strength and conditioning program should be based on scientific principles to enhance performance and increase injury resistance with intended outcomes specific to the sport (6). Program intensities should be within NSCA standards and guidelines. Please refer to chapters 14 to 21 and the NSCA's various position papers as resources for strength and conditioning training plan development. The director of strength and conditioning should oversee and monitor all performance training programs, including reconditioning. A copy of all programs designed by staff (i.e., the list of exercises to be performed) should be reviewed and on file in the director's office before a team begins their program (18).

Workout Sheet (Workout Card)

The process of generating a workout sheet is different for each strength and conditioning program. Strength and conditioning activities should be prearranged, and therefore athletes must have an approved workout sheet when training. Additional workouts should be approved by the overseeing strength and conditioning coach to ensure proper intensity and volume-load monitoring. Strength and conditioning staff members must be familiar with every exercise on each athlete's workout sheet and should not advise an athlete to perform exercises that are not listed on the workout sheet unless this has been suggested by the director or the sports medicine staff, which should be committed to writing as soon as possible after the session. For each exercise that is included on the sport teams' workout sheets, including plyometric, agility, and speed development drills, the director needs to inform the staff regarding how the exercise technique should be taught to athletes and also provide demonstrations and instruction. For additional supervision, practitioners may consider requiring the athletes' last set of foundational exercises to be seen by a staff member and checked off for proper execution. Establishing consistent verbiage across performance training programs is recommended.

Facility Administration

Strength and conditioning facility rules and guidelines are important for providing participants with guidance on conduct and behavior, keeping order, and keeping the program on course toward the goal of providing a safe, clean, and professional training environment. Refer to figure 24.6 for a list of common facility rules and guidelines. These should be posted in the training area where they can be easily seen.

Understand that the strength and conditioning facility is unique and that it may have certain characteristics that dictate the specific application of policies and activities. Equipment available and size of the facility or team can present the coach with a logistical challenge for scheduling and developing hours of operation. One should consider what workout format will affect the greatest number of athletes when making scheduling decisions. Particularly for small colleges or high schools, the goal is to organize the strength and conditioning program so as to allow the practitioner to work with the maximum number of athletes based on the equipment and time available while under a proper supervision ratio. In any case, the priority of a team's training time is dependent on the season they are in. In-season teams typically have priority over off-season teams, because often the training schedule revolves around the practice and game schedule. Off-season teams may have to compromise and train early in the morning if the facility cannot accommodate multiple teams at a time.

One potential solution is adopting a Monday-Wednesday-Friday format for off-season teams, which opens the facility to be used by in-season teams on Tuesday and Thursday. If Friday competitions interfere with this organization, a second scenario is scheduling some of the off-season teams on Monday-Tuesday-Thursday and some on Tuesday-Thursday-Friday. This will allow the facility to be used by in-season teams on Monday and Wednesday. Consider scheduling off-season teams during typical afternoon practice times. In-season teams can be scheduled early or late to reduce overcrowding in the facility (3).

For opening and closing procedures, policies are typically based on the daily operations, inspection, and cleaning of the strength and conditioning facility. Additionally, consider designating specific operating procedures for holidays or for the institution's academic calendar, stereo or music use, office hours, storage, and staff locker room activities. Again, these written principles are intended to enhance facility efficiency while promoting program effectiveness (19).

Emergency Planning and Response

Providing a standard of care is a shared responsibility including, but not limited to, medical personnel, sport coaches, strength and conditioning professionals, administrators, and the institution. Life safety is always the first priority when an emergency occurs. Keep in mind that an emergency, including athletic injuries, can occur anytime and anywhere during activity. Having a written response plan for environmental situations as well as life-threatening and non–life-threatening situations provides a guideline for proper procedures to be followed and practiced in case of an emergency. This **emergency action plan** is a written document that details the proper procedures for caring for injuries. All personnel in the strength and conditioning facility must know the emergency action plan and the proper procedures for dealing with emergencies.

Components of an Emergency Action Plan

The following are the typical items included or described in an emergency plan:

- EMS (emergency medical services) activation procedures
- Names and telephone numbers of primary, secondary, and tertiary individuals to contact
- Specific address of the strength and conditioning facility (to give directions to EMS)
- Locations of the telephones
- Locations of nearest exits
- Designated personnel qualified to care for injuries (i.e., sports medicine staff)
- Ambulance access
- Location of emergency supplies and first aid kit
- Plan of action in case of fire, tornado, life-threatening injury, crime, terrorism, and so forth

In addition to posting the emergency care plan in a clearly visible location, it is critical that all strength and conditioning professionals maintain current first aid and CPR certification and practice the emergency action plan at least quarterly.

Facility Rules and Guidelines

- Prior to participation, athletes must go through a preparticipation screening and clearance procedure (5).
- Prior to participation, all athletes must attend an orientation on common risks involved in resistance training, the proper execution of various exercises, and the possible consequences if proper technique is not used.
- Athletes must have a workout sheet, follow it, and record workout contents.
- If an athlete has an injury that inhibits a portion of the workout, the athlete must receive a modified program from the athletic medicine department that describes which exercises should be avoided and which ones may be substituted.
- Athletes are required to use locks on the ends of all barbells.
- No one should squat outside the squat or power rack.
- Bumper plates are required on the platforms for all power exercises.
- Athletes must not wear weight belts when the belts could contact equipment upholstery.
- Athletes should move weights from the racks to the bar only. They should never set plates on the floor or lean them against equipment or walls. Athletes should return dumbbells to the rack in the proper order. Athletes should not drop or throw weights or dumbbells.
- Athletes should show respect for equipment and facilities at all times; spitting in or defacing the facility is not tolerated and will result in immediate expulsion.
- The weight room requires concentration. Horseplay, loud or offensive language, or temper tantrums are not permitted.
- The staff offices and telephones are off limits to athletes unless permission to use them is given.
- Athletes should wear proper training attire, particularly shirts and athletic shoes, at all times.
- Athletes should use spotters for exercises that place the bar on the back or front shoulders and exercises that involve a bar or dumbbells moving over the face or above the head. Power exercises are not spotted.
- Athletes should immediately report any facility-related injury or facility or equipment irregularity to the supervisor on duty.
- Tobacco, food, chewing gum, glass bottles, cans, alcohol, drugs, and banned substances are not allowed in the strength and conditioning facility; plastic water bottles are acceptable.
- Supervisors are not responsible for users' personal belongings or lost or stolen items.
- Jewelry such as loose necklaces, bracelets, hanging earrings, and watches should not be worn.
- Athletes should keep feet off the walls.
- Athletes should minimize chalk and powder on the floor.
- All guests and visitors must report to the office for signing of the waiver form.
- Former athletes must have their programs preapproved by a staff supervisor and must sign a waiver form.
- Athletic department personnel can use these facilities for personal workouts if they do not interfere with the needs of the athletes.
- Non–athletic department personnel are allowed to use the facilities with permission of the athletic director after signing a waiver form. Recognized users may include athletes, students, guests, staff, faculty with permission, former athletes, family members, and visiting teams.
- Equipment leaving the weight room shall be checked out by the supervisor and recorded at the supervisor's desk.
- The on-duty supervisors have authority over all weight room conduct and use of equipment and may expel an athlete from the facility for failure to follow instructions.

FIGURE 24.6 A list of rules and policies should be posted in the training area where it can be easily seen.

Adapted from Earle 1993 (7); Epley, *Flight manual*, 1998 (8); Epley, *Make the play*, 1998 (9).

Emergency Personnel

Working collaboratively, establish a plan that allows for and determines the need for appropriate medical coverage to be in place. The emergency plan should include immediate access to or planned access to a physician for assessment of the circumstance in a timely manner. As a potential first responder, the strength and conditioning professional and any personnel associated with practices, skill instruction, and strength and conditioning should acquire and maintain a professional certification including standard first aid, CPR, and AED (6, 20).

Emergency Communication

Establish a direct line of communication and formulate a backup plan. Immediate communication is crucial to quick delivery of emergency care. Access to a telephone (land line or cellular) is a viable option if medical personnel are not on site. Ensure that participants in the strength and conditioning program and the overseeing supervisors know the location of the closest workable telephone, whether it is inside or outside (6, 20).

Emergency Equipment

Emergency equipment should be readily available in an emergency situation. Maintaining professional certifications for standard first aid, CPR, and AED means that personnel have been trained in advance on proper use. First responders should periodically rehearse. Additionally, emergency information for participants should be readily available for access by medical personnel (20).

Roles Within the Emergency Team

It is recommended that professionals develop an emergency plan specific to their own setting. Table 24.2 shows an example of an emergency procedures plan. An emergency plan should list strategies for handling emergency situations and provide names, titles, and telephone numbers of important individuals to contact as part of the emergency team. Each individual may have a different role, but understanding the roles allows the emergency team to function effectively.

Within the emergency team, four principal roles exist. The first is to provide immediate care of the athletes, as time is the most critical factor in emergency situations. The second involves emergency equipment retrieval, as users of the facility should be made aware of the types and locations of emergency equipment before participation. Next is the activation of the emergency medical system (EMS). Again, establish a method for a direct line of communication in cases in which emergency transportation is not already on site. Finally, the individual making the call should have been familiarized with the facility location during the orientation meeting. This will make it easier to direct EMS to the scene. Establish a cleared route and a direct line for transportation for quick entering and exiting of the facility.

Conclusion

Program goals give a strength and conditioning program direction and purpose, and program objectives help keep the program on task by providing steps toward these goals. Based on these goals and objectives, policies and

TABLE 24.2   Sample Emergency Procedures Protocol

FIRE
Step 1: Activate fire alarm
Step 2: Evacuate the building

Life-threatening situations	Environmental situations	Non–life-threatening situations
Step 1: call 911.	**Step 1:** Activate the appropriate alarm and get everyone directed to a predetermined safe location.	**Step 1:** Provide first aid.
Step 2: Do not move victim.	**Step 2:** Call 911 for medical help if necessary.	**Step 2:** Call 911 for medical help if necessary.
Step 3: If victim is conscious, ask permission to administer first aid.	**Step 3:** Account for all parties and notify rescue personnel.	**Step 3:** Activate the emergency communication plan to notify appropriate parties.
Step 4: Administer CPR or AED if necessary.	**Step 4:** Activate the emergency communication plan to notify appropriate parties.	**Step 4:** Document incident on injury report.
Step 5: Stay with victim until help arrives.	**Step 5:** Document incident on injury report.	
Step 6: Activate the emergency communication plan to notify appropriate parties.		
Step 7: Document incident on injury report.		

Adapted, by permission, from NSCA, 2011 (18).

procedures are developed to guide participant and staff conduct and to ensure a safe training environment. If appropriate documentation regarding the strength and conditioning facility is not properly collected and its equipment is not properly maintained, legal liability for injuries can occur. Claims of negligence may be made if injuries occur and appropriate precautions were not taken. Strength and conditioning professionals have a variety of responsibilities in the day-to-day operation of a strength and conditioning facility, including an awareness of the proper function and repair of all equipment to reduce the possibility of product liability. To provide direction to athletes and the strength and conditioning staff and to minimize the likelihood of litigation, each facility should have its own unique policies and procedures manual, with guidelines included for each topic covered in this chapter.

KEY TERMS

assumption of risk
breach of duty
damages
duty
emergency action plan
informed consent
liability

litigation
mission statement
negligence
policies
procedures
product liability
program goals

program objectives
proximate cause
risk management
scope of practice
standard of care
statute of limitations

STUDY QUESTIONS

1. What is the recommended coach-to-participant ratio during peak weight room usage time in a collegiate setting?
   a. 1:10
   b. 1:15
   c. 1:20
   d. 1:25

2. Which of the following individuals is responsible for allowing an athlete to begin formal involvement in a strength and conditioning program?
   a. athletic director
   b. athlete's parent or guardian
   c. team's certified athletic trainer
   d. strength and conditioning professional

3. Proper documentation is essential to the strength and conditioning facility. Which of the following is NOT part of the records that should be kept on file in the strength and conditioning facility?
   a. manufacturer's user's manual
   b. participant training logs
   c. written emergency plan
   d. medical health history

4. The strength and conditioning professional's knowledge and skill development includes competencies in all of the following EXCEPT
   a. exercise and sport science
   b. administration and management
   c. finance and appraisal
   d. teaching and coaching

5. Which of the following is NOT a component of an emergency plan?
   a. emergency medicine
   b. emergency communication
   c. emergency equipment
   d. emergency personnel

ANSWERS TO STUDY QUESTIONS

Chapter 1
1. b, 2. a, 3. b, 4. b, 5. b

Chapter 2
1. c, 2. d, 3. a, 4. a, 5. c

Chapter 3
1. b, 2. a, 3. a, 4. c, 5. d

Chapter 4
1. d, 2. a, 3. b, 4. b, 5. a

Chapter 5
1. d, 2. a, 3. c, 4. b, 5. c, 6. d

Chapter 6
1. d, 2. d, 3. d, 4. a, 5. c

Chapter 7
1. d, 2. a, 3. c, 4. d, 5. b

Chapter 8
1. a, 2. d, 3. b, 4. b, 5. c

Chapter 9
1. a, 2. b, 3. d, 4. c

Chapter 10
1. b, 2. a, 3. c, 4. c

Chapter 11
1. b, 2. d, 3. b, 4. c, 5. a

Chapter 12
1. a, 2. c, 3. b, 4. d, 5. b

Chapter 13
1. b, 2. c, 3. a, 4. c, 5. b

Chapter 14
1. c, 2. d, 3. c, 4. c, 5. a

Chapter 15
1. d, 2. b, 3. c, 4. b, 5. b

Chapter 16
1. b, 2. a, 3. b, 4. a, 5. c

Chapter 17
1. a, 2. c, 3. b, 4. a, 5. d

Chapter 18
1. d, 2. b, 3. c, 4. c, 5. a

Chapter 19
1. d, 2. c, 3. a, 4. c, 5. b

Chapter 20
1. c, 2. a, 3. b, 4. c, 5. d

Chapter 21
1. b, 2. c, 3. c, 4. b, 5. a

Chapter 22
1. c, 2. b, 3. b, 4. a, 5. d

Chapter 23
1. d, 2. a, 3. c, 4. d, 5. c

Chapter 24
1. c, 2. c, 3. d, 4. c, 5. a

REFERENCES

CHAPTER 1 Structure and Function of Body Systems

1. Billeter, R, and Hoppeler, H. Muscular basis of strength. In *The Encyclopaedia of Sports Medicine: Strength and Power in Sport.* 2nd ed. Komi, PV, ed. Oxford: Blackwell Science, 50-72, 2003.

2. Castro, MJ, Apple, DF, Staron, RS, Campos, GER, and Dudley, GA. Influence of complete spinal cord injury on skeletal muscle within six months of injury. *J Appl Physiol* 86:350-358, 1999.

3. Castro, MJ, Kent-Braun, JA, Ng, AV, Miller, RG, and Dudley, GA. Fiber-type specific Ca²⁺ actomyosin ATPase activity in multiple sclerosis. *Muscle Nerve* 21:547-549, 1998.

4. Dudley, GA, Czerkawski, J, Meinrod, A, Gillis, G, Baldwin, A, and Scarpone, M. Efficacy of naproxen sodium for exercise-induced dysfunction, muscle injury and soreness. *Clin J Sport Med* 7:3-10, 1997.

5. Dudley, GA, Harris, RT, Duvoisin, MR, Hather, BM, and Buchanan, P. Effect of voluntary versus artificial activation on the relation of muscle torque to speed. *J Appl Physiol* 69:2215-2221, 1990.

6. Harris, RT, and Dudley, GA. Factors limiting force during slow, shortening muscle actions in vivo. *Acta Physiol Scand* 152:63-71, 1994.

7. Hather, BM, Tesch, PA, Buchanan, P, and Dudley, GA. Influence of eccentric actions on skeletal muscle adaptations to resistance. *Acta Physiol Scand* 143:177-185, 1991.

8. Hunter, GR, Bamman, MM, Larson-Meyer, DE, Joanisse, DR, McCarthy, JP, Blaudeau, TE, and Newcomer, BR. Inverse relationship between exercise economy and oxidative capacity in muscle. *Eur J Appl Physiol* 94:558-568, 2005.

9. Kent-Braun, JA, Ng, AV, Castro, MJ, Weiner, MW, Dudley, GA, and Miller, RG. Strength, skeletal muscle size and enzyme activity in multiple sclerosis. *J Appl Physiol* 83:1998-2004, 1997.

10. Klug, GA, and Tibbits, GF. The effect of activity on calcium mediated events in striated muscle. In *Exercise and Sport Science Reviews.* Pandolf, KB, ed. New York: Macmillan, 1-60, 1988.

11. Mudd, LM, Fornetti, W, and Pivarnik, JM. Bone mineral density in collegiate female athletes: Comparisons among sports. *J Athl Train* 42:403-408, 2007.

12. Ploutz, LL, Biro, RL, Tesch, PA, and Dudley, GA. Effect of resistance training on muscle mass involvement in exercise. *J Appl Physiol* 76:1675-1681, 1994.

13. Tortora, GJ, and Derrickson, B. *Principles of Anatomy and Physiology.* Hoboken, NJ: Wiley, 259, 292-304, 692-699, 704-711, 730-737, 849-852, 857-860, 865-866, 2014.

CHAPTER 2 Biomechanics of Resistance Exercise

1. Almond, LM, Hamid, NA, and Wasserberg, J. Thoracic intradural disc herniation. *Br J Neurosurg* 21:32-34, 2007.

2. Anderson, CK, and Chaffin, DB. A biomechanical evaluation of five lifting techniques. *Appl Ergon* 17:2-8, 1986.

3. Bartelink, DL. The role of abdominal pressure in relieving the pressure on the lumbar intervertebral discs. *J Bone Joint Surg Br* 39-B:718-725, 1957.

4. Chou, LW, Kesar, TM, and Binder-Macleod, SA. Using customized rate-coding and recruitment strategies to maintain forces during repetitive activation of human muscles. *Phys Ther* 88:363-375, 2008.

5. Cleather, DJ. Adjusting powerlifting performances for differences in body mass. *J Strength Cond Res* 20:412-421, 2006.

6. Cormie, P, McCaulley, GO, Triplett, NT, and McBride, JM. Optimal loading for maximal power output during lower-body resistance exercises. *Med Sci Sports Exerc* 39:340-349, 2007.

7. Dolan, P, and Adams, MA. Recent advances in lumbar spinal mechanics and their significance for modelling. *Clin Biomech* 16 Suppl 1:S8-S16, 2001.

8. Ellenbecker, TS, Reinold, M, and Nelson, CO. Clinical concepts for treatment of the elbow in the adolescent overhead athlete. *Clin Sports Med* 29:705-724, 2010.

9. Folland, J, and Morris, B. Variable-cam resistance training machines: Do they match the angle-torque relationship in humans? *J Sports Sci* 26:163-169, 2008.

10. Frey-Law, LA, Laake, A, Avin, KG, Heitsman, J, Marler, T, and Abdel-Malek, K. Knee and elbow 3D strength surfaces: Peak torque-angle-velocity relationships. *J Appl Biomech* 28:726-737, 2012.

11. Funato, K, Kanehisa, H, and Fukunaga, T. Differences in muscle cross-sectional area and strength between elite senior and college Olympic weight lifters. *J Sports Med Phys Fitness* 40:312-318, 2000.

12. Gowitzke, BA, and Milner, M. *Scientific Bases of Human Movement.* Baltimore: Williams & Wilkins, 1988.

13. Gray, M, Di Brezzo, R, and Fort, IL. The effects of power and strength training on bone mineral density in premenopausal women. *J Sports Med Phys Fitness* 53:428-436, 2013.

14. Greenland, KO, Merryweather, AS, and Bloswick, DS. Prediction of peak back compressive forces as a function of lifting speed and compressive forces at lift origin and destination—a pilot study. *Saf Health Work* 2:236-242, 2011.

15. Hackett, DA, and Chow, CM. The Valsalva maneuver: Its effect on intra-abdominal pressure and safety issues during resistance exercise. *J Strength Cond Res* 27:2338-2345, 2013.

16. Harman, EA, Johnson, M, and Frykman, PN. A movement-oriented approach to exercise prescription. *NSCA J* 14:47-54, 1992.

17. Harman, EA, Rosenstein, RM, Frykman, PN, and Nigro, GA. Effects of a belt on intra-abdominal pressure during weight lifting. *Med Sci Sports Exerc* 21:186-190, 1989.

18. Hartmann, H, Wirth, K, and Klusemann, M. Analysis of the load on the knee joint and vertebral column with changes in squatting depth and weight load. *Sports Med* 43:993-1008, 2013.

19. Hill, TL, and White, GM. On the sliding-filament model of muscular contraction, IV. Calculation of force-velocity curves. *Proc Natl Acad Sci U S A* 61:889-896, 1968.

20. Ichinose, Y, Kanehisa, H, Ito, M, Kawakami, Y, and Fukunaga, T. Relationship between muscle fiber pennation and force generation capability in Olympic athletes. *Int J Sports Med* 19:541-546, 1998.

21. Ikegawa, S, Funato, K, Tsunoda, N, Kanehisa, H, Fukunaga, T, and Kawakami, Y. Muscle force per cross-sectional area is inversely related with pennation angle in strength trained athletes. *J Strength Cond Res* 22:128-131, 2008.

22. Jenkins, NH, and Mintowt-Czyz, WJ. Bilateral fracture-separations of the distal radial epiphyses during weight-lifting. *Br J Sports Med* 20:72-73, 1986.

23. Jorgensen, K. Force-velocity relationship in human elbow flexors and extensors. In *Biomechanics A-V.* PV Komi, ed. Baltimore: University Park Press, 1976.

24. Kahrizi, S, Parnianpour, M, Firoozabadi, SM, Kasemnejad, A, and Karimi, E. Evaluation of spinal internal loads and lumbar curvature under holding static load at different trunk and knee positions. *Pak J Biol Sci* 10:1036-1043, 2007.

25. Kanehisa, H, and Fukunaga, T. Velocity associated characteristics of force production in college weight lifters. *Br J Sports Med* 33:113-116, 1999.

26. Lake, JP, Carden, PJ, and Shorter, KA. Wearing knee wraps affects mechanical output and performance characteristics of back squat exercise. *J Strength Cond Res* 26:2844-2849, 2012.

27. Lander, JE, Bates, BT, Sawhill, JA, and Hamill, J. A comparison between free-weight and isokinetic bench pressing. *Med Sci Sports Exerc* 17:344-353, 1985.

28. Lander, JE, Simonton, RL, and Giacobbe, JK. The effectiveness of weight-belts during the squat exercise. *Med Sci Sports Exerc* 22:117-126, 1990.

29. Maffulli, N, and Bruns, W. Injuries in young athletes. *Eur J Pediatr* 159:59-63, 2000.

30. Mandell, PJ, Weitz, E, Bernstein, JI, Lipton, MH, Morris, J, Bradshaw, D, Bodkin, KP, and Mattmiller, B. Isokinetic trunk strength and lifting strength measures. Differences and similarities between low-back-injured and noninjured workers. *Spine* 18:2491-2501, 1993.

31. Maughan, RJ, Watson, JS, and Weir, J. Muscle strength and cross-sectional area in man: A comparison of strength-trained and untrained subjects. *Br J Sports Med* 18:149-157, 1984.

32. Milone, MT, Bernstein, J, Freedman, KB, and Tjoumakaris, F. There is no need to avoid resistance training (weight lifting) until physeal closure. *Phys Sportsmed* 41:101-105, 2013.

33. Moritani, T, and deVries, HA. Neural factors versus hypertrophy in the time course of muscle strength gain. *Am J Phys Med* 58:115-130, 1979.

34. Perrine, JJ, and Edgerton, VR. Muscle force-velocity and power-velocity relationships under isokinetic loading. *Med Sci Sports* 10:159-166, 1978.

35. Pierson, EH, Bantum, BM, and Schaefer, MP. Exertional rhabdomyolysis of the elbow flexor muscles from weight lifting. *Phys Med Rehabil* 6:556-559, 2014.

36. Raske, A, and Norlin, R. Injury incidence and prevalence among elite weight and power lifters. *Am J Sports Med* 30:248-256, 2002.

37. Reynolds, KL, Harman, EA, Worsham, RE, Sykes, MB, Frykman, PN, and Backus, VL. Injuries in women associated with a periodized strength training and running program. *J Strength Cond Res* 15:136-143, 2001.

38. Rokito, AS, and Lofin, I. Simultaneous bilateral distal biceps tendon rupture during a preacher curl exercise: A case report. *Bull NYU Hosp Jt Dis* 66:68-71, 2008.

39. Rutherford, OM, and Jones, DA. Measurement of fibre pennation using ultrasound in the human quadriceps in vivo. *Eur J Appl Physiol Occup Physiol* 65:433-437, 1992.

40. Scott, SH, and Winter, DA. A comparison of three muscle pennation assumptions and their effect on isometric and isotonic force. *J Biomech* 24:163-167, 1991.

41. Siewe, J, Rudat, J, Rollinghoff, M, Schlegel, UJ, Eysel, P, and Michael, JW. Injuries and overuse syndromes in powerlifting. *Int J Sports Med* 32:703-711, 2011.

42. Stone, MH, Sanborn, K, O'Bryant, HS, Hartman, M, Stone, ME, Proulx, C, Ward, B, and Hruby, J. Maximum strength-power-performance relationships in collegiate throwers. *J Strength Cond Res* 17:739-745, 2003.

43. Toji, H, and Kaneko, M. Effect of multiple-load training on the force-velocity relationship. *J Strength Cond Res* 18:792-795, 2004.

44. Zemper, ED. Four-year study of weight room injuries in a national sample of college football teams. *NSCA J* 12:32-34, 1990.

CHAPTER 3   Bioenergetics of Exercise and Training

1. Adeva-Andany, M, Lopez-Ojen, M, Funcasta-Calderon, R, Ameneiros-Rodriguez, E, Donapetry-Garcia, C, Vila-Altesor, M, and Rodriguez-Seijas, J. Comprehensive review on lactate metabolism in human health. *Mitochondrion* 17:76-100, 2014.

2. Ahlborg, G, and Felig, P. Influence of glucose ingestion on fuel-hormone response during prolonged exercise. *J Appl Physiol* 41:683-688, 1976.

3. Ahlborg, G, and Felig, P. Lactate and glucose exchange across the forearm, legs, and splanchnic bed during and after prolonged leg exercise. *J Clin Invest* 69:45-54, 1982.

4. Allen, DG, Lamb, GD, and Westerblad, H. Skeletal muscle fatigue: Cellular mechanisms. *Physiol Rev* 88:287-332, 2008.

5. Allen, DG, and Westerblad, H. Role of phosphate and calcium stores in muscle fatigue. *J Physiol* 536:657-665, 2001.

6. Altenburg, TM, Degens, H, van Mechelen, W, Sargeant, AJ, and de Haan, A. Recruitment of single muscle fibers during submaximal cycling exercise. *J Appl Physiol* 103:1752-1756, 2007.

7. Åstrand, P, Rodahl, K, Dahl, HA, and Stromme, SB. *Textbook of Work Physiology: Physiological Bases of Exercise.* Champaign, IL: Human Kinetics, 12-17, 2003.

8. Baker, JS, Thomas, N, Cooper, SM, Davies, B, and Robergs, RA. Exercise duration and blood lactate concentrations following high intensity cycle ergometry. *Res Sports Med* 20:129-141, 2012.

9. Barany, M, and Arus, C. Lactic acid production in intact muscle, as followed by ^{13}C and ^{1}H nuclear magnetic resonance. In *Human Muscle Power.* Jones, NL, McCartney, N, and McComas, AJ, eds. Champaign, IL: Human Kinetics, 153-164, 1986.

10. Barnard, RJ, Edgerton, VR, Furukawa, T, and Peter, JB. Histochemical, biochemical, and contractile properties of red, white, and intermediate fibers. *Am J Physiol* 220:410-414, 1971.

11. Barnett, C, Carey, M, Proietto, J, Cerin, E, Febbraio, MA, and Jenkins, D. Muscle metabolism during sprint exercise in man: Influence of sprint training. *J Sci Med Sport* 7:314-322, 2004.

12. Bastien, C, and Sanchez, J. Phosphagens and glycogen content in skeletal muscle after treadmill training in young and old rats. *Eur J Appl Physiol Occup Physiol* 52:291-295, 1984.

13. Berg, WE. Individual differences in respiratory gas exchange during recovery from moderate exercise. *Am J Physiol* 149:597-610, 1947.

14. Bogdanis, GC, Nevill, ME, Boobis, LH, and Lakomy, HK. Contribution of phosphocreatine and aerobic metabolism to energy supply during repeated sprint exercise. *J Appl Physiol* 80:876-884, 1996.

15. Bogdanis, GC, Nevill, ME, Boobis, LH, Lakomy, HK, and Nevill, AM. Recovery of power output and muscle metabolites following 30 s of maximal sprint cycling in man. *J Physiol* 482 (Pt 2):467-480, 1995.

16. Boobis, I, Williams, C, and Wooten, SN. Influence of sprint training on muscle metabolism during brief maximal exercise. *J Physiol* 342:36-37, 1983.

17. Borsheim, E, and Bahr, R. Effect of exercise intensity, duration and mode on post-exercise oxygen consumption. *Sports Med* 33:1037-1060, 2003.

18. Bridges, CR, Jr., Clark, BJ, 3rd, Hammond, RL, and Stephenson, LW. Skeletal muscle bioenergetics during frequency-dependent fatigue. *Am J Physiol* 260:C643-C651, 1991.

19. Brooks, GA. The lactate shuttle during exercise and recovery. *Med Sci Sports Exerc* 18:360-368, 1986.

20. Brooks, GA. Amino acid and protein metabolism during exercise and recovery. *Med Sci Sports Exerc* 19:S150-S156, 1987.

21. Brooks, GA, Brauner, KE, and Cassens, RG. Glycogen synthesis and metabolism of lactic acid after exercise. *Am J Physiol* 224:1162-1166, 1973.

22. Brooks, GA, Fahey, TD, and Baldwin, KM. *Exercise Physiology: Human Bioenergetics and Its Applications.* New York: McGraw-Hill, 102-108, 2005.

23. Buchheit, M, and Laursen, PB. High-intensity interval training, solutions to the programming puzzle: Part I: Cardiopulmonary emphasis. *Sports Med* 43:313-338, 2013.

24. Buchheit, M, and Laursen, PB. High-intensity interval training, solutions to the programming puzzle. Part II: Anaerobic energy, neuromuscular load and practical applications. *Sports Med* 43:927-954, 2013.

25. Burgomaster, KA, Heigenhauser, GJ, and Gibala, MJ. Effect of short-term sprint interval training on human skeletal muscle carbohydrate metabolism during exercise and time-trial performance. *J Appl Physiol* 100:2041-2047, 2006.

26. Burgomaster, KA, Hughes, SC, Heigenhauser, GJ, Bradwell, SN, and Gibala, MJ. Six sessions of sprint interval training increases muscle oxidative potential and cycle endurance capacity in humans. *Eur J Appl Physiol Occup Physiol* 98:1985-1990, 2005.

27. Busa, WB, and Nuccitelli, R. Metabolic regulation via intracellular pH. *Am J Physiol* 246:R409-R438, 1984.

28. Carling, D. AMP-activated protein kinase: Balancing the scales. *Biochimie* 87:87-91, 2005.

29. Cerretelli, P, Ambrosoli, G, and Fumagalli, M. Anaerobic recovery in man. *Eur J Appl Physiol Occup Physiol* 34:141-148, 1975.

30. Cerretelli, P, Rennie, D, and Pendergast, D. Kinetics of metabolic transients during exercise. *Int J Sports Med* 55:178-180, 1980.

31. Christensen, EH, Hedman, R, and Saltin, B. Intermittent and continuous running (A further contribution to the physiology of intermittent work). *Acta Physiol Scand* 50:269-286, 1960.

32. Coggan, AR, and Coyle, EF. Reversal of fatigue during prolonged exercise by carbohydrate infusion or ingestion. *J Appl Physiol* 63:2388-2395, 1987.

33. Constable, SH, Favier, RJ, McLane, JA, Fell, RD, Chen, M, and Holloszy, JO. Energy metabolism in contracting rat skeletal muscle: Adaptation to exercise training. *Am J Physiol* 253:C316-C322, 1987.

34. Constantin-Teodosiu, D, Greenhaff, PL, McIntyre, DB, Round, JM, and Jones, DA. Anaerobic energy production in human skeletal muscle in intense contraction: A comparison of 31P magnetic resonance spectroscopy and biochemical techniques. *Exp Physiol* 82:593-601, 1997.

35. Coyle, EF, Hagberg, JM, Hurley, BF, Martin, WH, Ehsani, AA, and Holloszy, JO. Carbohydrate feeding during prolonged strenuous exercise can delay fatigue. *J Appl Physiol Respir Environ Exerc Physiol* 55:230-235, 1983.

36. Craig, BW, Lucas, J, Pohlman, R, and Stelling, H. The effects of running, weightlifting and a combination of both on growth hormone release. *J Appl Sport Sci Res* 5:198-203, 1991.

37. Cramer, JT. Creatine supplementation in endurance sports. In *Essentials of Creatine in Sports and Health.* Stout, JR, Antonio, J, and Kalman, D, eds. Totowa, NJ: Humana, 45-100, 2008.

38. Creer, AR, Ricard, MD, Conlee, RK, Hoyt, GL, and Parcell, AC. Neural, metabolic, and performance adaptations to four weeks of high intensity sprint-interval training in trained cyclists. *Int J Sports Med* 25:92-98, 2004.

39. Davis, JA, Frank, MH, Whipp, BJ, and Wasserman, K. Anaerobic threshold alterations caused by endurance training in middle-aged men. *J Appl Physiol Respir Environ Exerc Physiol* 46:1039-1046, 1979.

40. di Prampero, PE, Peeters, L, and Margaria, R. Alactic O_2 debt and lactic acid production after exhausting exercise in man. *J Appl Physiol* 34:628-632, 1973.

41. Dohm, GL, Williams, RT, Kasperek, GJ, and Vanrij, AM. Increased excretion of urea and N-tau-methylhistidine by rats and humans after a bout of exercise. *J Appl Physiol* 52:27-33, 1982.

42. Donaldson, SK, Hermansen, L, and Bolles, L. Differential, direct effects of H^+ on Ca^{2+}-activated force of skinned fibers from the soleus, cardiac and adductor magnus muscles of rabbits. *Eur J Appl Physiol* 376:55-65, 1978.

43. Donovan, CM, and Brooks, GA. Endurance training affects lactate clearance, not lactate production. *Am J Physiol* 244:E83-E92, 1983.

44. Dudley, GA, and Djamil, R. Incompatibility of endurance- and strength-training modes of exercise. *J Appl Physiol* 59:1446-1451, 1985.

45. Dudley, GA, and Murray, TF. Energy for sport. *NSCA J* 3:14-15, 1982.

46. Dudley, GA, and Terjung, RL. Influence of aerobic metabolism on IMP accumulation in fast-twitch muscle. *Am J Physiol* 248:C37-C42, 1985.

47. Dufaux, B, Assmann, G, and Hollmann, W. Plasma lipoproteins and physical activity: A review. *Int J Sports Med* 3:123-136, 1982.

48. Edington, DW, and Edgerton, VR. *The Biology of Physical Activity.* Boston: Houghton Mifflin, 35-46, 1976.

49. Eriksson, BO, Gollnick, PD, and Saltin, B. Muscle metabolism and enzyme activities after training in boys 11-13 years old. *Acta Physiol Scand* 87:485-497, 1973.

50. Essen, B. Glycogen depletion of different fibre types in human skeletal muscle during intermittent and continuous exercise. *Acta Physiol Scand* 103:446-455, 1978.

51. Fabiato, A, and Fabiato, F. Effects of pH on the myofilaments and the sarcoplasmic reticulum of skinned cells from cardiac and skeletal muscles. *J Physiol* 276:233-255, 1978.

52. Farrell, PA, Wilmore, JH, Coyle, EF, Billing, JE, and Costill, DL. Plasma lactate accumulation and distance running performance. *Med Sci Sports* 11:338-344, 1979.

53. Fitts, RH. The cross-bridge cycle and skeletal muscle fatigue. *J Appl Physiol* 104:551-558, 2008.

54. Fleck, SJ, and Kraemer, WJ. *Designing Resistance Training Programs.* Champaign, IL: Human Kinetics, 65-73, 2003.

55. Freund, H, and Gendry, P. Lactate kinetics after short strenuous exercise in man. *Eur J Appl Physiol Occup Physiol* 39:123-135, 1978.

56. Friedman, JE, Neufer, PD, and Dohm, GL. Regulation of glycogen resynthesis following exercise: Dietary considerations. *Sports Med* 11:232-243, 1991.

57. Fuchs, F, Reddy, Y, and Briggs, FN. The interaction of cations with the calcium-binding site of troponin. *Biochim Biophys Acta* 221:407-409, 1970.

58. Gaesser, GA, and Brooks, GA. Metabolic bases of excess post-exercise oxygen consumption: A review. *Med Sci Sports Exerc* 16:29-43, 1984.

59. Ganong, WF. *Review of Medical Physiology.* New York: McGraw-Hill Medical, 8-10, 2005.

60. Garrett, R, and Grisham, C. *Biochemistry.* Belmont, CA: Brooks/Cole, 536, 2012.

61. Garrett, R, and Grisham, CM. *Biochemistry.* Fort Worth, TX: Saunders College, 618-619, 1999.

62. Gastin, PB. Energy system interaction and relative contribution during maximal exercise. *Sports Med* 31:725-741, 2001.

63. Gibala, MJ, Little, JP, van Essen, M, Wilkin, GP, Burgomaster, KA, Safdar, A, Raha, S, and Tarnopolsky, MA. Short-term sprint interval versus traditional endurance training: Similar initial adaptations in human skeletal muscle and exercise performance. *J Physiol* 575:901-911, 2006.

64. Gollnick, PD, Armstrong, RB, Saltin, B, Saubert, CW, Sembrowich, WL, and Shepherd, RE. Effect of training on enzyme activity and fiber composition of human skeletal muscle. *J Appl Physiol* 34:107-111, 1973.

65. Gollnick, PD, Armstrong, RB, Saubert, CW, Piehl, K, and Saltin, B. Enzyme activity and fiber composition in skeletal muscle of untrained and trained men. *J Appl Physiol* 33:312-319, 1972.

66. Gollnick, PD, and Bayly, WM. Biochemical training adaptations and maximal power. In *Human Muscle Power.* Jones, NL, McCartney, N, and McComas, AJ, eds. Champaign, IL: Human Kinetics, 255-267, 1986.

67. Gollnick, PD, Bayly, WM, and Hodgson, DR. Exercise intensity, training, diet, and lactate concentration in muscle and blood. *Med Sci Sports Exerc* 18:334-340, 1986.

68. Gollnick, PD, and Saltin, B. Significance of skeletal muscle oxidative enzyme enhancement with endurance training. *Clin Physiol* 2:1-12, 1982.

69. Graham, TE, Rush, JWE, and MacLean, DA. Skeletal muscle oxidative enzyme enhancement with endurance training. In *Exercise Metabolism.* Hargreaves, M, and Spriet, LL, eds. Champaign, IL: Human Kinetics, 41-72, 2006.

70. Grassi, B. Delayed metabolic activation of oxidative phosphorylation in skeletal muscle at exercise onset. *Med Sci Sports Exerc* 37:1567-1573, 2005.

71. Green, HJ, Duhamel, TA, Holloway, GP, Moule, J, Ouyang, J, Ranney, D, and Tupling, AR. Muscle metabolic responses during 16 hours of intermittent heavy exercise. *Can J Physiol Pharm* 85:634-645, 2007.

72. Greenwood, JD, Moses, GE, Bernardino, FM, Gaesser, GA, and Weltman, A. Intensity of exercise recovery, blood lactate disappearance, and subsequent swimming performance. *J Sports Sci* 26:29-34, 2008.

73. Häkkinen, K, Alen, M, Kraemer, WJ, Gorostiaga, E, Izquierdo, M, Rusko, H, Mikkola, J, Häkkinen, A, Valkeinen, H, Kaarakainen, E, Romu, S, Erola, V, Ahtiainen, J, and Paavolainen, L. Neuromuscular adaptations during concurrent strength and endurance training versus strength training. *Eur J Appl Physiol* 89:42-52, 2003.

74. Häkkinen, K, and Myllyla, E. Acute effects of muscle fatigue and recovery on force production and relaxation in endurance, power and strength athletes. *J Sports Med Phys Fitness* 30:5-12, 1990.

75. Harris, RC, Edwards, RH, Hultman, E, Nordesjo, LO, Nylind, B, and Sahlin, K. The time course of phosphorylcreatine resynthesis during recovery of the quadriceps muscle in man. *Eur J Appl Physiol* 367:137-142, 1976.

76. Hedman, R. The available glycogen in man and the connection between rate of oxygen intake and carbohydrate usage. *Acta Physiol Scand* 40:305-321, 1957.

77. Henry, FM. Aerobic oxygen consumption and alactic debt in muscular work. *J Appl Physiol* 3:427-438, 1951.

78. Hermansen, L. Effect of metabolic changes on force generation in skeletal muscle during maximal exercise. *Ciba Found Symp* 82:75-88, 1981.

79. Hermansen, L, and Stensvold, I. Production and removal of lactate during exercise in man. *Acta Physiol Scand* 86:191-201, 1972.

80. Hickson, RC. Interference of strength development by simultaneously training for strength and endurance. *Eur J Appl Physiol Occup Physiol* 45:255-263, 1980.

81. Hickson, RC, Dvorak, BA, Gorostiaga, EM, Kurowski, TT, and Foster, C. Potential for strength and endurance training to amplify endurance performance. *J Appl Physiol* 65:2285-2290, 1988.

82. Hickson, RC, Rosenkoetter, MA, and Brown, MM. Strength training effects on aerobic power and short-term endurance. *Med Sci Sports Exerc* 12:336-339, 1980.

83. Hill, AV, and Lupton, H. Muscular exercise, lactic acid, and the supply and utilization of oxygen. *Q J Med* 16:135-171, 1923.

84. Hirvonen, J, Rehunen, S, Rusko, H, and Harkonen, M. Breakdown of high-energy phosphate-compounds and lactate accumulation during short supramaximal exercise. *Eur J Appl Physiol Occup Physiol* 56:253-259, 1987.

85. Housh, TJ, Housh, DJ, and DeVries, HA. *Applied Exercise & Sport Physiology with Labs.* Scottsdale, AZ: Holcomb Hathaway, 39-43, 2012.

86. Hulsmann, WC. On the regulation of the supply of substrates for muscular activity. *Bibl Nutr Dieta* 11-15, 1979.

87. Hultman, E, and Sjoholm, H. Biochemical causes of fatigue. In *Human Muscle Power.* Jones, NL, McCartney, N, and McComas, AJ, eds. Champaign, IL: Human Kinetics, 215-235, 1986.

88. Hurley, BF, Seals, DR, Hagberg, JM, Goldberg, AC, Ostrove, SM, Holloszy, JO, Wiest, WG, and Goldberg, AP. High-density-lipoprotein cholesterol in bodybuilders v. powerlifters: Negative effects of androgen use. *JAMA* 252:507-513, 1984.

89. Jacobs, I. Blood lactate. Implications for training and sports performance. *Sports Med* 3:10-25, 1986.

90. Jacobs, I, Kaiser, P, and Tesch, P. Muscle strength and fatigue after selective glycogen depletion in human skeletal muscle fibers. *Eur J Appl Physiol Occup Physiol* 46:47-53, 1981.

91. Jacobs, I, Tesch, PA, Bar-Or, O, Karlsson, J, and Dotan, R. Lactate in human skeletal muscle after 10 and 30 s of supramaximal exercise. *J Appl Physiol Respir Environ Exerc Physiol* 55:365-367, 1983.

92. Jones, NL, and Ehrsam, RE. The anaerobic threshold. *Exerc Sport Sci Rev* 10:49-83, 1982.

93. Juel, C. Intracellular pH recovery and lactate efflux in mouse soleus muscles stimulated in vitro: The involvement of sodium/proton exchange and a lactate carrier. *Acta Physiol Scand* 132:363-371, 1988.

94. Kappenstein, J, Ferrauti, A, Runkel, B, Fernandez-Fernandez, J, Muller, K, and Zange, J. Changes in phosphocreatine concentration of skeletal muscle during high-intensity intermittent exercise in children and adults. *Eur J Appl Physiol* 113:2769-2779, 2013.

95. Karatzaferi, C, de Haan, A, Ferguson, RA, van Mechelen, W, and Sargeant, AJ. Phosphocreatine and ATP content in human single muscle fibres before and after maximum dynamic exercise. *Eur J Appl Physiol* 442:467-474, 2001.

96. Karlsson, J. Lactate and phosphagen concentrations in working muscle of man with special reference to oxygen deficit at the onset of work. *Acta Physiol Scand* 358 (Suppl): 1-72, 1971.

97. Karlsson, J, Nordesjo, LO, Jorfeldt, L, and Saltin, B. Muscle lactate, ATP, and CP levels during exercise after physical training in man. *J Appl Physiol* 33:199-203, 1972.

98. Kindermann, W, Simon, G, and Keul, J. The significance of the aerobic-anaerobic transition for the determination of work load intensities during endurance training. *Eur J Appl Physiol Occup Physiol* 42:25-34, 1979.

99. Knuttgen, HG, and Komi, PV. Basic definitions for exercise. In *The Encyclopaedia of Sports Medicine: Strength and Power in Sport.* Komi, PV, ed. Oxford, Boston: Blackwell Scientific, 3-8, 1991.

100. Lanza, IR, Wigmore, DM, Befroy, DE, and Kent-Braun, JA. In vivo ATP production during free-flow and ischaemic muscle contractions in humans. *J Physiol* 577:353-367, 2006.

101. Lehmann, M, and Keul, J. Free plasma catecholamines, heart rates, lactate levels, and oxygen uptake in competition weight lifters, cyclists, and untrained control subjects. *Int J Sports Med* 7:18-21, 1986.

102. Lemon, PW, and Mullin, JP. Effect of initial muscle glycogen levels on protein catabolism during exercise. *J Appl Physiol Respir Environ Exerc Physiol* 48:624-629, 1980.

103. MacDougall, JD. Morphological changes in human skeletal muscle following strength training and immobilization. In *Human Muscle Power.* Jones, NL, McCartney, N, and McComas, AJ, eds. Champaign, IL: Human Kinetics, 269-288, 1986.

104. MacDougall, JD, Ward, GR, Sale, DG, and Sutton, JR. Biochemical adaptation of human skeletal muscle to heavy resistance training and immobilization. *J Appl Physiol Respir Environ Exerc Physiol* 43:700-703, 1977.

105. Mainwood, GW, and Renaud, JM. The effect of acid-base balance on fatigue of skeletal-muscle. *Can J Physiol Pharm* 63:403-416, 1985.

106. Mazzeo, RS, Brooks, GA, Schoeller, DA, and Budinger, TF. Disposal of blood [1-C-13] lactate in humans during rest and exercise. *J Appl Physiol* 60:232-241, 1986.

107. McArdle, WD, Katch, FI, and Katch, VL. *Exercise Physiology: Energy, Nutrition, and Human Performance.* Philadelphia: Lippincott Williams & Wilkins, 143-144, 2007.

108. McCartney, N, Spriet, LL, Heigenhauser, GJ, Kowalchuk, JM, Sutton, JR, and Jones, NL. Muscle power and metabolism in maximal intermittent exercise. *J Appl Physiol* 60:1164-1169, 1986.

109. Medbo, JI, and Burgers, S. Effect of training on the anaerobic capacity. *Med Sci Sports Exerc* 22:501-507, 1990.

110. Medbo, JI, and Tabata, I. Relative importance of aerobic and anaerobic energy release during short-lasting exhausting bicycle exercise. *J Appl Physiol* 67:1881-1886, 1989.

111. Meyer, RA, and Terjung, RL. Differences in ammonia and adenylate metabolism in contracting fast and slow muscle. *Am J Physiol* 237:C111-C118, 1979.

112. Nader, GA. Concurrent strength and endurance training: From molecules to man. *Med Sci Sports Exerc* 38:1965-1970, 2006.

113. Nakamaru, Y, and Schwartz, A. The influence of hydrogen ion concentration on calcium binding and release by skeletal muscle sarcoplasmic reticulum. *J Gen Physiol* 59:22-32, 1972.

114. Nelson, CR, Debold, EP, and Fitts, RH. Phosphate and acidosis act synergistically to depress peak power in rat muscle fibers. *Am J Physiol* 307:C939-C950, 2014.

115. Nelson, CR, and Fitts, RH. Effects of low cell pH and elevated inorganic phosphate on the pCa-force relationship in single muscle fibers at near-physiological temperatures. *Am J Physiol* 306:C670-C678, 2014.

116. Neric, FB, Beam, WC, Brown, LE, and Wiersma, LD. Comparison of swim recovery and muscle stimulation on lactate removal after sprint swimming. *J Strength Cond Res* 23:2560-2567, 2009.

117. Nicolo, A, Bazzucchi, I, Lenti, M, Haxhi, J, Scotto di Palumbo, A, and Sacchetti, M. Neuromuscular and metabolic responses to high-intensity intermittent cycling protocols with different work-to-rest ratios. *Int J Sports Physiol Perform* 9:151-160, 2014.

118. Nielsen, JJ, Mohr, M, Klarskov, C, Kristensen, M, Krustrup, P, Juel, C, and Bangsbo, J. Effects of high-intensity intermittent training on potassium kinetics and performance in human skeletal muscle. *J Physiol* 554:857-870, 2004.

119. O'Reilly, KP, Warhol, MJ, Fielding, RA, Frontera, WR, Meredith, CN, and Evans, WJ. Eccentric exercise-induced muscle damage impairs muscle glycogen repletion. *J Appl Physiol* 63:252-256, 1987.

120. Opie, LH, and Newsholme, EA. The activities of fructose 1,6-diphosphatase, phosphofructokinase and phosphoenolpyruvate carboxykinase in white muscle and red muscle. *Biochem J* 103:391-399, 1967.

121. Pike, RL, and Brown, ML. *Nutrition: An Integrated Approach.* New York: Wiley, 463-465, 1984.

122. Poortmans, JR. Protein turnover and amino acid oxidation during and after exercise. *Med Sport Sci* 17:130-147, 1984.

123. Robergs, RA, Ghiasvand, F, and Parker, D. Biochemistry of exercise-induced metabolic acidosis. *Am J Physiol* 287:R502-R516, 2004.

124. Robergs, RA, Pearson, DR, Costill, DL, Fink, WJ, Pascoe, DD, Benedict, MA, Lambert, CP, and Zachweija, JJ. Muscle glycogenolysis during differing intensities of weight-resistance exercise. *J Appl Physiol* 70:1700-1706, 1991.

125. Roberts, AD, Billeter, R, and Howald, H. Anaerobic muscle enzyme changes after interval training. *Int J Sports Med* 3:18-21, 1982.

126. Ronnestad, BR, Hansen, EA, and Raastad, T. High volume of endurance training impairs adaptations to 12 weeks of strength training in well-trained endurance athletes. *Eur J Appl Physiol* 112:1457-1466, 2012.

127. Rozenek, R, Rosenau, L, Rosenau, P, and Stone, MH. The effect of intensity on heart rate and blood lactate response to resistance exercise. *J Strength Cond Res* 7:51-54, 1993.

128. Sahlin, K, and Ren, JM. Relationship of contraction capacity to metabolic changes during recovery from a fatiguing contraction. *J Appl Physiol* 67:648-654, 1989.

129. Sahlin, K, Tonkonogi, M, and Soderlund, K. Energy supply and muscle fatigue in humans. *Acta Physiol Scand* 162:261-266, 1998.

130. Saltin, B, and Gollnick, PD. Skeletal muscle adaptability: Significance for metabolism and performance. In *Handbook of Physiology.* Peachey, LD, Adrian, RH, and Geiger, SR, eds. Baltimore: Williams & Wilkins, 540-555, 1983.

131. Saltin, B, and Karlsson, J. Muscle glycogen utilization during work of different intensities. In *Muscle Metabolism During Exercise.* Pernow, B, and Saltin, B, eds. New York: Plenum Press, 289-300, 1971.

132. Sant'Ana Pereira, JA, Sargeant, AJ, Rademaker, AC, de Haan, A, and van Mechelen, W. Myosin heavy chain isoform expression and high energy phosphate content in human muscle fibres at rest and post-exercise. *J Physiol* 496:583-588, 1996.

133. Scala, D, McMillan, J, Blessing, D, Rozenek, R, and Stone, MH. Metabolic cost of a preparatory phase of training in weightlifting: A practical observation. *J Appl Sport Sci Res* 1:48-52, 1987.

134. Sedano, S, Marin, PJ, Cuadrado, G, and Redondo, JC. Concurrent training in elite male runners: The influence of strength versus muscular endurance training on performance outcomes. *J Strength Cond Res* 27:2433-2443, 2013.

135. Sherman, WM, and Wimer, GS. Insufficient dietary carbohydrate during training: Does it impair athletic performance? *Int J Sport Nutr* 1:28-44, 1991.

136. Sjodin, B, and Jacobs, I. Onset of blood lactate accumulation and marathon running performance. *Int J Sports Med* 2:23-26, 1981.

137. Skurvydas, A, Jascaninas, J, and Zachovajevas, P. Changes in height of jump, maximal voluntary contraction force and low-frequency fatigue after 100 intermittent or continuous jumps with maximal intensity. *Acta Physiol Scand* 169:55-62, 2000.

138. Smith, SA, Montain, SJ, Matott, RP, Zientara, GP, Jolesz, FA, and Fielding, RA. Creatine supplementation and age influence muscle metabolism during exercise. *J Appl Physiol* 85:1349-1356, 1998.

139. Stainsby, WN, and Barclay, JK. Exercise metabolism: O_2 deficit, steady level O_2 uptake and O2 uptake for recovery. *Med Sci Sports* 2:177-181, 1970.

140. Sugden, PH, and Newsholme, EA. The effects of ammonium, inorganic phosphate and potassium ions on the activity of phosphofructokinases from muscle and nervous tissues of vertebrates and invertebrates. *Biochem J* 150:113-122, 1975.

141. Sutton, JR. Hormonal and metabolic responses to exercise in subjects of high and low work capacities. *Med Sci Sports* 10:1-6, 1978.

142. Tanaka, K, Matsuura, Y, Kumagai, S, Matsuzaka, A, Hirakoba, K, and Asano, K. Relationships of anaerobic threshold and onset of blood lactate accumulation with endurance performance. *Eur J Appl Physiol Occup Physiol* 52:51-56, 1983.

143. Taylor, DJ, Styles, P, Matthews, PM, Arnold, DA, Gadian, DG, Bore, P, and Radda, GK. Energetics of human muscle: Exercise-induced ATP depletion. *Magn Reson Med* 3:44-54, 1986.

144. Tesch, P. Muscle fatigue in man. With special reference to lactate accumulation during short term intense exercise. *Acta Physiol Scand* 480 (Suppl):1-40, 1980.

145. Tesch, PA, Komi, PV, and Häkkinen, K. Enzymatic adaptations consequent to long-term strength training. *Int J Sports Med* 8 (Suppl 1):66-69, 1987.

146. Tesch, PA, Ploutz-Snyder, LL, Ystrom, L, Castro, MJ, and Dudley, GA. Skeletal muscle glycogen loss evoked by resistance exercise. *J Strength Cond Res* 12:67-73, 1998.

147. Thorstensson, A. Muscle strength, fibre types and enzyme activities in man. *Acta Physiol Scand* 443 (Suppl):1-45, 1976.

148. Thorstensson, A, Sjodin, B, Tesch, P, and Karlsson, J. Actomyosin ATPase, myokinase, CPK and LDH in human fast and slow twitch muscle fibres. *Acta Physiol Scand* 99:225-229, 1977.

149. Vandewalle, H, Peres, G, and Monod, H. Standard anaerobic exercise tests. *Sports Med* 4:268-289, 1987.

150. Vanhelder, WP, Radomski, MW, Goode, RC, and Casey, K. Hormonal and metabolic response to three types of exercise of equal duration and external work output. *Eur J Appl Physiol Occup Physiol* 54:337-342, 1985.

151. Vihko, V, Salminen, A, and Rantamaki, J. Oxidative and lysosomal capacity in skeletal-muscle of mice after endurance training of different intensities. *Acta Physiol Scand* 104:74-81, 1978.

152. Wakefield, BR, and Glaister, M. Influence of work-interval intensity and duration on time spent at a high percentage of VO2max during intermittent supramaximal exercise. *J Strength Cond Res* 23:2548-2554, 2009.

153. Walsh, B, Tonkonogi, M, Soderlund, K, Hultman, E, Saks, V, and Sahlin, K. The role of phosphorylcreatine and creatine in the regulation of mitochondrial respiration in human skeletal muscle. *J Physiol* 537:971-978, 2001.

154. Weir, JP, Beck, TW, Cramer, JT, and Housh, TJ. Is fatigue all in your head? A critical review of the central governor model. *Br J Sports Med* 40:573-586, 2006.

155. Weir, JP, and Cramer, JT. Principles of musculoskeletal exercise programming. In *ACSM Resource Manual for Exercise Testing and Prescription.* Kaminsky, LA, ed. Philadelphia: Lippincott Williams & Wilkins, 350-364, 2005.

156. Wells, JG, Balke, B, and Van Fossan, DD. Lactic acid accumulation during work: A suggested standardization of work classification. *J Appl Physiol* 10:51-55, 1957.

157. Whipp, BJ, Seard, C, and Wasserman, K. Oxygen deficit-oxygen debt relationships and efficiency of anaerobic work. *J Appl Physiol* 28:452-456, 1970.

158. Williams, JH, and Klug, GA. Calcium exchange hypothesis of skeletal-muscle fatigue—a brief review. *Muscle Nerve* 18:421-434, 1995.

159. Withers, RT, Sherman, WM, Clark, DG, Esselbach, PC, Nolan, SR, Mackay, MH, and Brinkman, M. Muscle metabolism during 30, 60 and 90 s of maximal cycling on an air-braked ergometer. *Eur J Appl Physiol Occup Physiol* 63:354-362, 1991.

160. York, JW, Oscai, LB, and Penney, DG. Alterations in skeletal-muscle lactate-dehydrogenase isoenzymes following exercise training. *Biochem Biophys Res Commun* 61:1387-1393, 1974.

161. Yoshida, T. Effect of dietary modifications on lactate threshold and onset of blood lactate accumulation during incremental exercise. *Eur J Appl Physiol* 53:200-205, 1984.

162. Zehnder, M, Muelli, M, Buchli, R, Kuehne, G, and Boutellier, U. Further glycogen decrease during early recovery after eccentric exercise despite a high carbohydrate intake. *Eur J Nutr* 43:148-159, 2004.

CHAPTER 4   Endocrine Responses to Resistance Exercise

1. Adem, A, Jossan, SS, d'Argy, R, Gillberg, PG, Nordberg, A, Winblad, B, and Sara, V. Insulin-like growth factor 1 (IGF-1) receptors in the human brain: Quantitative autoradiographic localization. *Brain Res* 503:299-303, 1989.

2. Allen, RE, Merkel, RA, and Young, RB. Cellular aspects of muscle growth: Myogenic cell proliferation. *J Anim Sci* 49:115-127, 1979.

3. Allen, RE, and Boxhorn, LK. Regulation of skeletal muscle satellite cell proliferation and differentiation by transforming growth factor-beta, insulin-like growth factor I, and fibroblast growth factor. *J Cell Physiol* 138:311-315, 1989.

4. Aristizabal, J, Freidenreich, D, Volk, B, Kupchak, B, Saenz, C, Maresh, C, Kraemer, W, and Volek, J. Effect of resistance training on resting metabolic rate and its estimation by a dual-energy X-ray absorptiometry metabolic map. *Eur J Clin Nutr,* 2014.

5. Atha, J. Strengthening muscle. *Exerc Sport Sci Rev* 9:1-73, 1981.

6. Bartalena, L. Recent achievements in studies on thyroid hormone-binding proteins. *Endocr Rev* 11:47-64, 1990.

7. Baxter, RC, and Martin, JL. Structure of the Mr 140,000 growth hormone-dependent insulin-like growth factor binding protein complex: Determination by reconstitution and affinity-labeling. *Proc Natl Acad Sci U S A* 86:6898-6902, 1989.

8. Baxter, RC, Martin, JL, and Beniac, VA. High molecular weight insulin-like growth factor binding protein complex. Purification and properties of the acid-labile subunit from human serum. *J Biol Chem* 264:11843-11848, 1989.

9. Beauloye, V, Muaku, SM, Lause, P, Portetelle, D, Renaville, R, Robert, AR, Ketelslegers, JM, and Maiter, D. Monoclonal antibodies to growth hormone (GH) prolong liver GH binding and GH-induced IGF-I/IGFBP-3 synthesis. *Am J Physiol* 277:E308-E315, 1999.

10. Ben-Ezra, V, McMurray, R, and Smith, A. Effects of exercise or diet on plasma somatomedin-C. *Med Sci Sports Exerc* 17:209, 1985.

11. Biro, J, and Endroczi, E. Nuclear RNA content and synthesis in anterior pituitary in intact, castrated and androgen sterilized rats. *Endocrinol Exp* 11:163-168, 1977.

12. Bleisch, W, Luine, VN, and Nottebohm, F. Modification of synapses in androgen-sensitive muscle. I. Hormonal regulation of acetylcholine receptor number in the songbird syrinx. *J Neurosci* 4:786-792, 1984.

13. Blum, WF, Jenne, EW, Reppin, F, Kietzmann, K, Ranke, MB, and Bierich, JR. Insulin-like growth factor I (IGF-I)-binding protein complex is a better mitogen than free IGF-I. *Endocrinology* 125:766-772, 1989.

14. Borer, KT, Nicoski, DR, and Owens, V. Alteration of pulsatile growth hormone secretion by growth-inducing exercise: Involvement of endogenous opiates and somatostatin. *Endocrinology* 118:844-850, 1986.

15. Boule, NG, Weisnagel, SJ, Lakka, TA, Tremblay, A, Bergman, RN, Rankinen, T, Leon, AS, Skinner, JS, Wilmore, JH, Rao, DC, Bouchard, C, and HERITAGE Family Study. Effects of exercise training on glucose homeostasis: The HERITAGE Family Study. *Diabetes Care* 28:108-114, 2005.

16. Buckler, JM. The effect of age, sex and exercise on the secretion of growth hormone. *Clin Sci* 37:765-774, 1969.

17. Buckler, JM. The relationship between exercise, body temperature and plasma growth hormone levels in a human subject. *J Physiol* 214 Suppl:25P-26P, 1971.

18. Bush, JA, Mastro, AM, and Kraemer, WJ. Proenkephalin peptide F immunoreactivity in different circulatory biocompartments after exercise. *Peptides* 27:1498-1506, 2006.

19. Chang, FE, Dodds, WG, Sullivan, M, Kim, MH, and Malarkey, WB. The acute effects of exercise on prolactin and growth hormone secretion: Comparison between sedentary women and women runners with normal and abnormal menstrual cycles. *J Clin Endocrinol Metab* 62:551-556, 1986.

20. Clarkson, PM, and Tremblay, I. Exercise-induced muscle damage, repair, and adaptation in humans. *J Appl Physiol* 65:1-6, 1988.

21. Clasen, BF, Krusenstjerna-Hafstrom, T, Vendelbo, MH, Thorsen, K, Escande, C, Moller, N, Pedersen, SB, Jorgensen, JO, and Jessen, N. Gene expression in skeletal muscle after an acute intravenous GH bolus in human subjects: Identification of a mechanism regulating ANGPTL4. *J Lipid Res* 54:1988-1997, 2013.

22. Clemmons, DR, Busby, HW, and Underwood, LE. Mediation of the growth promoting actions of growth hormone by somatomedin-C/insulin-like growth factor I and its binding protein. In *The Physiology of Human Growth*. Tanner, JM, and Preece, MA, eds. Cambridge: Cambridge University Press, 111-128, 1989.

23. Clemmons, DR, Thissen, JP, Maes, M, Ketelslegers, JM, and Underwood, LE. Insulin-like growth factor-I (IGF-I) infusion into hypophysectomized or protein-deprived rats induces specific IGF-binding proteins in serum. *Endocrinology* 125:2967-2972, 1989.

24. Coviello, AD, Lakshman, K, Mazer, NA, and Bhasin, S. Differences in the apparent metabolic clearance rate of testosterone in young and older men with gonadotropin suppression receiving graded doses of testosterone. *J Clin Endocrinol Metab* 91:4669-4675, 2006.

25. Craig, SK, Byrnes, WC, and Fleck, SJ. Plasma volume during weight lifting. *Int J Sports Med* 29:89-95, 2008.

26. Cumming, DC, Wall, SR, Galbraith, MA, and Belcastro, AN. Reproductive hormone responses to resistance exercise. *Med Sci Sports Exerc* 19:234-238, 1987.

27. Czech, MP. Signal transmission by the insulin-like growth factors. *Cell* 59:235-238, 1989.

28. Daughaday, WH, and Rotwein, P. Insulin-like growth factors I and II. Peptide, messenger ribonucleic acid and gene structures, serum, and tissue concentrations. *Endocr Rev* 10:68-91, 1989.

29. De Souza, MJ, Maguire, MS, Maresh, CM, Kraemer, WJ, Rubin, KR, and Loucks, AB. Adrenal activation and the prolactin response to exercise in eumenorrheic and amenorrheic runners. *J Appl Physiol* 70:2378-2387, 1991.

30. D'Ercole, AJ, Stiles, AD, and Underwood, LE. Tissue concentrations of somatomedin C: Further evidence for multiple sites of synthesis and paracrine or autocrine mechanisms of action. *Proc Natl Acad Sci U S A* 81:935-939, 1984.

31. Deschenes, MR, Maresh, CM, Armstrong, LE, Covault, J, Kraemer, WJ, and Crivello, JF. Endurance and resistance exercise induce muscle fiber type specific responses in androgen binding capacity. *J Steroid Biochem* 50:175-179, 1994.

32. Deschenes, MR, Kraemer, WJ, Bush, JA, Doughty, TA, Kim, D, Mullen, KM, and Ramsey, K. Biorhythmic influences on functional capacity of human muscle and physiological responses. *Med Sci Sports Exerc* 30:1399-1407, 1998.

33. Djarova, T, Ilkov, A, Varbanova, A, Nikiforova, A, and Mateev, G. Human growth hormone, cortisol, and acid-base balance changes after hyperventilation and breath-holding. *Int J Sports Med* 7:311-315, 1986.

34. Ekins, R. Measurement of free hormones in blood. *Endocr Rev* 11:5-46, 1990.

35. Elliot, DL, Goldberg, L, Watts, WJ, and Orwoll, E. Resistance exercise and plasma beta-endorphin/beta-lipotrophin immunoreactivity. *Life Sci* 34:515-518, 1984.

36. Estrada, M, Espinosa, A, Muller, M, and Jaimovich, E. Testosterone stimulates intracellular calcium release and mitogen-activated protein kinases via a G protein-coupled receptor in skeletal muscle cells. *Endocrinology* 144:3586-3597, 2003.

37. Fagin, JA, Fernandez-Mejia, C, and Melmed, S. Pituitary insulin-like growth factor-I gene expression: Regulation by triiodothyronine and growth hormone. *Endocrinology* 125:2385-2391, 1989.

38. Fahey, TD, Rolph, R, Moungmee, P, Nagel, J, and Mortara, S. Serum testosterone, body composition, and strength of young adults. *Med Sci Sports* 8:31-34, 1976.

39. Faria, AC, Veldhuis, JD, Thorner, MO, and Vance, ML. Half-time of endogenous growth hormone (GH) disappearance in normal man after stimulation of GH secretion by GH-releasing hormone and suppression with somatostatin. *J Clin Endocrinol Metab* 68:535-541, 1989.

40. Finkelstein, JW, Roffwarg, HP, Boyar, RM, Kream, J, and Hellman, L. Age-related change in the twenty-four-hour spontaneous secretion of growth hormone. *J Clin Endocrinol Metab* 35:665-670, 1972.

41. Fischer, E. Über die optischen isomeren des traubenzuckers, der gluconsäure und der zuckersäure. In *Untersuchungen Über Kohlenhydrate und Fermente (1884–1908)*. Anonymous. Berlin: Springer, 362-376, 1909.

42. Fleck, SJ. *Successful Long-Term Weight Training*. Indianapolis: Masters Press, 1999.

43. Fleck, SJ, and Kraemer, WJ. *Periodization Breakthrough*. Ronkonkoma, NY: Advanced Research Press, 1996.

44. Fleck, SJ, and Kraemer, WJ. *Designing Resistance Training Programs*. 3rd ed. Champaign, IL: Human Kinetics, 2003.

45. Florini, JR. Hormonal control of muscle growth. *Muscle Nerve* 10:577-598, 1987.

46. Florini, JR. Hormonal control of muscle cell growth. *J Anim Sci* 61:21-38, 1985.

47. Florini, JR, Prinz, PN, Vitiello, MV, and Hintz, RL. Somatomedin-C levels in healthy young and old men: Relationship to peak and 24-hour integrated levels of growth hormone. *J Gerontol* 40:2-7, 1985.

48. Fluckey, JD, Kraemer, WJ, and Farrell, PA. Arginine-stimulated insulin secretion from isolated rat pancreatic islets is increased following acute resistance exercise. *J Appl Physiol* 79:1100-1105, 1995.

49. Forbes, B, Szabo, L, Baxter, RC, Ballard, FJ, and Wallace, JC. Classification of the insulin-like growth factor binding proteins into three distinct categories according to their binding specificities. *Biochem Biophys Res Com* 157:196-202, 1988.

50. Fortunati, N, Catalano, MG, Boccuzzi, G, and Frairia, R. Sex Hormone-Binding Globulin (SHBG), estradiol and breast cancer. *Mol Cell Endocrinol* 316:86-92, 2010.

51. Fragala, MS, Kraemer, WJ, Denegar, CR, Maresh, CM, Mastro, AM, and Volek, JS. Neuroendocrine-immune interactions and responses to exercise. *Sports Med* 41:621-639, 2011.

52. Fragala, MS, Kraemer, WJ, Mastro, AM, Denegar, CR, Volek, JS, Kupchak, BR, Hakkinen, K, Anderson, JM, and Maresh, CM. Glucocorticoid receptor expression on human B cells in response to acute heavy resistance exercise. *Neuroimmunomodulation* 18:156-164, 2011.

53. French, DN, Kraemer, WJ, Volek, JS, Spiering, BA, Judelson, DA, Hoffman, JR, and Maresh, CM. Anticipatory responses of catecholamines on muscle force production. *J Appl Physiol* 102:94-102, 2007.

54. Fry, A, Schilling, B, Weiss, L, and Chiu, L. Beta2-adrenergic receptor downregulation and performance decrements during high-intensity resistance exercise overtraining. *J Appl Physiol* 101:1664-1672, 2006.

55. Fry, AC, Kraemer, WJ, Lynch, JM, Triplett, NT, and Koziris, LP. Does short-term near-maximal intensity machine resistance training induce overtraining? *J Strength Cond Res* 8:188-191, 1994.

56. Fry, AC, Kraemer, WJ, Stone, MH, Warren, BJ, Kearney, JT, Maresh, CM, Weseman, CA, and Fleck, SJ. Endocrine and performance responses to high volume training and amino acid supplementation in elite junior weightlifters. *Int J Sport Nutr* 3:306-322, 1993.

57. Fry, AC, Kraemer, WJ, Stone, MH, Warren, BJ, Fleck, SJ, Kearney, JT, and Gordon, SE. Endocrine responses to overreaching before and after 1 year of weightlifting. *Can J Appl Physiol* 19:400-410, 1994.

58. Fry, AC, Kraemer, WJ, van Borselen, F, Lynch, JM, Marsit, JL, Roy, EP, Triplett, NT, and Knuttgen, HG. Performance decrements with high-intensity resistance exercise overtraining. *Med Sci Sports Exerc* 26:1165-1173, 1994.

59. Fry, AC, Kraemer, WJ, and Ramsey, LT. Pituitary-adrenal-gonadal responses to high-intensity resistance exercise overtraining. *J Appl Physiol* 85:2352-2359, 1998.

60. Galbo, H. *Hormonal and Metabolic Adaptation to Exercise.* Stuttgart: Georg Thieme Verlag, 1983.

61. Gharib, SD, Wierman, ME, Shupnik, MA, and Chin, WW. Molecular biology of the pituitary gonadotropins. *Endocr Rev* 11:177-199, 1990.

62. Goldberg, AL, and Goodman, HM. Relationship between growth hormone and muscular work in determining muscle size. *J Physiol* 200:655-666, 1969.

63. Goldspink, G. Changes in muscle mass and phenotype and the expression of autocrine and systemic growth factors by muscle in response to stretch and overload. *J Anat* 194(Pt 3):323-334, 1999.

64. Gordon, SE, Kraemer, WJ, Vos, NH, Lynch, JM, and Knuttgen, HG. Effect of acid-base balance on the growth hormone response to acute high-intensity cycle exercise. *J Appl Physiol* 76:821-829, 1994.

65. Gordon, SE, Kraemer, WJ, Looney, DP, Flanagan, SD, Comstock, BA, and Hymer, WC. The influence of age and exercise modality on growth hormone bioactivity in women. *Growth Horm IGF Res* 24:95-103, 2014.

66. Gregory, SM, Headley, SA, Germain, M, Flyvbjerg, A, Frystyk, J, Coughlin, MA, Milch, CM, Sullivan, S, and Nindl, BC. Lack of circulating bioactive and immunoreactive IGF-I changes despite improved fitness in chronic kidney disease patients following 48 weeks of physical training. *Growth Horm IGF Res* 21:51-56, 2011.

67. Gregory, SM, Spiering, BA, Alemany, JA, Tuckow, AP, Rarick, KR, Staab, JS, Hatfield, DL, Kraemer, WJ, Maresh, CM, and Nindl, BC. Exercise-induced insulin-like growth factor I system concentrations after training in women. *Med Sci Sports Exerc* 45:420-428, 2013.

68. Guezennec, Y, Leger, L, Lhoste, F, Aymonod, M, and Pesquies, PC. Hormone and metabolite response to weight-lifting training sessions. *Int J Sports Med* 7:100-105, 1986.

69. Guma, A, Zierath, JR, Wallberg-Henriksson, H, and Klip, A. Insulin induces translocation of GLUT-4 glucose transporters in human skeletal muscle. *Am J Physiol* 268:E613-E622, 1995.

70. Hakkinen, K, Pakarinen, A, Alen, M, and Komi, PV. Serum hormones during prolonged training of neuromuscular performance. *Eur J Appl Physiol Occup Physiol* 53:287-293, 1985.

71. Hakkinen, K, Komi, PV, Alen, M, and Kauhanen, H. EMG, muscle fibre and force production characteristics during a 1 year training period in elite weight-lifters. *Eur J Appl Physiol Occup Physiol* 56:419-427, 1987.

72. Hakkinen, K, Pakarinen, A, Alen, M, Kauhanen, H, and Komi, PV. Relationships between training volume, physical performance capacity, and serum hormone concentrations during prolonged training in elite weight lifters. *Int J Sports Med* 8 Suppl 1:61-65, 1987.

73. Hakkinen, K, Pakarinen, A, Alen, M, Kauhanen, H, and Komi, PV. Neuromuscular and hormonal adaptations in athletes to strength training in two years. *J Appl Physiol* 65:2406-2412, 1988.

74. Hakkinen, K, Pakarinen, A, Alen, M, Kauhanen, H, and Komi, PV. Daily hormonal and neuromuscular responses to intensive strength training in 1 week. *Int J Sports Med* 9:422-428, 1988.

75. Hakkinen, K. Neuromuscular and hormonal adaptations during strength and power training. A review. *J Sports Med Phys Fitness* 29:9-26, 1989.

76. Hakkinen, K, Pakarinen, A, Kyrolainen, H, Cheng, S, Kim, DH, and Komi, PV. Neuromuscular adaptations and serum hormones in females during prolonged power training. *Int J Sports Med* 11:91-98, 1990.

77. Han, VK, D'Ercole, AJ, and Lund, PK. Cellular localization of somatomedin (insulin-like growth factor) messenger RNA in the human fetus. *Science* 236:193-197, 1987.

78. Hansen, S, Kvorning, T, Kjaer, M, and Sjogaard, G. The effect of short-term strength training on human skeletal muscle: The importance of physiologically elevated hormone levels. *Scand J Med Sci Sports* 11:347-354, 2001.

79. Hansson, HA, Brandsten, C, Lossing, C, and Petruson, K. Transient expression of insulin-like growth factor I immunoreactivity by vascular cells during angiogenesis. *Exp Mol Pathol* 50:125-138, 1989.

80. Henning, PC, Scofield, DE, Rarick, KR, Pierce, JR, Staab, JS, Lieberman, HR, and Nindl, BC. Effects of acute caloric restriction compared to caloric balance on the temporal response of the IGF-I system. *Metabolism* 62:179-187, 2013.

81. Hetrick, GA, and Wilmore, JH. Androgen levels and muscle hypertrophy during an eight-week training program for men/women. *Med Sci Sports Exerc* 11:102, 1979.

82. Hill, DJ, Camacho-Hubner, C, Rashid, P, Strain, AJ, and Clemmons, DR. Insulin-like growth factor (IGF)-binding protein release by human fetal fibroblasts: Dependency on cell density and IGF peptides. *J Endocrinol* 122:87-98, 1989.

83. Horikawa, R, Asakawa, K, Hizuka, N, Takano, K, and Shizume, K. Growth hormone and insulin-like growth factor I stimulate Leydig cell steroidogenesis. *Eur J Pharmacol* 166:87-94, 1989.

84. Housley, PR, Sanchez, ER, and Grippo, JF. Phosphorylation and reduction of glucocorticoid components. In *Receptor Phosphorylation.* Moudgil, VM, ed. Boca Raton, FL: CRC Press, 289-314, 1989.

85. Ikeda, T, Fujiyama, K, Takeuchi, T, Honda, M, Mokuda, O, Tominaga, M, and Mashiba, H. Effect of thyroid hormone on somatomedin-C release from perfused rat liver. *Experientia* 45:170-171, 1989.

86. Ishii, DN. Relationship of insulin-like growth factor II gene expression in muscle to synaptogenesis. *Proc Natl Acad Sci U S A* 86:2898-2902, 1989.

87. Jahreis, G, Hesse, V, Schmidt, HE, and Scheibe, J. Effect of endurance exercise on somatomedin-C/insulin-like growth factor I concentration in male and female runners. *Exp Clin Endocrinol* 94:89-96, 1989.

88. Jamurtas, AZ, Koutedakis, Y, Paschalis, V, Tofas, T, Yfanti, C, Tsiokanos, A, Koukoulis, G, Kouretas, D, and Loupos, D. The effects of a single bout of exercise on resting energy expenditure and respiratory exchange ratio. *Eur J Appl Physiol* 92:393-398, 2004.

89. Jensen, MD, Nielsen, S, Gupta, N, Basu, R, and Rizza, RA. Insulin clearance is different in men and women. *Metabolism* 61:525-530, 2012.

90. Kelly, A, Lyons, G, Gambki, B, and Rubinstein, N. Influences of testosterone on contractile proteins of the guinea pig temporalis muscle. *Adv Exp Med Biol* 182:155-168, 1985.

91. Kjaer, M, and Galbo, H. Effect of physical training on the capacity to secrete epinephrine. *J Appl Physiol* 64:11-16, 1988.

92. Kraemer, WJ, and Fleck, SJ. Resistance training: Exercise prescription. *Phys Sportsmed* 16:69-81, 1988.

93. Kraemer, WJ, Fleck, SJ, and Deschenes, M. A review: Factors in exercise prescription of resistance training. *NSCA J* 110:36-41, 1988.

94. Kraemer, WJ, and Baechle, TR. Development of a strength training program. In *Sports Medicine.* 2nd ed. Ryan, AJ, and Allman, FL, eds. San Diego: Academic Press, 113-127, 1989.

95. Kraemer, WJ, Patton, JF, Knuttgen, HG, Hannan, CJ, Kittler, T, Gordon, S, Dziados, JE, Fry, AC, Frykman, PN, and Harman, EA. The effects of high intensity cycle exercise on sympatho-adrenal medullary response patterns. *J Appl Physiol* 70:8-14, 1991.

96. Kraemer, WJ. Endocrine responses and adaptations to strength training. In *The Encyclopaedia of Sports Medicine: Strength and Power in Sport.* Komi, PV, ed. Oxford: Blackwell Scientific, 291-304, 1992.

97. Kraemer, WJ. Hormonal mechanisms related to the expression of muscular strength and power. In *The Encyclopaedia of Sports Medicine: Strength and Power in Sport.* Komi, PV, ed. Oxford: Blackwell Scientific, 64-76, 1992.

98. Kraemer, WJ. The physiological basis for strength training in midlife. In *Sports and Exercise in Midlife.* Gordon, SL, ed. Park Ridge, IL: American Academy of Orthopaedic Surgeons, 413-433, 1994.

99. Kraemer, WJ, Fleck, SJ, and Evans, WJ. Strength and power training: Physiological mechanisms of adaptation. In *Exercise and Sport Sciences Reviews, vol. 24.* Holloszy, JO, ed. Baltimore: Williams & Wilkins, 363-397, 1996.

100. Kraemer, WJ, Fry, AC, Frykman, PN, Conroy, B, and Hoffman, J. Resistance training and youth. *Pediatr Exerc Sci* 1:336-350, 1989.

101. Kraemer, WJ, and Koziris, LP. Olympic weightlifting and power lifting. In *Physiology and Nutrition for Competitive Sport.* Lamb, DR, and Knuttgen, HG, eds. Traverse City, MI: Cooper, 1-15, 1994.

102. Kraemer, WJ. A series of studies—the physiological basis for strength training in American football: Fact over philosophy. *J Strength Cond Res* 11:131-142, 1997.

103. Kraemer, WJ, and Nindl, BC. Factors involved with overtraining for strength and power. In *Overtraining in Sport.* Kreider, RB, Fry, AC, and O'Toole, ML, eds. Champaign, IL: Human Kinetics, 107-127, 1997.

104. Kraemer, WJ, Noble, B, Culver, B, and Lewis, RV. Changes in plasma proenkephalin peptide F and catecholamine levels during graded exercise in men. *Proc Natl Acad Sci U S A* 82:6349-6351, 1985.

105. Kraemer, WJ, Noble, BJ, Clark, MJ, and Culver, BW. Physiologic responses to heavy-resistance exercise with very short rest periods. *Int J Sports Med* 8:247-252, 1987.

106. Kraemer, WJ. Endocrine responses to resistance exercise. *Med Sci Sports Exerc* 20:S152-S157, 1988.

107. Kraemer, WJ, Armstrong, LE, Hubbard, RW, Marchitelli, LJ, Leva, N, Rock, PB, and Dziados, JE. Responses of plasma human atrial natriuretic factor to high intensity submaximal exercise in the heat. *Eur J Appl Physiol Occup Physiol* 57:399-403, 1988.

108. Kraemer, WJ, Deschenes, MR, and Fleck, SJ. Physiological adaptations to resistance exercise. Implications for athletic conditioning. *Sports Med* 6:246-256, 1988.

109. Kraemer, WJ, Rock, PB, Fulco, CS, Gordon, SE, Bonner, JP, Cruthirds, CD, Marchitelli, LJ, Trad, L, and Cymerman, A. Influence of altitude and caffeine during rest and exercise on plasma levels of proenkephalin peptide F. *Peptides* 9:1115-1119, 1988.

110. Kraemer, WJ, Fleck, SJ, Callister, R, Shealy, M, Dudley, GA, Maresh, CM, Marchitelli, L, Cruthirds, C, Murray, T, and Falkel, JE. Training responses of plasma beta-endorphin, adrenocorticotropin, and cortisol. *Med Sci Sports Exerc* 21:146-153, 1989.

111. Kraemer, WJ, Patton, JF, Knuttgen, HG, Marchitelli, LJ, Cruthirds, C, Damokosh, A, Harman, E, Frykman, P, and Dziados, JE. Hypothalamic-pituitary-adrenal responses to short-duration high-intensity cycle exercise. *J Appl Physiol* 66:161-166, 1989.

112. Kraemer, WJ, Dziados, JE, Gordon, SE, Marchitelli, LJ, Fry, AC, and Reynolds, KL. The effects of graded exercise on plasma proenkephalin peptide F and catecholamine responses at sea level. *Eur J Appl Physiol Occup Physiol* 61:214-217, 1990.

113. Kraemer, WJ, Marchitelli, L, Gordon, SE, Harman, E, Dziados, JE, Mello, R, Frykman, P, McCurry, D, and Fleck, SJ. Hormonal and growth factor responses to heavy resistance exercise protocols. *J Appl Physiol* 69:1442-1450, 1990.

114. Kraemer, WJ, Gordon, SE, Fleck, SJ, Marchitelli, LJ, Mello, R, Dziados, JE, Friedl, K, Harman, E, Maresh, C, and Fry, AC. Endogenous anabolic hormonal and growth factor responses to heavy resistance exercise in males and females. *Int J Sports Med* 12:228-235, 1991.

115. Kraemer, WJ, Fry, AC, Warren, BJ, Stone, MH, Fleck, SJ, Kearney, JT, Conroy, BP, Maresh, CM, Weseman, CA, and Triplett, NT. Acute hormonal responses in elite junior weightlifters. *Int J Sports Med* 13:103-109, 1992.

116. Kraemer, WJ, Dziados, JE, Marchitelli, LJ, Gordon, SE, Harman, EA, Mello, R, Fleck, SJ, Frykman, PN, and Triplett, NT. Effects of different heavy-resistance exercise protocols on plasma beta-endorphin concentrations. *J Appl Physiol* 74:450-459, 1993.

117. Kraemer, WJ, Fleck, SJ, Dziados, JE, Harman, EA, Marchitelli, LJ, Gordon, SE, Mello, R, Frykman, PN, Koziris, LP, and Triplett, NT. Changes in hormonal concentrations after different heavy-resistance exercise protocols in women. *J Appl Physiol* 75:594-604, 1993.

118. Kraemer, WJ, Aguilera, BA, Terada, M, Newton, RU, Lynch, JM, Rosendaal, G, McBride, JM, Gordon, SE, and Hakkinen, K. Responses of IGF-I to endogenous increases in growth hormone after heavy-resistance exercise. *J Appl Physiol* 79:1310-1315, 1995.

119. Kraemer, WJ, Patton, JF, Gordon, SE, Harman, EA, Deschenes, MR, Reynolds, K, Newton, RU, Triplett, NT, and Dziados, JE. Compatibility of high-intensity strength and endurance training on hormonal and skeletal muscle adaptations. *J Appl Physiol* 78:976-989, 1995.

120. Kraemer, WJ, Hakkinen, K, Newton, RU, McCormick, M, Nindl, BC, Volek, JS, Gotshalk, LA, Fleck, SJ, Campbell, WW, Gordon, SE, Farrell, PA, and Evans, WJ. Acute hormonal responses to heavy resistance exercise in younger and older men. *Eur J Appl Physiol Occup Physiol* 77:206-211, 1998.

121. Kraemer, WJ, Volek, JS, Bush, JA, Putukian, M, and Sebastianelli, WJ. Hormonal responses to consecutive days of heavy-resistance exercise with or without nutritional supplementation. *J Appl Physiol* 85:1544-1555, 1998.

122. Kraemer, WJ, Loebel, CC, Volek, JS, Ratamess, NA, Newton, RU, Wickham, RB, Gotshalk, LA, Duncan, ND, Mazzetti, SA, Gomez, AL, Rubin, MR, Nindl, BC, and Hakkinen, K. The effect of heavy resistance exercise on the circadian rhythm of salivary testosterone in men. *Eur J Appl Physiol* 84:13-18, 2001.

123. Kraemer, WJ, Rubin, MR, Hakkinen, K, Nindl, BC, Marx, JO, Volek, JS, French, DN, Gomez, AL, Sharman, MJ, Scheett, T, Ratamess, NA, Miles, MP, Mastro, A, VanHeest, J, Maresh, CM, Welsch, JR, and Hymer, WC. Influence of muscle strength and total work on exercise-induced plasma growth hormone isoforms in women. *J Sci Med Sport* 6:295-306, 2003.

124. Kraemer, WJ, and Ratamess, NA. Hormonal responses and adaptations to resistance exercise and training. *Sports Med* 35:339-361, 2005.

125. Kraemer, WJ, Nindl, BC, Marx, JO, Gotshalk, LA, Bush, JA, Welsch, JR, Volek, JS, Spiering, BA, Maresh, CM, Mastro, AM, and Hymer, WC. Chronic resistance training in women potentiates growth hormone in vivo bioactivity: Characterization of molecular mass variants. *Am J Physiol Endocrinol Metab* 291:E1177-E1187, 2006.

126. Kraemer, WJ, Spiering, BA, Volek, JS, Ratamess, NA, Sharman, MJ, Rubin, MR, French, DN, Silvestre, R, Hatfield, DL, Van Heest, JL, Vingren, JL, Judelson, DA, Deschenes, MR, and Maresh, CM. Androgenic responses to resistance exercise: Effects of feeding and L-carnitine. *Med Sci Sports Exerc* 38:1288-1296, 2006.

127. Kraemer, WJ, Nindl, BC, Volek, JS, Marx, JO, Gotshalk, LA, Bush, JA, Welsch, JR, Vingren, JL, Spiering, BA, Fragala, MS, Hatfield, DL, Ho, JY, Maresh, CM, Mastro, AM, and Hymer, WC. Influence of oral contraceptive use on growth hormone in vivo bioactivity following resistance exercise: Responses of molecular mass variants. *Growth Horm IGF Res* 18:238-244, 2008.

128. Kraemer, WJ, Dunn-Lewis, C, Comstock, BA, Thomas, GA, Clark, JE, and Nindl, BC. Growth hormone, exercise, and athletic performance: A continued evolution of complexity. *Curr Sports Med Rep* 9:242-252, 2010.

129. Kuoppasalmi, K, and Adlercreutz, H. Interaction between catabolic and anabolic steroid hormones in muscular exercise. In *Exercise Endocrinology.* Berlin: Walter de Gruyter, 65-98, 1985.

130. Kvorning, T, Andersen, M, Brixen, K, and Madsen, K. Suppression of endogenous testosterone production attenuates the response to strength training: A randomized, placebo-controlled, and blinded intervention study. *Am J Physiol Endocrinol Metab* 291:E1325-E1332, 2006.

131. Kvorning, T, Andersen, M, Brixen, K, Schjerling, P, Suetta, C, and Madsen, K. Suppression of testosterone does not blunt mRNA expression of myoD, myogenin, IGF, myostatin or androgen receptor post strength training in humans. *J Physiol* 578:579-593, 2007.

132. Lukaszewska, J, Biczowa, B, Bobilewixz, D, Wilk, M, and Bouchow-ixz-Fidelus, B. Effect of physical exercise on plasma cortisol and growth hormone levels in young weight lifters. *Endokrynol Pol* 2:149-158, 1976.

133. MacDougall, J. Morphological changes in human skeletal muscle following strength training and immobilization. In *Human Muscle Power*. Jones, NL, McCartney, N, and McComas, AJ, eds. Champaign, IL: Human Kinetics, 269-288, 1986.

134. Mahler, DA, Cunningham, LN, Skrinar, GS, Kraemer, WJ, and Colice, GL. Beta-endorphin activity and hypercapnic ventilatory responsiveness after marathon running. *J Appl Physiol* 66:2431-2436, 1989.

135. Maksay, G, and Toke, O. Asymmetric perturbations of signalling oligomers. *Prog Biophys Mol Biol* 114:153-169, 2014.

136. Martin, JB. Growth hormone releasing factor. In *Brain Peptides*. Krieger, DT, Brownstein, JJ, and Martin, JB, eds. New York: Wiley, 976-980, 1983.

137. Matheny, RW, Jr., and Nindl, BC. Loss of IGF-IEa or IGF-IEb impairs myogenic differentiation. *Endocrinology* 152:1923-1934, 2011.

138. Mauras, N, Rini, A, Welch, S, Sager, B, and Murphy, SP. Synergistic effects of testosterone and growth hormone on protein metabolism and body composition in prepubertal boys. *Metabolism* 52:964-969, 2003.

139. McCall, GE, Byrnes, WC, Fleck, SJ, Dickinson, A, and Kraemer, WJ. Acute and chronic hormonal responses to resistance training designed to promote muscle hypertrophy. *Can J Appl Physiol* 24:96-107, 1999.

140. McCusker, RH, Camacho-Hubner, C, and Clemmons, DR. Identification of the types of insulin-like growth factor-binding proteins that are secreted by muscle cells in vitro. *J Biol Chem* 264:7795-7800, 1989.

141. McKoy, G, Ashley, W, Mander, J, Yang, SY, Williams, N, Russell, B, and Goldspink, G. Expression of insulin growth factor-1 splice variants and structural genes in rabbit skeletal muscle induced by stretch and stimulation. *J Physiol* 516(Pt 2):583-592, 1999.

142. McMurray, RG, Eubank, TK, and Hackney, AC. Nocturnal hormonal responses to resistance exercise. *Eur J Appl Physiol Occup Physiol* 72:121-126, 1995.

143. Migiano, MJ, Vingren, JL, Volek, JS, Maresh, CM, Fragala, MS, Ho, JY, Thomas, GA, Hatfield, DL, Hakkinen, K, Ahtiainen, J, Earp, JE, and Kraemer, WJ. Endocrine response patterns to acute unilateral and bilateral resistance exercise in men. *J Strength Cond Res* 24:128-134, 2010.

144. Nindl, BC, Kraemer, WJ, Gotshalk, LA, Marx, JO, Volek, JS, Bush, FA, Hakkinen, K, Newton, RU, and Fleck, SJ. Testosterone responses after resistance exercise in women: Influence of regional fat distribution. *Int J Sport Nutr Exerc Metab* 11:451-465, 2001.

145. Nindl, BC. Insulin-like growth factor-I as a candidate metabolic biomarker: Military relevance and future directions for measurement. *J Diabetes Sci Technol* 3:371-376, 2009.

146. Nindl, BC. Insulin-like growth factor-I, physical activity, and control of cellular anabolism. *Med Sci Sports Exerc* 42:35-38, 2010.

147. Nindl, BC, Alemany, JA, Tuckow, AP, Rarick, KR, Staab, JS, Kraemer, WJ, Maresh, CM, Spiering, BA, Hatfield, DL, Flyvbjerg, A, and Frystyk, J. Circulating bioactive and immunoreactive IGF-I remain stable in women, despite physical fitness improvements after 8 weeks of resistance, aerobic, and combined exercise training. *J Appl Physiol* 109:112-120, 2010.

148. Nindl, BC, and Pierce, JR. Insulin-like growth factor I as a biomarker of health, fitness, and training status. *Med Sci Sports Exerc* 42:39-49, 2010.

149. Nindl, BC, McClung, JP, Miller, JK, Karl, JP, Pierce, JR, Scofield, DE, Young, AJ, and Lieberman, HR. Bioavailable IGF-I is associated with fat-free mass gains after physical training in women. *Med Sci Sports Exerc* 43:793-799, 2011.

150. Nindl, BC, Santtila, M, Vaara, J, Hakkinen, K, and Kyrolainen, H. Circulating IGF-I is associated with fitness and health outcomes in a population of 846 young healthy men. *Growth Horm IGF Res* 21:124-128, 2011.

151. Nindl, BC, Urso, ML, Pierce, JR, Scofield, DE, Barnes, BR, Kraemer, WJ, Anderson, JM, Maresh, CM, Beasley, KN, and Zambraski, EJ. IGF-I measurement across blood, interstitial fluid, and muscle biocompartments following explosive, high-power exercise. *Am J Physiol Regul Integr Comp Physiol* 303:R1080-R1089, 2012.

152. Okayama, T. Factors which regulate growth hormone secretion. *Med J* 17:13-19, 1972.

153. Pakarinen, A, Alen, M, Hakkinen, K, and Komi, P. Serum thyroid hormones, thyrotropin and thyroxine binding globulin during prolonged strength training. *Eur J Appl Physiol Occup Physiol* 57:394-398, 1988.

154. Perry, JK, Liu, DX, Wu, ZS, Zhu, T, and Lobie, PE. Growth hormone and cancer: An update on progress. *Curr Opin Endocrinol Diabetes Obes* 20:307-313, 2013.

155. Rance, NE, and Max, SR. Modulation of the cytosolic androgen receptor in striated muscle by sex steroids. *Endocrinology* 115:862-866, 1984.

156. Ratamess, NA, Kraemer, WJ, Volek, JS, Maresh, CM, Vanheest, JL, Sharman, MJ, Rubin, MR, French, DN, Vescovi, JD, Silvestre, R, Hatfield, DL, Fleck, SJ, and Deschenes, MR. Androgen receptor content following heavy resistance exercise in men. *J Steroid Biochem Mol Biol* 93:35-42, 2005.

157. Rogol, AD. Growth hormone: Physiology, therapeutic use, and potential for abuse. *Exerc Sport Sci Rev* 17:353-377, 1989.

158. Ronnestad, BR, Nygaard, H, and Raastad, T. Physiological elevation of endogenous hormones results in superior strength training adaptation. *Eur J Appl Physiol* 111:2249-2259, 2011.

159. Rosner, W. The functions of corticosteroid-binding globulin and sex hormone-binding globulin: Recent advances. *Endocr Rev* 11:80-91, 1990.

160. sRubin, MR, Kraemer, WJ, Maresh, CM, Volek, JS, Ratamess, NA, Vanheest, JL, Silvestre, R, French, DN, Sharman, MJ, Judelson, DA, Gomez, AL, Vescovi, JD, and Hymer, WC. High-affinity growth hormone binding protein and acute heavy resistance exercise. *Med Sci Sports Exerc* 37:395-403, 2005.

161. Sale, DG. Neural adaptation to resistance training. *Med Sci Sports Exerc* 20:S135-S145, 1988.

162. Schakman, O, Kalista, S, Barbe, C, Loumaye, A, and Thissen, JP. Glucocorticoid-induced skeletal muscle atrophy. *Int J Biochem Cell Biol* 45:2163-2172, 2013.

163. Sedliak, M, Finni, T, Cheng, S, Kraemer, WJ, and Hakkinen, K. Effect of time-of-day-specific strength training on serum hormone concentrations and isometric strength in men. *Chronobiol Int* 24:1159-1177, 2007.

164. Selye, H. A syndrome produced by diverse nocuous agents. *Nature* 138:32, 1936.

165. Selye, H. Stress and disease. *Geriatrics* 10:253-261, 1955.

166. Shaner, AA, Vingren, JL, Hatfield, DL, Budnar, RG, Jr., Duplanty, AA, and Hill, DW. The acute hormonal response to free weight and machine weight resistance exercise. *J Strength Cond Res* 28:1032-1040, 2014.

167. Skierska, E, Ustupska, J, Biczowa, B, and Lukaszewska, J. Effect of physical exercise on plasma cortisol, testosterone and growth hormone levels in weight lifters. *Endokrynol Pol* 2:159-165, 1976.

168. Skottner, A, Kanie, M, Jennische, E, Sjogren, J, and Fryklund, L. Tissue repair and IGF-1. *Acta Paediatr Scand* 347:110-112, 1988.

169. Smilios, I, Pilianidis, T, Karamouzis, M, and Tokmakidis, SP. Hormonal responses after various resistance exercise protocols. *Med Sci Sports Exerc* 35:644-654, 2003.

170. Sonntag, WE, Forman, LJ, Miki, N, and Meiters, J. Growth hormone secretion and neuroendocrine regulation. In *Handbook of Endocrinology.* Gass, GH, and Kaplan, HM, eds. Boca Raton, FL: CRC Press, 35-39, 1982.

171. Spiering, BA, Kraemer, WJ, Vingren, JL, Ratamess, NA, Anderson, JM, Armstrong, LE, Nindl, BC, Volek, JS, Hakkinen, K, and Maresh, CM. Elevated endogenous testosterone concentrations potentiate muscle androgen receptor responses to resistance exercise. *J Steroid Biochem Mol Biol* 114:195-199, 2009.

172. Staron, RS, Karapondo, DL, Kraemer, WJ, Fry, AC, Gordon, SE, Falkel, JE, Hagerman, FC, and Hikida, RS. Skeletal muscle adaptations during early phase of heavy-resistance training in men and women. *J Appl Physiol* 76:1247-1255, 1994.

173. Stone, MH, Byrd, R, and Johnson, C. Observations on serum androgen response to short term resistive training in middle age sedentary males. *NSCA J* 5:40-65, 1984.

174. Stone, MH, and O'Bryant, HS. *Weight Training: A Scientific Approach.* Minneapolis: Burgess International Group, 1987.

175. Suikkari, AM, Koivisto, VA, Koistinen, R, Seppala, M, and Yki-Jarvinen, H. Dose-response characteristics for suppression of low molecular weight plasma insulin-like growth factor-binding protein by insulin. *J Clin Endocrinol Metab* 68:135-140, 1989.

176. Suikkari, AM, Sane, T, Seppala, M, Yki-Jarvinen, H, Karonen, SL, and Koivisto, VA. Prolonged exercise increases serum insulin-like growth factor-binding protein concentrations. *J Clin Endocrinol Metab* 68:141-144, 1989.

177. Sutton, JR. Effect of acute hypoxia on the hormonal response to exercise. *J Appl Physiol* 42:587-592, 1977.

178. Szivak, TK, Hooper, DR, Dunn-Lewis, C, Comstock, BA, Kupchak, BR, Apicella, JM, Saenz, C, Maresh, CM, Denegar, CR, and Kraemer, WJ. Adrenal cortical responses to high-intensity, short rest, resistance exercise in men and women. *J Strength Cond Res* 27:748-760, 2013.

179. Tapperman, J. *Metabolic and Endocrine Physiology.* Chicago: Year Book Medical, 1980.

180. Terjung, R. Endocrine response to exercise. *Exerc Sport Sci Rev* 7:153-180, 1979.

181. Thomas, GA, Kraemer, WJ, Kennett, MJ, Comstock, BA, Maresh, CM, Denegar, CR, Volek, JS, and Hymer, WC. Immunoreactive and bioactive growth hormone responses to resistance exercise in men who are lean or obese. *J Appl Physiol* 111:465-472, 2011.

182. Triplett-McBride, NT, Mastro, AM, McBride, JM, Bush, JA, Putukian, M, Sebastianelli, WJ, and Kraemer, WJ. Plasma proenkephalin peptide F and human B cell responses to exercise stress in fit and unfit women. *Peptides* 19:731-738, 1998.

183. Turner, JD, Rotwein, P, Novakofski, J, and Bechtel, PJ. Induction of messenger RNA for IGF-I and -II during growth hormone-stimulated muscle hypertrophy. *Am J Physiol* 255:E513-E517, 1988.

184. Vanhelder, WP, Goode, RC, and Radomski, MW. Effect of anaerobic and aerobic exercise of equal duration and work expenditure on plasma growth hormone levels. *Eur J Appl Physiol Occup Physiol* 52:255-257, 1984.

185. Vanhelder, WP, Radomski, MW, and Goode, RC. Growth hormone responses during intermittent weight lifting exercise in men. *Eur J Appl Physiol Occup Physiol* 53:31-34, 1984.

186. Vicencio, JM, Ibarra, C, Estrada, M, Chiong, M, Soto, D, Parra, V, Diaz-Araya, G, Jaimovich, E, and Lavandero, S. Testosterone induces an intracellular calcium increase by a nongenomic mechanism in cultured rat cardiac myocytes. *Endocrinology* 147:1386-1395, 2006.

187. Vingren, JL, Koziris, LP, Gordon, SE, Kraemer, WJ, Turner, RT, and Westerlind, KC. Chronic alcohol intake, resistance training, and muscle androgen receptor content. *Med Sci Sports Exerc* 37:1842-1848, 2005.

188. Vingren, JL, Kraemer, WJ, Hatfield, DL, Volek, JS, Ratamess, NA, Anderson, JM, Hakkinen, K, Ahtiainen, J, Fragala, MS, Thomas, GA, Ho, JY, and Maresh, CM. Effect of resistance exercise on muscle steroid receptor protein content in strength-trained men and women. *Steroids* 74:1033-1039, 2009.

189. Vingren, JL, Kraemer, WJ, Ratamess, NA, Anderson, JM, Volek, JS, and Maresh, CM. Testosterone physiology in resistance exercise and training: The up-stream regulatory elements. *Sports Med* 40:1037-1053, 2010.

190. Weiss, LW, Cureton, KJ, and Thompson, FN. Comparison of serum testosterone and androstenedione responses to weight lifting in men and women. *Eur J Appl Physiol Occup Physiol* 50:413-419, 1983.

191. Westerlind, KC. Exercise and serum androgens in women. *Phys Sportsmed* 15:87-90, 1987.

192. Willoughby, DS, and Taylor, L. Effects of sequential bouts of resistance exercise on androgen receptor expression. *Med Sci Sports Exerc* 36:1499-1506, 2004.

193. Wolf, M, Ingbar, SH, and Moses, AC. Thyroid hormone and growth hormone interact to regulate insulin-like growth factor-I messenger ribonucleic acid and circulating levels in the rat. *Endocrinology* 125:2905-2914, 1989.

194. Yeoh, SI, and Baxter, RC. Metabolic regulation of the growth hormone independent insulin-like growth factor binding protein in human plasma. *Acta Endocrinol (Copenh)* 119:465-473, 1988.

195. Young, IR, Mesiano, S, Hintz, R, Caddy, DJ, Ralph, MM, Browne, CA, and Thorburn, GD. Growth hormone and testosterone can independently stimulate the growth of hypophysectomized prepubertal lambs without any alteration in circulating concentrations of insulin-like growth factors. *J Endocrinol* 121:563-570, 1989.

196. Zorzano, A, James, DE, Ruderman, NB, and Pilch, PF. Insulin-like growth factor I binding and receptor kinase in red and white muscle. *FEBS Lett* 234:257-262, 1988.

CHAPTER 5   Adaptations to Anaerobic Training Programs

1. Aagaard, P. Training-induced changes in neural function. *Exerc Sport Sci Rev* 31:61-67, 2003.

2. Aagaard, P, Andersen, JL, Dyhre-Poulsen, P, Leffers, A, Wagner, A, Magnusson, P, Halkjær-Kristensen, J, and Simonsen, EB. A mechanism for increased contractile strength of human pennate muscle in response to strength training: Changes in muscle architecture. *J Physiol* 534:613-623, 2001.

3. Aagaard, P, Simonsen, EB, Andersen, JL, Magnusson, P, and Dyhre-Poulsen, P. Neural adaptation to resistance training: Changes in evoked V-wave and H-reflex responses. *J Appl Physiol* 92:2309-2318, 2002.

4. Aagaard, P, Simonsen, EB, Andersen, JL, Magnusson, P, and Dyhre-Poulsen, P. Increased rate of force development and neural drive of human skeletal muscle following resistance training. *J Appl Physiol* 93:1318-1326, 2002.

5. Aagaard, P, Simonsen, EB, Andersen, JL, Magnusson, P, Halk-jaer-Kristensen, J, and Dyhre-Poulsen, P. Neural inhibition during maximal eccentric and concentric quadriceps contraction: Effects of resistance training. *J Appl Physiol* 89:2249-2257, 2000.

6. Abe, T, Kumagai, K, and Brechue, WF. Fascicle length of leg muscles is greater in sprinters than distance runners. *Med Sci Sports Exerc* 32:1125-1129, 2000.

7. Adams, GR, Harris, RT, Woodard, D, and Dudley, D. Mapping of electrical muscle stimulation using MRI. *J Appl Physiol* 74:532-537, 1993.

8. Allen, GD. Physiological and metabolic changes with six weeks of detraining. *Aust J Sci Med Sport* 21:4-9, 1989.

9. Always, SE, MacDougall, JD, and Sale, DG. Contractile adaptations in the human triceps surae after isometric exercise. *J Appl Physiol* 66:2725-2732, 1989.

10. Andersen, JL, and Aagaard, P. Myosin heavy chain IIX overshoot in human skeletal muscle. *Muscle Nerve* 23:1095-1104, 2000.

11. Baker, D, Nance, S, and Moore, M. The load that maximizes the average mechanical power output during explosive bench press throws in highly trained athletes. *J Strength Cond Res* 15:20-24, 2001.

12. Baker, D, Nance, S, and Moore, M. The load that maximizes the average mechanical power output during jump squats in power trained athletes. *J Strength Cond Res* 15:92-97, 2001.

13. Baty, JJ, Hwang, H, Ding, Z, Bernard, JR, Wang, B, Kwon, B, and Ivy, JL. The effect of a carbohydrate and protein supplement on resistance exercise performance, hormonal response, and muscle damage. *J Strength Cond Res* 21:321-329, 2007.

14. Beck, KC, and Johnson, BD. Pulmonary adaptations to dynamic exercise. In *ACSM's Resource Manual for Guidelines for Exercise Testing and Prescription.* Roitman, JL, ed. Baltimore: Williams & Wilkins, 305-313, 1998.

15. Behm, DG, Anderson, K, and Curnew, RS. Muscle force and activation under stable and unstable conditions. *J Strength Cond Res* 16:416-422, 2002.

16. Bell, GJ, Syrotuik, D, Martin, TP, Burnham, R, and Quinney, HA. Effect of concurrent strength and endurance training on skeletal muscle properties and hormone concentrations in humans. *Eur J Appl Physiol* 81:418-427, 2000.

17. Bell, GJ, and Wenger, HA. The effect of one-legged sprint training on intramuscular pH and nonbicarbonate buffering capacity. *Eur J Appl Physiol* 58:158-164, 1988.

18. Bickel, CS, Slade, J, Mahoney, E, Haddad, F, Dudley, GA, and Adams, GR. Time course of molecular responses of human skeletal muscle to acute bouts of resistance exercise. *J Appl Physiol* 98:482-488, 2005.

19. Biolo, G, Maggi, SP, Williams, BD, Tipton, KD, and Wolfe, RR. Increased rates of muscle protein turnover and amino acid transport after resistance exercise in humans. *J Physiol* 268:E514-E520, 1995.

20. Blazevich, AJ, Gill, ND, Bronks, R, and Newton, RU. Training-specific muscle architecture adaptations after 5-wk training in athletes. *Med Sci Sports Exerc* 35:2013-2022, 2003.

21. Budgett, R. Overtraining syndrome. *Br J Sports Med* 24:231-236, 1990.

22. Bush, JA, Kraemer, WJ, Mastro, AM, Triplett-McBride, T, Volek, JS, Putukian, M, Sebastianelli, WJ, and Knuttgen, HG. Exercise and recovery responses of adrenal medullary neurohormones to heavy resistance exercise. *Med Sci Sports Exerc* 31:554-559, 1999.

23. Callister, R, Callister, RJ, Fleck, SJ, and Dudley, GA. Physiological and performance responses to overtraining in elite judo athletes. *Med Sci Sports Exerc* 22:816-824, 1990.

24. Callister, R, Shealy, MJ, Fleck, SJ, and Dudley, GA. Performance adaptations to sprint, endurance and both modes of training. *J Appl Sport Sci Res* 2:46-51, 1988.

25. Campos, GE, Luecke, TJ, Wendeln, HK, Toma, K, Hagerman, FC, Murray, TF, Ragg, KE, Ratamess, NA, Kraemer, WJ, and Staron, RS. Muscular adaptations in response to three different resistance-training regimens: Specificity of repetition maximum training zones. *Eur J Appl Physiol* 88:50-60, 2002.

26. Carolan, B, and Cafarelli, E. Adaptations in coactivation after isometric resistance training. *J Appl Physiol* 73:911-917, 1992.

27. Chilibeck, PD, Calder, A, Sale, DG, and Webber, CE. Twenty weeks of weight training increases lean tissue mass but not bone mineral mass or density in healthy, active young women. *Can J Physiol Pharm* 74:1180-1185, 1996.

28. Colletti, LA, Edwards, J, Gordon, L, Shary, J, and Bell, NH. The effects of muscle-building exercise on bone mineral density of the radius, spine, and hip in young men. *Calcif Tissue Int* 45:12-14, 1989.

29. Conroy, BP, Kraemer, WJ, Maresh, CM, and Dalsky, GP. Adaptive responses of bone to physical activity. *Med Exerc Nutr Health* 1:64-74, 1992.

30. Conroy, BP, Kraemer, WJ, Maresh, CM, Fleck, SJ, Stone, MH, Fry, AC, Miller, PD, and Dalsky, GP. Bone mineral density in elite junior Olympic weightlifters. *Med Sci Sports Exerc* 25:1103-1109, 1993.

31. Cormie, P, McCaulley, GO, Triplett, NT, and McBride, JM. Optimal loading for maximal power output during lower-body resistance exercise. *Med Sci Sports Exerc* 39:340-349, 2007.

32. Cornelissen, VA, Fagard, RH, Coeckelberghs, E, and Vanhees, L. Impact of resistance training on blood pressure and other cardiovascular risk factors: A meta-analysis of randomized, controlled trials. *Hypertension* 58:950-958, 2011.

33. Costill, DL, Barnett, A, Sharp, R, Fink, WJ, and Katz, A. Leg muscle pH following sprint running. *Med Sci Sports Exerc* 15:325-329, 1983.

34. Craig, BW, Brown, R, and Everhart, J. Effects of progressive resistance training on growth hormone and testosterone levels in young and elderly subjects. *Mech Ageing Dev* 49:159-169, 1989.

35. Cussler, EC, Lohman, TG, Going, SB, Houtkooper, LB, Metcalfe, LL, Flint-Wagner, HG, Harris, RB, and Teixeira, PJ. Weight lifted in strength training predicts bone change in postmenopausal women. *Med Sci Sports Exerc* 35:10-17, 2003.

36. De Luca, CJ, and Contessa, P. Hierarchical control of motor units in voluntary contractions. *J Neurophysiol* 107:178-195, 2012.

37. Deligiannis, A, Zahopoulou, E, and Mandroukas, K. Echocardiographic study of cardiac dimensions and function in weight lifters and body builders. *Int J Sports Cardiol* 5:24-32, 1988.

38. Deschenes, MR, Covault, J, Kraemer, WJ, and Maresh, CM. The neuromuscular junction: Muscle fibre type differences, plasticity and adaptability to increased and decreased activity. *Sports Med* 17:358-372, 1994.

39. Deschenes, MR, Judelson, DA, Kraemer, WJ, Meskaitis, VJ, Volek, JS, Nindl, BC, Harman, FS, and Deaver, DR. Effects of resistance training on neuromuscular junction morphology. *Muscle Nerve* 23:1576-1581, 2000.

40. Deschenes, MR, Maresh, CM, Crivello, JF, Armstrong, LE, Kraemer, WJ, and Covault, J. The effects of exercise training of different intensities on neuromuscular junction morphology. *J Neurocytol* 22:603-615, 1993.

41. Dettmers, C, Ridding, MC, Stephan, KM, Lemon, RN, Rothwell, JC, and Frackowiak, RS. Comparison of regional cerebral blood flow with transcranial magnetic stimulation at different forces. *J Appl Physiol* 81:596-603, 1996.

42. Dook, JE, Henderson, JC, and Price, RI. Exercise and bone mineral density in mature female athletes. *Med Sci Sports Exerc* 29:291-296, 1997.

43. Duclos, M. A critical assessment of hormonal methods used in monitoring training status in athletes. *Int SportMed J* 9:56-66, 2008.

44. Dudley, GA, and Djamil, R. Incompatibility of endurance- and strength-training modes of exercise. *J Appl Physiol* 59:1446-1451, 1985.

45. Dupont, G, Millet, GP, Guinhouya, C, and Berthoin, S. Relationship between oxygen uptake kinetics and performance in repeated running sprints. *Eur J Appl Physiol* 95:27-34, 2005.

46. Eckstein, F, Hudelmaier, M, and Putz, R. The effects of exercise on human articular cartilage. *J Anat* 208:491-512, 2006.

47. Edge, J, Bishop, D, Hill-Haas, S, Dawson, B, and Goodman, C. Comparison of muscle buffer capacity and repeated-sprint ability of untrained, endurance-trained and team-sport athletes. *Eur J Appl Physiol* 96:225-234, 2006.

48. Enoka, RM. Neural adaptations with chronic physical activity. *J Biomech* 30:447-455, 1997.

49. Falkel, JE, Fleck, SJ, and Murray, TF. Comparison of central hemo-dynamics between power lifters and bodybuilders during exercise. *J Appl Sport Sci Res* 6:24-35, 1992.

50. Felici, F, Rosponi, A, Sbriccoli, P, Filligoi, C, Fattorini, L, and Marchetti, M. Linear and non-linear analysis of surface electromyograms in weightlifters. *Eur J Appl Physiol* 84:337-342, 2001.

51. Fisher, AG, Adams, TG, Yanowitz, FG, Ridges, JD, Orsmond, G, and Nelson, AG. Noninvasive evaluation of world class athletes engaged in different modes of training. *Am J Cardiol* 63:337-341, 1989.

52. Fleck, SJ. Cardiovascular adaptations to resistance training. *Med Sci Sports Exerc* 20:S146-S151, 1988.

53. Fleck, SJ. Cardiovascular responses to strength training. In *The Encyclopaedia of Sports Medicine: Strength and Power in Sport.* Komi, PV, ed. Oxford: Blackwell Scientific, 387-406, 2003.

54. Fleck, SJ, and Dean, LS. Resistance-training experience and the pressor response during resistance exercise. *J Appl Physiol* 63:116-120, 1987.

55. Fleck, SJ, Henke, C, and Wilson, W. Cardiac MRI of elite junior Olympic weight lifters. *Int J Sports Med* 10:329-333, 1989.

56. French, DN, Kraemer, WJ, Volek, JS, Spiering, BA, Judelson, DA, Hoffman, JR, and Maresh, CM. Anticipatory responses of catechol-amines on muscle force production. *J Appl Physiol* 102:94-102, 2007.

57. Frost, HM. Why do marathon runners have less bone than weight lifters? A vital-biomechanical view and explanation. *Bone* 20:183-189, 1997.

58. Fry, AC, and Kraemer, WJ. Resistance exercise overtraining and overreaching. *Sports Med* 23:106-129, 1997.

59. Fry, AC, Kraemer, WJ, Lynch, JM, Triplett, NT, and Koziris, LP. Does short-term near maximal intensity machine resistance training induce overtraining? *J Strength Cond Res* 8:188-191, 1994.

60. Fry, AC, Kraemer, WJ, and Ramsey, LT. Pituitary-adrenal-gonadal responses to high-intensity resistance exercise overtraining. *J Appl Physiol* 85:2352-2359, 1998.

61. Fry, AC, Kraemer, WJ, Stone, MH, Warren, BJ, Fleck, SJ, Kearney, JT, and Gordon, SE. Endocrine responses to over-reaching before and after 1 year of weightlifting training. *Can J Appl Physiol* 19:400-410, 1994.

62. Fry, AC, Kraemer, WJ, van Borselen, F, Lynch, JM, Marsit, JL, Roy, EP, Triplett, NT, and Knuttgen, HG. Performance decrements with high-intensity resistance exercise overtraining. *Med Sci Sports Exerc* 26:1165-1173, 1994.

63. Gabriel, DA, Kamen, G, and Frost, G. Neural adaptations to resistive exercise: Mechanisms and recommendations for training practices. *Sports Med* 36:133-149, 2006.

64. Gettman, LR, Culter, LA, and Strathman, T. Physiological changes after 20 weeks of isotonic vs isokinetic circuit training. *J Sports Med Phys Fitness* 20:265-274, 1980.

65. Glowacki, SP, Martin, SE, Maurer, A, Back, W, Green, JS, and Crouse, SF. Effects of resistance, endurance, and concurrent exercise on training outcomes in men. *Med Sci Sports Exerc* 36:2119-2127, 2004.

66. Goldspink, G. Changes in muscle mass and phenotype and the expression of autocrine and systemic growth factors by muscle in response to stretch and overload. *J Anat* 194:323-334, 1999.

67. Goldspink, G, and Yang, SY. Effects of activity on growth factor expression. *Int J Sport Nutr Exerc Metab* 11:S21-S27, 2001.

68. Gonyea, WJ. The role of exercise in inducing skeletal muscle fiber number. *J Appl Physiol* 48:421-426, 1980.

69. Gorassini, M, Yang, JF, Siu, M, and Bennett, DJ. Intrinsic activation of human motor units: Reduction of motor unit recruitment thresh-olds by repeated contractions. *J Neurophysiol* 87:1859-1866, 2002.

70. Granhed, H, Jonson, R, and Hansson, T. The loads on the lumbar spine during extreme weight lifting. *Spine* 12:146-149, 1987.

71. Green, H, Dahly, A, Shoemaker, K, Goreham, C, Bombardier, E, and Ball-Burnett, M. Serial effects of high-resistance and prolonged endurance training on Na+-K+ pump concentration and enzymatic activities in human vastus lateralis. *Acta Physiol Scand* 165:177-184, 1999.

72. Hakkinen, K, and Alen, M. Physiological performance, serum hor-mones, enzymes and lipids of an elite power athlete during training with and without androgens and during prolonged training. A case study. *J Sports Med Phys Fitness* 26:92-100, 1986.

73. Häkkinen, K, Alén, M, Kallinen, M, Izquierdo, M, Jokelainen, K, Lassila, H, Maikia, E, Kraemer, WJ, and Newton, RU. Muscle CSA, force production and activation of leg extensor during isometric and dynamic actions in middle-aged and elderly men and women. *J Aging Phys Act* 6:232-247, 1998.

74. Häkkinen, K, Alén, M, Kraemer, WJ, Gorostiaga, E, Izquierdo, M, Rusko, H, Mikkola, J, Häkkinen, A, Valkeinen, H, Kaarakainen, E, Romu, S, Erola, V, Ahtiainen, J, and Paavolainen, L. Neuromuscular adaptations during concurrent strength and endurance training versus strength training. *Eur J Appl Physiol* 89:42-52, 2003.

75. Häkkinen, K, Izquierdo, M, Aguado, X, Newton, RU, and Kraemer, WJ. Isometric and dynamic explosive force production of leg exten-sor muscles in men at different ages. *J Hum Mov Stud* 31:105-121, 1996.

76. Häkkinen, K, Kallinen, M, Izquierdo, M, Jokelainen, K, Lassila, H, Maikia, E, Kraemer, WJ, Newton, RU, and Alén, M. Changes in agonist-antagonist EMG, muscle CSA and force during strength training in middle-aged and older people. *J Appl Physiol* 84:1341-1349, 1998.

77. Häkkinen, K, Newton, RU, Gordon, SE, McCormick, M, Volek, JS, Nindl, BC, Gotshalk, LA, Campbell, WW, Evans, WJ, Häkkinen, A, Humphries, B, and Kraemer, WJ. Changes in muscle morphology, electromyographic activity, and force production characteristics during progressive strength training in young and older men. *J Gerontol Biol Sci* 53:415-423, 1998.

78. Häkkinen, K, and Pakarinen, A. Acute hormonal responses to two different fatiguing heavy-resistance protocols in male athletes. *J Appl Physiol* 74:882-887, 1993.

79. Häkkinen, K, Pakarinen, A, Alén, M, Kauhanen, H, and Komi, PV. Relationships between training volume, physical performance capac-ity, and serum hormone concentrations during prolonged training in elite weight lifters. *Int J Sports Med* 8:61-65, 1987.

80. Häkkinen, K, Pakarinen, A, Alén, M, Kauhanen, H, and Komi, PV. Neuromuscular and hormonal adaptations in athletes to strength training in two years. *J Appl Physiol* 65:2406-2412, 1988.

81. Halson, SL, and Jeukendrup, AE. Does overtraining exist? An analysis of overreaching and overtraining research. *Sports Med* 34:967-981, 2004.

82. Hansen, S, Kvorning, T, Kjaer, M, and Szogaard, G. The effect of short-term strength training on human skeletal muscle: The impor-tance of physiologically elevated hormone levels. *Scand J Med Sci Sports* 11:347-354, 2001.

83. Hather, BM, Tesch, PA, Buchanan, P, and Dudley, GA. Influence of eccentric actions on skeletal muscle adaptations to resistance. *Acta Physiol Scand* 143:177-185, 1991.

84. Henderson, NK, White, CP, and Eisman, JA. The role of exercise and fall risk reduction in prevention of osteoporosis. *Endocrin Metab Clin* 27:369-387, 1998.

85. Hibbs, AE, Thompson, KG, French, DN, Hodgson, D, and Spears, IR. Peak and average rectified EMG measures: Which method of data reduction should be used for assessing core training exercises? *J Electromyogr Kinesiol* 21:102-111, 2011.

86. Hickson, RC. Interference of strength development by simulta-neously training for strength and endurance. *Eur J Appl Physiol* 45:255-263, 1980.

87. Ho, K, Roy, R, Taylor, J, Heusner, W, Van Huss, W, and Carrow, R. Muscle fiber splitting with weightlifting exercise. *Med Sci Sports Exerc* 9:65, 1977.

88. Hortobagyi, T, Houmard, JA, Stevenson, JR, Fraser, DD, Johns, RA, and Israel, RG. The effects of detraining on power athletes. *Med Sci Sports Exerc* 25:929-935, 1993.

89. Howatson, GI, Zult, T, Farthing, JP, Ziidewind, I, and Hortobagyi, T. Mirror training to augment cross-education during resistance training: A hypothesis. *Front Hum Neurosci* 24:394, 2013.

90. Hurley, BF. Effects of resistance training on lipoprotein-lipid profiles: A comparison to aerobic exercise training. *Med Sci Sports Exerc* 21:689-693, 1989.

91. Kanehisa, H, and Fukunaga, T. Profiles of musculoskeletal development in limbs of college Olympic weightlifters and wrestlers. *Eur J Appl Physiol* 79:414-420, 1999.

92. Kannus, P, Jozsa, L, Natri, A, and Jarvinen, M. Effects of training, immobilization and remobilization on tendons. *Scand J Med Sci Sports* 7:67-71, 1997.

93. Karlsson, TS, Johnell, O, and Obrandt, KJ. Is bone mineral advantage maintained long-term in previous weightlifters? *Calcif Tissue Int* 57:325-328, 1995.

94. Kearns, CF, Abe, T, and Brechue, WF. Muscle enlargement in sumo wrestlers includes increased muscle fascicle length. *Eur J Appl Physiol* 83:289-296, 2000.

95. Kelley, GA, and Kelley, KS. Progressive resistance exercise and resting blood pressure: A meta-analysis of randomized controlled trials. *Hypertension* 35:838-843, 2000.

96. Kellis, E, Arabatzi, F, and Papadopoulos, C. Muscle co-activation around the knee in drop jumping using the co-contraction index. *J Electromyogr Kinesiol* 13:229-238, 2003.

97. Khaled, MB. Effect of traditional aerobic exercises versus sprint interval training on pulmonary function tests in young sedentary males: A randomised controlled trial. *J Clin Diagn Res* 7:1890-1893, 2013.

98. Kim, JS, Cross, JM, and Bamman, MM. Impact of resistance loading on myostatin expression and cell cycle regulation in young and older men and women. *Am J Physiol Endocrinol Metab* 288:E1110-1119, 2005.

99. Kjaer, MJ. Role of extracellular matrix in adaptation of tendon and skeletal muscle to mechanical loading. *Physiol Rev* 84, 649-698, 2004.

100. Konig, D, Huonker, M, Schmid, A, Halle, M, Berg, A, and Keul, J. Cardiovascular, metabolic, and hormonal parameters in professional tennis players. *Med Sci Sports Exerc* 33:654-658, 2001.

101. Kosek, DJ, Kim, JS, Petrella, JK, Cross, JM, and Bamman, MM. Efficacy of 3 days/wk resistance training on myofiber hypertrophy and myogenic mechanisms in young vs. older adults. *J Appl Physiol* 101:531-544, 2006.

102. Kraemer, WJ. Endocrine responses to resistance exercise. *Med Sci Sports Exerc* 20:152-157, 1998.

103. Kraemer, WJ, Adams, K, Cafarelli, E, Dudley, GA, Dooly, C, Feigenbaum, MS, Fleck, SJ, Franklin, B, Fry, AC, Hoffman, JR, Newton, RU, Potteiger, J, Stone, MH, Ratamess, NA, Triplett-McBride, T, and American College of Sports Medicine. American College of Sports Medicine position stand. Progression models in resistance training for healthy adults. *Med Sci Sports Exerc* 34:364-380, 2002.

104. Kraemer, WJ, Fleck, SJ, Dziados, JE, Harman, EA, Marchitelli, LJ, Gordon, SE, Mello, R, Frykman, PN, Koziris, LP, and Triplett, NT. Changes in hormonal concentrations after different heavy-resistance exercise protocols in women. *J Appl Physiol* 75:594-604, 1993.

105. Kraemer, WJ, Fleck, SJ, Maresh, CM, Ratamess, NA, Gordon, SE, Goetz, KL, Harman, EA, Frykman, PN, Volek, JS, Mazzetti, SA, Fry, AC, Marchitelli, LJ, and Patton, JF. Acute hormonal responses to a single bout of heavy resistance exercise in trained power lifters and untrained men. *Can J Appl Physiol* 24:524-537, 1999.

106. Kraemer, WJ, Gordon, SE, Fleck, SJ, Marchitelli, LJ, Mello, R, Dziados, JE, Friedl, K, Harman, E, Maresh, CM, and Fry, AC. Endogenous anabolic hormonal and growth factor responses to heavy resistance exercise in males and females. *Int J Sports Med* 12:228-235, 1991.

107. Kraemer, WJ, and Koziris, LP. Olympic weightlifting and power lifting. In *Physiology and Nutrition for Competitive Sport.* Lamb, DR, Knuttgen, HG, and Murray, R, eds. Carmel, IN: Cooper, 1-54, 1994.

108. Kraemer, WJ, Koziris, LP, Ratamess, NA, Häkkinen, K, Triplett-McBride, NT, Fry, AC, Gordon, SE, Volek, JS, French, DN, Rubin, MR, Gómez, AL, Sharman, MJ, Lynch, JM, Izquierdo, M, Newton, RU, and Fleck, SJ. Detraining produces minimal changes in physical performance and hormonal variables in recreationally strength-trained men. *J Strength Cond Res* 16:373-382, 2002.

109. Kraemer, WJ, Marchitelli, L, McCurry, D, Mello, R, Dziados, JE, Harman, E, Frykman, P, Gordon, SE, and Fleck, SJ. Hormonal and growth factor responses to heavy resistance exercise. *J Appl Physiol* 69:1442-1450, 1990.

110. Kraemer, WJ, and Nindl, BC. Factors involved with overtraining for strength and power. In *Overtraining in Sport.* Kreider, RB, Fry, AC, and O'Toole, ML, eds. Champaign, IL: Human Kinetics, 69-86, 1998.

111. Kraemer, WJ, Noble, BJ, Culver, BW, and Clark, MJ. Physiologic responses to heavy-resistance exercise with very short rest periods. *Int J Sports Med* 8:247-252, 1987.

112. Kraemer, WJ, Patton, J, Gordon, SE, Harman, EA, Deschenes, MR, Reynolds, K, Newton, RU, Triplett, NT, and Dziados, JE. Compatibility of high intensity strength and endurance training on hormonal and skeletal muscle adaptations. *J Appl Physiol* 78:976-989, 1995.

113. Kraemer, WJ, and Ratamess, NA. Physiology of resistance training: Current issues. *Orthop Phys Ther Clin N Am* 4:467-513, 2000.

114. Kraemer, WJ, and Ratamess, NA. Fundamentals of resistance training: Progression and exercise prescription. *Med Sci Sports Exerc* 36:674-678, 2004.

115. Kraemer, WJ, and Ratamess, NA. Hormonal responses and adaptations to resistance exercise and training. *Sports Med* 35:339-361, 2005.

116. Kraemer, WJ, Ratamess, NA, and French, DN. Resistance training for health and performance. *Curr Sport Med Rep* 1:165-171, 2002.

117. Kraemer, WJ, Rubin, MR, Häkkinen, K, Nindl, BC, Marx, JO, Volek, JS, French, DN, Gómez, AL, Sharman, MJ, Scheett, TP, Ratamess, NA, Miles, MP, Mastro, AM, Van Heest, JL, Maresh, CM, Welsch, JR, and Hymer, WC. Influence of muscle strength and total work on exercise-induced plasma growth hormone isoforms in women. *J Sci Med Sport* 6:295-306, 2003.

118. Kraemer, WJ, Spiering, BA, Volek, JS, Ratamess, NA, Sharman, MJ, Rubin, MR, French, DN, Silvestre, R, Hatfield, DL, Van Heest, JL, Vingren, JL, Judelson, DA, Deschenes, MR, and Maresh, CM. Androgenic responses to resistance exercise: Effects of feeding and L-carnitine. *Med Sci Sports Exerc* 38:1288-1296, 2006.

119. Kraemer, WJ, Staron, RS, Karapondo, D, Fry, AC, Gordon, SE, Volek, JS, Nindl, BC, Gotshalk, L, Newton, RU, and Häkkinen, K. The effects of short-term resistance training on endocrine function in men and women. *Eur J Appl Physiol* 78:69-76, 1998.

120. Kraemer, WJ, Volek, JS, Clark, KL, Gordon, SE, Incledon, T, Puhl, SM, Triplett-McBride, NT, McBride, JM, Putukian, M, and Sebastianelli, WJ. Physiological adaptations to a weight-loss dietary regimen and exercise programs in women. *J Appl Physiol* 83:270-279, 1997.

121. Kubo, K, Kanehisa, H, and Fukunaga, T. Effects of resistance and stretching training programmes on the viscoelastic properties of human tendon structures in vivo. *J Physiol* 538:219-226, 2002.

122. Kubo, K, Komuro, T, Ishiguro, N, Tsunoda, N, and Sato, Y. Effects of low-load resistance training with vascular occlusion on the mechanical properties of muscle and tendon. *J Appl Biomech* 22:112-119, 2006.

123. Kubo, K, Yata, H, Kanehisa, H, and Fukunaga, T. Effects of isometric squat training on the tendon stiffness and jump performance. *Eur J Appl Physiol* 96:305-314, 2006.

124. Kuipers, H, and Keizer, HA. Overtraining in elite athletes: Review and directions for the future. *Sports Med* 6:79-92, 1988.

125. Langberg, H, Rosendal, L, and Kjaer, M. Training-induced changes in peritendinous type I collagen turnover determined by microdialysis in humans. *J Physiol* 534:297-302, 2001.

126. Leveritt, M, and Abernethy, PJ. Acute effects of high-intensity endurance exercise on subsequent resistance activity. *J Strength Cond Res* 13:47-51, 1999.

127. Leveritt, M, Abernethy, PJ, Barry, B, and Logan, PA. Concurrent strength and endurance training: The influence of dependent variable selection. *J Strength Cond Res* 17:503-508, 2003.

128. Luthi, JM, Howald, H, Claassen, H, Rosler, K, Vock, P, and Hoppeler, H. Structural changes in skeletal muscle tissue with heavy-resistance exercise. *Int J Sports Med* 7:123-127, 1986.

129. MacDougall, JD, Elder, GCB, Sale, DG, and Sutton, JR. Effects of strength training and immobilization on human muscle fibers. *Eur J Appl Physiol* 43:25-34, 1980.

130. MacDougall, JD, Gibala, MJ, Tarnopolsky, MA, MacDonald, JR, Interisano, SA, and Yarasheski, KE. The time course for elevated muscle protein synthesis following heavy resistance exercise. *Can J Appl Physiol* 20:480-486, 1995.

131. MacDougall, JD, Sale, DG, Always, SE, and Sutton, JR. Muscle fiber number in biceps brachii in bodybuilders and control subjects. *J Appl Physiol* 57:1399-1403, 1984.

132. MacDougall, JD, Sale, DG, Elder, GC, and Sutton, JR. Muscle ultrastructural characteristics of elite powerlifters and bodybuilders. *Eur J Appl Physiol* 48:117-126, 1982.

133. MacDougall, JD, Sale, DG, Moroz, JR, Elder, GCB, Sutton, JR, and Howald, H. Mitochondrial volume density in human skeletal muscle following heavy resistance training. *Med Sci Sports Exerc* 11:164-166, 1979.

134. MacDougall, JD, Tuxen, D, Sale, DG, Moroz, JR, and Sutton, JR. Arterial blood pressure response to heavy resistance exercise. *J Appl Physiol* 58:785-790, 1985.

135. MacDougall, JD, Ward, GR, Sale, DG, and Sutton, JR. Biochemical adaptation of human skeletal muscle to heavy resistance training and immobilization. *J Appl Physiol* 43:700-703, 1977.

136. McCall, GE, Byrnes, WC, Fleck, SJ, Dickinson, A, and Kraemer, WJ. Acute and chronic hormonal responses to resistance training designed to promote muscle hypertrophy. *Can J Appl Physiol* 24:96-107, 1999.

137. McCarthy, JP, Agre, JC, Graf, BK, Pozniak, MA, and Vailas, AC. Compatibility of adaptive responses with combining strength and endurance training. *Med Sci Sports Exerc* 27:429-436, 1995.

138. McCarthy, JP, Pozniak, MA, and Agre, JC. Neuromuscular adaptations to concurrent strength and endurance training. *Med Sci Sports Exerc* 34:511-519, 2002.

139. McCartney, N, McKelvie, RS, Martin, J, Sale, DG, and MacDougall, JD. Weight-training induced attenuation of the circulatory response of older males to weight lifting. *J Appl Physiol* 74:1056-1060, 1993.

140. Meeusen, R, Duclos, M, Foster, C, Fry, A, Gleeson, M, Nieman, D, Raglin, J, Rietjens, G, Steinacker, J, and Urhausen, A. Prevention, diagnosis, and treatment of the over training syndrome: Joint consensus statement of the European College of Sport Science and the American College of Sports Medicine. *Med Sci Sports Exerc* 45:186-205, 2013.

141. Meeusen, R, Piacentini, MF, Busschaert, B, Buyse, L, De Schutter, G, and Stray-Gundersen, J. Hormonal responses in athletes: The use of a two bout exercise protocol to detect subtle differens in (over) training status. *Eur J Appl Physiol* 91:140-146, 2004.

142. Miller, BF, Olesen, JL, Hansen, M, Døssing, S, Crameri, RM, Welling, RJ, Langberg, H, Flyvbjerg, A, Kjaer, M, Babraj, JA, Smith, K, and Rennie, MJ. Coordinated collagen and muscle protein synthesis in human patella tendon and quadriceps muscle after exercise. *J Physiol* 15:1021-1033, 2005.

143. Minchna, H, and Hantmann, G. Adaptation of tendon collagen to exercise. *Int Orthop* 13:161-165, 1989.

144. Moore, CA, and Fry, AC. Nonfunctional overreaching during off-season training for skill position players in collegiate American football. *J Strength Cond Res* 21:793-800, 2007.

145. Moritani, T, and deVries, HA. Neural factors versus hypertrophy in the time course of muscle strength gain. *Am J Phys Med* 58:115-130, 1979.

146. Mujika, I, and Padilla, S. Muscular characteristics of detraining in humans. *Med Sci Sports Exerc* 33:1297-1303, 2001.

147. Munn, J, Herbert, RC, and Gandevia, SC. Contralateral effects of unilateral resistance training: A meta-analysis. *J Appl Physiol* 96:1861-1866, 2004.

148. Nardone, A, Romano, C, and Schieppati, M. Selective recruitment of high-threshold human motor units during voluntary isotonic lengthening of active muscles. *J Physiol* 409:451-471, 1989.

149. Newton, RU, Kraemer, WJ, Häkkinen, K, Humphries, BJ, and Murphy, AJ. Kinematics, kinetics, and muscle activation during explosive upper body movements: Implications for power development. *J Appl Biomech* 12:31-43, 1996.

150. Ortenblad, N, Lunde, PK, Levin, K, Andersen, JL, and Pedersen, PK. Enhanced sarcoplasmic reticulum Ca(2+) release following intermittent sprint training. *Am J Physiol* 279:R152-R160, 2000.

151. Pensini, M, Martin, A, and Maffiuletti, MA. Central versus peripheral adaptations following eccentric resistance training. *Int J Sports Med* 23:567-574, 2002.

152. Perry, J, Schmidt Easterday, C, and Antonelli, DJ. Surface versus intramuscular electrodes for electromyography of superficial and deep muscles. *Phys Ther* 61:7-15, 1981.

153. Pette, D, and Staron, RS. Mammalian skeletal muscle fiber type transitions. *Int Rev Cytol* 170:143-223, 1997.

154. Pette, D, and Staron, RS. Cellular and molecular diversities of mammalian skeletal muscle fibers. *Rev Physiol Biochem Pharmacol* 116:1-76, 1990.

155. Pette, D, and Staron, RS. Myosin isoforms, muscle fiber types, and transitions. *Microsc Res Tech* 50:500-509, 2002.

156. Phillips, S, Tipton, K, Aarsland, A, Wolf, S, and Wolfe, R. Mixed muscle protein synthesis and breakdown after resistance exercise in humans. *Am J Physiol Endocrinol Metab* 273:E99-E107, 1997.

157. Ploutz, LL, Tesch, PA, Biro, RL, and Dudley, GA. Effect of resistance training on muscle use during exercise. *J Appl Physiol* 76:1675-1681, 1994.

158. Pocock, NA, Eisman, J, Gwinn, T, Sambrook, P, Kelley, P, Freund, J, and Yeates, M. Muscle strength, physical fitness, and weight but not age to predict femoral neck bone mass. *J Bone Min Res* 4:441-448, 1989.

159. Raastad, T, Glomsheller, T, Bjoro, T, and Hallen, J. Changes in human skeletal muscle contractility and hormone status during 2 weeks of heavy strength training. *Eur J Appl Physiol* 84:54-63, 2001.

160. Ratamess, NA, Falvo, MJ, Mangine, GT, Hoffman, JR, Faigenbaum, AD, and Kang, J. The effect of rest interval length on metabolic responses to the bench press exercise. *Eur J Appl Physiol* 100:1-17, 2007.

161. Ratamess, NA, and Izquierdo, M. Neuromuscular adaptations to training. In *The Olympic Textbook of Medicine in Sport.* Hoboken, NJ: Wiley, 67-78, 2008.

162. Ratamess, NA, Kraemer, WJ, Volek, JS, Maresh, CM, Van Heest, JL, Sharman, MS, Rubin, MR, French, DN, Vescovi, JD, Silvestre, R, Hatfield, DL, Fleck, SJ, and Deschenes, MR. Effects of heavy resistance exercise volume on post-exercise androgen receptor content in resistance-trained men. *J Steroid Biochem* 93:35-42, 2005.

163. Ratamess, NA, Kraemer, WJ, Volek, JS, Rubin, MR, Gómez, AL, French, DN, Sharman, MJ, McGuigan, MM, Scheett, TP, Häkkinen, K, and Dioguardi, F. The effects of amino acid supplementation on muscular performance during resistance training overreaching: Evidence of an effective overreaching protocol. *J Strength Cond Res* 17:250-258, 2003.

164. Sabo, D, Bernd, L, Pfeil, J, and Reiter, A. Bone quality in the lumbar spine in high-performance athletes. *Eur Spine J* 5:258-263, 1996.

165. Sadusky, TJ, Kemp, TJ, Simon, M, Carey, N, and Coulton, GR. Identification of Serhl, a new member of the serine hydrolase family induced by passive stretch of skeletal muscle in vivo. *Genomics* 73:38-49, 2001.

166. Sale, DG. Influence of exercise and training on motor unit activation. *Exerc Sport Sci Rev* 15:95-151, 1987.

167. Sale, DG. Neural adaptations to strength training. In *The Encyclopaedia of Sports Medicine: Strength and Power in Sport.* Komi, PV, ed. Oxford: Blackwell Scientific, 281-314, 2003.

168. Sale, DG, Jacobs, I, MacDougall, JD, and Garner, S. Comparison of two regimens of concurrent strength and endurance training. *Med Sci Sports Exerc* 22:348-356, 1990.

169. Sale, DG, Moroz, DE, McKelvie, RS, MacDougall, JD, and McCartney, N. Effect of training on the blood pressure response to weight lifting. *Can J Appl Physiol* 19:60-74, 1994.

170. Sale, DG, Upton, ARM, McComas, AJ, and MacDougall, JD. Neuromuscular functions in weight-trainers. *Exp Neurol* 82:521-531, 1983.

171. Santana, JC, Vera-Garcia, FJ, and McGill, SM. A kinetic and electromyographic comparison of the standing cable press and bench press. *J Strength Cond Res* 21:1271-1277, 2007.

172. Sedano, S, Marín, PJ, Cuadrado, G, and Redondo, JC. Concurrent training in elite male runners: The influence of strength versus muscular endurance training on performance outcomes. *J Strength Cond Res* 27:2433-2443, 2013.

173. Semmler, J. Motor unit synchronization and neuromuscular performance. *Exerc Sport Sci Rev* 30:8-14, 2002.

174. Semmler, JG, Sale, MV, Meyer, FG, and Nordstrom, MA. Motor-unit coherence and its relation with synchrony are influenced by training. *J Neurophysiol* 92:3320-3331, 2004.

175. Sharp, RL, Costill, DL, Fink, WJ, and King, DS. Effects of eight weeks of bicycle ergometer sprint training on human muscle buffer capacity. *Int J Sports Med* 7, 13-17, 1986.

176. Shima, SN, Ishida, K, Katayama, K, Morotome, Y, Sato, Y, and Miyamura, M. Cross education of muscular strength during unilateral resistance training and detraining. *Eur J Appl Physiol* 86:287-294, 2002.

177. Shinohara, M, Kouzaki, M, Yoshihisa, T, and Fukunaga, T. Efficacy of tourniquet ischemia for strength training with low resistance. *Eur J Appl Physiol* 77:189-191, 1998.

178. Skerry, TM. Mechanical loading and bone: What sort of exercise is beneficial to the skeleton? *Bone* 20:179-181, 1997.

179. Spiering, BA, Kraemer, WJ, Anderson, JM, Armstrong, LE, Nindl, BC, Volek, JS, and Maresh, CM. Resistance exercise biology. Manipulation of resistance exercise programme variables determines the response of cellular and molecular signaling pathways. *Sports Med* 38:527-540, 2008.

180. Staff, PH. The effects of physical activity on joints, cartilage, tendons, and ligaments. *Scand J Med Sci Sports* 29:59-63, 1982.

181. Staron, RS. The classification of human skeletal muscle fiber types. *J Strength Cond Res* 11:67, 1997.

182. Staron, RS, Hagerman, FC, and Hikida, RS. The effects of detraining on an elite power lifter. A case study. *J Neurol Sci* 51:247-257, 1981.

183. Staron, RS, Karapondo, DL, Kraemer, WJ, Fry, AC, Gordon, SE, Falkel, JE, Hagerman, FC, and Hikida, RS. Skeletal muscle adaptations during the early phase of heavy-resistance training in men and women. *J Appl Physiol* 76:1247-1255, 1994.

184. Staron, RS, Malicky, ES, Leonardi, MJ, Falkel, JE, Hagerman, FC, and Dudley, GA. Muscle hypertrophy and fast fiber type conversions in heavy resistance-trained women. *Eur J Appl Physiol* 60:71-79, 1989.

185. Stone, MH, Keith, RE, Kearney, JT, Fleck, SE, Wilson, GD, and Triplett, NT. Overtraining: A review of the signs, symptoms and possible causes. *J Appl Sport Sci Res* 5:35-50, 1991.

186. Strope, MA, Nigh, P, Carter, MI, Lin, N, Jiang, J, and Hinton, PS. Physical activity-associated bone loading during adolescence and young adulthood is positively associated with adult bone mineral density in men. *Am J Mens Health,* 2014 [e-pub ahead of print].

187. Taaffe, DR, Robinson, TL, Snow, CM, and Marcus, R. High impact exercise promotes bone gain in well-trained female athletes. *J Bone Min Res* 12:255-260, 1997.

188. Takarada, Y, Sato, Y, and Ishii, N. Effects of resistance exercise combined with vascular occlusion on muscle function in athletes. *Eur J Appl Physiol* 86:308-314, 2002.

189. Ter Haar Romeny, BM, Dernier Van Der Goen, JJ, and Gielen, CCAM. Changes in recruitment order of motor units in the human biceps muscle. *Exp Neurol* 78:360-368, 1982.

190. Tesch, PA. Skeletal muscle adaptations consequent to long-term heavy-resistance exercise. *Med Sci Sports Exerc* 20:S124-S132, 1988.

191. Tesch, PA, and Larsson, L. Muscle hypertrophy in bodybuilders. *Eur J Appl Physiol* 49:310, 1982.

192. Tipton, KD, and Ferrando, AA. Improving muscle mass: Response of muscle metabolism to exercise, nutrition and anabolic agents. *Essays Biochem* 44:85-98, 2008.

193. Tremblay, MS, Copeland, JL, and Van Helder, W. Effect of training status and exercise mode on endogenous steroid hormones in men. *J Appl Physiol* 96, 531-539, 2003.

194. Urhausen, A, and Kinderman, W. Diagnosis of overtraining: What tools do we have? *Sports Med* 32:95-102, 2002.

195. Vanwanseele, B, Lucchinetti, E, and Stüssi, E. The effects of immobilization on the characteristics of articular cartilage: Current concepts and future directions. *Osteoarthritis Cartilage* 10:408-419, 2002.

196. Virvidakis, K, Georgion, E, Konkotsidis, A, Ntalles, K, and Proukasis, C. Bone mineral content of junior competitive weightlifters. *Int J Sports Med* 11:244-246, 1990.

197. Wilson, JM, Marin, PJ, Rhea, MR, Wilson, SM, Loenneke, JP, and Anderson, JC. Concurrent training: A meta-analysis examining interference of aerobic and resistance exercises. *J Strength Cond Res* 26:2293-2307, 2012.

198. Wittich, A, Mautalen, CA, Oliveri, MB, Bagur, A, Somoza, F, and Rotemberg, E. Professional football (soccer) players have a markedly greater skeletal mineral content, density, and size than age- and BMI-matched controls. *Calcif Tissue Int* 63:112-117, 1998.

CHAPTER 6   Adaptations to Aerobic Endurance Training Programs

1. Andersen, P. Capillary density in skeletal muscle of man. *Acta Physiol Scand* 95:203-205, 1975.

2. Andersen, P, and Henriksson, J. Training induced changes in the subgroups of human type II skeletal muscle fibres. *Acta Physiol Scand* 99:123-125, 1977.

3. Astrand, PO. Physical performance as a function of age. *JAMA* 205:729-733, 1968.

4. Astrand, PO, Cuddy, TE, Saltin, B, and Stenberg, J. Cardiac output during submaximal and maximal work. *J Appl Physiol* 19:268-274, 1964.

5. Åstrand, PO, Rodahl, K, Dahl, HA, and Strømme, SB. *Textbook of Work Physiology: Physiological Basis of Exercise.* Champaign, IL: Human Kinetics, 313-368, 2003.

6. Barcroft, H, and Swan, HJC. Sympathetic control of human blood vessels. *California Medicine* 79:337, 1953.

7. Beck, KC, and Johnson, BD. Pulmonary adaptations to dynamic exercise. In *ACSM's Resource Manual for Guidelines for Exercise Testing and Prescription*. Roitman, JL, ed. Baltimore: Williams and Wilkins, 305-313, 1998.

8. Blaauw, B, Schiaffino, S, and Reggiani, C. Mechanisms modulating skeletal muscle phenotype. *Compr Physiol* 3:1645-1687, 2013.

9. Bompa, TO, and Haff, GG. *Periodization: Theory and Methodology of Training*. Champaign, IL: Human Kinetics, 156-160, 2009.

10. Borer, KT. Physical activity in the prevention and amelioration of osteoporosis in women: Interaction of mechanical, hormonal and dietary factors. *Sports Med* 35:779-830, 2005.

11. Borresen, J, and Lambert, MI. Autonomic control of heart rate during and after exercise: Measurements and implications for monitoring training status. *Sports Med* 38:633-646, 2008.

12. Boudenot, A, Presle, N, Uzbekov, R, Toumi, H, Pallu, S, and Lespessailles, E. Effect of interval-training exercise on subchondral bone in a chemically-induced osteoarthritis model. *Osteoarthritis Cartilage* 22:1176-1185, 2014.

13. Brooks, GA, Fahey, TD, and Baldwin, KM. *Exercise Physiology: Human Bioenergetics and Its Applications*. 4th ed. Mountain View, CA: Mayfield, 2004.

14. Buchheit, M, and Laursen, PB. High-intensity interval training, solutions to the programming puzzle: Part I: Cardiopulmonary emphasis. *Sports Med* 43:313-338, 2013.

15. Buckwalter, JA. Osteoarthritis and articular cartilage use, disuse, and abuse: Experimental studies. *J Rheumatol Suppl* 43:13-15, 1995.

16. Burke, LM, Hawley, JA, Wong, SH, and Jeukendrup, AE. Carbohydrates for training and competition. *J Sports Sci* 29(Suppl 1):S17-S27, 2011.

17. Callister, R, Shealy, MJ, Fleck, SJ, and Dudley, GA. Performance adaptations to sprint, endurance and both modes of training. *J Appl Sport Sci Res* 2:46-51, 1988.

18. Charkoudian, N, and Joyner, MJ. Physiologic considerations for exercise performance in women. *Clin Chest Med* 25:247-255, 2004.

19. Costill, DL, Daniels, J, Evans, W, Fink, W, Krahenbuhl, G, and Saltin, B. Skeletal muscle enzymes and fiber composition in male and female track athletes. *J Appl Physiol* 40:149-154, 1976.

20. Coyle, EF, Hemmert, MK, and Coggan, AR. Effects of detraining on cardiovascular responses to exercise: Role of blood volume. *J Appl Physiol* 60:95-99, 1986.

21. Coyle, EF, Martin, WH, Bloomfield, SA, Lowry, OH, and Holloszy, JO. Effects of detraining on responses to submaximal exercise. *J Appl Physiol* 59:853-859, 1985.

22. Coyle, EF, Martin, WH, Sinacore, DR, Joyner, MJ, Hagberg, JM, and Holloszy, JO. Time course of loss of adaptations after stopping prolonged intense endurance training. *J Appl Physiol Respir Environ Exerc Physiol* 57:1857-1864, 1984.

23. Drinkwater, BL, and Horvath, SM. Detraining effects on young women. *Medicine and Science in Sports* 4:91-95, 1972.

24. Durstine, JL, and Davis, PG. Specificity of exercise training and testing. In *ACSM's Resource Manual for Guidelines for Exercise Testing and Prescription*. Roitman, JL, ed. Baltimore: Williams and Wilkins, 472-479, 1998.

25. Fardy, PS. Effects of soccer training and detraining upon selected cardiac and metabolic measures. *Res Q* 40:502-508, 1969.

26. Fardy, PS. Training for aerobic power. In *Toward an Understanding of Human Performance*. Burke, EJ, ed. Ithaca, NY: Mouvement, 10-14, 1977.

27. Fink, WJ, Costill, DL, and Pollock, ML. Submaximal and maximal working capacity of elite distance runners: Part II. Muscle fiber composition and enzyme activities. *Ann N Y Acad Sci* 301:323-327, 1977.

28. Fleck, SJ, and Kraemer, WJ. The overtraining syndrome. *NSCA J* 4:50-51, 1982.

29. Fleck, SJ, and Kraemer, WJ. *Periodization Breakthrough: The Ultimate Training System*. Ronkonkoma, NY: Advanced Research Press, 1996.

30. Flynn, MG, Pizza, FX, Boone, JB, Jr., Andres, FF, Michaud, TA, and Rodriguez-Zayas, JR. Indices of training stress during competitive running and swimming seasons. *Int J Sports Med* 15:21-26, 1994.

31. Franch, J, Madsen, K, Djurhuus, MS, and Pedersen, PK. Improved running economy following intensified training correlates with reduced ventilatory demands. *Med Sci Sports Exerc* 30:1250-1256, 1998.

32. Franklin, BA. Normal cardiorespiratory responses to acute exercise. In *ACSM's Resource Manual for Guidelines for Exercise Testing and Prescription*. Roitman, JL, ed. Baltimore: Williams and Wilkins, 137-145, 1998.

33. Franklin, BA, and Roitman, JL. Cardiorespiratory adaptations to exercise. In *ACSM's Resource Manual for Guidelines for Exercise Testing and Prescription*. Roitman, JL, ed. Baltimore: Williams and Wilkins, 146-155, 1998.

34. Frost, HM. Why do marathon runners have less bone than weight lifters? A vital-biomechanical view and explanation. *Bone* 20:183-189, 1997.

35. Fry, AC, and Kraemer, WJ. Resistance exercise overtraining and overreaching: Neuroendocrine responses. *Sports Med* 23:106-129, 1997.

36. Fry, AC, Kraemer, WJ, and Ramsey, LT. Pituitary-adrenal-gonadal responses to high-intensity resistance exercise overtraining. *J Appl Physiol* 85:2352-2359, 1998.

37. Gaesser, GA, and Wilson, LA. Effects of continuous and interval training on the parameters of the power-endurance time relationship for high-intensity exercise. *Int J Sports Med* 9:417-421, 1988.

38. Galbo, H. Endocrinology and metabolism in exercise. *Curr Probl Clin Biochem* 11:26-44, 1982.

39. Galbo, H. *Hormonal and Metabolic Adaptation to Exercise*. New York: Thieme-Stratton, 1983.

40. Gibala, MJ, and Mcgee, SL. Metabolic adaptations to short-term high-intensity interval training: A little pain for a lot of gain? *Exerc Sport Sci Rev* 36:58-63, 2008.

41. Gollnick, PD. Relationship of strength and endurance with skeletal muscle structure and metabolic potential. *Int J Sports Med* 3(Suppl 1):26-32, 1982.

42. Gollnick, PD, Armstrong, RB, Saltin, B, Saubert, CWT, Sembrowich, WL, and Shepherd, RE. Effect of training on enzyme activity and fiber composition of human skeletal muscle. *J Appl Physiol* 34:107-111, 1973.

43. Gollnick, PD, Armstrong, RB, Saubert, CWT, Piehl, K, and Saltin, B. Enzyme activity and fiber composition in skeletal muscle of untrained and trained men. *J Appl Physiol* 33:312-319, 1972.

44. Gonzalez-Alonso, J, Mortensen, SP, Jeppesen, TD, Ali, L, Barker, H, Damsgaard, R, Secher, NH, Dawson, EA, and Dufour, SP. Haemodynamic responses to exercise, ATP infusion and thigh compression in humans: Insight into the role of muscle mechanisms on cardiovascular function. *J Physiol* 586:2405-2417, 2008.

45. Green, HJ, Jones, LL, and Painter, DC. Effects of short-term training on cardiac function during prolonged exercise. *Med Sci Sports Exerc* 22:488-493, 1990.

46. Guyton, AC, and Hall, JE. *Textbook of Medical Physiology*. 10th ed. Philadelphia: Saunders, 101-114, 2000.

47. Halson, SL, and Jeukendrup, AE. Does overtraining exist? An analysis of overreaching and overtraining research. *Sports Med* 34:967-981, 2004.

48. Harber, M, and Trappe, S. Single muscle fiber contractile properties of young competitive distance runners. *J Appl Physiol* 105:629-636, 2008.

49. Havenith, G, and Holewijn, M. Environmental considerations: Altitude and air pollution. In *ACSM's American College of Sports Medicine Resource Manual for Guidelines for Exercise Testing and Prescription.* Roitman, JL, ed. Baltimore: Williams and Wilkins, 215-222, 1998.

50. Hedelin, R, Kentta, G, Wiklund, U, Bjerle, P, and Henriksson-Larsen, K. Short-term overtraining: Effects on performance, circulatory responses, and heart rate variability. *Med Sci Sports Exerc* 32:1480-1484, 2000.

51. Hermansen, L, and Wachtlova, M. Capillary density of skeletal muscle in well-trained and untrained men. *J Appl Physiol* 30:860-863, 1971.

52. Hickson, RC. Skeletal muscle cytochrome c and myoglobin, endurance, and frequency of training. *J Appl Physiol Respir Environ Exerc Physiol* 51:746-749, 1981.

53. Hickson, RC, Bomze, HA, and Holloszy, JO. Linear increase in aerobic power induced by a strenuous program of endurance exercise. *J Appl Physiol Respir Environ Exerc Physiol* 42:372-376, 1977.

54. Hickson, RC, Dvorak, BA, Gorostiaga, EM, Kurowski, TT, and Foster, C. Potential for strength and endurance training to amplify endurance performance. *J Appl Physiol* 65:2285-2290, 1988.

55. Hickson, RC, Hagberg, JM, Ehsani, AA, and Holloszy, JO. Time course of the adaptive responses of aerobic power and heart rate to training. *Med Sci Sports Exerc* 13:17-20, 1981.

56. Holloszy, JO. Adaptation of skeletal muscle to endurance exercise. *Med Sci Sports* 7:155-164, 1975.

57. Holloszy, JO. Biochemical adaptations in muscle: Effects of exercise on mitochondrial oxygen uptake and respiratory enzyme activity in skeletal muscle. *J Biol Chem* 242:2278-2282, 1967.

58. Holloszy, JO. Regulation by exercise of skeletal muscle content of mitochondria and GLUT4. *J Physiol Pharmacol* 59(Suppl 7):5-18, 2008.

59. Holloszy, JO, Kohrt, WM, and Hansen, PA. The regulation of carbohydrate and fat metabolism during and after exercise. *Front Biosci* 3:D1011-D1027, 1998.

60. Houston, ME, Bentzen, H, and Larsen, H. Interrelationships between skeletal muscle adaptations and performance as studied by detraining and retraining. *Acta Physiol Scand* 105:163-170, 1979.

61. Howald, H. Training-induced morphological and functional changes in skeletal muscle. *Int J Sports Med* 3:1-12, 1982.

62. Jones, AM, and Carter, H. The effect of endurance training on parameters of aerobic fitness. *Sports Med* 29:373-386, 2000.

63. Jones, M, and Tunstall Pedoe, DS. Blood doping—a literature review. *Br J Sports Med* 23:84-88, 1989.

64. Joseph, V, and Pequignot, JM. Breathing at high altitude. *Cell Mol Life Sci* 66:3565-3573, 2009.

65. Kim, V, and Criner, GJ. Chronic bronchitis and chronic obstructive pulmonary disease. *Am J Respir Crit Care Med* 187:228-237, 2013.

66. Kiviranta, I, Tammi, M, Jurvelin, J, Arokoski, J, Saamanen, AM, and Helminen, HJ. Articular cartilage thickness and glycosaminoglycan distribution in the canine knee joint after strenuous running exercise. *Clin Orthop Relat Res*:302-308, 1992.

67. Kiviranta, I, Tammi, M, Jurvelin, J, Saamanen, AM, and Helminen, HJ. Moderate running exercise augments glycosaminoglycans and thickness of articular cartilage in the knee joint of young beagle dogs. *J Orthop Res* 6:188-195, 1988.

68. Konopka, AR, and Harber, MP. Skeletal muscle hypertrophy after aerobic exercise training. *Exerc Sport Sci Rev* 42:53-61, 2014.

69. Kraemer, WJ, and Baechle, TR. Development of a strength training program. In *Sports Medicine.* Allman, FL, and Ryan, AJ, eds. Orlando, FL: Academic Press, 113-127, 1989.

70. Kraemer, WJ, and Fleck, SJ. Aerobic metabolism, training, and evaluation. *NSCA J* 5:52-54, 1982.

71. Kraemer, WJ, Fry, AC, Warren, BJ, Stone, MH, Fleck, SJ, Kearney, JT, Conroy, BP, Maresh, CM, Weseman, CA, Triplett, NT, et al. Acute hormonal responses in elite junior weightlifters. *Int J Sports Med* 13:103-109, 1992.

72. Kraemer, WJ, Marchitelli, L, Gordon, SE, Harman, E, Dziados, JE, Mello, R, Frykman, P, McCurry, D, and Fleck, SJ. Hormonal and growth factor responses to heavy resistance exercise protocols. *J Appl Physiol* 69:1442-1450, 1990.

73. Kraemer, WJ, and Nindl, BC. Factors involved with overtraining for strength and power. In *Overtraining in Sport.* Kreider, RB, Fry, AC, and O'Toole, ML, eds. Champaign, IL: Human Kinetics, 69-86, 1998.

74. Kraemer, WJ, Patton, JF, Knuttgen, HG, Marchitelli, LJ, Cruthirds, C, Damokosh, A, Harman, E, Frykman, P, and Dziados, JE. Hypothalamic-pituitary-adrenal responses to short-duration high-intensity cycle exercise. *J Appl Physiol* 66:161-166, 1989.

75. Kraemer, WJ, and Ratamess, NA. Endocrine responses and adaptations to strength training. In *The Encyclopedia of Sports Medicine: Strength and Power in Sport.* Komi, PV, ed. Malden, MA: Blackwell Scientific, 361-386, 1992.

76. Kraemer, WJ, Volek, JS, and Fleck, SJ. Chronic musculoskeletal adaptations to resistance training. In *ACSM's Resource Manual for Guidelines for Exercise Testing and Prescription.* Roitman, JL, ed. Baltimore: Williams and Wilkins, 174-181, 1998.

77. Kuipers, H, and Keizer, HA. Overtraining in elite athletes: Review and directions for the future. *Sports Med* 6:79-92, 1988.

78. Kyle, UG, Genton, L, Hans, D, Karsegard, L, Slosman, DO, and Pichard, C. Age-related differences in fat-free mass, skeletal muscle, body cell mass and fat mass between 18 and 94 years. *Eur J Clin Nutr* 55:663-672, 2001.

79. Landi, F, Marzetti, E, Martone, AM, Bernabei, R, and Onder, G. Exercise as a remedy for sarcopenia. *Curr Opin Clin Nutr Metab Care* 17:25-31, 2014.

80. Laursen, PB. Training for intense exercise performance: High-intensity or high-volume training? *Scand J Med Sci Sports* 20(Suppl 2):1-10, 2010.

81. Lehmann, MJ, Lormes, W, Opitz-Gress, A, Steinacker, JM, Netzer, N, Foster, C, and Gastmann, U. Training and overtraining: An overview and experimental results in endurance sports. *J Sports Med Phys Fitness* 37:7-17, 1997.

82. Lemon, PW, and Nagle, FJ. Effects of exercise on protein and amino acid metabolism. *Med Sci Sports Exerc* 13:141-149, 1981.

83. Lester, M, Sheffield, LT, Trammell, P, and Reeves, TJ. The effect of age and athletic training on the maximal heart rate during muscular exercise. *Am Heart J* 76:370-376, 1968.

84. Lewis, DA, Kamon, E, and Hodgson, JL. Physiological differences between genders: Implications for sports conditioning. *Sports Med* 3:357-369, 1986.

85. Louie, D. The effects of cigarette smoking on cardiopulmonary function and exercise tolerance in teenagers. *Can Respir J* 8:289-291, 2001.

86. Lovasi, GS, Diez Roux, AV, Hoffman, EA, Kawut, SM, Jacobs, DR, Jr., and Barr, RG. Association of environmental tobacco smoke exposure in childhood with early emphysema in adulthood among nonsmokers: The MESA-lung study. *Am J Epidemiol* 171:54-62, 2010.

87. Luger, A, Deuster, PA, Kyle, SB, Gallucci, WT, Montgomery, LC, Gold, PW, Loriaux, DL, and Chrousos, GP. Acute hypothalamic-pituitary-adrenal responses to the stress of treadmill exercise: Physiologic adaptations to physical training. *N Engl J Med* 316:1309-1315, 1987.

88. Lundback, B, Lindberg, A, Lindstrom, M, Ronmark, E, Jonsson, AC, Jonsson, E, Larsson, LG, Andersson, S, Sandstrom, T, and Larsson, K. Not 15 but 50% of smokers develop COPD? Report from the Obstructive Lung Disease in Northern Sweden Studies. *Respir Med* 97:115-122, 2003.

89. Madsen, K, Pedersen, PK, Djurhuus, MS, and Klitgaard, NA. Effects of detraining on endurance capacity and metabolic changes during prolonged exhaustive exercise. *J Appl Physiol* 75:1444-1451, 1993.

90. Martin, WH, Coyle, EF, Bloomfield, SA, and Ehsani, AA. Effects of physical deconditioning after intense endurance training on left ventricular dimensions and stroke volume. *J Am Coll Cardiol* 7:982-989, 1986.

91. McArdle, WD, Katch, FI, and Katch, VI. *Exercise Physiology.* Philadelphia: Lea and Febiger, 2014.

92. Meeusen, R, Duclos, M, Foster, C, Fry, A, Gleeson, M, Nieman, D, Raglin, J, Rietjens, G, Steinacker, J, and Urhausen, A. Prevention, diagnosis, and treatment of the overtraining syndrome: Joint consensus statement of the European College of Sport Science and the American College of Sports Medicine. *Med Sci Sports Exerc* 45:186-205, 2013.

93. Moreno, AH, Burchell, AR, Van Der Woude, R, and Burke, JH. Respiratory regulation of splanchnic and systemic venous return. *Am J Physiol* 213:455-465, 1967.

94. Morgan, T, Cobb, L, Short, F, Ross, R, and Gunn, D. Effects of long-term exercise on human muscle mitochondria. In *Muscle Metabolism During Exercise.* Pernow, B, and Saltin, B, eds. New York: Plenum Press, 87-95, 1971.

95. Mujika, I, and Padilla, S. Detraining: Loss of training-induced physiological and performance adaptations: Part I. Short term insufficient training stimulus. *Sports Med.* 30:79-87, 2000.

96. Mujika, I. and Padilla, S. Detraining: Loss of training-induced physiological and performance adaptations: Part II. Long term insufficient training stimulus. *Sports Med.* 30:145-154, 2000.

97. Muza, SR, Sawka, MN, Young, AJ, Dennis, RC, Gonzalez, RR, Martin, JW, Pandolf, KB, and Valeri, CR. Elite special forces: Physiological description and ergogenic influence of blood reinfusion. *Aviat Space Environ Med* 58:1001-1004, 1987.

98. Oettmeier, R, Arokoski, J, Roth, AJ, Helminen, HJ, Tammi, M, and Abendroth, K. Quantitative study of articular cartilage and subchondral bone remodeling in the knee joint of dogs after strenuous running training. *J Bone Miner Res* 7(Suppl 2):S419-S424, 1992.

99. Ogawa, T, Spina, RJ, Martin, WH, Kohrt, WM, Schechtman, KB, Holloszy, JO, and Ehsani, AA. Effects of aging, sex, and physical training on cardiovascular responses to exercise. *Circulation* 86:494-503, 1992.

100. Oliveira, CD, Bairros, AV, and Yonamine, M. Blood doping: Risks to athletes' health and strategies for detection. *Subst Use Misuse* 49:1168-1181, 2014.

101. Papathanasiou, G, Georgakopoulos, D, Georgoudis, G, Spyropoulos, P, Perrea, D, and Evangelou, A. Effects of chronic smoking on exercise tolerance and on heart rate-systolic blood pressure product in young healthy adults. *Eur J Cardiovasc Prev Rehabil* 14:646-652, 2007.

102. Pette, D, and Staron, RS. Transitions of muscle fiber phenotypic profiles. *Histochem Cell Biol* 115:359-372, 2001.

103. Ploutz-Snyder, LL, Simoneau, JA, Gilders, RM, Staron, RS, and Hagerman, FC. Cardiorespiratory and metabolic adaptations to hyperoxic training. *Eur J Appl Physiol Occup Physiol* 73:38-48, 1996.

104. Pollock, ML. Submaximal and maximal working capacity of elite distance runners: Part I. Cardiorespiratory aspects. *Ann N Y Acad Sci* 301:310-322, 1977.

105. Raglin, J, and Wilson, G. Overtraining and staleness in athletes. In *Emotions in Sports.* Hanin, YL, ed. Champaign, IL: Human Kinetics, 191-207, 2000.

106. Rankinen, T, Sung, YJ, Sarzynski, MA, Rice, TK, Rao, DC, and Bouchard, C. Heritability of submaximal exercise heart rate response to exercise training is accounted for by nine SNPs. *J Appl Physiol* 112:892-897, 2012.

107. Robertson, RJ, Gilcher, R, Metz, KF, Skrinar, GS, Allison, TG, Bahnson, HT, Abbott, RA, Becker, R, and Falkel, JE. Effect of induced erythrocythemia on hypoxia tolerance during physical exercise. *J Appl Physiol Respir Environ Exerc Physiol* 53:490-495, 1982.

108. Sale, DG. Influence of exercise and training on motor unit activation. *Exerc Sport Sci Rev* 15:95-151, 1987.

109. Saltin, B, Blomqvist, G, Mitchell, JH, Johnson, RL, Jr., Wildenthal, K, and Chapman, CB. Response to exercise after bed rest and after training. *Circulation* 38:1-78, 1968.

110. Saltin, B, Nazar, K, Costill, D.L, Stein, E, Jansson, E, Essen, B, and Gollnick, D. The nature of the training response: Peripheral and central adaptations of one-legged exercise. *Acta Physiol Scand* 96:289-305, 1976.

111. Sawka, MN, Dennis, RC, Gonzalez, RR, Young, AJ, Muza, SR, Martin, JW, Wenger, CB, Francesconi, RP, Pandolf, KB, and Valeri, CR. Influence of polycythemia on blood volume and thermoregulation during exercise-heat stress. *J Appl Physiol* 62:912-918, 1987.

112. Sawka, MN, Gonzalez, RR, Young, AJ, Muza, SR, Pandolf, KB, Latzka, WA, Dennis, RC, and Valeri, CR. Polycythemia and hydration: Effects on thermoregulation and blood volume during exercise-heat stress. *Am J Physiol* 255:R456-R463, 1988.

113. Sawka, MN, Joyner, MJ, Miles, DS, Robertson, RJ, Spriet, LL, and Young, AJ. American College of Sports Medicine position stand: The use of blood doping as an ergogenic aid. *Med Sci Sports Exerc* 28:i-viii, 1996.

114. Seene, T, Alev, K, Kaasik, P, Pehme, A, and Parring, AM. Endurance training: Volume-dependent adaptational changes in myosin. *Int J Sports Med* 26:815-821, 2005.

115. Silverman, HG, and Mazzeo, RS. Hormonal responses to maximal and submaximal exercise in trained and untrained men of various ages. *J Gerontol A Biol Sci Med Sci* 51:B30-B37, 1996.

116. Skoluda, N, Dettenborn, L, Stalder, T, and Kirschbaum, C. Elevated hair cortisol concentrations in endurance athletes. *Psychoneuroendocrinology* 37:611-617, 2012.

117. Sperlich, B, Zinner, C, Krueger, M, Wegrzyk, J, Achtzehn, S, and Holmberg, HC. Effects of hyperoxia during recovery from 5×30-s bouts of maximal-intensity exercise. *J Sports Sci* 30:851-858, 2012.

118. Sperlich, B, Zinner, C, Krueger, M, Wegrzyk, J, Mester, J, and Holmberg, HC. Ergogenic effect of hyperoxic recovery in elite swimmers performing high-intensity intervals. *Scand J Med Sci Sports* 21:e421-e429, 2011.

119. Staff, PH. The effects of physical activity on joints, cartilage, tendons and ligaments. *Scand J Soc Med Suppl* 29:59-63, 1982.

120. Staton, GW. Chronic obstructive diseases of the lung. In *ACP Medicine.* Dale, DC, and Federman, DD, eds. New York: WebMD Professional, 2720-2743, 2007.

121. Stone, MH, Keith, RE, Kearney, JT, Fleck, SJ, Wilson, GD, and Triplett, NT. Overtraining: A review of the signs, symptoms and possible causes. *Journal of Strength and Conditioning Research* 5:35-50, 1991.

122. Tamaki, H, Kitada, K, Akamine, T, Murata, F, Sakou, T, and Kurata, H. Alternate activity in the synergistic muscles during prolonged low-level contractions. *J Appl Physiol* 84:1943-1951, 1998.

123. Tanaka, H, Monahan, KD, and Seals, DR. Age-predicted maximal heart rate revisited. *J Am Coll Cardiol* 37:153-156, 2001.

124. Tipton, KD, and Wolfe, RR. Exercise-induced changes in protein metabolism. *Acta Physiol Scand* 162:377-387, 1998.

125. Tomlin, DL, and Wenger, HA. The relationship between aerobic fitness and recovery from high intensity intermittent exercise. *Sports Med* 31:1-11, 2001.

126. Trappe, S, Harber, M, Creer, A, Gallagher, P, Slivka, D, Minchev, K, and Whitsett, D. Single muscle fiber adaptations with marathon training. *J Appl Physiol* 101:721-727, 2006.

127. Triplett-McBride, NT, Mastro, AM, McBride, JM, Bush, JA, Putukian, M, Sebastianelli, WJ, and Kraemer, WJ. Plasma proenkephalin peptide F and human B cell responses to exercise stress in fit and unfit women. *Peptides* 19:731-738, 1998.

128. Tuna, Z, Güzel, NA, Aral, AL, Elbeg, S, Özer, C, Erikoglu, G, Atak, A, and Pinar, L. Effects of an acute exercise up to anaerobic threshold on serum anabolic and catabolic factors in trained and sedentary young males. *Gazi Med J* 25:47-51, 2014.

129. Urhausen, A, Gabriel, H, and Kindermann, W. Blood hormones as markers of training stress and overtraining. *Sports Med* 20:251-276, 1995.

130. Urhausen, A, and Kindermann, W. Diagnosis of overtraining: What tools do we have? *Sports Med* 32:95-102, 2002.

131. Vogel, JA, Patton, JF, Mello, RP, and Daniels, WL. An analysis of aerobic capacity in a large United States population. *J Appl Physiol* 60:494-500, 1986.

132. Vollaard, NB, Constantin-Teodosiu, D, Fredriksson, K, Rooyackers, O, Jansson, E, Greenhaff, PL, Timmons, JA, and Sundberg, CJ. Systematic analysis of adaptations in aerobic capacity and submaximal energy metabolism provides a unique insight into determinants of human aerobic performance. *J Appl Physiol* 106:1479-1486, 2009.

133. Wilkinson, SB, Phillips, SM, Atherton, PJ, Patel, R, Yarasheski, KE, Tarnopolsky, MA, and Rennie, MJ. Differential effects of resistance and endurance exercise in the fed state on signalling molecule phosphorylation and protein synthesis in human muscle. *J Physiol* 586:3701-3717, 2008.

134. Wilson, JM, Loenneke, JP, Jo, E, Wilson, GJ, Zourdos, MC, and Kim, JS. The effects of endurance, strength, and power training on muscle fiber type shifting. *J Strength Cond Res* 26:1724-1729, 2012.

135. Wilt, F. Training for competitive running. In *Exercise Physiology.* Fall, HB, ed. New York: Academic Press, 395-414, 1968.

136. Wyatt, FB, Donaldson, A, and Brown, E. The overtraining syndrome: A meta-analytic review. *J Exerc Physiol Online* 16:12-23, 2013.

137. Zhou, B, Conlee, RK, Jensen, R, Fellingham, GW, George, JD, and Fisher, AG. Stroke volume does not plateau during graded exercise in elite male distance runners. *Med Sci Sports Exerc* 33:1849-1854, 2001.

138. Zouhal, H, Jacob, C, Delamarche, P, and Gratas-Delamarche, A. Catecholamines and the effects of exercise, training and gender. *Sports Med* 38:401-423, 2008.

CHAPTER 7   Age- and Sex-Related Differences and Their Implications for Resistance Exercise

1. Alentorn-Geli, E, Myer, GD, Silvers, HJ, Samitier, G, Romero, D, Lázaro-Haro, C, and Cugat, R. Prevention of non-contact anterior cruciate ligament injuries in soccer players. Part 2: A review of prevention programs aimed to modify risk factors and to reduce injury rates. *Knee Surg Sports Traumatol Arthrosc* 17:859-879, 2009.

2. American Academy of Pediatrics. Intensive training and sports specialization in young athletes. *Pediatrics* 106:154-157, 2000.

3. American Academy of Pediatrics. Strength training by children and adolescents. *Pediatrics* 121:835-840, 2008.

4. American College of Sports Medicine. *ACSM's Guidelines for Exercise Testing and Prescription.* 9th ed. Philadelphia: Lippincott Williams & Wilkins, 184, 2014.

5. American College of Sports Medicine position stand. Exercise and physical activity for older adults. *Med Sci Sports Exerc* 41:1510-1530, 2009.

6. American College of Sports Medicine position stand. The female athlete triad. *Med Sci Sports Exerc* 39:1867-1882, 2007.

7. American Orthopaedic Society for Sports Medicine. *Proceedings of the Conference on Strength Training and the Prepubescent.* Chicago: American Orthopaedic Society for Sports Medicine, 1-14, 1988.

8. Annesi, J, Westcott, W, Faigenbaum, AD, and Unruh, JL. Effects of a 12 week physical activity program delivered by YMCA after-school counselors (Youth Fit for Life) on fitness and self-efficacy changes in 5-12 year old boys and girls. *Res Q Exerc Sport* 76:468-476, 2005.

9. Arendt, E, and Dick, R. Knee injury patterns among men and women in collegiate basketball and soccer: NCAA data and review of literature. *Am J Sports Med* 23:694-701, 1995.

10. Bailey, D, and Martin, A. Physical activity and skeletal health in adolescents. *Pediatr Exerc Sci* 6:330-347, 1994.

11. Bassey, E, Fiatarone, M, O'Neill, E, Kelly, M, Evans, W, and Lipsitz, L. Leg extensor power and functional performance in very old men and women. *Clin Sci* 82:321-327, 1992.

12. Behm, DG, Faigenbaum, AD, Falk, B, and Klentrou, P. Canadian Society for Exercise Physiology position paper: Resistance training in children and adolescents. *Appl Physiol Nutr Metab* 33:547-561, 2008.

13. Behringer, M, vom Heede, A, Matthews, M, and Mester, J. Effects of strength training on motor performance skills in children and adolescents: A meta-analysis. *Pediatr Exerc Sci* 23:186-206, 2011.

14. Behringer, M, vom Heede, A, Yue, Z, and Mester, J. Effects of resistance training in children and adolescents: A meta-anlaysis. *Pediatrics* 126:e1199-e1210, 2010.

15. Benson, AC, Torode, ME, and Fiatarone Singh, MA. The effect of high intensity progressive resistance training on adiposity in children: A randomized controlled trial. *Int J Obes* 32:1016-1027, 2008.

16. Binzoni, T, Bianchi, S, Hanquinet, S, Kaelin, A, Sayegh, Y, Dumont, M, and Jéquier, S. Human gastrocnemius medialis pennation angle as a function of age: From newborn to the elderly. *J Physiol Anthropol* 20:293-298, 2001.

17. Bishop, P, Cureton, K, and Collins, M. Sex difference in muscular strength in equally-trained men and women. *Ergonomics* 30:675-687, 1987.

18. Blanksby, B, and Gregor, J. Anthropometric, strength, and physiological changes in male and female swimmers with progressive resistance training. *Aust J Sport Sci* 1:3-6, 1981.

19. Blimkie, C. Benefits and risks of resistance training in youth. In *Intensive Participation in Children's Sports.* Cahill, B, and Pearl, A, eds. Champaign, IL: Human Kinetics, 133-167, 1993.

20. Boden, BP, Dean, GS, Feagin, JA, and Garrett, WE. Mechanisms of anterior cruciate ligament injury. *Orthopedics* 23:573-578, 2000.

21. Brenner, JS. Overuse injuries, overtraining, and burnout in child and adolescent athletes. *Pediatrics* 119:1242-1245, 2007.

22. British Association of Exercise and Sport Sciences. BASES position statement on guidelines for resistance exercise in young people. *J Sports Sci* 22:383-390, 2004.

23. Buenen, G, and Malina, R. Growth and physical performance relative to the timing of the adolescent growth spurt. In *Exercise and Sport Science Reviews.* Pandolf, K, ed. New York: Macmillan, 503-540, 1988.

24. Bulgakova, N, Vorontsov, A, and Fomichenko, T. Improving the technical preparedness of young swimmers by using strength training. *Soviet Sports Rev* 25:102-104, 1990.

25. Byrd, R, Pierce, K, Rielly, L, and Brady, J. Young weightlifters' performance across time. *Sports Biomech* 2:133-140, 2003.

26. Campbell, AJ, Borrie, MJ, Spears, GF, Jackson, SL, Brown, JS, and Fitzgerald, JL. Circumstances and consequences of falls experienced by a community population 70 years and over during a prospective study. *Age Ageing* 19:136-141, 1990.

27. Campbell, W, Crim, M, Young, V, and Evans, W. Increased energy requirements and changes in body composition with resistance training in older adults. *Am J Clin Nutr* 60:167-175, 1994.

28. Campbell, W, Crim, M, Young, V, Joseph, J, and Evans, W. Effects of resistance training and dietary protein intake on protein metabolism in older adults. *Am J Appl Physiol* 268:E1143-E1153, 1995.

29. Castro, M, McCann, D, Shaffrath, J, and Adams, W. Peak torque per unit cross-sectional area differs between strength-training and untrained adults. *Med Sci Sports Exerc* 27:397-403, 1995.

30. Castro-Piñero, J, Ortega, FB, Artero, EG, Girela-Rejón, MJ, Sjöström, M, and Ruiz, JR. Assessing muscular strength in youth: Usefulness of standing long jump as a general index of muscular fitness. *J Strength Cond Res* 24:1810-1817, 2010.

31. Centers for Disease Control and Prevention. Strength training among adults >65 years United States, 2001. *MMWR* 53:1-4, 2004.

32. Charette, S, McEvoy, L, Pyka, G, Snow-Harter, C, Guido, D, Wiswell, R, and Marcus, R. Muscle hypertrophy response to resistance training in older women. *J Appl Physiol* 70:1912-1916, 1991.

33. Chilibeck, P, Calder, A, Sale, D, and Webber, C. A comparison of strength and muscle mass increases during resistance training in young women. *Eur J Appl Physiol* 77:170-175, 1998.

34. Christmas, C, and Andersen, R. Exercise and older patients. Guidelines for the clinician. *J Am Geriatr Soc* 48:318-324, 2000.

35. Chu, D, Faigenbaum, A, and Falkel, J. *Progressive Plyometrics for Kids.* Monterey, CA: Healthy Learning, 15-19, 2006.

36. Cohen, DD, Voss, C, Taylor, MJD, Delextrat, A, Ogunleye, AA, and Sandercock, G. Ten-year secular changes in muscular fitness in English children. *Acta Paediatr* 100:e175-e177, 2011.

37. Colliander, E, and Tesch, P. Bilateral eccentric and concentric torque of quadriceps and hamstrings in females and males. *Eur J Appl Physiol* 59:227-232, 1989.

38. Colliander, E, and Tesch, P. Responses to eccentric and concentric resistance training in females and males. *Acta Physiol Scand* 141:149-156, 1990.

39. Comstock, RD, Collins, CL, Corlette, JD, Fletcher, EN, and Center for Injury Research and Policy of the Research Institute at Nationwide Children's Hospital. National high-school sports-related injury surveillance study, 2011-2012 school year. www.nationwide childrens.org/cirp-rio-study-reports. Accessed June 10, 2014.

40. Conroy, B, Kraemer, W, Maresh, C, Fleck, S, Stone, M, Fry, A, Miller, P, and Dalsky, G. Bone mineral density in elite junior Olympic weightlifters. *Med Sci Sports Exerc* 25:1103-1109, 1993.

41. Cooper, R, Kuh, D, and Hardy, R. Objectively measured physical capability levels and mortality: Systematic review and meta-analysis. *Br Med J* 341:c4467, 2010.

42. Cumming, D, Wall, S, Galbraith, M, and Belcastro, A. Reproductive hormone responses to resistance exercise. *Med Sci Sports Exerc* 19:234-238, 1987.

43. Cureton, K, Collins, M, Hill, D, and McElhannon, F. Muscle hypertrophy in men and women. *Med Sci Sports Exerc* 20:338-344, 1988.

44. Dalsky, G, Stocke, K, Ehasani, A, Slatopolsky, E, Lee, W, and Birge, S. Weight-bearing exercise training and lumbar bone mineral content in post menopausal women. *Ann Intern Med* 108:824-828, 1988.

45. Davies, B, Greenwood, E, and Jones, S. Gender differences in the relationship of performance in the handgrip and standing long jump tests to lean limb volume in young athletes. *Eur J Appl Physiol* 58:315-320, 1988.

46. De Loes, M, Dahlstedt, L, and Thomeé, R. A 7-year study on risks and costs of knee injuries in male and female youth participants in 12 sports. *Scand J Med Sci Sports* 10:90-97, 2000.

47. De Souza, MJ, Nattiv, A, Joy, E, Misra, M, Williams, NI, Mallinson, RJ, Gibbs, JC, Olmstead, M, Goolsby, M, and Matheson, G. Female athlete triad coalition consensus statement on treatment and return to play of the female athlete triad. *Clin J Sports Med* 24:96-119, 2014.

48. De Vos, N, Singh, N, Ross, D, Stavrinos, T, Orr, R, and Singh, M. Optimal load for increasing muscle power during explosive resistance training in older adults. *J Gerontol A Biol Sci Med Sci* 60:638-647, 2005.

49. DiFiori, JP, Benjamin, HJ, Brenner, J, Gregory, A, Jayanthi, N, Landry, G, and Luke, A. Overuse injuries and burnout in youth sports:

50. A position statement from the American Medical Society for Sports Medicine. *Clin J Sports Med* 24:3-20, 2014.

51. Docherty, D, Wenger, H, Collis, M, and Quinney, H. The effects of variable speed resistance training on strength development in prepubertal boys. *J Hum Mov Stud* 13:377-382, 1987.

52. Drinkwater, B. Weight-bearing exercise and bone mass. *Phys Med Rehabil Clin* 6:567-578, 1995.

53. Emery, C. Injury prevention and future research. *Med Sci Sports Exerc* 48:179-200, 2005.

54. Evans, W. Exercise training guidelines for the elderly. *Med Sci Sports Exerc* 31:12-17, 1999.

55. Faigenbaum, A. Strength training for children and adolescents. *Clin Sports Med* 19:593-619, 2000.

56. Faigenbaum, AD, Farrell, A, Fabiano, M, Radler, T, Naclerio, F, Ratamess, NA, Kang, J, and Myer, GD. Effects of integrative neuromuscular training on fitness performance in children. *Pediatr Exerc Sci* 23:573-584, 2011.

57. Faigenbaum, AD, Farrell, A, Fabiano, M, Radler, T, Naclerio, F, Ratamess, NA, Kang, J, and Myer, GD. Effects of detraining on fitness performance in 7-year-old children. *J Strength Cond Res* 27:323-330, 2013.

58. Faigenbaum, AD, Kraemer, WJ, Blimkie, CJ, Jeffreys, I, Micheli, LJ, Nitka, M, and Rowland, TW. Youth resistance training: Updated position statement paper from the National Strength and Conditioning Association. *J Strength Cond Res* 23:S60-S79, 2009.

59. Faigenbaum, AD, Lloyd, RS, and Myer, GD. Youth resistance training: Past practices, new perspectives and future directions. *Pediatr Exerc Sci* 25:591-604, 2013.

60. Faigenbaum, AD, Lloyd, RS, Sheehan, D, and Myer, GD. The role of the pediatric exercise specialist in treating exercise deficit disorder in youth. *Strength Cond J* 35:34-41, 2013.

61. Faigenbaum, AD, and McFarland, JE. Criterion repetition maximum testing. *Strength Cond J* 36:88-91, 2014.

62. Faigenbaum, AD, McFarland, JE, Herman, RE, Naclerio, F, Ratamess, NA, Kang, J, and Myer, GD. Reliability of the one-repetition-maximum power clean test in adolescent athletes. *J Strength Cond Res* 26:432-437, 2012.

63. Faigenbaum, A, and Mediate, P. The effects of medicine ball training on fitness performance of high school physical education students. *Physical Educator* 63:160-167, 2006.

64. Faigenbaum, A, Milliken, L, LaRosa-Loud, R, Burak, B, Doherty, C, and Westcott, W. Comparison of 1 and 2 days per week of strength training in children. *Res Q Exerc Sport* 73:416-424, 2002.

65. Faigenbaum, A, Milliken, L, Moulton, L, and Westcott, W. Early muscular fitness adaptations in children in response to two different resistance training regimens. *Pediatr Exerc Sci* 17:237-248, 2005.

66. Faigenbaum, A, Milliken, L, and Westcott, W. Maximal strength testing in healthy children. *J Strength Cond Res* 17:162-166, 2003.

67. Faigenbaum, AD, and Myer, GD. Resistance training among young athletes: Safety, efficacy and injury prevention effects. *Br J Sports Med* 44:56-63, 2010.

68. Faigenbaum, A, and Polakowski, C. Olympic-style weightlifting, kid style. *Strength Cond J* 21:73-76, 1999.

69. Faigenbaum, A, and Schram, J. Can resistance training reduce injuries in youth sports? *Strength Cond J* 26:16-21, 2004.

70. Faigenbaum, A, Westcott, W, Long, C, LaRosa-Loud, R, Delmonico, M, and Micheli, L. Relationship between repetitions and selected percentages of the one repetition maximum in healthy children. *Pediatr Phys Ther* 10:110-113, 1998.

71. Faigenbaum, A, Westcott, W, Micheli, L, Outerbridge, A, Long, C, LaRosa-Loud, R, and Zaichkowsky, L. The effects of strength training and detraining on children. *J Strength Cond Res* 10:109-114, 1996.

71. Faigenbaum, A, Zaichkowsky, L, Westcott, W, Micheli, L, and Fehlandt, A. The effects of a twice per week strength training program on children. *Pediatr Exerc Sci* 5:339-346, 1993.

72. Falk, B, and Eliakim, A. Resistance training, skeletal muscle and growth. *Pediatr Endocrinol Rev* 1:120-127, 2003.

73. Falk, B, and Mor, G. The effects of resistance and martial arts training in 6 to 8 year old boys. *Pediatr Exerc Sci* 8:48-56, 1996.

74. Falk, B, and Tenenbaum, G. The effectiveness of resistance training in children. A meta-analysis. *Sports Med* 22:176-186, 1996.

75. Fiatarone, M, Marks, E, Ryan, N, Meredith, C, Lipsitz, L, and Evans, W. High-intensity strength training in nonagenarians: Effects on skeletal muscle. *JAMA* 263:3029-3034, 1990.

76. Fiatarone, M, O'Neill, E, Ryan, N, Clements, K, Solares, G, Nelson, M, Roberts, S, Kehayias, J, Lipsitz, L, and Evans, W. Exercise training and nutritional supplementation for physical frailty in very elderly people. *New Engl J Med* 330:1769-1775, 1994.

77. Fielding, RA, LeBrasseur, NK, Cuoco, A, Bean, J, Mizer, K, and Fiatarone Singh, MA. High-velocity resistance training increases skeletal muscle peak power in older women. *J Am Geriatr Soc* 50:655-662, 2002.

78. Ford, H, and Puckett, J. Comparative effects of prescribed weight training and basketball programs on basketball test scores of ninth grade boys. *Percept Mot Skills* 56:23-26, 1983.

79. Fransen, J, Pion, J, Vandendriessche, J, Vandorpe, B, Vaeyens, R, Lenoir, M, and Philippaerts, RM. Differences in physical fitness and gross motor coordination in boys aged 6-12 years specializing in one versus sampling more than one sport. *J Sports Sci* 30:379-386, 2012.

80. Frontera, W, Meredith, C, O'Reilly, K, Knuttgen, H, and Evans, W. Strength conditioning of older men: Skeletal muscle hypertrophy and improved function. *J Appl Physiol* 42:1038-1044, 1988.

81. Fukunga, T, Funato, K, and Ikegawa, S. The effects of resistance training on muscle area and strength in prepubescent age. *Ann Physiol Anthropol* 11:357-364, 1992.

82. Galvao, D, and Taaffe, D. Resistance training for the older adult: Manipulating training variables to enhance muscle strength. *J Strength Cond Res* 27:48-54, 2005.

83. Garhammer, J. A comparison of maximal power outputs between elite male and female weightlifters in competition. *Int J Sports Biomech* 7:3-11, 1991.

84. Garhammer, J. A review of power output studies of Olympic and powerlifting: Methodology, performance prediction and evaluation tests. *J Strength Cond Res* 7:76-89, 1993.

85. Gonzalez-Badillo, JJ, Gorostiaga, EM, Arellano, R, and Izquierdo, M. Moderate resistance training volume produces more favorable strength gains than high or low volumes during a short-term training cycle. *J Strength Cond Res* 19:689-697, 2005.

86. Gonzalez-Badillo, JJ, Izquierdo, M, and Gorostiaga, EM. Moderate volume of high relative training intensity produces greater strength gains compared with low and high volume in competitive weightlifters. *J Strength Cond Res* 20:73-81, 2006.

87. Granacher, U, Goesele, A, Roggo, K, Wischer, T, Fischer, S, Zuerny, C, Gollhofer, A, and Kriemler, S. Effects and mechanisms of strength training in children. *Int J Sports Med* 32:357-364, 2011.

88. Granacher, U, Muehlbauer, T, Zahner, L, Gollhofer, A, and Kressig, RW. Comparison of traditional and recent approaches in the promotion of balance and strength in older adults. *Sports Med* 41:377-400, 2011.

89. Greulich, WW, and Pyle, SI. *Radiographic Atlas of Skeletal Development of the Hand and Wrist.* 2nd ed. Los Angeles: Stanford University Press, 1959.

90. Gumbs, V, Segal, D, Halligan, J, and Lower, G. Bilateral distal radius and ulnar fractures in adolescent weight lifters. *Am J Sports Med* 10:375-379, 1982.

91. Gunter, K, Almstedt, H, and Janz, K. Physical activity in childhood may be the key to optimizing lifespan skeletal health. *Exerc Sport Sci Rev* 40:13-21, 2012.

92. Häkkinen, K, and Häkkinen, A. Muscle cross-sectional area, force production and relaxation characteristics in women at different ages. *Eur J Appl Physiol* 62:410-414, 1991.

93. Häkkinen, K, Pakarinen, A, and Kallinen, M. Neuromuscular adaptations and serum hormones in women during short-term intensive strength training. *Eur J Appl Physiol* 64:106-111, 1992.

94. Häkkinen, K, Pakarinen, A, Kyrolainen, H, Cheng, S, Kim, D, and Komi, P. Neuromuscular adaptations and serum hormones in females during prolonged power training. *Int J Sports Med* 11:91-98, 1990.

95. Hamill, B. Relative safety of weight lifting and weight training. *J Strength Cond Res* 8:53-57, 1994.

96. Hardy, LL, King, L, Farrell, L, Macniven, R, and Howlett, S. Fundamental movement skills among Australian preschool children. *J Sci Med Sport* 13:503-508, 2010.

97. Harries, SK, Lubans, DR, and Callister, R. Resistance training to improve power and sports performance in adolescent athletes: A systematic review and meta-analysis. *J Sci Med Sport* 15:532-540, 2012.

98. Henwood, T, and Taaffe, D. Improved physical performance in older adults undertaking a short-term programme of high-velocity resistance training. *Gerontology* 51:108-115, 2005.

99. Hetherington, M. Effect of isometric training on the elbow flexion force torque of grade five boys. *Res Q* 47:41-47, 1976.

100. Hetzler, R, DeRenne, C, Buxton, B, Ho, KW, Chai, DX, and Seichi, G. Effects of 12 weeks of strength training on anaerobic power in prepubescent male athletes. *J Strength Cond Res* 11:174-181, 1997.

101. Hewett, T. Neuromuscular and hormonal factors associated with knee injuries in female athletes: Strategies for intervention. *Sports Med* 29:313-327, 2000.

102. Hewett, TE, and Myer, GD. The mechanistic connection between the trunk, hip, knee, and anterior cruciate ligament injury. *Exerc Sport Sci Rev* 39:161-166, 2011.

103. Hewett, T, Myer, G, and Ford, K. Reducing knee and anterior cruciate ligament injuries among female athletes. *J Knee Surg* 18:82-88, 2005.

104. Hind, K, and Burrows, M. Weight-bearing exercise and bone mineral accrual in children and adolescents: A review of controlled trials. *Bone* 40:14-27, 2007.

105. Holloway, J. A summary chart: Age related changes in women and men and their possible improvement with training. *J Strength Cond Res* 12:126-128, 1998.

106. Hurley, B, and Hagberg, J. Optimizing health in older persons: Aerobic or strength training? In *Exercise and Sport Sciences Reviews.* Holloszy, J, ed. Philadelphia: Williams & Wilkins, 61-89, 1998.

107. Imamura, K, Ashida, H, Ishikawa, T, and Fujii, M. Human major psoas muscle and sacrospinalis muscle in relation to age: A study by computed tomography. *J Gerontol* 38:678-681, 1983.

108. Ingle, L, Sleap, M, and Tolfrey, K. The effect of a complex training and detraining programme on selected strength and power variables in early pubertal boys. *J Sports Sci* 24:987-997, 2006.

109. Iwamoto, J, Takeda, T, and Ichimura, S. Effect of exercise training and detraining on bone mineral density in postmenopausal women with osteoporosis. *J Orthop Sci* 6:128-132, 2001.

110. Jette, A, and Branch, L. The Framingham disability study: II. Physical disability among the aging. *Am J Public Health* 71:1211-1216, 1981.

111. Joseph, AM, Collins, CL, Henke, NM, Yard, EE, Fields, SK, and Comstock, DA. A multisport epidemiological comparison of anterior cruciate ligament injuries in high school athletes. *J Athl Train* 48:810-817, 2013.

112. Kanis, J, Melton, L, Christiansen, C, Johnson, C, and Khaltaev, N. The diagnosis of osteoporosis. *J Bone Miner Res* 9:1137-1141, 1994.

113. Karlsson, MK, Vonschewelov, T, Karlsson, C, Cöster, M, and Rosengen, BE. Prevention of falls in elderly: A review. *Scand J Public Health* 41:442-454, 2013.

114. Katzmarzyk, P, Malina, R, and Beunen, G. The contribution of biologic maturation to the strength and motor fitness of children. *Ann Hum Biol* 24:493-505, 1997.

115. Kaufman, LB, and Schilling, DL. Implementation of a strength training program for a 5-year-old child with poor body awareness and developmental coordination disorder. *Phys Ther* 87:455-467, 2007.

116. Kelley, GA, Kelley, KS, and Tran, ZV. Resistance training and bone mineral density in women: A meta-analysis of controlled trials. *Am J Phys Med Rehabil* 80:65-77, 2001.

117. Kinugasa, T, and Kilding, AE. A comparison of post-match recovery strategies in youth soccer players. *J Strength Cond Res* 23:1402-1407, 2009.

118. Komi, P, and Karlsson, J. Skeletal muscle fibre types, enzyme activities and physical performance in young males and females. *Acta Physiol Scand* 103:210-218, 1978.

119. Kraemer, W. Endocrine responses to resistance exercise. *Med Sci Sports Exerc* 20(Suppl):152-157, 1988.

120. Kraemer, W, Adams, K, Cafarelli, E, Dudley, G, Dooly, C, Feigenbaum, M, Fleck, S, Franklin, B, Newtown, R, Potteiger, J, Stone, M, Ratamess, N, and Triplett-McBride, T. Progression models in resistance training for healthy adults. *Med Sci Sports Exerc* 34:364-380, 2002.

121. Kraemer, W, Fry, A, Frykman, P, Conroy, B, and Hoffman, J. Resistance training and youth. *Pediatr Exerc Sci* 1:336-350, 1989.

122. Kraemer, W, Mazzetti, S, Nindl, B, Gotshalk, L, Bush, J, Marx, J, Dohi, K, Gomez, A, Miles, M, Fleck, S, Newton, R, and Häkkinen, K. Effect of resistance training on women's strength/power and occupational performances. *Med Sci Sports Exerc* 33:1011-1025, 2001.

123. Kravitz, L, Akalan, C, Nowicki, K, and Kinzey, SJ. Prediction of 1 repetition maximum in high-school power lifters. *J Strength Cond Res* 17:167-172, 2003.

124. Lauback, L. Comparative muscle strength of men and women: A review of the literature. *Aviat Space Environ Med* 47:534-542, 1976.

125. Layne, J, and Nelson, M. The effects of progressive resistance training on bone density: A review. *Med Sci Sports Exerc* 31:25-30, 1999.

126. Lexell, J, and Downham, D. What is the effect of ageing on Type II muscle fibers? *J Neurol Sci* 107:250-251, 1992.

127. Lillegard, W, Brown, E, Wilson, D, Henderson, R, and Lewis, E. Efficacy of strength training in prepubescent to early postpubescent males and females: Effects of gender and maturity. *Pediatr Rehabil* 1:147-157, 1997.

128. Ling, CHY, Taekema, D, de Craen, AJM, Gussekloo, J, Westendorp, RGJ, and Maier, AB. Handgrip strength and mortality in the oldest old population: The Leiden 85-plus study. *Can Med Assoc J* 182:429-435, 2010.

129. Lloyd, RS, Faigenbaum, AD, Stone, MH, Oliver, JL, Jeffreys, I, Moody, JA, Brewer, C, Pierce, K, McCambridge, TM, Howard, R, Herrington, L, Hainline, B, Micheli, LJ, Jaques, R, Kraemer, WJ, McBride, MG, Best, TM, Chu, DA, Alvar, BA, and Myer, GD. Position statement on youth resistance training: The 2014 international consensus. *Br J Sports Med* 48:498-505, 2014.

130. Lloyd, RS, and Oliver, JL. The Youth Physical Development model: A new approach to long-term athletic development. *Strength Cond J* 34:61-72, 2012.

131. Lloyd, RS, Oliver, JL, Faigenbaum, AD, Myer, GD, and De Ste Croix, M. Chronological age versus biological maturation: Implications for exercise programming in youth. *J Strength Cond Res* 28:1454-1464, 2014.

132. Lopopolo, R, Greco, M, Sullivan, D, Craik, R, and Mangione, K. Effect of therapeutic exercise on gait speed in community-dwelling elderly people: A meta analysis. *Phys Ther* 86:520-540, 2006.

133. Maddalozzo, GF, and Snow, CM. High intensity resistance training: Effects of bone in older men and women. *Calcif Tissue Int* 66:399-404, 2000.

134. Magill, R, and Anderson, D. Critical periods as optimal readiness for learning sports skills. In *Children and Youth in Sport: A Biopsychosocial Perspective.* Smoll, F, and Smith, R, eds. Madison, WI: Brown & Benchmark, 57-72, 1995.

135. Malina, R. Physical activity and training: Effects on stature and the adolescent growth spurt. *Med Sci Sports Exerc* 26:759-766, 1994.

136. Malina, R, Bouchard, C, and Bar-Or, O. *Growth, Maturation, and Physical Activity.* Champaign, IL: Human Kinetics, 2004.

137. Mayhew, J, and Salm, P. Gender differences in anaerobic power tests. *Eur J Appl Physiol* 60:133-138, 1990.

138. McCartney, N. Acute responses to resistance training and safety. *Med Sci Sports Exerc* 31:31-37, 1999.

139. McKay, H, MacLean, L, Petit, M, MacKelvie-O'Brien, K, Janssen, P, Beck, T, and Khan, K. "Bounce at the Bell": A novel program of short bursts of exercise improves proximal femur bone mass in early pubertal children. *Br J Sports Med* 39:521-526, 2005.

140. Meltzer, D. Age dependence of Olympic weightlifting ability. *Med Sci Sports Exerc* 26:1053-1067, 1994.

141. Meredith, C, Frontera, W, and Evans, W. Body composition in elderly men: Effect of dietary modification during strength training. *J Am Geriatr Soc* 40:155-162, 1992.

142. Metter, E, Conwit, R, Tobin, J, and Fozard, J. Age-associated loss of power and strength in the upper extremities in women and men. *J Gerontol Biol Sci Med* 52:B267-B276, 1997.

143. Micheli, L. The child athlete. In *ACSM's Guidelines for the Team Physician.* Cantu, R, and Micheli, L, eds. Philadelphia: Lea & Febiger, 228-241, 1991.

144. Micheli, L, and Natsis, KI. Preventing injuries in sports: What the team physician needs to know. In *F.I.M.S. Team Physician Manual.* 3rd ed. Micheli, LJ, Pigozzi, F, Chan, KM, Frontera, WR, Bachl, N, Smith, AD, and Alenabi, T, eds. London: Routledge, 505-520, 2013.

145. Micheli, L. Strength training in the young athlete. In *Competitive Sports for Children and Youth.* Brown, E, and Branta, C, eds. Champaign, IL: Human Kinetics, 99-105, 1988.

146. Micheli, L, Glassman, R, and Klein, M. The prevention of sports injuries in children. *Clin Sports Med* 19:821-834, 2000.

147. Mihata, LC, Beutler, AI, and Boden, BP. Comparing the incidence of anterior cruciate ligament injury in collegiate lacrosse, soccer, and basketball players: Implications for anterior cruciate ligament mechanism and prevention. *Am J Sports Med* 34:899-904, 2006.

148. Miller, A, MacDougall, J, Tarnopolsky, M, and Sale, D. Gender differences in strength and muscle fiber characteristics. *Eur J Appl Physiol* 66:254-262, 1992.

149. Milliken, LA, Faigenbaum, AD, and LaRousa-Loud, R. Correlates of upper and lower body muscular strength in children. *J Strength Cond Res* 22:1339-1346, 2008.

150. Moeller, J, and Lamb, M. Anterior cruciate ligament injuries in female athletes. *Phys Sportsmed* 25:31-48, 1997.

151. Moesch, K, Elbe, AM, Hauge, MLT, and Wikman, JM. Late specialization: The key to success in centimeters, grams, or seconds (cgs) sports. *Scand J Med Sci Sports* 21:e282-e290, 2011.

152. Moliner-Urdiales, D, Ruiz, JR, Ortega, FB, Jiménez-Pavón, D, Vicente-Rodriguez, G, Rey-López, JP, Martinez-Gómez, D, Casajus, JA, Mesana, MI, Marcos, A, Noriega-Borge, MJ, Sjöström, M, Castillo, MJ, and Moreno, LA. Secular trends in health-related physical fitness in Spanish adolescents: The AVENA and HELENA studies. *J Sci Med Sport* 13:584-588, 2010.

153. Morris, F, Naughton, G, Gibbs, J, Carlson, J, and Wark, J. Prospective ten-month exercise intervention in premenarcheal girls: Positive effects on bone and lean mass. *J Bone Miner Res* 12:1453-1462, 1997.

154. Myer, GD, Ford, KR, Divine, JG, Wall, EJ, Kahanov, L, and Hewett, TE. Longitudinal assessment of noncontact anterior cruciate ligament injury risk factors during maturation in a female athlete: A case report. *J Athl Train* 44:101-109, 2009.

155. Myer, GD, Ford, KR, Brent, JL, and Hewett, TE. The effects of plyometric versus dynamic balance training on power, balance and landing force in female athletes. *J Strength Cond Res* 20:345-353, 2006.

156. Myer, GD, Ford, KR, Palumbo, JP, and Hewett, TE. Neuromuscular training improves performance and lower-extremity biomechanics in female athletes. *J Strength Cond Res* 19:51-60, 2005.

157. Myer, GD, Lloyd, RS, Brent, JL, and Faigenbaum, AD. How young is "too young" to start training? *ACSM Health Fit J* 17:14-23, 2013.

158. Myer, GD, Quatman, CE, Khoury, J, Wall, EJ, and Hewett, TE. Youth versus adult "weightlifting" injuries presenting to United States emergency rooms: Accidental versus nonaccidental injury mechanisms. *J Strength Cond Res* 23:2054-2060, 2009.

159. Myer, GD, Sugimoto, D, Thomas, S, and Hewett, TE. The influence of age on the effectiveness of neuromuscular training to reduce anterior cruciate ligament injury in female athletes: A meta-analysis. *Am J Sports Med* 41:203-215, 2013.

160. National Collegiate Athletic Association. Injury rate for women's basketball increases sharply. *NCAA News* 31(May 11):9, 13, 1994.

161. National Strength and Conditioning Association. Strength training for female athletes. *NSCA J* 11:43-55, 29-36, 1989.

162. Naylor, LH, Watts, K, Sharpe, JA, Jones, TW, Davis, EA, Thompson, A, George, K, Ramsay, JM, O'Driscoll, G, and Green, DJ. Resistance training and diastolic myocardial tissue velocities in obese children. *Med Sci Sports Exerc* 40:2027-2032, 2008.

163. Nelson, M, Fiatarone, M, Morganti, C, Trice, I, Greenberg, R, and Evans, W. Effects of high intensity strength training on multiple risk factors for osteoporotic fractures. *JAMA* 272:1909-1914, 1994.

164. Nelson-Wong, E, Appell, R, McKay, M, Nawaz, H, Roth, J, Sigler, R, 3rd, and Walker, M. Increased fall risk is associated with elevated co-contraction about the ankle during static balance challenges in older adults. *Eur J Appl Physiol* 112:1379-1389, 2012.

165. Ng, M, Fleming, T, Robinson, M, Thomson, B, Graetz, N, Margano, C, et al. Global, regional and national prevalence of overweight and obesity in children and adults during 1980-2013: A systematic analysis for the Global Burden of Disease study 2013. *Lancet* 384:766-781, 2014.

166. Nichols, D, Sanborn, C, and Love, A. Resistance training and bone mineral density in adolescent females. *J Pediatr* 139:494-500, 2001.

167. Nielsen, B, Nielsen, K, Behrendt-Hansen, M, and Asmussen, E. Training of "functional muscular strength" in girls 7-19 years old. In *Children and Exercise IX.* Berg, K, and Eriksson, B, eds. Baltimore: University Park Press, 69-77, 1980.

168. Ogden, CL, Carroll, MD, Kit, BK, and Flegal, KM. Prevalence of childhood and adult obesity in the United States, 2011-2012. *JAMA* 311:806-814, 2014.

169. Ormsbee, MJ, Pdaro, CM, Ilich, JZ, Purcell, S, Siervo, M, Folsom, A, and Panton, L. Osteosarcopenic obesity: The role of bone, muscle, and fat on health. *J Cachexia Sarcopenia Muscle* 5:183-192, 2014.

170. Orr, R, de Vos, N, Singh, N, Ross, D, Stavrinos, T, and Fiatarone-Singh, M. Power training improves balance in healthy older adults. *J Gerontol A Biol Sci Med Sci* 61:78-85, 2006.

171. Otis, C, Drinkwater, B, and Johnson, M. ACSM position stand: The female athlete triad. *Med Sci Sports Exerc* 29:i-ix, 1997.

172. Ozmun, J, Mikesky, A, and Surburg, P. Neuromuscular adaptations following prepubescent strength training. *Med Sci Sports Exerc* 26:510-514, 1994.

173. Padua, DA, Carcia, CR, Arnold, BL, and Granata, KP. Sex differences in leg stiffness and stiffness recruitment strategy during two-legged hopping. *J Mot Behav* 37:111-125, 2005.

174. Park, CH, Elavsky, S, and Koo, KM. Factors influencing physical activity in older adults. *J Exerc Rehabil* 10:45-52, 2014.

175. Pfeiffer, R, and Francis, R. Effects of strength training on muscle development in prepubescent, pubescent and postpubescent males. *Phys Sportsmed* 14:134-143, 1986.

176. Piirainen, JM, Cronin, NJ, Avela, J, and Linnamo, V. Effects of plyometric and pneumatic explosive strength training on neuromuscular function and dynamic balance control in 60-70 year old males. *J Electromyogr Kinesiol* 24:246-252, 2014.

177. Pizzigalli, L, Filippini, A, Ahmaidi, S, Jullien, H, and Rainoldi, A. Prevention of falling risk in elderly people: The relevance of muscular strength and symmetry of lower limbs in postural stability. *J Strength Cond Res* 25:567-574, 2011.

178. Pollock, ML, Franklin, BA, Balady, GJ, Chaitman, BL, Fleg, JL, Fletcher, B, Limacher, M, Piña, IL, Stein, RA, Williams, M, and Bazzare, T. Resistance exercise in individuals with and without cardiovascular disease: Benefits, rationale, safety, and prescription. *Circulation* 101:828-833, 2000.

179. Porter, MM. Power training for older adults. *Appl Physiol Nutr Metab* 31:87-94, 2006.

180. Potdevin, FJ, Alberty, ME, Chevutschi, A, Pelayo, P, and Sidney, MC. Effects of a 6-week plyometric training program on performances in pubescent swimmers. *J Strength Cond Res* 25:80-86, 2011.

181. Purves-Smith, FM, Sgarioto, N, and Hepple, RT. Fiber typing in aging muscle. *Exerc Sport Sci Rev* 42:45-52, 2014.

182. Quatman, CE, Ford, KR, Myer, GD, and Hewett, TE. Maturation leads to gender differences in landing force and vertical jump performance. *Am J Sports Med* 34:806-813, 2006.

183. Quatman-Yates, CC, Myer, GD, Ford, KR, and Hewett, TE. A longitudinal evaluation of maturational effects on lower extremity strength in female adolescent athletes. *Pediatr Phys Ther* 25:271-276, 2013.

184. Ramsay, J, Blimkie, C, Smith, K, Garner, S, and MacDougall, J. Strength training effects in prepubescent boys. *Med Sci Sports Exerc* 22:605-614, 1990.

185. Reid, KF, Callahan, DM, Carabello, RJ, Phillips, EM, Frontera, WR, and Fielding, RA. Lower extremity power training in elderly subjects with mobility limitations: A randomized controlled trial. *Aging Clin Exp Res* 20:337-343, 2008.

186. Roche, AF, Chumlea, WC, and Thissen, D. *Assessing the Skeletal Maturity of the Hand-Wrist: Fels Method.* Springfield, IL: Charles C Thomas, 1988.

187. Rowe, P. Cartilage fracture due to weight lifting. *Br J Sports Med* 13:130-131, 1979.

188. Rubenstein, LZ. Falls in older people: Epidemiology, risk factors and strategies for prevention. *Age Ageing* 35:ii37-ii41, 2006.

189. Runhaar, J, Collard, DCM, Kemper, HCG, van Mechelen, W, and Chinapaw, M. Motor fitness in Dutch youth: Differences over a 26-year period (1980-2006). *J Sci Med Sport* 13:323-328, 2010.

190. Ryan, J, and Salciccioli, G. Fractures of the distal radial epiphysis in adolescent weight lifters. *Am J Sports Med* 4:26-27, 1976.

191. Ryushi, T, Häkkinen, K, Kauhanen, H, and Komi, P. Muscle fiber characteristics, muscle cross sectional area and force production in strength athletes, physically active males and females. *Scand J Sports Sci* 10:7-15, 1988.

192. Sadres, E, Eliakim, A, Constantini, N, Lidor, R, and Falk, B. The effect of long term resistance training on anthropometric measures, muscle strength and self-concept in pre-pubertal boys. *Pediatr Exerc Sci* 13:357-372, 2001.

193. Shaibi, G, Cruz, M, Ball, G, Weigensberg, MJ, Salem, GJ, Crespo, NC, and Goran, MI. Effects of resistance training on insulin sensitivity in overweight Latino adolescent males. *Med Sci Sports Exerc* 38:1208-1215, 2006.

194. Shambaugh, J, Klein, A, and Herbert, J. Structural measures as predictors of injury in basketball players. *Med Sci Sports Exerc* 23:522-527, 1991.

195. Shaw, C, McCully, K, and Posner, J. Injuries during the one repetition maximum assessment in the elderly. *J Cardiopulm Rehabil* 15:283-287, 1995.

196. Shephard, R. Exercise and training in women, part 1: Influence of gender on exercise and training response. *Can J Appl Physiol* 25:19-34, 2000.

197. Sherrington, C, Whitney, JC, Lord, SR, Herbert, RD, Cumming, RG, and Close, JCT. Effective exercise for the prevention of falls: A systematic review and meta-analysis. *J Am Geriatr Soc* 56:2234-2243, 2008.

198. Smith, JJ, Eather, N, Morgan, PJ, Plotnikoff, RC, Faigenbaum, AD, and Lubans, DR. The health benefits of muscular fitness for children and adolescents: A systematic review and meta-analysis. *Sports Med* 44:1209-1223, 2014.

199. Society of Health and Physical Educators. *National Standards & Grade-Level Outcomes for K-12 Physical Education.* Champaign, IL: Human Kinetics, 11-13, 2014.

200. Steib, S, Schoene, D, and Pfeifer, K. Dose–response relationship of resistance training in older adults: A meta-analysis. *Med Sci Sports Exerc* 42:902-914, 2010.

201. Stewart, CHE, and Rittweger, J. Adaptive processes in skeletal muscle: Molecular and genetic influences. *J Musculoskelt Neuronal Interact* 6:73-86, 2006.

202. Straight, CR, Lofgren, IE, and Delmonico, MJ. Resistance training in older adults: Are community-based interventions effective for improving health outcomes? *Am J Lifestyle Med* 6:407-414, 2012.

203. Strong, W, Malina, R, Blimkie, C, Daniels, S, Dishman, R, Gutin, B, Hergenroeder, A, Must, A, Nixon, P, Pivarnik, J, Rowland, T, Trost, S, and Trudeau, F. Evidence based physical activity for school-age youth. *J Pediatr* 46:732-737, 2005.

204. Sugimoto, D, Myer, GD, Foss, KD, and Hewett, TE. Dosage effects of neuromuscular training intervention to reduce anterior cruciate ligament injuries in female athletes: Meta- and sub-group analyses. *Sports Med* 44:551-562, 2014.

205. Tanner, JM, Healy, MJR, Goldstein, H, and Cameron, N. *Assessment of Skeletal Maturity and Prediction of Adult Height (TW3 Method).* 3rd ed. London: Saunders, 2001.

206. Tanner, JM, Whitehouse, RH, Cameron, N, Marshall, WA, Healy, MJR, and Goldstein, H. *Assessment of Skeletal Maturity and Prediction of Adult Height (TW2 Method).* New York: Academic Press, 1975.

207. Tanner, JM, Whitehouse, RH, and Healy, MJR. *A New System for Estimating Skeletal Maturity From the Hand and Wrist, with Standards Derived From a Study of 2,600 Healthy British Children.* Paris: International Children's Centre, 1962.

208. Telama, R, Yang, X, Viikari, J, Valimaki, I, Wanne, O, and Raitakari, O. Physical activity from childhood to adulthood: A 21 year tracking study. *Am J Prev Med* 28:267-273, 2005.

209. Tiedemann, A, Sherrington, C, Close, JCT, and Lord, SR. Exercise and Sports Science Australia position statement on exercise and falls prevention in older people. *J Sci Med Sport* 14:489-495, 2011.

210. Tremblay, MS, Gray, CE, Akinroye, K, Harrington, DM, Katzmarzyk, PT, Lambert, EV, Liukkonen, J, Maddison, R, Ocansey, RT, Onywera, VO, Prista, A, Reilly, JJ, Martínez, MDPR, Duenas, OLS, Standage, M, and Tomkinson, G. Physical activity of children: A global matrix of grades comparing 15 countries. *J Phys Act Health* 11 (Suppl 1):s113-s125, 2014.

211. Tsolakis, C, Vagenas, G, and Dessypris, A. Strength adaptations and hormonal responses to resistance training and detraining in preadolescent males. *J Strength Cond Res* 18:625-629, 2004.

212. Valovich-McLeod, TC, Decoster, LC, Loud, KJ, Micheli, LJ, Parker, T, Sandrey, MA, and White, C. National Athletic Trainers' Association position statement: Prevention of pediatric overuse injuries. *J Athl Train* 46:206-220, 2011.

213. Van der Sluis, A, Elferink-Gemser, MT, Coelho-e-Silva, MJ, Nijboer, JA, Brink, MS, and Visscher, C. Sports injuries aligned to peak height velocity in talented pubertal soccer players. *Int J Sports Med* 35:351-355, 2014.

214. Vandervoot, A, and McComas, A. Contractile changes in opposing muscle of the human ankle joint with aging. *J Appl Physiol* 61:361-367, 1986.

215. Vicente-Rodriguez, G. How does exercise affect bone development during growth? *Sports Med* 36:561-569, 2006.

216. Virvidakis, K, Georgiu, E, Korkotsidis, A, Ntalles, K, and Proukakis, C. Bone mineral content of junior competitive weightlifters. *Int J Sports Med* 11:244-246, 1990.

217. Wallerstein, LF, Tricoli, V, Barroso, R, Rodacki, ALF, Russo, L, Aihara, AY, Fernandes, ARC, de Mello, MT, and Ugrinowitsch, C. Effects of strength and power training on neuromuscular variables in older adults. *J Aging Phys Act* 20:171-185, 2012.

218. Watts, K, Beye, P, and Siafarikas, A. Exercise training normalizes vascular dysfunction and improves central adiposity in obese adolescents. *J Am Coll Cardiol* 43:1823-1827, 2004.

219. Watts, K, Jones, T, Davis, E, and Green, D. Exercise training in obese children and adolescents. *Sports Med* 35:375-392, 2005.

220. Weltman, A, Janney, C, Rians, C, Strand, K, Berg, B, Tippet, S, Wise, J, Cahill, B, and Katch, F. The effects of hydraulic resistance strength training in pre-pubertal males. *Med Sci Sports Exerc* 18:629-638, 1986.

221. West, R. The female athlete: The triad of disordered eating, amenorrhoea and osteoporosis. *Sports Med* 26:63-71, 1998.

222. Westcott, W, and Baechle, T. *Strength Training for Seniors.* Champaign, IL: Human Kinetics, 1-13, 1999.

223. Winter, DA. *Biomechanics and Motor Control of Human Movement.* 3rd ed. New York: Wiley, 151-152, 2005.

224. Wojtys, E, Huston, L, Lindenfeld, T, Hewett, T, and Greenfield, M. Association between the menstrual cycle and anterior cruciate injuries in female athletes. *Am J Sports Med* 26:614-619, 1998.

225. Yarasheski, K, Zachwieja, J, and Bier, D. Acute effects of resistance exercise on muscle protein synthesis in young and elderly men and women. *Am J Appl Physiol* 265:210-214, 1993.

CHAPTER 8 Psychology of Athletic Preparation and Performance

1. Bandura, A. Self-efficacy: Toward a unifying theory of behavioral change. *Psychol Rev* 84:191-215, 1977.

2. Burton, D, Naylor, S, and Holliday, B. Goal setting in sport: Investigating the goal effectiveness paradox. In *Handbook of Sport Psychology.* Singer, R, Hausenblas, H, and Janelle, C, eds. New York: Wiley, 497-528, 2001.

3. Cahill, L, McGaugh, JL, and Weinberger, NM. The neurobiology of learning and memory: Some reminders to remember. *Trends Neurosci* 24:578-581, 2001.

4. Chiviacowsky, S, and Wulf, G. Self-controlled feedback is effective if it is based on the learner's performance. *Res Q Exerc Sport* 76:42-48, 2005.

5. Chiviacowsky, S, Wulf, G, and Lewthwaite, R. Self-controlled learning: The importance of protecting perceptions of competence. *Front Psychol* 3:458, 2012.

6. Chiviacowsky, S, Wulf, G, Lewthwaite, R, and Campos, T. Motor learning benefits of self-controlled practice in persons with Parkinson's disease. *Gait Posture* 35:601-605, 2012.

7. Deci, EL. Intrinsic motivation: Theory and application. In *Psychology of Motor Behavior and Sport.* Landers, DM, and Christina, RW, eds. Champaign, IL: Human Kinetics, 388-396, 1978.

8. Feltz, DL, and Landers, DM. The effects of mental practice on motor skill learning and performance: A meta-analysis. *J Sport Psychol* 5,1:25-57, 1983.

9. Fitts, PM, and Posner, MI. *Human Performance.* Belmont, CA: Brooks/Cole, 1967.

10. Gill, D, and Williams, L. *Psychological Dynamics of Sport and Exercise.* Champaign, IL: Human Kinetics, 2008.

11. Gould, D, and Udry, E. Psychological skills for enhancing performance: Arousal regulation strategies. *Med Sci Sports Exerc* 26:478-485, 1994.

12. Hanin, YL. Interpersonal and intragroup anxiety in sports. In *Anxiety in Sports: An International Perspective.* Hackfort, D, and Spielberger, CD, eds. New York: Taylor & Francis, 19-28, 1989.

13. Hardy, L. Testing the predictions of the cusp catastrophe model of anxiety and performance. *Sport Psychol* 10:140-156, 1996.

14. Hatfield, BD, and Walford, GA. Understanding anxiety: Implications for sport performance. *NSCA J* 9:60-61, 1987.

15. Jacobson, E. *Progressive Relaxation.* Chicago: University of Chicago Press, 1929.

16. Kantak, SS, and Winstein, CJ. Learning-performance distinction and memory processes for motor skills: A focused review and perspective. *Behav Brain Res* 228:219-231, 2012.

17. Kerr, JH. *Motivation and Emotion in Sport: Reversal Theory.* East Sussex, UK: Psychology Press, 1999.

18. Landin, D, and Hebert, EP. A comparison of three practice schedules along the contextual interference continuum. *Res Q Exerc Sport* 68:357-361, 1997.

19. Landin, DK, Hebert, EP, and Fairweather, M. The effects of variable practice on the performance of a basketball skill. *Res Q Exerc Sport* 64:232-237, 1993.

20. Lewthwaite, R, and Wulf, G. Social-comparative feedback affects motor skill learning. *Q J Exp Psychol* 63:738-749, 2010.

21. Locke, EA, and Latham, GP. The application of goal setting to sports. *J Sport Psychol* 7:205-222, 1985.

22. Martens, R. *Social Psychology and Physical Activity.* New York: Harper & Row, 1975.

23. McClelland, DC, Atkinson, JW, Clark, RA, and Lowell, EL. *The Achievement Motive.* New York: Appleton-Century-Crofts, 1953.

24. Naylor, JC, and Briggs, GE. Effects of task complexity and task organization on the relative efficiency of part and whole training methods. *J Exp Psychol* 65:217-224, 1963.

25. Nideffer, RM. Test of attentional and interpersonal style. *J Pers Soc Psychol* 34:394-404, 1976.

26. Oxendine, JB. Emotional arousal and motor performance. *Quest* 13:23-32, 1970.

27. Plautz, EJ, Milliken, GW, and Nudo, RJ. Effects of repetitive motor training on movement representations in adult squirrel monkeys: Role of use versus learning. *Neurobiol Learn Mem* 74:27-55, 2000.

28. Porges, S, McCabe, P, and Yongue, B. Respiratory-heart rate interactions: Psychophysiological implications for pathophysiology and behavior. In *Perspectives in Cardiovascular Psychophysiology.* Caccioppo, JT, and Petty, RE, eds. New York: Guilford, 223-264, 1982.

29. Sakadjian, A, Panchuk, D, and Pearce, AJ. Kinematic and kinetic improvements associated with action observation facilitated learning of the power clean in Australian footballers. *J Strength Cond Res* 28:1613-1625, 2014.

30. Schmidt, RA, and Lee, T. *Motor Control and Learning.* 5th ed. Champaign, IL: Human Kinetics, 327-329, 1988.

31. Selye, H. The stress concept: Past, present and future. In *Stress Research: Issues for the Eighties.* Cooper, CL, ed. New York: Wiley, 1983.

32. Shea, CH, Wright, DL, Wulf, G, and Whitacre, C. Physical and observational practice afford unique learning opportunities. *J Mot Behav* 32:27-36, 2000.

33. Shea, JB, and Morgan, RL. Contextual interference effects on the acquisition, retention, and transfer of a motor skill. *J Exp Psychol Hum Learn* 5:179, 1979.

34. Smeeton, NJ, Williams, AM, Hodges, NJ, and Ward, P. The relative effectiveness of various instructional approaches in developing anticipation skill. *J Exp Psychol Appl* 11:98-110, 2005.

35. Spence, JT, and Spence, KW. The motivational components of manifest anxiety: Drive and drive stimuli. In *Anxiety and Behavior.* Spielberger, CD, ed. New York: Academic Press, 291-326, 1966.

36. Spielberger, CD. *Understanding Stress and Anxiety.* London: Harper & Row, 1979.

37. Spielberger, CD, Gorsuch, RL, and Lushene, RE. *Manual for the State-Trait Anxiety Inventory.* Palo Alto, CA: Consulting Psychologists Press, 1970.

38. Van Raalte, JL. Self talk. In *Routledge Handbook of Applied Psychology.* Anderson, SHM, ed. New York: Routledge, 210-517, 2010.

39. Weinberg, RS. Activation/arousal control. In *Routledge Handbook of Applied Sport Psychology.* Anderson, SHM, ed. New York: Routledge, 471-480, 2010.

40. Weinberg, RS, and Gould, D. *Foundations of Sport and Exercise Psychology.* 3rd ed. Champaign, IL: Human Kinetics, 2015.

41. Wightman, DC, and Lintern, G. Part-task training for tracking and manual control. *Hum Factors* 27:267-283, 1985.

42. Williams, JM, and Krane, V. Psychological characteristics of peak performance. In *Applied Sport Psychology: Personal Growth to Peak Performance.* Williams, JM, ed. Mountain View, CA: Mayfield, 158-170, 1998.

43. Winstein, CJ, Pohl, PS, Cardinale, C, Green, A, Scholtz, L, and Waters, CS. Learning a partial-weight-bearing skill: Effectiveness of two forms of feedback. *Phys Ther* 76:985-993, 1996.

44. Winstein, CJ, and Schmidt, RA. Reduced frequency of knowledge of results enhances motor skill learning. *J Exp Psychol Learn Mem Cogn* 16:677-691, 1990.

45. Wolpe, J. Psychotherapy by reciprocal inhibition. *Cond Reflex* 3:234-240, 1968.

46. Wood, JV, Perunovic, WE, and Lee, JW. Positive self-statements: Power for some, peril for others. *Psychol Sci* 20:860-866, 2009.

47. Wulf, G, Shea, C, and Lewthwaite, R. Motor skill learning and performance: A review of influential factors. *Med Educ* 44:75-84, 2010.

48. Wulf, G, Shea, CH, and Matschiner, S. Frequent feedback enhances complex motor skill learning. *J Mot Behav* 30:180-192, 1998.

49. Wulf, G, and Weigelt, C. Instructions about physical principles in learning a complex motor skill: To tell or not to tell. *Res Q Exerc Sport* 68:362-367, 1997.

50. Yerkes, RM, and Dodson, JD. The relation of strength of stimulus to rapidity of habit-formation. *J Comp Neurol Psychol* 18:459-482, 1908.

CHAPTER 9   Basic Nutritional Factors in Health

1. Acheson, KJ, Schutz, Y, Bessard, T, Anantharaman, K, Flatt, JP, and Jequier, E. Glycogen storage capacity and de novo lipogenesis during massive carbohydrate overfeeding in man. *Am J Clin Nutr* 48:240-247, 1988.

2. Akermark, C, Jacobs, I, Rasmusson, M, and Karlsson, J. Diet and muscle glycogen concentration in relation to physical performance in Swedish elite ice hockey players. *Int J Sport Nutr* 6:272-284, 1996.

3. Allen, S, McBride, WT, Young, IS, MacGowan, SW, McMurray, TJ, Prabhu, S, Penugonda, SP, and Armstrong, MA. A clinical, renal and immunological assessment of surface modifying additive treated (SMART) cardiopulmonary bypass circuits. *Perfusion* 20:255-262, 2005.

4. Almond, CS, Shin, AY, Fortescue, EB, Mannix, RC, Wypij, D, Binstadt, BA, Duncan, CN, Olson, DP, Salerno, AE, Newburger, JW, and Greenes, DS. Hyponatremia among runners in the Boston Marathon. *New Engl J Med* 352:1550-1556, 2005.

5. Anderson, GH, Tecimer, SN, Shah, D, and Zafar, TA. Protein source, quantity, and time of consumption determine the effect of proteins on short-term food intake in young men. *J Nutr* 134:3011-3015, 2004.

6. Arieff, AI, Llach, F, and Massry, SG. Neurological manifestations and morbidity of hyponatremia: Correlation with brain water and electrolytes. *Medicine* 55:121-129, 1976.

7. Armstrong, LE, Maresh, CM, Castellani, JW, Bergeron, MF, Kenefick, RW, LaGasse, KE, and Riebe, D. Urinary indices of hydration status. *Int J Sport Nutr* 4:265-279, 1994.

8. Atkinson, FS, Foster-Powell, K, and Brand-Miller, JC. International tables of glycemic index and glycemic load values: 2008. *Diabetes Care* 31:2281-2283, 2008.

9. Bailey, RL, Dodd, KW, Goldman, JA, Gahche, JJ, Dwyer, JT, Moshfegh, AJ, Sempos, CT, and Picciano, MF. Estimation of total usual calcium and vitamin D intakes in the United States. *J Nutr* 140:817-822, 2010.

10. Balsom, PD, Wood, K, Olsson, P, and Ekblom, B. Carbohydrate intake and multiple sprint sports: With special reference to football (soccer). *Int J Sports Med* 20:48-52, 1999.

11. Bangsbo, J, Graham, TE, Kiens, B, and Saltin, B. Elevated muscle glycogen and anaerobic energy production during exhaustive exercise in man. *J Physiol* 451:205-227, 1992.

12. Bar-Or, O, Blimkie, CJ, Hay, JA, MacDougall, JD, Ward, DS, and Wilson, WM. Voluntary dehydration and heat intolerance in cystic fibrosis. *Lancet* 339:696-699, 1992.

13. Bardis, CN, Kavouras, SA, Kosti, L, Markousi, M, and Sidossis, LS. Mild hypohydration decreases cycling performance in the heat. *Med Sci Sports Exerc* 45:1782-1789, 2013.

14. Batchelder, BC, Krause, BA, Seegmiller, JG, and Starkey, CA. Gastrointestinal temperature increases and hypohydration exists after collegiate men's ice hockey participation. *J Strength Cond Res* 24:68-73, 2010.

15. Bermejo, F, and Garcia-Lopez, S. A guide to diagnosis of iron deficiency and iron deficiency anemia in digestive diseases. *World J Gastroenterol* 15:4638-4643, 2009.

16. Borzoei, S, Neovius, M, Barkeling, B, Teixeira-Pinto, A, and Rossner, S. A comparison of effects of fish and beef protein on satiety in normal weight men. *Eur J Clin Nutr* 60:897-902, 2006.

17. Bozian, RC, Ferguson, JL, Heyssel, RM, Meneely, GR, and Darby, WJ. Evidence concerning the human requirement for vitamin B12. Use of the whole body counter for determination of absorption of vitamin B12. *Am J Clin Nutr* 12:117-129, 1963.

18. Brownlie, T, 4th, Utermohlen, V, Hinton, PS, Giordano, C, and Haas, JD. Marginal iron deficiency without anemia impairs aerobic adaptation among previously untrained women. *Am J Clin Nutr* 75:734-742, 2002.

19. Buyken, AE, Goletzke, J, Joslowski, G, Felbick, A, Cheng, G, Herder, C, and Brand-Miller, JC. Association between carbohydrate quality and inflammatory markers: Systematic review of observational and interventional studies. *Am J Clin Nutr* 99:813-833, 2014.

20. Cahill, GF, Jr. Starvation in man. *Clin Endocrinol Metab* 5:397-415, 1976.

21. Campbell, B, Kreider, RB, Ziegenfuss, T, La Bounty, P, Roberts, M, Burke, D, Landis, J, Lopez, H, and Antonio, J. International Society of Sports Nutrition position stand: Protein and exercise. *J Int Soc Sports Nutr* 4:8, 2007.

22. Casa, DJ, Armstrong, LE, Hillman, SK, Montain, SJ, Reiff, RV, Rich, BS, Roberts, WO, and Stone, JA. National Athletic Trainers' Association position statement: Fluid replacement for athletes. *J Athl Train* 35:212-224, 2000.

23. Cermak, NM, and van Loon, LJ. The use of carbohydrates during exercise as an ergogenic aid. *Sports Med* 43:1139-1155, 2013.

24. Chen, HY, Cheng, FC, Pan, HC, Hsu, JC, and Wang, MF. Magnesium enhances exercise performance via increasing glucose availability in the blood, muscle, and brain during exercise. *PLoS One* 9:e85486, 2014.

25. Cheuvront, SN, Carter, R, 3rd, Castellani, JW, and Sawka, MN. Hypohydration impairs endurance exercise performance in temperate but not cold air. *J Appl Physiol* 99:1972-1976, 2005.

26. Cheuvront, SN, Carter R, 3rd, and Sawka, MN. Fluid balance and endurance exercise performance. *Curr Sports Med Rep* 2:202-208, 2003.

27. Chiu, YT, and Stewart, ML. Effect of variety and cooking method on resistant starch content of white rice and subsequent postprandial glucose response and appetite in humans. *Asia Pac J Clin Nutr* 22:372-379, 2013.

28. Churchward-Venne, TA, Burd, NA, and Phillips, SM. Nutritional regulation of muscle protein synthesis with resistance exercise: Strategies to enhance anabolism. *Nutr Metab* 9:40, 2012.

29. Cogswell, ME, Zhang, Z, Carriquiry, AL, Gunn, JP, Kuklina, EV, Saydah, SH, Yang, Q, and Moshfegh, AJ. Sodium and potassium intakes among US adults: NHANES 2003-2008. *Am J Clin Nutr* 96:647-657, 2012.

30. Committee on Sports Medicine and Fitness. Climatic heat stress and the exercising child and adolescent. *Pediatrics* 106:158-159, 2000.

31. Coris, EE, Ramirez, AM, and Van Durme, DJ. Heat illness in athletes: The dangerous combination of heat, humidity and exercise. *Sports Med* 34:9-16, 2004.

32. Costabile, A, Kolida, S, Klinder, A, Gietl, E, Bauerlein, M, Frohberg, C, Landschutze, V, and Gibson, GR. A double-blind, placebo-controlled, cross-over study to establish the bifidogenic effect of a very-long-chain inulin extracted from globe artichoke (Cynara scolymus) in healthy human subjects. *Br J Nutr* 104:1007-1017, 2010.

33. Currell, K, and Jeukendrup, AE. Superior endurance performance with ingestion of multiple transportable carbohydrates. *Med Sci Sports Exerc* 40:275-281, 2008.

34. Davis, SE, Dwyer, GB, Reed, K, Bopp, C, Stosic, J, and Shepanski, M. Preliminary investigation: The impact of the NCAA Wrestling Weight Certification Program on weight cutting. *J Strength Cond Res* 16:305-307, 2002.

35. DeMarco, HM, Sucher, KP, Cisar, CJ, and Butterfield, GE. Pre-exercise carbohydrate meals: Application of glycemic index. *Med Sci Sports Exerc* 31:164-170, 1999.

36. Devaney, BL, and Frazão, E. *Review of Dietary Reference Intakes for Selected Nutrients: Challenges and Implications for Federal Food and Nutrition Policy.* Washington, DC: U.S. Department of Agriculture, Economic Research Service, 1, 2007.

37. Distefano, LJ, Casa, DJ, Vansumeren, MM, Karslo, RM, Huggins, RA, Demartini, JK, Stearns, RL, Armstrong, LE, and Maresh, CM. Hypohydration and hyperthermia impair neuromuscular control after exercise. *Med Sci Sports Exerc* 45:1166-1173, 2013.

38. Djousse, L, Pankow, JS, Eckfeldt, JH, Folsom, AR, Hopkins, PN, Province, MA, Hong, Y, and Ellison, RC. Relation between dietary linolenic acid and coronary artery disease in the National Heart, Lung, and Blood Institute Family Heart Study. *Am J Clin Nutr* 74:612-619, 2001.

39. Drewnowski, A. Concept of a nutritious food: Toward a nutrient density score. *Am J Clin Nutr* 82:721-732, 2005.

40. Drinkwater, BL, Kupprat, IC, Denton, JE, Crist, JL, and Horvath, SM. Response of prepubertal girls and college women to work in the heat. *J Appl Physiol* 43:1046-1053, 1977.

41. Duraffourd, C, De Vadder, F, Goncalves, D, Delaere, F, Penhoat, A, Brusset, B, Rajas, F, Chassard, D, Duchampt, A, Stefanutti, A, Gautier-Stein, A, and Mithieux, G. Mu-opioid receptors and dietary protein stimulate a gut-brain neural circuitry limiting food intake. *Cell* 150:377-388, 2012.

42. Esmarck, B, Andersen, JL, Olsen, S, Richter, EA, Mizuno, M, and Kjaer, M. Timing of postexercise protein intake is important for muscle hypertrophy with resistance training in elderly humans. *J Physiol* 535:301-311, 2001.

43. Evans, WJ, and Hughes, VA. Dietary carbohydrates and endurance exercise. *Am J Clin Nutr* 41:1146-1154, 1985.

44. Fan, J, and Watanabe, T. Inflammatory reactions in the pathogenesis of atherosclerosis. *J Atheroscler Thromb* 10:63-71, 2003.

45. Foster-Powell, K, Holt, SH, and Brand-Miller, JC. International table of glycemic index and glycemic load values: 2002. *Am J Clin Nutr* 76:5-56, 2002.

46. Fulgoni, VL, 3rd, Keast, DR, Auestad, N, and Quann, EE. Nutrients from dairy foods are difficult to replace in diets of Americans: Food pattern modeling and an analyses of the National Health and Nutrition Examination Survey 2003-2006. *Nutr Res* 31:759-765, 2011.

47. Garfinkel, D, and Garfinkel, L. Magnesium and regulation of carbohydrate metabolism at the molecular level. *Magnesium* 7:249-261, 1988.

48. Geigy, LC. *Units of Measurement, Body Fluids, Composition of the Body, Nutrition.* West Caldwell, NJ: Ciba-Geigy Corporation, 217, 1981.

49. Gerber, GS, and Brendler, CB. Evaluation of the urologic patient: History, physical examination, and urinalysis. In *Campbell-Walsh Urology.* 10th ed. Wein, AJ, Kavoussi, LR, Novick, AC, Partin, AW, and Peters, CA, eds. Philadelphia: Elsevier Saunders, 73-98, 2011.

50. Godek, SF, Godek, JJ, and Bartolozzi, AR. Hydration status in college football players during consecutive days of twice-a-day preseason practices. *Am J Sports Med* 33:843-851, 2005.

51. Godek, SF, Peduzzi, C, Burkholder, R, Condon, S, Dorshimer, G, and Bartolozzi, AR. Sweat rates, sweat sodium concentrations, and sodium losses in 3 groups of professional football players. *J Athl Train* 45:364-371, 2010.

52. Gonzalez-Alonso, J, Calbet, JA, and Nielsen, B. Muscle blood flow is reduced with dehydration during prolonged exercise in humans. *J Physiol* 513:895-905, 1998.

53. Hall, KD. What is the required energy deficit per unit weight loss? *Int J Obes* 32:573-576, 2008.

54. Hawley, JA, Schabort, EJ, Noakes, TD, and Dennis, SC. Carbohydrate-loading and exercise performance. An update. *Sports Med* 24:73-81, 1997.

55. Hayes, LD, and Morse, CI. The effects of progressive dehydration on strength and power: Is there a dose response? *Eur J Appl Physiol* 108:701-707, 2010.

56. Heaney, RP, and Layman, DK. Amount and type of protein influences bone health. *Am J Clin Nutr* 87:1567S-1570S, 2008.

57. Helge, JW, Watt, PW, Richter, EA, Rennie, MJ, and Kiens, B. Fat utilization during exercise: Adaptation to a fat-rich diet increases utilization of plasma fatty acids and very low density lipoprotein-triacylglycerol in humans. *J Physiol* 537:1009-1020, 2001.

58. Henry, YM, Fatayerji, D, and Eastell, R. Attainment of peak bone mass at the lumbar spine, femoral neck and radius in men and women: Relative contributions of bone size and volumetric bone mineral density. *Osteoporos Int* 15:263-273, 2004.

59. Henson, S, Blandon, J, Cranfield, J, and Herath, D. Understanding the propensity of consumers to comply with dietary guidelines directed at heart health. *Appetite* 54:52-61, 2010.

60. Hermansen, K, Rasmussen, O, Gregersen, S, and Larsen, S. Influence of ripeness of banana on the blood glucose and insulin response in type 2 diabetic subjects. *Diabet Med* 9:739-743, 1992.

61. Hinton, PS, Giordano, C, Brownlie, T, and Haas, JD. Iron supplementation improves endurance after training in iron-depleted, nonanemic women. *J Appl Physiol* 88:1103-1111, 2000.

62. Hornick, BA. *Job Descriptions: Models for the Dietetics Profession.* Chicago: American Dietetic Association, 9-14, 2008.

63. Hosseinpour-Niazi, S, Sohrab, G, Asghari, G, Mirmiran, P, Moslehi, N, and Azizi, F. Dietary glycemic index, glycemic load, and cardiovascular disease risk factors: Tehran Lipid and Glucose Study. *Arch Iran Med* 16:401-407, 2013.

64. Howarth, KR, Phillips, SM, MacDonald, MJ, Richards, D, Moreau, NA, and Gibala, MJ. Effect of glycogen availability on human skeletal muscle protein turnover during exercise and recovery. *J Appl Physiol* 109:431-438, 2010.

65. Huang, PC, and Chiang, A. Effects of excess protein intake on nitrogen utilization in young men. *J Formos Med Assoc* 91:659-664, 1992.

66. Hulston, CJ, Venables, MC, Mann, CH, Martin, C, Philp, A, Baar, K, and Jeukendrup, AE. Training with low muscle glycogen enhances fat metabolism in well-trained cyclists. *Med Sci Sports Exerc* 42:2046-2055, 2010.

67. Institute of Medicine (U.S.). Panel on Dietary Antioxidants and Related Compounds. *Dietary Reference Intakes for Vitamin C, Vitamin E, Selenium, and Carotenoids.* Washington, DC: National Academy Press, 2000.

68. Institute of Medicine (U.S.). Panel on Dietary Reference Intakes for Electrolytes and Water. *Dietary Reference Intakes for Water, Potassium, Sodium, Chloride, and Sulfate.* Washington, DC: National Academies Press, 1-405, 2005.

69. Institute of Medicine (U.S.). Panel on Macronutrients. *Dietary Reference Intakes for Energy, Carbohydrate, Fiber, Fat, Fatty Acids, Cholesterol, Protein, and Amino Acids.* Washington, DC: National Academies Press, 589-738, 2005.

70. Institute of Medicine (U.S.). Panel on Micronutrients. *Dietary Reference Intakes for Vitamin A, Vitamin K, Arsenic, Boron, Chromium, Copper, Iodine, Iron, Manganese, Molybdenum, Nickel, Silicon, Vanadium, and Zinc.* Washington, DC: National Academy Press, 82-161, 290-393, 2001.

71. Institute of Medicine (U.S.). Standing Committee on the Scientific Evaluation of Dietary Reference Intakes. *Dietary Reference Intakes for Calcium, Phosphorus, Magnesium, Vitamin D, and Fluoride.* Washington, DC: National Academy Press, 71-145, 1997.

72. Institute of Medicine (U.S.). Panel on Folate, Other B Vitamins, and Choline. *Dietary Reference Intakes for Thiamin, Riboflavin, Niacin, Vitamin B_6, Folate, Vitamin B_12, Pantothenic Acid, Biotin, and Choline.* Washington, DC: National Academy Press, 1-400, 1998.

73. Institute of Medicine (U.S.). Committee on Military Nutrition Research. *Fluid Replacement and Heat Stress.* Washington, DC: National Academy Press, 8, 1994.

74. Ivy, JL. Glycogen resynthesis after exercise: Effect of carbohydrate intake. *Int J Sports Med* 19 (Suppl):S142-S145, 1998.

75. Jacobs, KA, and Sherman, WM. The efficacy of carbohydrate supplementation and chronic high-carbohydrate diets for improving endurance performance. *Int J Sport Nutr* 9:92-115, 1999.

76. Jenkins, DJ, Wolever, TM, Taylor, RH, Barker, H, Fielden, H, Baldwin, JM, Bowling, AC, Newman, HC, Jenkins, AL, and Goff, DV. Glycemic index of foods: A physiological basis for carbohydrate exchange. *Am J Clin Nutr* 34:362-366, 1981.

77. Jensen, J, Rustad, PI, Kolnes, AJ, and Lai, YC. The role of skeletal muscle glycogen breakdown for regulation of insulin sensitivity by exercise. *Front Physiol* 2:112, 2011.

78. Jequier, E, and Schutz, Y. Long-term measurements of energy expenditure in humans using a respiration chamber. *Am J Clin Nutr* 38:989-998, 1983.

79. Jeukendrup, AE. Regulation of fat metabolism in skeletal muscle. *Ann NY Acad Sci* 967:217-235, 2002.

80. Jeukendrup, AE, Jentjens, RL, and Moseley, L. Nutritional considerations in triathlon. *Sports Med* 35:163-181, 2005.

81. Jones, LC, Cleary, MA, Lopez, RM, Zuri, RE, and Lopez, R. Active dehydration impairs upper and lower body anaerobic muscular power. *J Strength Cond Res* 22:455-463, 2008.

82. Joy, JM, Lowery, RP, Wilson, JM, Purpura, M, De Souza, EO, Wilson, SM, Kalman, DS, Dudeck, JE, and Jager, R. The effects of 8 weeks of whey or rice protein supplementation on body composition and exercise performance. *Nutr J* 12:86, 2013.

83. Judelson, DA, Maresh, CM, Anderson, JM, Armstrong, LE, Casa, DJ, Kraemer, WJ, and Volek, JS. Hydration and muscular performance: Does fluid balance affect strength, power and high-intensity endurance? *Sports Med* 37:907-921, 2007.

84. Katsanos, CS, Kobayashi, H, Sheffield-Moore, M, Aarsland, A, and Wolfe, RR. A high proportion of leucine is required for optimal stimulation of the rate of muscle protein synthesis by essential amino acids in the elderly. *Am J Physiol* 291:E381-E387, 2006.

85. Kerksick, C, Harvey, T, Stout, J, Campbell, B, Wilborn, C, Kreider, R, Kalman, D, Ziegenfuss, T, Lopez, H, Landis, J, Ivy, JL, and Antonio, J. International Society of Sports Nutrition position stand: Nutrient timing. *J Int Soc Sports Nutr* 5:17, 2008.

86. Kerstetter, JE, O'Brien, KO, and Insogna, KL. Dietary protein affects intestinal calcium absorption. *Am J Clin Nutr* 68:859-865, 1998.

87. Kerstetter, JE, O'Brien, KO, and Insogna, KL. Dietary protein, calcium metabolism, and skeletal homeostasis revisited. *Am J Clin Nutr* 78:584S-592S, 2003.

88. Kilding, AE, Tunstall, H, Wraith, E, Good, M, Gammon, C, and Smith, C. Sweat rate and sweat electrolyte composition in international female soccer players during game specific training. *Int J Sports Med* 30:443-447, 2009.

89. Kim, SK, Kang, HS, Kim, CS, and Kim, YT. The prevalence of anemia and iron depletion in the population aged 10 years or older. *Korean J Hematol* 46:196-199, 2011.

90. Kirwan, JP, Barkoukis, H, Brooks, LM, Marchetti, CM, Stetzer, BP, and Gonzalez, F. Exercise training and dietary glycemic load may have synergistic effects on insulin resistance in older obese adults. *Ann Nutr Metab* 55:326-333, 2009.

91. Krieger, JW, Sitren, HS, Daniels, MJ, and Langkamp-Henken, B. Effects of variation in protein and carbohydrate intake on body mass and composition during energy restriction: A meta-regression. *Am J Clin Nutr* 83:260-274, 2006.

92. Kurnik, D, Loebstein, R, Rabinovitz, H, Austerweil, N, Halkin, H, and Almog, S. Over-the-counter vitamin K1-containing multivitamin supplements disrupt warfarin anticoagulation in vitamin K1-depleted patients. A prospective, controlled trial. *Thromb Haemost* 92:1018-1024, 2004.

93. Layman, DK. Dietary Guidelines should reflect new understandings about adult protein needs. *Nutr Metab* 6:12, 2009.

94. Layman, DK, Clifton, P, Gannon, MC, Krauss, RM, and Nuttall, FQ. Protein in optimal health: Heart disease and type 2 diabetes. *Am J Clin Nutr* 87:1571S-1575S, 2008.

95. Lemon, PW, and Mullin, JP. Effect of initial muscle glycogen levels on protein catabolism during exercise. *J Appl Physiol* 48:624-629, 1980.

96. Lemon, PW, Tarnopolsky, MA, MacDougall, JD, and Atkinson, SA. Protein requirements and muscle mass/strength changes during intensive training in novice bodybuilders. *J Appl Physiol* 73:767-775, 1992.

97. Levenhagen, DK, Gresham, JD, Carlson, MG, Maron, DJ, Borel, MJ, and Flakoll, PJ. Postexercise nutrient intake timing in humans is critical to recovery of leg glucose and protein homeostasis. *Am J Physiol* 280:E982-E993, 2001.

98. Levine, E, Abbatangelo-Gray, J, Mobley, AR, McLaughlin, GR, and Herzog, J. Evaluating MyPlate: An expanded framework using traditional and nontraditional metrics for assessing health communication campaigns. *J Nutr Educ Behav* 44:S2-S12, 2012.

99. Liu, S, Willett, WC, Stampfer, MJ, Hu, FB, Franz, M, Sampson, L, Hennekens, CH, and Manson, JE. A prospective study of dietary glycemic load, carbohydrate intake, and risk of coronary heart disease in US women. *Am J Clin Nutr* 71:1455-1461, 2000.

100. Ludwig, DS. Dietary glycemic index and obesity. *J Nutr* 130:280S-283S, 2000.

101. Luhovyy, BL, Akhavan, T, and Anderson, GH. Whey proteins in the regulation of food intake and satiety. *J Am Coll Nutr* 26:704S-712S, 2007.

102. Malczewska, J, Raczynski, G, and Stupnicki, R. Iron status in female endurance athletes and in non-athletes. *Int J Sport Nutr Exerc Metab* 10:260-276, 2000.

103. Manoguerra, AS, Erdman, AR, Booze, LL, Christianson, G, Wax, PM, Scharman, EJ, Woolf, AD, Chyka, PA, Keyes, DC, Olson, KR, Caravati, EM, and Troutman, WG. Iron ingestion: An evidence-based consensus guideline for out-of-hospital management. *Clin Toxicol* 43:553-570, 2005.

104. Marlett, JA, Hosig, KB, Vollendorf, NW, Shinnick, FL, Haack, VS, and Story, JA. Mechanism of serum cholesterol reduction by oat bran. *Hepatology* 20:1450-1457, 1994.

105. Martin, WF, Armstrong, LE, and Rodriguez, NR. Dietary protein intake and renal function. *Nutr Metab* 2:25, 2005.

106. Martini, WZ, Chinkes, DL, and Wolfe, RR. The intracellular free amino acid pool represents tracer precursor enrichment for calculation of protein synthesis in cultured fibroblasts and myocytes. *J Nutr* 134:1546-1550, 2004.

107. Mattar, M, and Obeid, O. Fish oil and the management of hypertriglyceridemia. *Nutr Health* 20:41-49, 2009.

108. Maughan, RJ, and Leiper, JB. Sodium intake and post-exercise rehydration in man. *Eur J Appl Physiol Occup Physiol* 71:311-319, 1995.

109. Maughan, RJ, Watson, P, and Shirreffs, SM. Heat and cold: What does the environment do to the marathon runner? *Sports Med* 37:396-399, 2007.

110. Millward, DJ, Layman, DK, Tome, D, and Schaafsma, G. Protein quality assessment: Impact of expanding understanding of protein and amino acid needs for optimal health. *Am J Clin Nutr* 87:1576S-1581S, 2008.

111. Monsen, ER. Iron nutrition and absorption: Dietary factors which impact iron bioavailability. *J Am Diet Assoc* 88:786-790, 1988.

112. Montain, SJ, and Coyle, EF. Influence of graded dehydration on hyperthermia and cardiovascular drift during exercise. *J Appl Physiol* 73:1340-1350, 1992.

113. Mori, TA. Omega-3 fatty acids and hypertension in humans. *Clin Exp Pharmacol Physiol* 33:842-846, 2006.

114. Moshfegh, AJ, Goldman, JA, Jaspreet, A, Rhodes, D, and LaComb, R. *What We Eat in America: NHANES 2005-2006: Usual Nutrient Intakes From Food and Water Compared to 1997 Dietary Reference Intakes for Vitamin D, Calcium, Phosphorus, and Magnesium.* U.S. Department of Agriculture, Agricultural Research Service, 6-16, 2009.

115. Murphy, SP. Using DRIs for dietary assessment. *Asia Pac J Clin Nutr* 17 (Suppl):299-301, 2008.

116. Musunuru, K. Atherogenic dyslipidemia: Cardiovascular risk and dietary intervention. *Lipids* 45:907-914, 2010.

117. Nadel, ER. Control of sweating rate while exercising in the heat. *Med Sci Sports* 11:31-35, 1979.

118. Naghii, MR, and Fouladi, AI. Correct assessment of iron depletion and iron deficiency anemia. *Nutr Health* 18:133-139, 2006.

119. Neale, RJ, and Waterlow, JC. The metabolism of 14C-labelled essential amino acids given by intragastric or intravenous infusion to rats on normal and protein-free diets. *Br J Nutr* 32:11-25, 1974.

120. Osterberg, KL, Horswill, CA, and Baker, LB. Pregame urine specific gravity and fluid intake by National Basketball Association players during competition. *J Athl Train* 44:53-57, 2009.

121. Paddon-Jones, D, Short, KR, Campbell, WW, Volpi, E, and Wolfe, RR. Role of dietary protein in the sarcopenia of aging. *Am J Clin Nutr* 87:1562S-1566S, 2008.

122. Paddon-Jones, D, Westman, E, Mattes, RD, Wolfe, RR, Astrup, A, and Westerterp-Plantenga, M. Protein, weight management, and satiety. *Am J Clin Nutr* 87:1558S-1561S, 2008.

123. Parr, EB, Camera, DM, Areta, JL, Burke, LM, Phillips, SM, Hawley, JA, and Coffey, VG. Alcohol ingestion impairs maximal post-exercise rates of myofibrillar protein synthesis following a single bout of concurrent training. *PLoS One* 9:e88384, 2014.

124. Pastori, D, Carnevale, R, Cangemi, R, Saliola, M, Nocella, C, Bartimoccia, S, Vicario, T, Farcomeni, A, Violi, F, and Pignatelli, P. Vitamin E serum levels and bleeding risk in patients receiving oral anticoagulant therapy: A retrospective cohort study. *J Am Heart Assoc* 2:e000364, 2013.

125. Pejic, RN, and Lee, DT. Hypertriglyceridemia. *J Am Board Fam Med* 19:310-316, 2006.

126. Pendergast, DR, Horvath, PJ, Leddy, JJ, and Venkatraman, JT. The role of dietary fat on performance, metabolism, and health. *Am J Sports Med* 24:S53-S58, 1996.

127. Phillips, SM. A brief review of critical processes in exercise-induced muscular hypertrophy. *Sports Med* 44 (Suppl):71-77, 2014.

128. Phillips, SM, Moore, DR, and Tang, JE. A critical examination of dietary protein requirements, benefits, and excesses in athletes. *Int J Sport Nutr Exerc Metab* 17 (Suppl):S58-S76, 2007.

129. Pitsiladis, YP, Duignan, C, and Maughan, RJ. Effects of alterations in dietary carbohydrate intake on running performance during a 10 km treadmill time trial. *Br J Sports Med* 30:226-231, 1996.

130. Plourde, M, and Cunnane, SC. Extremely limited synthesis of long chain polyunsaturates in adults: Implications for their dietary essentiality and use as supplements. *Appl Physiol Nutr Metab* 32:619-634, 2007.

131. Poole, C, Wilborn, C, Taylor, L, and Kerksick, C. The role of post-exercise nutrient administration on muscle protein synthesis and glycogen synthesis. *J Sport Sci Med* 9:354-363, 2010.

132. Poortmans, JR, and Dellalieux, O. Do regular high protein diets have potential health risks on kidney function in athletes? *Int J Sport Nutr Exerc Metab* 10:28-38, 2000.

133. Popowski, LA, Oppliger, RA, Patrick Lambert, G, Johnson, RF, Kim Johnson, A, and Gisolf, CV. Blood and urinary measures of hydration status during progressive acute dehydration. *Med Sci Sports Exerc* 33:747-753, 2001.

134. Raben, A, Agerholm-Larsen, L, Flint, A, Holst, JJ, and Astrup, A. Meals with similar energy densities but rich in protein, fat, carbohydrate, or alcohol have different effects on energy expenditure and substrate metabolism but not on appetite and energy intake. *Am J Clin Nutr* 77:91-100, 2003.

135. Ramnani, P, Gaudier, E, Bingham, M, van Bruggen, P, Tuohy, KM, and Gibson, GR. Prebiotic effect of fruit and vegetable shots containing Jerusalem artichoke inulin: A human intervention study. *Br J Nutr* 104:233-240, 2010.

136. Reimers, KJ. Evaluating a healthy, high performance diet. *Strength Cond* 16:28-30, 1994.

137. Risser, WL, Lee, EJ, Poindexter, HB, West, MS, Pivarnik, JM, Risser, JM, and Hickson, JF. Iron deficiency in female athletes: Its prevalence and impact on performance. *Med Sci Sports Exerc* 20:116-121, 1988.

138. Rivera-Brown, AM, Ramirez-Marrero, FA, Wilk, B, and Bar-Or, O. Voluntary drinking and hydration in trained, heat-acclimatized girls exercising in a hot and humid climate. *Eur J Appl Physiol* 103:109-116, 2008.

139. Robins, AL, Davies, DM, and Jones, GE. The effect of nutritional manipulation on ultra-endurance performance: A case study. *Res Sports Med* 13:199-215, 2005.

140. Romijn, JA, Coyle, EF, Sidossis, LS, Gastaldelli, A, Horowitz, JF, Endert, E, and Wolfe, RR. Regulation of endogenous fat and carbohydrate metabolism in relation to exercise intensity and duration. *Am J Physiol* 265:E380-E391, 1993.

141. Ross, AC. *Modern Nutrition in Health and Disease.* Philadelphia: Wolters Kluwer Health/Lippincott Williams & Wilkins, 17-18, 2014.

142. Ross, AC, and Institute of Medicine (U.S.). Committee to Review Dietary Reference Intakes for Vitamin D and Calcium. *Dietary Reference Intakes: Calcium, Vitamin D.* Washington, DC: National Academies Press, 1-512, 2011.

143. Rowlands, DS, and Hopkins, WG. Effects of high-fat and high-carbohydrate diets on metabolism and performance in cycling. *Metabolism* 51:678-690, 2002.

144. Ryan, MF. The role of magnesium in clinical biochemistry: An overview. *Ann Clin Biochem* 28:19-26, 1991.

145. Saunders, MJ, Kane, MD, and Todd, MK. Effects of a carbohydrate-protein beverage on cycling endurance and muscle damage. *Med Sci Sports Exerc* 36:1233-1238, 2004.

146. Sawka, MN, Burke, LM, Eichner, ER, Maughan, RJ, Montain, SJ, and Stachenfeld, NS. American College of Sports Medicine position stand. Exercise and fluid replacement. *Med Sci Sports Exerc* 39:377-390, 2007.

147. Sawka, MN, and Coyle, EF. Influence of body water and blood volume on thermoregulation and exercise performance in the heat. *Exerc Sport Sci Rev* 27:167-218, 1999.

148. Sawka, MN, Latzka, WA, Matott, RP, and Montain, SJ. Hydration effects on temperature regulation. *Int J Sports Med* 19 (Suppl):S108-S110, 1998.

149. Schoffstall, JE, Branch, JD, Leutholtz, BC, and Swain, DE. Effects of dehydration and rehydration on the one-repetition maximum bench press of weight-trained males. *J Strength Cond Res* 15:102-108, 2001.

150. Schrauwen-Hinderling, VB, Hesselink, MK, Schrauwen, P, and Kooi, ME. Intramyocellular lipid content in human skeletal muscle. *Obesity* 14:357-367, 2006.

151. Schurch, MA, Rizzoli, R, Slosman, D, Vadas, L, Vergnaud, P, and Bonjour, JP. Protein supplements increase serum insulin-like growth factor-I levels and attenuate proximal femur bone loss in patients with recent hip fracture. A randomized, double-blind, placebo-controlled trial. *Ann Int Med* 128:801-809, 1998.

152. Schwingshackl, L, and Hoffmann, G. Long-term effects of low glycemic index/load vs. high glycemic index/load diets on parameters of obesity and obesity-associated risks: A systematic review and meta-analysis. *Nutr Metab Cardiovasc Dis* 23:699-706, 2013.

153. Sherman, WM, Doyle, JA, Lamb, DR, and Strauss, RH. Dietary carbohydrate, muscle glycogen, and exercise performance during 7 d of training. *Am J Clin Nutr* 57:27-31, 1993.

154. Shils, ME, and Shike, M. *Modern Nutrition in Health and Disease.* Philadelphia: Lippincott Williams & Wilkins, 141-156, 2006.

155. Shirreffs, SM, and Maughan, RJ. Volume repletion after exercise-induced volume depletion in humans: Replacement of water and sodium losses. *Am J Physiol* 274:F868-F875, 1998.

156. Shirreffs, SM, Taylor, AJ, Leiper, JB, and Maughan, RJ. Post-exercise rehydration in man: Effects of volume consumed and drink sodium content. *Med Sci Sports Exerc* 28:1260-1271, 1996.

157. Siraki, AG, Deterding, LJ, Bonini, MG, Jiang, J, Ehrenshaft, M, Tomer, KB, and Mason, RP. Procainamide, but not N-acetylprocainamide, induces protein free radical formation on myeloperoxidase: A potential mechanism of agranulocytosis. *Chem Res Toxicol* 21:1143-1153, 2008.

158. Smith, MF, Newell, AJ, and Baker, MR. Effect of acute mild dehydration on cognitive-motor performance in golf. *J Strength Cond Res* 26:3075-3080, 2012.

159. Soetan, KO, and Oyewole, OE. The need for adequate processing to reduce the antinutritional factors in plants used as human foods and animal feeds: A review. *Afr J Food Sci* 3:223-232, 2009.

160. Sparks, MJ, Selig, SS, and Febbraio, MA. Pre-exercise carbohydrate ingestion: Effect of the glycemic index on endurance exercise performance. *Med Sci Sports Exerc* 30:844-849, 1998.

161. Stoltzfus, R. Defining iron-deficiency anemia in public health terms: A time for reflection. *J Nutr* 131:565S-567S, 2001.

162. Stone, NJ, Robinson, JG, Lichtenstein, AH, Bairey Merz, CN, Blum, CB, Eckel, RH, Goldberg, AC, Gordon, D, Levy, D, Lloyd-Jones, DM, McBride, P, Schwartz, JS, Shero, ST, Smith, SC, Jr., Watson, K, and Wilson, PW. Guideline on the treatment of blood cholesterol to reduce atherosclerotic cardiovascular risk in adults: A report of the American College of Cardiology/American Heart Association Task Force on Practice Guidelines. *J Am Coll Cardiol* 63:2889-2934, 2014.

163. Sugiura, K, and Kobayashi, K. Effect of carbohydrate ingestion on sprint performance following continuous and intermittent exercise. *Med Sci Sports Exerc* 30:1624-1630, 1998.

164. Tapiero, H, Gate, L, and Tew, KD. Iron: Deficiencies and requirements. *Biomed Pharmacother* 55:324-332, 2001.

165. Tarnopolsky, M. Protein requirements for endurance athletes. *Nutrition* 20:662-668, 2004.

166. Taylor, R, Magnusson, I, Rothman, DL, Cline, GW, Caumo, A, Cobelli, C, and Shulman, GI. Direct assessment of liver glycogen storage by 13C nuclear magnetic resonance spectroscopy and regulation of glucose homeostasis after a mixed meal in normal subjects. *J Clin Invest* 97:126-132, 1996.

167. Thomas, DE, Brotherhood, JR, and Brand, JC. Carbohydrate feeding before exercise: Effect of glycemic index. *Int J Sports Med* 12:180-186, 1991.

168. Tripette, J, Loko, G, Samb, A, Gogh, BD, Sewade, E, Seck, D, Hue, O, Romana, M, Diop, S, Diaw, M, Brudey, K, Bogui, P, Cisse, F, Hardy-Dessources, MD, and Connes, P. Effects of hydration and dehydration on blood rheology in sickle cell trait carriers during exercise. *Am J Physiol* 299:H908-H914, 2010.

169. Trumbo, P, Schlicker, S, Yates, AA, and Poos, M. Dietary reference intakes for energy, carbohydrate, fiber, fat, fatty acids, cholesterol, protein and amino acids. *J Am Diet Assoc* 102:1621-1630, 2002.

170. Tsuji, T, Fukuwatari, T, Sasaki, S, and Shibata, K. Twenty-four-hour urinary water-soluble vitamin levels correlate with their intakes in free-living Japanese schoolchildren. *Public Health Nutr* 14:327-333, 2011.

171. U.S. Department of Agriculture. http://choosemyplate.gov/food-groups/oils.html.

172. U.S. Department of Agriculture, Agricultural Research Service. *Nutrient Intakes From Food: Mean Amounts and Percentages of Calories From Protein, Carbohydrate, Fat, and Alcohol, One Day, 2005-2006.* www.ars.usda.gov/ba/bhnrc/fsrg, 2008. Accessed February 15, 2015.

173. U.S. Department of Agriculture, Agricultural Research Service. *Nutrient Intakes From Food: Mean Amounts Consumed per Individual, by Gender and Age.* What We Eat in America, NHANES 2009-2010, 2012.

174. U.S. Department of Agriculture, Agricultural Research Service. *Report of the Dietary Guidelines Advisory Committee on the Dietary Guidelines for Americans, 2010.* Washington, DC: U.S. Department of Agriculture, 2010.

175. U.S. Department of Agriculture, Agricultural Research Service. *USDA National Nutrient Database for Standard Reference, Release 27.* Washington, DC: U.S. Department of Agriculture, 2014.

176. U.S. Department of Health and Human Services. *Scientific Report of the 2015 Dietary Guidelines Advisory Committee.* Washington, DC: U.S. Department of Health and Human Services, 2015.

177. Valko, M, Rhodes, CJ, Moncol, J, Izakovic, M, and Mazur, M. Free radicals, metals and antioxidants in oxidative stress-induced cancer. *Chem Biol Interact* 160:1-40, 2006.

178. Volpe, SL, Poule, KA, and Bland, EG. Estimation of prepractice hydration status of National Collegiate Athletic Association Division I athletes. *J Athl Train* 44:624-629, 2009.

179. Wallace, KL, Curry, SC, LoVecchio, F, and Raschke, RA. Effect of magnesium hydroxide on iron absorption after ferrous sulfate. *Ann Emerg Med* 34:685-687, 1999.

180. Wee, SL, Williams, C, Gray, S, and Horabin, J. Influence of high and low glycemic index meals on endurance running capacity. *Med Sci Sports Exerc* 31:393-399, 1999.

181. Wenos, DL, and Amato, HK. Weight cycling alters muscular strength and endurance, ratings of perceived exertion, and total body water in college wrestlers. *Percept Mot Skills* 87:975-978, 1998.

182. Wilk, B, and Bar-Or, O. Effect of drink flavor and NaCl on voluntary drinking and hydration in boys exercising in the heat. *J Appl Physiol* 80:1112-1117, 1996.

183. World Health Organization. Worldwide prevalence of anaemia 1993-2005. WHO Global Database on Anaemia. www.who.int/vmnis/database/anaemia/en. Accessed February 15, 2015.

184. Young, VR, and Pellett, PL. Plant proteins in relation to human protein and amino acid nutrition. *Am J Clin Nutr* 59:1203S-1212S, 1994.

185. Zawila, LG, Steib, CS, and Hoogenboom, B. The female collegiate cross-country runner: Nutritional knowledge and attitudes. *J Athl Train* 38:67-74, 2003.

CHAPTER 10   Nutritional Strategies to Maximize Performance

1. Acheson, KJ, Schutz, Y, Bessard, T, Anantharaman, K, Flatt, JP, and Jequier, E. Glycogen storage capacity and de novo lipogenesis during massive carbohydrate overfeeding in man. *Am J Clin Nutr* 48:240-247, 1988.

2. Ainsworth, BE, Haskell, WL, Herrmann, SD, Meckes, N, Bassett, DR, Jr., Tudor-Locke, C, Greer, JL, Vezina, J, Whitt-Glover, MC, and Leon, AS. 2011 Compendium of Physical Activities: A second update of codes and MET values. *Med Sci Sports Exerc* 43:1575-1581, 2011.

3. Ali, A, and Williams, C. Carbohydrate ingestion and soccer skill performance during prolonged intermittent exercise. *J Sports Sci* 27:1499-1508, 2009.

4. American Academy of Pediatrics. Climatic heat stress and the exercising child and adolescent. *Pediatrics* 106:158-159, 2000.

5. American College of Sports Medicine, American Dietetic Association, and Dietitians of Canada. Joint position statement: Nutrition and athletic performance. *Med Sci Sports Exerc* 41:709-731, 2009.

6. American Psychiatric Association, DSM-5 Task Force. *Diagnostic and Statistical Manual of Mental Disorders.* Washington, DC: American Psychiatric Association, 329-354, 2013.

7. Andrews, JL, Sedlock, DA, Flynn, MG, Navalta, JW, and Ji, H. Carbohydrate loading and supplementation in endurance-trained women runners. *J Appl Physiol* 95:584-590, 2003.

8. Aragon, AA, and Schoenfeld, BJ. Nutrient timing revisited: Is there a post-exercise anabolic window? *J Int Soc Sports Nut* 10:5, 2013.

9. Asp, S, Rohde, T, and Richter, EA. Impaired muscle glycogen resynthesis after a marathon is not caused by decreased muscle GLUT-4 content. *J Appl Physiol* 83:1482-1485, 1997.

10. Balsom, PD, Gaitanos, GC, Soderlund, K, and Ekblom, B. High-intensity exercise and muscle glycogen availability in humans. *Acta Physiol Scand* 165:337-345, 1999.

11. Bangsbo, J, Norregaard, L, and Thorsoe, F. The effect of carbohydrate diet on intermittent exercise performance. *Int J Sports Med* 13:152-157, 1992.

12. Bennett, CB, Chilibeck, PD, Barss, T, Vatanparast, H, Vandenberg, A, and Zello, GA. Metabolism and performance during extended high-intensity intermittent exercise after consumption of low- and high-glycaemic index pre-exercise meals. *Br J Nutr* 108 (Suppl):S81-S90, 2012.

13. Bergeron, M, Devore, C, and Rice, S. Climatic heat stress and exercising children and adolescents. *Pediatrics* 128:e741-e747, 2011.

14. Biolo, G, Maggi, SP, Williams, BD, Tipton, KD, and Wolfe, RR. Increased rates of muscle protein turnover and amino acid transport after resistance exercise in humans. *Am J Physiol* 268:E514-E520, 1995.

15. Boisseau, N, and Delamarche, P. Metabolic and hormonal responses to exercise in children and adolescents. *Sports Med* 30:405-422, 2000.

16. Borsheim, E, Cree, MG, Tipton, KD, Elliott, TA, Aarsland, A, and Wolfe, RR. Effect of carbohydrate intake on net muscle protein synthesis during recovery from resistance exercise. *J Appl Physiol* 96:674-678, 2004.

17. Bradley, U, Spence, M, Courtney, CH, McKinley, MC, Ennis, CN, McCance, DR, McEneny, J, Bell, PM, Young, IS, and Hunter, SJ. Low-fat versus low-carbohydrate weight reduction diets: Effects on weight loss, insulin resistance, and cardiovascular risk: A randomized control trial. *Diabetes* 58:2741-2748, 2009.

18. Breen, L, Philp, A, Witard, OC, Jackman, SR, Selby, A, Smith, K, Baar, K, and Tipton, KD. The influence of carbohydrate-protein co-ingestion following endurance exercise on myofibrillar and mitochondrial protein synthesis. *J Physiol* 589:4011-4025, 2011.

19. Burke, LM. Nutrition strategies for the marathon: Fuel for training and racing. *Sports Med* 37:344-347, 2007.

20. Burke, LM. Fueling strategies to optimize performance: Training high or training low? *Scand J Med Sci Sports* 20 (Suppl):48-58, 2010.

21. Centers for Disease Control. Body Mass Index: Considerations for Practitioners. www.cdc.gov/obesity/downloads/BMIforPactitioners.pdf, 2010. Accessed February 6, 2015.

22. Cermak, NM, Res, PT, de Groot, LC, Saris, WH, and van Loon, LJ. Protein supplementation augments the adaptive response of skeletal muscle to resistance-type exercise training: A meta-analysis. *Am J Clin Nutr* 96:1454-1464, 2012.

23. Chryssanthopoulos, C, and Williams, C. Pre-exercise carbohydrate meal and endurance running capacity when carbohydrates are ingested during exercise. *Int J Sports Med* 18:543-548, 1997.

24. Chryssanthopoulos, C, Williams, C, Nowitz, A, Kotsiopoulou, C, and Vleck, V. The effect of a high carbohydrate meal on endurance running capacity. *Int J Sport Nutr Exerc Metab* 12:157-171, 2002.

25. Coyle, EF. Timing and method of increased carbohydrate intake to cope with heavy training, competition and recovery. *J Sports Sci* 9:29-52, 1991.

26. Coyle, EF, Coggan, AR, Hemmert, MK, and Ivy, JL. Muscle glycogen utilization during prolonged strenuous exercise when fed carbohydrate. *J Appl Physiol* 61:165-172, 1986.

27. Coyle, EF, Coggan, AR, Hemmert, MK, Lowe, RC, and Walters, TJ. Substrate usage during prolonged exercise following a preexercise meal. *J Appl Physiol* 59:429-433, 1985.

28. Currell, K, and Jeukendrup, AE. Superior endurance performance with ingestion of multiple transportable carbohydrates. *Med Sci Sports Exerc* 40:275-281, 2008.

29. Fletcher, GO, Dawes, J, and Spano, M. The potential dangers of using rapid weight loss techniques. *Strength Cond J* 36:45-48, 2014.

30. Foster, GD, Wyatt, HR, Hill, JO, Makris, AP, Rosenbaum, DL, Brill, C, Stein, RI, Mohammed, BS, Miller, B, Rader, DJ, Zemel, B, Wadden, TA, Tenhave, T, Newcomb, CW, and Klein, S. Weight and metabolic outcomes after 2 years on a low-carbohydrate versus low-fat diet: A randomized trial. *Ann Int Med* 153:147-157, 2010.

31. Frost, E, Redman, L, and Bray, G. Effect of dietary protein intake on diet-induced thermogenesis during overfeeding [abstract]. The 32nd Annual Scientific Meeting of The Obesity Society, 2014. www.obesity.org/news-center/study-suggests-the-human-body-cannot-be-trained-to-maintain-a-higher-metabolism.htm.

32. Garby, L, Lammert, O, and Nielsen, E. Changes in energy expenditure of light physical activity during a 10 day period at 34 degrees C environmental temperature. *Eur J Clin Nutr* 44:241-244, 1990.

33. Garthe, I, Raastad, T, and Sundgot-Borgen, J. Long-term effect of nutritional counselling on desired gain in body mass and lean body mass in elite athletes. *Appl Physiol Nutr Metab* 36:547-554, 2011.

34. Gilson, SF, Saunders, MJ, Moran, CW, Moore, RW, Womack, CJ, and Todd, MK. Effects of chocolate milk consumption on markers of muscle recovery following soccer training: A randomized cross-over study. *J Int Soc Sports Nutr* 7:19, 2010.

35. Glynn, EL, Fry, CS, Drummond, MJ, Dreyer, HC, Dhanani, S, Volpi, E, and Rasmussen, BB. Muscle protein breakdown has a minor role in the protein anabolic response to essential amino acid and carbohydrate intake following resistance exercise. *Am J Physiol* 299:R533-R540, 2010.

36. Goh, Q, Boop, CA, Luden, ND, Smith, AG, Womack, CJ, and Saunders, MJ. Recovery from cycling exercise: Effects of carbohydrate and protein beverages. *Nutrients* 4:568-584, 2012.

37. Goltz, FR, Stenzel, LM, and Schneider, CD. Disordered eating behaviors and body image in male athletes. *Rev Bras Psiquiatr* 35:237-242, 2013.

38. Gomes, RV, Moreira, A, Coutts, AJ, Capitani, CD, and Aoki, MS. Effect of carbohydrate supplementation on the physiological and perceptual responses to prolonged tennis match play. *J Strength Cond Res* 28:735-741, 2014.

39. Haff, GG, Lehmkuhl, MJ, McCoy, LB, and Stone, MH. Carbohydrate supplementation and resistance training. *J Strength Cond Res* 17:187-196, 2003.

40. Hansen, M, Bangsbo, J, Jensen J, Bibby, BM, and Madsen, K. Effect of whey protein hydrolysate on performance and recovery of top-class orienteering runners. *Int J Sport Nutr Exerc Metab*, 2014. [e-pub ahead of print].

41. Harris, EC, and Barraclough, B. Excess mortality of mental disorder. *Br J Psychiatry* 173:11-53, 1998.

42. Harris, J, and Benedict, F. *A Biometric Study of Basal Metabolism in Man.* Washington, DC: Carnegie Institution, 370-373, 1919.

43. Harvie, M, Wright, C, Pegington, M, McMullan, D, Mitchell, E, Martin, B, Cutler, RG, Evans, G, Whiteside, S, Maudsley, S, Camandola, S, Wang, R, Carlson, OD, Egan, JM, Mattson, MP, and Howell, A. The effect of intermittent energy and carbohydrate restriction v. daily energy restriction on weight loss and metabolic disease risk markers in overweight women. *Br J Nutr* 110:1534-1547, 2013.

44. Hatfield, DL, Kraemer, WJ, Volek, JS, Rubin, MR, Grebien, B, Gomez, AL, French, DN, Scheett, TP, Ratamess, NA, Sharman, MJ, McGuigan, MR, Newton, RU, and Hakkinen, K. The effects of carbohydrate loading on repetitive jump squat power performance. *J Strength Cond Res* 20:167-171, 2006.

45. Helge, JW, Watt, PW, Richter, EA, Rennie, MJ, and Kiens, B. Fat utilization during exercise: Adaptation to a fat-rich diet increases

utilization of plasma fatty acids and very low density lipoprotein-tri-acylglycerol in humans. *J Physiol* 537:1009-1020, 2001.

46. Hession, M, Rolland, C, Kulkarni, U, Wise, A, and Broom, J. Systematic review of randomized controlled trials of low-carbohydrate vs. low-fat/low-calorie diets in the management of obesity and its comorbidities. *Obes Rev* 10:36-50, 2009.

47. Hill, RJ, and Davies, PS. The validity of self-reported energy intake as determined using the doubly labelled water technique. *Br J Nutr* 85:415-430, 2001.

48. Hoek, HW. Classification, epidemiology and treatment of DSM-5 feeding and eating disorders. *Curr Opin Psychiatry* 26:529-531, 2013.

49. Howarth, KR, Moreau, NA, Phillips, SM, and Gibala, MJ. Coingestion of protein with carbohydrate during recovery from endurance exercise stimulates skeletal muscle protein synthesis in humans. *J Appl Physiol* 106:1394-1402, 2009.

50. Hudson, JI, Hiripi, E, Pope, HG, Jr., and Kessler, RC. The prevalence and correlates of eating disorders in the National Comorbidity Survey Replication. *Biol Psychiatry* 61:348-358, 2007.

51. Institute of Medicine (U.S.). Panel on Dietary Reference Intakes for Electrolytes and Water. *Dietary Reference Intakes for Water, Potassium, Sodium, Chloride, and Sulfate.* Washington, DC: National Academies Press, 2005.

52. Institute of Medicine (U.S.). Panel on Macronutrients. *Dietary Reference Intakes for Energy, Carbohydrate, Fiber, Fat, Fatty Acids, Cholesterol, Protein, and Amino Acids.* Washington, DC: National Academies Press, 111-121, 2005.

53. Institute of Medicine (U.S.). Committee on Military Nutrition Research. *Fluid Replacement and Heat Stress.* Washington, DC: National Academy Press, 8, 1994.

54. Jacobs, I, Kaiser, P, and Tesch, P. Muscle strength and fatigue after selective glycogen depletion in human skeletal muscle fibers. *Eur J Appl Physiol Occup Physiol* 46:47-53, 1981.

55. Jacobs, I, Westlin, N, Karlsson, J, Rasmusson, M, and Houghton, B. Muscle glycogen and diet in elite soccer players. *Eur J Appl Physiol Occup Physiol* 48:297-302, 1982.

56. Jensen, J, Rustad, PI, Kolnes, AJ, and Lai, YC. The role of skeletal muscle glycogen breakdown for regulation of insulin sensitivity by exercise. *Front Physiol* 2:112, 2011.

57. Jentjens, R, and Jeukendrup, A. Determinants of post-exercise glycogen synthesis during short-term recovery. *Sports Med* 33:117-144, 2003.

58. Jentjens, RL, Achten, J, and Jeukendrup, AE. High oxidation rates from combined carbohydrates ingested during exercise. *Med Sci Sports Exerc* 36:1551-1558, 2004.

59. Jequier, E, and Schutz, Y. Long-term measurements of energy expenditure in humans using a respiration chamber. *Am J Clin Nutr* 38:989-998, 1983.

60. Jeukendrup, AE. Oral carbohydrate rinse: Placebo or beneficial? *Curr Sports Med Rep* 12:222-227, 2013.

61. Jeukendrup, AE, and Jentjens, R. Oxidation of carbohydrate feedings during prolonged exercise: Current thoughts, guidelines and directions for future research. *Sports Med* 29:407-424, 2000.

62. Jeukendrup, AE, Wagenmakers, AJ, Stegen, JH, Gijsen, AP, Brouns, F, and Saris, WH. Carbohydrate ingestion can completely suppress endogenous glucose production during exercise. *Am J Physiol* 276:E672-E683, 1999.

63. Joy, JM, Lowery, RP, Wilson, JM, Purpura, M, De Souza, EO, Wilson, SM, Kalman, DS, Dudeck, JE, and Jager, R. The effects of 8 weeks of whey or rice protein supplementation on body composition and exercise performance. *Nutr J* 12:86, 2013.

64. Khan, Y, and Tisman, G. Pica in iron deficiency: A case series. *J Med Case Rep* 4:86, 2010.

65. Kovacs, MS. A review of fluid and hydration in competitive tennis. *Int J Sports Physiol Perform* 3:413-423, 2008.

66. Kreider, RB. Physiological considerations of ultraendurance performance. *Int J Sport Nutr* 1:3-27, 1991.

67. Kreitzman, SN, Coxon, AY, and Szaz, KF. Glycogen storage: Illusions of easy weight loss, excessive weight regain, and distortions in estimates of body composition. *Am J Clin Nutr* 56:292S-293S, 1992.

68. Krustrup, P, Mohr, M, Ellingsgaard, H, and Bangsbo, J. Physical demands during an elite female soccer game: Importance of training status. *Med Sci Sports Exerc* 37:1242-1248, 2005.

69. Kutz, MR, and Gunter, MJ. Creatine monohydrate supplementation on body weight and percent body fat. *J Strength Cond Res* 17:817-821, 2003.

70. Lambert, BS, Oliver, JM, Katts, GR, Green, JS, Martin, SE, and Crouse, SF. DEXA or BMI: Clinical considerations for evaluating obesity in collegiate division I-A American football athletes. *Clin J Sport Med* 22:436-438, 2012.

71. Lee, JD, Sterrett, LE, Guth, LM, Konopka, AR, and Mahon, AD. The effect of pre-exercise carbohydrate supplementation on anaerobic exercise performance in adolescent males. *Pediatr Exerc Sci* 23:344-354, 2011.

72. Lemon, PW, and Mullin, JP. Effect of initial muscle glycogen levels on protein catabolism during exercise. *J Appl Physiol* 48:624-629, 1980.

73. Levenhagen, DK, Gresham, JD, Carlson, MG, Maron, DJ, Borel, MJ, and Flakoll, PJ. Postexercise nutrient intake timing in humans is critical to recovery of leg glucose and protein homeostasis. *Am J Physiol* 280:E982-E993, 2001.

74. MacDougall, JD, Ray, S, Sale, DG, McCartney, N, Lee, P, and Garner, S. Muscle substrate utilization and lactate production. *Can J Appl Physiol* 24:209-215, 1999.

75. Maclean, WC, Jr., Placko, RP, and Graham, GC. Plasma free amino acids of children consuming a diet with uneven distribution of protein relative to energy. *J Nutr* 106:241-248, 1976.

76. Makris, A, and Foster, GD. Dietary approaches to the treatment of obesity. *Psychiatr Clin North Am* 34:813-827, 2011.

77. Mamerow, MM, Mettler, JA, English, KL, Casperson, SL, Arentson-Lantz, E, Sheffield-Moore, M, Layman, DK, and Paddon-Jones, D. Dietary protein distribution positively influences 24-h muscle protein synthesis in healthy adults. *J Nutr* 144:876-880, 2014.

78. Marmy-Conus, N, Fabris, S, Proietto, J, and Hargreaves, M. Pre-exercise glucose ingestion and glucose kinetics during exercise. *J Appl Physiol* 81:853-857, 1996.

79. Maughan, RJ, and Shirreffs, SM. Development of individual hydration strategies for athletes. *Int J Sport Nutr Exerc Metab* 18:457-472, 2008.

80. Millard-Stafford, M, Warren, GL, Thomas, LM, Doyle, JA, Snow, T, and Hitchcock, K. Recovery from run training: Efficacy of a carbohydrate-protein beverage? *Int J Sport Nutr Exerc Metab* 15:610-624, 2005.

81. Mitchell, CJ, Churchward-Venne, TA, Parise, G, Bellamy, L, Baker, SK, Smith, K, Atherton, PJ, and Phillips, SM. Acute post-exercise myofibrillar protein synthesis is not correlated with resistance training-induced muscle hypertrophy in young men. *PLoS One* 9:e89431, 2014.

82. Mitchell, JB, Costill, DL, Houmard, JA, Fink, WJ, Roberg, RA, and Davis, JA. Gastric emptying: Influence of prolonged exercise and carbohydrate concentration. *Med Sci Sports Exerc* 21:269-274, 1989.

83. Muller, MJ, Bosy-Westphal, A, Klaus, S, Kreymann, G, Luhrmann, PM, Neuhauser-Berthold, M, Noack, R, Pirke, KM, Platte, P, Selberg, O, and Steiniger, J. World Health Organization equations have

shortcomings for predicting resting energy expenditure in persons from a modern, affluent population: Generation of a new reference standard from a retrospective analysis of a German database of resting energy expenditure. *Am J Clin Nutr* 80:1379-1390, 2004.

84. Murphy, CH, Hector, AJ, and Phillips, SM. Considerations for protein intake in managing weight loss in athletes. *Eur J Sport Sci* 15:1-8, 2014.

85. Murray, R, Paul, GL, Seifert, JG, and Eddy, DE. Responses to varying rates of carbohydrate ingestion during exercise. *Med Sci Sports Exerc* 23:713-718, 1991.

86. National Heart, Lung, and Blood Institute. Clinical guidelines on the identification, evaluation, and treatment of overweight and obesity in adults. The evidence report. *Obes Res* 6:464, 1998.

87. National Institute of Mental Health. What are eating disorders? www.nimh.nih.gov/health/publications/eating-disorders-new-trifold/index.shtml, 2014. Accessed February 7, 2015.

88. Nelson, KM, Weinsier, RL, Long, CL, and Schutz, Y. Prediction of resting energy expenditure from fat-free mass and fat mass. *Am J Clin Nutr* 56:848-856, 1992.

89. Nicholas, CW, Green, PA, Hawkins, RD, and Williams, C. Carbohydrate intake and recovery of intermittent running capacity. *Int J Sport Nutr* 7:251-260, 1997.

90. Nieman, DC. Influence of carbohydrate on the immune response to intensive, prolonged exercise. *Exerc Immunol Rev* 4:64-76, 1998.

91. Norton, LE, Layman, DK, Bunpo, P, Anthony, TG, Brana, DV, and Garlick, PJ. The leucine content of a complete meal directs peak activation but not duration of skeletal muscle protein synthesis and mammalian target of rapamycin signaling in rats. *J Nutr* 139:1103-1109, 2009.

92. Ogden, CL, Carroll, MD, Kit, BK, and Flegal, KM. Prevalence of childhood and adult obesity in the United States, 2011-2012. *JAMA* 311:806-814, 2014.

93. Okano, G, Takeda, H, Morita, I, Katoh, M, Mu, Z, and Miyake, S. Effect of pre-exercise fructose ingestion on endurance performance in fed men. *Med Sci Sports Exerc* 20:105-109, 1988.

94. Oosthuyse, T, and Bosch, AN. The effect of the menstrual cycle on exercise metabolism: Implications for exercise performance in eumenorrhoeic women. *Sports Med* 40:207-227, 2010.

95. Ormsbee, MJ, Bach, CW, and Baur, DA. Pre-exercise nutrition: The role of macronutrients, modified starches and supplements on metabolism and endurance performance. *Nutrients* 6:1782-1808, 2014.

96. Ostojic, SM, and Mazic, S. Effects of a carbohydrate-electrolyte drink on specific soccer tests and performance. *J Sports Sci Med* 1:47-53, 2002.

97. Paddon-Jones, D, Sheffield-Moore, M, Zhang, XJ, Volpi, E, Wolf, SE, Aarsland, A, Ferrando, AA, and Wolfe, RR. Amino acid ingestion improves muscle protein synthesis in the young and elderly. *Am J Physiol* 286:E321-E328, 2004.

98. Parkin, JA, Carey, MF, Martin, IK, Stojanovska, L, and Febbraio, MA. Muscle glycogen storage following prolonged exercise: Effect of timing of ingestion of high glycemic index food. *Med Sci Sports Exerc* 29:220-224, 1997.

99. Pascoe, DD, Costill, DL, Fink, WJ, Robergs, RA, and Zachwieja, JJ. Glycogen resynthesis in skeletal muscle following resistive exercise. *Med Sci Sports Exerc* 25:349-354, 1993.

100. Paul, D, Jacobs, KA, Geor, RJ, and Hinchcliff, KW. No effect of pre-exercise meal on substrate metabolism and time trial performance during intense endurance exercise. *Int J Sport Nutr Exerc Metab* 13:489-503, 2003.

101. Perez-Schindler, J, Hamilton, DL, Moore, DR, Baar, K, and Philp, A. Nutritional strategies to support concurrent training. *Eur J Sport Sci*, 2014. [e-pub ahead of print].

102. Pettersson, S, Ekstrom, MP, and Berg, CM. Practices of weight regulation among elite athletes in combat sports: A matter of mental advantage? *J Athl Train* 48:99-108, 2013.

103. Phillips, SM. A brief review of critical processes in exercise-induced muscular hypertrophy. *Sports Med* 44 (Suppl):S71-S77, 2014.

104. Phillips, SM, Tipton, KD, Aarsland, A, Wolf, SE, and Wolfe, RR. Mixed muscle protein synthesis and breakdown after resistance exercise in humans. *Am J Physiol* 273:E99-E107, 1997.

105. Pizza, FX, Flynn, MG, Duscha, BD, Holden, J, and Kubitz, ER. A carbohydrate loading regimen improves high intensity, short duration exercise performance. *Int J Sport Nutr* 5:110-116, 1995.

106. Rankin, JW. Weight loss and gain in athletes. *Curr Sports Med Rep* 1:208-213, 2002.

107. Ravussin, E, Burnand, B, Schutz, Y, and Jequier, E. Twenty-four-hour energy expenditure and resting metabolic rate in obese, moderately obese, and control subjects. *Am J Clin Nutr* 35:566-573, 1982.

108. Ravussin, E, Lillioja, S, Anderson, TE, Christin, L, and Bogardus, C. Determinants of 24-hour energy expenditure in man. Methods and results using a respiratory chamber. *J Clin Invest* 78:1568-1578, 1986.

109. Rico-Sanz, J, Zehnder, M, Buchli, R, Dambach, M, and Boutellier, U. Muscle glycogen degradation during simulation of a fatiguing soccer match in elite soccer players examined noninvasively by 13C-MRS. *Med Sci Sports Exerc* 31:1587-1593, 1999.

110. Rowlands, DS, Nelson, AR, Phillips, SM, Faulkner, JA, Clarke, J, Burd, NA, Moore, D, and Stellingwerff, T. Protein-leucine fed dose effects on muscle protein synthesis after endurance exercise. *Med Sci Sports Exerc*, 2014. [e-pub ahead of print].

111. Saunders, MJ, Luden, ND, and Herrick, JE. Consumption of an oral carbohydrate-protein gel improves cycling endurance and prevents postexercise muscle damage. *J Strength Cond Res* 21:678-684, 2007.

112. Sawka, MN, Burke, LM, Eichner, ER, Maughan, RJ, Montain, SJ, and Stachenfeld, NS. American College of Sports Medicine position stand: Exercise and fluid replacement. *Med Sci Sports Exerc* 39:377-390, 2007.

113. Schabort, EJ, Bosch, AN, Weltan, SM, and Noakes, TD. The effect of a preexercise meal on time to fatigue during prolonged cycling exercise. *Med Sci Sports Exerc* 31:464-471, 1999.

114. Schoeller, DA. Limitations in the assessment of dietary energy intake by self-report. *Metabolism* 44:18-22, 1995.

115. Schoenfeld, BJ, Aragon, AA, and Krieger, JW. The effect of protein timing on muscle strength and hypertrophy: A meta-analysis. *J Int Soc Sports Nutr* 10:53, 2013.

116. Shepherd, SJ, and Gibson, PR. Fructose malabsorption and symptoms of irritable bowel syndrome: Guidelines for effective dietary management. *J Am Diet Assoc* 106:1631-1639, 2006.

117. Sherman, WM, Costill, DL, Fink, WJ, Hagerman, FC, Armstrong, LE, and Murray, TF. Effect of a 42.2-km footrace and subsequent rest or exercise on muscle glycogen and enzymes. *J Appl Physiol* 55:1219-1224, 1983.

118. Shirreffs, SM, and Maughan, RJ. Volume repletion after exercise-induced volume depletion in humans: Replacement of water and sodium losses. *Am J Physiol* 274:F868-F875, 1998.

119. Skoog, SM, and Bharucha, AE. Dietary fructose and gastrointestinal symptoms: A review. *Am J Gastroenterol* 99:2046-2050, 2004.

120. Stearns, RL, Emmanuel, H, Volek, JS, and Casa, DJ. Effects of ingesting protein in combination with carbohydrate during exercise on endurance performance: A systematic review with meta-analysis. *J Strength Cond Res* 24:2192-2202, 2010.

121. Sundgot-Borgen, J, and Torstveit, MK. Prevalence of eating disorders in elite athletes is higher than in the general population. *Clin J Sport Med* 14:25-32, 2004.

122. Tarnopolsky, M, Bosman, M, Macdonald, J, Vandeputte, D, Martin, J, and Roy, B. Postexercise protein-carbohydrate and carbohydrate supplements increase muscle glycogen in men and women. *J Appl Physiol* 83:1877-1883, 1997.

123. Tarnopolsky, MA, Atkinson, SA, Phillips, SM, and MacDougall, JD. Carbohydrate loading and metabolism during exercise in men and women. *J Appl Physiol* 78:1360-1368, 1995.

124. Tarnopolsky, MA, Gibala, M, Jeukendrup, AE, and Phillips, SM. Nutritional needs of elite endurance athletes. Part I: Carbohydrate and fluid requirements. *Eur J Sport Sci* 5:3-14, 2005.

125. Tarnopolsky, MA, Zawada, C, Richmond, LB, Carter, S, Shearer, J, Graham, T, and Phillips, SM. Gender differences in carbohydrate loading are related to energy intake. *J Appl Physiol* 91:225-230, 2001.

126. Thompson, J, and Manore, MM. Predicted and measured resting metabolic rate of male and female endurance athletes. *J Am Diet Assoc* 96:30-34, 1996.

127. Tipton, KD, Ferrando, AA, Phillips, SM, Doyle, D, Jr., and Wolfe, RR. Postexercise net protein synthesis in human muscle from orally administered amino acids. *Am J Physiol* 276:E628-E634, 1999.

128. Triplett, D, Doyle, JA, Rupp, JC, and Benardot, D. An isocaloric glucose-fructose beverage's effect on simulated 100-km cycling performance compared with a glucose-only beverage. *Int J Sport Nutr Exerc Metab* 20:122-131, 2010.

129. U.S. Department of Agriculture, Agricultural Research Service. *National Nutrient Database for Standard Reference, Release 26*, 2013. http://ndb.nal.usda.gov/ndb/search. Accessed February 15, 2015.

130. U.S. Department of Agriculture, Human Nutrition Information Service. *Report of the Dietary Guidelines Advisory Committee on the Dietary Guidelines for Americans, 2010.* Washington, DC: U.S. Department of Agriculture, 40-41, 2010.

131. U.S. Food and Drug Administration. Part 180—Food additives permitted in food or in contact with food on an interim basis pending additional study. Subpart B—Specific requreiments for certain food additives. www.accessdata.fda.gov/scripts/cdrh/cfdocs/cfcfr/CFRSearch.cfm?fr=180.30, 2014. Accessed February 7, 2015.

132. Vergauwen, L, Brouns, F, and Hespel, P. Carbohydrate supplementation improves stroke performance in tennis. *Med Sci Sports Exerc* 30:1289-1295, 1998.

133. Walker, JL, Heigenhauser, GJ, Hultman, E, and Spriet, LL. Dietary carbohydrate, muscle glycogen content, and endurance performance in well-trained women. *J Appl Physiol* 88:2151-2158, 2000.

134. Warhol, MJ, Siegel, AJ, Evans, WJ, and Silverman, LM. Skeletal muscle injury and repair in marathon runners after competition. *Am J Pathol* 118:331-339, 1985.

135. Weinheimer, EM, Sands, LP, and Campbell, WW. A systematic review of the separate and combined effects of energy restriction and exercise on fat-free mass in middle-aged and older adults: Implications for sarcopenic obesity. *Nutr Rev* 68:375-388, 2010.

136. Welsh, RS, Davis, JM, Burke, JR, and Williams, HG. Carbohydrates and physical/mental performance during intermittent exercise to fatigue. *Med Sci Sports Exerc* 34:723-731, 2002.

137. Widrick, JJ, Costill, DL, Fink, WJ, Hickey, MS, McConell, GK, and Tanaka, H. Carbohydrate feedings and exercise performance: Effect of initial muscle glycogen concentration. *J Appl Physiol* 74:2998-3005, 1993.

138. Wilk, B, and Bar-Or, O. Effect of drink flavor and NaCl on voluntary drinking and hydration in boys exercising in the heat. *J Appl Physiol* 80:1112-1117, 1996.

139. Williams, C, Brewer, J, and Walker, M. The effect of a high carbohydrate diet on running performance during a 30-km treadmill time trial. *Eur J Appl Physiol Occup Physiol* 65:18-24, 1992.

140. Wilson, JM, Marin, PJ, Rhea, MR, Wilson, SM, Loenneke, JP, and Anderson, JC. Concurrent training: A meta-analysis examining interference of aerobic and resistance exercises. *J Strength Cond Res* 26:2293-2307, 2012.

141. Yamada, Y, Uchida, J, Izumi, H, Tsukamoto, Y, Inoue, G, Watanabe, Y, Irie, J, and Yamada, S. A non-calorie-restricted low-carbohydrate diet is effective as an alternative therapy for patients with type 2 diabetes. *Int Med* 53:13-19, 2014.

142. Zeederberg, C, Leach, L, Lambert, EV, Noakes, TD, Dennis, SC, and Hawley, JA. The effect of carbohydrate ingestion on the motor skill proficiency of soccer players. *Int J Sport Nutr* 6:348-355, 1996.

143. Zucker, NL, Womble, LG, Milliamson, DA, and Perrin, LA. Protective factors for eating disorders in female college athletes. *Eat Disord* 7:207-218, 2007.

CHAPTER 11 Performance-Enhancing Substances and Methods

1. Abrahamsen, B, Nielsen, TL, Hangaard, J, Gregersen, G, Vahl, N, Korsholm, L, Hansen, TB, Andersen, M, and Hagen, C. Dose-, IGF-I- and sex-dependent changes in lipid profile and body composition during GH replacement therapy in adult onset GH deficiency. *Eur J Endocrinol* 150:671-679, 2004.

2. Alén, M, and Häkkinen, K. Physical health and fitness of an elite bodybuilder during 1 year of self-administration of testosterone and anabolic steroids: A case study. *Int J Sports Med* 6:24-29, 1985.

3. Alén, M, Häkkinen, K, and Komi, PV. Changes in neuromuscular performance and muscle fiber characteristics of elite power athletes self-administering androgenic and anabolic steroids. *Acta Physiol Scand* 122:535-544, 1984.

4. Alford, C, Cox, H, and Wescott, R. The effects of red bull energy drink on human performance and mood. *Amino Acids* 21:139-150, 2001.

5. Alvares, TS, Conte-Junior, CA, Silva, JT, and Paschoalin, VM. Acute L-arginine supplementation does not increase nitric oxide production in healthy subjects. *Nutr Metab* 9:54, 2012.

6. Anderson, RL, Wilmore, JH, Joyner, MJ, Freund, BJ, Hartzell, AA, Todd, CA, and Ewy, GA. Effects of cardioselective and nonselective beta-adrenergic blockade on the performance of highly trained runners. *Am J Cardiol* 55:149D-154D, 1985.

7. Antal, LC, and Good, CS. Effects of oxprenolol on pistol shooting under stress. *Practitioner* 224:755-760, 1980.

8. Arenas, J, Ricoy, JR, Encinas, AR, Pola, P, D'Iddio, S, Zeviani, M, Didonato, S, and Corsi, M. Carnitine in muscle, serum, and urine of nonprofessional athletes: Effects of physical exercise, training, and L-carnitine administration. *Muscle Nerve* 14:598-604, 1991.

9. Artioli, GG, Gualano, B, Smith, A, Stout, J, and Lancha, AH, Jr. Role of beta-alanine supplementation on muscle carnosine and exercise performance. *Med Sci Sports Exerc* 42:1162-1173, 2010.

10. Aschenbach, W, Ocel, J, Craft, L, Ward, C, Spangenburg, E, and Williams, J. Effect of oral sodium loading on high-intensity arm ergometry in college wrestlers. *Med Sci Sports Exerc* 32:669-675, 2000.

11. Astorino, TA, Matera, AJ, Basinger, J, Evans, M, Schurman, T, and Marquez, R. Effects of red bull energy drink on repeated sprint performance in women athletes. *Amino Acids* 42:1803-1808, 2012.

12. Astrup, A, Breum, L, Toubro, S, Hein, P, and Quaade, F. The effect and safety of an ephedrine/caffeine compound compared to ephedrine, caffeine and placebo in obese subjects on an energy restricted diet. A double blind trial. *Int J Obes Relat Metab Disord* 16:269-277, 1992.

13. Bacurau, RF, Navarro, F, Bassit, RA, Meneguello, MO, Santos, RV, Almeida, AL, and Costa Rosa, LF. Does exercise training interfere with the effects of L-carnitine supplementation? *Nutrition* 19:337-341, 2003.

14. Bahrke, MS, and Yesalis, CE. Abuse of anabolic androgenic steroids and related substances in sport and exercise. *Curr Opin Pharmacol* 4:614-620, 2004.

15. Ball, D, and Maughan, RJ. The effect of sodium citrate ingestion on the metabolic response to intense exercise following diet manipulation in man. *Exp Physiol* 82:1041-1056, 1997.

16. Barnett, C, Costill, DL, Vukovich, MD, Cole, KJ, Goodpaster, BH, Trappe, SW, and Fink, WJ. Effect of L-carnitine supplementation on muscle and blood carnitine content and lactate accumulation during high-intensity sprint cycling. *Int J Sport Nutr* 4:280-288, 1994.

17. Baumann, GP. Growth hormone doping in sports: A critical review of use and detection strategies. *Endocrinol Rev* 33:155-186, 2012.

18. Behre, H, and Nieschlag, E. Testosterone buciclate (20 Aet-1) in hypogonadal men: Pharmacokinetics and pharmacodynamics of the new long-acting androgen ester. *J Clin Endocrinol Metab* 75:1204-1210, 1992.

19. Bell, DG, and Jacobs, I. Combined caffeine and ephedrine ingestion improves run times of Canadian forces warrior test. *Aviat Space Environ Med* 70:325-329. 1999.

20. Bell, DG, Jacobs, I, McLellan, TM, and Zamecnik, J. Reducing the dose of combined caffeine and ephedrine preserves the ergogenic effect. *Aviat Space Environ Med* 71:415-419, 2000.

21. Bell, DG, Jacobs, I, and Zamecnik, J. Effects of caffeine, ephedrine and their combination on time to exhaustion during high-intensity exercise. *Eur J Appl Physiol Occup Physiol* 77:427-433, 1998.

22. Bell, GJ, and Wenger, HA. The effect of one-legged sprint training on intramuscular pH and nonbicarbonate buffering capacity. *Eur J Appl Physiol Occup Physiol* 58:158-164, 1988.

23. Bemben, MG, Bemben, DA, Loftiss, DD, and Knehans, AW. Creatine supplementation during resistance training in college football athletes. *Med Sci Sports Exerc* 33:1667-1673, 2001.

24. Bergen, WG, and Merkel, RA. Body composition of animals treated with partitioning agents: Implications for human health. *FASEB J* 5:2951-2957, 1991.

25. Berglund, B, and Ekblom, B. Effect of recombinant human erythropoietin treatment on blood pressure and some haematological parameters in healthy men. *J Intern Med* 229:125-130, 1991.

26. Berning, JM, Adams, KJ, and Stamford, BA. Anabolic steroid usage in athletics: Facts, fiction, and public relations. *J Strength Cond Res* 18:908-917, 2004.

27. Bhasin, S, Storer, TW, Berman, N, Callegari, C, Clevenger, B, Phillips, J, Bunnell, TJ, Tricker, R, Shirazi, A, and Casaburi, R. The effects of supraphysiologic doses of testosterone on muscle size and strength in normal men. *New Engl J Med* 335:1-7, 1996.

28. Bishop, D, Edge, J, Davis, C, and Goodman, C. Induced metabolic alkalosis affects muscle metabolism and repeated-sprint ability. *Med Sci Sports Exerc* 36:807-813, 2004.

29. Bishop, D, Lawrence, S, and Spencer, M. Predictors of repeated-sprint ability in elite female hockey players. *J Sci Med Sport* 6:199-209, 2003.

30. Bode-Böger, SM, Böger, RH, Schröder, EP, and Frölich, JC. Exercise increases systemic nitric oxide production in men. *J Cardiovasc Risk* 1:173-178, 1994.

31. Bogdanis, GC, Nevill, ME, Boobis, LH, and Lakomy, HK. Contribution of phosphocreatine and aerobic metabolism to energy supply during repeated sprint exercise. *J Appl Physiol* 80:876-884, 1996.

32. Børsheim, E, Cree, MG, Tipton, KD, Elliott, TA, Aarsland, A, and Wolfe, RR. Effect of carbohydrate intake on net muscle protein synthesis during recovery from resistance exercise. *J Appl Physiol* 96:674-678, 2004.

33. Brandsch, C, and Eder, K. Effect of L-carnitine on weight loss and body composition of rats fed a hypocaloric diet. *Ann Nutr Metab* 46:205-210, 2002.

34. Broeder, CE, Quindry, J, Brittingham, K, Panton, L, Thomson, J, Appakondu, S, Breuel, K, Byrd, R, Douglas, J, Earnest, C, Mitchell, C, Olson, M, Roy, T, and Yarlagadda, C. The Andro Project: Physiological and hormonal influences of androstenedione supplementation in men 35 to 65 years old participating in a high-intensity resistance training program. *Arch Intern Med* 160:3093-3104, 2000.

35. Brown, CM, McGrath, JC, Midgley, JM, Muir, AG, O'Brien, JW, Thonoor, CM, Williams, CM, and Wilson, VG. Activities of octopamine and synephrine stereoisomers on alpha-adrenoceptors. *Br J Pharmacol* 93:417-429, 1988.

36. Brown, GA, Vukovich, M, and King, DS. Testosterone prohormone supplements. *Med Sci Sports Exerc* 38:1451-1461, 2006.

37. Brown, GA, Vukovich, MD, Sharp, RL, Reifenrath, TA, Parsons, KA, and King, DS. Effect of oral DHEA on serum testosterone and adaptations to resistance training in young men. *J Appl Physiol* 87:2274-2283, 1999.

38. Bruce, CR, Anderson, ME, Fraser, SF, Stepto, NK, Klein, R, Hopkins, WG, and Hawley, JA. Enhancement of 2000-m rowing performance after caffeine ingestion. *Med Sci Sports Exerc* 32:1958-1963, 2000.

39. Buckley, WE, Yesalis, CE, Friedl, KE, Anderson, WA, Streit, AL, and Wright, JE. Estimated prevalence of anabolic steroid use among male high school seniors. *JAMA* 260:3441-3445, 1988.

40. Buford, TW, Kreider, RB, Stout, JR, Greenwood, M, Campbell, B, Spano, M, Ziegenfuss, T, Lopez, H, Landis, J, and Antonio, J. International Society of Sports Nutrition position stand: Creatine supplementation and exercise. *J Int Soc Sports Nutr* 4:6, 2007.

41. Cafri, G, Thompson, JK, Ricciardelli, L, McCabe, M, Smolak, L, and Yesalis, C. Pursuit of the muscular ideal: Physical and psychological consequences and putative risk factors. *Clin Psychol Rev* 25:215-239, 2005.

42. Campbell, B. Dietary protein strategies for performance enhancement. In *Sports Nutrition: Enhancing Athletic Performance.* Campbell, B, ed. Boca Raton, FL: CRC Press, 163-164, 2014.

43. Campbell, B, Wilborn, C, La Bounty, P, Taylor, L, Nelson, MT, Greenwood, M, Ziegenfuss, TN, Lopez, HL, Hoffman, JR, Stout, JR, Schmitz, S, Collins, R, Kalman, DS, Antonio, J, and Kreider, RB. International Society of Sports Nutrition position stand: Energy drinks. *J Int Soc Sports Nutr* 10:1, 2013.

44. Candow, DG, Kleisinger, AK, Grenier, S, and Dorsch, KD. Effect of sugar-free Red Bull energy drink on high-intensity run time-to-exhaustion in young adults. *J Strength Cond Res* 23:1271-1275, 2009.

45. Carpene, C, Galitzky, J, Fontana, E, Atgie, C, Lafontan, M, and Berlan, M. Selective activation of beta3-adrenoreceptors by octopamine: Comparative studies in mammalian fat cells. *Naunyn Schmiedebergs Arch Pharmacol* 359:310-321, 1999.

46. Casal, DC, and Leon, AS. Failure of caffeine to affect substrate utilization during prolonged running. *Med Sci Sports Exerc* 17:174-179, 1985.

47. Cazzola, M. A global strategy for prevention and detection of blood doping with erythropoietin and related drugs. *Haematologica* 85:561-563, 2000.

48. Cheetham, ME, Boobis, LH, Brooks, S, and Williams, C. Human muscle metabolism during sprint running. *J Appl Physiol* 61:54-60, 1986.

49. Choong, K, Lakshman, KM, and Bhasin, S. The physiological and pharmacological basis for the ergogenic effects of androgens in elite sports. *Asian J Androl* 10:351-363, 2008.

50. Cohen, PA, Travis, JC, and Venhuis, BJ. A synthetic stimulant never tested in humans, 1,3-dimethylbutylamine (DMBA), is identified in multiple dietary supplements. *Drug Test Anal,* 2014. [e-pub ahead of print].

51. Collier, SR, Casey, DP, and Kanaley, JA. Growth hormone responses to varying doses of oral arginine. *Growth Horm IGF Res* 15:136-139, 2005.

52. Collomp, K, Ahmaidi, S, Audran, M, Chanal, JL, and Prefaut, C. Effects of caffeine ingestion on performance and anaerobic metabolism during the Wingate test. *Int J Sports Med* 12:439-443, 1991.

53. Collomp, K, Ahmaidi, S, Chatard, JC, Audran, M, and Prefaut, C. Benefits of caffeine ingestion on sprint performance in trained and untrained swimmers. *Eur J Appl Physiol* 64:377-380, 1992.

54. Cooke, RR, McIntosh, RP, McIntosh, JG, and Delahunt, JW. Serum forms of testosterone in men after an hCG stimulation: Relative increase in non-protein bound forms. *Clin Endocrinol* 32:165-175, 1990.

55. Coombes, J, and McNaughton, L. Effects of bicarbonate ingestion on leg strength and power during isokinetic knee flexion and extension. *J Strength Cond Res* 7:241-249, 1993.

56. Costill, DL, Dalsky, GP, and Fink, WJ. Effects of caffeine ingestion on metabolism and exercise performance. *Med Sci Sports* 10:155-158, 1978.

57. Cox, G, and Jenkins, DG. The physiological and ventilatory responses to repeated 60 s sprints following sodium citrate ingestion. *J Sports Sci* 12:469-475, 1994.

58. Crist, DM, Peake, GT, Loftfield, RB, Kraner, JC, and Egan, PA. Supplemental growth hormone alters body composition, muscle protein metabolism and serum lipids in fit adults: Characterization of dose-dependent and response-recovery effects. *Mech Ageing Dev* 58:191-205, 1991.

59. Curry, LA, and Wagman, DF. Qualitative description of the prevalence and use of anabolic androgenic steroids by United States powerlifters. *Percept Mot Skills* 88:224-233, 1999.

60. Dalbo, VJ, Roberts, MD, Stout, JR, and Kerksick, CM. Putting to rest the myth of creatine supplementation leading to muscle cramps and dehydration. *Br J Sports Med* 42:567-573, 2008.

61. David, KG, Dingemanse, E, Freud, J, Laqueur, E. Über krystallinisches mannliches Hormon aus Hoden (Testosteron) wirksamer als aus harn oder aus Cholesterin bereitetes Androsteron [On crystalline male hormone from testicles (testosterone) effective as from urine or from cholesterol]. *Hoppe Seylers Z Physiol Chem* 233:281, 1935.

62. Dawson, B, Cutler, M, Moody, A, Lawrence, S, Goodman, C, and Randall, N. Effects of oral creatine loading on single and repeated maximal short sprints. *Aust J Sci Med Sport* 27:56-61, 1995.

63. Del Coso, J, Salinero, JJ, González-Millán, C, Abián-Vicén, J, and Pérez-González, B. Dose response effects of a caffeine-containing energy drink on muscle performance: A repeated measures design. *J Int Soc Sports Nutr* 9:21, 2012.

64. Deutz, NE, Pereira, SL, Hays, NP, Oliver, JS, Edens, NK, Evans, CM, and Wolfe, RR. Effect of β-hydroxy-β-methylbutyrate (HMB) on lean body mass during 10 days of bed rest in older adults. *Clin Nutr* 32:704-712, 2013.

65. Dickman, S. East Germany: Science in the disservice of the state. *Science* 254:26-27, 1991.

66. Dodge, T, and Hoagland, MF. The use of anabolic androgenic steroids and polypharmacy: A review of the literature. *Drug Alcohol Depend* 114:100-109, 2011.

67. Duncan, MJ, and Oxford, SW. The effect of caffeine ingestion on mood state and bench press performance to failure. *J Strength Cond Res* 25:178-185, 2011.

68. Dunnett, M, and Harris, RC. Influence of oral beta-alanine and L-histidine supplementation on the carnosine content of the gluteus medius. *Equine Vet J* (Suppl) 30:499-504, 1999.

69. Dvorak, J, Baume, N, Botre, F, Broseus, J, Budgett, R, Frey, WO, Geyer, H, Harcourt, PR, Ho, D, Howman, D, Isola, V, Lundby, C, Marclay, F, Peytavin, A, Pipe, A, Pitsiladis, YP, Reichel, C, Robinson, N, Rodchenkov, G, Saugy, M, Sayegh, S, Segura, J, Thevis, M, Vernec, A, Viret, M, Vouillamoz, M, and Zorzoli, M. Time for change: A roadmap to guide the implementation of the World Anti-Doping Code 2015. *Br J Sports Med* 48:801-806, 2014.

70. Edge, J, Bishop, D, and Goodman, C. The effects of training intensity on muscle buffer capacity in females. *Eur J Appl Physiol* 96:97-105, 2006.

71. Edge, J, Bishop, D, Goodman, C, and Dawson, B. Effects of high- and moderate-intensity training on metabolism and repeated sprints. *Med Sci Sports Exerc* 37:1975-1982, 2005.

72. Eichner, ER. Blood doping: Infusions, erythropoietin and artificial blood. *Sports Med* 37:389-391, 2007.

73. Ekblom, B, and Berglund, B. Effect of erythropoietin administration on mammal aerobic power. *Scand J Med Sci Sports* 1:88-93, 1991.

74. Eley, HL, Russell, ST, Baxter, JH, Mukerji, P, and Tisdale, MJ. Signaling pathways initiated by beta-hydroxy-beta-methylbutyrate to attenuate the depression of protein synthesis in skeletal muscle in response to cachectic stimuli. *Am J Physiol* 293:E923-E931, 2007.

75. Fahey, TD, and Brown, CH. The effects of an anabolic steroid on the strength, body composition, and endurance of college males when accompanied by a weight training program. *Med Sci Sports* 5:272-276, 1973.

76. Fahs, CA, Heffernan, KS, and Fernhall, B. Hemodynamic and vascular response to resistance exercise with L-arginine. *Med Sci Sports Exerc* 41:773-779, 2009.

77. Fayh, AP, Krause, M, Rodrigues-Krause, J, Ribeiro, JL, Ribeiro, JP, Friedman, R, Moreira, JC, and Reischak-Oliveira, A. Effects of L-arginine supplementation on blood flow, oxidative stress status and exercise responses in young adults with uncomplicated type I diabetes. *Eur J Nutr* 52:975-983, 2013.

78. Febbraio, MA, Flanagan, TR, Snow, RJ, Zhao, S, and Carey, MF. Effect of creatine supplementation on intramuscular TCr, metabolism and performance during intermittent, supramaximal exercise in humans. *Acta Physiol Scand* 155:387-395, 1995.

79. Finkelstein, BS, Imperiale, TF, Speroff, T, Marrero, U, Radcliffe, DJ, and Cuttler, L. Effect of growth hormone therapy on height in children with idiopathic short stature: A meta-analysis. *Arch Pediatr Adolesc Med* 156:230-240, 2002.

80. Fong, Y, Rosenbaum, M, Tracey, KJ, Raman, G, Hesse, DG, Matthews, DE, Leibel, RL, Gertner, JM, Fischman, DA, and Lowry, SF. Recombinant growth hormone enhances muscle myosin heavy-chain mRNA accumulation and amino acid accrual in humans. *Proc Natl Acad Sci U S A* 86:3371-3374, 1989.

81. Forbes, G. The effect of anabolic steroids on lean body mass: The dose response curve. *Metabolism* 34:571-573, 1985.

82. Forbes, GB, Porta, CR, Herr, BE, and Griggs, RC. Sequence of changes in body composition induced by testosterone and reversal of changes after drug is stopped. *JAMA* 267:397-399, 1992.

83. Forbes, SC, Candow, DG, Little, JP, Magnus, C, and Chilibeck, PD. Effect of Red Bull energy drink on repeated Wingate cycle performance and bench-press muscle endurance. *Int J Sport Nutr Exerc Metab* 17:433-444, 2007.

84. Foster, ZJ, and Housner, JA. Anabolic-androgenic steroids and testosterone precursors: Ergogenic aids and sport. *Curr Sports Med Rep* 3:234-241, 2004.

85. Fowler, WM, Jr., Gardner, GW, and Egstrom, GH. Effect of an anabolic steroid on physical performance of young men. *J Appl Physiol* 20:1038-1040, 1965.

86. Franke, WW, and Berendonk, B. Hormonal doping and androgenization of athletes: A secret program of the German Democratic Republic government. *Clin Chem* 43:1262-1279, 1997.

87. Frankos, VH, Street, DA, and O'Neill, RK. FDA regulation of dietary supplements and requirements regarding adverse event reporting. *Clin Pharmacol Ther* 87:239-244, 2010.

88. Friedl, K, Dettori, J, Hannan, C, Jr., Patience, T, and Plymate, S. Comparison of the effects of high dose testosterone and 19-nortestosterone to a replacement dose of testosterone on strength and body composition in normal men. *J Steroid Biochem* 40:607-612, 1991.

89. Frishman, WH. Beta-adrenergic receptor blockers. Adverse effects and drug interactions. *Hypertension* 11:1121-1129, 1988.

90. Froiland, K, Koszewski, W, Hingst, J, and Kopecky, L. Nutritional supplement use among college athletes and their sources of information. *Int J Sport Nutr Exerc Metab* 14:104-120, 2004.

91. Fudala, PJ, Weinrieb, RM, Calarco, JS, Kampman, KM, and Boardman, C. An evaluation of anabolic-androgenic steroid abusers over a period of 1 year: Seven case studies. *Ann Clin Psychiatry* 15:121-130, 2003.

92. Fugh-Berman, A, and Myers, A. Citrus aurantium, an ingredient of dietary supplements marketed for weight loss: Current status of clinical and basic research. *Exp Biol Med* 229:698-704, 2004.

93. Gaitanos, GC, Williams, C, Boobis, LH, and Brooks, S. Human muscle metabolism during intermittent maximal exercise. *J Appl Physiol* 75:712-719, 1993.

94. Gallagher, PM, Carrithers, JA, Godard, MP, Schulze, KE, and Trappe, SW. Beta-hydroxy-beta-methylbutyrate ingestion, part I: Effects on strength and fat free mass. *Med Sci Sports Exerc* 32:2109-2115, 2000.

95. Gareau, R, Audran, M, Baynes, RD, Flowers, CH, Duvallet, A, Senécal, L, and Brisson, GR. Erythropoietin abuse in athletes. *Nature* 380:113, 1996.

96. Garlick, PJ, and Grant, I. Amino acid infusion increases the sensitivity of muscle protein synthesis in vivo to insulin. Effect of branched-chain amino acids. *Biochem J* 254:579-584, 1988.

97. Giamberardino, MA, Dragani, L, Valente, R, Di Lisa, F, Saggini, R, and Vecchiet, L. Effects of prolonged L-carnitine administration on delayed muscle pain and CK release after eccentric effort. *Int J Sports Med* 17:320-324, 1996.

98. Goldstein, ER, Ziegenfuss, T, Kalman, D, Kreider, R, Campbell, B, Wilborn, C, Taylor, L, Willoughby, D, Stout, J, Graves, BS, Wildman, R, Ivy, JL, Spano, M, Smith, AE, and Antonio, J. International Society of Sports Nutrition position stand: Caffeine and performance. *J Int Soc Sports Nutr* 7:5, 2010.

99. Goodbar, NH, Foushee, JA, Eagerton, DH, Haynes, KB, and Johnson, AA. Effect of the human chorionic gonadotropin diet on patient outcomes. *Ann Pharmacother* 47:e23, 2013.

100. Gonzalez, AM, Walsh, AL, Ratamess, NA, Kang, J, and Hoffman, JR. Effect of a pre-workout energy supplement on acute multi-joint resistance exercise. *J Sports Sci Med* 10:261-266, 2011.

101. Graham, TE, Hibbert, E, and Sathasivam, P. Metabolic and exercise endurance effects of coffee and caffeine ingestion. *J Appl Physiol* 85:883-889, 1998.

102. Greenhaff, PL. Creatine and its application as an ergogenic aid. *Int J Sport Nutr* 5 (Suppl):S100-S110, 1995.

103. Greenwood, M, Kreider, RB, Melton, C, Rasmussen, C, Lancaster, S, Cantler, E, Milnor, P, and Almada, A. Creatine supplementation during college football training does not increase the incidence of cramping or injury. *Mol Cell Biochem* 244:83-88, 2003.

104. Greer, BK, and Jones, BT. Acute arginine supplementation fails to improve muscle endurance or affect blood pressure responses to resistance training. *J Strength Cond Res* 25:1789-1794, 2011.

105. Greer, F, McLean, C, and Graham, TE. Caffeine, performance, and metabolism during repeated Wingate exercise tests. *J Appl Physiol* 85:1502-1508, 1998.

106. Griggs, RC, Kingston, W, Jozefowicz, RF, Herr, BE, Forbes, G, and Halliday, D. Effect of testosterone on muscle mass and muscle protein synthesis. *J Appl Physiol* 66:498-503, 1989.

107. Haaz, S, Fontaine, KR, Cutter, G, Limdi, N, Perumean-Chaney, S, and Allison, DB. Citrus aurantium and synephrine alkaloids in the treatment of overweight and obesity: An update. *Obes Rev* 7:79-88, 2006.

108. Haff, GG, Kirksey, KB, Stone, MH, Warren, BJ, Johnson, RL, Stone, M, O'Bryant, H, and Proulx, C. The effect of 6 weeks of creatine monohydrate supplementation on dynamic rate of force development. *J Strength Cond Res* 14:426-433, 2000.

109. Haller, CA, Benowitz, NL, and Jacob, P. Hemodynamic effects of ephedra-free weight-loss supplements in humans. *Am J Med* 118:998-1003, 2005.

110. Harris, RC, Tallon, MJ, Dunnett, M, Boobis, L, Coakley, J, Kim, HJ, Fallowfield, JL, Hill, CA, Sale, C, and Wise, JA. The absorption of orally supplied beta-alanine and its effect on muscle carnosine synthesis in human vastus lateralis. *Amino Acids* 30:279-289, 2006.

111. Hartgens, F, Van Marken Lichtenbelt, WD, Ebbing, S, Vollaard, N, Rietjens, G, and Kuipers, H. Body composition and anthropometry in bodybuilders: Regional changes due to nandrolone decanoate administration. *Int J Sports Med* 22:235-241, 2001.

112. Hausswirth, C, Bigard, AX, Lepers, R, Berthelot, M, and Guezennec, CY. Sodium citrate ingestion and muscle performance in acute hypobaric hypoxia. *Eur J Appl Physiol Occup Physiol* 71:362-368, 1995.

113. Hervey, GR, Knibbs, AV, Burkinshaw, L, Morgan, DB, Jones, PR, Chettle, DR, and Vartsky, D. Effects of methandienone on the performance and body composition of men undergoing athletic training. *Clin Sci* 60:457-461, 1981.

114. Hill, CA, Harris, RC, Kim, HJ, Harris, BD, Sale, C, Boobis, LH, Kim, CK, and Wise, JA. Influence of beta-alanine supplementation on skeletal muscle carnosine concentrations and high intensity cycling capacity. *Amino Acids* 32:225-233, 2007.

115. Hirvonen, J, Nummela, A, Rusko, H, Rehunen, S, and Härkönen, M. Fatigue and changes of ATP, creatine phosphate, and lactate during the 400-m sprint. *Can J Sport Sci* 17:141-144, 1992.

116. Ho, JY, Kraemer, WJ, Volek, JS, Fragala, MS, Thomas, GA, Dunn-Lewis, C, Coday, M, Häkkinen, K, and Maresh, CM. l-Carnitine l-tartrate supplementation favorably affects biochemical markers of recovery from physical exertion in middle-aged men and women. *Metabolism* 59:1190-1199, 2010.

117. Hobson, RM, Harris, RC, Martin, D, Smith, P, Macklin, B, Elliott-Sale, KJ, and Sale, C. Effect of sodium bicarbonate supplementation on 2000-m rowing performance. *Int J Sports Physiol Perform* 9:139-144, 2014.

118. Hoffman, JR, Kang, J, Ratamess, NA, Hoffman, MW, Tranchina, CP, and Faigenbaum, AD. Examination of a pre-exercise, high energy supplement on exercise performance. *J Int Soc Sports Nutr* 6:2, 2009.

119. Hoffman, JR, Kang, J, Ratamess, NA, Jennings, PF, Mangine, G, and Faigenbaum, AD. Thermogenic effect from nutritionally enriched coffee consumption. *J Int Soc Sports Nutr* 3:35-41, 2006.

120. Hoffman, AR, Kuntze, JE, Baptista, J, Baum, HB, Baumann, GP, Biller, BM, Clark, RV, Cook, D, Inzucchi, SE, Kleinberg, D, Klibanski, A, Phillips, LS, Ridgway, EC, Robbins, RJ, Schlechte, J, Sharma, M, Thorner, MO, and Vance, ML. Growth hormone (GH) replacement therapy in adult-onset GH deficiency: Effects on body composition in men and women in a double-blind, randomized, placebo-controlled trial. *J Clin Endocrinol Metab* 89:2048-2056, 2004.

121. Hoffman, JR, Kraemer, WJ, Bhasin, S, Storer, T, Ratamess, NA, Haff, GG, Willoughby, DS, and Rogol, AD. Position stand on androgen and human growth hormone use. *J Strength Cond Res* 23 (Suppl):S1-S59, 2009.

122. Hoffman, J, Ratamess, N, Kang, J, Mangine, G, Faigenbaum, A, and Stout, J. Effect of creatine and beta-alanine supplementation on performance and endocrine responses in strength/power athletes. *Int J Sport Nutr Exerc Metab* 16:430-446, 2006.

123. Hoffman, J, Ratamess, NA, Ross, R, Kang, J, Magrelli, J, Neese, K, Faigenbaum, AD, and Wise, JA. Beta-alanine and the hormonal response to exercise. *Int J Sports Med* 29:952-958, 2008.

124. Holmgren, P, Nordén-Pettersson, L, and Ahlner, J. Caffeine fatalities—four case reports. *Forensic Sci Int* 139:71-73, 2004.

125. Horn, S, Gregory, P, and Guskiewicz, KM. Self-reported anabolic-androgenic steroids use and musculoskeletal injuries: Findings from the center for the study of retired athletes health survey of retired NFL players. *Am J Phys Med Rehabil* 88:192-200, 2009.

126. Horswill, CA, Costill, DL, Fink, WJ, Flynn, MG, Kirwan, JP, Mitchell, JB, and Houmard, JA. Influence of sodium bicarbonate on sprint performance: Relationship to dosage. *Med Sci Sports Exerc* 20:566-569, 1988.

127. Howland, J, and Rohsenow, DJ. Risks of energy drinks mixed with alcohol. *JAMA* 309:245-246, 2013.

128. Hsu, KF, Chien, KY, Chang-Chien, GP, Lin, SF, Hsu, PH, and Hsu, MC. Liquid chromatography-tandem mass spectrometry screening method for the simultaneous detection of stimulants and diuretics in urine. *J Anal Toxicol* 35:665-674, 2011.

129. Huang, A, and Owen, K. Role of supplementary L-carnitine in exercise and exercise recovery. *Med Sport Sci* 59:135-142, 2012.

130. Hülsmann, WC, and Dubelaar, ML. Carnitine requirement of vascular endothelial and smooth muscle cells in imminent ischemia. *Mol Cell Biochem* 116:125-129, 1992.

131. Hultman, E, Cederblad, G, and Harper, P. Carnitine administration as a tool of modify energy metabolism during exercise. *Eur J Appl Physiol Occup Physiol* 62:450, 1991.

132. Hultman, E, Söderlund, K, Timmons, JA, Cederblad, G, and Greenhaff, PL. Muscle creatine loading in men. *J Appl Physiol* 81:232-237, 1996.

133. Irving, LM, Wall, M, Neumark-Sztainer, D, and Story, M. Steroid use among adolescents: Findings from Project EAT. *J Adolesc Health* 30:243-252, 2002.

134. Ivy, JL, Kammer, L, Ding, Z, Wang, B, Bernard, JR, Liao, YH, and Hwang, J. Improved cycling time-trial performance after ingestion of a caffeine energy drink. *Int J Sport Nutr Exerc Metab* 19:61-78, 2009.

135. Jabłecka, A, Bogdański, P, Balcer, N, Cieślewicz, A, Skołuda, A, and Musialik, K. The effect of oral L-arginine supplementation on fasting glucose, HbA1c, nitric oxide and total antioxidant status in diabetic patients with atherosclerotic peripheral arterial disease of lower extremities. *Eur Rev Med Pharmacol* 16:342-350, 2012.

136. Jabłecka, A, Checiński, P, Krauss, H, Micker, M, and Ast, J. The influence of two different doses of L-arginine oral supplementation on nitric oxide (NO) concentration and total antioxidant status (TAS) in atherosclerotic patients. *Med Sci Monit* 10:CR29-CR32, 2004.

137. Jacobs, I, Pasternak, H, and Bell, DG. Effects of ephedrine, caffeine, and their combination on muscular endurance. *Med Sci Sports Exerc* 35:987-994, 2003.

138. Kamalakkannan, G, Petrilli, CM, George, I, LaManca, J, McLaughlin, BT, Shane, E, Mancini, DM, and Maybaum, S. Clenbuterol increases lean muscle mass but not endurance in patients with chronic heart failure. *J Heart Lung Transpl* 27:457-461, 2008.

139. Katsanos, CS, Kobayashi, H, Sheffield-Moore, M, Aarsland, A, and Wolfe, RR. A high proportion of leucine is required for optimal stimulation of the rate of muscle protein synthesis by essential amino acids in the elderly. *Am J Physiol* 291:E381-E387, 2006.

140. Kendrick, IP, Harris, RC, Kim, HJ, Kim, CK, Dang, VH, Lam, TQ, Bui, TT, Smith, M, and Wise, JA. The effects of 10 weeks of resistance training combined with beta-alanine supplementation on whole body strength, force production, muscular endurance and body composition. *Amino Acids* 34:547-554, 2008.

141. Kerksick, CM, Wilborn, CD, Campbell, B, Harvey, TM, Marcello, BM, Roberts, MD, Parker, AG, Byars, AG, Greenwood, LD, Almada, AL, Kreider, RB, and Greenwood, M. The effects of creatine monohydrate supplementation with and without D-pinitol on resistance training adaptations. *J Strength Cond Res* 23:2673-2682, 2009.

142. Kerner, J, and Hoppel, C. Fatty acid import into mitochondria. *Biochim Biophys Acta* 1486:1-17, 2000.

143. Kerrigan, S, and Lindsey, T. Fatal caffeine overdose: Two case reports. *Forensic Sci Int* 153:67-69, 2005.

144. King, DS, Sharp, RL, Vukovich, MD, Brown, GA, Reifenrath, TA, Uhl, NL, and Parsons, KA. Effect of oral androstenedione on serum testosterone and adaptations to resistance training in young men: A randomized controlled trial. *JAMA* 281:2020-2028, 1999.

145. Kinugasa, R, Akima, H, Ota, A, Ohta, A, and Kuno, SY. Short-term creatine supplementation does not improve muscle activation or sprint performance in humans. *Eur J Appl Physiol* 91:230-237, 2004.

146. Knitter, AE, Panton, L, Rathmacher, JA, Petersen, A, and Sharp, R. Effects of beta-hydroxy-beta-methylbutyrate on muscle damage after a prolonged run. *J Appl Physiol* 89:1340-1344, 2000.

147. Kraemer, WJ, Spiering, BA, Volek, JS, Ratamess, NA, Sharman, MJ, Rubin, MR, French, DN, Silvestre, R, Hatfield, DL, Van Heest, JL, Vingren, JL, Judelson, DA, Deschenes, MR, and Maresh, CM. Androgenic responses to resistance exercise: Effects of feeding and L-carnitine. *Med Sci Sports Exerc* 38:1288-1296, 2006.

148. Kraemer, WJ, Volek, JS, French, DN, Rubin, MR, Sharman, MJ, Gómez, AL, Ratamess, NA, Newton, RU, Jemiolo, B, Craig, BW, and Häkkinen, K. The effects of L-carnitine L-tartrate supplementation on hormonal responses to resistance exercise and recovery. *J Strength Cond Res* 17:455-462, 2003.

149. Kreider, RB. Effects of creatine supplementation on performance and training adaptations. *Mol Cell Biochem* 244:89-94, 2003.

150. Kreider, RB, Ferreira, M, Wilson, M, and Almada, AL. Effects of calcium beta-hydroxy-beta-methylbutyrate (HMB) supplementation during resistance-training on markers of catabolism, body composition and strength. *Int J Sports Med* 20:503-509, 1999.

151. Kreider, RB, Melton, C, Rasmussen, CJ, Greenwood, M, Lancaster, S, Cantler, EC, Milnor, P, and Almada, AL. Long-term creatine supplementation does not significantly affect clinical markers of health in athletes. *Mol Cell Biochem* 244:95-104, 2003.

152. Kruse, P, Ladefoged, J, Nielsen, U, Paulev, PE, and Sørensen, JP. Beta-blockade used in precision sports: Effect on pistol shooting performance. *J Appl Physiol* 61:417-420, 1986.

153. Kuipers, H, Wijnen, JA, Hartgens, F, and Willems, SM. Influence of anabolic steroids on body composition, blood pressure, lipid profile and liver functions in body builders. *Int J Sports Med* 12:413-418, 1991.

154. LaBotz, M, and Smith, BW. Creatine supplement use in an NCAA Division I athletic program. *Clin J Sport Med* 9:167-169, 1999.

155. Liddle, DG, and Connor, DJ. Nutritional supplements and ergogenic AIDS. *Prim Care* 40:487-505, 2013.

156. Linderman, JK, and Gosselink, KL. The effects of sodium bicarbonate ingestion on exercise performance. *Sports Med* 18:75-80, 1994.

157. Lindh, AM, Peyrebrune, MC, Ingham, SA, Bailey, DM, and Folland, JP. Sodium bicarbonate improves swimming performance. *Int J Sports Med* 29:519-523, 2008.

158. Linossier, MT, Dormois, D, Brégère, P, Geyssant, A, and Denis, C. Effect of sodium citrate on performance and metabolism of human skeletal muscle during supramaximal cycling exercise. *Eur J Appl Physiol Occup Physiol* 76:48-54, 1997.

159. Liu, TH, Wu, CL, Chiang, CW, Lo, YW, Tseng, HF, and Chang, CK. No effect of short-term arginine supplementation on nitric oxide production, metabolism and performance in intermittent exercise in athletes. *J Nutr Biochem* 20:462-468, 2009.

160. Llewellyn, W. *Anabolics 2005: Anabolic Steroid Reference Manual.* Jupiter, FL: Body of Science, 267-331, 2005.

161. Loughton, SJ, and Ruhling, RO. Human strength and endurance responses to anabolic steroid and training. *J Sports Med Phys Fitness* 17:285-296, 1977.

162. MacRae, JC, Skene, PA, Connell, A, Buchan, V, and Lobley, GE. The action of the beta-agonist clenbuterol on protein and energy metabolism in fattening wether lambs. *Br J Nutr* 59:457-465, 1988.

163. Mahesh, VB, and Greenblatt, RB. The in vivo conversion of dehydroepiandrosterone and androstenedione to testosterone in the human. *Acta Endrocrinol* 41:400-406, 1962.

164. Maltin, CA, Delday, MI, Hay, SM, Smith, FG, Lobley, GE, and Reeds, PJ. The effect of the anabolic agent, clenbuterol, on overloaded rat skeletal muscle. *Biosci Rep* 7:143-149, 1987.

165. Maltin, CA, Delday, MI, Watson, JS, Heys, SD, Nevison, IM, Ritchie, IK, and Gibson, PH. Clenbuterol, a beta-adrenoceptor agonist, increases relative muscle strength in orthopaedic patients. *Clin Sci* 84:651-654, 1993.

166. Martineau, L, Horan, MA, Rothwell, NJ, and Little, RA. Salbutamol, a beta 2-adrenoceptor agonist, increases skeletal muscle strength in young men. *Clin Sci* 83:615-621, 1992.

167. McCabe, SE, Brower, KJ, West, BT, Nelson, TF, and Wechsler, H. Trends in non-medical use of anabolic steroids by U.S. college students: Results from four national surveys. *Drug Alcohol Depend* 90:243-251, 2007.

168. McCartney, N, Spriet, LL, Heigenhauser, GJ, Kowalchuk, JM, Sutton, JR, and Jones, NL. Muscle power and metabolism in maximal intermittent exercise. *J Appl Physiol* 60:1164-1169, 1986.

169. McNaughton, L, Backx, K, Palmer, G, and Strange, N. Effects of chronic bicarbonate ingestion on the performance of high-intensity work. *Eur J Appl Physiol Occup Physiol* 80:333-336, 1999.

170. McNaughton, L, and Cedaro, R. Sodium citrate ingestion and its effects on maximal anaerobic exercise of different durations. *Eur J Appl Physiol Occup Physiol* 64:36-41, 1992.

171. McNaughton, LR, Ford, S, and Newbold, C. Effect of sodium bicarbonate ingestion on high intensity exercise in moderately trained women. *J Strength Cond Res* 11:98-102, 1997.

172. McNaughton, LR, Siegler, J, and Midgley, A. Ergogenic effects of sodium bicarbonate. *Curr Sports Med Rep* 7:230-236, 2008.

173. Menon, DK. Successful treatment of anabolic steroid-induced azoospermia with human chorionic gonadotropin and human menopausal gonadotropin. *Fertil Steril* 79:1659-1661, 2003.

174. Midgley, SJ, Heather, N, and Davies, JB. Levels of aggression among a group of anabolic-androgenic steroid users. *Med Sci Law* 41:309-314, 2001.

175. Migeon, CJ. Adrenal androgens in man. *Am J Med* 53:606-626, 1972.

176. Moss, JL, Crosnoe, LE, and Kim, ED. Effect of rejuvenation hormones on spermatogenesis. *Fertil Steril* 99:1814-1820, 2013.

177. Mujika, I, Chatard, JC, Lacoste, L, Barale, F, and Geyssant, A. Creatine supplementation does not improve sprint performance in competitive swimmers. *Med Sci Sports Exerc* 28:1435-1441, 1996.

178. Nevill, ME, Boobis, LH, Brooks, S, and Williams, C. Effect of training on muscle metabolism during treadmill sprinting. *J Appl Physiol* 67:2376-2382, 1989.

179. Nissen, S, Sharp, R, Ray, M, Rathmacher, JA, Rice, D, Fuller, JC, Jr., Connelly, AS, and Abumrad, N. Effect of leucine metabolite beta-hydroxy-beta-methylbutyrate on muscle metabolism during resistance-exercise training. *J Appl Physiol* 81:2095-2104, 1996.

180. Norton, LE, Wilson, GJ, Layman, DK, Moulton, CJ, and Garlick, PJ. Leucine content of dietary proteins is a determinant of postprandial skeletal muscle protein synthesis in adult rats. *Nutr Metab* 9:67, 2012.

181. O'Connor, DM, and Crowe, MJ. Effects of beta-hydroxy-beta-methylbutyrate and creatine monohydrate supplementation on the aerobic and anaerobic capacity of highly trained athletes. *J Sports Med Phys Fitness* 43:64-68, 2003.

182. Oöpik, V, Saaremets, I, Medijainen, L, Karelson, K, Janson, T, and Timpmann, S. Effects of sodium citrate ingestion before exercise on endurance performance in well trained college runners. *Br J Sports Med* 37:485-489, 2003.

183. Pagonis, TA, Angelopoulos, NV, Koukoulis, GN, and Hadjichristodoulou, CS. Psychiatric side effects induced by supraphysiological

doses of combinations of anabolic steroids correlate to the severity of abuse. *Eur Psychiatry* 21:551-562, 2006.

184. Panton, LB, Rathmacher, JA, Baier, S, and Nissen, S. Nutritional supplementation of the leucine metabolite beta-hydroxy-beta-methylbutyrate (HMB) during resistance training. *Nutrition* 16:734-739, 2000.

185. Pasiakos, SM, McClung, HL, McClung, JP, Margolis, LM, Andersen, NE, Cloutier, GJ, Pikosky, MA, Rood, JC, Fielding, RA, and Young, AJ. Leucine-enriched essential amino acid supplementation during moderate steady state exercise enhances postexercise muscle protein synthesis. *Am J Clin Nutr* 94:809-818, 2011.

186. Pearson, DR, Hamby, DG, Russel, W, and Harris, T. Long-term effects of creatine monohydrate on strength and power. *J Strength Cond Res* 13:187-192, 1999.

187. Perry, P, Lund, B, Deninger, M, Kutscher, E, and Schneider, J. Anabolic steroid use in weightlifters and bodybuilders: An internet survey of drug utilization. *Clin J Sport Med* 15:326-330, 2005.

188. Petroczi, A, Naughton, D, Pearce, G, Bailey, R, Bloodworth, A, and McNamee, M. Nutritional supplement use by elite young UK athletes: Fallacies of advice regarding efficacy. *J Int Soc Sports Nutr* 5:22, 2008.

189. Poortmans, JR, Auquier, H, Renaut, V, Durussel, A, Saugy, M, and Brisson, GR. Effect of short-term creatine supplementation on renal responses in men. *Eur J Appl Physiol Occup Physiol* 76:566-567, 1997.

190. Poortmans, J, and Francaux, M. Long-term oral creatine supplementation does not impair renal function in healthy athletes. *Med Sci Sports Exerc* 31:1108-1110, 1999.

191. Pope, HG, Jr., Gruber, AJ, Choi, P, Olivardia, R, and Phillips, KA. Muscle dysmorphia. An underrecognized form of body dysmorphic disorder. *Psychosomatics* 38:548-557, 1997.

192. Pope, HG, Jr., and Katz, DL. Psychiatric and medical effects of anabolic-androgenic steroid use. A controlled study of 160 athletes. *Arch Gen Psychiatry* 51:375-382, 1994.

193. Pope, HG, Jr., Katz, DL, and Hudson, JI. Anorexia nervosa and "reverse anorexia" among 108 male bodybuilders. *Comp Psychiatry* 34:406-409, 1993.

194. Pope, HG, Jr., Kouri, EM, and Hudson, JI. Effects of supraphysiologic doses of testosterone on mood and aggression in normal men: A randomized controlled trial. *Arch Gen Psychiatry* 57:133-140, 2000.

195. Prather, ID, Brown, DE, North, P, and Wilson, JR. Clenbuterol: A substitute for anabolic steroids? *Med Sci Sports Exerc* 27:1118-1121, 1995.

196. Ransone, J, Neighbors, K, Lefavi, R, and Chromiak, J. The effect of beta-hydroxy beta-methylbutyrate on muscular strength and body composition in collegiate football players. *J Strength Cond Res* 17:34-39, 2003.

197. Rasmussen, BB, Tipton, KD, Miller, SL, Wolf, SE, and Wolfe, RR. An oral essential amino acid-carbohydrate supplement enhances muscle protein anabolism after resistance exercise. *J Appl Physiol* 88:386-392, 2000.

198. Reardon, CL, and Creado, S. Drug abuse in athletes. *Subst Abuse Rehabil* 14:95-105, 2014.

199. Rieu, I, Balage, M, Sornet, C, Giraudet, C, Pujos, E, Grizard, J, Mosoni, L, and Dardevet, D. Leucine supplementation improves muscle protein synthesis in elderly men independently of hyper-aminoacidaemia. *J Physiol* 575:305-315, 2006.

200. Roberts, RA, Ghiasvand, F, and Parker, D. Biochemistry of exercise-induced metabolic acidosis. *Am J Physiol* 287:R502-R516, 2004.

201. Roy, BD, Tarnopolsky, MA, MacDougall, JD, Fowles, J, and Yarasheski, KE. Effect of glucose supplement timing on protein metabolism after resistance training. *J Appl Physiol* 82:1882-1888, 1997.

202. Rubin, MR, Volek, JS, Gómez, AL, Ratamess, NA, French, DN, Sharman, MJ, and Kraemer, WJ. Safety measures of L-carnitine L-tartrate supplementation in healthy men. *J Strength Cond Res* 15:486-490, 2001.

203. Russell, C, Papadopoulos, E, Mezil, Y, Wells, GD, Plyley, MJ, Greenway, M, and Klentrou, P. Acute versus chronic supplementation of sodium citrate on 200 m performance in adolescent swimmers. *J Int Soc Sports Nutr* 11:26, 2014.

204. Salomon, F, Cuneo, RC, Hesp, R, and Sönksen, PH. The effects of treatment with recombinant human growth hormone on body composition and metabolism in adults with growth hormone deficiency. *New Engl J Med* 321:1797-1803, 1989.

205. Schabort, EJ, Wilson, G, and Noakes, TD. Dose-related elevations in venous pH with citrate ingestion do not alter 40-km cycling time-trial performance. *Eur J Appl Physiol* 83:320-327, 2000.

206. Schilling, BK, Stone, MH, Utter, A, Kearney, JT, Johnson, M, Coglianese, R, Smith, L, O'Bryant, HS, Fry, AC, Starks, M, Keith, R, and Stone, ME. Creatine supplementation and health variables: A retrospective study. *Med Sci Sports Exerc* 33:183-188, 2001.

207. Schwarz, S, Onken, D, and Schubert, A. The steroid story of Jenapharm: From the late 1940s to the early 1970s. *Steroids* 64:439-445, 1999.

208. Schwedhelm, E, Maas, R, Freese, R, Jung, D, Lukacs, Z, Jambrecina, A, Spickler, W, Schulze, F, and Böger, RH. Pharmacokinetic and pharmacodynamic properties of oral L-citrulline and L-arginine: Impact on nitric oxide metabolism. *Br J Clin Pharmacol* 65:51-59, 2008.

209. Sepkowitz, KA. Energy drinks and caffeine-related adverse effects. *JAMA* 309:243-244, 2013.

210. Shekelle, P, Hardy, M, Morton, S, Maglione, M, Suttorp, M, Roth, E, and Jungvig, L. Ephedra and ephedrine for weight loss and athletic performance enhancement: Clinical efficacy and side effects. *Evid Rep Technol Assess (Summ)* 76:1-4, 2003.

211. Smith, HJ, Mukerji, P, and Tisdale, MJ. Attenuation of proteasome-induced proteolysis in skeletal muscle by {beta}-hydroxy-{beta}-methylbutyrate in cancer-induced muscle loss. *Cancer Res* 65:277-283, 2005.

212. Snow, RJ, McKenna, MJ, Selig, SE, Kemp, J, Stathis, CG, and Zhao, S. Effect of creatine supplementation on sprint exercise performance and muscle metabolism. *J Appl Physiol* 84:1667-1673, 1998.

213. Souissi, M, Abedelmalek, S, Chtourou, H, Atheymen, R, Hakim, A, and Sahnoun, Z. Effects of morning caffeine ingestion on mood states, simple reaction time, and short-term maximal performance on elite judoists. *Asian J Sports Med* 3:161-168, 2012.

214. Spiering, BA, Kraemer, WJ, Vingren, JL, Hatfield, DL, Fragala, MS, Ho, JY, Maresh, CM, Anderson, JM, and Volek, JS. Responses of criterion variables to different supplemental doses of L-carnitine L-tartrate. *J Strength Cond Res* 21:259-264, 2007.

215. Spriet, LL. Caffeine and performance. *Int J Sport Nutr* 5:S84-S99, 1995.

216. Spriet, LL, MacLean, DA, Dyck, DJ, Hultman, E, Cederblad, G, and Graham, TE. Caffeine ingestion and muscle metabolism during prolonged exercise in humans. *Am J Physiol* 262:E891-E898, 1992.

217. Stamford, BA, and Moffatt, R. Anabolic steroid: Effectiveness as an ergogenic aid to experienced weight trainers. *J Sports Med Phys Fitness* 14:191-197, 1974.

218. Stein, MR, Julis, RE, Peck, CC, Hinshaw, W, Sawicki, JE, and Deller, JJ, Jr. Ineffectiveness of human chorionic gonadotropin in weight reduction: A double-blind study. *Am J Clin Nutr* 29:940-948, 1976.

219. Stephens, TJ, McKenna, MJ, Canny, BJ, Snow, RJ, and McConell, GK. Effect of sodium bicarbonate on muscle metabolism during intense endurance cycling. *Med Sci Sports Exerc* 34:614-621, 2002.

220. Stohs, SJ, Preuss, HG, and Shara, M. A review of the human clinical studies involving Citrus aurantium (bitter orange) extract and its primary protoalkaloid p-synephrine. *Int J Med Sci* 9:527-538, 2012.

221. Stout, JR, Cramer, JT, Zoeller, RF, Torok, D, Costa, P, Hoffman, JR, Harris, RC, and O'Kroy, J. Effects of beta-alanine supplementation on the onset of neuromuscular fatigue and ventilatory threshold in women. *Amino Acids* 32:381-386, 2007.

222. Striley, CL, Griffiths, RR, and Cottler, LB. Evaluating dependence criteria for caffeine. *J Caffeine Res* 1:219-225, 2011.

223. Stromme, SB, Meen, HD, and Aakvaag, A. Effects of an androgenic-anabolic steroid on strength development and plasma testosterone levels in normal males. *Med Sci Sports* 6:203-208, 1974.

224. Suzuki, Y, Ito, O, Mukai, N, Takahashi, H, and Takamatsu, K. High level of skeletal muscle carnosine contributes to the latter half of exercise performance during 30-s maximal cycle ergometer sprinting. *Jpn J Physiol* 52:199-205, 2002.

225. Swirzinski, L, Latin, RW, Berg, K, and Grandjean, A. A survey of sport nutrition supplements in high school football players. *J Strength Cond Res* 14:464-469, 2000.

226. Tang, JE, Lysecki, PJ, Manolakos, JJ, MacDonald, MJ, Tarnopolsky, MA, and Phillips, SM. Bolus arginine supplementation affects neither muscle blood flow nor muscle protein synthesis in young men at rest or after resistance exercise. *J Nutr* 141:195-200, 2011.

227. Tarnopolsky, MA. Caffeine and endurance performance. *Sports Med* 18:109-125, 1994.

228. Tavares, AB, Micmacher, E, Biesek, S, Assumpção, R, Redorat, R, Veloso, U, Vaisman, M, Farinatti, PT, and Conceição, F. Effects of growth hormone administration on muscle strength in men over 50 years old. *Int J Endocrinol* 2013:942030, 2013.

229. Tesch, PA. Exercise performance and beta-blockade. *Sports Med* 2:389-412, 1985.

230. Tipton, KD, Ferrando, AA, Phillips, SM, Doyle, D, Jr., and Wolfe, RR. Postexercise net protein synthesis in human muscle from orally administered amino acids. *Am J Physiol* 276:E628-E634, 1999.

231. Tipton, KD, Gurkin, BE, Matin, S, and Wolfe, RR. Nonessential amino acids are not necessary to stimulate net muscle protein synthesis in healthy volunteers. *J Nutr Biochem* 10:89-95, 1999.

232. Tipton, KD, Rasmussen, BB, Miller, SL, Wolf, SE, Owens-Stovall, SK, Petrini, BE, and Wolfe, RR. Timing of amino acid-carbohydrate ingestion alters anabolic response of muscle to resistance exercise. *Am J Physiol* 281:E197-E206, 2001.

233. Tiryaki, GR, and Atterbom, HA. The effects of sodium bicarbonate and sodium citrate on 600 m running time of trained females. *J Sports Med Phys Fitness* 35:194-198, 1995.

234. Torpy, JM, and Livingston, EH. JAMA patient page. Energy drinks. *JAMA* 309:297, 2013.

235. Transparency Market Research. Sports nutrition market—global industry analysis, size, share, growth, trends and forecast, 2013-2019. www.transparencymarketresearch.com/sports-nutrition-market.html. Accessed January 9, 2015.

236. Trice, I, and Haymes, EM. Effects of caffeine ingestion on exercise-induced changes during high-intensity, intermittent exercise. *Int J Sport Nutr* 5:37-44, 1995.

237. Underwood, LE, Attie, KM, and Baptista, J. Growth hormone (GH) dose-response in young adults with childhood-onset GH deficiency: A two-year, multicenter, multiple-dose, placebo-controlled study. *J Clin Endocrinol Metab* 88:5273-5280, 2003.

238. vandenBerg, P, Neumark-Sztainer, D, Cafri, G, and Wall, M. Steroid use among adolescents: Longitudinal findings from Project EAT. *Pediatrics* 119:476-486, 2007.

239. Vanhatalo, A, Bailey, SJ, DiMenna, FJ, Blackwell, JR, Wallis, GA, and Jones, AM. No effect of acute L-arginine supplementation on O_2 cost or exercise tolerance. *Eur J Appl Physiol* 113:1805-1819, 2013.

240. van Marken Lichtenbelt, WD, Hartgens, F, Vollaard, NB, Ebbing, S, and Kuipers, H. Bodybuilders' body composition: Effect of nandrolone decanoate. *Med Sci Sports Exerc* 36:484-489, 2004.

241. van Someren, K, Edwards, AJ, Howatson, G. Supplementation with beta-hydroxy-beta-methylbutyrate (HMB) and alpha-ketoisocaproic acid (KIC) reduces signs and symptoms of exercise-induced muscle damage in man. *Int J Sport Nutr Exerc Metab* 15:413-424, 2005.

242. van Someren, K, Fulcher, K, McCarthy, J, Moore, J, Horgan, G, and Langford, R. An investigation into the effects of sodium citrate ingestion on high-intensity exercise performance. *Int J Sport Nutr* 8:356-363, 1998.

243. Volek, JS, Duncan, ND, Mazzetti, SA, Staron, RS, Putukian, M, Gómez, AL, Pearson, DR, Fink, WJ, and Kraemer, WJ. Performance and muscle fiber adaptations to creatine supplementation and heavy resistance training. *Med Sci Sports Exerc* 31:1147-1156, 1999.

244. Volek, JS, and Kraemer, WJ. Creatine supplementation: Its effect on human muscular performance and body composition. *J Strength Cond Res* 10:200-210, 1996.

245. Volek, JS, Kraemer, WJ, Rubin, MR, Gómez, AL, Ratamess, NA, and Gaynor, P. L-carnitine L-tartrate supplementation favorably affects markers of recovery from exercise stress. *Am J Physiol* 282:E474-E482, 2002.

246. Volek, JS, Ratamess, NA, Rubin, MR, Gómez, AL, French, DN, McGuigan, MM, Scheett, TP, Sharman, MJ, Häkkinen, K, and Kraemer, WJ. The effects of creatine supplementation on muscular performance and body composition responses to short-term resistance training overreaching. *Eur J Appl Physiol* 91:628-637, 2004.

247. Wächter, S, Vogt, M, Kreis, R, Boesch, C, Bigler, P, Hoppeler, H, and Krähenbühl, S. Long-term administration of L-carnitine to humans: Effect on skeletal muscle carnitine content and physical performance. *Clin Chim Acta* 318:51-61, 2002.

248. Wallace, MB, Lim, J, Cutler, A, and Bucci, L. Effects of dehydroepiandrosterone vs androstenedione supplementation in men. *Med Sci Sports Exerc* 31:1788-1792, 1999.

249. Walsh, AL, Gonzalez, AM, Ratamess, NA, Kang, J, and Hoffman, JR. Improved time to exhaustion following ingestion of the energy drink Amino Impact. *J Int Soc Sports Nutr* 7:14, 2010.

250. Ward, P. The effect of an anabolic steroid on strength and lean body mass. *Med Sci Sports* 5:277-282, 1973.

251. Webster, MJ, Webster, MN, Crawford, RE, and Gladden, LB. Effect of sodium bicarbonate ingestion on exhaustive resistance exercise performance. *Med Sci Sports Exerc* 25:960-965, 1993.

252. Welle, S, Jozefowicz, R, Forbes, G, and Griggs, RC. Effect of testosterone on metabolic rate and body composition in normal men and men with muscular dystrophy. *J Clin Endocrinol Metab* 74:332-335, 1992.

253. Wiles, JD, Bird, SR, Hopkins, J, and Riley, M. Effect of caffeinated coffee on running speed, respiratory factors, blood lactate and perceived exertion during 1500-m treadmill running. *Br J Sports Med* 26:116-120, 1992.

254. Williams, AD, Cribb, PJ, Cooke, MB, and Hayes, A. The effect of ephedra and caffeine on maximal strength and power in resistance-trained athletes. *J Strength Cond Res* 22:464-470, 2008.

255. Willoughby, DS, and Rosene, J. Effects of oral creatine and resistance training on myosin heavy chain expression. *Med Sci Sports Exerc* 33:1674-1681, 2001.

256. Wilson, J. Androgen abuse by athletes. *Endocr Rev* 9:181-199, 1988.

257. Wilson, JM, Lowery, RP, Joy, JM, Andersen, JC, Wilson, SM, Stout, JR, Duncan, N, Fuller, JC, Baier, SM, Naimo, MA, and Rathmacher, J. The effects of 12 weeks of beta-hydroxy-beta-methylbutyrate free acid supplementation on muscle mass, strength, and power in resistance-trained individuals: A randomized, double-blind, placebo-controlled study. *Eur J Appl Physiol* 114:1217-1227, 2014.

258. Windsor, RE, and Dumitru, D. Anabolic steroid use by athletes. How serious are the health hazards? *Postgrad Med* 84:37-38, 41-43, 47-49, 1988.

259. Zoeller, RF, Stout, JR, O'Kroy, JA, Torok, DJ, and Mielke, M. Effects of 28 days of beta-alanine and creatine monohydrate supplementation on aerobic power, ventilatory and lactate thresholds, and time to exhaustion. *Amino Acids* 33:505-510, 2007.

CHAPTER 12   Principles of Test Selection and Administration

1. Anastasi, A. *Psychological Testing.* 7th ed. Upper Saddle River, NJ: Prentice Hall, 113-139, 1997.

2. Baumgartner, TA, and Jackson, AS. *Measurement for Evaluation in Physical Education and Exercise Science.* 8th ed. Madison, WI: Brown & Benchmark, 69-107, 2007.

3. Ben Abdelkrim, N, Castagna, C, Jabri, I, Battikh, T, El Fazaa, S, and El Ati, J. Activity profile and physiological requirements of junior elite basketball players in relation to aerobic-anaerobic fitness. *J Strength Cond Res* 24:2330-2342, 2010.

4. Bergeron, MF, Bahr, R, Bartsch, P, Bourdon, L, Calbet, JA, Carlsen, KH, Castagna, O, Gonzalez-Alonso, J, Lundby, C, Maughan, RJ, Millet, G, Mountjoy, M, Racinais, S, Rasmussen, P, Singh, DG, Subudhi, AW, Young, AJ, Soligard, T, and Engebretsen, L. International Olympic Committee consensus statement on thermoregulatory and altitude challenges for high-level athletes. *Br J Sports Med* 46:770-779, 2012.

5. Bogdanis, GC, Nevill, ME, Boobis, LH, Lakomy, HK, and Nevill, AM. Recovery of power output and muscle metabolites following 30 s of maximal sprint cycling in man. *J Physiol* 482 (Pt 2):467-480, 1995.

6. Brukner, P, and Khan, K. *Clinical Sports Medicine.* 4th ed. New York: McGraw-Hill, 1142-1143, 2012.

7. Buchheit, M, and Laursen, PB. High-intensity interval training, solutions to the programming puzzle. Part II: Anaerobic energy, neuromuscular load and practical applications. *Sports Med* 43:927-954, 2013.

8. Chu, D, and Vermeil, A. The rationale for field testing. *NSCA J* 5:35-36, 1983.

9. Dawson, B, Goodman, C, Lawrence, S, Preen, D, Polglaze, T, Fitzsimons, M, and Fournier, P. Muscle phosphocreatine repletion following single and repeated short sprint efforts. *Scand J Med Sci Sports* 7:206-213, 1997.

10. Fox, EL, Bowers, RW, and Foss, ML. *The Physiological Basis for Exercise and Sport.* 5th ed. Dubuque, IL: Brown, 338-340, 1993.

11. Fulco, CS, Rock, PB, and Cymerman, A. Maximal and submaximal exercise performance at altitude. *Aviat Space Environ Med* 69:793-801, 1998.

12. Gillam, GM, and Marks, M. 300 yard shuttle run. *NSCA J* 5:46, 1983.

13. Hayes, M, Castle, PC, Ross, EZ, and Maxwell, NS. The influence of hot humid and hot dry environments on intermittent-sprint exercise performance. *Int J Sports Physiol Perform* 9:387-396, 2014.

14. Heyward, VH. *Advanced Fitness Assessment and Exercise Prescription.* 7th ed. Champaign, IL: Human Kinetics, 47-78, 2014.

15. Hopkins, WG. Measures of reliability in sports medicine and science. *Sports Med* 30:1-15, 2000.

16. Joyce, D, and Lewindon, D. *High-Performance Training for Sports.* Champaign, IL: Human Kinetics, 3-5, 2014.

17. Kraning, KK, and Gonzalez, RR. A mechanistic computer simulation of human work in heat that accounts for physical and physiological effects of clothing, aerobic fitness, and progressive dehydration. *J Therm Biol* 22:331-342, 1997.

18. Larsen, GE, George, JD, Alexander, JL, Fellingham, GW, Aldana, SG, and Parcell, AC. Prediction of maximum oxygen consumption from walking, jogging, or running. *Res Q Exerc Sport* 73:66-72, 2002.

19. Matuszak, ME, Fry, AC, Weiss, LW, Ireland, TR, and McKnight, MM. Effect of rest interval length on repeated 1 repetition maximum back squats. *J Strength Cond Res* 17:634-637, 2003.

20. McArdle, WD, Katch, FI, and Katch, VL. *Exercise Physiology: Energy, Nutrition, and Human Performance.* 7th ed. Baltimore: Lippincott Williams & Wilkins, 648-661, 2007.

21. Messick, S. Validity. In *Educational Measurement,* Linn, R, ed. New York: Macmillan, 13-104, 1989.

22. Morrow, JR. *Measurement and Evaluation in Human Performance.* 4th ed. Champaign, IL: Human Kinetics, 102-108, 2011.

23. Narazaki, K, Berg, K, Stergiou, N, and Chen, B. Physiological demands of competitive basketball. *Scand J Med Sci Sports* 19:425-432, 2009.

24. Negrete, RJ, Hanney, WJ, Pabian, P, and Kolber, MJ. Upper body push and pull strength ratio in recreationally active adults. *Int J Sports Phys Ther* 8:138-144, 2013.

25. Newton, R, and Dugan, E. Application of strength diagnosis. *Strength Cond J* 24:50-59, 2002.

26. Parkin, JM, Carey, MF, Zhao, S, and Febbraio, MA. Effect of ambient temperature on human skeletal muscle metabolism during fatiguing submaximal exercise. *J Appl Physiol* 86:902-908, 1999.

27. Pescatello, LS, ed. *ACSM's Guidelines for Exercise Testing and Prescription.* 9th ed. Philadelphia: Wolters Kluwer Health/Lippincott Williams & Wilkins, 201-202, 216-223, 2014.

28. Ratamess, NA. *ACSM's Foundations of Strength Training and Conditioning.* Philadelphia: Lippincott Williams & Wilkins, 451-454, 2012.

29. Read, PJ, Hughes, J, Stewart, P, Chavda, S, Bishop, C, Edwards, M, and Turner, AN. A needs analysis and field-based testing battery for basketball. *J Strength Cond Res* 36:13-20, 2014.

30. Reilly, T, and Waterhouse, J. Sports performance: Is there evidence that the body clock plays a role? *Eur J Appl Physiol* 106:321-332, 2009.

31. Schuler, B, Thomsen, JJ, Gassmann, M, and Lundby, C. Timing the arrival at 2340 m altitude for aerobic performance. *Scand J Med Sci Sports* 17:588-594, 2007.

32. Sparks, SA, Cable, NT, Doran, DA, and Maclaren, DP. Influence of environmental temperature on duathlon performance. *Ergonomics* 48:1558-1567, 2005.

33. Turner, AN, and Stewart, PF. Repeat sprint ability. *Strength Cond J* 35:37-41, 2013.

34. Wisloff, U, Castagna, C, Helgerud, J, Jones, R, and Hoff, J. Strong correlation of maximal squat strength with sprint performance and vertical jump height in elite soccer players. *Br J Sports Med* 38:285-288, 2004.

CHAPTER 13   Administration, Scoring, and Interpretation of Selected Tests

1. Andersson, H, Raastad, T, Nilsson, J, Paulsen, G, Garthe, I, and Kadi, F. Neuromuscular fatigue and recovery in elite female soccer: Effects of active recovery. *Med Sci Sports Exerc* 40:372-380, 2008.

2. Arnason, A, Sigurdsson, SB, Gudmundsson, A, Holme, I, Engebretsen, L, and Bahr, R. Physical fitness, injuries, and team performance in soccer. *Med Sci Sports Exerc* 36:278-285, 2004.

3. Atkins, S, Hesketh, C, and Sinclair, J. The presence of bilateral imbalance of the lower limbs in elite youth soccer players of different ages. *J Strength Cond Res,* 2013.

4. Atkins, SJ. Performance of the Yo-Yo intermittent recovery test by elite professional and semiprofessional rugby league players. *J Strength Cond Res* 20:222-225, 2006.

5. Baker, D. 10-year changes in upper body strength and power in elite professional rugby league players: The effect of training age, stage, and content. *J Strength Cond Res* 27:285-292, 2013.

6. Baker, D, and Newton, RU. Discriminative analyses of various upper body tests in professional rugby-league players. *Int J Sports Physiol Perform* 1:347-360, 2006.

7. Baker, D, and Newton, RU. Comparison of lower body strength, power, acceleration, speed, agility, and sprint momentum to describe and compare playing rank among professional rugby league players. *J Strength Cond Res* 22:153-158, 2008.

8. Baker, DG, and Newton, RU. An analysis of the ratio and relationship between upper body pressing and pulling strength. *J Strength Cond Res* 18:594-598, 2004.

9. Bangsbo, J, Iaia, FM, and Krustrup, P. The Yo-Yo intermittent recovery test: A useful tool for evaluation of physical performance in intermittent sports. *Sports Med* 38:37-51, 2008.

10. Barr, MJ, and Nolte, VW. The importance of maximal leg strength for female athletes when performing drop jumps. *J Strength Cond Res* 28:373-380, 2014.

11. Baumgartner, TA, and Jackson, AS. *Measurement for Evaluation in Physical Education and Exercise Science.* 8th ed. Madison, WI: Brown & Benchmark, 255-256, 2007.

12. Black, W, and Roundy, E. Comparisons of size, strength, speed, and power in NCAA Division 1-A football players. *J Strength Cond Res* 8:80-85, 1994.

13. Bradley, PS, Bendiksen, M, Dellal, A, Mohr, M, Wilkie, A, Datson, N, Orntoft, C, Zebis, M, Gomez-Diaz, A, Bangsbo, J, and Krustrup, P. The application of the Yo-Yo intermittent endurance level 2 test to elite female soccer populations. *Scand J Med Sci Sports* 24:43-54, 2014.

14. Bressel, E, Yonker, JC, Kras, J, and Heath, EM. Comparison of static and dynamic balance in female collegiate soccer, basketball, and gymnastics athletes. *J Athl Train* 42:42-46, 2007.

15. Burr, JF, Jamnik, RK, Baker, J, Macpherson, A, Gledhill, N, and McGuire, EJ. Relationship of physical fitness test results and hockey playing potential in elite-level ice hockey players. *J Strength Cond Res* 22:1535-1543, 2008.

16. Butler, RJ, Plisky, PJ, Southers, C, Scoma, C, and Kiesel, KB. Biomechanical analysis of the different classifications of the Functional Movement Screen deep squat test. *Sports Biomech* 9:270-279, 2010.

17. Castagna, C, and Castellini, E. Vertical jump performance in Italian male and female national team soccer players. *J Strength Cond Res* 27:1156-1161, 2013.

18. Church, JB. Basic statistics for the strength and conditioning professional. *Strength Cond J* 30:51-53, 2008.

19. Cohen, JA. *Statistical Power Analysis for the Behavioural Sciences.* Hillsdale, NJ: Erlbaum, 273-379, 1988.

20. Comfort, P, Graham-Smith, P, Matthews, MJ, and Bamber, C. Strength and power characteristics in English elite rugby league players. *J Strength Cond Res* 25:1374-1384, 2011.

21. Crewther, BT, McGuigan, MR, and Gill, ND. The ratio and allometric scaling of speed, power, and strength in elite male rugby union players. *J Strength Cond Res* 25:1968-1975, 2011.

22. Cullen, BD, Cregg, CJ, Kelly, DT, Hughes, SM, Daly, PG, and Moyna, NM. Fitness profiling of elite level adolescent Gaelic football players. *J Strength Cond Res* 27:2096-2103, 2013.

23. Davlin, CD. Dynamic balance in high level athletes. *Percept Mot Skills* 98:1171-1176, 2004.

24. Department of the Army. *Physical Fitness Training: Field Manual No. 21-20.* Washington, DC: Headquarters, Department of the Army, 1998.

25. Deprez, D, Coutts, AJ, Lenoir, M, Fransen, J, Pion, J, Philippaerts, R, and Vaeyens, R. Reliability and validity of the Yo-Yo intermittent recovery test level 1 in young soccer players. *J Sports Sci* 32:903-910, 2014.

26. Desgorces, FD, Berthelot, G, Dietrich, G, and Testa, MS. Local muscular endurance and prediction of 1 repetition maximum for bench in 4 athletic populations. *J Strength Cond Res* 24:394-400, 2010.

27. Driss, T, and Vandewalle, H. The measurement of maximal (anaerobic) power output on a cycle ergometer: A critical review. *Biomed Res Int* 2013:589361, 2013.

28. Evans, EM, Rowe, DA, Misic, MM, Prior, BM, and Arngrímsson, SA. Skinfold prediction equation for athletes developed using a four-component model. *Med Sci Sports Exerc* 37:2006-2011, 2005.

29. Flanagan, E. The effect size statistic-applications for the strength and conditioning coach. *Strength Cond J* 35:37-40, 2013.

30. Fox, EL, Bowers, RW, and Foss, ML. *The Physiological Basis for Exercise and Sport*. 5th ed. Dubuque, IL: Brown, 676, 1993.

31. Fry, AC, and Kraemer, WJ. Physical performance characteristics of American collegiate football players. *J Appl Sport Sci Res* 5:126-138, 1991.

32. Fry, AC, Schilling, BK, Staron, RS, Hagerman, FC, Hikida, RS, and Thrush, JT. Muscle fiber characteristics and performance correlates of male Olympic-style weightlifters. *J Strength Cond Res* 17:746-754, 2003.

33. Gabbett, T, and Georgieff, B. Physiological and anthropometric characteristics of Australian junior national, state, and novice volleyball players. *J Strength Cond Res* 21:902-908, 2007.

34. Gabbett, T, Jenkins, D, and Abernethy, B. Relationships between physiological, anthropometric, and skill qualities and playing performance in professional rugby league players. *J Sports Sci* 29:1655-1664, 2011.

35. Gabbett, T, Kelly, J, and Pezet, T. Relationship between physical fitness and playing ability in rugby league players. *J Strength Cond Res* 21:1126-1133, 2007.

36. Gabbett, T, Kelly, J, Ralph, S, and Driscoll, D. Physiological and anthropometric characteristics of junior elite and sub-elite rugby league players, with special reference to starters and non-starters. *J Sci Med Sport* 12:215-222, 2009.

37. Garcia-Lopez, J, Morante, JC, Ogueta-Alday, A, and Rodriguez-Marroyo, JA. The type of mat (Contact vs. Photocell) affects vertical jump height estimated from flight time. *J Strength Cond Res* 27:1162-1167, 2013.

38. Gillam, GM, and Marks, M. 300 yard shuttle run. *NSCA J* 5:46, 1983.

39. Gorostiaga, EM, Granados, C, Ibanez, J, Gonzalez-Badillo, JJ, and Izquierdo, M. Effects of an entire season on physical fitness changes in elite male handball players. *Med Sci Sports Exerc* 38:357-366, 2006.

40. Granados, C, Izquierdo, M, Ibanez, J, Ruesta, M, and Gorostiaga, EM. Effects of an entire season on physical fitness in elite female handball players. *Med Sci Sports Exerc* 40:351-361, 2008.

41. Gribble, PA, Hertel, J, and Plisky, P. Using the Star Excursion Balance Test to assess dynamic postural-control deficits and outcomes in lower extremity injury: A literature and systematic review. *J Athl Train* 47:339-357, 2012.

42. Haugen, TA, Tonnessen, E, and Seiler, S. Speed and countermovement-jump characteristics of elite female soccer players, 1995-2010. *Int J Sports Physiol Perform* 7:340-349, 2012.

43. Hertel, J, Braham, RA, Hale, SA, and Olmsted-Kramer, LC. Simplifying the star excursion balance test: Analyses of subjects with and without chronic ankle instability. *J Orthop Sports Phys Ther* 36:131-137, 2006.

44. Hetzler, RK, Stickley, CD, Lundquist, KM, and Kimura, IF. Reliability and accuracy of handheld stopwatches compared with electronic timing in measuring sprint performance. *J Strength Cond Res* 22:1969-1976, 2008.

45. Heyward, VH. *Advanced Fitness Assessment and Exercise Prescription*. Champaign, IL: Human Kinetics, 47-56, 222, 235-244, 2014.

46. Heyward, VH, and Stolarczyk, LM. *Applied Body Composition Assessment*. Champaign, IL: Human Kinetics, 106-134, 1996.

47. Hoffman, J. *Norms for Fitness, Performance, and Health*. Champaign, IL: Human Kinetics, 36-38, 55-58, 113, 2006.

48. Hoffman, JR, Ratamess, NA, Klatt, M, Faigenbaum, AD, Ross, RE, Tranchina, NM, McCurley, RC, Kang, J, and Kraemer, WJ. Comparison between different off-season resistance training programs in Division III American college football players. *J Strength Cond Res* 23:11-19, 2009.

49. Hoffman, JR, Ratamess, NA, Neese, KL, Ross, RE, Kang, J, Magrelli, JF, and Faigenbaum, AD. Physical performance characteristics in National Collegiate Athletic Association Division III champion female lacrosse athletes. *J Strength Cond Res* 23:1524-1529, 2009.

50. Hoffman, JR, Vazquez, J, Pichardo, N, and Tenenbaum, G. Anthropometric and performance comparisons in professional baseball players. *J Strength Cond Res* 23:2173-2178, 2009.

51. Hopkins, WG. Progressive statistics for studies in sports medicine and exercise science. *Med Sci Sports Exerc* 41:3-13, 2009.

52. Hrysomallis, C. Balance ability and athletic performance. *Sports Med* 41:221-232, 2011.

53. Hrysomallis, C. Injury incidence, risk factors and prevention in Australian rules football. *Sports Med* 43:339-354, 2013.

54. Iverson, GL, and Koehle, MS. Normative data for the balance error scoring system in adults. *Rehabil Res Pract* 2013:846418, 2013.

55. Jackson, AS, and Pollock, ML. Generalized equations for predicting body density of men. *Br J Nutr* 40:497-504, 1978.

56. Jackson, AS, Pollock, ML, and Gettman, LR. Intertester reliability of selected skinfold and circumference measurements and percent fat estimates. *Res Q* 49:546-551, 1978.

57. Jackson, AS, Pollock, ML, and Ward, A. Generalized equations for predicting body density of women. *Med Sci Sports Exerc* 12:175-181, 1980.

58. Krustrup, P, Bradley, PS, Christensen, JF, Castagna, C, Jackman, S, Connolly, L, Randers, MB, Mohr, M, and Bangsbo, J. The Yo-Yo IE2 Test: Physiological response for untrained men vs trained soccer players. *Med Sci Sports Exerc* 47, 100-108, 2015.

59. Krustrup, P, Zebis, M, Jensen, JM, and Mohr, M. Game-induced fatigue patterns in elite female soccer. *J Strength Cond Res* 24:437-441, 2010.

60. Leger, L, and Boucher, R. An indirect continuous running multistage field test: The Université de Montréal track test. *Can J Appl Sport Sci* 5:77-84, 1990.

61. Leger, L, and Mercier, D. Gross energy cost of horizontal treadmill and track running. *Sports Med* 1:270-277, 1984.

62. Lloyd, RS, Oliver, JL, Hughes, MG, and Williams, CA. Reliability and validity of field-based measures of leg stiffness and reactive strength index in youths. *J Sports Sci* 27:1565-1573, 2009.

63. Magal, M, Smith, RT, Dyer, JJ, and Hoffman, JR. Seasonal variation in physical performance-related variables in male NCAA Division III soccer players. *J Strength Cond Res* 23:2555-2559, 2009.

64. Mann, JB, Stoner, JD, and Mayhew, JL. NFL-225 test to predict 1RM bench press in NCAA Division I football players. *J Strength Cond Res* 26:2623-2631, 2012.

65. McArdle, WD, Katch, FI, and Katch, VL. *Exercise Physiology: Energy, Nutrition, and Human Performance*. 8th ed. Baltimore: Lippincott Williams & Wilkins, 236-237, 749-752, 2015.

66. McCurdy, K, and Langford, G. The relationship between maximum unilateral squat strength and balance in young adult men and women. *J Sports Sci Med* 5:282-288, 2006.

67. McCurdy, K, Walker, JL, Langford, GA, Kutz, MR, Guerrero, JM, and McMillan, J. The relationship between kinematic determinants of jump and sprint performance in division I women soccer players. *J Strength Cond Res* 24:3200-3208, 2010.

68. McGill, SM, Andersen, JT, and Horne, AD. Predicting performance and injury resilience from movement quality and fitness scores in a basketball team over 2 years. *J Strength Cond Res* 26:1731-1739, 2012.

69. McGuigan, MR, Doyle, TL, Newton, M, Edwards, DJ, Nimphius, S, and Newton, RU. Eccentric utilization ratio: Effect of sport and phase of training. *J Strength Cond Res* 20:992-995, 2006.

70. McGuigan, MR, Sheppard, JM, Cormack, SJ, and Taylor, K. Strength and power assessment protocols. In *Physiological Tests for Elite Athletes.* Tanner, RK, and Gore, CJ, eds. Champaign, IL: Human Kinetics, 207-230, 2013.

71. McMaster, DT, Gill, N, Cronin, J, and McGuigan, M. A brief review of strength and ballistic assessment methodologies in sport. *Sports Med* 44:603-623, 2014.

72. Meir, R, Newton, R, Curtis, E, Fardell, M, and Butler, B. Physical fitness qualities of professional rugby league football players: Determination of positional differences. *J Strength Cond Res* 15:450-458, 2001.

73. Miller, T. *NSCA's Guide to Tests and Assessments.* Champaign, IL: Human Kinetics, 10-29, 193-199, 229-247, 295-315, 2012.

74. Mohr, M, Krustrup, P, and Bangsbo, J. Match performance of top-level soccer players with special reference to development of fatigue. *J Sports Sci* 21:519-528, 2003.

75. Moresi, MP, Bradshaw, EP, Greene, D, and Naughton, G. The assessment of adolescent female athletes using standing and reactive long jumps. *Sports Biomech* 10:73-84, 2011.

76. Mujika, I, Santisteban, J, Impellizzeri, FM, and Castagna, C. Fitness determinants of success in men's and women's football. *J Sports Sci* 27:107-114, 2009.

77. Newton, R, and Dugan, E. Application of strength diagnosis. *Strength Cond J* 24:50-59, 2002.

78. Nieman, DC. *Fitness and Sports Medicine.* 3rd ed. Palo Alto, CA: Bull, 504, 1995.

79. Nieman, DC. *Exercise Testing and Prescription: A Health-Related Approach.* 7th ed. New York: McGraw-Hill, 148-150, 2011.

80. Nimphius, S, McGuigan, MR, and Newton, RU. Relationship between strength, power, speed, and change of direction performance of female softball players. *J Strength Cond Res* 24:885-895, 2010.

81. Nimphius, S, McGuigan, MR, and Newton, RU. Changes in muscle architecture and performance during a competitive season in female softball players. *J Strength Cond Res* 26:2655-2666, 2012.

82. Oba, Y, Hetzler, RK, Stickley, CD, Tamura, K, Kimura, IF, and Heffernan, T. Allometric scaling of strength scores in NCAA Division IA football athletes. *J Strength Cond Res* 28:3330-3337, 2014.

83. Olmsted, LC, Carcia, CR, Hertel, J, and Shultz, SJ. Efficacy of the star excursion balance tests in detecting reach deficits in subjects with chronic ankle instability. *J Athl Train* 37:501-506, 2002.

84. Parchmann, CJ, and McBride, JM. Relationship between functional movement screen and athletic performance. *J Strength Cond Res* 25:3378-3384, 2011.

85. Parsonage, JR, Williams, RS, Rainer, P, McKeown, I, and Williams, MD. Assessment of conditioning-specific movement tasks and physical fitness measures in talent identified under 16-year-old rugby union players. *J Strength Cond Res* 28:1497-1506, 2014.

86. Pauole, K, Madole, K, Garhammer, J, Lacourse, M, and Rozenek, R. Reliability and validity of the t-test as a measure of agility, leg power, and leg speed in college-aged men and women. *J Strength Cond Res* 14:443-450, 2000.

87. Pearson, SN, Cronin, JB, Hume, PA, and Slyfield, D. Kinematics and kinetics of the bench-press and bench-pull exercises in a strength-trained sporting population. *Sports Biomech* 8:245-254, 2009.

88. Pescatello, LS, ed. *ACSM's Guidelines for Exercise Testing and Prescription.* 9th ed. Philadelphia: Wolters Kluwer Health/Lippincott Williams & Wilkins, 62-109, 2014.

89. Ransdell, LB, and Murray, T. A physical profile of elite female ice hockey players from the USA. *J Strength Cond Res* 25:2358-2363, 2011.

90. Ratamess, NA. *ACSM's Foundations of Strength Training and Conditioning.* Philadelphia: Lippincott Williams & Wilkins, 451-486, 2012.

91. Reid, DD, and Sandland, RL. New lamps for old? *J Roy Statist Soc Ser C* 32:86-87, 1983.

92. Reilly, T, and Waterhouse, J. Sports performance: Is there evidence that the body clock plays a role? *Eur J Appl Physiol* 106:321-332, 2009.

93. Reiman, MP, and Manske, R. *Functional Testing in Human Performance.* Champaign, IL: Human Kinetics, 108-109, 2009.

94. Rhea, MR. Determining the magnitude of treatment effects in strength training research through the use of the effect size. *J Strength Cond Res* 18:918-920, 2004.

95. Riemann, BL, Guskiewicz, KM, and Shields, EW. Relationship between clinical and forceplate measures of postural stability. *J Sport Rehabil* 8:71-82, 1999.

96. Sanchez-Medina, L, Gonzalez-Badillo, JJ, Perez, CE, and Pallares, JG. Velocity- and power-load relationships of the bench pull vs. bench press exercises. *Int J Sports Med* 35:209-216, 2014.

97. Sassi, RH, Dardouri, W, Yahmed, MH, Gmada, N, Mahfoudhi, ME, and Gharbi, Z. Relative and absolute reliability of a modified agility T-test and its relationship with vertical jump and straight sprint. *J Strength Cond Res* 23:1644-1651, 2009.

98. Schaal, M, Ransdell, LB, Simonson, SR, and Gao, Y. Physiologic performance test differences in female volleyball athletes by competition level and player position. *J Strength Cond Res* 27:1841-1850, 2013.

99. Sedano, S, Vaeyens, R, Philippaerts, RM, Redondo, JC, and Cuadrado, G. Anthropometric and anaerobic fitness profile of elite and non-elite female soccer players. *J Sports Med Phys Fitness* 49:387-394, 2009.

100. Semenick, D. The T-test. *NSCA J* 12:36-37, 1990.

101. Sheppard, JM, and Young, WB. Agility literature review: Classifications, training and testing. *J Sports Sci* 24:919-932, 2006.

102. Silvestre, R, West, C, Maresh, CM, and Kraemer, WJ. Body composition and physical performance in men's soccer: A study of a National Collegiate Athletic Association Division I team. *J Strength Cond Res* 20:177-183, 2006.

103. Slaughter, MH, Lohman, TG, Boileau, RA, Horswill, CA, Stillman, RJ, Van Loan, MD, and Bemben, DA. Skinfold equations for estimation of body fatness in children and youth. *Hum Biol* 60:709-723, 1988.

104. Sloan, AW, and Weir, JB. Nomograms for prediction of body density and total body fat from skinfold measurements. *J Appl Physiol* 28:221-222, 1970.

105. Spiteri, T, Nimphius, S, Hart, NH, Specos, C, Sheppard, JM, and Newton, RU. The contribution of strength characteristics to change of direction and agility performance in female basketball players. *J Strength Cond Res* 28:2415-2423, 2014.

106. Sporis, G, Jukic, I, Ostojic, SM, and Milanovic, D. Fitness profiling in soccer: Physical and physiologic characteristics of elite players. *J Strength Cond Res* 23:1947-1953, 2009.

107. Sporis, G, Ruzic, L, and Leko, G. The anaerobic endurance of elite soccer players improved after a high-intensity training intervention in the 8-week conditioning program. *J Strength Cond Res* 22:559-566, 2008.

108. Stewart, PF, Turner, AN, and Miller, SC. Reliability, factorial validity, and interrelationships of five commonly used change of direction speed tests. *Scand J Med Sci Sports* 24:500-506, 2014.

109. Stockbrugger, BA, and Haennel, RG. Contributing factors to performance of a medicine ball explosive power test: A comparison between jump and nonjump athletes. *J Strength Cond Res* 17:768-774, 2003.

110. Thomas, JR, Nelson, JK, and Silverman, SJ. *Research Methods in Physical Activity.* 6th ed. Champaign, IL: Human Kinetics, 99-112, 2011.

111. Thorpe, JL, and Ebersole, KT. Unilateral balance performance in female collegiate soccer athletes. *J Strength Cond Res* 22:1429-1433, 2008.

112. Till, K, Cobley, S, O'Hara, J, Brightmore, A, Cooke, C, and Chapman, C. Using anthropometric and performance characteristics to predict selection in junior UK Rugby League players. *J Sci Med Sport* 14:264-269, 2011.

113. Till, K, Cobley, S, O'Hara, J, Morley, D, Chapman, C, and Cooke, C. Retrospective analysis of anthropometric and fitness characteristics associated with long-term career progression in Rugby League. *J Sci Med Sport* 18:310-314, 2015.

114. Till, K, Tester, E, Jones, B, Emmonds, S, Fahey, J, and Cooke, C. Anthropometric and physical characteristics of English academy rugby league players. *J Strength Cond Res* 28:319-327, 2014.

115. Turner, AN, and Stewart, PF. Repeat sprint ability. *Strength Cond J* 35:37-41, 2013.

116. Vernillo, G, Silvestri, A, and Torre, AL. The yo-yo intermittent recovery test in junior basketball players according to performance level and age group. *J Strength Cond Res* 26:2490-2494, 2012.

117. Vescovi, JD, Brown, TD, and Murray, TM. Descriptive characteristics of NCAA Division I women lacrosse players. *J Sci Med Sport* 10:334-340, 2007.

118. Vescovi, JD, and McGuigan, MR. Relationships between sprinting, agility, and jump ability in female athletes. *J Sports Sci* 26:97-107, 2008.

119. Volek, JS, Ratamess, NA, Rubin, MR, Gomez, AL, French, DN, McGuigan, MM, Scheett, TP, Sharman, MJ, Hakkinen, K, and Kraemer, WJ. The effects of creatine supplementation on muscular performance and body composition responses to short-term resistance training overreaching. *Eur J Appl Physiol* 91:628-637, 2004.

120. Walklate, BM, O'Brien, BJ, Paton, CD, and Young, W. Supplementing regular training with short-duration sprint-agility training leads to a substantial increase in repeated sprint-agility performance with national level badminton players. *J Strength Cond Res* 23:1477-1481, 2009.

121. Whitehead, PN, Schilling, BK, Peterson, DD, and Weiss, LW. Possible new modalities for the Navy physical readiness test. *Mil Med* 177:1417-1425, 2012.

122. Whitmer, T, Fry, AC, Forsythe, C, Andre, MJ, Lane, MT, Hudy, A, and Honnold, D. Accuracy of a vertical jump contact mat for determining jump height and flight time. *J Strength Cond Res* 29:877-881, 2015.

123. Wisloff, U, Castagna, C, Helgerud, J, Jones, R, and Hoff, J. Strong correlation of maximal squat strength with sprint performance and vertical jump height in elite soccer players. *Br J Sports Med* 38:285-288, 2004.

124. Wisloff, U, Helgerud, J, and Hoff, J. Strength and endurance of elite soccer players. *Med Sci Sports Exerc* 30:462-467, 1998.

125. YMCA. *YMCA Fitness Testing and Assessment Manual.* Champaign, IL: Human Kinetics, 2000.

126. Young, W, Russell, A, Burge, P, Clarke, A, Cormack, S, and Stewart, G. The use of sprint tests for assessment of speed qualities of elite Australian rules footballers. *Int J Sports Physiol Perform* 3:199-206, 2008.

127. Young, WB, and Pryor, L. Relationship between pre-season anthropometric and fitness measures and indicators of playing performance in elite junior Australian Rules football. *J Sci Med Sport* 10:110-118, 2007.

CHAPTER 14   Warm-Up and Flexibility Training

1. Andersen, JC. Stretching before and after exercise: Effect on muscle soreness and injury risk. *J Athl Train* 40:218-220, 2005.

2. Anthony, CP, and Kolthoff, NJ. *Textbook of Anatomy and Physiology.* 9th ed. St. Louis: Mosby, 1975.

3. Asmussen, E, Bonde-Peterson, F, and Jorgenson, K. Mechano-elastic properties of human muscles at different temperatures. *Acta Physiol Scand* 96:86-93, 1976.

4. Bandy, WD, and Irion, JM. The effect of time on static stretch on the flexibility of the hamstring muscles. *Phys Ther* 74:845-852, 1994.

5. Bandy, WD, Irion, JM, and Briggler, M. The effect of static stretch and dynamic range of motion training on the flexibility of the hamstring muscles. *J Orthop Sports Phys Ther* 27:295-300, 1998.

6. Bandy, WD, Irion, JM, and Briggler, M. The effect of time and frequency of static stretching on flexibility of the hamstring muscles. *Phys Ther* 77:1090-1096, 1997.

7. Behm, DG, Bambury, A, Cahill, F, and Power, K. Effect of acute static stretching on force, balance, reaction time, and movement time. *Med Sci Sports Exerc* 36:1397-1402, 2004.

8. Behm, DG, Button, DC, and Butt, JC. Factors affecting force loss with prolonged stretching. *Can J Appl Physiol* 26:261-272, 2001.

9. Bergh, U, and Ekblom, B. Influence of muscle temperature on maximal strength and power output in human muscle. *Acta Physiol Scand* 107:332-337, 1979.

10. Bishop, D. Warm-up. Potential mechanisms and the effects of passive warm-up on performance. *Sports Med* 33:439-454, 2003.

11. Bishop, D. Warm up II. Performance changes following active warm-up and how to structure the warm-up. *Sports Med* 33:483-498, 2003.

12. Blazevich, AJ, Cannavan, D, Waugh, CM, Fath, F, Miller, SC, and Kay, AD. Neuromuscular factors influencing the maximum stretch limit of the human plantar flexors. *J Appl Physiol* 113(9):1446-1455, 2012

13. Brodowicz, GR, Welsh, R, and Wallis, J. Comparison of stretching with ice, stretching with heat, or stretching alone on hamstring flexibility. *J Athl Train* 31:324-327, 1996.

14. Burkett, LN, Phillips, WT, and Ziuraitis, J. The best warm-up for the vertical jump in college-age athletic men. *J Strength Cond Res* 19:673-676, 2005.

15. Cherry, DB. Review of physical therapy alternatives for reducing muscle contracture. *Phys Ther* 60:877-881, 1980.

16. Church, JB, Wiggins, MS, Moode, FM, and Crist, R. Effect of warm-up and flexibility treatments on vertical jump performance. *J Strength Cond Res* 15:332-336, 2001.

17. Cipriani, D, Abel, B, and Pirrwitz, D. A comparison of two stretching protocols on hip range of motion: Implications for total daily stretch duration. *J Strength Cond Res* 17:274-278, 2003.

18. Condon, SM, and Hutton, RS. Soleus muscle electromyographic activity and ankle dorsiflexion range of motion during four stretching procedures. *Phys Ther* 67:24-30, 1987.

19. Cook, G. *Movement: Functional Movement Systems: Screening Assessment and Corrective Strategies.* Aptos, CA: On Target, 19, 2010.

20. Corbin, CB, Dowell, LJ, Lindsey, R, and Tolson, H. *Concepts in Physical Education.* Dubuque, IA: Brown, 1-320, 1978.

21. Cornelius, WJ. The effective way. *NSCA J* 7:62-64, 1985.

22. Cornelius, WJ, and Hinson, MM. The relationship between isometric contractions of hip extensors and subsequent flexibility in males. *Sports Med Phys Fitness* 20:75-80, 1980.

23. Cornwell, A, Nelson, AG, and Sidaway, B. Acute effects of stretching on the neuromechanical properties of the triceps surae muscle complex. *Eur J Appl Physiol* 86:428-434, 2002.

24. Covert, CA, Alexander, MP, Petronis, JJ, and Davis, DS. Comparison of ballistic and static stretching on hamstring muscle length using an equal stretching dose. *J Strength Cond Res* 24:3008-3014, 2010.

25. Cramer, JT, Housh, TJ, Coburn, JW, Beck, TW, and Johnson, GO. Acute effects of static stretching on maximal eccentric torque production in women. *J Strength Cond Res* 20:354-358, 2006.

26. Cramer, JT, Housh, TJ, Johnson, GO, Miller, JM, Coburn, JW, and Beck, TW. Acute effects of static stretching on peak torque in women. *J Strength Cond Res* 18:236-241, 2004.

27. Cramer, JT, Housh, TJ, Weir, JP, Johnson, GO, Coburn, JW, and Beck, TW. The acute effects of static stretching on peak torque, mean power output, electromyography, and mechanomyography. *Eur J Appl Physiol* 93:530-539, 2005.

28. Davis, DS, Ashby, PE, McCale, KL, McQuain, JA, and Wine, JM. The effectiveness of 3 stretching techniques on hamstring flexibility using consistent stretching parameters. *J Strength Cond Res* 19:27-32, 2005.

29. Depino, GM, Webright, WG, and Arnold, BL. Duration of maintained hamstring flexibility after cessation of an acute static stretching protocol. *J Athl Train* 35:56-59, 2000.

30. deVries, HA, and Housh, TJ. *Physiology of Exercise for Physical Education, Athletics and Exercise Science.* 5th ed. Dubuque, IA: Brown, 1995.

31. de Weijer, VC, Gorniak, GC, and Shamus, E. The effect of static stretch and warm-up exercise on hamstring length over the course of 24 hours. *J Orthop Sports Phys Ther* 33:727-733, 2003.

32. Earle, RW, and Baechle, TR, eds. *NSCA's Essentials of Personal Training.* Champaign, IL: Human Kinetics, 267-294, 2004.

33. Enoka, RM. *Neuromechanics of Human Movement.* 4th ed. Champaign, IL: Human Kinetics, 305-309, 2008.

34. Etnyre, BR, and Abraham, LD. Gains in range of ankle dorsiflexion using three popular stretching techniques. *Am J Phys Med* 65:189-196, 1986.

35. Evetovich, TK, Nauman, NJ, Conley, DS, and Todd, JB. Effect of static stretching of the biceps brachii on torque, electromyography, and mechanomyography during concentric isokinetic muscle actions. *J Strength Cond Res* 17:484-488, 2003.

36. Faigenbaum, AD, Bellucci, M, Bernieri, A, Bakker, B, and Hoorens, K. Acute effects of different warm-up protocols on fitness performance in children. *J Strength Cond Res* 19:376-381, 2005.

37. Fleck, SJ, and Kraemer, WJ. *Designing Resistance Training Programs.* 3rd ed. Champaign, IL: Human Kinetics, 142, 2004.

38. Fletcher, IM, and Jones, B. The effect of different warm-up stretch protocols on 20 meter sprint performance in trained rugby union players. *J Strength Cond Res* 18:885-888, 2004.

39. Flexibility: Roundtable. *NSCA J* 6:10-22, 71-73, 1984.

40. Fox, EL. *Sports Physiology.* Philadelphia: Saunders, 240-350, 1979.

41. Fradkin, AJ, Gabbe, BJ, and Cameron, PA. Does warming up prevent injury in sport? The evidence from randomised controlled trials. *J Sci Med Sport* 9:214-220, 2006.

42. Fradkin, AJ, Zazryn, TR, and Smoliga, JM. Effects of warming up on physical performance: A systematic review with meta analysis. *J Strength Cond Res* 24:140-148, 2010.

43. Funk, DC, Swank, AM, Mikla, BM, Fagan, TA, and Farr, BK. Impact of prior exercise on hamstring flexibility: A comparison of proprioceptive neuromuscular facilitation and static stretching. *J Strength Cond Res* 17:489-492, 2003.

44. Getchell, B. *Physical Fitness: A Way of Life.* New York: Wiley, 1-53, 1979.

45. Gleim, GW, and McHugh, MP. Flexibility and its effects on sports injury and performance [review]. *Sports Med* 24:289-299, 1997.

46. Gremion, G. Is stretching for sports performance still useful? A review of the literature. *Rev Med Suisse* 27:1830-1834, 2005.

47. Hart, L. Effect of stretching on sport injury risk: A review. *Med Sci Sports Exerc* 36:371-378, 2004.

48. Hedrick, A. Dynamic flexibility training. *Strength Cond J* 22:33-38, 2000.

49. Hedrick, A. Flexibility, body-weight and stability ball exercises. In *NSCA's Essentials of Personal Training.* Earle, RW, and Baechle, TR, eds. Champaign, IL: Human Kinetics, 268-294, 2004.

50. Herbert, RD, and Gabriel, M. Effects of stretching before and after exercise on muscle soreness and risk of injury: A systematic review. *Br Med J* 325:468-470, 2002.

51. Hoffman, J. *Physiological Aspects of Sports Training and Performance.* Champaign, IL: Human Kinetics, 156, 2002.

52. Holland, GJ. The physiology of flexibility: A review of the literature. *Kinesthesiol Rev* 1:49-62, 1966.

53. Holt, LE, Travis, TM, and Okia, T. Comparative study of three stretching techniques. *Percept Mot Skills* 31:611-616, 1970.

54. Jeffreys, I. Warm-up revisited: The ramp method of optimizing warm-ups. *Prof Strength Cond* 6:12-18, 2007.

55. Johansson, PH, Lindstrom, L, Sundelin, G, and Lindstrom, B. The effects of pre-exercise stretching on muscular soreness, tenderness and force loss following heavy eccentric exercise. *Scand J Med Sci Sports* 9:219-225, 1999.

56. Kay, AD, and Blazevich, AJ. Effect of acute static stretching on maximal muscle performance: A systematic review. *Med Sci Sports Exerc* 44:154-164, 2012.

57. Knapik, JJ, Bauman, CL, and Jones, BH. Preseason strength and flexibility imbalances associated with athletic injuries in female collegiate athletes. *Am J Orthop Soc Sports Med* 19:76-81, 1991.

58. Knapik, JJ, Jones, BH, Bauman, CL, and Harris, JM. Strength, flexibility and athletic injuries. *Sports Med* 14:277-288, 1992.

59. Knudson, DV, Magnusson, P, and McHugh, M. Current issues in flexibility fitness. *Pres Counc Phys Fit Sports Res Dig* 3:1-6, 2000.

60. Leighton, JR. A study of the effect of progressive weight training on flexibility. *J Assoc Phys Ment Rehabil* 18:101, 1964.

61. Lund, H, Vestergaard-Poulsen, P, Kanstrup, IL, and Sejrsen, P. The effect of passive stretching on delayed onset muscle soreness, and other detrimental effects following eccentric exercise. *Scand J Med Sci Sports* 8:216-221, 1998.

62. Magnusson, SP, Simonsen, EB, Aagaard, P, Boesen, J, Johannsen, F, and Kjaer, M. Determinants of musculoskeletal flexibility: Viscoelastic properties, cross-sectional area, EMG and stretch tolerance. *Scand J Med Sci Sports* 7:195-202, 1997.

63. Mahieu, NN, McNair, P, De Muynck, M, Stevens, V, Blanckaert, I, Smits, N, and Witvrouw, E. Effect of static and ballistic stretching on the muscle-tendon tissue properties. *Med Sci Sports Exerc* 39:494-501, 2007.

64. Mann, DP, and Jones, MT. Guidelines to the implementation of a dynamic stretching program. *Strength Cond J* 21:53-55, 1999.

65. Marek, SM, Cramer, JT, Fincher, AL, Massey, LL, Dangelmaier, SM, Purkayastha, S, Fitz, KA, and Culbertson, JY. Acute effects of static and proprioceptive neuromuscular facilitation stretching on muscle strength and power output. *J Athl Train* 40:94-103, 2005.

66. Marshall, JL, Johanson, N, Wickiewicz, TL, Tishler, HM, Koslin, BL, Zeno, S, and Myers, A. Joint looseness: A function of the person and the joint. *Med Sci Sports Exerc* 12:189-194, 1980.

67. Massis, M. Flexibility: The missing link in the Power Jigsaw. *Prof Strength Cond* 14:16-19, 2009.

68. McArdle, WD, Katch, FI, and Katch, VL. *Exercise Physiology: Energy, Nutrition and Human Performance.* 6th ed. Baltimore: Lippincott Williams & Wilkins, 574-575, 2007.

69. McAtee, RE, and Charland, J. *Facilitated Stretching.* 3rd ed. Champaign, IL: Human Kinetics, 13-20, 2007.

70. McFarland, B. Developing maximum running speed. *NSCA J* 6:24-28, 1984.

71. McNeal, JR, and Sands, WA. Stretching for performance enhancement. *Curr Sports Med Rep* 5:141-146, 2006.

72. Moore, MA, and Hutton, RS. Electromyographic investigation of muscle stretching techniques. *Med Sci Sports Exerc* 12:322-329, 1980.

73. Nelson, AG, Kokkonen, J, and Arnall, DA. Acute muscle stretching inhibits muscle strength endurance performance. *J Strength Cond Res* 19:338-343, 2005.

74. Nelson, RT, and Bandy, WD. Eccentric training and static stretching improve hamstring flexibility of high school males. *J Athl Train* 39:254-258, 2004.

75. Pope, RP, Herbert, RD, Kirwan, JD, and Graham, BJ. A randomised trial of pre-exercise stretching for prevention of lower limb injury. *Med Sci Sports Exerc* 32:271-277, 2000.

76. Power, K, Behm, D, Cahill, F, Carroll, M, and Young, W. An acute bout of static stretching: Effects on force and jumping performance. *Med Sci Sports Exerc* 36:1389-1396, 2004.

77. Prentice, WE. A comparison of static stretching and PNF stretching for improving hip joint flexibility. *Athl Train* 18(1):56-59, 1983.

78. Riewald, S. Stretching the limits of knowledge on stretching. *Strength Cond J* 26:58-59, 2004.

79. Roberts, JM, and Wilson, K. Effect of stretching duration on active and passive range of motion in the lower extremity. *Br J Sports Med* 33:259-263, 1999.

80. Sady, SP, Wortman, M, and Blanket, D. Flexibility training: Ballistic, static or proprioceptive neuromuscular facilitation? *Arch Phys Med Rehabil* 63:261-263, 1992.

81. Safran, MR, Garrett, WE, Seaber, AV, Glisson, RR, and Ribbeck, BM. The role of warm-up in muscular injury prevention. *Am J Sports Med* 16:123-129, 1988.

82. Sands, WA. Flexibility. In *Strength and Conditioning: Biological Principles and Practical Applications.* Cardinale, M, Newton, R, and Nosaka, K, eds. Hoboken, NJ: Wiley, 389-398, 2011.

83. Shrier, I. Does stretching improve performance? A systematic and critical review of the literature [review]. *Clin J Sport Med* 14:267-273, 2004.

84. Shrier, I. Meta-analysis on pre-exercise stretching. *Med Sci Sports Exerc* 36:1832, 2004.

85. Shrier, I. Stretching before exercise: An evidence based approach. *Br J Sports Med* 34:324-325, 2000.

86. Shrier, I. Stretching before exercise does not reduce the risk of local muscle injury: A critical review of the clinical and basic science literature. *Clin J Sport Med* 9:221-227, 1999.

87. Simic, L, Sarabon, N, and Markovic, G. Does pre-exercise static stretching inhibit maximal muscular performance? A meta-analytical review. *Scand J Med Sci Sports* 23:131-148, 2013.

88. Tanigawa, MC. Comparison of the hold relax procedure and passive mobilization on increasing muscle length. *Phys Ther* 52:725-735, 1972.

89. Thacker, SB, Gilchrist, J, Stroup, DF, and Kimsey, CD, Jr. The impact of stretching on sports injury risk: A systematic review of the literature. *Med Sci Sports Exerc* 36:371-378, 2004.

90. Todd, T. Historical perspective: The myth of the muscle-bound lifter. *NSCA J* 6:37-41, 1985.

91. Voss, DE, Ionta, MK, and Myers, BJ. *Proprioceptive Neuromuscular Facilitation: Patterns and Techniques.* 3rd ed. Philadelphia: Harper & Row, 1-370, 1985.

92. Wallmann, HW, Mercer, JA, and McWhorter, JW. Surface electromyographic assessment of the effect of static stretching of the gastrocnemius on vertical jump performance. *J Strength Cond Res* 19:684-688, 2005.

93. Walter, SD, Figoni, SF, Andres, FF, and Brown, E. Training intensity and duration in flexibility. *Clin Kinesthesiol* 50:40-45, 1996.

94. Weiss, LW, Cureton, KJ, and Thompson, FN. Comparison of serum testosterone and androstenedione responses to weight lifting in men and women. *Eur J Appl Physiol* 50:413-419, 1983.

95. Wilmore, JH, Parr, RB, Girandola, RN, Ward, P, Vodak, PA, Barstow, TJ, Pipes, TV, Romero, GT, and Leslie, P. Physiological alterations consequent to circuit weight training. *Med Sci Sport* 10:79-84, 1978.

96. Winters, MV, Blake, CG, Trost, JS, Marcello-Brinker, TB, Lowe, LM, Garber, MB, and Wainner, RS. Passive versus active stretching of hip flexor muscles in subjects with limited hip extension: A randomized clinical trial. *Phys Ther* 84:800-807, 2004.

97. Witvrouw, E, Mahieu, N, Danneels, L, and McNair, P. Stretching and injury prevention: An obscure relationship. *Sports Med* 34:443-449, 2004.

98. Yamaguchi, T, and Ishii, K. Effects of static stretching for 30 seconds and dynamic stretching on leg extension power. *J Strength Cond Res* 19:677-683, 2005.

99. Young, WB, and Behm, DG. Effects of running, static stretching and practice jumps on explosive force production and jumping performance. *J Sports Med Phys Fitness* 43:21-27, 2003.

100. Young, WB, and Behm, DG. Should static stretching be used during a warm up for strength and power activities? *Strength Cond J* 24:33-37, 2002.

CHAPTER 15   Free Weight and Machine Exercise Technique

1. Bartelink, DL. The role of abdominal pressure in relieving the pressure on the lumbar intervertebral discs. *J Bone Joint Surg* 39B:718-725, 1957.

2. Bauer, JA, Fry, A, and Carter, C. The use of lumbar-supporting weight belts while performing squats: Erector spinae electromyographic activity. *J Strength Cond Res* 13:384-388, 1999.

3. Hackett, DA, and Chow, C. The Valsalva maneuver: Its effect on intra-abdominal pressure and safety issues during resistance exercise. *J Strength Cond Res* 27:2338-2345, 2013.

4. Harman, EA, Rosenstein, RM, Frykman, PN, and Nigro, GA. Effects of a belt on intra-abdominal pressure during weight lifting. *Med Sci Sports Exerc* 21:186-190, 1989.

5. Herbert, L, and Miller, G. Newer heavy load lifting methods help firms reduce back injuries. *Occup Health Saf* (February):57-60, 1987.

6. Ikeda, ER, Borg, A, Brown, D, Malouf, J, Showers, KM, and Li, SL. The Valsalva maneuver revisited: The influence of voluntary breathing on isometric muscle strength. *J Strength Cond Res* 23:127-132, 2009.

7. Lander, JE, Hundley, JR, and Simonton, RL. The effectiveness of weight belts during multiple repetitions of the squat exercise. *Med Sci Sports Exerc* 24:603-609, 1992.

8. Morris, JM, Lucas, BD, and Bresler, B. Role of the trunk in stability of the spine. *J Bone Joint Surg* 43A:327-351, 1961.

9. Sogabe, A, Iwasaki, S, Gallager, PM, Edinger, S, and Fry, A. Influence of stance width on power production during the barbell squat. *J Strength Cond Res* 24(Suppl):1, 2010.

10. Tillaar, RVD, and Saeterbakken, A. The sticking region in three chest-press exercises with increasing degrees of freedom. *J Strength Cond Res* 26:2962-2969, 2012.

CHAPTER 16   Alternative Modes and Nontraditional Implement Exercise Technique

1. Anderson, CE, Sforzo, GA, and Sigg, JA. The effects of combining elastic and free weight resistance on strength and power in athletes. *J Strength Cond Res* 22:567-574, 2008.

2. Anderson, K, and Behm, DG. Trunk muscle activity increases with unstable squat movements. *Can J Appl Physiol* 30:33-45, 2005.

3. Ariel, G. Variable resistance versus standard resistance training. *Scholastic Coach* 46:68-69, 74, 1976.

4. Baker, D. Using strength platforms for explosive performance. In *High Performance Training for Sports.* Joyce, D, and Lewindon, D, eds. Champaign, IL: Human Kinetics, 127-144, 2014.

5. Baker, D, and Newton, RU. Methods to increase the effectiveness of maximal power training for the upper body. *Strength Cond J* 27:24-32, 2005.

6. Baker, DG, and Newton, RU. Effect of kinetically altering a repetition via the use of chain resistance on velocity during the bench press. *J Strength Cond Res* 23:1941-1946, 2009.

7. Beardsley, C, and Contreras, B. The role of kettlebells in strength and conditioning: A review of the literature. *Strength Cond J* 36:64-70, 2014.

8. Behm, DG, Anderson, K, and Curnew, RS. Muscle force and activation under stable and unstable conditions. *J Strength Cond Res* 16:416-422, 2002.

9. Behm, DG, Drinkwater, EJ, Willardson, JM, and Cowley, PM. Canadian Society for Exercise Physiology position stand: The use of instability to train the core in athletic and nonathletic conditioning. *Appl Physiol Nutr Metab* 35:109-112, 2010.

10. Behm, DG, Drinkwater, EJ, Willardson, JM, and Cowley, PM. The use of instability to train the core musculature. *Appl Physiol Nutr Metab* 35:91-108, 2010.

11. Bennett, S. Using "Strongman" exercises in training. *Strength Cond J* 30:42-43, 2008.

12. Berning, JM, Adams, KJ, Climstein, M, and Stamford, BA. Metabolic demands of "junkyard" training: Pushing and pulling a motor vehicle. *J Strength Cond Res* 21:853-856, 2007.

13. Berning, JM, Coker, CA, and Adams, KJ. Using chains for strength and conditioning. *Strength Cond J* 26:80-84, 2004.

14. Berning, JM, Coker, CA, and Briggs, D. The biomechanical and perceptual influence of chain resistance on the performance of the Olympic clean. *J Strength Cond Res* 22:390-395, 2008.

15. Bobbert, MF, and Van Soest, AJ. Effects of muscle strengthening on vertical jump height: A simulation study. *Med Sci Sports Exerc* 26:1012-1020, 1994.

16. Bullock, JB, and Aipa, DMM. Coaching considerations for the tire flip. *Strength Cond J* 32:75-78, 2010.

17. Campbell, BI, and Otto, WHI. Should kettlebells be used in strength and conditioning? *Strength Cond J* 35:27-29, 2013.

18. Caraffa, A, Cerulli, G, Projetti, M, Aisa, G, and Rizzo, A. Prevention of anterior cruciate ligament injuries in soccer. A prospective controlled study of proprioceptive training. *Knee Surg Sports Traumatol Arthrosc* 4:19-21, 1996.

19. Cosio-Lima, LM, Reynolds, KL, Winter, C, Paolone, V, and Jones, MT. Effects of physioball and conventional floor exercises on early phase adaptations in back and abdominal core stability and balance in women. *J Strength Cond Res* 17:721-725, 2003.

20. Cotter, S. *Kettlebell Training.* Champaign, IL: Human Kinetics, 1-24, 2014.

21. Cressey, EM, West, CA, Tiberio, DP, Kraemer, WJ, and Maresh, CM. The effects of ten weeks of lower-body unstable surface training on markers of athletic performance. *J Strength Cond Res* 21:561-567, 2007.

22. DeGarmo, R. University of Nebraska in-season resistance training for horizontal jumpers. *Strength Cond J* 22:23, 2000.

23. Drinkwater, EJ, Prichett, EJ, and Behm, DG. Effect of instability and resistance on unintentional squat-lifting kinetics. *Int J Sports Physiol Perform* 2:400-413, 2007.

24. Ebben, WP, and Jensen, RL. Electromyographic and kinetic analysis of traditional, chain, and elastic band squats. *J Strength Cond Res* 16:547-550, 2002.

25. Escamilla, RF, Zheng, N, Imamura, R, Macleod, TD, Edwards, WB, Hreljac, A, Fleisig, GS, Wilk, KE, Moorman, CT, 3rd, and Andrews, JR. Cruciate ligament force during the wall squat and the one-leg squat. *Med Sci Sports Exerc* 41:408-417, 2009.

26. Farrar, RE, Mayhew, JL, and Koch, AJ. Oxygen cost of kettlebell swings. *J Strength Cond Res* 24:1034-1036, 2010.

27. Findley, BW. Training with rubber bands. *Strength Cond J* 26:68-69, 2004.

28. Fitzgerald, GK, Axe, MJ, and Snyder-Mackler, L. The efficacy of perturbation training in nonoperative anterior cruciate ligament rehabilitation programs for physically active individuals. *Phys Ther* 80:128-140, 2000.

29. Fleck, SJ, and Kraemer, WJ. *Designing Resistance Training Programs.* 4th ed. Champaign, IL: Human Kinetics, 15-61, 2014.

30. Frost, DM, Cronin, J, and Newton, RU. A biomechanical evaluation of resistance: Fundamental concepts for training and sports performance. *Sports Med* 40:303-326, 2010.

31. Grimm, NL, Shea, KG, Leaver, RW, Aoki, SK, and Carey, JL. Efficacy and degree of bias in knee injury prevention studies: A systematic review of RCTs. *Clin Orthop Relat Res* 471:308-316, 2013.

32. Hackett, DA, and Chow, CM. The Valsalva maneuver: Its effect on intra-abdominal pressure and safety issues during resistance exercise. *J Strength Cond Res* 27:2338-2345, 2013.

33. Haff, GG. Roundtable discussion: Machines versus free weights. *Strength Cond J* 22:18-30, 2000.

34. Hakkinen, K, Pastinen, UM, Karsikas, R, and Linnamo, V. Neuromuscular performance in voluntary bilateral and unilateral contraction and during electrical stimulation in men at different ages. *Eur J Appl Physiol Occup Physiol* 70:518-527, 1995.

35. Hamlyn, N, Behm, DG, and Young, WB. Trunk muscle activation during dynamic weight-training exercises and isometric instability activities. *J Strength Cond Res* 21:1108-1112, 2007.

36. Harman, E. Resistance training modes: A biomechanical perspective. *Strength Cond* 16:59-65, 1994.

37. Harrison, JS. Bodyweight training: A return to basics. *Strength Cond J* 32:52-55, 2010.

38. Harrison, JS, Schoenfeld, B, and Schoenfeld, ML. Applications of kettlebells in exercise program design. *Strength Cond J* 33:86-89, 2011.

39. Hedrick, A. Implement training. In *Conditioning for Strength and Human Performance.* Chandler, TJ, and Brown, LE, eds. Philadelphia: Lippincott Williams & Wilkins, 537-558, 2013.

40. Hulsey, CR, Soto, DT, Koch, AJ, and Mayhew, JL. Comparison of kettlebell swings and treadmill running at equivalent rating of perceived exertion values. *J Strength Cond Res* 26:1203-1207, 2012.

41. Israetel, MA, McBride, JM, Nuzzo, JL, Skinner, JW, and Dayne, AM. Kinetic and kinematic differences between squats performed with and without elastic bands. *J Strength Cond Res* 24:190-194, 2010.

42. Jakobi, JM, and Chilibeck, PD. Bilateral and unilateral contractions: Possible differences in maximal voluntary force. *Can J Appl Physiol* 26:12-33, 2001.

43. Jay, K, Frisch, D, Hansen, K, Zebis, MK, Andersen, CH, Mortensen, OS, and Andersen, LL. Kettlebell training for musculoskeletal and

cardiovascular health: A randomized controlled trial. *Scand J Work Environ Health* 37:196-203, 2011.

44. Keogh, JW, Payne, AL, Anderson, BB, and Atkins, PJ. A brief description of the biomechanics and physiology of a strongman event: The tire flip. *J Strength Cond Res* 24:1223-1228, 2010.

45. Kobayashi, Y, Kubo, J, Matsuo, A, Matsubayashi, T, Kobayashi, K, and Ishii, N. Bilateral asymmetry in joint torque during squat exercise performed by long jumpers. *J Strength Cond Res* 24:2826-2830, 2010.

46. Kozub, FM, and Voorhis, T. Using bands to create technique-specific resistance training for developing explosive power in wrestlers. *Strength Cond J* 34:92-95, 2012.

47. Lederman, E. The myth of core stability. *J Bodyw Mov Ther* 14:84-98, 2010.

48. Matthews, M, and Cohen, D. The modified kettlebell swing. *Strength Cond J* 35:79-81, 2013.

49. McBride, JM, Cormie, P, and Deane, R. Isometric squat force output and muscle activity in stable and unstable conditions. *J Strength Cond Res* 20:915-918, 2006.

50. McCurdy, KW, Langford, GA, Doscher, MW, Wiley, LP, and Mallard, KG. The effects of short-term unilateral and bilateral lower-body resistance training on measures of strength and power. *J Strength Cond Res* 19:9-15, 2005.

51. McGill, SM, Cannon, J, and Andersen, JT. Analysis of pushing exercises: Muscle activity and spine load while contrasting techniques on stable surfaces with a labile suspension strap training system. *J Strength Cond Res* 28:105-116, 2014.

52. McGill, SM, and Marshall, LW. Kettlebell swing, snatch, and bottoms-up carry: Back and hip muscle activation, motion, and low back loads. *J Strength Cond Res* 26:16-27, 2012.

53. McGill, SM, McDermott, A, and Fenwick, CM. Comparison of different strongman events: Trunk muscle activation and lumbar spine motion, load, and stiffness. *J Strength Cond Res* 23:1148-1161, 2009.

54. McMaster, DT, Cronin, J, and McGuigan, M. Forms of variable resistance training. *Strength Cond J* 31:50-64, 2009.

55. McMaster, DT, Cronin, J, and McGuigan, MR. Quantification of rubber and chain-based resistance modes. *J Strength Cond Res* 24:2056-2064, 2010.

56. Moffroid, MT, Haugh, LD, Haig, AJ, Henry, SM, and Pope, MH. Endurance training of trunk extensor muscles. *Phys Ther* 73:10-17, 1993.

57. Morriss, CJ, Tolfrey, K, and Coppack, RJ. Effects of short-term isokinetic training on standing long-jump performance in untrained men. *J Strength Cond Res* 15:498-502, 2001.

58. Myer, GD, Ford, KR, and Hewett, TE. New method to identify athletes at high risk of ACL injury using clinic-based measurements and freeware computer analysis. *Br J Sports Med* 45:238-244, 2011.

59. Myer, GD, Paterno, MV, Ford, KR, and Hewett, TE. Neuromuscular training techniques to target deficits before return to sport after anterior cruciate ligament reconstruction. *J Strength Cond Res* 22:987-1014, 2008.

60. Nuzzo, JL, McCaulley, GO, Cormie, P, Cavill, MJ, and McBride, JM. Trunk muscle activity during stability ball and free weight exercises. *J Strength Cond Res* 22:95-102, 2008.

61. Otto, WH, 3rd, Coburn, JW, Brown, LE, and Spiering, BA. Effects of weightlifting vs. kettlebell training on vertical jump, strength, and body composition. *J Strength Cond Res* 26:1199-1202, 2012.

62. Patterson, RM, Stegink Jansen, CW, Hogan, HA, and Nassif, MD. Material properties of Thera-Band Tubing. *Phys Ther* 81:1437-1445, 2001.

63. Pipes, TV. Variable resistance versus constant resistance strength training in adult males. *Eur J Appl Physiol* 39:27-35, 1978.

64. Ratamess, N. *ACSM's Foundations of Strength and Conditioning.* Philadelphia: Lippincott Williams & Wilkins, 229-253, 2012.

65. Reed, CA, Ford, KR, Myer, GD, and Hewett, TE. The effects of isolated and integrated "core stability" training on athletic performance measures: A systematic review. *Sports Med* 42:697-706, 2012.

66. Santana, JC, and Fukuda, DH. Unconventional methods, techniques, and equipment for strength and conditioning in combat sports. *Strength Cond J* 33:64-70, 2011.

67. Santana, JC, Vera-Garcia, FJ, and McGill, SM. A kinetic and electromyographic comparison of the standing cable press and bench press. *J Strength Cond Res* 21:1271-1277, 2007.

68. Schoenfeld, BJ, and Contreras, BM. The long-lever posterior-tilt plank. *Strength Cond J* 35:98-99, 2013.

69. Simmons, LP. Chain reaction: Accomodating leverages. *Powerlifting USA* 19:2-3, 1996.

70. Simmons, LP. Bands and chains. *Powerlifting USA* 22:26-27, 1999.

71. Snarr, R, and Esco, MR. Push-up with knee tuck using a suspension device. *Strength Cond J* 35:30-32, 2013.

72. Snarr, RL, and Esco, MR. Electromyographic comparison of traditional and suspension push-ups. *J Hum Kinet* 39:75-83, 2013.

73. Stanton, R, Reaburn, PR, and Humphries, B. The effect of short-term Swiss ball training on core stability and running economy. *J Strength Cond Res* 18:522-528, 2004.

74. Stevenson, MW, Warpeha, JM, Dietz, CC, Giveans, RM, and Erdman, AG. Acute effects of elastic bands during the free-weight barbell back squat exercise on velocity, power, and force production. *J Strength Cond Res* 24:2944-2954, 2010.

75. Stone, MH, Plisk, S, and Collins, D. Training principles: Evaluation of modes and methods of resistance-training—a coaching perspective. *Sports Biomech* 1:79-104, 2002.

76. Thomas, JF, Larson, KL, Hollander, DB, and Kraemer, RR. Comparison of two-hand kettlebell exercise and graded treadmill walking: Effectiveness as a stimulus for cardiorespiratory fitness. *J Strength Cond Res* 28:998-1006, 2014.

77. Tobin, DP. Advanced strength and power training for the elite athlete. *Strength Cond J* 36:59-65, 2014.

78. Tvrdy, D. The reverse side plank/bridge: An alternate exercise for core training. *Strength Cond J* 34:86-88, 2012.

79. Wallace, BJ, Winchester, JB, and McGuigan, MR. Effects of elastic bands on force and power characteristics during the back squat exercise. *J Strength Cond Res* 20:268-272, 2006.

80. Waller, M, Piper, T, and Townsend, R. Strongman events and strength and conditioning programs. *Strength Cond J* 25:44-52, 2003.

81. Willardson, JM. Core stability training: Applications to sports conditioning programs. *J Strength Cond Res* 21:979-985, 2007.

82. Willson, JD, Dougherty, CP, Ireland, ML, and Davis, IM. Core stability and its relationship to lower extremity function and injury. *J Am Acad Orthop Surg* 13:316-325, 2005.

83. Winwood, PW, Cronin, JB, Posthumus, LR, Finlayson, S, Gill, ND, and Keogh, JW. Strongman versus traditional resistance training effects on muscular function and performance. *J Strength Cond Res*, 2015. [e-pub ahead of print].

84. Winwood, PW, Keogh, JW, and Harris, NK. The strength and conditioning practices of strongman competitors. *J Strength Cond Res* 25:3118-3128, 2011.

85. Zatsiorsky, VM, and Kraemer, WJ. *Science and Practice of Strength Training.* 2nd ed. Champaign, IL: Human Kinetics, 109-136, 2006.

86. Zemke, B, and Wright, G. The use of strongman type implements and training to increase sport performance in collegiate athletes. *Strength Cond J* 33:1-7, 2011.

CHAPTER 17   Resistance Training Program Design

1. Anderson, T, and Kearney, JT. Muscular strength and absolute and relative endurance. *Res Q Exerc Sport* 53:1-7, 1982.

2. Baechle, TR, and Earle, RW. Learning how to manipulate training variables to maximize results. In *Weight Training: Steps to Success.* 4th ed. Champaign, IL: Human Kinetics, 177-188, 2011.

3. Baker, D, and Newton, RU. Acute effect of power output of alternating an agonist and antagonist muscle exercise during complex training. *J Strength Cond Res* 19(1):202-205, 2005.

4. Baker, D, Wilson, G, and Carlyon, R. Periodization: The effect on strength of manipulating volume and intensity. *J Strength Cond Res* 8:235-242, 1994.

5. Berger, RA. Comparative effects of three weight training programs. *Res Q* 34:396-398, 1963.

6. Berger, RA. Effect of varied weight training programs on strength. *Res Q* 33:168-181, 1962.

7. Berger, RA. Optimum repetitions for the development of strength. *Res Q* 33:334-338, 1962.

8. Bompa, TA, and Haff, GG. *Periodization: Theory and Methodology of Training.* 5th ed. Champaign, IL: Human Kinetics, 31-122, 259-286, 2009.

9. Chapman, PP, Whitehead, JR, and Binkert, RH. The 225-lb reps-to-fatigue test as a submaximal estimate of 1RM bench press performance in college football players. *J Strength Cond Res* 12(4):258-261, 1998.

10. Cormie, P, McBride, JM, and McCaulley, GO. The influence of body mass on calculation of power during lower-body resistance exercises. *J Strength Cond Res* 21(4):1042-1049, 2007.

11. Cormie, P, McCaulley, GO, Triplett, NT, and McBride, JM. Optimal loading for maximal power output during lower-body resistance exercises. *Med Sci Sports Exerc* 39(2):340-349, 2007.

12. Cormie, P, McBride, JM, and McCaulley, GO. Power-time, force-time, and velocity-time curve analysis during the jump squat: Impact of load. *J Appl Biomech* 24(2):112-120, 2008.

13. Craig, BW, Lucas, J, Pohlman, R, and Schilling, H. The effect of running, weightlifting and a combination of both on growth hormone release. *J Appl Sport Sci Res* 5(4):198-203, 1991.

14. DeLorme, TL. Restoration of muscle power by heavy-resistance exercises. *J Bone Joint Surg* 27:645, 1945.

15. DeLorme, TL, and Watkins, AL. Technics of progressive resistance exercise. *Arch Phys Med Rehabil* 29:263-273, 1948.

16. DeRenne, C, Hetzler, RK, Buxton, BP, and Ho, KW. Effects of training frequency on strength maintenance in pubescent baseball players. *J Strength Cond Res* 10:8-14, 1996.

17. Dudley, GA, Tesch, PA, Miller, BJ, and Buchanan, P. Importance of eccentric actions in performance adaptations to resistance training. *Aviat Space Environ Med* 62:543-550, 1991.

18. Earle, RW. Weight training exercise prescription. In *Essentials of Personal Training Symposium Workbook.* Lincoln, NE: NSCA Certification Commission, 3-39, 2006.

19. Edgerton, VR. Neuromuscular adaptation to power and endurance work. *Can J Appl Sport Sci* 1:49-58, 1976.

20. Fleck, SJ, and Kraemer, WJ. *Designing Resistance Training Programs.* 4th ed. Champaign, IL: Human Kinetics, 1-62, 179-296, 2014.

21. Garhammer, J. A review of power output studies of Olympic and powerlifting: Methodology, performance prediction and evaluation tests. *J Strength Cond Res* 7(2):76-89, 1993.

22. Garhammer, J, and McLaughlin, T. Power output as a function of load variation in Olympic and power lifting [abstract]. *J Biomech* 13(2):198, 1980.

23. Gettman, LR, and Pollock, ML. Circuit weight training: A critical review of its physiological benefits. *Phys Sportsmed* 9:44-60, 1981.

24. Graves, JE, Pollock, ML, Leggett, SH, Braith, RW, Carpenter, DM, and Bishop, LE. Effect of reduced training frequency on muscular strength. *Int J Sports Med* 9:316-319, 1988.

25. Häkkinen, K. Factors affecting trainability of muscular strength during short-term and prolonged training. *NSCA J* 7(2):32-37, 1985.

26. Häkkinen, K. Neuromuscular responses in male and female athletes to two successive strength training sessions in one day. *J Sports Med Phys Fitness* 32:234-242, 1992.

27. Häkkinen, K, Pakarinen, A, Alén, M, Kauhanen, H, and Komi, PV. Daily hormonal and neuromuscular responses to intensive strength training in 1 week. *Int J Sports Med* 9:422-428, 1988.

28. Häkkinen, K, Pakarinen, A, Alén, M, Kauhanen, H, and Komi, PV. Neuromuscular and hormonal responses in elite athletes to two successive strength training sessions in one day. *Eur J Appl Physiol* 57:133-139, 1988.

29. Harman, E, and Frykman, P. CSCS coaches' school: Order of exercise: The multiple mini-circuit weight-training program. *NSCA J* 14(1):57-61, 1992.

30. Harman, E, Johnson, M, and Frykman, P. CSCS coaches' school: Program design: A movement-oriented approach to exercise prescription. *NSCA J* 14(1):47-54, 1992.

31. Hather, BM, Tesch, PA, Buchanan, P, and Dudley, GA. Influence of eccentric actions on skeletal muscle adaptations to resistance training. *Acta Physiol Scand* 143:177-185, 1992.

32. Hedrick, A. Training for hypertrophy. *Strength Cond* 17(3):22-29, 1995.

33. Herrick, AR, and Stone, MH. The effects of periodization versus progressive resistance exercise on upper and lower body strength in women. *J Strength Cond Res* 10(2):72-76, 1996.

34. Hickson, R, Rosenkoetter, MA, and Brown, MM. Strength training effects on aerobic power and short-term endurance. *Med Sci Sports Exerc* 12:336-339, 1980.

35. Hoeger, W, Barette, SL, Hale, DF, and Hopkins, DR. Relationship between repetitions and selected percentages of one repetition maximum. *J Appl Sport Sci Res* 1(1):11-13, 1987.

36. Hoeger, W, Hopkins, DR, Barette, SL, and Hale, DF. Relationship between repetitions and selected percentages of one repetition maximum: A comparison between untrained and trained males and females. *J Appl Sport Sci Res* 4:47-54, 1990.

37. Hoffman, JR, Kraemer, WJ, Fry, AC, Deschenes, M, and Kemp, M. The effects of self-selection for frequency of training in a winter conditioning program for football. *J Appl Sport Sci Res* 4:76-82, 1990.

38. Hoffman, JR, Maresh, CM, Armstrong, LE, and Kraemer, WJ. Effects of off-season and in-season resistance training programs on a collegiate male basketball team. *J Hum Muscle Perform* 1:48-55, 1991.

39. Hunter, GR. Changes in body composition, body build, and performance associated with different weight training frequencies in males and females. *NSCA J* 7(1):26-28, 1985.

40. Ikai, M, and Fukunaga, T. Calculation of muscle strength per unit cross-sectional area of human muscle by means of ultrasonic measurement. *Int Z Angew Physiol* 26:26-32, 1968.

41. Komi, PV. Neuromuscular performance: Factors influencing force and speed production. *Scand J Sports Sci* 1:2-15, 1979.

42. Kraemer, WJ. Endocrine responses and adaptations to strength and power training. In *The Encyclopaedia of Sports Medicine: Strength and Power in Sport.* 2nd ed. Komi, PV, ed. Malden, MA: Blackwell Scientific, 361-386, 2003.

43. Kraemer, WJ. Exercise prescription in weight training: A needs analysis. *NSCA J* 5(1):64-65, 1983.

44. Kraemer, WJ. A series of studies: The physiological basis for strength training in American football: Fact over philosophy. *J Strength Cond Res* 11(3):131-142, 1997.

45. Kraemer, WJ, and Koziris, LP. Muscle strength training: Techniques and considerations. *Phys Ther Pract* 2:54-68, 1992.

46. Kraemer, WJ, Newton, RU, Bush, J, Volek, J, Triplett, NT, and Koziris, LP. Varied multiple set resistance training program produces greater gain than single set program. *Med Sci Sports Exerc* 27:S195, 1995.

47. Kraemer, WJ, Noble, BJ, Clark, MJ, and Culver, BW. Physiologic responses to heavy resistance exercise with very short rest periods. *Int J Sports Med* 8:247-252, 1987.

48. Kramer, JB, Stone, MH, O'Bryant, HS, Conley, MS, Johnson, RL, Nieman, DC, Honeycutt, DR, and Hoke, TP. Effects of single vs. multiple sets of weight training: Impact of volume, intensity, and variation. *J Strength Cond Res* 11(3):143-147, 1997.

49. Lander, J. Maximum based on reps. *NSCA J* 6(6):60-61, 1984.

50. Larson, GD, Jr., and Potteiger, JA. A comparison of three different rest intervals between multiple squat bouts. *J Strength Cond Res* 11(2):115-118, 1997.

51. LeSuer, DA, McCormick, JH, Mayhew, JL, Wasserstein, RL, and Arnold, MD. The accuracy of predicting equations for estimating 1RM performance in the bench press, squat, and deadlift. *J Strength Cond Res* 11(4):211-213, 1997.

52. Luthi, JM, Howald, H, Claassen, H, Rosler, K, Vock, P, and Hoppler, H. Structural changes in skeletal muscle tissue with heavy-resistance exercise. *Int J Sports Med* 7:123-127, 1986.

53. Marcinik, EJ, Potts, J, Schlabach, G, Will, S, Dawson, P, and Hurley, BF. Effects of strength training on lactate threshold and endurance performance. *Med Sci Sports Exerc* 23:739-743, 1991.

54. Mayhew, JL, Ball, TE, Arnold, ME, and Bowen, JC. Relative muscular endurance performance as a predictor of bench press strength in college men and women. *J Appl Sport Sci Res* 6(4):200-206, 1992.

55. Mayhew, JL, Ware, JS, Bemben, MG, Wilt, B, Ward, TE, Farris, B, Juraszek, J, and Slovak, JP. The NFL-225 test as a measure of bench press strength in college football players. *J Strength Cond Res* 13(2):130-134, 1999.

56. Mayhew, JL, Ware, JS, and Prinster, JL. Using lift repetitions to predict muscular strength in adolescent males. *NSCA J* 15(6):35-38, 1993.

57. McBride, JM, Triplett-McBride, T, Davie, A, and Newton, RU. The effect of heavy- vs. light-load jump squats on the development of strength, power, and speed. *J Strength Cond Res* 16(1):75-82, 2002.

58. McBride, JM, McCaulley, GO, Cormie, P, Nuzzo, JL, Cavill, MJ, and Triplett, NT. Comparison of methods to quantify volume during resistance exercise. *J Strength Cond Res* 23(1):106-110, 2009.

59. McBride, JM, Kirby, TJ, Haines, TL, and Skinner, J. Relationship between relative net vertical impulse and jump height in jump squats performed to various squat depths and with various loads. *Int J Sports Physiol Perform* 5(4):484-496, 2010.

60. McBride, JM, Skinner, JW, Schafer, PC, Haines, TL, and Kirby, TJ. Comparison of kinetic variables and muscle activity during a squat vs. a box squat. *J Strength Cond Res* 24(12):3195-3199, 2010.

61. McBride, JM, Haines, TL, and Kirby, TJ. Effect of loading on peak power of the bar, body, and system during power cleans, squats, and jump squats. *J Sports Sci* 29(11):1215-1221, 2011.

62. McBride, JM, and Snyder, JG. Mechanical efficiency force–time curve variation during repetitive jumping in trained and untrained jumpers. *Eur J Appl Physiol* 112(10):3469-3477, 2012.

63. McDonagh, MJN, and Davies, CTM. Adaptive response of mammalian skeletal muscle to exercise with high loads. *Eur J Appl Physiol* 52:139-155, 1984.

64. McGee, D, Jessee, TC, Stone, MH, and Blessing, D. Leg and hip endurance adaptations to three weight-training programs. *J Appl Sport Sci Res* 6:92-95, 1992.

65. Morales, J, and Sobonya, S. Use of submaximal repetition tests for predicting 1-RM strength in class athletes. *J Strength Cond Res* 10(3):186-189, 1996.

66. Newton, RU, and Kraemer, WJ. Developing explosive muscular power: Implications for a mixed methods training strategy. *NSCA J* 16(5):20-31, 1994.

67. Newton, RU, Kraemer, WJ, Häkkinen, K, Humphries, BJ, and Murphy, AJ. Kinematics, kinetics, and muscle activation during explosive upper body movements: Implications for power development. *J Appl Biomech* 12:31-43, 1996.

68. Nuzzo, JL, and McBride, JM. The effect of loading and unloading on muscle activity during the jump squat. *J Strength Cond Res* 27(7):1758-1764, 2013.

69. O'Bryant, HS, Byrd, R, and Stone, MH. Cycle ergometer performance and maximum leg and hip strength adaptations to two different methods of weight training. *J Appl Sport Sci Res* 2:27-30, 1988.

70. O'Shea, P. Effects of selected weight training programs on the development of strength and muscle hypertrophy. *Res Q* 37:95-102, 1966.

71. Ostrowski, KJ, Wilson, GJ, Weatherby, R, Murphy, PW, and Lyttle, AD. The effect of weight training volume on hormonal output and muscular size and function. *J Strength Cond Res* 11(3):148-154, 1997.

72. Pauletto, B. Choice and order of exercise. *NSCA J* 8(2):71-73, 1986.

73. Pauletto, B. Intensity. *NSCA J* 8(1):33-37, 1986.

74. Pauletto, B. Rest and recuperation. *NSCA J* 8(3):52-53, 1986.

75. Pauletto, B. Sets and repetitions. *NSCA J* 7(6):67-69, 1985.

76. Richardson, T. Program design: Circuit training with exercise machines. *NSCA J* 15(5):18-19, 1993.

77. Robinson, JM, Stone, MH, Johnson, RL, Penland, CM, Warren, BJ, and Lewis, RD. Effects of different weight training exercise/rest intervals on strength, power, and high intensity exercise endurance. *J Strength Cond Res* 9(4):216-221, 1995.

78. Roundtable: Circuit training. *NSCA J* 12(2):16-27, 1990.

79. Roundtable: Circuit training—part II. *NSCA J* 12(3):10-21, 1990.

80. Sale, DG, MacDougall, JD, Jacobs, I, and Garner, S. Interaction between concurrent strength and endurance training. *J Appl Physiol* 68:260-270, 1990.

81. Santa Maria, DL, Grzybinski, P, and Hatfield, B. Power as a function of load for a supine bench press exercise. *NSCA J* 6(6):58, 1984.

82. Sewall, LP, and Lander, JE. The effects of rest on maximal efforts in the squat and bench press. *J Appl Sport Sci Res* 5:96-99, 1991.

83. Sforzo, GA, and Touey, PR. Manipulating exercise order affects muscular performance during a resistance exercise training session. *J Strength Cond Res* 10(1):20-24, 1996.

84. Sobonya, S, and Morales, J. The use of maximal repetition test for prediction of 1 repetition maximum loads [abstract]. *Sports Med Train Rehabil* 4:154, 1993.

85. Staron, RS, Malicky, ES, Leonardi, MJ, Falkel, JE, Hagerman, FC, and Dudley, GA. Muscle hypertrophy and fast fiber type conversions in heavy resistance-trained women. *Eur J Appl Physiol Occup Physiol* 60:71-79, 1989.

86. Stone, MH, and O'Bryant, HS. *Weight Training: A Scientific Approach.* Minneapolis: Burgess, 104-190, 1987.

87. Stone, MH, O'Bryant, HS, Garhammer, J, McMillan, J, and Rozenek, R. A theoretical model of strength training. *NSCA J* 4(4):36-40, 1982.

88. Stone, MH, and Wilson, D. Resistive training and selected effects. *Med Clin N Am* 69:109-122, 1985.

89. Stowers, T, McMillan, J, Scala, D, Davis, V, Wilson, D, and Stone, MH. The short-term effects of three different strength-power training methods. *NSCA J* 5(3):24-27, 1983.

90. Tan, B. Manipulating resistance training program variables to optimize maximum strength in men. *J Strength Cond Res* 13(3):289-304, 1999.

91. Tesch, PA. Training for bodybuilding. In *The Encyclopaedia of Sports Medicine: Strength and Power in Sport.* 1st ed. Komi, PV, ed. Malden, MA: Blackwell Scientific, 370-380, 1992.

92. Tesch, PA, and Larson, L. Muscle hypertrophy in body builders. *Eur J Appl Physiol* 49:301-306, 1982.

93. Wagner, LL, Evans, SA, Weir, JP, Housh, TJ, and Johnson, GO. The effect of grip width on bench press performance. *Int J Sport Biomech* 8:1-10, 1992.

94. Ware, JS, Clemens, CT, Mayhew, JL, and Johnston, TJ. Muscular endurance repetitions to predict bench press and squat strength in college football players. *J Strength Cond Res* 9(2):99-103, 1995.

95. Weir, JP, Wagner, LL, and Housh, TJ. The effect of rest interval length on repeated maximal bench presses. *J Strength Cond Res* 8(1):58-60, 1994.

96. Weiss, L. The obtuse nature of muscular strength: The contribution of rest to its development and expression. *J Appl Sport Sci Res* 5(4):219-227, 1991.

97. Wilk, KE, Escamilla, RF, Fleisig, GS, Barrentine, SW, Andrews, JR, and Boyd, ML. A comparison of tibiofemoral joint forces and electromyographic activity during open and closed chain exercises. *Am J Sports Med* 24(4):518-527, 1996.

98. Wilk, KE, Yenchak, AJ, Arrigo, CA, and Andrews, JR. The advanced throwers ten exercise program: A new exercise series for enhanced dynamic shoulder control in the overhead throwing athlete. *Phys Sportsmed* 39:90-97, 2011.

99. Willoughby, DS. The effects of mesocycle-length weight training programs involving periodization and partially equated volumes on upper and lower body strength. *J Strength Cond Res* 7:2-8, 1993.

100. Wilson, G, Elliott, B, and Kerr, G. Bar path and force profile characteristics for maximal and submaximal loads in the bench press. *Int J Sport Biomech* 5:390-402, 1989.

CHAPTER 18 Plyometric Training Program Design and Technique

1. Albert, M. *Eccentric Muscle Training in Sports and Orthopaedics.* New York: Churchill Livingstone, 1995.

2. Allerheilegen, B, and Rogers, R. Plyometrics program design. *Strength Cond* 17:26-31, 1995.

3. Asmussen, E, and Bonde-Peterson, F. Storage of elastic energy in skeletal muscles in man. *Acta Physiol Scand* 91:385-392, 1974.

4. Aura, O, and Viitasalo, JT. Biomechanical characteristics of jumping. *Int J Sports Biomech* 5:89-97, 1989.

5. Bobbert, MF. Drop jumping as a training method for jumping ability. *Sports Med* 9:7-22, 1990.

6. Bobbert, MF, Gerritsen, KGM, Litjens, MCA, and Van Soest, AJ. Why is countermovement jump height greater than squat jump height? *Med Sci Sports Exerc* 28:1402-1412, 1996.

7. Borkowski, J. Prevention of pre-season muscle soreness: Plyometric exercise [abstract]. *Athl Train* 25:122, 1990.

8. Bosco, C, Ito, A, Komi, PV, Luhtanen, P, Rahkila, P, Rusko, H, and Viitasalo, JT. Neuromuscular function and mechanical efficiency of human leg extensor muscles during jumping exercises. *Acta Physiol Scand* 114:543-550, 1982.

9. Bosco, C, and Komi, PV. Potentiation of the mechanical behavior of the human skeletal muscle through prestretching. *Acta Physiol Scand* 106:467-472, 1979.

10. Bosco, C, Komi, PV, and Ito, A. Prestretch potentiation of human skeletal muscle during ballistic movement. *Acta Physiol Scand* 111:135-140, 1981.

11. Bosco, C, Viitasalo, JT, Komi, PV, and Luhtanen, P. Combined effect of elastic energy and myoelectrical potentiation during stretch shortening cycle exercise. *Acta Physiol Scand* 114:557-565, 1982.

12. Cavagna, GA. Storage and utilization of elastic energy in skeletal muscle. In *Exercise and Sport Science Reviews,* vol. 5. Hutton, RS, ed. Santa Barbara, CA: Journal Affiliates, 80-129, 1977.

13. Cavagna, GA, Dusman, B, and Margaria, R. Positive work done by a previously stretched muscle. *J Appl Physiol* 24:21-32, 1968.

14. Cavagna, GA, Saibere, FP, and Margaria, R. Effect of negative work on the amount of positive work performed by an isolated muscle. *J Appl Physiol* 20:157-158, 1965.

15. Chambers, C, Noakes, TD, Lambert, EV, and Lambert, MI. Time course of recovery of vertical jump height and heart rate versus running speed after a 90-km foot race. *J Sports Sci* 16:645-651, 1998.

16. Chu, D. *Jumping Into Plyometrics.* 2nd ed. Champaign, IL: Human Kinetics, 1998

17. Chu, D, Faigenbaum, A, and Falkel, J. *Progressive Plyometrics for Kids.* Monterey, CA: Healthy Learning, 2006.

18. Chu, D, and Plummer, L. Jumping into plyometrics: The language of plyometrics. *NSCA J* 6:30-31, 1984.

19. Dillman, CJ, Fleisig, GS, and Andrews, JR. Biomechanics of pitching with emphasis upon shoulder kinematics. *J Orthop Sports Phys Ther* 18:402-408, 1993.

20. Dursenev, L, and Raeysky, L. Strength training for jumpers. *Soviet Sports Rev* 14:53-55, 1979.

21. Enoka, RM. *Neuromechanical Basis of Kinesiology.* 2nd ed. Champaign, IL: Human Kinetics, 1994.

22. Escamilla, RF, Fleisig, GS, Barrentine, SW, and Andrews, JR. Kinematic comparisons of throwing different types of baseball pitches. *J Appl Biomech* 14:1-23, 1998.

23. Feltner, M, and Dapena, J. Dynamics of the shoulder and elbow joints of the throwing arm during a baseball pitch. *Int J Sports Biomech* 2:235, 1986.

24. Fowler, NE, Lees, A, and Reilly, T. Changes in stature following plyometric drop-jump and pendulum exercises. *Ergonomics* 40:1279-1286, 1997.

25. Fowler, NE, Lees, A, and Reilly, T. Spinal shrinkage in unloaded and loaded drop-jumping. *Ergonomics* 37:133-139, 1994.

26. Gambetta, V. Plyometric training. *Track Field Q Rev* 80:56-57, 1978.

27. Guyton, AC, and Hall, JE. *Textbook of Medical Physiology.* 10th ed. Philadelphia: Saunders, 2000.

28. Halling, AH, Howard, ME, and Cawley, PW. Rehabilitation of anterior cruciate ligament injuries. *Clin Sports Med* 12:329-348, 1993.

29. Harman, EA, Rosenstein, MT, Frykman, PN, and Rosenstein, RM. The effects of arms and countermovement on vertical jumping. *Med Sci Sports Exerc* 22:825-833, 1990.

30. Hewett, TE, Stroupe, AL, Nance, TA, and Noyes, FR. Plyometric training in female athletes. *Am J Sports Med* 24:765-773, 1996.

31. Hill, AV. *First and Last Experiments in Muscle Mechanics.* Cambridge: Cambridge University Press, 1970.

32. Holcomb, WR, Kleiner, DM, and Chu, DA. Plyometrics: Considerations for safe and effective training. *Strength Cond* 20:36-39, 1998.

33. Kaeding, CC, and Whitehead, R. Musculoskeletal injuries in adolescents. *Prim Care* 25:211-223, 1998.

34. Karst, GM, and Willett, GM. Onset timing of electromyographic activity in the vastus medialis oblique and vastus lateralis muscles in subjects with and without patellofemoral pain syndrome. *Phys Ther* 75:813-823, 1995.

35. Kilani, HA, Palmer, SS, Adrian, MJ, and Gapsis, JJ. Block of the stretch reflex of vastus lateralis during vertical jump. *Hum Mov Sci* 8:247-269, 1989.

36. Knowlton, GC, and Britt, LP. Relation of height and age to reflex time [abstract]. *Am J Physiol* 159:576, 1949.

37. Korchemny, R. Evaluation of sprinters. *NSCA J* 7:38-42, 1985.

38. Kroll, W. Patellar reflex time and reflex latency under Jendrassik and crossed extensor facilitation. *Am J Phys Med* 47:292-301, 1968.

39. LaChance, P. Plyometric exercise. *Strength Cond* 17:16-23, 1995.

40. Lipp, EJ. Athletic physeal injury in children and adolescents. *Orthop Nurs* 17:17-22, 1998.

41. Luhtanen, P, and Komi, P. Mechanical factors influencing running speed. In *Biomechanics VI-B*. Asmussen, E, ed. Baltimore: University Park Press, 23-29, 1978.

42. Matthews, PBC. The knee jerk: Still an enigma? *Can J Physiol Pharm* 68:347-354, 1990.

43. Myer, GD, Paterno, MV, Ford, KR, and Hewett, TE. Neuromuscular training techniques to target deficits before return to sport after anterior cruciate ligament reconstruction. *J Strength Cond Res* 22:987-1014, 2008.

44. National Strength and Conditioning Association. Position statement: Explosive/plyometric exercises. *NSCA J* 15:16, 1993.

45. Newton, RU, Murphy, AJ, Humphries, BJ, Wilson, GJ, Kraemer, WJ, and Häkkinen, K. Influence of load and stretch shortening cycle on the kinematics, kinetics and muscle activation that occurs during explosive upper-body movements. *Eur J Appl Physiol* 75:333-342, 1997.

46. Pappas, AM, Zawacki, RM, and Sullivan, TJ. Biomechanics of baseball pitching: A preliminary report. *Am J Sports Med* 13:216-222, 1985.

47. Potach, DH, Katsavelis, D, Karst, GM, Latin, RW, and Stergiou, N. The effects of a plyometric training program on the latency time of the quadriceps femoris and gastrocnemius short-latency responses. *J Sports Med Phys Fitness* 49:35-43, 2009.

48. Radcliffe, JC, and Osternig, LR. Effects on performance of variable eccentric loads during depth jumps. *J Sport Rehabil* 4:31-41, 1995.

49. Stone, MH, and O'Bryant, HS. *Weight Training: A Scientific Approach*. Minneapolis: Burgess International, 1987.

50. Svantesson, U, Grimby, G, and Thomeé, R. Potentiation of concentric plantar flexion torque following eccentric and isometric muscle actions. *Acta Physiol Scand* 152:287-293, 1994.

51. Voight, ML, Draovitch, P, and Tippett, S. Plyometrics. In *Eccentric Muscle Training in Sports and Orthopaedics*. Albert, M, ed. New York: Churchill Livingstone, 61-88, 1995.

52. Wathen, D. Literature review: Plyometric exercise. *NSCA J* 15:17-19, 1993.

53. Wilk, KE, Voight, ML, Keirns, MA, Gambetta, V, Andrews, JR, and Dillman, CJ. Stretch-shortening drills for the upper extremities: Theory and clinical applications. *J Orthop Sports Phys Ther* 17:225-239, 1993.

54. Wilson, GJ, Murphy, AJ, and Giorgi, A. Weight and plyometric training: Effects on eccentric and concentric force production. *Can J Appl Physiol* 21:301-315, 1996.

55. Wilson, GJ, Newton, RU, Murphy, AJ, and Humphries, BJ. The optimal training load for the development of dynamic athletic performance. *Med Sci Sports Exerc* 25:1279-1286, 1993.

56. Wilt, F. Plyometrics: What it is and how it works. *Athl J* 55:76, 89-90, 1975.

CHAPTER 19 Speed and Agility Program Design and Technique

1. Aagaard, P, Simonsen, EB, Andersen, JL, Magnusson, P, and Dyhre-Poulsen, P. Increased rate of force development and neural drive of human skeletal muscle following resistance training. *J Appl Physiol* 93:1318-1326, 2002.

2. Alcaraz, PE, Palao, JM, and Elvira, JLL. Determining the optimal load for resisted sprint training with sled towing. *J Strength Cond Res* 23:480-485, 2009.

3. Alexander, RM. Mechanics of skeleton and tendons. In *Handbook of Physiology, Section 1: The Nervous System*. Brookhardt, JM, Mountcastle, VB, Brooks, VB, and Greiger, SR, eds. Bethesda, MD: American Physiological Society, 17-42, 1981.

4. Alexander, RM. *Principles of Animal Locomotion*. Princeton, NJ: Princeton University Press, 2003.

5. Angelozzi, M, Madama, M, Corsica, C, Calvisi, V, Properzi, G, McCaw, ST, and Cacchio, A. Rate of force development as an adjunctive outcome measure for return-to-sport decisions after anterior cruciate ligament reconstruction. *J Orthop Sports Phys Ther* 42:772-780, 2012.

6. Arabatzi, F, and Kellis, E. Olympic weightlifting training causes different knee muscle-coactivation adaptations compared with traditional weight training. *J Strength Cond Res* 26:2192-2201, 2012.

7. Åstrand, PO, Rodahl, K, Dahl, HA, and Stromme, SB. *Textbook of Work Physiology*. Champaign, IL: Human Kinetics, 2003.

8. Barnes, JL, Schilling, BK, Falvo, MJ, Weiss, LW, Creasy, AK, and Fry, AC. Relationship of jumping and agility performance in female volleyball athletes. *J Strength Cond Res* 21:1192-1196, 2007.

9. Biewener, AA. *Animal Locomotion*. Oxford: Oxford University Press, 230-262, 2003.

10. Blickhan, R. The spring-mass model for running and hopping. *J Biomech* 22:1217-1227, 1989.

11. Bloomfield, J, Polman, R, O'Donoghue, P, and McNaughton, L. Effective speed and agility conditioning methodology for random intermittent dynamic type sports. *J Strength Cond Res* 21:1093-1100, 2007.

12. Bosquet, L, Berryman, N, and Dupuy, O. A comparison of 2 optical timing systems designed to measure flight time and contact time during jumping and hopping. *J Strength Cond Res* 23:2660-2665, 2009.

13. Bundle, MW, Hoyt, RW, and Weyand, PG. High-speed running performance: A new approach to assessment and prediction. *J Appl Physiol* 95:1955-1962, 2003.

14. Burke, RE. Motor units: Anatomy, physiology, and functional organization. In *Handbook of Physiology, Section 1: The Nervous System*. Brookhart, JM, Mountcastle, VB, Brooks, VB, and Greiger, SR, eds. Bethesda, MD: American Physiological Society, 345-422, 1981.

15. Castillo-Rodríguez, A, Fernández-García, JC, Chinchilla-Minguet, JL, and Carnero, EÁ. Relationship between muscular strength and sprints with changes of direction. *J Strength Cond Res* 26:725-732, 2012.

16. Chaouachi, A, Brughelli, M, Chamari, K, Levin, GT, Abdelkrim, NB, Laurencelle, L, and Castagna, C. Lower limb maximal dynamic strength and agility determinants in elite basketball players. *J Strength Cond Res* 23:1570-1577, 2009.

17. Clark, KP, and Weyand, PG. Are running speeds maximized with simple-spring stance mechanics? *J Appl Physiol* 117:604-615, 2014.

18. Comfort, P, Udall, R, and Jones, PA. The effect of loading on kinematic and kinetic variables during the midthigh clean pull. *J Strength Cond Res* 26:1208-1214, 2012.

19. Cormie, P, McGuigan, MR, and Newton, RU. Influence of strength on magnitude and mechanisms of adaptation to power training. *Med Sci Sports Exerc* 42:1566-1581, 2010.

20. Cottle, CA, Carlson, LA, and Lawrence, MA. Effects of sled towing on sprint starts. *J Strength Cond Res* 28:1241-1245, 2014.

21. Dalleau, G, Belli, A, Bourdin, M, and Lacour, JR. The spring-mass model and the energy cost of treadmill running. *Eur J Appl Physiol Occup Physiol* 77:257-263, 1998.

22. DeWeese, BH, Grey, HS, Sams, ML, Scruggs, SK, and Serrano, AJ. Revising the definition of periodization: Merging historical principles with modern concern. *Olympic Coach* 24:5-19, Winter 2013.

23. DeWeese, BH, Sams, ML, and Serrano, AJ. Sliding toward Sochi—part 1: A review of programming tactics used during the 2010-2014 Quadrennial. *NSCA Coach* 1:30-43, 2014.

24. DeWeese, BH, Serrano, AJ, Scruggs, SK, and Burton, JK. The mid-thigh pull: Proper application and progressions of a weightlifting movement derivative. *Strength Cond J* 35:54-58, 2013.

25. Dietz, V. Neuronal control of functional movement. In *The Encyclopedia of Sports Medicine: Strength and Power in Sport.* Komi, PV, ed. Oxford: Blackwell Science, 11-26, 2003.

26. Dillman, CJ. Kinematic analyses of running. *Exerc Sport Sci Rev* 3:193-218, 1975.

27. Dutto, DJ, and Smith, GA. Changes in spring-mass characteristics during treadmill running to exhaustion. *Med Sci Sports Exerc* 34:1324-1331, 2002.

28. Enoka, RM. Eccentric contractions require unique activation strategies by the nervous system. *J Appl Physiol* 81:2339-2346, 1996.

29. Farley, CT, and Gonzalez, O. Leg stiffness and stride frequency in human running. *J Biomech* 29:181-186, 1996.

30. Fry, AC, Schilling, BK, Staron, RS, Hagerman, FC, Hikida, RS, and Thrush, JT. Muscle fiber characteristics and performance correlates of male Olympic-style weightlifters. *J Strength Cond Res* 17:746-754, 2003.

31. Gabbett, TJ, Kelly, JN, and Sheppard, JM. Speed, change of direction speed, and reactive agility of rugby league players. *J Strength Cond Res* 22:174-181, 2008.

32. Haff, GG, and Nimphius, S. Training principles for power. *Strength Cond J* 34:2-12, 2012.

33. Hakkinen, K. Neuromuscular adaptation during strength training, age, detraining, and immobilization. *Crit Rev Phys Rehabil Med* 6:161-198, 1994.

34. Hakkinen, K, and Komi, PV. Changes in electrical and mechanical behavior of leg extensor muscle during heavy resistance strength training. *Scand J Sport Sci* 7:55-64, 1985.

35. Hartmann, J, and Tunneemann, H. *Fitness and Strength Training.* Berlin: Sportverlag, 50-69, 1989.

36. Hawley, JA, ed. *Running.* Oxford: Blackwell Science, 28-43, 2000.

37. Hodgson, M, Docherty, D, and Robbins, D. Post-activation potentiation: Underlying physiology and implications for motor performance. *Sports Med* 35:585-595, 2005.

38. Houck, J. Muscle activation patterns of selected lower extremity muscles during stepping and cutting tasks. *J Electromyogr Kinesiol* 13:545-554, 2003.

39. Houk, JC, and Rymer, WZ. Neural control of muscle length and tension. In *Handbook of Physiology, Section 1: The Nervous System.* Brookhart, JM, Mountcastle, VB, Brooks, VB, and Greiger, SR, eds. Bethesda, MD: American Physiological Society, 257-323, 1981.

40. Jakalski, K. The pros and cons of using resisted and assisted training methods with high school sprinters parachutes, tubing, and towing. *Track Coach,* 4585-4589, 1998.

41. Jones, P, Bampouras, T, and Marrin, K. An investigation into the physical determinants of change of direction speed. *J Sports Med Phys Fitness* 49:97-104, 2009.

42. Kawamori, N, Newton, RU, Hori, N, and Nosaka, K. Effects of weighted sled towing with heavy versus light load on sprint acceleration ability. *J Strength Cond Res* 28:2738-2745, 2014.

43. Komi, PV. Neuromuscular performance: Factors inflencing force and speed production. *Scand J Sport Sci* 1:2-15, 1979.

44. Komi, PV. Training of muscle strength and power: Interaction of neuromotoric, hypertrophic, and mechanical factors. *Int J Sports Med* 7 suppl 1:10-15, 1986.

45. Komi, PV. Stretch-shortening cycle. In *The Encyclopedia of Sports Medicine: Strength and Power in Sport.* Komi, PV, ed. Oxford: Blackwell Science, 184-202, 2003.

46. Komi, PV, and Nicol, C. Stretch-shortening cycle of muscle function. In *Biomechanics in Sport.* Zatsiorsky, VM, ed. Oxford: Blackwell Science, 87-102, 2000.

47. Kraemer, WJ, and Looney, D. Underlying mechanisms and physiology of muscular power. *Strength Cond J* 34:13-19, 2012.

48. Kyröläinen, H, Komi, PV, and Belli, A. Changes in muscle activity patterns and kinetics with increasing running speed. *J Strength Cond Res* 13:400-406, 1999.

49. Letzelter, M, Sauerwein, G, and Burger, R. Resistance runs in speed development. *Modern Coach and Athlete* 33:7-12, 1995.

50. Lloyd, RS, Read, P, Oliver, JL, Meyers, RW, Nimphius, S, and Jeffreys, I. Considerations for the development of agility during childhood and adolescence. *Strength Cond J* 35:2-11, 2013.

51. Lockie, RG, Murphy, AJ, and Spinks, CD. Effects of resisted sled towing on sprint kinematics in field sport athletes. *J Strength Cond Res* 17:760-767, 2003.

52. Mann, RV. *The Mechanics of Sprinting and Hurdling.* Lexington, KY: CreateSpace, 89-125, 2011.

53. Mann, RV, and Herman, J. Kinematic analysis of Olympic sprint performance: Men's 200 meters. *Int J Sports Biomech* 1:151-162, 1985.

54. Marshall, BM, Franklyn-Miller, AD, King, EA, Moran, KA, Strike, SC, and Falvey, EC. Biomechanical factors associated with time to complete a change of direction cutting maneuver. *J Strength Cond Res* 28:2845-2851, 2014.

55. Mero, A, and Komi, PV. Electromyographic activity in sprinting at speeds ranging from sub-maximal to supra-maximal. *Med Sci Sports Exerc* 19:266-274, 1987.

56. Moolyk, AN, Carey, JP, and Chiu, LZ. Characteristics of lower extremity work during the impact phase of jumping and weightlifting. *J Strength Cond Res* 27:3225-3232, 2013.

57. Naczk, M, Naczk, A, Brzenczek-Owczarzak, W, Arlet, J, and Adach, Z. Relationship between maximal rate of force development and maximal voluntary contractions. *Studies in Physical Culture and Tourism* 17:301-306, 2010.

58. Nimphius, S. Increasing agility. In *High-Performance Training for Sports.* Joyce, D, and Lewindon, D, eds. Champaign, IL: Human Kinetics, 185-198, 2014.

59. Nimphius, S, Geib, G, Spiteri, T, and Carlisle, D. "Change of direction deficit" measurement in Division I American football players. *Journal of Australian Strength and Conditioning* 21:115-117, 2013.

60. Nimphius, S, McGuigan, MR, and Newton, RU. Changes in muscle architecture and performance during a competitive season in female softball players. *J Strength Cond Res* 26:2655-2666, 2012.

61. Nimphius, S, Spiteri, T, Seitz, L, Haff, E, and Haff, G. Is there a pacing strategy during a 505 change of direction test in adolescents? *J Strength Cond Res* 27:S104-S105, 2013.

62. Paddon-Jones, D, Leveritt, M, Lonergan, A, and Abernethy, P. Adaptation to chronic eccentric exercise in humans: The influence of contraction velocity. *Eur J Appl Physiol* 85:466-471, 2001.

63. Pauole, K, Madole, K, Garhammer, J, Lacourse, M, and Rozenek, R. Reliability and validity of the T-test as a measure of agility, leg power, and leg speed in college-aged men and women. *J Strength Cond Res* 14:443-450, 2000.

64. Porter, JM, Nolan, RP, Ostrowski, EJ, and Wulf, G. Directing attention externally enhances agility performance: A qualitative and quantitative analysis of the efficacy of using verbal instructions to focus attention. *Front Psychol* 1:216, 2010.

65. Putnam, CA, and Kozey, JW. Substantive issues in running. In *Biomechanics of Sport.* Vaughn, CL, ed. Boca Raton, FL: CRC Press, 1-33, 1989.

66. Robbins, DW. Postactivation potentiation and its practical applicability: A brief review. *J Strength Cond Res* 19:453-458, 2005.

67. Ross, A, and Leveritt, M. Long-term metabolic and skeletal muscle adaptations to short-sprint training: Implications for sprint training and tapering. *Sports Med* 31:1063-1082, 2001.

68. Ross, A, Leveritt, M, and Riek, S. Neural influences on sprint running: Training adaptations and acute responses. *Sports Med* 31:409-425, 2001.

69. Sale, DG. Postactivation potentiation: Role in human performance. *Exerc Sport Sci Rev* 30:138-143, 2002.

70. Sasaki, S, Nagano, Y, Kaneko, S, Sakurai, T, and Fukubayashi, T. The relationship between performance and trunk movement during change of direction. *J Sports Sci Med* 10:112, 2011.

71. Schmidtbleicher, D. Strength training (part 1): Structural analysis of motor strength qualities and its application to training. *Sci Per Res Tech Sport: Phys Training/Strength* W-4:1-12, 1985.

72. Schmidtbleicher, D. Strength training (part 2): Structural analysis of motor strength qualities and its applications to training. *Sci Per Res Tech Sport: Phys Training/Strength* W-4:1-10, 1985.

73. Schmidtbleicher, D. Training for power events. In *The Encyclopaedia of Sports Medicine: Strength and Power in Sport.* Komi, PV, ed. Oxford, UK: Blackwell, 169-179, 1992.

74. Schmolinsky, G. *Track and Field: The East German Textbook of Athletics.* Toronto: Sports Book, 1993.

75. Serpell, BG, Young, WB, and Ford, M. Are the perceptual and decision-making components of agility trainable? A preliminary investigation. *J Strength Cond Res* 25:1240-1248, 2011.

76. Sheppard, J, Dawes, J, Jeffreys, I, Spiteri, T, and Nimphius, S. Broadening the view of agility: A scientific review of the literature. *Journal of Australian Strength and Conditioning* 22:6-25, 2014.

77. Sheppard, JM, and Young, W. Agility literature review: Classifications, training and testing. *J Sports Sci* 24:919-932, 2006.

78. Shimokochi, Y, Ide, D, Kokubu, M, and Nakaoji, T. Relationships among performance of lateral cutting maneuver from lateral sliding and hip extension and abduction motions, ground reaction force, and body center of mass height. *J Strength Cond Res* 27:1851-1860, 2013.

79. Sierer, SP, Battaglini, CL, Mihalik, JP, Shields, EW, and Tomasini, NT. The National Football League combine: Performance differences between drafted and nondrafted players entering the 2004 and 2005 drafts. *J Strength Cond Res* 22:6-12, 2008.

80. Siff, MC. *Supertraining.* Denver: Supertraining Institute, 267-284, 2003.

81. Spiteri, T, Cochrane, JL, Hart, NH, Haff, GG, and Nimphius, S. Effect of strength on plant foot kinetics and kinematics during a change of direction task. *Eur J Sport Sci* 13:646-652, 2013.

82. Spiteri, T, Cochrane, JL, and Nimphius, S. The evaluation of a new lower-body reaction time test. *J Strength Cond Res* 27:174-180, 2013.

83. Spiteri, T, Hart, NH, and Nimphius, S. Offensive and defensive agility: A sex comparison of lower body kinematics and ground reaction forces. *J Appl Biomech* 30:514-520, 2014.

84. Spiteri, T, and Nimphius, S. Relationship between timing variables and plant foot kinetics during change of direction movements. *Journal of Australian Strength and Conditioning* 21:73-77, 2013.

85. Spiteri, T, Nimphius, S, and Cochrane, JL. Comparison of running times during reactive offensive and defensive agility protocols. *Journal of Australian Strength and Conditioning* 20:73-78, 2012.

86. Spiteri, T, Nimphius, S, Hart, NH, Specos, C, Sheppard, JM, and Newton, RU. The contribution of strength characteristics to change of direction and agility performance in female basketball athletes. *J Strength Cond Res* 28:2415-2423, 2014.

87. Stone, M, Stone, M, and Sands, WA. *Principles and Practice of Resistance Training.* Champaign, IL: Human Kinetics, 45-62, 2007.

88. Stone, MH, O'Bryant, HS, McCoy, L, Coglianese, R, Lehmkuhl, M, and Schilling, B. Power and maximum strength relationships during performance of dynamic and static weighted jumps. *J Strength Cond Res* 17:140-147, 2003.

89. Stone, MH, Sanborn, K, O'Bryant, HS, Hartman, M, Stone, ME, Proulx, C, Ward, B, and Hruby, J. Maximum strength-power-performance relationships in collegiate throwers. *J Strength Cond Res* 17:739-745, 2003.

90. Vescovi, JD, and McGuigan, MR. Relationships between sprinting, agility, and jump ability in female athletes. *J Sports Sci* 26:97-107, 2008.

91. Vescovi, JD, Rupf, R, Brown, TD, and Marques, MC. Physical performance characteristics of high-level female soccer players 12-21 years of age. *Scand J Med Sci Sports* 21:670-678, 2011.

92. Weyand, PG, Bundle, MW, McGowan, CP, Grabowski, A, Brown, MB, Kram, R, and Herr, H. The fastest runner on artificial legs: Different limbs, similar function? *J Appl Physiol* 107:903-911, 2009.

93. Weyand, PG, Sandell, RF, Prime, DN, and Bundle, MW. The biological limits to running speed are imposed from the ground up. *J Appl Physiol* 108:950-961, 2010.

94. Weyand, PG, Sternlight, DB, Bellizzi, MJ, and Wright, S. Faster top running speeds are achieved with greater ground forces not more rapid leg movements. *J Appl Physiol* 89:1991-1999, 2000.

95. Wood, GA. Biomechanical limitations to sprint running. In *Medicine and Sport Science.* Hebbelink, M, Shephard, RJ, Van Gheluwe, B, and Atha, J, eds. Basel: Karger, 58-71, 1987.

96. Young, WB. Transfer of strength and power training to sports performance. *Int J Sports Physiol Perform* 1:74-83, 2006.

97. Young, W, and Farrow, D. The importance of a sport-specific stimulus for training agility. *Strength Cond J* 35:39-43, 2013.

98. Young, W, Farrow, D, Pyne, D, McGregor, W, and Handke, T. Validity and reliability of agility tests in junior Australian football players. *J Strength Cond Res* 25:3399-3403, 2011.

99. Zatsiorsky, VM, and Kraemer, WJ. *Science and Practice of Strength Training.* Champaign, IL: Human Kinetics, 47-66, 2006.

CHAPTER 20 Aerobic Endurance Exercise Training

1. Åstrand, PO, Rodahl, K, Dahl, HA, and Stromme, SB. *Textbook of Work Physiology.* 4th ed. Champaign, IL: Human Kinetics, 242-243, 2003.

2. Banister, EW. Modeling elite athletic performance. In *Physiological Testing of the High-Performance Athlete.* 2nd ed. MacDougall, JD, Wenger, HA, and Green, HJ, eds. Champaign, IL: Human Kinetics, 403-424, 1991.

3. Beck, TW. Cardiovascular training methods. In *NSCA's Essentials of Personal Training.* 2nd ed. Coburn, JW, and Malek, MH, eds. Champaign, IL: Human Kinetics, 329-346, 2012.

4. Beneke, R. Anaerobic threshold, individual anaerobic threshold, and maximal lactate steady state in rowing. *Med Sci Sports Exerc* 27:863-867, 1995.

5. Boulay, MR, Simoneau, JA, Lortie, G, and Bouchard, C. Monitoring high-intensity endurance exercise with heart rate and thresholds. *Med Sci Sports Exerc* 29:125-132, 1997.

6. Boutcher, SH, Seip, RL, Hetzler, RK, Pierce, EF, Snead, D, and Weltman, A. The effects of specificity of training on rating of perceived exertion at the lactate threshold. *Eur J Appl Physiol Occup Physiol* 59:365-369, 1989.

7. Brooks, GA, and Mercier, J. Balance of carbohydrate and lipid utilization during exercise: The "crossover" concept. *J Appl Physiol* 76:2253-2261, 1994.

8. Buchheit, M, and Laursen, PB. High-intensity interval training, solutions to the programming puzzle. Part I: Cardiopulmonary emphasis. *Sports Med* 43:313-338, 2013.

9. Buchheit, M, and Laursen, PB. High-intensity interval training, solutions to the programming puzzle: Part II: Anaerobic energy, neuromuscular load and practical applications. *Sports Med* 43:927-954, 2013.

10. Burke, EJ. Physiological effects of similar training programs in males and females. *Res Q* 48:510-517, 1977.

11. Burke, ER, Cerny, F, Costill, D, and Fink, W. Characteristics of skeletal muscle in competitive cyclists. *Med Sci Sports Exerc* 9:109-112, 1977.

12. Cavanagh, PR, Pollock, ML, and Landa, J. Biomechanical comparison of elite and good distance runners. *Ann NY Acad Sci* 301:328-345, 1977.

13. Ceci, R, and Hassmén, P. Self-monitored exercise at three different RPE intensities in treadmill vs. field running. *Med Sci Sports Exerc* 23:732-738, 1991.

14. Conley, DL, and Krahenbuhl, GS. Running economy and distance running performance of highly trained athletes. *Med Sci Sports Exerc* 12:357-360, 1980.

15. Costill, DL. *Inside Running: Basics of Sports Physiology.* Indianapolis: Benchmark Press, 101-103, 117-118, 1986.

16. Costill, DL, Fink, WJ, and Pollock, ML. Muscle fiber composition and enzyme activities of elite distance runners. *Med Sci Sports Exerc* 8:96-100, 1976.

17. Costill, DL, King, R, Thomas, DC, and Hargreaves, M. Effects of reduced training on muscular power in swimmers. *Phys Sportsmed* 13:94-101, 1985.

18. Costill, DL, Thomas, R, Roberts, RA, Pascoe, D, Lambert, C, Barr, S, and Fink, WJ. Adaptations to swimming training: Influence of training volume. *Med Sci Sports Exerc* 23:371-377, 1991.

19. Costill, DL, Thomason, H, and Roberts, E. Fractional utilization of the aerobic capacity during distance running. *Med Sci Sports Exerc* 5:248-252, 1973.

20. Coyle, EF, Coggan, AR, Hemmert, MK, and Ivy, JL. Muscle glycogen utilization during prolonged strenuous exercise when fed carbohydrate. *J Appl Physiol* 61:165-172, 1986.

21. Coyle, EF, Coggan, AR, Hopper, MK, and Walters, TJ. Determinants of endurance in well-trained cyclists. *J Appl Physiol* 64:2622-2630, 1988.

22. Coyle, EF, Feltner, ME, Kautz, SA, Hamilton, MT, Montain, SJ, Baylor, AM, Abraham, LD, and Petrek, GW. Physiological and biomechanical factors associated with elite endurance cycling performance. *Med Sci Sports Exerc* 23:93-107, 1991.

23. Coyle, EF, Hagberg, JM, Hurley, BF, Martin, WH, Ehsani, AA, and Holloszy, JO. Carbohydrate feeding during prolonged strenuous exercise can delay fatigue. *J Appl Physiol* 55:230-235, 1983.

24. Daniels, J. Training distance runners—primer. *Gatorade Sports Science Exchange* 1:1-5, 1989.

25. Davidson, CJ, Pardyjak, ER, and Martin, JC. Training with power measurement: A new era in cycling training. *Strength Cond J* 25:28-29, 2003.

26. Dishman, RK, Patton, RW, Smith, J, Weinberg, R, and Jackson, A. Using perceived exertion to prescribe and monitor exercise training heart rate. *Int J Sports Med* 8:208-213, 1987.

27. Drinkwater, BL, and Horvath, SM. Detraining effects on young women. *Med Sci Sports* 4:91-95, 1972.

28. Dudley, GA, Abraham, WM, and Terjung, RL. Influence of exercise intensity and duration on biochemical adaptations in skeletal muscle. *J Appl Physiol* 53:844-850, 1982.

29. Ehsani, AA, Hagberg, JM, and Hickson, RC. Rapid changes in left ventricular dimensions and mass in response to physical conditioning and deconditioning. *Am J Cardiol* 42:52-56, 1978.

30. Epthorp, JA. Altitude training and its effects on performance: Systematic review. *J Aust Strength Cond* 22:78-88, 2014.

31. Farrell, PA, Wilmore, JH, Coyle, EF, Billing, JE, and Costill, DL. Plasma lactate accumulation and distance running performance. *Med Sci Sports Exerc* 11:338-344, 1979.

32. Foster, C, Daniels, JT, and Yarbrough, RA. Physiological and training correlates of marathon running performance. *Aust J Sports Med* 9:58-61, 1977.

33. Foster, C, Hector, LL, Welsh, R, Schrager, M, Green, MA, and Snyder, AC. Effects of specific versus cross-training on running performance. *Eur J Appl Physiol Occup Physiol* 70:367-372, 1995.

34. Foxdal, P, Sjödin, B, Sjödin, A, and Ostman, B. The validity and accuracy of blood lactate measurements for prediction of maximal endurance running capacity. Dependency of analyzed blood media in combination with different designs of the exercise test. *Int J Sports Med* 15:89-95, 1994.

35. Garber, CE, Blissmer, B, Deschenes, MR, Franklin, BA, Lamonte, MJ, Lee, IM, Nieman, DC, and Swain, DP. American College of Sports Medicine position stand. Quantity and quality of exercise for developing and maintaining cardiorespiratory, musculoskeletal, and neuromotor fitness in apparently healthy adults: Guidance for prescribing exercise. *Med Sci Sports Exerc* 43:1334-1359, 2011.

36. Gardner, AS, Stephens, S, Martin, DT, Lawton, E, Lee, H, and Jenkins, D. Accuracy of SRM and power tap power monitoring systems for bicycling. *Med Sci Sports Exerc* 36:1252-1258, 2004.

37. Gergley, TJ, McArdle, WD, DeJesus, P, Toner, MM, Jacobowitz, S, and Spina, RJ. Specificity of arm training on aerobic power during swimming and running. *Med Sci Sports Exerc* 16:349-354, 1984.

38. Gettman, LR, Pollock, ML, Durstine, JL, Ward, A, Ayres, J, and Linnerud, AC. Physiological responses of men to 1, 3, and 5 day per week training programs. *Res Q* 47:638-646, 1976.

39. Glass, SC, Knowlton, RG, and Becque, MD. Accuracy of RPE from graded exercise to establish exercise training intensity. *Med Sci Sports Exerc* 24:1303-1307, 1992.

40. Gollnick, PD. Metabolism of substrates: Energy substrate metabolism during exercise and as modified by training. *Fed Proc* 44:353-357, 1985.

41. Haddad, M, Padulo, J, and Chamari, K. The usefulness of session rating of perceived exertion for monitoring training load despite several influences on perceived exertion. *Int J Sport Physiol Perform* 9:882-883, 2014.

42. Hagerman, PS. Aerobic endurance training program design. In *NSCA's Essentials of Personal Training.* 2nd ed. Coburn, JW, and Malek, MH, eds. Champaign, IL: Human Kinetics, 389-410, 2012.

43. Hansen, AK, Fischer, CP, Plomgaard, P, Andersen, JL, Saltin, B, and Pedersen, BK. Skeletal muscle adaptation: Training twice every second day vs. training once daily. *J Appl Physiol* 98:93-99, 2005.

44. Hermansen, L, Hultman, E, and Saltin, B. Muscle glycogen during prolonged severe exercise. *Acta Physiol Scand* 71:129-139, 1967.

45. Hickson, RC, Dvorak, BA, Gorostiaga, EM, Kurowski, TT, and Foster, C. Potential for strength and endurance training to amplify endurance performance. *J Appl Physiol* 65:2285-2290, 1988.

46. Hickson, RC, and Rosenkoetter, MA. Reduced training frequencies and maintenance of increased aerobic power. *Med Sci Sports Exerc* 13:13-16, 1981.

47. Holloszy, JO, and Booth, FW. Biochemical adaptations to endurance exercise in muscle. *Annu Rev Physiol* 38:273-291, 1976.

48. Holloszy, JO, and Coyle, EF. Adaptations of skeletal muscle to endurance exercise and their metabolic consequences. *J Appl Physiol* 56:831-838, 1984.

49. Hootman, JM, Macera, CA, Ainsworth, BE, Martin, M, Addy, CL, and Blair, SN. Association among physical activity level, cardiorespiratory fitness, and risk of musculoskeletal injury. *Am J Epidemiol* 154:251-258, 2001.

50. Hoppeler, H. Exercise-induced ultrastructural changes in skeletal muscle. *Int J Sports Med* 7:187-204, 1986.

51. Humberstone-Gough, CE, Saunders, PU, Bonetti, DL, Stephens, S, Bullock, N, Anson, JM, and Gore, CJ. Comparison of live high: train low altitude and intermittent hypoxic exposure. *J Sports Sci Med* 12:394-401, 2013.

52. Klausen, K, Andersen, LB, and Pelle, I. Adaptive changes in work capacity, skeletal muscle capillarization and enzyme levels during training and detraining. *Acta Physiol Scand* 113:9-16, 1981.

53. Kohrt, WM, Morgan, DW, Bates, B, and Skinner, JS. Physiological responses of triathletes to maximal swimming, cycling, and running. *Med Sci Sports Exerc* 19:51-55, 1987.

54. Lamb, DR. Basic principles for improving sport performance. *Gatorade Sports Science Exchange* 8:1-5, 1995.

55. Laursen, PB, and Jenkins, DG. The scientific basis for high-intensity interval training: Optimising training programmes and maximising performance in highly trained endurance athletes. *Sports Med* 32:53-73, 2002.

56. Magel, JR, Foglia, GF, McArdle, WD, Gutin, B, Pechar, GS, and Katch, FI. Specificity of swim training on maximum oxygen uptake. *J Appl Physiol* 38:151-155, 1975.

57. Martin, JC, Milliken, DL, Cobb, JE, McFadden, KL, and Coggan, AR. Validation of a mathematical model for road cycling power. *J Appl Biomech* 14:276-291, 1998.

58. Matoba, H, and Gollnick, PD. Response of skeletal muscle to training. *Sports Med* 1:240-251, 1984.

59. Maughan, RJ. Physiology and biochemistry of middle distance and long distance running. In *Handbook of Sports Medicine and Science: Running*. Hawley, JA, ed. Oxford, UK: Blackwell Science, 14-27, 2000.

60. Maughan, RJ, and Leiper, JB. Aerobic capacity and fractional utilisation of aerobic capacity in elite and non-elite male and female marathon runners. *Eur J Appl Physiol Occup Physiol* 52:80-87, 1983.

61. McCole, SD, Claney, K, Conte, JC, Anderson, R, and Hagberg, JM. Energy expenditure during bicycling. *J Appl Physiol* 68:748-753, 1990.

62. Mikkola, J, Vesterinen, V, Taipale, R, Capostagno, B, Häkkinen, K, and Nummela, A. Effect of resistance training regimens on treadmill running and neuromuscular performance in recreational endurance runners. *J Sports Sci* 29:1359-1371, 2011.

63. Mujika, I, Padilla, S, Pyne, D, and Busso, T. Physiological changes associated with the pre-event taper in athletes. *Sports Med* 34:891-927, 2004.

64. Neary, JP, Martin, TP, Reid, DC, Burnham, R, and Quinney, HA. The effects of a reduced exercise duration taper programme on performance and muscle enzymes of endurance cyclists. *Eur J Appl Physiol Occup Physiol* 65:30-36, 1992.

65. O'Toole, ML, Douglas, PS, and Hiller, WDB. Use of heart rate monitors by endurance athletes: Lessons from triathletes. *J Sports Med Phys Fitness* 38:181-187, 1998.

66. Peacock, AJ. ABC of oxygen: Oxygen at high altitude. *Br Med J* 317:1063-1066, 1998.

67. Perrault, H. Cardiorespiratory function. In *Exercise and the Female: A Life Span Approach (Perspectives in Exercise Science and Sports Medicine series, vol. 9)*. Carmel, IN: Cooper Publishing Group, 147-214, 1996.

68. Pette, D. Historical perspectives: Plasticity of mammalian skeletal muscle. *J Appl Physiol* 90:1119-1124, 2001.

69. Pollock, ML, Gettman, LR, Milesis, CA, Bah, MD, Durstine, L, and Johnson, RB. Effects of frequency and duration of training on attrition and incidence of injury. *Med Sci Sports Exerc* 9:31-36, 1977.

70. Potteiger, JA, and Evans, BW. Using heart rate and ratings of perceived exertion to monitor intensity in runners. *J Sport Med Phys Fit* 35:181-186, 1995.

71. Potteiger, JA, and Weber, SF. Rating of perceived exertion and heart rate as indicators of exercise intensity in different environmental temperatures. *Med Sci Sports Exerc* 26:791-796, 1994.

72. Powers, SK, and Howley, ET. *Exercise Physiology: Theory and Application to Fitness and Performance*. 8th ed. New York: McGraw-Hill, 283-284, 2011.

73. Saltin, B, Henriksson, J, Nygaard, E, Andersen, P, and Jansson, E. Fiber types and metabolic potentials of skeletal muscles in sedentary man and endurance runners. *Ann NY Acad Sci* 301:3-29, 1977.

74. Sharkey, BJ. Intensity and duration of training and the development of cardiorespiratory endurance. *Med Sci Sports Exerc* 2:197-202, 1970.

75. Shepley, B, MacDougall, JD, Cipriano, N, Sutton, JR, Tarnopolsky, MA, and Coates, G. Physiological effects of tapering in highly trained athletes. *J Appl Physiol* 72:706-711, 1992.

76. Short, KR, Vittone, JL, Bigelow, ML, Proctor, DN, Coenen-Schimke, JM, Rys, P, and Nair, KS. Changes in myosin heavy chain mRNA and protein expression in human skeletal muscle with age and endurance exercise training. *J Appl Physiol* 99:95-102, 2005.

77. Svedenhag, J. Endurance conditioning. In *Endurance in Sport (Encyclopaedia of Sports Medicine Series)*. 2nd ed. Shephard, RJ, and Åstrand, PO, eds. London: Blackwell Science, 402-408, 2008.

78. Swain, DP, Coast, JR, Clifford, PS, Milliken, MC, and Stray-Gundersen, J. Influence of body size on oxygen consumption during bicycling. *J Appl Physiol* 62:668-672, 1987.

79. Thomas, L, Mujika, I, and Busso, T. A model study of optimal training reduction during pre-event taper in elite swimmers. *J Sports Sci* 26:643-652, 2008.

80. Troup, JP. The physiology and biomechanics of competitive swimming. *Clin Sports Med* 18:267-285, 1999.

81. Van Handel, PJ, Katz, A, Troup, JP, and Bradley, PW. Aerobic economy and competitive swim performance of U.S. elite swimmers. In *Swimming Science V*. Ungerechts, BE, Wilke, K, and Reischle, K, eds. Champaign, IL: Human Kinetics, 219-227, 1988.

82. Wells, CL, and Pate, RR. Training for performance of prolonged exercise. In *Perspectives in Exercise Science and Sports Medicine*. Lamb, DL, and Murray, R, eds. Indianapolis: Benchmark Press, 357-388, 1995.

83. Wenger, HA, and Bell, GJ. The interactions of intensity, frequency and duration of exercise training in altering cardiorespiratory fitness. *Sports Med* 3:346-356, 1986.

84. Wilber, RL. Application of altitude/hypoxic training by elite athletes. *Med Sci Sports Exerc* 39:1610-1624, 2007.

85. Wilber, RL, Moffatt, RJ, Scott, BE, Lee, DT, and Cucuzzo, NA. Influence of water run training on the maintenance of aerobic performance. *Med Sci Sports Exerc* 28:1056-1062, 1996.

86. Wyatt, FB. Physiological responses to attitude: A brief review. *J Exerc Physiol Online* 17:90-96, 2014.

87. Zupan, MF, and Petosa, PS. Aerobic and resistance cross-training for peak triathlon performance. *Strength Cond J* 17:7-12, 1995.

CHAPTER 21   Periodization

1. Baker, D, Wilson, G, and Carlyon, R. Periodization: The effect on strength of manipulating volume and intensity. *J Strength Cond Res* 8:235-242, 1994.

2. Bompa, TO. Antrenamentul in perooda, pregatitoare. *Caiet Pentre Sporturi Nautice* 3:22-24, 1956.

3. Bompa, TO, and Haff, GG. *Periodization: Theory and Methodology of Training*. Champaign, IL: Human Kinetics, 1-424, 2009.

4. Bondarchuk, AP. Track and field training. *Legkaya Atletika* 12:8-9, 1986.

5. Bondarchuk, AP. Constructing a training system. *Track Tech* 102:254-269, 1988.

6. Bondarchuk, AP. The role and sequence of using different training-load intensities. *Fit Sports Rev Inter* 29:202-204, 1994.

7. Bosquet, L, Montpetit, J, Arvisais, D, and Mujika, I. Effects of tapering on performance: A meta-analysis. *Med Sci Sports Exerc* 39:1358-1365, 2007.

8. Bradley-Popovich, GE, and Haff, GG. Nonlinear versus linear periodization models. *Strength Cond J* 23:42-44, 2001.

9. Bruin, G, Kuipers, H, Keizer, HA, and Vander Vusse, GJ. Adaptation and overtraining in horses subjected to increasing training loads. *J Appl Physiol* 76:1908-1913, 1994.

10. Buford, TW, Rossi, SJ, Smith, DB, and Warren, AJ. A comparison of periodization models during nine weeks with equated volume and intensity for strength. *J Strength Cond Res* 21:1245-1250, 2007.

11. Charniga, A, Gambetta, V, Kraemer, W, Newton, H, O'Bryant, HS, Palmieri, G, Pedemonte, J, Pfaff, D, and Stone, MH. Periodization: Part 1. *NSCA J* 8:12-22, 1986.

12. Charniga, A, Gambetta, V, Kraemer, W, Newton, H, O'Bryant, HS, Palmieri, G, Pedemonte, J, Pfaff, D, and Stone, MH. Periodization: Part 2. *NSCA J* 8:17-24, 1986.

13. Charniga, A, Gambetta, V, Kraemer, W, Newton, H, O'Bryant, HS, Palmieri, G, Pedemonte, J, Pfaff, D, and Stone, MH. Periodization: Part 3. *NSCA J* 9:16-26, 1987.

14. Chiu, LZF, and Barnes, JL. The fitness-fatigue model revistited: Implications for planning short- and long-term training. *NSCA J* 25:42-51, 2003.

15. Counsilman, JE, and Counsilman, BE. *The New Science of Swimming.* Englewood Cliffs, NJ: Prentice Hall, 229-244, 1994.

16. de Lima, C, Boullosa, DA, Frollini, AB, Donatto, FF, Leite, RD, Gonelli, PR, Montebello, MI, Prestes, J, and Cesar, MC. Linear and daily undulating resistance training periodizations have differential beneficial effects in young sedentary women. *Int J Sports Med* 33:723-727, 2012.

17. Edington, DW, and Edgerton, VR. *The Biology of Physical Activity.* Boston: Houghton Mifflin, 1-120, 1976.

18. Fleck, S, and Kraemer, WJ. *Designing Resistance Training Programs.* 4th ed. Champaign, IL: Human Kinetics, 1-375, 2004.

19. Foster, C. Monitoring training in athletes with reference to overtraining syndrome. *Med Sci Sports Exerc* 30:1164-1168, 1998.

20. Fry, AC. The role of training intensity in resistance exercise overtraining and overreaching. In *Overtraining in Sport.* Kreider, RB, Fry, AC, and O'Toole, ML, eds. Champaign, IL: Human Kinetics, 107-127, 1998.

21. Garhammer, J. Periodization of strength training for athletes. *Track Tech* 73:2398-2399, 1979.

22. Haff, GG. Periodization of training. In *Conditioning for Strength and Human Performance.* 2nd ed. Brown, LE, and Chandler, J, eds. Philadelphia: Wolters-Kluwer/Lippincott Williams & Wilkins, 326-345, 2012.

23. Haff, GG. Peaking for competition in individual sports. In *High-Performance Training for Sports.* Joyce, D, and Lewindon, D, eds. Champaign, IL: Human Kinetics, 524-540, 2014.

24. Haff, GG. Periodization strategies for youth development. In *Strength and Conditioning for Young Athletes: Science and Application.* Lloyd, RS, and Oliver, JL, eds. London: Routledge, Taylor & Francis, 149-168, 2014.

25. Haff, GG. The essentials of periodization. In *Strength and Conditioning for Sports Performance.* Jeffreys, I, and Moody, J, eds. London: Routledge, Taylor & Francis, in press

26. Haff, GG, and Burgess, SJ. Resistance training for endurance sports. In *Developing Endurance.* Reuter, BH, ed. Champaign, IL: Human Kinetics, 135-180, 2012.

27. Haff, GG, and Haff, EE. Resistance training program design. In *Essentials of Periodization.* Malek, MH, and Coburn, JW, eds. Champaign, IL: Human Kinetics, 359-401, 2012.

28. Haff, GG, and Haff, EE. Training integration and periodization. In *Strength and Conditioning Program Design.* Hoffman, J, ed. Champaign, IL: Human Kinetics, 209-254, 2012.

29. Haff, GG, Kraemer, WJ, O'Bryant, HS, Pendlay, G, Plisk, S, and Stone, MH. Roundtable discussion: Periodization of training—part 1. *NSCA J* 26 (Pt 1):50-69, 2004.

30. Haff, GG, Kraemer, WJ, O'Bryant, HS, Pendlay, G, Plisk, S, and Stone, MH. Roundtable discussion: Periodization of training—part 2. *NSCA J* 26 (Pt 2):56-70, 2004.

31. Haff, GG, and Nimphius, S. Training principles for power. *Strength Cond J* 34:2-12, 2012.

32. Harre, D. Principles of athletic training. In *Principles of Sports Training: Introduction to the Theory and Methods of Training.* Harre, D, ed. Berlin: Sportverlag, 73-94, 1982.

33. Harre, D. *Principles of Sports Training.* Berlin: Sportverlag, 10-94, 1982.

34. Hartmann, H, Bob, A, Wirth, K, and Schmidtbleicher, D. Effects of different periodization models on rate of force development and power ability of the upper extremity. *J Strength Cond Res* 23:1921-1932, 2009.

35. Hoffman, JR, Ratamess, NA, Klatt, M, Faigenbaum, AD, Ross, RE, Tranchina, NM, McCurley, RC, Kang, J, and Kraemer, WJ. Comparison between different off-season resistance training programs in Division III American college football players. *J Strength Cond Res* 23:11-19, 2009.

36. Issurin, V. *Block Periodization: Breakthrough in Sports Training.* Muskegon, MI: Ultimate Athlete Concepts, 1-213, 2008.

37. Issurin, VB. New horizons for the methodology and physiology of training periodization. *Sports Med* 40:189-206, 2010.

38. Kawamori, N, Crum, AJ, Blumert, P, Kulik, J, Childers, J, Wood, J, Stone, MH, and Haff, GG. Influence of different relative intensities on power output during the hang power clean: Identification of the optimal load. *J Strength Cond Res* 19:698-708, 2005.

39. Kawamori, N, and Haff, GG. The optimal training load for the development of muscular power. *J Strength Cond Res* 18:675-684, 2004.

40. Komi, PV. Training of muscle strength and power: Interaction of neuromotoric, hypertrophic, and mechanical factors. *Int J Sports Med* 7:10-15, 1986.

41. Kraemer, WJ. A series of studies: The physiological basis for strength training in American football: Fact over philosophy. *J Strength Cond Res* 11:131-142, 1997.

42. Kraemer, WJ, and Fleck, SJ. *Optimizing Strength Training: Designing Nonlinear Periodization Workouts.* Champaign, IL: Human Kinetics, 1-245, 2007.

43. Matveyev, L. *Periodization of Sports Training.* Moscow: Fizkultura i Sport, 1965.

44. Matveyev, LP. *Fundamentals of Sports Training.* Moscow: Fizkultua i Sport, 86-298, 1977.

45. McNamara, JM, and Stearne, DJ. Flexible nonlinear periodization in a beginner college weight training class. *J Strength Cond Res* 24:17-22, 2010.

46. Meeusen, R, Duclos, M, Foster, C, Fry, A, Gleeson, M, Nieman, D, Raglin, J, Rietjens, G, Steinacker, J, and Urhausen, A. Prevention, diagnosis, and treatment of the overtraining syndrome: Joint consensus statement of the European College of Sport Science and the American College of Sports Medicine. *Med Sci Sports Exerc* 45:186-205, 2013.

47. Miranda, F, Simao, R, Rhea, M, Bunker, D, Prestes, J, Leite, RD, Miranda, H, de Salles, BF, and Novaes, J. Effects of linear vs. daily undulatory periodized resistance training on maximal and submaximal strength gains. *J Strength Cond Res* 25:1824-1830, 2011.

48. Nádori, L. *Training and Competition.* Budapest: Sport, 1962.

49. Nádori, L, and Granek, I. *Theoretical and Methodological Basis of Training Planning With Special Considerations Within a Microcycle.* Lincoln, NE: NSCA, 1-63,1989.

50. Painter, KB, Haff, GG, Ramsey, MW, McBride, J, Triplett, T, Sands, WA, Lamont, HS, Stone, ME, and Stone, MH. Strength gains: Block vs daily undulating periodization weight-training among track and field athletes. *Int J Sports Physiol Perform* 7:161-169, 2012.

51. Plisk, SS, and Stone, MH. Periodization strategies. *Strength Cond* 25:19-37, 2003.

52. Prestes, J, Frollini, AB, de Lima, C, Donatto, FF, Foschini, D, de Cassia, Marqueti, R, Figueira, A, Jr., and Fleck, SJ. Comparison between linear and daily undulating periodized resistance training to increase strength. *J Strength Cond Res* 23:2437-2442, 2009.

53. Rhea, MR, Ball, SD, Phillips, WT, and Burkett, LN. A comparison of linear and daily undulating periodized programs with equated volume and intensity for strength. *J Strength Cond Res* 16:250-255, 2002.

54. Selye, H. *The Stress of Life.* New York: McGraw-Hill, 1-324, 1956.

55. Selye, H. A syndrome produced by diverse nocuous agents. 1936. *J Neuropsych Clin Neurosci* 10:230-231, 1998.

56. Stone, MH, and O'Bryant, HO. *Weight Training: A Scientific Approach.* Edina, MN: Burgess, 1-361, 1987.

57. Stone, MH, O'Bryant, H, and Garhammer, J. A hypothetical model for strength training. *J Sports Med* 21:342-351, 1981.

58. Stone, MH, O'Bryant, HS, and Garhammer, J. A theoretical model of strength training. *NSCA J* 3:36-39, 1982.

59. Stone, MH, Stone, ME, and Sands, WA. *Principles and Practice of Resistance Training.* Champaign, IL: Human Kinetics, 241-287, 2007.

60. Stone, MH, and Wathen, D. Letter to the editor. *NSCA J* 23:7-9, 2001.

61. Tschiene, P. Finally a theory of training to overcome doping. *Athletics Science Bulletin* 1:30-34, 1989.

62. Tschiene, P. A necessary direction in training: The integration of biological adaptation in the training program. *Coach Sport Sci J* 1:2-14, 1995.

63. Verkhoshansky, YU. Theory and methodology of sport preparation: Block training system for top-level athletes. *Teoria i Practica Physicheskoj Culturi* 4:2-14, 2007.

64. Verkhoshansky, YU, and Verkhoshansky, N. *Special Strength Training Manual for Coaches.* Rome: Verkhosansky STM, 27-142, 2011.

65. Zatsiorsky, VM. *Science and Practice of Strength Training.* Champaign, IL: Human Kinetics, 3-18, 108-133, 1995.

66. Zatsiorsky, VM, and Kraemer, WJ. *Science and Practice of Strength Training.* 2nd ed. Champaign, IL: Human Kinetics, 3-14, 89-108, 2006.

CHAPTER 22   Rehabilitation and Reconditioning

1. Adams, D, Logerstedt, DS, Hunter-Giordano, A, Axe, MJ, and Snyder-Mackler, L. Current concepts for anterior cruciate ligament reconstruction: A criterion-based rehabilitation progression. *J Orthop Sports Phys Ther* 42:601-614, 2012.

2. Alentorn-Geli, E, Myer, G, Silvers, H, Samitier, G, Romero, D, Lázaro-Haro, C, and Cugat, R. Prevention of non-contact anterior cruciate ligament injuries in soccer players. Part 1: Mechanisms of injury and underlying risk factors. *Knee Surg Sports Traumatol Arthrosc* 17:705-729, 2009.

3. Behrens, SB, Deren, ME, Matson, A, Fadale, PD, and Monchik, KO. Stress fractures of the pelvis and legs in athletes: A review. *Sports Health* 5:165-174, 2013.

4. Burkhart, SS, Johnson, TC, Wirth, MA, and Athanasiou, KA. Cyclic loading of transosseous rotator cuff repairs: Tension overload as a possible cause of failure. *Arthroscopy* 13:172-176, 1997.

5. Byl, NN, McKenzie, AL, West, JM, Whitney, JD, Hunt, TK, and Scheuenstuhl, HA. Low-dose ultrasound effects on wound healing: A controlled study with yucatan pigs. *Arch Phys Med Rehabil* 73:656-664, 1992.

6. Byram, IR, Bushnell, BD, Dugger, K, Charron, K, Harrell, FE, and Noonan, TJ. Preseason shoulder strength measurements in professional baseball pitchers: Identifying players at risk for injury. *Am J Sports Med* 38:1375-1382, 2010.

7. Clarsen, B, Bahr, R, Andersson, SH, Munk, R, and Myklebust, G. Reduced glenohumeral rotation, external rotation weakness and scapular dyskinesis are risk factors for shoulder injuries among elite male handball players: A prospective cohort study. *Br J Sports Med* 48:1327-1333, 2014.

8. Courson, R, Goldenberg, M, Adams, KG, Anderson, SA, Colgate, B, Cooper, L, Dewald, L, Floyd, RT, Gregory, DB, Indelicato, PA, Klossner, D, O'Leary, R, Ray, T, Selgo, T, Thompson, C, and Turbak, G. Inter-association consensus statement on best practices for sports medicine management for secondary schools and colleges. *J Athl Train* 49:128-137, 2014.

9. De Lorme, TL. Restoration of muscle power by heavy resistance exercise. *J Bone Joint Surg* 27:645-667, 1945.

10. De Lorme, TL, and Watkins, AL. Technics of progressive resistance exercise. *Arch Phys Med* 29:263-273, 1948.

11. Dwelly, PM, Tripp, BL, Tripp, PA, Eberman, LE, and Gorin, S. Glenohumeral rotational range of motion in collegiate overhead-throwing athletes during an athletic season. *J Athl Train* 44:611-616, 2009.

12. Fleck, SJ, and Kraemer, WJ. *Designing Resistance Training Programs.* Champaign, IL: Human Kinetics, 2014.

13. Freeman, MAR, and Wybe, B. Articular contributions to limb muscle reflexes: The effects of a partial neurectomy of the knee joint on postural reflexes. *Br J Surg* 53:61, 1966.

14. Fukuda, TY, Melo, WP, Zaffalon, BM, Rossetto, FM, Magalhaes, E, Bryk, FF, and Martin, RL. Hip posterolateral musculature strengthening in sedentary women with patellofemoral pain syndrome: A randomized controlled clinical trial with 1-year follow-up. *J Orthop Sports Phys Ther* 42:823-830, 2012.

15. Gilchrist, J, Mandelbaum, BR, Melancon, H, Ryan, GW, Silvers, HJ, Griffin, LY, Watanabe, DS, Dick, RW, and Dvorak, J. A randomized controlled trial to prevent noncontact anterior cruciate ligament injury in female collegiate soccer players. *Am J Sports Med* 36:1476-1483, 2008.

16. Grindstaff, TL, and Potach, DH. Prevention of common wrestling injuries. *Strength Cond J* 28:20-28, 2006.

17. Grooms, DR, Palmer, T, Onate, JA, Myer, GD, and Grindstaff, T. Soccer-specific warm-up and lower extremity injury rates in collegiate male soccer players. *J Athl Train* 48:782-789, 2013.

18. Gross, MT. Chronic tendinitis: Pathomechanics of injury, factors affecting the healing response, and treatment. *J Orthop Sports Phys Ther* 16:248-261, 1992.

19. Hägglund, M, Waldén, M, and Ekstrand, J. Previous injury as a risk factor for injury in elite football: A prospective study over two consecutive seasons. *Br J Sports Med* 40:767-772, 2006.

20. Herring, SA, Kibler, WB, and Putukian, M. Team physician consensus statement: 2013 update. *Med Sci Sports Exerc* 45:1618-1622, 2013.

21. Hewett, TE, Lindenfeld, TN, Riccobene, JV, and Noyes, FR. The effect of neuromuscular training on the incidence of knee injury in female athletes: A prospective study. *Am J Sports Med* 27:699-706, 1999.

22. Hildebrand, KA, Gallant-Behm, CL, Kydd, AS, and Hart, DA. The basics of soft tissue healing and general factors that influence such healing. *Sports Med Arthrosc* 13:136-144, 2005.

23. Hillman, S. Principles and techniques of open kinetic chain rehabilitation: The upper extremity. *J Sport Rehabil* 3:319-330, 1994.

24. Houglum, PA. Soft tissue healing and its impact on rehabilitation *J Sport Rehabil* 1:19-39, 1992.

25. Hurd, WJ, Kaplan, KM, Eiattrache, NS, Jobe, FW, Morrey, BF, and Kaufman, KR. A profile of glenohumeral internal and external rotation motion in the uninjured high school baseball pitcher, part I: Motion. *J Athl Train* 46:282-288, 2011.

26. Ireland, ML, Willson, JD, Ballantyne, BT, and Davis, IM. Hip strength in females with and without patellofemoral pain. *J Orthop Sports Phys Ther* 33:671-676, 2003.

27. Jackson, BA, Schwane, JA, and Starcher, BC. Effect of ultrasound therapy on the repair of achilles tendon injuries in rats. *Med Sci Sports Exerc* 23:171-176, 1991.

28. Knapik, JJ, Mawdsley, RH, and Ramos, MU. Angular specificity and test mode specificity of isometric and isokinetic strength training. *J Orthop Sports Phys Ther* 5:58-65, 1983.

29. Knight, KL. Knee rehabilitation by the daily adjustable progressive resistive exercise technique. *Am J Sports Med* 7:336-337, 1979.

30. Knight, KL. Quadriceps strengthening with the dapre technique: Case studies with neurological implications. *Med Sci Sports Exerc* 17:646-650, 1985.

31. Lankhorst, NE, Bierma-Zeinstra, SMA, and Middelkoop, MV. Risk factors for patellofemoral pain syndrome: A systematic review. *J Orthop Sports Phys Ther* 42:81-94, 2012.

32. Leadbetter, WB. Cell-matrix response in tendon injury. *Clin Sports Med* 11:533-578, 1992.

33. Lee, M, and Carroll, TJ. Cross education: Possible mechanisms for the contralateral effects of unilateral resistance training. *Sports Med* 37:1-14, 2007.

34. Lee, M, Gandevia, SC, and Carroll, TJ. Unilateral strength training increases voluntary activation of the opposite untrained limb. *Clin Neurophysiol* 120:802-808, 2009.

35. Leggin, BG, Sheridan, S, and Eckenrode, BJ. Rehabilitation after surgical management of the thrower's shoulder. *Sports Med Arthrosc* 20:49-55, 2012.

36. Leighton, JR, Holmes, D, Benson, J, Wooten, B, and Schmerer, R. A study of the effectiveness of ten different methods of progressive resistance exercise on the development of strength, flexibility, girth, and body weight. *J Assoc Phys Ment Rehabil* 21:78-81, 1967.

37. Logerstedt, D, Lynch, A, Axe, M, and Snyder-Mackler, L. Symmetry restoration and functional recovery before and after anterior cruciate ligament reconstruction. *Knee Surg Sports Traumatol Arthrosc* 21:859-868, 2013.

38. Lorenz, D, and Reiman, M. The role and implementation of eccentric training in athletic rehabilitation: Tendinopathy, hamstring strains, and ACL reconstruction. *Int J Sports Phys Ther* 6:27-44, 2011.

39. Mandelbaum, BR, Silvers, HJ, Watanabe, DS, Knarr, JF, Thomas, SD, Griffin, LY, Kirkendall, DT, and Garrett, W Jr. Effectiveness of a neuromuscular and proprioceptive training program in preventing anterior cruciate ligament injuries in female athletes: 2-year follow-up. *Am J Sports Med* 33:1003-1010, 2005.

40. Martimbianco, ALC, Gomes-da Silva, BN, de Carvalho, APV, Silva, V, Torloni, MR, and Peccin, MS. Effectiveness and safety of cryotherapy after arthroscopic anterior cruciate ligament reconstruction. A systematic review of the literature. *Phys Ther Sport* 15:261-268, 2014.

41. Mascal, CL, Landel, R, and Powers, C. Management of patellofemoral pain targeting hip, pelvis, and trunk muscle function: 2 case reports. *J Orthop Sports Phys Ther* 33:647-660, 2003.

42. McMorris, RO, and Elkins, EC. A study of production and evaluation of muscular hypertrophy. *Arch Phys Med Rehabil* 35:420-426, 1954.

43. Mellion, MB, Walsh, WM, and Shelton, GL. *The Team Physician's Handbook*. Philadelphia: Hanley & Belfus, 1-150, 1997.

44. Mueller, MJ, and Maluf, KS. Tissue adaptation to physical stress: A proposed "physical stress theory" to guide physical therapist practice, education, and research. *Phys Ther* 82:383-403, 2002.

45. Myer, GD, Martin, L, Ford, KR, Paterno, MV, Schmitt, LC, Heidt, RS, Colosimo, A, and Hewett, TE. No association of time from surgery with functional deficits in athletes after anterior cruciate ligament reconstruction: Evidence for objective return-to-sport criteria. *Am J Sports Med* 40:2256-2263, 2012.

46. Nichols, AW. Does eccentric training of hamstring muscles reduce acute injuries in soccer? *Clin J Sport Med* 23:85-86, 2013.

47. Nilstad, A, Andersen, TE, Bahr, R, Holme, I, and Steffen, K. Risk factors for lower extremity injuries in elite female soccer players. *Am J Sports Med* 42:940-948, 2014.

48. Olsen, OE, Myklebust, G, Engebretsen, L, Holme, I, and Bahr, R. Exercises to prevent lower limb injuries in youth sports: Cluster randomised controlled trial. *Br Med J* 330:449, 2005.

49. Paterno, MV, Rauh, MJ, Schmitt, LC, Ford, KR, and Hewett, TE. Incidence of second ACL injuries 2 years after primary ACL reconstruction and return to sport. *Am J Sports Med*, 42:1567-1573, 2014.

50. Petersen, J, Thorborg, K, Nielsen, MB, Budtz-Jørgensen, E, and Hölmich, P. Preventive effect of eccentric training on acute hamstring injuries in men's soccer: A cluster-randomized controlled trial. *Am J Sports Med* 39:2296-2303, 2011.

51. Ramirez, A, Schwane, JA, McFarland, C, and Starcher, BC. The effect of ultrasound on collagen synthesis and fibroblast proliferation in vitro. *Med Sci Sports Exerc* 29:326-332, 1997.

52. Rees, JD, Maffulli, N, and Cook, J. Management of tendinopathy. *Am J Sports Med* 37:1855-1867, 2009.

53. Riemann, BL, and Lephart, SM. The sensorimotor system, part II: The role of proprioception in motor control and functional joint stability. *J Athl Train* 37:80-84, 2002.

54. Saragiotto, B, Yamato, T, Hespanhol, L, Jr., Rainbow, M, Davis, I, and Lopes, A. What are the main risk factors for running-related injuries? *Sports Med* 44:1153-1163, 2014.

55. Schmitt, LC, Paterno, MV, and Hewett, TE. The impact of quadriceps femoris strength asymmetry on functional performance at return to sport following anterior cruciate ligament reconstruction. *J Orthop Sports Phys Ther* 42:750-759, 2012.

56. Steindler, A. *Kinesiology of the Human Body Under Normal and Pathological Conditions*. Springfield, IL: Charles C Thomas, 82, 1955.

57. Stone, M, and O'Bryant, H. *Weight Training: A Scientific Approach*. Minneapolis: Burgess International, 1987.

58. Sugimoto, D, Myer, G, Barber-Foss, K, and Hewett, T. Dosage effects of neuromuscular training intervention to reduce anterior cruciate ligament injuries in female athletes: Meta- and sub-group analyses. *Sports Med* 44:551-562, 2014.

59. Tate, A, Turner, GN, Knab, SE, Jorgensen, C, Strittmatter, A, and Michener, LA. Risk factors associated with shoulder pain and disability across the lifespan of competitive swimmers. *J Athl Train* 47:149-158, 2012.

60. Tippett, SR. *Coaches Guide to Sport Rehabilitation*. Champaign, IL: Leisure Press, 1990.

61. Tordi, N, Belli, A, Mougin, F, Rouillon, JD, and Gimenez, M. Specific and transfer effects induced by arm or leg training. *Int J Sports Med* 22:517-524, 2001.

62. van den Bekerom, MP, Struijs, PA, Blankevoort, L, Welling, L, van Dijk, CN, and Kerkhoffs, GM. What is the evidence for rest, ice, compression, and elevation therapy in the treatment of ankle sprains in adults? *J Athl Train* 47:435-443, 2012.

63. Voight, ML, and Cook, G. Clinical application of closed kinetic chain exercises. *J Sport Rehabil* 5:25-44, 1996.

64. Voight, ML, and Thomson, BC. The role of the scapula in the rehabilitation of shoulder injuries. *J Athl Train* 35:364-372, 2000.

65. Wathen, D. Communication: Athletic trainer/conditioning coach relations—communication is the key. *NSCA J* 6:32-33, 1984.

66. Wilder, RP, and Sethi, S. Overuse injuries: Tendinopathies, stress fractures, compartment syndrome, and shin splints. *Clin Sports Med* 23:55-81, 2004.

67. Wilk, KE, and Arrigo, CA. An integrated approach to upper extremity exercises. *Orthop Phys Ther Clin N Am* 1:337, 1992.

68. Wilk, KE, Arrigo, CA, and Andrews, JR. The rehabilitation program of the thrower's elbow. *J Orthop Sports Phys Ther* 17:225-239, 1993.

69. Wilk, KE, Macrina, LC, Cain, EL, Dugas, JR, and Andrews, JR. Rehabilitation of the overhead athlete's elbow. *Sports Health* 4:404-414, 2012.

70. Wilk, KE, Macrina, LC, Fleisig, GS, Aune, KT, Porterfield, RA, Harker, P, Evans, TJ, and Andrews, JR. Deficits in glenohumeral passive range of motion increase risk of elbow injury in professional baseball pitchers: A prospective study. *Am J Sports Med* 42:2075-2081, 2014.

71. Wilk, KE, Yenchak, AJ, Arrigo, CA, and Andrews, JR. The advanced throwers ten exercise program: A new exercise series for enhanced dynamic shoulder control in the overhead throwing athlete. *Phys Sportsmed* 39:90-97, 2011.

72. Willems, TM, Witvrouw, E, Delbaere, K, Mahieu, N, De Bourdeaudhuij, I, and De Clercq, D. Intrinsic risk factors for inversion ankle sprains in male subjects: A prospective study. *Am J Sports Med* 33:415-423, 2005.

73. Zinovieff, AN. Heavy resistance exercise: The Oxford technique. *Br J Phys Med* 14:129, 1951.

CHAPTER 23 Facility Design, Layout, and Organization

1. Abbott, AA. Fitness facility orientation. *ACSMs Health Fit J* 15(3):38-40, 2011.

2. *ACSM's Health/Fitness Facility Standards and Guidelines.* Champaign, IL: Human Kinetics, 49-72, 2012.

3. Armitage-Johnson, S. Providing a safe training environment for participants, part I. *Strength Cond* 16(1):64, 1994.

4. Armitage-Johnson, S. Providing a safe training environment, part II. *Strength Cond* 16(2):34, 1994.

5. Hypes, MG. Planning and designing facilities. *JOPHERD* 77(4):18-22, 2006.

6. Kroll, B. Facility design: Developing the strength training facility. *NSCA J* 11(6):53, 1989.

7. Kroll, W. Structural and functional considerations in designing the facility, part I. *NSCA J* 13(1):51-58, 1991.

8. Kroll, W. Structural and functional considerations in designing the facility, part II. *NSCA J* 13(3):51-57, 1991.

CHAPTER 24 Policies, Procedures and Legal Issues

1. Baley, JA, and Matthews, DL. *Law and Liability in Athletics, Physical Education, and Recreation.* Boston: Allyn & Bacon, 1984.

2. Bart, CK. Industrial firms and the power of mission. *Industrial Marketing Management* 26(4):371-383, 1997.

3. Boyle, M. Creating efficient and effective workouts. In *Designing Strength Training Programs and Facilities.* Reading, MA: Elite Conditioning, 219-227, 2006.

4. Brown, VA. *Boston University Strength and Conditioning Internship Manual.* Boston: Boston University, 4-13, 2014.

5. Bucher, CA, and Krotee, ML. *Management of Physical Education & Sport,* 11th ed. Boston: McGraw-Hill, 1998.

6. Casa, DJ, Anderson, SA, Baker, L, Bennett, S, Bergeron, MF, Connolly, D, Courson, R, Drezner, JA, Eichner, R, Epley, B, Fleck, S, Franks, R, Gilchrist, J, Guskiewicz, KM, Harmon, KG, Hoffman, J, Holschen, J, Indelicato, P, Jost, J, Kinniburgh, A, Klossner, D, Lawless, C, Lopez, RM, Martin, G, McDermott, BP, Mihalik, JP, Moreau, B, Myslinski, T, Pagnotta, K, Poddar, S, Robinson, B, Rogers, G, Russell, A, Sales, L, Sandler, D, Stearns, RL, Stiggins, C, Thompson, C, and Washington, R. The Inter-Association Task Force for Preventing Sudden Death in Collegiate Conditioning Sessions: Best practices recommendations. *J Athl Train* 47(4):477-480, 2012.

7. Earle, RW. *Staff and Facility Policies and Procedures Manual.* Omaha, NE: Creighton University, 1993.

8. Epley, BD. *Flight Manual.* Lincoln, NE: University of Nebraska Printing, 1998.

9. Epley, BD. *Make the Play.* Lincoln, NE: University of Nebraska Printing, 1998.

10. Gentil, P, and Bottaro, M. Influence of supervision ratio on muscle adaptations to resistance training in nontrained subjects. *J Strength Cond Res* 24(3):639-643, 2010.

11. Halling, D. Legal terminology for the strength and conditioning specialist. *NSCA J* 13(4):59-61, 1991.

12. Herbert, DL. A good reason for keeping records. *Strength Cond* 16(3):64, 1994.

13. Herbert, DL. Legal aspects of strength and conditioning. *NSCA J* 15(4):79, 1993.

14. Kleiner, DM, Holcomb, W, and Worley, M. Role of the strength and conditioning professional in rehabilitating an injured athlete. *Strength Cond* 18(2):49-54, 1996.

15. Kroll, B. Liability considerations for strength training facilities. *Strength Cond* 17(6):16-17, 1995.

16. NCAA. *Proposal Number 2013-18.* Indianapolis: NCAA, 2014.

17. NSCA. *National Strength and Conditioning Association Code of Ethics.* Colorado Springs, CO: NSCA, 2008.

18. NSCA. *NSCA Performance Center Emergency Policies and Procedures.* Colorado Springs, CO: NSCA, 2011.

19. NSCA. *Strength and Conditioning Professional Standards and Guidelines.* Colorado Springs, CO: NSCA, 2001.

20. NSCA. *Strength and Conditioning Professional Standards and Guidelines (Revised).* Colorado Springs, CO: NSCA, 1-26, 2009.

21. Rabinoff, R. Weight room litigation: What's it all about. *Strength Cond* 16(2):10-12, 1994.

22. Stern, GJ. *The Drucker Foundation Self-Assessment Tool: Process Guide.* San Francisco: Jossey-Bass, 133-140, 1999.

23. Taylor, JH. *Performance Training Program Manual.* Las Cruces, NM: New Mexico State University, 2006.

INDEX

Page numbers ending in an *f* or a *t* indicate a figure or a table, respectively.

G. Gregory Haff, PhD, CSCS,*D, FNSCA is the course coordinator for the postgraduate degree in strength and conditioning at Edith Cowan University in Joondalup, Australia. He is the president of the National Strength and Conditioning Association (NSCA) and a senior associate editor for the *Journal of Strength and Conditioning Research*. Dr. Haff was the United Kingdom Strength and Conditioning Association (UKSCA) Strength and Conditioning Coach of the Year for Research and Education in 2014 and the 2011 NSCA William J. Kraemer Outstanding Sport Scientist award winner. He is a certified strength and conditioning specialist with distinction, a 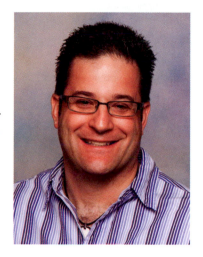 UKSCA-accredited strength and conditioning coach, and an accredited Australian Strength and Conditioning Association level 2 strength and conditioning coach. Additionally, he is a national-level weightlifting coach in the United States and Australia. He serves as a consultant for numerous sporting bodies, including teams in the Australian Football League, Australian Rugby Union, Australian Basketball Association, and National Football League in the United States.

N. Travis Triplett, PhD, CSCS,*D, FNSCA, is a professor and chairperson of the department of health and exercise science at Appalachian State University in Boone, North Carolina. She has served as the secretary-treasurer of the board of directors for the National Strength and Conditioning Association (NSCA) and was the 2010 NSCA William J. Kraemer Outstanding Sport Scientist award winner. She has served on two panels for NASA, one for developing resistance exercise countermeasures to microgravity environments for the International Space Station, and was a sports physiology research assistant at the U.S. Olympic Training Center in Colorado Springs, Colorado. Dr. Triplett is 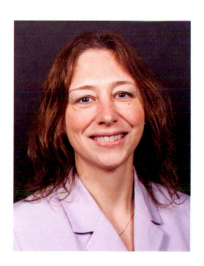 currently a senior associate editor for the *Journal of Strength and Conditioning Research* and is a certified strength and conditioning specialist with distinction as well as a USA Weightlifting club coach.

CONTRIBUTORS

Douglas Berninger, MEd, CSCS,*D, RSCC
National Strength and Conditioning Association

Victor Brown, III, MS, ATC, CSCS, NSCA-CPT
Ithaca College

Bill Campbell, PhD, CSCS, FISSN
University of South Florida

Scott Caulfield, BS, CSCS,*D, RSCC*D
National Strength and Conditioning Association

Donald Chu, PhD, PT, ATC, CSCS,*D, NSCA-CPT,*D, FNSCA
Athercare Fitness & Rehabilitation and Rocky Mountain University of Health Professions

Joel Cramer, PhD, CSCS,*D, NSCA-CPT,*D, FNSCA
University of Nebraska-Lincoln

Jay Dawes, PhD, CSCS,*D, NSCA-CPT,*D, FNSCA
University of Colorado-Colorado Springs

Brad H. DeWeese, EdD, CSCS, NSCA-CPT, USATF
East Tennessee State University

Andrea DuBois, MS, HSF
University of Southern California

Avery Faigenbaum, EdD, CSCS,*D, CSPS, FACSM, FNSCA
The College of New Jersey

Duncan French, PhD, CSCS
University of Northumbria at Newcastle

Terry Grindstaff, PhD, PT, ATC, SCS, CSCS
Creighton University

G. Gregory Haff, PhD, CSCS,*D, FNSCA
Edith Cowan University

Trent Herda, PhD
University of Kansas

Andrea Hudy, MA, CSCS, RSCC*D
University of Kansas

Ian Jeffreys, PhD, CSCS,*D, NSCA-CPT,*D, RSCC*D, FNSCA
University of South Wales

William J. Kraemer, PhD, CSCS,*D, FACSM, FNSCA
The Ohio State University

Rhodri Lloyd, PhD, CSCS,*D
Cardiff Metropolitan University

Jeffrey McBride, PhD, CSCS, FNSCA
Appalachian State University

Michael McGuigan, PhD, CSCS
Auckland University of Technology, New Zealand

Sophia Nimphius, PhD, CSCS,*D
Edith Cowan University

David Potach, MS, PT, SCS, CSCS,*D, NSCA-CPT,*D
Specialized Physical Therapy

Benjamin Reuter, PhD, ATC, CSCS,*D
California University of Pennsylvania

Carwyn Sharp, PhD, CSCS,*D
National Strength and Conditioning Association

Jeremy Sheppard, PhD, CSCS,*D, RSCC*E
Edith Cowan University

Marie Spano, MS, RD, CSCS, CSSD
Spano Sports Nutrition Consulting

Barry Spiering, PhD, CSCS
Nike Sport Research Lab

Traci Statler, PhD, CSCS, CC-AASP
California State University, Fullerton

Ann Swank, PhD, CSCS, FACSM
University of Louisville

N. Travis Triplett, PhD, CSCS,*D, FNSCA
Appalachian State University

Jakob Vingren, PhD, CSCS,*D, FACSM
University of North Texas

CONTRIBUTORS TO PREVIOUS EDITIONS

William B. Allerheiligen, MS, CSCS,*D, NSCA-CPT,*D, FNSCA

Stephanie Armitage-Kerr, PhD, CSCS

Thomas R. Baechle, EdD, CSCS,*D, Retired, NSCA-CPT,*D, Retired

Richard A. Borden, PhD, PT, CSCS, Retired, FNSCA

Evan B. Brody, PhD

Donald A. Chu, PhD, PT, ATC, CSCS,*D, NSCA-CPT,*D, FNSCA

Mike Conley, MD, PhD

Brian Conroy, MD, PhD, CSCS

Joel T. Cramer, PhD, CSCS,*D, NSCA-CPT,*D, FNSCA

Gary Dudley, PhD, CSCS, FACSM

Roger W. Earle, MA, CSCS,*D, NSCA-CPT,*D

Boyd Epley, MEd, CSCS,*D, RSCC*E, FNSCA

Avery D. Faigenbaum, EdD, CSCS,*D, CSPS, FACSM, FNSCA

Karl E. Friedl, PhD

John Garhammer, PhD, CSCS, NSCA-CPT, FNSCA

Lori Greenwood, PhD, ATC, LAT

Michael Greenwood, PhD, CSCS,*D, RSCC*D, FACSM, FNSCA

Terry L. Grindstaff, PhD, PT, ATC, SCS, CSCS

Patrick S. Hagerman, EdD, CSCS, NSCA-CPT, FNSCA

Everett Harman, PhD, CSCS, NSCA-CPT, TSAC-F

Robert T. Harris, PhD

Bradley D. Hatfield, PhD, FACSM

Jay R. Hoffman, PhD, CSCS,*D, RSCC*D, FACSM, FNSCA

William R. Holcomb, PhD, ATC/L, CSCS,*D, FNSCA

Jean Barrett Holloway, MA, CSCS

Gary R. Hunter, PhD, CSCS, FACSM

Ian Jeffreys, PhD, CSCS,*D, NSCA-CPT,*D, RSCC*D, FNSCA

William J. Kraemer, PhD, CSCS,*D, FACSM, FNSCA

Clay Pandorf, BS

Steven S. Plisk, MS

David H. Potach, MS, PT, SCS, CSCS,*D, NSCA-CPT,*D

Jeffrey A. Potteiger, PhD, FACSM

Nicholas A. Ratamess, PhD, CSCS,*D, FNSCA

Kristin Reimers, PhD, RD

Benjamin H. Reuter, PhD, ATC, CSCS,*D

Fred Roll, BS

Jaime Ruud, MS, RD

Douglas M. Semenick, EdD

Barry A. Spiering, PhD, CSCS

Michael H. Stone, PhD, FNSCA

Jeffrey R. Stout, PhD, CSCS, FACSM, FNSCA

Ann Swank, PhD, CSCS, FACSM

John Taylor, MS, FNSCA

Jakob L. Vingren, PhD, CSCS,*D

Dan Wathen, MS, ATC, CSCS,*D, NSCA-CPT,*D, FNSCA

Mark A. Williams, PhD, FACSM

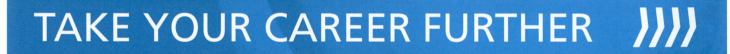
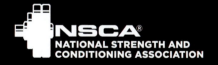
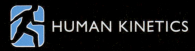